Medical Microbiology

Commissioning Editor: Inta Ozols
Project Development Manager: Siân Jarman
Project Managers: Camilla Rockwood, Susan Stuart
Designer: Judith Wright
Illustrators: Richard Morris and David Gardner

Medical Microbiology

Cedric Mims
BSc MD FRCPath
Emeritus Professor, Department of Microbiology
Guy's Hospital Medical School, London, UK

Hazel M Dockrell
BA PhD
Professor of Immunology, Department of Infectious and Tropical Diseases
London School of Hygiene & Tropical Medicine, London, UK

Richard V Goering
BA MS PhD
Professor and Associate Chair, Department of Medical Microbiology and Immunology
Creighton University, School of Medicine, Omaha, Nebraska, USA

Ivan Roitt
DSc HonFRCP FRCPath FRS
Emeritus Professor of Immunology, Windeyer Institute of Medical Sciences
University College London, London, UK

Derek Wakelin
BSc PhD DSc FRCPath
Emeritus Professor, School of Life and Environmental Sciences
University of Nottingham, Nottingham, UK

Mark Zuckerman
BSc (Hons) MB BS MRCP MSc FRCPath
Consultant Virologist and Honorary Senior Lecturer;
Health Protection Agency, London;
Department of Infectious Diseases
London South Specialist Virology Centre
Guy's, King's and St Thomas' School of Medicine
King's College Hospital NHS Trust, London, UK

THIRD EDITION

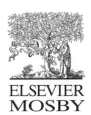

ELSEVIER
MOSBY

Edinburgh London New York Oxford Philadelphia St Louis Sydney Toronto 2004

MOSBY
An imprint of Elsevier Limited

First edition published by Mosby-Year Book Europe Ltd., 1993
Second edition published by Mosby-Year Book Europe Ltd., 1998
Third edition published 2004
  Reprinted 2005

ISBN 0 3230 3575 2 (Main Edition)
ISBN 0 7234 3403 4 (International Student Edition)

British Library Cataloguing in Publication Data
A catalogue record for this book is available from the British Library

Library of Congress Cataloging in Publication Data
A catalog record for this book is available from the Library of Congress

Notice
Medical knowledge is constantly changing. Standard safety precautions must be
followed, but as new research and clinical experience broaden our knowledge,
changes in treatment and drug therapy may become necessary or appropriate.
Readers are advised to check the most current product information provided by the
manufacturer of each drug to be administered to verify the recommended dose, the
method and duration of administration, and contraindications. It is the
responsibility of the practitioner, relying on experience and knowledge of the
patient, to determine dosages and the best treatment for each individual patient.
Neither the Publisher nor the editors/contributor assumes any liability for any
injury and/or damage to persons or property arising from this publication.

The Publisher

The
Publisher's
policy is to use
**paper manufactured
from sustainable forests**

Printed in Spain

Contents

Preface   ix
Acknowledgements   x
Contributors   x

A contemporary approach to microbiology
Microbes and parasites   1

The context for contemporary
  medical microbiology   1
Microbiology past, present and future   2
The approach adopted in this book   4

SECTION 1 THE ADVERSARIES: MICROBES

1. Microbes as parasites
The varieties of microbes   7
Living inside or outside cells   8
Systems of classification   9

2. The bacteria
Structure   11
Nutrition   13
Growth and division   13
Gene expression   14
Extrachromosomal elements   17
Mutation and gene transfer   19
Survival under adverse conditions   24
The genomics of medically important bacteria   24

3. The viruses
Infection of host cells   29
Replication   31
Outcome of viral infection   33
Major groups of viruses   35

4. The fungi
Major groups of disease-causing fungi   39

5. The protozoa   43

6. The helminths and arthropods
The helminths   47
The arthropods   49

7. Prions
'Rogue protein' pathogenesis   53
Development and transmission of prion
  diseases   54
Medical problems posed by prion disease   54

8. The host–parasite relationship
The normal flora   57
Symbiotic associations   60
The characteristics of parasitism   62
The evolution of parasitism   63

SECTION 2 THE ADVERSARIES: HOST DEFENSES

9. The innate defenses of the body
Defense against entry into the body   72
Defenses once the microorganism penetrates the
  body   72

10. Adaptive responses provide a 'quantum leap' in effective defense
The role of antibodies   87
The role of T lymphocytes   89
Extracellular attack on large infectious agents   93
Local defenses at mucosal surfaces   94

11. The cellular basis of adaptive immune responses
B and T cell receptors   100
Clonal expansion of lymphocytes   102
The role of memory cells   103
Stimulation of lymphocytes   104
Cytokines   104
Regulatory mechanisms   106
Tolerance mechanisms   106

SECTION 3 THE CONFLICTS

12. Background to the infectious diseases
Host–parasite relationships *117*
Causes of infectious diseases *118*
The biologic response gradient *120*

13. Entry, exit and transmission
Sites of entry *123*
Exit and transmission *130*
Types of transmission between humans *132*
Transmission from animals *137*

14. Immune defenses in action
Complement *143*
Acute phase proteins and pattern recognition receptors *144*
Fever *144*
Natural killer cells *144*
Phagocytosis *145*
Cytokines *147*
Antibody-mediated immunity *148*
Cell-medited immunity *151*
Recovery from infection *154*

15. Spread and replication
Features of surface and systemic infections *157*
Mechanisms of spread through the body *159*
Genetic determinants of spread and replication *162*
Other factors affecting spread and replication *163*

16. Parasite survival strategies and persistent infections
Parasite survival strategies *167*
Concealment of antigens *169*
Antigenic variation *172*
Immunosuppression *173*
Persistent infections *176*

17. Pathologic consequences of infection
Pathology caused directly by the microorganism *184*
Pathologic activation of natural immune mechanisms *187*
Pathologic consequences of the immune response *189*
Skin rashes *193*
Viruses and cancer *194*

SECTION 4 CLINICAL MANIFESTATION AND DIAGNOSIS OF INFECTIONS BY BODY SYSTEM

Introduction to Section 4: The Clinical Manifestations of Infection *199*

18. Upper respiratory tract infections
The common cold *201*
Pharyngitis and tonsillitis *202*
Parotitis *210*
Otitis and sinusitis *211*
Acute epiglottitis *213*
Oral cavity infections *213*
Laryngitis and tracheitis *214*
Diphtheria *214*

19. Lower respiratory tract infections
Acute infections *217*
Chronic infections *232*
Parasitic infections *237*

20. Urinary tract infections
Acquisition and etiology *241*
Pathogenesis *242*
Clinical features and complications *244*
Laboratory diagnosis *245*

Treatment *247*
Prevention *248*

21. Sexually transmitted diseases
STDs and sexual behavior *251*
Syphilis *251*
Gonorrhea *256*
Chlamydial infection *258*
Other causes of inguinal lymphadenopathy *261*
Mycoplasmas and non-gonococcal urethritis *262*
Other causes of vaginitis and urethritis *262*
Genital herpes *263*
Human papillomavirus infection *264*
Human immunodeficiency virus *264*
Opportunistic STDs *273*
Arthropod infestations *275*

22. Gastrointestinal tract infections
Diarrheal diseases caused by bacterial or viral infection *277*
Food poisoning *292*
Helicobacter pylori and gastric ulcer disease *293*

Parasites and the gastrointestinal tract *293*
Systemic infection initiated in the gastrointestinal tract *300*

23. Obstetric and perinatal infections
Infections occurring in pregnancy *313*
Congenital infections *313*
Infections occurring around the time of birth *318*

24. Central nervous system infections
Invasion of the central nervous system *323*
The body's response to invasion *324*
Meningitis *325*
Encephalitis *331*
Neurologic diseases of possible viral etiology *337*
Spongiform encephalopathy caused by scrapie-type agents *337*
CNS disease caused by parasites *338*
Brain abscesses *339*
Tetanus and botulism *339*

25. Infections of the eye
Conjunctivitis *343*
Infection of the deeper layers of the eye *345*

26. Infections of the skin, soft tissue, muscle and associated systems
Bacterial infections of skin, soft tissue and muscle *350*
Mycobacterial diseases of the skin *357*
Fungal infections of the skin *359*
Parasitic infections of the skin *264*
Mucocutaneous lesions caused by viruses *366*
Smallpox *373*
Measles *374*
Rubella *375*
Other infections producing skin lesions *376*
Kawasaki syndrome *377*
Viral infections of muscle *377*
Parasitic infections of muscle *377*

Joint and bone infections *378*
Infections of the hemopoietic system *380*

27. Vector-borne infections
Arboviruses infections *383*
Infections caused by Rickettsiae *386*
Borrelia infections *389*
Protozoal infections *391*
Helminth infections *397*

28. Multisystem zoonoses
Arenavirus infections *401*
Korean hemorrhagic fever *402*
Marburg and Ebola hemorrhagic fevers *402*
Q fever *403*
Anthrax *404*
Plague *405*
Yersinia enterocolitica infection *407*
Tularemia *407*
Pasteurella multocida infection *407*
Leptospirosis *407*
Rat bite fever *408*
Brucellosis *409*
Helminth infections *410*

29. Fever of unknown origin
Definitions of fever of unknown origin *413*
Causes of FUO *413*
Investigation of classical FUO *414*
Treatment of FUO *415*
FUO in specific patient groups *415*
Infective endocarditis *416*

30. Infections in the compromised host
The compromised host *423*
Infections of the host with deficient innate immunity due to physical factors *426*
Infections associated with secondary adaptive immunodeficiency *429*
Other important opportunist pathogens *431*

SECTION 5 DIAGNOSIS AND CONTROL

31. Strategies for control: an introduction
Epidemiologic considerations *441*
Detection and diagnosis *447*
Chemotherapy versus vaccination *447*
Control versus eradication *450*

32. Diagnosis of infection and assessment of host defense mechanisms
Aims of the clinical microbiology laboratory *453*
Specimen processing *453*
Non-cultural techniques for the laboratory diagnosis of infection *455*
Cultivation (culture) of microorganisms *462*

Identification of microorganisms grown in culture   464

Antibody detection methods for the diagnosis of infection   466

Assessment of host defense systems   468

Protocols for specimen processing   471

33. Attacking the enemy: antimicrobial agents and chemotherapy

Selective toxicity   473

Discovery and design of antibacterial agents   473

Classification of antibacterial agents   474

Resistance to antibacterial agents   475

Classes of antibacterial agents   477

Inhibitors of cell wall synthesis   478

Inhibitors of protein synthesis   485

Inhibitors of nucleic acid synthesis   492

Antimetabolites affecting nucleic acid synthesis   494

Other agents that affect DNA   496

Inhibitors of cytoplastic membrane function   496

Urinary tract antiseptics   496

Antituberculous agents   496

Antibacterial agents in practice   497

Antibiotic assays   499

Antiviral therapy   499

Antifungal agents   504

Antiparasitic agents   505

Use and misuse of antimicrobial agents   507

34. Vaccination

The aims of vaccination   513

Requirements of a good vaccine   514

Types of vaccine   516

Special considerations   520

Community-based control by vaccination   524

Factors influencing the success of vaccination   527

Current vaccine practice   528

35. Passive and non-specific immunotherapy

Passive immunization with antibody   539

Non-specific cellular immunostimulation   542

Correction of host immunodeficiency   543

36. Hospital infection, sterilization and disinfection

Common hospital-acquired infections   546

Important causes of hospital infection   546

Sources and routes of spread of hospital infection   548

Host factors and hospital infection   549

Consequences of hospital infection   551

Prevention of hospital infection   551

Investigating hospital infection   555

Sterilization and disinfection   556

Appendix – Pathogen parade   567

Answers   631

Index   640

Preface

The third edition of Medical Microbiology keeps to the pattern of earlier editions, focusing on the conflict between host and parasite. It has been extensively updated, with improved layout and illustrations, but the basic principles and the central role of immunology have not changed. It continues to be clinically oriented.

This time we are privileged to have Richard Goering as a major author, and as a result the book is now more closely adapted to the curriculum and needs of American students. We also welcome Hazel Dockrell (immunology) and Mark Zuckerman (virology) as principal authors. Rosamund Williams and John Playfair, who played such a major part in earlier editions, have relinquished their roles as main authors, and we gratefully acknowledge their contributions.

Medical school curricula are changing, and often microbiology is no longer taught as a separate discipline but is integrated with pathology, immunology and clinical studies. Organ-based infectious disease themes are becoming popular. There is nevertheless a need for a foundation text such as this one. The system-based treatment is retained and for ready reference details about each microbe are included in a 'Pathogen Parade' at the end of the book.

The number of fully sequenced microbes increases inexorably, and we are beginning to understand how a given gene product contributes to disease and pathogenicity. Wherever possible we have referred to the molecular basis for microbial pathogenicity and disease.

Each chapter ends with Key Facts and Questions (mostly case-based, in USMLE format), and chapters now have a 'Lessons in Microbiology' drawer to flesh out the subject with historical, epidemiological, or other aspects of the subject.

We believe Medical Microbiology continues to give students a readable, exciting and informative insight into the causation, diagnosis, prevention and treatment of infectious diseases.

Cedric Mims, Hazel M Dockrell, Richard V Goering,
Ivan Roitt, Derek Wakelin, Mark Zuckerman
2004

Acknowledgements

We wish to express our appreciation of the generosity of many colleagues throughout the world who supplied illustrative material, particularly W Edmund Farrar, Martin J Wood, John A Innes, Hugh Tubbs, James S Bingham, Ralph Muller, John R Baker, John Oxford and Dilip K Banerjee. We would also like to thank the library of The Wellcome Institute for the History of Medicine for providing portrait photographs for the historical profiles.

CM, HMD, RVG, IR, DW, MZ

Contributors

Roy M Anderson FRS
Linacre Professor and Head of Department
Director of Wellcome Trust Centre for Epidemiology of Infectious Disease
Department of Zoology
University of Oxford
Oxford, UK

Gillian Urwin MSc MB BS MRCPath
Consultant Microbiologist
Department of Microbiology
Essex Rivers Healthcare NHS Trust
Colchester, UK

John Playfair MB BChir PhD DSc
Emeritus Professor
Department of Immunology
University College and Middlesex School of Medicine
London, UK

Rosamund Williams PhD FRCPath
Division of Emerging and other Communicable Diseases,
Surveillance and Control
World Health Organization
Geneva, Switzerland

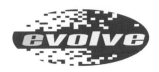

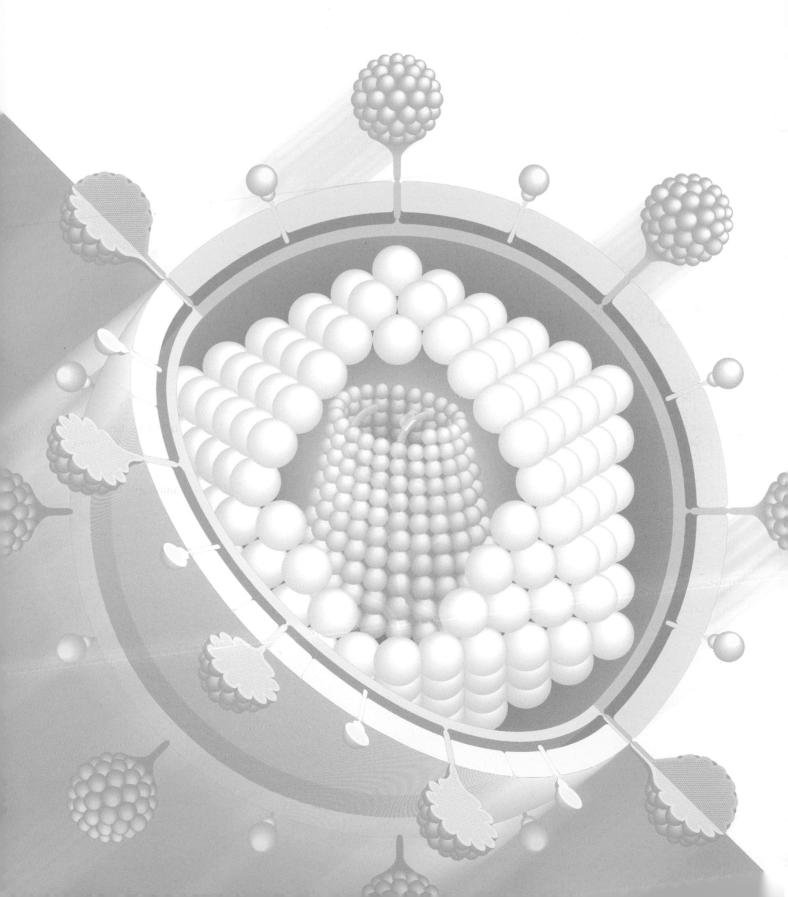

A contemporary approach to microbiology

MICROBES AND PARASITES

The conventional distinction between 'microbes' and 'parasites' is essentially arbitrary

Microbiology is sometimes defined as the biology of microscopic organisms, its subject being the 'microbes'. Traditionally, clinical microbiology has been concerned with those organisms responsible for the major infectious diseases of humans and whose size makes them invisible to the naked eye. It is not surprising that the range of organisms included has reflected those diseases that have been (or continue to be) of greatest importance in those countries where the scientific and clinical discipline of microbiology developed, notably Europe and the USA. The term 'microbes' has usually been applied in a restricted fashion, primarily to viruses, bacteria and related organisms. Fungi and protozoans ('parasites') have sometimes been included as relatively minor contributors, but in general they have been treated as the subjects of other disciplines (mycology and parasitology).

Although there can be no argument that viruses and bacteria are the most numerous and most important pathogens, the conventional distinction between these as 'microbes' and the other infectious agents (fungi, protozoan, worm and arthropod parasites) is essentially arbitrary, not least because the criterion of microscopic visibility cannot be applied rigidly *(Fig. 00.1)*. Perhaps we should remember that the first 'microbe' to be associated with a specific clinical condition was a parasitic worm—the nematode *Trichinella spiralis*—whose larval stages are just visible to the naked eye (though microscopy is needed for certain identification). *T. spiralis* was first identified in 1835 and causally related to the disease trichinellosis in the 1860s.

THE CONTEXT FOR CONTEMPORARY MEDICAL MICROBIOLOGY

Many microbiology texts deal with infectious organisms as agents of disease in isolation—isolated both from other infectious organisms and from the biologic context in which they live and in which disease is caused. It is certainly convenient to list and deal with organisms group by group, to summarize the diseases they cause, and to review the forms of control available, but this approach produces a static picture of what is a dynamic relationship between the organism and its host.

Host response is the outcome of the complex interplay between host and parasite

Host response can be discussed in terms of pathologic signs and symptoms and in terms of immune control, but it is better treated as the outcome of the complex interplay between two organisms—host and parasite; without this dimension a distorted view of infectious disease results. It simply is not true that 'microbe + host = disease', and clinicians are well aware of this. Understanding why it is that most host–microbe contacts do not result in disease, and what changes so that disease does arise, is as important as the identification of infectious organisms and a knowledge of the ways in which they can be controlled.

We therefore believe that our approach to microbiology, both in terms of the organisms that might usefully be considered within a textbook and also in terms of the contexts in which they and the diseases they cause are discussed,

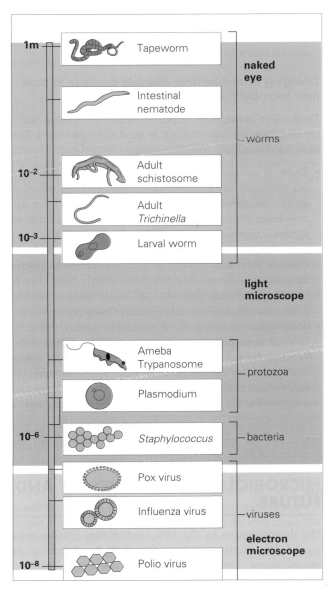

Fig. 00.1 Relative sizes of the organisms covered in this book.

THE APPROACH ADOPTED IN THIS BOOK

The factors outlined above indicate the need for a text with a dual function:

- First, it should provide a more inclusive treatment of the organisms responsible for infectious disease.
- Second, the purely clinical/laboratory approach to microbiology should be replaced with an approach that will stress the biologic context in which clinical/laboratory studies are to be undertaken.

The approach we have adopted in this book is to look at microbiology from the viewpoint of the conflicts inherent in all host–pathogen relationships. We first describe the adversaries: the infectious organisms on the one hand, and the innate and adaptive defense mechanisms of the host on the other. The outcome of the conflicts between the two is then amplified and discussed system by system. Rather than taking each organism or each disease manifestation in turn, we look at the major environments available for infectious organisms in the human body, such as the respiratory system, the gut, the urinary tract, the blood and the central nervous system. The organisms that invade and establish in each of these are examined in terms of the pathologic responses they provoke. Finally, we look at how the conflicts we have described can be controlled or eliminated, both at the level of the individual patient and at the level of the community. We hope that such an approach will provide readers with a dynamic view of host–pathogen interactions and allow them to develop a more creative understanding of infection and disease.

KEY FACTS

- Our approach is to provide a comprehensive account of the organisms that cause infectious disease in humans, from the viruses to the worms, and to cover the biologic bases of infection, disease, host–pathogen interactions, disease control and epidemiology.

- The diseases caused by microbial pathogens will be placed in the context of the conflict that exists between them and the innate and adaptive defenses of their hosts.

- Infections will be described and discussed in terms of the major body systems, treating these as environments in which microbes can establish themselves, flourish and give rise to pathologic changes.

QUESTIONS

1. What are the major groups of pathogenic organisms that cause disease in humans?
2. What infections are responsible for more than one million deaths each year?
3. Name four infectious agents identified in the 1990s.
4. What factors are likely to influence the prevalence of infectious diseases in the 21st century?

FURTHER READING

Mims CA, Nash A, Stephen J. *Pathogenesis of Infectious Disease*, 5th edition. London: Academic Press, 2001.

The adversaries—microbes

1

1. Microbes as parasites   *7*

2. The bacteria   *11*

3. The viruses   *29*

4. The fungi   *39*

5. The protozoa   *43*

6. The helminths and arthropods   *47*

7. Prions   *53*

8. The host—parasite relationship   *57*

Microbes as parasites

THE VARIETIES OF MICROBES

Prokaryotes and eukaryotes

A number of important and distinctive biologic characteristics must be taken into account when considering any organism in relation to infectious disease. One of these is the way in which the organism is constructed, particularly the way in which genetic material and cellular components are organized.

All organisms other than viruses and prions are made up of cells

Viruses are not cells—they do have genetic material (DNA or RNA) but lack cell membranes, cytoplasm and the machinery for synthesizing macromolecules, depending instead upon host cells for this process. Conventional viruses have their genetic material packed in capsules. The agents (prions) which cause diseases such as Creutzfeldt–Jakob disease, kuru, scrapie and bovine spongiform encephalopathy (BSE) appear to lack nucleic acid and consist only of proteinaceous infectious particles.

All other organisms have a cellular organization, their bodies being made up of single cells (most 'microbes') or of many cells. Each cell has genetic material (DNA) and cytoplasm with synthetic machinery, and is bounded by a cell membrane.

Bacteria are prokaryotes, all other organisms are eukaryotes

There are many differences between the two major divisions —prokaryotes and eukaryotes—of cellular organisms *(Fig. 1.1)*. These include the following.

In prokaryotes:

- A distinct nucleus is absent.
- DNA is in the form of a single circular chromosome. Additional DNA is carried in plasmids.
- Transcription and translation can be carried out simultaneously.

In eukaryotes:

- DNA is carried on several chromosomes within a nucleus.
- The nucleus is bounded by a nuclear membrane.
- Transcription requires formation of messenger RNA (mRNA) and movement of mRNA out of the nucleus into the cytoplasm.
- Translation takes place on ribosomes.
- The cytoplasm is rich in membrane-bound organelles (mitochondria, endoplasmic reticulum, Golgi apparatus, lysosomes) which are absent in prokaryotes.

Gram-negative bacteria have an outer lipopolysaccharide-rich layer

Another important difference between prokaryotes and the majority of eukaryotes is that the cell membrane (plasma membrane) of prokaryotes is covered by a thick protective cell wall. In Gram-positive bacteria, this wall, made of peptido-glycan, forms the external surface of the cell, while in Gram-negative bacteria there is an additional outer layer rich in lipopolysaccharides. These layers play an important role in protecting the cell against the immune system and chemo-therapeutic agents, and in stimulating certain pathologic responses. They also confer antigenicity.

Micro- and macroparasites

Microparasites replicate within the host

There is an important distinction between micro- and macroparasites that overrides their differences in size. Microparasites (viruses, bacteria, protozoa, fungi) replicate within the host and can, theoretically, multiply to produce a very large number of progeny, thereby causing an over-whelming infection. In contrast, macroparasites (worms, arthropods), even those that are microscopic, do not have this ability: one infectious stage matures into one reproducing stage, and the resulting progeny leave the host to continue the

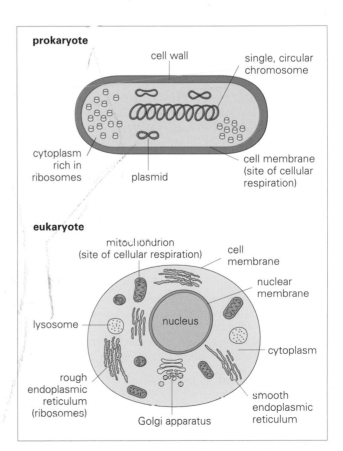

Fig. 1.1 Prokaryote and eukaryote cells. The major features of cellular organization are shown diagrammatically.

cycle. The level of infection is therefore determined by the numbers of organisms that enter the body. This distinction between micro- and macroparasites has important clinical and epidemiologic implications

Of course the boundary between micro- and macroparasites is not always clear. The progeny of some macroparasites do remain within the host, and infections can lead to the build-up of overwhelming numbers, particularly in immune-suppressed patients. The roundworms *Trichinella*, *Strongyloides stercoralis* and some filarial nematodes, and *Sarcoptes scabiei* (the itch mite), are examples of this type of parasite.

Organisms that are small enough can live inside cells

Absolute size has other biologically significant implications for the host–pathogen relationship, which cut across the divisions between micro- and macroparasites. Perhaps the most important of these is the relative size of a pathogen and its host's cells. Organisms that are small enough can live inside cells and by doing so establish a biologic relationship with the host that is quite different from that of an extracellular organism—one that influences both disease and control.

LIVING INSIDE OR OUTSIDE CELLS

The basis of all host–pathogen relationships is the exploitation by one organism (the pathogen) of the environment provided by another (the host). The nature and degree of exploitation varies from relationship to relationship, but the pathogen's primary requirement is a supply of metabolic materials from the host, whether provided in the form of nutrients or (as in the case of viruses) in the form of nuclear synthetic machinery. The reliance of viruses upon host synthetic machinery requires an obligatory intracellular habit: viruses must live within host cells. Some other groups of pathogens (*Chlamydia*, *Rickettsia*) also live only within cells. In the remaining groups of pathogens, different species have adopted either the intracellular or the extracellular habit, or, in a few cases, both. Intracellular microparasites other than viruses take their metabolic requirements directly from the pool of nutrients available in the cell itself, whereas extracellular organisms take theirs from the nutrients present in tissue fluids, or, occasionally, by feeding directly on host cells (e.g. *Entamoeba histolytica*, the organism associated with amebic dysentery). Macroparasites are almost always extracellular (though *Trichinella* is intracellular), and many feed by ingesting and digesting host cells; others can take up nutrients directly from tissue fluids or intestinal contents.

Pathogens within cells are protected from many of the host's defense mechanisms

As will be discussed in greater detail in Chapter 13, the intracellular pathogens pose problems for the host that are quite different from those posed by extracellular organisms. Pathogens that live within cells are largely protected against many of the host's defense mechanisms while they remain there, particularly against the action of specific antibodies. Control of these infections depends therefore on the activities of intracellular killing mechanisms, short range mediators or cytotoxic agents, although the latter may destroy both the pathogen and the host cell, leading to tissue damage. This problem, of targeting activity against the pathogen when it lives within a vulnerable cell, also arises when using drugs or antibiotics, as it is difficult to achieve selective action against the pathogen while leaving the host cell intact. Even more problematic is the fact that many intracellular pathogens live inside the very cells responsible for the host's immune and inflammatory mechanisms and therefore depress the host's defensive abilities. For example, a variety of viral, bacterial and protozoal pathogens live inside macrophages, and several viruses (including HIV) are specific for lymphocytes.

Intracellular life has many advantages for the pathogen. It provides access to the host's nutrient supply and its genetic machinery and allows escape from host surveillance and antimicrobial defenses. However, no organism can be wholly intracellular at all times: if it is to replicate successfully, transmission must occur between the host's cells, and this inevitably involves some exposure to the extracellular environment. As far as the host is concerned, this extracellular phase in the development of the pathogen provides an opportunity to control infection through defense mechanisms such as phagocytosis, antibody and complement. However, transmission between cells can involve destruction of the initially infected cell and so contribute to tissue damage and general host pathology.

Living outside cells provides opportunities for growth, reproduction and dissemination

Extracellular pathogens can grow and reproduce freely, and may move extensively within the tissues of the body. However, they also face constraints on their survival and development. The most important is continuous exposure to components of the host's defense mechanisms, particularly antibody, complement and phagocytic cells.

The characteristics of extracellular organisms lead to pathologic consequences that are quite different from those associated with intracellular species. These are seen most dramatically with the macroparasites, whose sheer physical size, reproductive capacity and mobility can result in extensive destruction of host tissues. Many extracellular pathogens have the ability to spread rapidly through extracellular fluids or to move rapidly over surfaces, resulting in a widespread infection within a relatively short time. The rapid colonization of the entire mucosal surface of the small bowel by *Vibrio cholerae* is a good example. Successful host defense against extracellular parasites requires mechanisms that differ from those used in defense against intracellular parasites. The variety of locations and tissues occupied by extracellular parasites also poses problems for the host in ensuring effective deployment of defense mechanisms. Defense against intestinal parasites requires components of the innate and adaptive immune systems that are quite distinct from those effective against parasites in other sites, and those living in the lumen may be unaffected by responses operating in the mucosa. These problems in mounting effective defense are most acute where large macroparasites are concerned, because their size often renders them insusceptible to defense mechanisms that can be used against smaller organisms. For example, worms cannot be phagocytosed, they often have protected external layers, and can actively move away from areas where the host response is activated.

SYSTEMS OF CLASSIFICATION

Infectious diseases are caused by organisms belonging to a very wide range of different groups—prions, viruses, bacteria, fungi, protozoa, helminths (worms) and arthropods. Each has its own system of classification, making it possible to identify and categorize the organisms concerned. Correct identification is an essential requirement for accurate diagnosis and effective treatment. Identification is achieved by a variety of means, from simple observation to molecular analysis. The approaches used vary between the major groups. For the protozoa, fungi, worms and arthropods, the basic unit of classification is the species, essentially defined as a group of organisms capable of reproducing sexually with one another. Species provide the basis for the binomial system of classification, used for eukaryote and some prokaryote organisms. Species are in turn grouped into a 'genus' (closely related but non-interbreeding species). Each organism is identified by two names, indicating the 'genus' and the 'species', respectively. For example, *Homo sapiens* and *Escherichia coli*. Related genera are grouped into progressively broader and more inclusive categories.

Classification of bacteria and viruses

The concept of 'species' is a basic difficulty in classifying prokaryotes and viruses. Classification of bacteria uses a mixture of easily determined practical characteristics, based on size, shape, color, staining properties, respiration and reproduction, and a more sophisticated analysis of immunologic, biochemical and molecular criteria. The former characteristics can be used to divide the organisms into conventional taxonomic groupings, as shown for the Gram-positive bacteria in *Figure 1.2* (see also Chapter 2).

Correct identification of bacteria below the species level is often vital to differentiate pathogenic and non-pathogenic forms

Correct treatment requires correct identification. For some bacteria the important subspecies groups are identified on the basis of their immunologic properties. Cell wall, flagellar and capsule antigens are used in tests with specific antisera to define serogroups and serotypes (e.g. in salmonellae, streptococci, shigellae, *E. coli*). In others, biochemical characteristics are used to define other subspecies groupings (biotypes, strains, groups). For example, certain strains of *Staphylococcus aureus* release a β-hemolysin (causing red blood cells to lyse). Production of other toxins is also important in differentiating between groups, as in *E. coli*. Bacteria can also be classified below species level by their susceptibility to particular bacteriophage viruses. Phage typing is used, for example, in differentiating between isolates of *Staph. aureus, Vibrio cholerae* and *Salmonella typhi*.

Direct genetic approaches are also used in identification and classification. These include:

- measuring total genome size (the molecular weight of the DNA present);
- determining the ratio of the bases guanine and cytosine in the DNA;
- using specific probes to identify particular sequences of DNA in the genome.

Classification of viruses departs even further from the binomial system

For viruses, families and, sometimes, genera are used, but not species. Groupings are based on characteristics such as the type of nucleic acid present (DNA or RNA), the mode of replication, the symmetry of the virus particle (icosahedral, helical or complex) and the presence or absence of an external envelope, as shown for the DNA viruses in *Figure 1.3* (see also Chapter 3). The equivalents of subspecies categories are also used, and indeed are more easily determined than species

staining	shape	respiration	shape/reproduction	genus	species
Gram-positive	cocci	aerobic	clusters	*Staphylococcus*	*S. aureus*
		aerobic	chains/pairs	*Streptococcus*	*S. faecalis*
		anaerobic		*Peptococcus*	*P. magnus*
	bacilli	aerobic	sporing	*Bacillus*	*B. anthracis*
		aerobic	non-sporing	*Listeria*	*L. monocytogenes*
		anaerobic	sporing	*Clostridium*	*C. tetani*
		anaerobic	non-sporing	*Propionibacterium*	*P. acnes*

Fig. 1.2 How the structural and biological characteristics of bacteria can be used in classification, taking Gram-positive bacteria as an example.

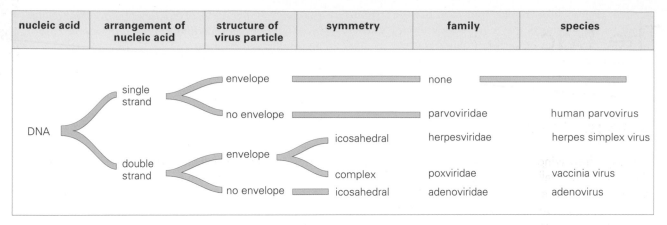

nucleic acid	arrangement of nucleic acid	structure of virus particle	symmetry	family	species
DNA	single strand	envelope		none	
		no envelope		parvoviridae	human parvovirus
	double strand	envelope	icosahedral	herpesviridae	herpes simplex virus
			complex	poxviridae	vaccinia virus
		no envelope	icosahedral	adenoviridae	adenovirus

Fig. 1.3 How the characteristics of viruses can be used in classification, taking DNA viruses as an example.

could be, given the peculiar biologic characteristics of viruses. These categories include serotypes, strains, variants and isolates and are determined primarily by serologic reactivity of virus material. The influenza virus, for example, can be considered as the equivalent of a genus containing three types (A, B, C). Identification can be carried out using the stable nucleoprotein antigen, which differs between the three types. The neuraminidase and hemagglutinin antigens are not stable and show variation within types. Characterization of these antigens in an isolate enables the particular variant to be identified (see Chapter 19). A further example is seen in adenoviruses, for which the various antigens associated with a component of the capsid can be used to define groups, types and finer subdivisions.

Classification assists diagnosis and the understanding of pathogenicity

Prompt identification of organisms is necessary clinically so that diagnoses can be made and appropriate treatments advised. To understand host–parasite interactions, however, not only should the identity of an organism be known, but as much as possible of its general biology; useful predictions can then be made about the consequences of infection. For these reasons, in subsequent chapters we have included outline classifications of the important pathogens, accompanied by brief accounts of their structure (gross and microscopic), modes of life, molecular biology, biochemistry, replication and reproduction.

KEY FACTS

- Organisms that cause infectious diseases can be grouped into seven major categories: prions, viruses, bacteria, fungi, protozoa, helminths and arthropods.

- Identification and classification of these organisms is an important part of microbiology and essential for correct diagnosis, treatment and control.

- Each group has distinctive characteristics (structural and molecular make-up, biochemical and metabolic strategies, reproductive processes) which determine how the organisms interact with their hosts and how they cause disease.

- Many pathogens live within cells, where they are protected from many components of the host's protective responses.

QUESTIONS

1. List the key differences between prokaryotes and eukaryotes.
2. What are the important differences between micro- and macroparasites?
3. List three advantages that organisms gain by living within cells.
4. What approaches can be used to identify and classify bacteria?

FURTHER READING

Collier LH, ed. *Topley and Wilson's Microbiology and Microbial Infections*, 9th edition. London: Edward Arnold, 1998.

The bacteria

INTRODUCTION

Although free-living bacteria exist in huge numbers, relatively few species cause disease. The majority of these are now well known and well studied; however, new pathogens continue to emerge and the significance of previously unrecognized infections becomes apparent. A good example is infection with *Legionella*, the cause of Legionnaires' disease.

Bacteria are single-celled prokaryotes, their DNA forming a long circular molecule, but not contained within a defined nucleus. Many are motile, using a unique pattern of flagella. The bacterial cell is surrounded by a complex cell wall and often a thick capsule. They reproduce by binary fission, often at very high rates, and show a wide range of metabolic patterns, both aerobic and anaerobic. Classification of bacteria uses both phenotypic and genotypic data. For clinical purposes the phenotypic data are of most practical value, and rest on an understanding of bacterial structure and biology (see *Figure 32.20*). Detailed summaries of members of the major bacterial groups are given in the Appendix (Pathogen Parade).

STRUCTURE

Bacteria are 'prokaryotes' and have a characteristic cellular organization

The genetic information of bacteria is carried in a long, double-stranded (ds), circular molecule of DNA *(Fig. 2.1)*. By analogy with eukaryotes (see Chapter 1) this can be termed a 'chromosome', but there are no introns; instead, the DNA comprises a continuous coding sequence of genes. The chromosome is not localized within a distinct nucleus; no nuclear membrane is present, and the DNA is tightly coiled into a region known as the 'nucleoid'. Genetic information in the cell may also be extrachromosomal, present as small circular DNA molecules termed plasmids. The cytoplasm contains no organelles other than ribosomes for protein synthesis. Although ribosomal function is the same in both pro- and eukaryotic cells, organelle structure is different. Ribosomes are characterized as 70S in prokaryotes and 80S in eukaryotes (the 'S' unit relates to how a particle behaves when studied under extreme centrifugal force in an ultracentrifuge). The bacterial 70S ribosome is specifically targeted by antimicrobials such as the aminoglycosides (see Chapter 33). Many of the metabolic functions performed in eukaryote cells by membrane-bound organelles such as mitochondria are carried out by the prokaryotic cell membrane. In all bacteria except mycoplasmas the cell is surrounded by a complex cell wall. External to this wall may be capsules, flagella and pili. Knowledge of the cell wall and these external structures is important in diagnosis and pathogenicity and for understanding bacterial biology.

Bacteria are classified according to their cell wall as Gram positive or Gram negative

Gram staining is a basic microbiologic procedure for detection and identification of bacteria (see Chapter 32). The main structural component of the cell wall is a 'peptidoglycan' (mucopeptide or murein), a mixed polymer of hexose sugars (*N*-acetylglucosamine and *N*-acetylmuramic acid) and amino acids.

- In Gram-positive bacteria the peptidoglycan forms a thick (20–80 nm) layer external to the cell membrane, and may contain other macromolecules.
- In Gram-negative species the peptidoglycan layer is thin (5–10 nm) and is overlaid by an outer membrane, anchored to lipoprotein molecules in the peptidoglycan layer. The principal molecules of the outer membrane are lipopolysaccharides and lipoprotein *(Fig. 2.2)*.

The polysaccharides and charged amino acids in the peptidoglycan layer make it highly polar, providing the bacterium with a thick hydrophilic surface. This property allows Gram-positive organisms to resist the activity of bile in the intestine. Conversely, the layer is digested by lysozyme, an enzyme present in body secretions, which therefore has bactericidal properties. Synthesis of peptidoglycan is disrupted by penicillin and cephalosporin antibiotics (see Chapter 33).

In Gram-negative bacteria the outer membrane is also hydrophilic, but the lipid components of the constituent molecules give hydrophobic properties as well. Entry of hydrophilic molecules such as sugars and amino acids is necessary for nutrition and is achieved through special channels or pores formed by proteins called 'porins'. The lipopolysaccharide (LPS) in the membrane confers both antigenic properties (the 'O antigens' from the carbohydrate chains) and toxic properties (the 'endotoxin' from the lipid A component; see Chapter 17).

In the Gram-positive mycobacteria the peptidoglycan layer has a different chemical basis for cross-linking to the lipoprotein layer, and the outer envelope contains a variety of complex lipids (mycolic acids). These create a waxy layer, which alters both the staining properties of these organisms (the so-called acid-fast bacteria) and gives considerable

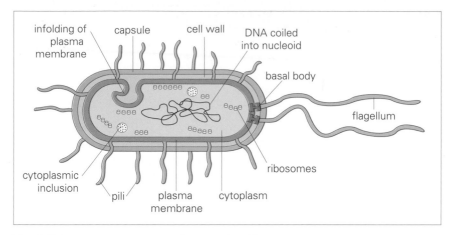

Fig. 2.1 Diagrammatic structure of a generalized bacterium.

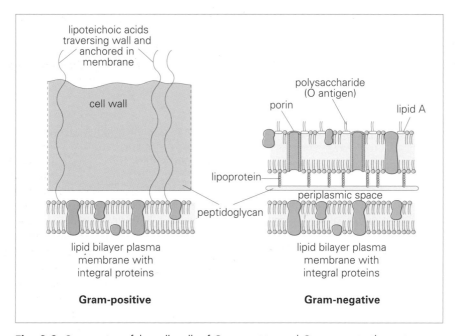

Fig. 2.2 Construction of the cell walls of Gram-positive and Gram-negative bacteria.

resistance to drying and other environmental factors. Myco-bacterial cell wall components also have a pronounced adjuvant activity (i.e. they promote immunologic responsiveness).

External to the cell wall may be an additional capsule of high molecular weight polysaccharides (or amino acids in anthrax bacilli) that give a slimy surface. This provides protection against phagocytosis by host cells and is important in determining virulence. With *Streptococcus pneumoniae* infection, only a few capsulated organisms can cause a fatal infection, but unencapsulated mutants cause no disease.

The cell wall is a major contributor to the ultimate shape of the organism, an important characteristic for bacterial identification. In general, bacterial shapes are categorized as either spherical (cocci), rods (bacilli) or helical (spirilla), although there are variations on these themes.

Many bacteria possess flagella

Flagella are long helical filaments extending from the cell surface, which enable bacteria to move in their environment.

These may be restricted to the poles of the cell, singly (polar) or in tufts (lophotrichous), or distributed over the general surface of the cell (peritrichous). Bacterial flagella are quite different from eukaryote flagella, and the forces that result in movement are generated quite differently (being independent of adenosine triphosphate, ATP). Motility allows positive and negative responses to chemical stimuli (chemotaxis). Flagella are built of protein components (flagellins), which are strongly antigenic. These antigens, the H antigens, are important targets of protective antibody responses.

Pili are another form of bacterial surface projection

Pili (fimbriae) are more rigid than flagella and function in attachment, either to other bacteria (the 'sex' pili) or to host cells (the 'common' pili). Adherence to host cells involves specific interactions between component molecules of the pili (adhesins) and molecules in host cell membranes. For example, the adhesins of *Escherichia coli* interact with fucose/mannose molecules on the surface of intestinal epithelial cells (see Chapter 22). The presence of many pili may help to prevent phagocytosis, reducing host resistance to bacterial infection. Although immunogenic, their antigens can be changed, allowing the bacteria to avoid immune recognition. The mechanism of 'antigenic variation' has been elucidated in the gonococci and is known to involve recombination of genes coding for 'constant' and 'variable' regions of pili molecules.

NUTRITION

All pathogenic bacteria are heterotrophic

All bacteria obtain energy by oxidizing preformed organic molecules (carbohydrates, lipids and proteins) from their environment. Metabolism of these molecules yields ATP as an energy source. Metabolism may be aerobic, where the final electron acceptor is oxygen, or anaerobic, where the final acceptor may be an organic or inorganic molecule other than oxygen.

- In aerobic metabolism (i.e. aerobic respiration), complete utilization of an energy source such as glucose produces 38 molecules of ATP.
- Anaerobic metabolism utilizing an inorganic molecule other than oxygen as the final hydrogen acceptor (anaerobic respiration) is incomplete and produces fewer ATP molecules than aerobic respiration.
- Anaerobic metabolism utilizing an organic final hydrogen acceptor (fermentation) is much less efficient and produces only two molecules of ATP.

Anaerobic metabolism, while less efficient, can thus be used in the absence of oxygen when appropriate substrates are available, as they usually are in the host's body. The requirement for oxygen in respiration may be 'obligate' or it may be 'facultative', some organisms being able to switch between aerobic and anaerobic metabolism. Those that use fermentation pathways often use the major product pyruvate in secondary fermentations by which additional energy can be generated.

Bacteria obtain nutrients mainly by taking up small molecules across the cell wall

Bacteria take up small molecules such as amino acids, oligosaccharides and small peptides across the cell wall. Gram-negative species can also take up and use larger molecules after preliminary digestion in the periplasmic space. Uptake and transport of nutrients into the cytoplasm is achieved by the cell membrane using a variety of transport mechanisms, including facilitated diffusion which utilizes a carrier to move compounds to equalize their intra- and extracellular concentrations, and active transport where energy is expended to deliberately increase intracellular concentrations of a substrate. Oxidative metabolism also takes place at the membrane–cytoplasm interface.

Some species require only minimal nutrients in their environment, having considerable synthetic powers, whereas others have complex nutritional requirements. *E. coli*, for example, can be grown in media providing only glucose and inorganic salts; streptococci, on the other hand, will grow only in complex media providing them with many organic compounds.

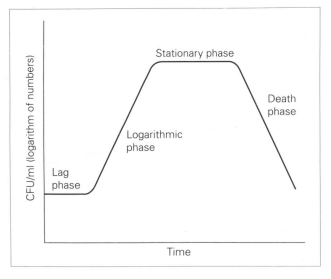

Fig. 2.3 The bacterial growth curve. (CFU, colony-forming units.)

GROWTH AND DIVISION

The rate at which bacteria grow and divide depends in large part on the nutritional status of the environment. The growth and division of a single *E. coli* cell into identical 'daughter cells' may occur in as little as 20–30 minutes in rich laboratory media, whereas the same process is much slower (1–2 hours) in a nutritionally depleted environment. Conversely, even in the best environment, other bacteria such as *Mycobacterium tuberculosis* may grow much more slowly, dividing every 24 hours. When introduced into a new environment, bacterial growth follows a characteristic pattern depicted in *Figure 2.3*. After an initial period of adjustment (lag phase), cell division rapidly occurs, with the population doubling at a constant rate (generation time), for a period termed log or exponential phase. As nutrients are depleted and toxic products accumulate, cell growth slows to a stop (stationary phase) and eventually enters a phase of decline (death).

A bacterial cell must duplicate its genomic DNA before it can divide

All bacterial genomes are circular, and their replication begins at a single site known as the origin of replication (termed OriC). A multienzyme replication complex binds to the origin and initiates unwinding and separation of the two DNA strands, using enzymes called helicases and topoisomerases (e.g. DNA gyrase). The separated DNA strands each serves as a template for DNA polymerase. The polymerization reaction involves incorporation of deoxyribonucleotides, which correctly base pair with the template DNA. Two characteristic replication forks are formed, which proceed in opposite directions around the chromosome. The two copies of the total genetic information (genome) produced during replication each comprises one parental strand and one newly synthesized strand of DNA.

Replication of the genome takes approximately 40 minutes in *E. coli*, so when these bacteria grow and divide every 20–30 minutes they need to initiate new rounds of DNA replication before an existing round of replication has finished. In such instances daughter cells inherit DNA that has already initiated its own replication.

Replication must be accurate

Accurate replication is essential because DNA carries the information that defines the properties and processes of a cell. It is achieved because DNA polymerase is capable of proofreading newly incorporated deoxyribonucleotides and excising those that are incorrect. This reduces the frequency of errors to approximately one mistake (an incorrect base pair) per 10^{10} nucleotides copied.

Cell division is preceded by genome segregation and septum formation

The process of cell division (or septation) involves:

- segregation of the replicated genomes;
- formation of a septum in the middle of the cell;
- division of the cell to give separate daughter cells.

The septum is formed by an invagination of the cytoplasmic membrane and ingrowth of the peptidoglycan cell wall (and outer membrane in Gram-negative bacteria). Septation and DNA replication and genome segregation are not tightly coupled, but are sufficiently well coordinated to ensure that very few daughter cells do not have the correct complement of genomic DNA.

The mechanics of cell division result in reproducible cellular arrangements when viewed by microscopic examination. For example, cocci dividing in one plane may appear chained (streptococci) or paired (diplococci), while division in multiple planes results in clusters (staphylococci). As with cell shape, these arrangements have served as an important characteristic for bacterial identification.

Bacterial growth and division are important targets for antimicrobial agents

Antimicrobials that target the processes involved in bacterial growth and division include:

- quinolones (nalidixic acid and norfloxacin), which inhibit the unwinding of DNA by DNA gyrase during DNA replication;
- the many inhibitors of peptidoglycan cell wall synthesis (e.g. beta-lactams such as the penicillins, cephalosporins and carbapenems, and glycopeptides such as vancomycin).

These are considered in more detail in Chapter 33.

GENE EXPRESSION

Gene expression describes the processes involved in decoding the 'genetic information' contained within a gene to produce a functional protein or RNA molecule.

Most genes are transcribed into messenger RNA (mRNA)

The overwhelming majority of genes (e.g. up to 98% in *E. coli*) are transcribed into mRNA, which is then translated into proteins. Certain genes, however, are transcribed to produce ribosomal RNA species (5S, 16S, 23S), which provide a scaffold for assembling ribosomal subunits; others are transcribed into transfer RNA (tRNA) molecules, which together with the ribosome participate in decoding mRNA into functional proteins.

Transcription

The DNA is copied by a DNA-dependent RNA polymerase to yield an RNA transcript. The polymerization reaction involves incorporation of ribonucleotides, which correctly base pair with the template DNA.

Transcription is initiated at promoters

Promoters are nucleotide sequences in DNA that can bind the RNA polymerase. The frequency of transcription initiation can be influenced by many factors, for example:

- the exact DNA sequence of the promoter site;
- the overall topology (supercoiling) of the DNA;
- the presence or absence of regulatory proteins that bind adjacent to and may overlap the promoter site.

Consequently, different promoters have widely different rates of transcriptional initiation (of up to 3000-fold). Their activities can be altered by regulatory proteins. Sigma factor (a component RNA polymerase) plays an important role in promoter recognition. The presence of several different sigma factors in bacteria enables sets of genes to be switched on simply by altering the level of expression of a particular sigma factor. This is particularly important in controlling the expression of genes involved in spore formation in Gram-positive bacteria.

Transcription usually terminates at specific termination sites

These termination sites are characterized by a series of uracil residues in the mRNA following an inverted repeat sequence, which can adopt a stem-loop structure (which forms as a result of the base-pairing of ribonucleotides) and interfere with RNA polymerase activity. In addition, certain transcripts terminate following interaction of RNA polymerase with the transcription termination protein, rho.

mRNA transcripts often encode more than one protein in bacteria

The bacterial arrangement seen for single genes (promoter–structural-gene–transcriptional-terminator) is described as monocistronic. However, a single promoter and terminator may flank multiple structural genes, a polycistronic arrangement known as an operon. Operon transcription thus results in polycistronic mRNA encoding more than one protein (*Fig. 2.4*). Operons provide a way of ensuring that protein subunits that make up particular enzyme complexes or are required for a specific biological process are synthesized simultaneously and in the correct stoichiometry. For example, the proteins required for the uptake and metabolism of lactose are encoded by the *lac* operon. Many of the proteins responsible for the pathogenic properties of medically

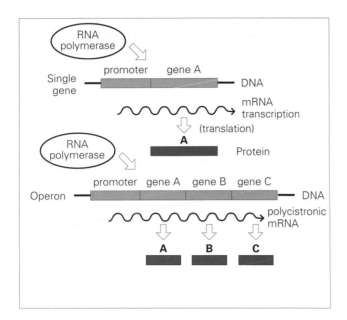

Fig. 2.4 Bacterial genes are present on DNA as separate discrete units (single genes) or as operons (multigenes), which are transcribed from promoters to give, respectively, monocistronic or polycistronic messenger RNA (mRNA) molecules. mRNA is then translated into protein.

important microorganisms are likewise encoded by operons, for example:

- cholera toxin from *Vibrio cholerae*;
- fimbriae (pili) of uropathogenic *E. coli,* which mediate colonization.

Translation

The exact sequence of amino acids in a protein (polypeptide) is specified by the sequence of nucleotides found in the mRNA transcripts. Decoding this information to produce a protein is achieved by ribosomes and tRNA molecules in a process known as translation. Each set of three bases (triplet) in the mRNA sequence corresponds to a codon for a specific amino acid.

Translation begins with formation of an initiation complex and terminates at a STOP codon

The initiation complex comprises mRNA, ribosome and an initiator transfer RNA molecule (tRNA) carrying formyl-methionine. Ribosomes bind to specific sequences in mRNA (Shine–Dalgarno sequences) and begin translation at an initiation (START) codon, AUG, which hybridizes with a specific complementary sequence (the anti-codon loop) of the initiator tRNA molecule. The polypeptide chain elongates as a result of movement of the ribosome along the mRNA molecule and the recruitment of further tRNA molecules (carrying different amino acids), which recognize the subsequent codon triplets. Ribosomes carry out a condensation reaction, which couples the incoming amino acid (carried on the tRNA) to the growing polypeptide chain.

Translation is terminated when the ribosome encounters one of three termination (STOP) codons: UGA, UAA or UAG.

Transcription and translation are important targets for antimicrobial agents

Such antimicrobial agents include:

- inhibitors of RNA polymerase, such as rifampicin;
- an array of bacterial protein synthesis inhibitors including macrolides (e.g. erythromycin), aminoglycosides, tetracycline, streptomycin and chloramphenicol (see Chapter 33).

Regulation of gene expression

Bacteria adapt to their environment by controlling gene expression

Bacteria show a remarkable ability to adapt to changes in their environment. This is predominantly achieved by controlling gene expression, thereby ensuring that proteins are only produced when and if they are required. For example:

- Bacteria may encounter a new source of carbon or nitrogen and as a consequence switch on new metabolic pathways that enable them to transport and use such compounds.
- When compounds such as amino acids are depleted from a bacterium's environment the bacterium may be able to switch on the production of enzymes that enable it to synthesize the particular molecule it requires de novo.

Expression of many virulence determinants by pathogenic bacteria is highly regulated

This makes sense since it conserves metabolic energy and ensures that virulence determinants are only produced when their particular property is needed. For example, entero-bacterial pathogens are often transmitted in contaminated water supplies. The temperature of such water will probably be lower than 25°C and low in nutrients. However, upon entering the human gut there will be a striking change in the bacterium's environment—the temperature will rise to 37°C, there will be an abundant supply of carbon and nitrogen and a low availability of both oxygen and free iron (an essential nutrient). Bacteria adapt to such changes by switching on or off a range of metabolic and virulence-associated genes.

The analysis of virulence gene expression is one of the fastest growing aspects of the study of microbial pathogenesis. It provides an important insight into how bacteria adapt to the many changes they encounter as they initiate infection and spread into different host tissues.

The most common way of altering gene expression is to change the amount of mRNA transcription

The level of mRNA transcription can be altered by altering the efficiency of binding of RNA polymerase to promoter sites. Environmental changes such as shifts in growth temperature (from 25°C to 37°C) or the availability of oxygen can change the extent of supercoiling in DNA, thereby altering the overall topology of promoters and the efficiency of transcription initiation. However, most instances of transcriptional regulation are mediated by regulatory proteins, which bind specifically to the DNA adjacent to or overlapping the promoter site and alter RNA polymerase binding and trans-

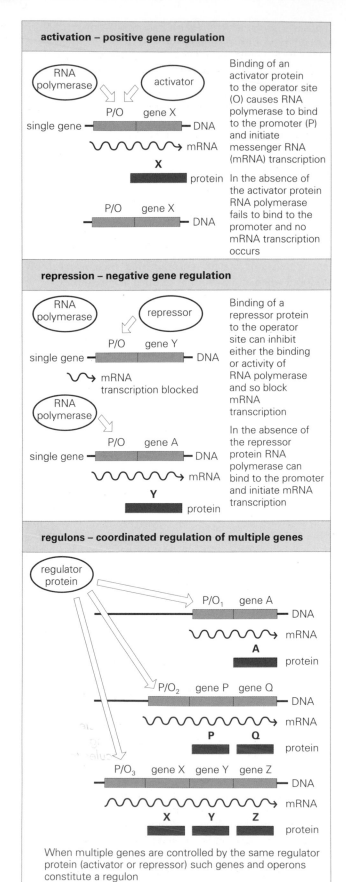

Fig. 2.5 Expression of genes in bacteria is highly regulated, enabling them to switch genes on or off in response to changes in available nutrients or other changes in their environment. Genes and operons controlled by the same regulator constitute a regulon.

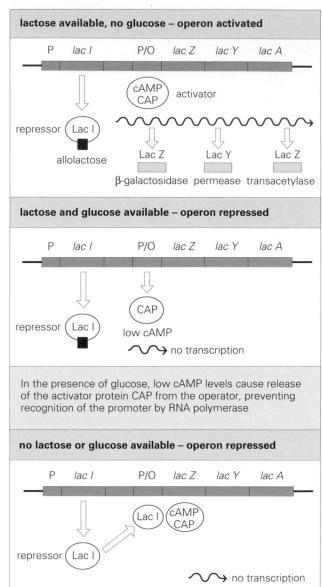

Fig. 2.6 Control of the *lac* operon. Transcription is controlled by the lactose repressor protein (Lac I, negative regulation) and by the catabolite activator protein (CAP, positive regulation). In the presence of lactose as the sole carbon source for growth the *lac* operon is switched on. Bacteria prefer to use glucose rather than lactose, so if glucose is also present the *lac* operon is switched off until the glucose has been used.

cription. The regions of DNA to which regulatory proteins bind are known as operators or operator sites. Regulatory proteins fall into two distinct classes:

• those that increase the rate of transcription initiation (activators);
• those that inhibit transcription (repressors) *(Fig. 2.5)*.

Genes subject to negative regulation bind repressor proteins. Genes subject to positive regulation need to bind activated regulatory protein(s) to promote transcription initiation.

The principles of gene regulation in bacteria can be illustrated by the regulation of genes involved in sugar metabolism

Bacteria use sugars as a carbon source for growth and prefer to use glucose rather than other less well-metabolized sugars. When growing in an environment containing both glucose and lactose, bacteria such as *E. coli* preferentially metabolize glucose and at the same time prevent the expression of the *lac* operon, the products of which transport and metabolize lactose *(Fig. 2.6)*. This is known as catabolite repression. It occurs because the transcriptional initiation of the *lac* operon is dependent upon a positive regulator, the cAMP-dependent catabolite activator protein (CAP), which is only activated when cAMP is bound. When bacteria grow on glucose the cytoplasmic levels of cAMP are low and so CAP is not activated. CAP is therefore unable to bind to its DNA binding site adjacent to the *lac* promoter and facilitate transcription initiation by RNA polymerase. When the glucose is depleted, the cAMP concentration rises, resulting in the formation of activated cAMP–CAP complexes, which bind the appropriate site on the DNA, increasing RNA polymerase binding and transcription.

CAP is an example of a global regulatory protein that controls the expression of multiple genes; it controls the expression of over 100 genes in *E. coli*. All genes controlled by the same regulator are considered to constitute a regulon *(Fig. 2.5)*. In addition to the influence of CAP on the *lac* operon, the operon is also subject to negative regulation by the lactose repressor protein (Lac I, *Fig. 2.6*). Lac I is encoded by the *lac I* gene, which is located immediately upstream of the lactose operon and transcribed by a separate promoter. In the absence of lactose, Lac I binds specifically to the operator region of the *lac* promoter and blocks transcription. An inducer molecule, allolactose (or its non-metabolizable homologue, isopropyl-thiogalactoside—IPTG) is able to bind to Lac I, causing an allosteric change in its structure. This releases it from the DNA, thereby alleviating the repression. The *lac* operon therefore illustrates the fine tuning of gene regulation in bacteria—the operon is switched on only if lactose is available as a carbon source for cell growth, but remains unexpressed if glucose, the cell's preferred carbon source, is also present.

Expression of bacterial virulence genes is often controlled by regulatory proteins

An example of such regulation is the production of diphtheria toxin by *Corynebacterium diphtheriae* (see Chapter 18), which is subject to negative regulation if there is free iron in the growth environment. A repressor protein, DtxR, binds iron and undergoes a conformational change that allows it to bind with high affinity to the operator site of the toxin gene and inhibit transcription. When *C. diphtheriae* grow in an environment with a very low concentration of iron (i.e. similar to that of human secretions), DtxR is unable to bind iron, and toxin production occurs.

Many bacterial virulence genes are subject to positive regulation by 'two-component regulators'

These two-component regulators usually comprise two separate proteins:

- one acting as a sensor to detect environmental changes (such as alterations in temperature);
- the other acting as a DNA-binding protein capable of activating (or repressing in some cases) transcription.

In *Bordetella pertussis*, the causative agent of whooping cough (see Chapter 19), a two-component regulator (encoded by the *bvg* locus) controls expression of a large number virulence genes. The sensor protein, BvgS, is a cytoplasmic membrane-located histidine kinase, which senses environmental signals (temperature, Mg^{2+}, nicotinic acid), leading to an alteration in its autophosphorylating activity. In response to positive regulatory signals such as an elevation in temperature, BvgS undergoes autophosphorylation and then phosphorylates, so activating the DNA-binding protein BvgA. BvgA then binds to the operators of the pertussis toxin operon and other virulence-associated genes and activates their transcription.

In *Staphylococcus aureus* a variety of virulence genes are influenced by global regulatory systems, the best studied and most important of which is a two-component regulator termed accessory gene regulator (agr). Agr control is complex in that it serves as a positive regulator for exotoxins secreted late in the bacterial lifecycle (post-exponential phase) but behaves as a negative regulator for virulence factors associated with the cell surface.

Regulation of virulence genes often involves a cascade of activators

For example:

- In *B. pertussis*, BvgA appears to activate the expression of another regulatory protein, which in turn activates the expression of filamentous hemagglutinin, the major adherence factor produced by *B. pertussis*.
- The control of virulence gene expression in *V. cholerae* is under the control of ToxR, a cytoplasmic membrane-located protein, which senses environmental changes. ToxR activates both the transcription of the cholera toxin operon and another regulatory protein, ToxT, which in turn activates the transcription of other virulence genes such as toxin-co-regulated pili, an essential virulence factor required for colonization of the human small intestine.

EXTRACHROMOSOMAL ELEMENTS

In addition to the chromosome, many bacteria possess smaller, independently replicating (extrachromosomal) nucleic acid molecules termed plasmids and bacteriophages

Plasmids are independent, self-replicating, circular units of dsDNA, some of which are relatively large (60–120 kb) while others are quite small (1.5–15 kb). Plasmid replication is similar to the replication of genomic DNA, though there may be some differences. Not all plasmids are replicated bidirectionally—some have a single replication fork, others are replicated like a 'rolling circle'. The number of plasmids per bacterial cell (copy number) varies for different plasmids, ranging from 1–1000 copies/cell. The rate of initiation of plasmid replication determines the plasmid copy number;

however, larger plasmids generally tend to have lower copy numbers than smaller plasmids. Some plasmids (broad-host range plasmids) are able to replicate in many different bacterial species, others have a more restricted host range.

Plasmids contain genes for replication, and in some cases for mediating their own transfer between bacteria (*tra* genes). Plasmids may additionally carry a wide variety of genes (up to 100 on larger plasmids) which can confer phenotypic advantages to the host bacterial cell.

Widespread use of antimicrobials has applied a strong selection pressure in favor of bacteria able to resist them

In the majority of cases, resistance to antimicrobials is due to the presence of resistance genes on conjugative plasmids (R plasmids; see Chapter 33). These are known to have existed before the era of mass antibiotic treatments, but they have become widespread in many species as a result of selection. R plasmids may carry genes for resistance to several antimicrobials. For example, the common R plasmid, R1, confers resistance to ampicillin, chloramphenicol, fusidic acid, kanamycin, streptomycin and sulfonamides, and there are many others conferring resistance to a wide spectrum of antimicrobials. R plasmids can recombine so that individual plasmids can be responsible for new combinations of multiple drug resistance.

Plasmids can carry virulence genes

Plasmids may encode toxins and other proteins that increase the virulence of microorganisms. For example:

- The virulent enterotoxinogenic strains of *E. coli* that cause diarrhea produce one of two different types of plasmid-encoded enterotoxin. The enterotoxin alters the secretion of fluid and electrolytes by the intestinal epithelium (see Chapter 22).
- In *Staphylococcus aureus* both an enterotoxin and a number of enzymes involved in bacterial virulence (hemolysin, fibrinolysin) are encoded by plasmid genes.

The production of toxins by bacteria, and their pathologic effects, are discussed in detail in Chapter 17.

Plasmids are valuable tools for cloning and manipulating genes

Molecular biologists have generated a wealth of recombinant plasmids to use as vectors for genetic engineering (*Fig. 2.7*). Plasmids can be used to transfer genes across species barriers

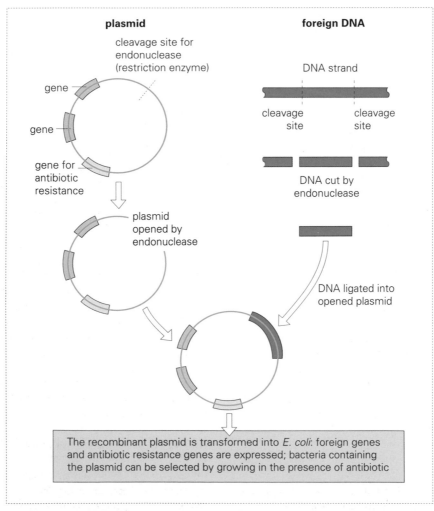

Fig. 2.7 The use of plasmid vectors to introduce foreign DNA in *Escherichia coli*—a basic step in gene cloning.

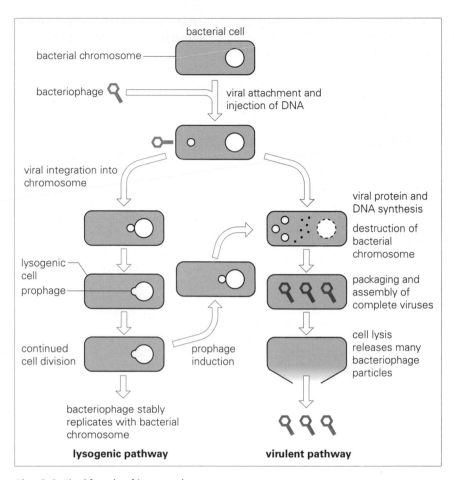

Fig. 2.8 The lifecycle of bacteriophages.

so that defined gene products can be studied or synthesized in large quantities in different recipient organisms.

Bacteriophages are bacterial viruses that can survive outside as well as inside the bacterial cell

Bacteriophages differ from plasmids in that their reproduction usually leads to destruction of the bacterial cell. In general, bacteriophages consists of a protein coat or head (capsid) which surrounds nucleic acid which may be either DNA or RNA but not both. Some bacteriophages may also possess a tail-like structure which aids them in attaching to and infecting their bacterial host. As illustrated in *Figure 2.8* for DNA-containing bacteriophages, the virus attaches and injects its DNA into the bacterium, leaving the protective protein coat behind. Virulent bacteriophages instigate a form of molecular mutiny to commandeer cellular nucleic acid and protein to produce new virus DNA and protein. Many new virus particles (virions) are then assembled and released into the environment as the bacterial cell ruptures (lyses) thus allowing the cycle to begin again.

While destruction of the host is always the direct consequence of virulent bacteriophage infection, temperate bacteriophages may exercise a 'choice'. Following infection, they may immediately reproduce in a manner similar to their virulent counterparts. However, in some instances they may insert into the bacterial chromosome. This process, termed lysogeny, does not kill the cell since the integrated viral DNA (now called a prophage) is quiescently carried and replicated within the bacterial chromosome. New characteristics may be expressed by the cell as a result of prophage presence (prophage conversion) which, in some instances, may increase bacterial virulence (e.g. the gene for diphtheria toxin resides on a prophage). Nevertheless, this latent state is eventually destined to end, often in response to some environmental stimulus inactivating the bacteriophage repressor which normally maintains the lysogenic condition. During this induction process the viral DNA is excised from the chromosome and proceeds to active replication and assembly, resulting in cell lysis and viral release.

Whether virulent or temperate, bacteriophage infection ultimately results in death of the host cell which, given current problems with multiple resistance, has sparked a renewed interest in their use as 'natural' antimicrobial agents. However, a variety of issues related to dosing, delivery, quality control, etc. have impeded the use of 'bacteriophage therapy' in routine clinical practice.

MUTATION AND GENE TRANSFER

Bacteria are haploid organisms, their chromosomes containing one copy of each gene. Replication of the DNA is a precise process resulting in each daughter cell acquiring an exact copy of the parental genome. Changes in the genome can occur by two processes:

- mutation;
- recombination.

These processes result in progeny with phenotypic characteristics that may differ from those of the parent. This is of considerable significance in terms of virulence and drug resistance.

Mutation

Changes in the nucleotide sequence of DNA can occur spontaneously or under the influence of external agents

While mutations may spontaneously occur as a result of errors in the DNA replication process, a variety of chemicals (mutagens) bring about direct changes in the DNA molecule. A classic example of such an interaction involves compounds known as nucleotide-base analogues. These agents mimic normal nucleotides during DNA synthesis but are capable of multiple pairing with a counterpart on the opposite strand. While 5-bromouracil is considered a thymine analogue, for example, it may also behave as a cytosine, thus allowing the potential for a change from T-A to C-G in a replicating DNA duplex. Other agents may cause changes by inserting (intercalating) and distorting the DNA helix or by interacting directly with nucleotide bases to chemically alter them.

Regardless of their cause, changes in DNA may generally be characterized as follows.

- Point mutations—changes in single nucleotides which alter the triplet code. Such mutations may result in:
  - no change in the amino acid sequence of the protein encoded by the gene, because the different codons specify the same amino acid and are therefore silent mutations;
  - an amino acid substitution in the translated protein (missense mutation), which may or may not alter its stability or functional properties;
  - the formation of a STOP codon, causing premature termination and production of a truncated protein (nonsense mutation).
- More comprehensive changes in the DNA, which involve deletion, replacement, insertion or inversion of several or many bases. The majority of these changes are likely to harm the organism, but a few may be beneficial and confer a selective advantage through the production of different proteins.

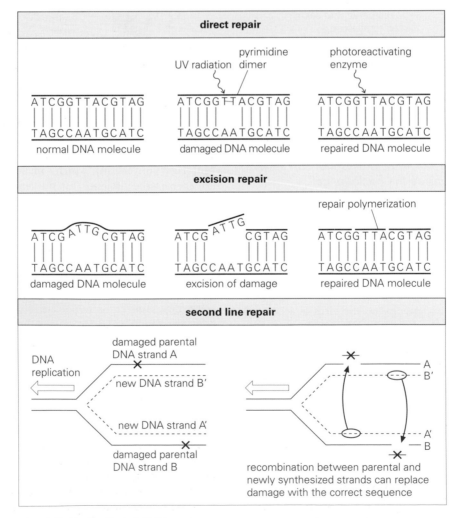

Fig. 2.9 Mechanisms of DNA repair.

Bacterial cells are not defenseless against genetic damage

Since the bacterial genome is the most fundamental molecule of identity in the cell, enzymatic machinery is in place to protect it against both spontaneously occurring and induced mutational damage. As illustrated in *Figure 2.9* these DNA repair processes include the following.

- Direct repair which either reverses or simply removes the damage. This may be regarded as 'first line' defense. For example, abnormally linked pyrimidine bases in DNA (pyrimidine dimers) resulting from ultraviolet radiation are directly reversed by a light-dependent enzyme through a repair process known as photoreactivation.
- Excision repair where damage in a DNA strand is recognized by an enzymatic 'housekeeping' process and excised, followed by repair polymerization to fill the gap using the intact complementary DNA strand as a template. This is also a primary form of defense since the goal is to correct damage before it encounters and potentially interferes with the moving DNA replication fork. Some of these housekeeping genes are also part of an inducible system (SOS repair) which is activated by the presence of DNA damage to quickly respond and effect repair.
- 'Second line' repair which operates when DNA damage has reached a point where it is more difficult to correct. When normal DNA replication processes are blocked, permissive systems may allow the interfering damage to be inaccurately corrected, allowing errors to occur but improving the probability of cell survival. In other instances, where damage has passed the replication fork, post-replication or recombinational repair processes may 'cut and paste' to construct error-free DNA from multiple copies of the sequence found in parental and daughter strands.

Bacterial DNA repair has provided a model for understanding similar, more complex processes in humans

DNA repair mechanisms appear to be present in all living organisms as a defense against environmental damage. The study of these processes in bacteria has led to an important understanding of general principles that apply to higher organisms, including issues of cancer and aging in humans. For example, several human disorders are now known to be DNA-repair related, including:

- xeroderma pigmentosum, characterized by extreme sensitivity to the sun, with great risk for development of a variety of skin cancers such as basal cell carcinoma, squamous cell carcinoma and melanoma;
- Cockayne syndrome, characterized by progressive neurologic degeneration, growth retardation, and sun sensitivity not associated with cancer;
- trichothiodystrophy, characterized by mental and growth retardation, fragile hair deficient in sulfur, and sun sensitivity not associated with cancer.

Gene transfer and recombination

New genotypes arise when genetic material is transferred from one bacterium to another. In such instances, the transferred DNA either:

- recombines with the genome of the recipient cell;
- or is on a plasmid capable of replication in the recipient without recombination.

Recombination can bring about large changes in the genetic material, and since these events usually involve functional genes, they are likely to be expressed phenotypically. DNA can be transferred from a donor cell to a recipient cell by:

- transformation;
- transduction;
- conjugation;
- transposition *(Fig. 2.10)*.

Transformation

Some bacteria can be transformed by DNA present in their environment

Certain bacteria such as *Streptococcus pneumoniae*, *Bacillus subtilis*, *Haemophilus influenzae* and *Neisseria gonorrhoeae* are naturally 'competent' to take up DNA fragments from related species across their cell walls. Such DNA fragments may be present in the environment of the competent cell as a result of lysis of other organisms, the release of their DNA and its cleavage into smaller fragments. Once taken into the cell, chromosomal DNA must recombine with an homologous segment of the recipient's chromosome to be stably maintained and inherited. If the DNA is completely unrelated, the absence of homology prevents recombination and the DNA is degraded. However, plasmid DNA may be transformed into a cell and expressed without recombination. Thus, transformation has served as a powerful tool for molecular genetic analysis of bacteria *(Fig. 2.7)*

Most bacteria are not naturally competent to be transformed by DNA, but competence can be induced artificially by either treating cells with certain bivalent cations and then subjecting them to a heat shock at 42°C or by electric shock treatment (electroporation).

Prior to uptake by competent cells, DNA is extracellular, unprotected, and thus vulnerable to destruction by environmental extremes (e.g. DNA-degrading enzymes—DNases). Thus, it is the least important mechanism of gene transfer from the standpoint of clinical relevance (e.g. probability of transfer within a patient).

Transduction

Transduction involves the transfer of genetic material by infection with a bacteriophage

During the process of virulent bacteriophage replication (or temperate bacteriophages exercising the direct lysis option), other DNA in the cell (genomic or plasmid) is occasionally erroneously packaged into the virus head, resulting in a 'transducing particle', which can attach to and transfer the DNA into a recipient cell. If chromosomal, the DNA must be incorporated into the recipient genome by homologous recombination to be stably inherited and expressed. As with transformation, plasmid DNA may be transduced and expressed in a recipient without recombination. In either case, this type of gene transfer is known as generalized transduction *(Fig. 2.10)*.

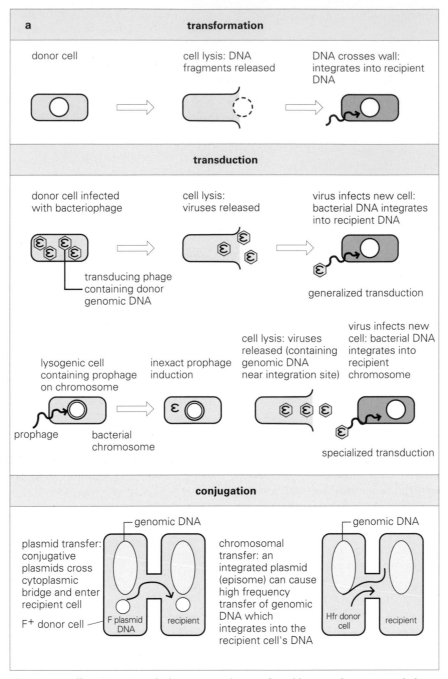

Fig. 2.10 Different ways in which genes can be transferred between bacteria. With the exception of plasmid transfer, donor DNA integrates into the recipient's genome by a process of either homologous or illegitimate (in the case of transposons) recombination.

Another form of transduction occurs with 'temperate' bacteriophages, since they integrate at specialized attachment sites in the bacterial genome. As these prophages prepare to enter the lytic cycle, they occasionally incorrectly excise from the site of attachment. This can result in phages containing a piece of bacterial genomic DNA adjacent to the attachment site. Infection of a recipient cell then results in a high frequency of recombinants where donor DNA has recombined with the recipient genome in the vicinity of the attachment site. Since this 'specialized transduction' is based on specific chromosome–prophage interaction, only genomic DNA, and not plasmids, is transferred by this process.

In contrast to transformation, transduced DNA is always protected, thus increasing its probability of successful transfer and potential clinical relevance. However, bacteriophages are extremely host-specific 'parasites' and therefore unable to move any DNA between bacteria of different species.

Conjugation

Conjugation is a type of bacterial 'mating' in which DNA is transferred from one bacterium to another

Conjugation is dependent upon the *tra* genes found in 'conjugative' plasmids which, among other things, encode instructions for the bacterial cell to produce a sex pilus—a

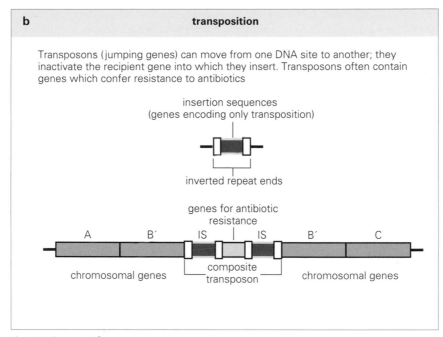

b   **transposition**

Transposons (jumping genes) can move from one DNA site to another; they inactivate the recipient gene into which they insert. Transposons often contain genes which confer resistance to antibiotics

insertion sequences
(genes encoding only transposition)

inverted repeat ends

genes for antibiotic
resistance

A   B′   IS   IS   B′   C

chromosomal genes   composite   chromosomal genes
                        transposon

Fig. 2.10, cont'd.

tube-like appendage which allows cell-to-cell contact to insure the protected transfer of a plasmid DNA copy from a donor cell to a recipient *(Fig. 2.10)*. Since the *tra* genes take up genetic space, 'conjugative' plasmids are generally larger than non-conjugative ones.

Occasionally, conjugative plasmids such as the fertility plasmid (F plasmid or F factor) of *E. coli* integrate into the bacterial genome, and such integrated plasmids are called episomes. When an integrated F episome attempts conjugative transfer, the duplication–transfer process eventually moves into regions of adjacent genomic DNA which are carried along from the donor cell into the recipient. Such strains, in contrast to cells containing the unintegrated F plasmid, mediate high frequency transfer and recombination of genomic DNA (Hfr strains). However, conjugation with Hfr donor cells does not result in complete transfer of the integrated plasmid. Thus, the recipient cell does not become Hfr and is incapable of serving as a conjugation donor. The circular nature of the bacterial genome and the relative 'map' positions of different genes were established using interrupted mating of Hfr strains.

When a non-conjugative plasmid is present in the same cell as a conjugative plasmid, they are sometimes transferred together into the recipient cell by a process known as mobilization. Conjugative transfer of plasmids with resistance genes has been an important cause of the spread of resistance to commonly used antibiotics within and between many bacterial species, since no recombination is required for expression in the recipient. Of all the mechanisms for gene transfer, this rapid and highly efficient movement of genetic information through bacterial populations is clearly of the highest clinical relevance.

Transposition

Transposable elements are DNA sequences that can jump (transpose) from a site in one DNA molecule to another in a cell

While plasmid transfer involves the movement of genetic information between bacterial cells, transposition is the movement of such information between DNA molecules. The most extensively studied transposable elements are those found in *E. coli* and other Gram-negative bacteria, although examples are also found in Gram-positive bacteria, yeast, plants and other organisms.

Insertion sequences are the smallest and simplest 'jumping genes'

Insertion sequence elements (ISs) are less than 2 kb in length and only encode functions such as the transposase enzyme, which is required for transposition from one DNA site to another. At the ends of ISs there are usually short inverted repeat sequences (23 nucleotides long in IS1), which are also important in the process of locating and inserting into a DNA target *(Fig. 2.10)*. During the transposition process, a portion of the target sequence is duplicated, resulting in short direct repeat sequences (the same sequence in the same orientation) on each side of the newly inserted IS element. Many aspects of the target selection process remain unclear. While A/T-rich regions of DNA appear to be preferred, some ISs are highly selective whereas others are generally indiscriminate. Transposition does not rely on enzymatic processes typically used by the cell for homologous recombination (recombination between highly related DNA molecules) and is thus termed 'illegitimate recombination'. The result is a typically small number of ISs in bacterial genomes. In *E. coli*, IS1 is found in 6 to 10 copies; IS2 and 3 around 5 copies. Multiple IS copies serve an important function as 'portable regions of homology' throughout a bacterial genome where homologous recombinaton may occur between different DNA regions or molecules (e.g. chromosome and plasmid) carrying the same IS sequence. It is this process that allows chromosomal integration of the F plasmid to produce Hfr strains. Two IS elements inserting relatively near to each other allow the entire region to become transposable, further promoting the potential for genetic exchange in bacterial populations.

Transposons are larger, more complex elements which encode multiple genes

Transposons are larger than 2 kb in size and contain genes in addition to those required for transposition (often encoding resistance to one or more antibiotics) *(Fig. 2.10)*. Furthermore, virulence genes, such as those encoding heat-stable enterotoxin from *E. coli*, have been found on transposons.

Transposons can be divided into two classes:

- composite transposons where two copies of an identical IS element flank antibiotic-resistance genes (kanamycin resistance in Tn5);
- simple transposons, such as Tn3 (encoding resistance to beta-lactams).

ISs at the ends of composite transposons may be in either the same or inverted orientation (i.e. direct or indirect repeats). Although part of the composite transposon structure, the terminal IS elements are fully intact and capable of independent transposition.

Simple transposons move only as a single unit, containing genes for transposition and other functions (e.g. antibiotic resistance) with short, inversely oriented sequences (indirect repeats) at each end.

Mobile genetic elements promote a variety of DNA rearrangements which may have important clinical consequences

The ease with which transposons move into or out of DNA sequences means that transposition can occur:

- from host genomic DNA harboring a transposon to a plasmid;
- from one plasmid to another plasmid;
- from a plasmid to genomic DNA.

Transposition onto a broad-host range conjugative plasmid can lead to the rapid dissemination of resistance among different bacteria. The transposition process (whether by ISs or transposons) can be deleterious if insertion occurs within, and disrupts, a functional gene. However, transpositional mutagenesis has been effectively utilized in the molecular biology laboratory to produce extremely specific mutations without the harmful secondary effects often seen with more generally acting chemical mutagens.

Pathogenicity islands are a special class of mobile genetic elements containing groups of coordinately controlled virulence genes, often with ISs, direct repeat sequences, etc. at their ends. Though originally observed in uropathogenic *E.*

coli (encoding hemolysins and pili), pathogenicity islands have now been found in a number of additional bacterial species including *Helicobacter pylori*, *Vibrio cholerae*, *Salmonella* spp., *Staphylococcus aureus*, and *Yersinia* spp. Such regions are not found in non-pathogenic bacteria, may be quite large (up to hundreds of kilobases), and tend to be unstable (spontaneously lost). Differences in DNA sequence (G+C content) between such elements and their host genomes support speculation regarding their origin and movement from unrelated bacterial species.

SURVIVAL UNDER ADVERSE CONDITIONS

Some bacteria form endospores

Certain bacteria can form highly resistant spores—endospores—within their cells, and these enable them to survive adverse conditions. They are formed when the cells are unable to grow (e.g. when environmental conditions change or when nutrients are exhausted), but never by actively growing cells. The spore has a complex multilayered coat surrounding a new bacterial cell. There are many differences in composition between endospores and normal cells, notably the presence of dipicolinic acid and a high calcium content, both of which are thought to confer the endospore's extreme resistance to heat and chemicals.

Because of their resistance, spores can remain viable in a dormant state for many years, reconverting rapidly to normal existence when conditions improve. When this occurs a new bacterial cell grows out from the spore and resumes vegetative life. Endospores are abundant in soils, and those of the *Clostridium* and *Bacillus* are a particular hazard *(Fig. 2.11)*. Tetanus and anthrax caused by these bacteria are both associated with endospore infection of wounds, the bacteria developing from the spores once in appropriate conditions.

THE GENOMICS OF MEDICALLY IMPORTANT BACTERIA

Advances in DNA sequencing techniques are leading to an ever-increasing number of bacterial pathogens for which the total genomic sequence is known *(Fig. 2.12)*. This evolving database represents a powerful resource with enormous potential application for the understanding and treatment of

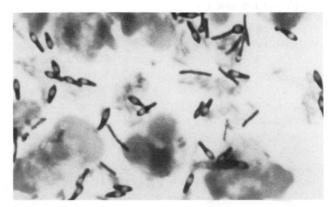

Fig. 2.11 *Clostridium tetani* with terminal spores.

Acinetobacter baumannii, Bacillus anthracis, Bacteroides fragilis, Bordetella bronchiseptica, Bordetella parpertussis, Bordetella pertussis, Borrelia burgdorferi, Brucella abortus, Burkholderia cepacia, Burkholderia mallei, Burkholderia pseudomallei, Campylobacter jejuni, Chlamydophila pneumoniae, Chlamydophila psittaci, Chlamydia trachomatis, Clostridium botulinum, Clostridium difficile, Corynebacterium diphtheriae, Coxiella burnetii, Enterobacter cloacae, Enterococcus faecalis, Enterococcus faecium, Escherichia coli, Francisella tularensis, Haemophilus influenzae, Helicobacter pylori, Klebsiella pneumoniae, Legionella pneumophila, Listeria monocytogenes, Moraxella catarrhalis, Mycobacterium avium, Mycobacterium bovis, Mycobacterium leprae, Mycobacterium tuberculosis, Mycoplasma genitalium, Mycoplasma pneumoniae, Neisseria gonorrhoeae, Neisseria meningitidis, Pasteurella multocida, Proteus mirabilis, Pseudomonas aeruginosa, Rickettsia prowazekii, Salmonella dublin, Salmonella enteritidis, Salmonella paratyphi, Salmonella typhi, Salmonella typhimurium, Staphylococcus aureus, Staphylococcus epidermidis, Streptococcus agalactiae, Streptococcus pneumoniae, Streptococcus pyogenes, Treponema pallidum, Ureaplasma urealyticum, Vibrio cholerae, Yersinia enterocolitica, Yersinia pestis

Fig. 2.12 Representative bacterial pathogens whose genomic sequence is entirely or largely known.

infectious disease. At present the utilization of this information is in its infancy; nevertheless, several instances where sequence-based information will be extremely useful in the study of clinically important microorganisms have already emerged, as described below.

Application of genomics facilitates identification

- *Identification and classification.* The genes encoding ribosomal RNA (16S, 23S and 5S) are typically found together in an operon where their transcription is coordinated *(Fig. 2.13).* This rDNA operon is found at least once and often in multiple copies distributed around the chromosome, depending on the bacterial species (*Borrelia burgdorferi* has one copy; *Staphylococcus aureus* has 5–6).

While the rDNA operon contains many conserved sequences (identical in different bacterial species), a portion of the 16S- and 23S-encoding regions have been found to be species specific. In between them, an 'internally transcribed spacer' (ITS) region exhibits variability that may have utility in differentiating closely-related bacterial isolates. Such information clearly has potential for future application in approaches to the rapid identification, classification and epidemiology of clinically important microorganisms (see Chapters 31 and 36).

- *Resistance to antimicrobial agents.* Genes specifically mediating antimicrobial resistance are well known (see Chapter 33). However, total genome sequencing provides more detailed information to insure their detection and allows a global overview where multiple loci may interact to effect resistance. For example, methicillin resistance in *Staphylococcus aureus* is influenced by a number of genes (e.g. *mecA, femA, femB, murE,* etc.) at different chromosomal locations.

- *Molecular epidemiology.* While a variety of phenotypic and genotypic methods have been employed to assess interrelationships in clinical isolates (see Chapter 36), epidemiologic analysis is now moving toward a more sequence-based approach. In contrast to earlier methods, sequence data are highly portable (internet transfer, etc.), less ambiguous (encoded entirely in the characters A, T, G and C, corresponding to the four bases adenine, thymine, guanine and cytosine, respectively), and easily stored in databases. In one approach, sequences from the internal regions of six or seven 'housekeeping' (essential) genes are compared to assess the epidemiologic relatedness of different isolates (multi-locus sequence typing, MLST). However, which chromosomal regions will ultimately provide the most epidemiologically relevant information in different bacterial pathogens will become clearer as additional genomes are sequenced.

Various approaches to the detection and utilization of genomic sequence information exist

Methods such as the polymerase chain reaction (PCR) and nucleic acid probes have clearly had a pivotal role in providing sequence-based answers to clinical microbiology questions (see Chapter 36). Nevertheless, the massive amounts of genomic sequence currently being generated have spawned innovative approaches aimed at extracting the maximum amount of information from the large databases which have been created.

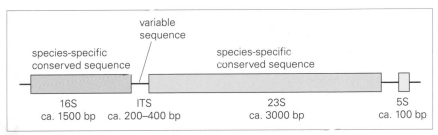

Fig. 2.13 Typical arrangement of the bacterial operon encoding ribosomal RNA. Sizes of the genes for 16S, 23S, 5S rRNA, and the internally transcribed spacer (ITS) region are indicated in nucleotide base pairs (bp). Regions encoding sequences helpful for species identification or epidemiology are indicated.

DNA microarrays provide a means for the 'parallel processing' of genomic information

Traditionally, molecular biology has operated by analyzing one gene in one experiment. While yielding important information, this approach is time consuming and does not afford ready access to the information (chromosomal organization and multiple-gene interaction) contained within genomic-sequence databases. Microarrays represent a new approach to this issue where information may be obtained from multiple queries simultaneously posed to a genomic-sequence database (parallel processing). DNA microarrays are based on the principles of nucleic hybridization (A pairs with T; G pairs with C). While there are a number of variations on the theme, the general format is the arrangement of samples (e.g. gene sequences) in a known matrix on a solid support (nylon, glass, etc.). Using specialized robotics, individual 'spots' may be less than 200 µm in diameter, allowing a single array (often called a DNA chip) to contain thousands of spots. Different fluorescently labeled probes of known sequence may then be simultaneously applied followed by monitoring to detect whether complementary binding has occurred.

At present, DNA microarrays are finding use in two main applications: identification of mutations and studies on gene expression

In a number of instances, specific point mutations are clinically important in pathogenic bacteria. Since these changes involve only one nucleotide base they are often referred to as single nucleotide polymorphisms (SNPs). Resistance to the quinolone class of antibiotics, for example, may result from a single base change within the bacterial *gyrA* gene (Chapter 33). In the past, such mutations have been

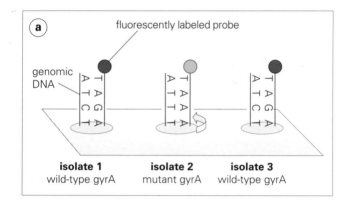

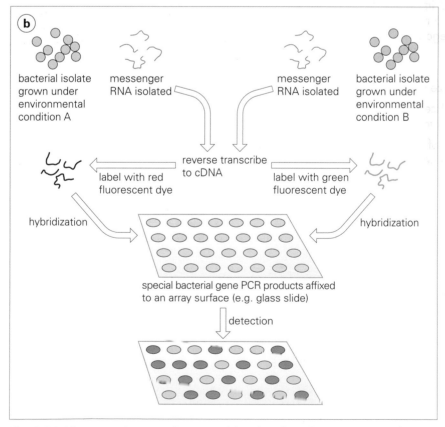

Fig. 2.14 Microarray detection of mutations (a) and analysis of gene expression (b).

detected by PCR amplification of the desired *gyrA* region followed by DNA sequencing and analysis. As illustrated in *Figure 2.14a*, DNA microarrays allow *gyrA* amplicons from different bacterial isolates to be applied to the same chip. Two *gyrA* probes (wild type, fluorescently labeled red; mutant, fluorescently labeled green) are applied to the array under conditions so stringent that only 100% homology will result in hybridization. In this manner the presence or absence of the specific mutation may be quickly and accurately assessed in a large number of isolates simultaneously.

Studies of gene expression are extremely important to the understanding of numerous bacterial processes, including virulence. For example, analysis might involve a comparison of gene expression (transcription) in an organism under different environmental conditions *(Fig. 2.14b)*. In such an experiment, genomics can provide data allowing sequences from every known chromosomal gene of the organism to be applied to a unique position on the chip. Messenger RNA (the result of gene expression) may be isolated from the same bacteria grown under either environmental condition A or B.

Using the enzyme reverse transcriptase in a process similar to that naturally employed by retroviruses (see Chapter 3), the mRNA is copied into complementary DNA (termed cDNA). Different fluorescent dyes (red or green) are bound to the A or B cDNA, respectively, which is then allowed to hybridize to complementary sequences on the chip. Array spots with red fluorescence will indicate genes expressed in environment A. Those appearing green will correspond to genes active in environment B, while yellow spots (red + green) will indicate genes active under both conditions.

Through innovative technologies such as DNA microarrays, and other approaches which may as yet only exist in an inquisitive mind, genomics will clearly play a major role in our understanding and treatment of infectious disease in the years ahead.

Major groups of bacteria

Detailed summaries of members of the major bacterial groups are given in the Appendix (Pathogen Parade).

KEY FACTS

- Bacteria are prokaryotes. Their DNA is not contained within a nucleus and there are relatively few cytoplasmic organelles.

- The cell wall is a key structure in metabolism, virulence and immunity. Its staining characteristics define the two major divisions: the Gram-positive and Gram-negative bacteria. Flagella may be present and confer motility.

- Bacteria metabolize aerobically and anaerobically and can utilize a range of substrates.

- The bacterial cell wall and their reproductive processes are targets for antimicrobial agents.

- Transcription of bacterial DNA may involve single or multiple genes. The arrangement of promoter and terminal sequences flanking multiple genes forms an operon.

- Bacteria can regulate gene expression to optimize exploitation of their environment.

- Plasmids and bacteriophages are independently replicating extrachromosomal agents. Plasmids may carry genes that affect resistance to antimicrobials or virulence.

- Genetic material can be carried from one bacterium to another in several ways; this can result in the rapid spread of resistance to antimicrobials.

- Genomics is revolutionizing the study and the control of bacterial infections.

? QUESTIONS

1. Which of the following is a distinctive component of the cell wall of Gram-negative bacteria?
   A. Capsule
   B. Lipopolysaccharide
   C. Peptidoglycan
   D. Plasma membrane
   E. Murein

2. Which of the following is a Gram-positive bacterium?
   A. *Salmonella*
   B. *Campylobacter*
   C. *Staphylococcus*
   D. *Neisseria*
   E. *Shigella*

3. At its fastest, *Escherichia coli* can divide:
   A. Every 24 hours
   B. Every 12 hours
   C. Every 6 hours
   D. Every hour
   E. Every 30 minutes

4. Bacteria can be killed by antimicrobial agents that:
   A. Inhibit unwinding of DNA prior to division
   B. Inhibit RNA polymerase
   C. Inhibit cell wall synthesis
   D. Inhibit protein synthesis
   E. All of these

5. Which process is not involved in transfer of genetic information between bacteria?
   A. Transduction
   B. Transformation
   C. Conjugation
   D. Mutation
   E. Transposition

6. Which are sometimes referred to as 'jumping genes'?
   A. Plasmids
   B. Transposons
   C. Bacteriophages
   D. Operons
   E. Two-component regulators

FURTHER READING

Collier L, Balows A, Sussman M, eds. *Topley and Wilson's Microbiology and Microbial Infections,* 9th edition. London: Edward Arnold, 1998.

Lewin B. *Genes VII.* Oxford: Oxford University Press, 2000.

The viruses

INTRODUCTION

Viruses differ from all other infectious organisms in their structure and biology, particularly in their reproduction. Although viruses carry conventional genetic information in their DNA or RNA, they lack the synthetic machinery necessary for this information to be processed into new virus material. A virus by itself is metabolically inert—it can replicate only after infection of a host cell, when it can parasitize the host's ability to transcribe and/or translate genetic information. Viruses infect every form of life. They cause some of the commonest and many of the most serious diseases of humans. Some insert their genetic material into the human genome and can cause cancer. Viruses are difficult targets for chemotherapy, but many can be controlled by effective vaccines.

Viruses share some common structural features

Viruses range from very small (poliovirus, at 30 nm) to quite large (vaccinia virus, at 400 nm, is as big as small bacteria). Their organization varies considerably between the different groups, but there are some general characteristics common to all:

- The genetic material, in the form of single-stranded (ss) or double-stranded (ds), linear or circular RNA or DNA, is contained within a capsule or capsid, made up of a number of individual protein molecules (capsomeres).
- The complete unit of nucleic acid and capsid is called the 'nucleocapsid', and often has a distinctive symmetry depending upon the ways in which the individual capsomeres are assembled *(Fig. 3.1)*. Symmetry can be icosahedral, helical or complex.
- In many cases the entire 'virus particle' or 'virion' consists only of a nucleocapsid. In others the virion consists of the nucleocapsid surrounded by an outer envelope or membrane *(Fig. 3.2)*. This is generally a lipid bilayer of host cell origin, into which virus proteins and glycoproteins are inserted.

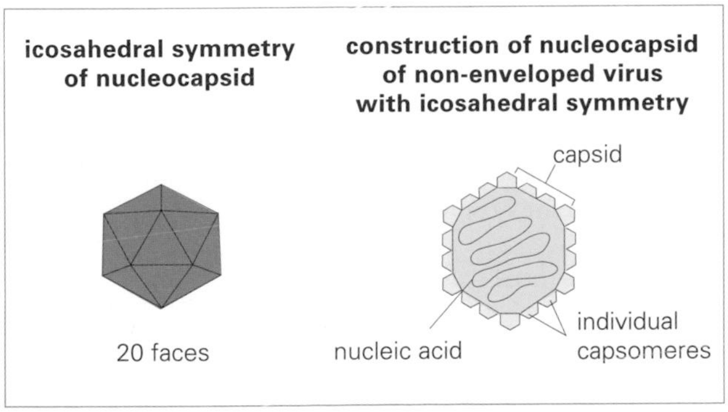

The outer surface of the virus particle is the part that first makes contact with the membrane of the host cell

The structure and properties of the outer surface of the virus particle are therefore of vital importance in understanding the process of infection. In general, naked (envelope-free) viruses are resistant and survive well in the outside world; they may also be bile-resistant, allowing infection through the alimentary canal. Enveloped viruses are more susceptible to environmental factors such as drying, gastric acidity and bile. These differences in susceptibility influence the ways in which these viruses can be transmitted.

INFECTION OF HOST CELLS

The stages involved in infection of host cells are summarized in *Figure 3.3* (see also *Fig. 2.3*).

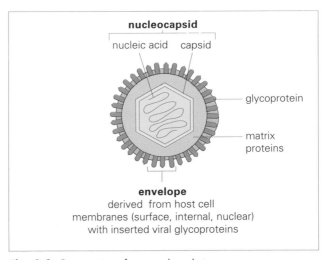

Fig. 3.2 Construction of an enveloped virus.

Fig. 3.1 Symmetry and construction of the viral nucleocapsid.

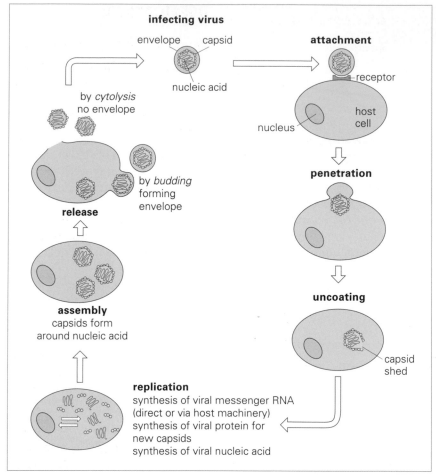

Fig. 3.3 Stages in the infection of a host's cell and replication of a virus. Several thousand virus particles may be formed from each cell.

Virus particles enter the body of the host in many ways

The commonest forms of virus transmission (*Fig. 3.4;* see Chapter 13) are:

- via inhaled droplets (e.g. rhinovirus);
- in food or water (e.g. hepatitis A);
- by direct transfer from other infected hosts (e.g. HIV);
- from bites of vector arthropods (e.g. yellow fever).

Viruses show host specificity, which is initially based upon an ability to attach to the host cell

Like all pathogens, viruses usually infect only one or a restricted range of host species. The initial basis of specificity is the ability of the virus particle to attach to the host cell.

The process of attachment to, or adsorption by, a host cell depends first upon the operation of general intermolecular forces, then upon more specific interactions between the molecules of the nucleocapsid (in naked viruses) or the virus membrane (in enveloped viruses) and the molecules of the host cell membrane. In many cases there is a specific interaction with a particular host molecule, which therefore acts as a receptor. Influenza virus, for example, attaches by its hemagglutinin to a glycoprotein (sialic acid) found on cells of mucous membranes and on red blood cells; other examples

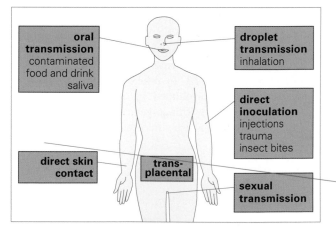

Fig. 3.4 Routes by which viruses enter the body.

are given in *Figure 3.5*. Attachment to the receptor is followed by entry into the host cell.

Once in the host's cytoplasm the virus is no longer infective

After fusion of viral and host membranes, or uptake into a phagosome, the virus particle is carried into the cytoplasm across the plasma membrane. At this stage, the envelope

CELL MEMBRANE RECEPTORS FOR VIRUSES	
virus	**receptor molecule**
influenza	sialic acid on glycoproteins, including the glycophorin A molecule
rabies	acetylcholine receptor
HIV	CD4 and CXCR4, molecules on T cells, CCR5 on macrophages
Epstein–Barr	C3d receptor on B cells
vaccinia	epidermal growth factor receptor
reovirus type 3	β-adrenergic hormone receptor
encephalomyocarditis	glycophorin A molecule
rhinovirus	intercellular adhesion molecule-1

Fig. 3.5 Molecules used by viruses in attaching to host cells.

and/or the capsid are shed and the viral nucleic acids released. The virus is now no longer infective: this 'eclipse phase' persists until new complete virus particles reform after replication. The way in which replication occurs is determined by the nature of the nucleic acid concerned.

REPLICATION

Viruses must first synthesize messenger RNA (mRNA)

Viruses contain either DNA or RNA, never both. The nucleic acids are present as single or double strands in a linear (DNA or RNA) or circular (DNA) form. The genome of the virus may be carried on a single molecule of nucleic acid or on several molecules. With this diversity it is not surprising that the process of replication in the host cell is also diverse. In viruses containing DNA, mRNA can be formed using the host's own RNA polymerase to transcribe directly from the viral DNA. The RNA of viruses cannot be transcribed in this way, as host polymerases do not work from RNA. If transcription is necessary, the virus must provide its own polymerases. These may be carried in the nucleocapsid or may be synthesized after infection.

RNA viruses produce mRNA by several different routes

In dsRNA viruses, one strand is first transcribed by viral polymerase into mRNA (*Fig. 3.6*). In ssRNA viruses there are three distinct routes to the formation of mRNA:

- Where the single strand has the positive sense configuration (i.e. has the same base sequence as that required for translation), it can be used directly as mRNA.
- Where the strand has the negative sense configuration, it must first be transcribed, using viral polymerase, into a positive sense strand, which can then act as mRNA.
- Retroviruses follow a completely different route. Their positive sense ssRNA is first made into a negative sense ssDNA, using the viral reverse transcriptase enzyme carried

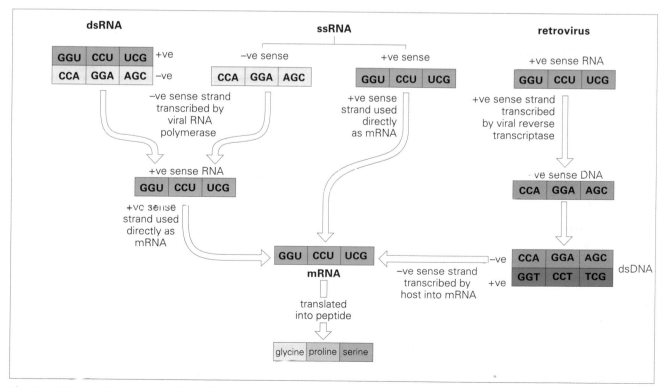

Fig. 3.6 Ways in which genomic RNA of RNA viruses can be transcribed into messenger RNA (mRNA) before translation into proteins. (+ve, positive sense; –ve, negative sense; ds, double stranded; ss, single stranded.)

MAJOR GROUPS OF VIRUSES						
DNA viruses						
virus family	**envelope present**	**capsid symmetry**	**particle size (nm)**	**DNA molecular weight (×10⁻⁶)**	**DNA structure***	**medically important viruses**
Parvoviridae	no	icosahedral	18–26	2	ss linear	B19 virus
Papovaviridae	no	icosahedral	45–55	3–5	ds circular, supercoiled	papilloma viruses polyomavirus (JC, BK)
Adenoviridae	no	icosahedral	70–90	23	ds linear	adenoviruses
Hepadnaviridae	yes	icosahedral	42	1.5	ds incomplete, circular	hepatitis B virus
Herpesviridae	yes	icosahedral	100**	100–150	ds linear	herpes simplex virus varicella-zoster virus cytomegalovirus Epstein–Barr virus human herpes virus (HHV)-6 human herpes virus (HHV)-7 human herpes virus (HHV)-8
Poxviridae	yes	complex	250 × 300	125–185	ds linear	smallpox virus vaccinia virus
RNA viruses						
virus family	**envelope present**	**capsid symmetry**	**particle size (nm)**	**DNA mol. wt (×10⁻⁶)**	**RNA structure***	**medically important viruses**
Picornaviridae	no	icosahedral	25–30	2–3	ss linear, non-segmented, +ve sense	poliovirus, rhinovirus hepatitis A virus enteroviruses
Reoviridae	no	icosahedral	75	15	ds linear, 10 segments	reovirus, rotavirus Colorado tick fever
Togaviridae	yes	icosahedral	60–70	4	ss linear, non-segmented, +ve sense	rubella virus Western equine encephalitis virus Chikunganya virus
Flaviviridae	yes	?	40–60	3–4.4	ssRNA, +ve sense	yellow fever virus hepatitis C virus dengue virus West Nile virus Japanese encephalitis virus
Retroviridae	yes	icosahedral	80–120	7†	ss linear, 2 segments, >+ve sense	HIV types 1 and 2 human T cell lymphotropic virus types 1 and 2

Fig. 3.12 Summary of major families of viruses.

MAJOR GROUPS OF VIRUSES						
RNA viruses						
virus family	**envelope present**	**capsid symmetry**	**particle size (nm)**	**DNA mol. wt ($\times 10^{-6}$)**	**RNA structure***	**medically important viruses**
Coronaviridae	yes	helical	120–160	5	ss linear, non-segmented, +ve sense	coronavirus, SARS coronavirus (SARS CoV)
Caliciviridae	no	icosahedral	35–40	2.6	ssRNA, +ve sense	noroviruses (formerly SRSV or Norwalk-like viruses)
Orthomyxoviridae	yes	helical	80–120	4	ss linear, 8 segments, –ve sense	influenza virus
Paramyxoviridae	yes	helical	120–250	6	ss linear, non-segmented, –ve sense	measles, mumps, parainfluenza, respiratory syncytial viruses
Rhabdoviridae	yes	helical	75 × 180	3–4	ss linear, non-segmented, –ve sense	rabies virus
Arenaviridae	yes	helical	50–300	5	ss circular, 2 segments with cohesive ends, –ve sense	lymphocytic choriomeningitis virus Lassa virus
Bunyaviridae	yes	helical	80–120	5	ss circular, 3 segments with cohesive ends, –ve sense	California encephalitis sandfly fever viruses Crimean–Congo haemorrhagic fever virus Hantaan-like viruses Sin Nombre-like viruses
Filoviridae	yes	complex	80 × 14000	4.2	ssRNA, –ve sense	Marburg, Ebola virus

*ss, single stranded; ds, double stranded
**the herpesvirus nucleocapsid is 100 nm, but the envelope varies in size; the entire virus can be as large as 200 nm in diameter
†retrovirus RNA contains 2 identical molecules of molecular weight 3.5×10^{6}
SARS, severe acute respiratory syndrome; SRSV, small round structured viruses.

Fig. 3.12, cont'd.

? QUESTIONS

1. Which of the following is an RNA virus?
A. Papilloma virus
B. Influenza virus
C. Hepatitis B virus
D. Epstein–Barr virus
E. Herpes simplex virus

2. Which of the following is a DNA virus?
A. Poliovirus
B. Rubella virus
C. Vaccinia virus
D. Measles virus
E. HIV 1

3. The cellular receptor used by influenza virus is:
A. Sialic acid
B. Acetylcholine
C. CD4
D. Glycophorin A
E. C3d receptor

4. Which of the following viruses can cause cancer?
A. HIV
B. Herpes simplex
C. Hepatitis A
D. Human T cell lymphotropic viruses
E. Rotavirus

FURTHER READING

Cann AJ. *Principles of Molecular Virology*, 2nd edition. London: Academic Press, 1997.

Collier LH, ed. *Topley and Wilson's Microbiology and Microbial Infections*, 9th edition. London: Edward Arnold, 1998.

The fungi

INTRODUCTION

Fungi are eukaryotes, but are quite distinct from plants and animals. Characteristically, they are multinucleate or multicellular organisms with a thick chitin-containing cell wall. They may grow as thread-like filaments (hyphae), but many other growth forms occur. Of these the single-celled yeasts and the mushroom are most familiar. Fungi are ubiquitous as free-living organisms and are of enormous importance commercially in baking, brewing and in pharmaceuticals. Some form part of the body's normal flora, and others are common causes of local infections on skin and hair. A number of fungi are associated with significant disease and many of these are acquired from the external environment. Pathogenic species invade tissues and digest material externally by releasing enzymes; they also take up nutrients directly from host tissues. The study of fungi is known as mycology.

MAJOR GROUPS OF DISEASE-CAUSING FUNGI

Fungal pathogens can be classified on the basis of their growth forms or the type of infection they cause

Fungal pathogens may exist as branched filamentous forms or as yeasts *(Fig. 4.1)*; some show both growth forms in their cycle and are known as 'dimorphic' fungi. In filamentous forms (e.g. *Trichophyton*), the mass of hyphae forms a 'mycelium'. Asexual reproduction results in the formation of sporangia, which liberate the spores by which the fungus is dispersed; spores are a common cause of infection after inhalation. In yeast-like forms (e.g. *Cryptococcus*) the characteristic form is the single cell, which reproduces by division. Budding may also occur, with the 'bud' remaining attached, forming pseudohyphae. Dimorphic forms (e.g. *Histoplasma*) form hyphae at environmental temperatures, but occur as yeast cells in the body, the switch being temperature-induced. *Candida* is an important exception in the dimorphic group, showing the reverse and forming hyphae within the body.

Three types of infection (mycoses) are recognized:

- *superficial mycoses* where the fungus grows at the body surface on skin or hair;
- *cutaneous and subcutaneous mycoses* where nails and deeper layers of the skin are involved;
- *systemic or deep mycoses* with involvement of internal organs. This category includes the *opportunistic* fungi that cause disease in patients with compromised immune systems.

The first two are usually mild, but the third can be life-threatening. The superficial pathogens are spread by direct contact, whereas the deep mycoses often result from the opportunistic growth of fungi in individuals with impaired immune competence (see Chapter 30). Free-living fungi can also cause disease. This occurs indirectly when toxins produced by fungi are present in items used as food (e.g. the aflatoxins from *Aspergillus flavus*) or when their spores are

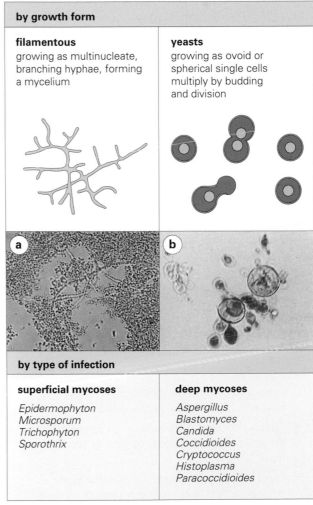

by growth form	
filamentous growing as multinucleate, branching hyphae, forming a mycelium	**yeasts** growing as ovoid or spherical single cells multiply by budding and division
a	b

by type of infection	
superficial mycoses	**deep mycoses**
Epidermophyton *Microsporum* *Trichophyton* *Sporothrix*	*Aspergillus* *Blastomyces* *Candida* *Coccidioides* *Cryptococcus* *Histoplasma* *Paracoccidioides*

Fig. 4.1. Two ways to classify fungi that cause disease: by growth form and by type of infection. (a) Hyphae in skin scraping from ringworm lesion. (Courtesy of DK Banerjee.) (b) Spherical yeasts of *Histoplasma*. (Courtesy of Y Clayton and G Midgley.)

IMPORTANT FUNGAL DISEASES				
type	anatomic location	representative disease	causative organisms	growth form
superficial	hair shaft, dead layer of skin	ptyriasis versicolor, tinea nigra, piedra	*Trichosporon, Malassezia, Exophiala*	Y/F
cutaneous	epidermis, hair, nails	tinea (ringworm)	*Microsporum, Trichophyton, Epidermophyton*	F
subcutaneous	dermis, subcutis	spirotrichosis mycetoma	*Sporothrix* several genera	Y* F
systemic	internal organs	coccidioidomycosis histoplasmosis blastomycosis paracoccioidomycosis	*Coccidioides* *Histoplasma* *Blastomyces* *Paracoccidioides*	** Y Y Y
opportunisitc	internal organs	cryptococcosis candidiasis aspergillosis pneumocystis pneumonia	*Cryptococcus* *Candida* *Aspergillus* *Pneumocystis*	Y Y† F* N/A

Y, yeast; F, filamentous, *growth form in the body; †also forms pseudohyphae
**Coccidioides* has an unusual growth form with yeast-like endospores within a spherule
N/A, Y/F growth forms are not applicable

Fig. 4.2 Summary of fungi that cause important human diseases.

inhaled, an immune response occurs and a hypersensitivity pneumonitis develops

Many of the fungi that cause disease are normally free-living in the environment, but can survive in the body if acquired by inhalation or by entry through wounds. Some fungi are part of the normal flora (e.g. *Candida*) and are innocuous unless the body's defenses are compromised. The filamentous forms grow extracellularly, but yeasts can survive and multiply within macrophages and neutrophils. Neutrophils can play a major role in controlling the establishment of invading fungi. Species that are too large for phagocytosis can be killed by extracellular factors released from phagocytes as well as by other components of the immune response. Some species, notably *Cryptococcus neoformans*, prevent phagocytic uptake because they are surrounded by a polysaccharide capsule (see Chapter 24). Until, recently, *Pneumocystis,* an important opportunistic infection in AIDS patients, was classified as a protozoan, but it is now regarded as an atypical fungus. It attaches to lung cells (pneumocytes) and can give rise to a fatal pneumonia-like disease.

The major groups of fungi causing human disease are shown in *Figure 4.2*.

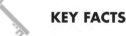

KEY FACTS

- Fungi are distinct from plants and animals, have a thick chitinous cell wall, and grow as filaments (hyphae) or single-celled yeasts.

- Species causing disease may be acquired from the environment or occur as part of the normal flora.

- Infections may be located superficially, in cutaneous and subcutaneous sites, or in deep tissues.

- Infections are most serious in immunocompromised individuals.

QUESTIONS

1. Which is a fungus that forms part of the normal flora, but which can cause disease?
   A. *Histoplasma*
   B. *Blastomyces*
   C. *Candida*
   D. *Aspergillus*
   E. *Cryptococcus*

2. Superficial fungi invade?
   A. Epidermis
   B. Nails
   C. Vagina
   D. Dead skin
   E. Dermis

FURTHER READING

Hay RJ. Medical mycology. In: Collier LH et al., eds. *Topley and Wilson's Microbiology and Microbial Infections*, 9th edition. London: Edward Arnold, 1998.

Kwon-Chung KJ, Bennett JE. *Medical Mycology.* Philadelphia: Lea & Febiger, 1992.

Sternberg S. The emerging fungal threat. *Science* 1995; 266:1632.

The protozoa

INTRODUCTION

Protozoa are single-celled animals, ranging in size from 2 μm to 100 μm. Many species are free-living, but others are important parasites of humans. Some free-living species can infect humans opportunistically, and some parasites cause severe disease only in immunocompromised individuals. Infections are most prevalent in tropical and subtropical regions, but also occur in temperate regions. Protozoa may cause disease directly (e.g. the rupture of red cells in malaria), but more often the pathology is caused by the host's response. Most infections are not life threatening (except in immunocompromised patients), but malaria kills more than 1.5 million people each year, mostly young children.

Protozoa can infect all the major tissues and organs of the body

Protozoa infect body tissues and organs as:

- intracellular parasites in a wide variety of cells (red cells, macrophages, epithelial cells, brain, muscle);
- extracellular parasites in the blood, intestine or urinogenital system.

The locations of the species of greatest importance are shown in *Figure. 5.1*.

Intracellular species obtain nutrients from the host cell by direct uptake or by ingestion of cytoplasm. Extracellular species feed by direct nutrient uptake or by ingestion of host cells. Reproduction in humans is usually asexual, by binary or multiple division of growing stages (trophozoites). Sexual reproduction is normally absent or occurs in the insect vector phase; *Cryptosporidium* is exceptional in undergoing both asexual and sexual reproduction in humans. Asexual reproduction gives the potential for a rapid increase in number, particularly where host defense mechanisms are impaired. For this reason some protozoans are most pathogenic in the very young (e.g. *Toxoplasma* in neonates). The AIDS epidemic has focused attention on a number of protozoa formerly unrecognized as human pathogens, which give rise to opportunistic infections in immunocompromised individuals. These include *Cryptosporidium*, *Isospora*, *Blastocystis* and members of the Microsporidia. New parasites continue to emerge: e.g. *Cyclospora cayetanensis*, a food-transmitted cause of diarrhea, identified in 1994.

Protozoa have evolved many sophisticated strategies to avoid host responses

Extracellular species evade immune recognition of their plasma membrane. The interface between host and extracellular protozoa is the parasite's plasma membrane, and examples of strategies to avoid immune recognition of this surface include the following.

- Trypanosomes undergo repeated antigenic variation of surface antigens.
- Malaria parasites show polymorphisms in dominant surface antigens.
- Amebae can consume complement at the cell surface.

Intracellular species evade host defense mechanisms. Although intracellular stages are removed from direct contact with antibody, complement and phagocytes, their antigens may be expressed at the surface of the host cell, which can then be a target for cytotoxic effectors. Survival within cells, particularly within macrophages (*Leishmania, Toxoplasma*), involves a variety of devices to evade or inactivate the harmful effects of intracellular enzymes or reactive oxygen and nitrogen metabolites.

Protozoa use a variety of routes to infect humans

Many extracellular protozoa are transmitted by ingestion of food or water contaminated with transmission stages such as

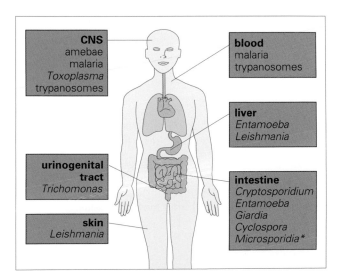

Fig. 5.1 The occurrence of protozoan parasites in the body.
*Can also occur in other sites. (CNS, central nervous system.)

FEATURES OF MEDICALLY IMPORTANT PROTOZOA			
location	**species**	**mode of transmission**	**disease**
intestinal tract	*Entamoeba histolytica* *Giardia lamblia* *Cryptosporidium* spp. *Cyclospora cayetanensis* *Microsporidia*	ingestion of cysts in food	amebiasis giardiasis cryptosporidiosis cyclosporiasis microsporidiosis
urinogenital tract	*Trichomonas vaginalis*	sexual	trichomoniasis

blood and tissue	*Trypanosoma* spp.
	    T. cruzi
	
	    T. gambiense
	    T. rhodesiense
		reduviid bug
		
		tsetse fly
			trypanosomiasis
			Chagas' disease
			
			sleeping sickness

	Leishmania spp.
	    L. donovani
	
	    L. tropica, L. mexicana
	    L. braziliensis
		sand fly
		
		sand fly
			visceral leishmaniasis (kala-azar)
			
			cutaneous leishmaniasis
			mucocutaneous leishmaniasis

	Plasmodium spp.
	    P. vivax, P. ovale
	    P. malariae
	
	    P. falciparum
		Anopheles mosquito
		
		Anopheles mosquito
			malaria
			
			malaria

	Toxoplasma gondii	ingestion of cysts in raw meat; contact with soil contaminated by cat feces	toxoplasmosis

Fig. 5.2 Summary of the location, transmission and diseases caused by protozoan parasites.

cysts, but *Trichomonas vaginalis* is transmitted through sexual activity, and the trypanosomes by insect vectors. The most important intracellular species—*Plasmodium* and *Leishmania* —are also insect transmitted, but others *(Toxoplasma)* can be acquired by ingestion or from the mother in utero *(Fig. 5.2.)*.

KEY FACTS

- Protozoa are single-celled animals, occurring both as free-living organisms and as parasites. Both can cause disease in humans.

- The single most important protozoan disease is malaria, which causes some 1.5 million deaths each year.

- Protozoa live both outside and within cells, and have complex ways of avoiding the responses of their hosts.

- Most infections are acquired through ingestion of contaminated water or food, or via insect vectors. A few are transmitted from mother to fetus.

QUESTIONS

1. The most important parasitic infection is:
A. Leishmaniasis
B. Malaria
C. Cryptosporidiosis
D. Amebiasis
E. Trypanosomiasis

2. Which of these parasites does not occur in the human intestine?
A. *Giardia*
B. *Entamoeba*
C. *Cyclospora*
D. *Toxoplasma*
E. *Cryptosporidium*

3. Which of these parasites is an extracellular organism?
A. *Cryptosporidium*
B. *Leishmania*
C. *Toxoplasma*
D. *Giardia*
E. *Plasmodium*

FURTHER READING

Cox FEG, Wakelin D. Parasitology. In: Collier LH et al., eds. *Topley and Wilson's Microbiology and Microbial Infections*, 9th edition. London: Edward Arnold, 1998.

Despommier DD et al. *Parasitic Diseases*, 4th edition. New York: Apple Trees Productions, 2000.

The helminths and arthropods

6

INTRODUCTION

The term 'helminth' is used for all groups of parasitic worms. Three main groups are important in humans: the tapeworms (Cestoda), the flukes (Trematoda or Digenea) and the roundworms (Nematoda). The first two belong to the Platyhelminths or flatworms, the third are included in a separate phylum. Platyhelminths have flattened bodies with muscular suckers and/or hooks for attachment to the host. Nematodes (roundworms) have long cylindrical bodies and generally lack specialized attachment organs. Helminths are generally large organisms with a complex body organization. Although invading larval stages may measure only 100–200 μm, adult worms may be centimeters or even meters long. Infections are commonest in warmer countries, but intestinal species also occur in temperate regions. The arthropods are the largest and arguably most successful single group of animals. Those of most relevance to human disease are the insects, ticks and mites. Many of these have adapted to live on humans or use humans as sources of food (blood and tissue fluid). Linked with these feeding habits is the ability of many arthropods to transmit a very wide variety of microbial pathogens. Others, acting as intermediate hosts, may transmit helminth parasites when eaten, and yet other species can inflict dangerous bites and stings.

THE HELMINTHS

Transmission of helminths occurs in four distinct ways

Transmission routes are summarized in *Figure 6.1*. Infection can occur after:

- swallowing infective eggs or larvae via the fecal–oral route;
- swallowing infective larvae in the tissues of another host;
- active penetration of the skin by larval stages;
- the bite of an infected blood-sucking insect vector.

The greater frequency of helminths in tropical and subtropical regions reflects the climatic conditions that favor survival of infective stages, the socioeconomic conditions that facilitate fecal–oral contact, the practices involved in food preparation and consumption, and the availability of suitable vectors. Elsewhere, infections are commonest in children, in individuals closely associated with domestic animals and in individuals with particular food preferences.

Many helminths live in the intestine, while others live in the deeper tissues. Almost all organs of the body can be parasitized. Flukes and nematodes actively feed on host tissues or on the intestinal contents; tapeworms have no digestive system and absorb pre-digested nutrients.

The majority of helminths do not replicate within the host. In its simplest form, as in many intestinal worms, sexual reproduction results in the production of eggs, which are released from the host in fecal material. In others, reproductive stages may accumulate within the host, but do not mature. Certain tapeworm larval stages can reproduce asexually in man. The nematode *Strongyloides* is exceptional in that eggs produced in the intestine can hatch there, releasing infective larvae, which reinvade the body—the process of

'autoinfection'. A similar phenomenon occurs with the tapeworm *Taenia solium*.

The outer surfaces of helminths provide the primary host–parasite interface

In tapeworms and flukes the surface is a complex plasma membrane, and in both there are protective mechanisms to prevent the host damaging the outer surface. The nematode

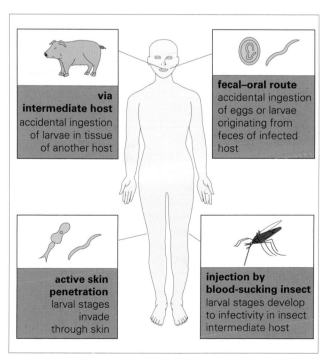

Fig. 6.1 How helminth parasites enter the body.

via **intermediate host**
accidental ingestion of larvae in tissue of another host

fecal–oral route
accidental ingestion of eggs or larvae originating from feces of infected host

active skin penetration
larval stages invade through skin

injection by blood-sucking insect
larval stages develop to infectivity in insect intermediate host

47

HUMAN NEMATODE INFECTIONS		
species	**acquired by**	**site in humans**
transmitted person-to-person		
Ascaris lumbricoides	ingestion of eggs	small intestine
Enterobius vermicularis	ingestion of eggs	large intestine
Hookworms		
Ancylostoma duodenale	skin penetration by infective larvae	small intestine
Necator americanus		small intestine
Strongyloides stercoralis	skin penetration by infective larvae; autoinfection	small intestine (adults) general tissues (larvae)
Trichuris trichiura	ingestion of eggs	large intestine
transmitted person-to-person via arthropod vector		
Brugia malayi	bite of mosquito carrying infective larvae	lymphatics (adults) blood (larvae)
Onchocerca volvulus	bite of *Simulium* fly carrying infective larvae	skin (larvae, adults) eye (larvae)
Wuchereria bancrofti	bite of mosquito carrying infective larvae	lymphatics (adults) blood (larvae)
Loa loa	bite of deer fly carrying infective larvae	tissues
zoonoses transmitted from animals		
Angiostrongylus cantonensis	ingestion of larvae in snails, crustacea	CNS (larvae)
Anisakis simplex	ingestion of larvae in fish	stomach, small intestine (larvae)
Capillaria phillipinensis	ingestion of larvae in fish	small intestine (adults, larvae)
*Toxocara canis**	ingestion of eggs passed by dogs	tissues, CNS (larvae)
*Trichinella spiralis**	ingestion of larvae in pork, wild mammals	small intestine (adults) muscles (larvae)
*these species are the commonest in this group		

Fig. 6.4 Summary of the location and transmission of nematodes that infect humans.

INFECTIOUS DISEASES TRANSMITTED BY ARTHROPODS		
	disease	**arthropod vector**
viruses		
arboviruses	dengue fever	mosquitoes
	yellow fever	mosquitoes
	encephalitides	mosquitoes, ticks
	hemorrhagic fevers	ticks, mosquitoes
bacteria		
Yersinia pestis	plague	fleas
Borrelia recurrentis	relapsing fever	soft ticks
Borrelia burgdorferi	Lyme disease	hard ticks
rickettsias		
R. prowazeki	epidemic typhus	lice, ticks
R. mooseri	endemic (murine) typhus	fleas
R. rickettsia	spotted fever	ticks
R. akari	rickettsial pox	mites
protozoa		
Trypanosome cruzi	American trypanosomiasis (Chagas' disease)	reduviid bugs
T.b. rhodesiense	African trypanosomiasis (sleeping sickness)	tsetse flies
T.b. gambiense		
Plasmodium spp.	malaria	mosquitoes
Leishmania spp.	leishmaniasis	sandflies
worms		
Wuchereria and Brugia	lymphatic filariasis	mosquitoes
Onchocerca	onchocerciasis	*Simulium* flies

Fig. 6.5 Summary of infectious diseases transmitted by arthropods.

KEY FACTS

- Helminths are multicellular worms that parasitize many organs of the body, most commonly the gastrointestinal tract.

- Transmission may be direct, through swallowing infective stages or by larvae penetrating the skin, or indirect via intermediate hosts or insect vectors.

- The most serious helminth infection is schistosomiasis, caused by infection with blood flukes. The pathology is primarily due to hypersensitivity reactions to eggs as they pass through the tissues.

- Arthropods of importance in human disease are those that feed on blood or body tissues (insects, ticks, mites) and those which transmit other infections, particularly viruses, bacteria and protozoa.

The host–parasite relationship

INTRODUCTION

The preceding chapters have focused primarily on organisms that are quite clearly disease agents. Small numbers may be found in healthy individuals, but their presence in large numbers is usually associated with pathologic changes. The organisms covered in the first section of this chapter may cause disease under certain circumstances (e.g. in the newborn or in stressed, traumatized or immunocompromised individuals), but usually coexist quite peacefully with their host. Many of these form what is termed the 'indigenous' or 'normal' flora of the body—a collection of species routinely found in the normal healthy individual. Their relationship with the host makes an interesting comparison with that of species that are considered as true parasites or pathogens and is discussed later in this chapter in the broader context of symbiotic relationships and the evolution of host–parasite relationships.

THE NORMAL FLORA

Why is it called the normal flora?

The term *flora* is used because the majority of the organisms concerned are bacteria. It has been estimated that humans have approximately 10^{13} cells in the body and something like 10^{14} bacteria associated with them, the majority in the large bowel. Members of groups such as viruses, fungi and protozoa are also regularly found in healthy individuals, but form only a minor component of the total population of resident organisms.

The organisms occur in those parts of the body that are exposed to, or communicate with, the external environment, namely the skin, nose and mouth, and intestinal and urino-genital tracts. Internal organs and tissues are normally sterile. The main organisms found in these sites are shown in *Figure 8.1*.

The normal flora is acquired rapidly during and shortly after birth and changes continuously throughout life

The organisms present at any given time reflect the age, nutrition and environment of the individual. It is therefore difficult to define the normal flora very precisely because it is to a large extent environmentally determined. This is well illustrated by data from NASA astronauts who were rendered relatively bacteriologically sterile by antibiotic treatment before their space flights. It took only 6 weeks after the flight for their flora to repopulate, and the repopulating species were precisely those of their immediate neighbors. The bowel flora of children in developing countries is quite different from that of children in developed countries. In addition, breastfed infants have lactic acid streptococci and lactobacilli in their gastrointestinal tract, whereas bottlefed children show a much greater variety of organisms.

Different regions of the skin support different flora

Exposed dry areas have relatively few resident organisms on the surface, whereas moister areas (axillae, perineum, between the toes, scalp) support much larger populations. *Staphylococcus epidermidis* is one of the commonest species, making up some 90% of the aerobes and occurring in densities of 10^3–10^4/cm^2; *Staph. aureus* may be present in the moister regions.

Anaerobic diphtheroids occur below the skin surface in hair follicles, sweat and sebaceous glands, *Propionibacterium acnes* being a familiar example. Changes in the skin occurring during puberty often lead to increased numbers of this species, which can be associated with acne.

A number of fungi, including *Candida*, occur on the scalp and around the nails. They are infrequent on dry skin, but can cause infection in moist skin folds (intertrigo).

Both the nose and mouth can be heavily colonized by bacteria

The majority of bacteria here are anaerobes. Common species colonizing these areas include streptococci, staphylococci, diphtheroids and Gram-negative cocci. Some of the aerobic bacteria found in healthy individuals are potentially pathogenic (e.g. *Staph. aureus*, *Streptococcus pneumoniae*, *Strep. pyogenes*, *Neisseria meningitidis*); *Candida* is also a potential pathogen.

The mucous membranes of the mouth can have the same microbial density as the large intestine, numbers approaching 10^{11}/g wet weight of tissue.

Dental caries is one of the commonest infectious diseases in developed countries

The surfaces of the teeth and the gingival crevices carry large numbers of anaerobic bacteria. Plaque is a film of bacterial cells anchored in a polysaccharide matrix, which the organisms secrete. When teeth are not cleaned regularly, plaque can accumulate rapidly and the activities of certain bacteria, notably *Streptococcus mutans*, can lead to dental decay (caries), as acid fermented from carbohydrates can attack

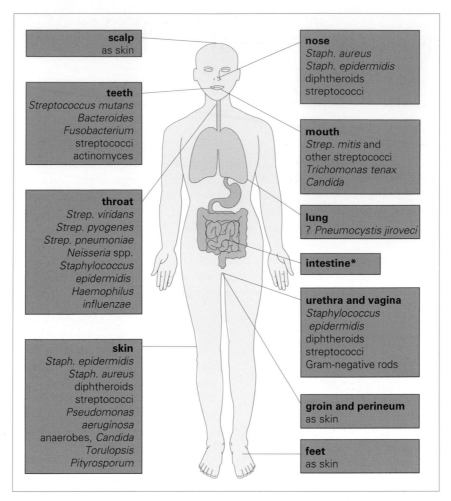

Fig. 8.1 Examples of organisms that occur as members of the normal flora and their location on the body. (*Those found in the intestine are detailed in *Figure 8.2*.)

dental enamel. The prevalence of dental decay is linked to diet.

The pharynx and trachea carry their own normal flora

The flora of the pharynx and trachea may include both α- and β-hemolytic streptococci as well as a number of anaerobes, staphylococci (including *Staph. aureus*), *Neisseria* and diphtheroids. The respiratory tract is normally quite sterile, despite the regular intake of organisms by breathing. However substantial numbers of clinically normal people may carry the fungus *Pneumocystis jiroveci* (previously known as *P. carinii*) in their lungs.

In the gut the density of microorganisms increases from the stomach to the large intestine

Stomach contents harbor only transient organisms, the acidic pH providing an effective barrier. However, the gastric mucosa may be colonized by acid-tolerant lactobacilli and streptococci. The upper intestine is only lightly colonized (10^4 organisms/g), but populations increase markedly in the ileum, where streptococci, lactobacilli, enterobacteriaceae and *Bacteroides* may all be present. Bacterial numbers are very high

(estimated at 10^{11}/g) in the large bowel, and many species can be found *(Fig. 8.2)*. The vast majority (95–99%) are anaerobes, *Bacteroides* being especially common and a major component of fecal material. Harmless protozoans can also occur in the intestine (e.g. *Entamoeba coli*) and these can be considered as part of the normal flora, despite being animals.

The urethra is lightly colonized in both sexes, but the vagina supports an extensive flora of bacteria and fungi

The urethra in both sexes is relatively lightly colonized, although *Staph. epidermidis*, *Strep. faecalis* and diphtheroids may be present. In the vagina the composition of the bacterial and fungal flora undergoes age-related changes:

- Before puberty the predominant organisms are staphylococci, streptococci, diphtheroids and *Escherichia coli*.
- Subsequently, *Lactobacillus aerophilus* predominates, its fermentation of glycogen being responsible for the maintenance of an acid pH, which prevents overgrowth by other vaginal organisms.

A number of fungi occur, including *Candida*, which can overgrow to cause the pathogenic condition 'thrush' if the

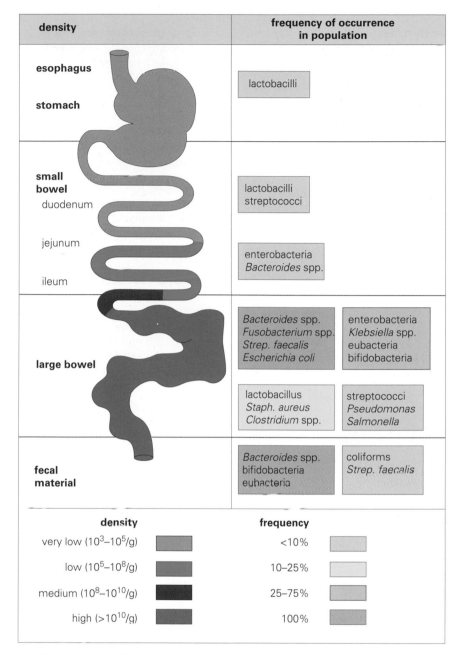

density	frequency of occurrence in population	
esophagus **stomach**	lactobacilli	
small bowel duodenum jejunum ileum	lactobacilli streptococci enterobacteria *Bacteroides* spp.	
large bowel	*Bacteroides* spp. *Fusobacterium* spp. *Strep. faecalis* *Escherichia coli* lactobacillus *Staph. aureus* *Clostridium* spp.	enterobacteria *Klebsiella* spp. eubacteria bifidobacteria streptococci *Pseudomonas* *Salmonella*
fecal material	*Bacteroides* spp. bifidobacteria eubacteria	coliforms *Strep. faecalis*

density		frequency	
very low (10^3–10^5/g)		<10%	
low (10^5–10^8/g)		10–25%	
medium (10^8–10^{10}/g)		25–75%	
high (>10^{10}/g)		100%	

Fig. 8.2 The longitudinal distribution, frequency of occurrence and densities of the bacteria making up the normal flora of the human gastrointestinal tract.

vaginal pH rises and competing bacteria diminish. The protozoan *Trichomonas vaginalis* may also be present in healthy individuals.

Advantages and disadvantages of the normal flora

Some of the species of the normal flora are positively beneficial to the host

The importance of these species for health is sometimes revealed quite dramatically under stringent antibiotic therapy. This can drastically reduce their numbers to a minimum, and the host may then be overrun by introduced pathogens or by overgrowth of organisms normally present in small numbers.

After treatment with clindamycin, overgrowth by *Clostridium difficile*, which survives treatment, can give rise to antibiotic-associated diarrhea or, more seriously, pseudomembranous colitis.

Ways in which the normal flora prevents colonization by potential pathogens include the following.

- Skin bacteria produce fatty acids, which discourage other species from invading.
- Gut bacteria release a number of factors with antibacterial activity (bacteriocins, colicins) as well as metabolic waste products that help prevent the establishment of other species.
- Vaginal lactobacilli maintain an acid environment, which suppresses growth of other organisms.

- The sheer number of bacteria present in the normal flora of the intestine means that almost all of the available ecologic niches become occupied; these species therefore outcompete others for living space.

Gut bacteria also release organic acids, which may have some metabolic value to the host; they also produce B vitamins and vitamin K in amounts that are large enough to be valuable if the diet is deficient. The antigenic stimulation provided by the intestinal flora helps to ensure the normal development of the immune system.

What happens when the normal flora is absent?

Germ-free animals tend to live longer, presumably because of the complete absence of pathogens, and develop no caries (see Chapter 18). However, their immune system is less well developed and they are vulnerable to introduced microbial pathogens. At the time of birth, humans are germ free, but acquire the normal flora during and immediately after birth, with the accompaniment of intense immunologic activity.

The disadvantages of the normal flora lie in the potential for spread into previously sterile parts of the body

This may happen:

- when the intestine is perforated or the skin is broken;
- during extraction of teeth (when viridans streptococci may enter the bloodstream);
- when organisms from the perianal skin ascend the urethra and cause urinary tract infection.

Members of the normal flora are important causes of hospital-acquired infection when patients are exposed to invasive treatments. Patients suffering burns are also at risk.

Overgrowth by potentially pathogenic members of the normal flora can occur when the composition of the flora changes (e.g. after antibiotics) or when:

- the local environment changes (e.g. increases in stomach or vaginal pH);
- the immune system becomes ineffective (e.g. AIDS, clinical immunosuppression).

Under these conditions, the potential pathogens take the opportunity to increase their population size or invade tissues, so becoming harmful to the host. An account of diseases associated with such opportunistic infections is given in Chapter 30.

SYMBIOTIC ASSOCIATIONS

All living animals are used as habitats by other organisms; none is exempt from such invasion—even protozoans have their own flora and fauna. As evolution has produced larger, more complex and better regulated bodies, it has increased the number and variety of habitats for other organisms to colonize. The most complex bodies, those of birds and mammals (including humans), provide the most diverse environments, and are the most heavily colonized.

As the normal flora demonstrates, pathogenesis is not the inevitable consequence of host–microbe associations. Many factors influence the outcome of a particular association, and organisms may be pathogenic in one situation but harmless

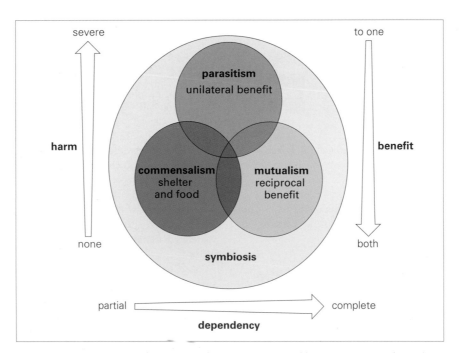

Fig. 8.3 The relationships between symbiotic associations. Most species are independent of other species or rely on them only temporarily for food (e.g. predators and their prey). Some species form closer associations termed 'symbioses' and there are three major categories—commensalism, parasitism and mutualism—though each merges with the other and no definition separates one absolutely from the others.

in another. To understand the microbiologic basis of infectious disease, host–microbe associations that can be pathogenic need to be placed firmly in the context of other symbiotic (interspecies) associations, such as commensalism or mutualism, where the outcome for the host does not normally involve any damage or disadvantage.

Commensalism, mutualism and parasitism are categories of symbiotic association

All associations in which one species lives in or on the body of another can be grouped under the general term 'symbiosis' (literally 'living together'). Symbiosis has no overtones of benefit or harm and includes a wide diversity of associations. Attempts have been made to categorize types of association very specifically, but these have failed because all associations form part of a continuum (Fig. 8.3). Three broad categories of symbiosis—commensalism, mutualism and parasitism—can be identified on the basis of the relative benefit obtained by each partner. None of these categories of association is restricted to any particular taxonomic group. Indeed some

organisms fit into each category depending upon the circumstances in which they live (Fig. 8.4).

Commensalism

In commensalism one species of organism uses the body of a larger species

At its simplest, a commensal association is one in which one species of organism uses the body of a larger species as its physical environment and may make use of that environment to acquire nutrients.

Like all animals, humans support an extensive commensal microbial flora on the skin, in the mouth and in the alimentary tract. The majority of these microbes are bacteria, and their relationship with the host may be highly specialized, with specific attachment mechanisms and precise environmental requirements. Normally such microbes are harmless, but they can become harmful if their environmental conditions change in some way (e.g. *Bacteroides, Escherichia coli, Staphylococcus aureus*). Conversely, commensal microbes can benefit the host:

- by preventing colonization by more pathogenic species (e.g. the intestinal flora);
- by producing metabolites that are used by the host (e.g. the bacteria and protozoa in the ruminant stomach).

It follows that the normal definition of commensalism is merely one of convenience, as the association can merge into either mutualism or parasitism.

Mutualism

Mutualistic relationships provide reciprocal benefits for the two organisms involved

Frequently the relationship is obligatory for at least one member, and may be for both. Good examples are the bacteria and protozoa living in the stomachs of domestic ruminants, which play an essential role in the digestion and utilization of cellulose, receiving in return both the environment and the nutrition essential for their survival. The dividing line between commensalism and mutualism can be hard to draw. In humans, good health and resistance to colonization by pathogens can depend upon the integrity of the normal commensal enteric bacteria, many of which are highly specialized for life in the human intestine, but there is certainly no strict mutual dependence in this relationship.

Parasitism

In parasitism the symbiotic relationship benefits only the parasite

The terms 'parasites' and 'parasitism' are sometimes thought to apply only to protozoans and worms, but all pathogens are parasites. Parasitism is a one-sided relationship in which the benefits go only to the parasite, the host providing parasites with their physicochemical environment, their food, respiratory and other metabolic needs, and even the signals that regulate their development. Although parasites are thought of as necessarily harmful, this is a view colored by human and veterinary clinical medicine, and by the results of

---

commensalism – large intestine of man

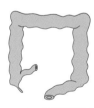

Bacteroides spp.

Host provides environment. Bacteria ferment digested food. Present in large numbers (10^{10}/g) but usually harmless. May be harmful if tissues damaged (surgery), gut flora changes (antibiotics), or immunity reduced

parasitism – large intestine of man

Entamoeba histolytica

Host provides environment. Protozoa feed on mucosa causing ulcers and dysentery

mutualism –rumen of cattle

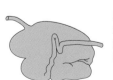

Bacteroides spp.

Host provides environment. Bacteria metabolize host food to fatty acids and gases. Host uses fatty acids as energy source

Fig. 8.4 Examples of commensalism, parasitism and mutualism. The first two examples show how difficult it is to categorize any organism as entirely harmless, entirely harmful or entirely beneficial.

laboratory experimentation. In fact many 'parasites' establish quite innocuous associations with their natural hosts and are not at all pathogenic under normal circumstances (e.g. when their natural host is in good health); the rabies virus, for example, coexists with many wild mammals but can cause fatal disease in humans. This state of 'balanced pathogenicity' is sometimes explained as the outcome of selective pressures acting upon a relationship over a long period of evolutionary time. It may reflect selection of an increased level of genetically determined resistance in the host population and decreased pathogenicity in the parasite (as has happened with myxomatosis in rabbits). Alternatively, it may be the evolutionary norm, and 'unbalanced pathogenicity' may simply be the consequence of organisms becoming established in 'unnatural' (i.e. new) hosts. So, like the other categories of symbiosis, parasitism is impossible to define exclusively except in the context of clearcut and highly pathogenic organisms. The belief that 'harmfulness' is a necessary characteristic of a parasite is difficult to sustain in any broader view, and the reasons for this are discussed in more detail below.

THE CHARACTERISTICS OF PARASITISM

Many different groups of organisms are parasitic, and all animals are parasitized

Parasitism as a way of life has been adopted by many different groups of organisms. Some groups, such as viruses, are exclusively parasitic (see below), but the majority include both parasitic and free-living representatives. Parasites occur in all animals, from the simplest to the most complex, and are an almost inevitable accompaniment of organized animal existence. We can see, then, that parasitism has been an evolutionary success; as a way of life it must confer very considerable advantages.

Parasitism has metabolic, nutritional and reproductive advantages

The most obvious advantage of parasitism is metabolic. The parasite is provided with a variety of metabolic requirements by the host, at no energy cost to itself, so it can devote a large proportion of its own resources to replication or reproduction. This one-sided metabolic relationship shows a broad spectrum of dependence, both within and between the various groups of parasites. Some parasites are totally dependent upon the host, while others are only partly dependent.

Viruses are completely dependent upon the host for all their metabolic needs

Viruses are at one extreme of the 'parasite dependency' spectrum. They are obligate parasites, possessing the genetic information required for production of new viruses, but none of the cellular machinery necessary to transcribe or translate this information, to assemble new virus particles or to produce the energy for these processes. The host provides not only the basic building blocks for the production of new viruses, but also the synthetic machinery and the energy required (Fig. 8.5). Retroviruses go one stage further in

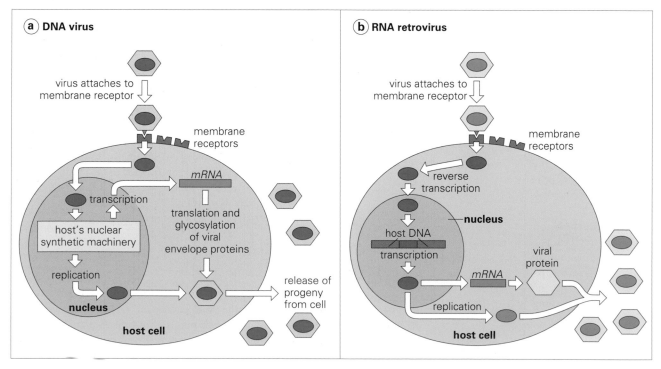

Fig. 8.5 How DNA and RNA viruses invade and infect cells. (a) DNA viruses such as the herpesviruses have their own DNA, and use only the host's cellular machinery to make more DNA and more virus protein and glycoprotein. These are then reassembled into new virus particles before they are released from the cell. (b) RNA retroviruses (e.g. HIV) first make viral DNA, using their reverse transcriptase, insert this DNA into the host's genetic material so that viral RNA can be transcribed, and then translate some of the RNA into virus protein. The viral protein and RNA are then reassembled into new particles and released.

dependence, inserting their own genetic information into the host's DNA in order to parasitize the transcription process. Viruses therefore represent the ultimate parasitic condition and are qualitatively different from all other parasites in the nature of their relationship with the host.

The basis for the fundamental difference between viruses and other parasites is the difference between virus organization and the cellular organization of prokaryotic and eukaryotic parasites. Non-viral parasites have their own genetic and cellular machinery, and multi-enzyme systems for independent metabolic activity and macromolecular synthesis. The degree of reliance on the host for nutritional requirements varies considerably and follows no consistent pattern between the various groups, nor does it follow that smaller parasites tend to be more dependent; for example, some of the largest parasites, the tapeworms, are wholly reliant upon the host's digestive machinery to provide their nutritional needs. All, of course, receive nutrition from the host, but whereas some use macromolecular material (proteins, polysaccharides) of host origin and digest it using their own enzyme systems, others rely on the host for the process of digestion as well, being able to take up only low molecular weight materials (amino acids, monosaccharides). Nutritional dependence may also include host provision of growth factors that the parasite is unable to synthesize itself. All internal parasites rely upon the host's respiratory and transport systems to provide oxygen, although some respire anaerobically in either a facultative or obligate manner.

Parasite development can be controlled by the host

The advantage that parasitism confers in reproductive terms makes it vital to coordinate parasite development with the availability of suitable hosts. Indeed, one of the characteristic features of parasites is that their development may be controlled partly or completely by the host, the parasite having lost the ability to initiate or to regulate its own development. At its simplest, host control is limited to providing the cell surface molecules necessary for parasite attachment and internalization. Many parasites, from viruses to protozoa, rely on the recognition of such molecular signals for their entry into host cells, and this process provides the trigger for their replicative or reproductive cycles.

Other parasites, primarily the eukaryotes, require more comprehensive and sophisticated signals, often a complex of signals, to initiate and regulate their entire developmental cycle. The complexity of the signal required for development is one of the factors determining the specificity of the host–parasite relationship. Where the availability of one of the signals entails that parasite development can occur in only one species, host specificity is high. Where many host species are capable of providing the necessary signals for a parasite, specificity is low.

Disadvantages of parasitism

The most obvious disadvantage of parasitism arises from the fact that the host controls the development of the parasite. No development is possible without a suitable host, and many parasites will die if no host becomes available. For this reason, several adaptations have evolved to promote prolonged survival in the outside world and so maximize the chances of successful host contact (e.g. virus particles, bacterial spores, protozoan cysts and worm eggs). The prolific replication of parasites is another device to achieve the same end. Nevertheless, where parasites fail to make contact with a host, their powers of survival are ultimately limited. Adaptation to host signals can therefore have a reproductive cost (i.e. the loss of many potential parasites).

THE EVOLUTION OF PARASITISM

As so many organisms are parasitic and every group of animals is subject to invasion by parasites, the development of parasitism as a way of life must have occurred at an early stage in evolution and at frequent intervals thereafter. How this occurred is not fully understood, and it may well have been different in different groups of organisms. In many, parasitism most probably arose as a consequence of accidental contacts between organism and host. Of many such contacts some would have resulted in prolonged survival, and under favorable nutritional circumstances prolonged survival would have been associated with enhanced replication, giving the organism a selective advantage within the environment.

Bacterial parasites evolved through accidental contact

In the case of bacteria, it is easy to see how accidental contact in environments rich in free-living bacteria could lead to successful colonization of the gastrointestinal tract and external orifices. Initially the organisms concerned would have had to be facultative parasites, capable of life both within or outside host organisms (many pathogenic bacteria still have this property, e.g. *Legionella, Vibrio*), but selective pressures would have forced others into obligatory parasitism. Such events are of course speculative, but are supported by the close relationship of enteric bacteria such as *E. coli* with free-living photosynthetic purple bacteria.

Many bacteria and related parasites of humans and other mammals may have originated via the route of accidental contact, but it is clear that others have become adapted to these hosts after initially becoming parasitic in other species. Blood-feeding arthropods provide an example of the most obvious route for this, as their parasites have ready access to the tissues of the animals on which the arthropods feed.

Many bacterial parasites have evolved to live inside host cells

Bacteria that became parasitic by accidental contact would have lived outside host cells at first and would not have had the advantages of being intracellular. The evolution of the intracellular habit required further modifications to allow survival within host cells, but could easily have been initiated by passive phagocytic uptake. Subsequent survival of the microbe would depend upon the possession of surface or metabolic properties that prevented digestion and destruction by the host cell. The success of intracellular life can be measured not only by the large number of bacteria that have adopted this habit, but also by the extent to which some organisms have integrated their biology with that of the host

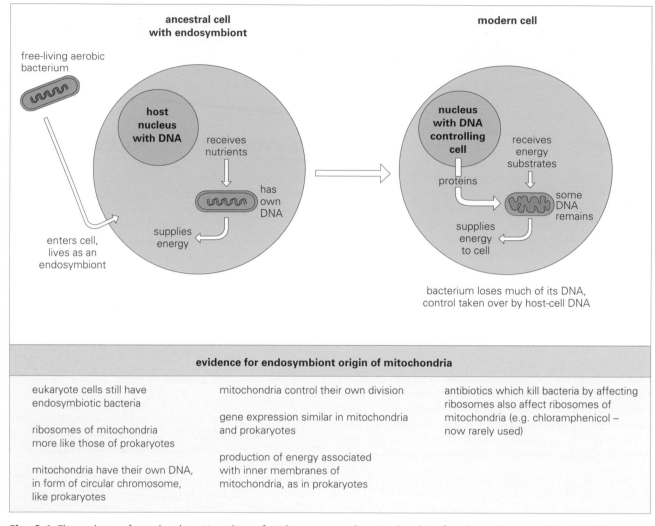

ancestral cell with endosymbiont

modern cell

free-living aerobic bacterium

host nucleus with DNA

receives nutrients

has own DNA

enters cell, lives as an endosymbiont

supplies energy

nucleus with DNA controlling cell

receives energy substrates

proteins

some DNA remains

supplies energy to cell

bacterium loses much of its DNA, control taken over by host-cell DNA

evidence for endosymbiont origin of mitochondria

eukaryote cells still have endosymbiotic bacteria

ribosomes of mitochondria more like those of prokaryotes

mitochondria have their own DNA, in form of circular chromosome, like prokaryotes

mitochondria control their own division

gene expression similar in mitochondria and prokaryotes

production of energy associated with inner membranes of mitochondria, as in prokaryotes

antibiotics which kill bacteria by affecting ribosomes also affect ribosomes of mitochondria (e.g. chloramphenicol – now rarely used)

Fig. 8.6 The evolution of mitochondria. Many lines of evidence suggest that mitochondria of modern eukaryote cells evolved from bacteria that established symbiotic (mutualistic) relationships with ancestral cells.

cell. The endpoint of such integration is perhaps to be seen in the evolution of the eukaryote mitochondrion, which is widely considered to be the product of symbiotically associated heterotrophic purple bacteria (*Fig. 8.6*).

The pathway of virus evolution is uncertain

Clearly, parasitism by bacteria, which are undoubtedly ancient organisms (they can be traced back 3–5 billion years in the fossil record), depended upon the evolution of higher organisms to act as hosts. Whether the same is true of viruses is open to question, and depends upon whether viruses are considered primarily or secondarily simple. If viruses evolved from cellular ancestors by a process of secondary simplification, then parasitism must have evolved long after the evolution of prokaryotes and eukaryotes. If viruses are primitively non-cellular then it is possible that they became parasitic at a very early stage in the evolution of cellular life, at some point when, because of environmental change, independent existence became impossible. A third alternative is that viruses were never anything other than fragments of the nuclear material of other organisms and have in effect always been parasitic. Modern viruses may, in fact, have arisen by all three pathways.

Eukaryote parasites have evolved through accidental contact

The evolution of parasitism by eukaryotes is likely to have arisen much as it may have done in prokaryotes (i.e. through accidental contact and via blood-feeding arthropods). Examples can be found among both protozoan and worm parasites to support this view:

- There are protozoa such as the free-living ameba *Naegleria*, which can opportunistically invade the human body and cause severe and sometimes fatal disease.
- There are several species of nematode worms that can live either as parasites or as free-living organisms, *Strongyloides stercoralis* being the most important in humans.
- It is likely that trypanosomes (the protozoans responsible for sleeping sickness) were primarily adapted as parasites of blood-feeding flies and only secondarily became established as parasites of mammals.

Parasite adaptations to overcome host inflammatory and immune responses

We can view the evolution of parasitism and the adaptations necessary for life within another animal as being exactly analogous to the adaptations necessary for life within any other specialized habitat: the environment in which parasites live is merely one of the many to which organisms have become adapted in evolution (comparable with life in soil, freshwater, salt water, decaying material and so on). However, it is always necessary to remember that in one major respect parasitism is quite different from any other specialist mode of life. This difference is that the environment in which a parasite lives, the body of the host, is not passive; on the contrary it is capable of an active response to the presence of the parasite.

The attractiveness of animal bodies as environments for parasites means that hosts are under continual pressures from infection, and these pressures are increased when hosts live:

- close together;
- in insanitary conditions;
- in climates that favor the survival of parasite stages in the external world.

Pressure of infection has been a major influence in evolution

Pressure of infection has been a major selective influence in evolution, and there is little doubt that it has been largely responsible for the development of the sophisticated inflammatory and immune responses we see in humans and other mammals. In evolutionary terms all infection has its costs to the host because it diverts valuable resources from the activities of survival and reproduction; there has therefore been pressure to develop means of overcoming infection whether or not it causes disease. Of course, this is not the focus of clinical microbiology, which legitimately places emphasis on the costs of infection in terms of frank disease, but it should be remembered because it explains more fully the nature of the continuing battle between host and parasite—the former attempting to contain or destroy, the latter attempting to evade or suppress—and why the emergence of new, and the return of old, infectious diseases are a constant threat.

Parasites are faced not only with the problems of surviving within the environment they experience initially, but also of surviving in that environment as it changes in ways that are likely to be harmful to them. The inflammatory and immune responses that follow the establishment of infection are the most important means by which the host can control infections by those organisms able to penetrate its natural barriers and survive within its body. These responses represent formidable obstacles to the continued survival of parasites, forcing them to evolve strategies to cope with harmful changes in their environment. The successful parasite is therefore one that can cope with, or evade, the host's response in one of the ways shown in *Figure 8.7*.

All of these adaptations are known to exist within different groups of parasites and they are well documented in the case of some of the major human pathogens. Indeed they are often the very reason why such organisms are major pathogens. Nevertheless, transmission and survival of many parasites depends upon the existence of particularly susceptible host individuals (e.g. children) to provide a continuing reservoir of infective stages.

EVASION STRATEGIES	
strategy	**example**
elicit minimal response	herpes simplex virus—survives in host cells for long periods in a latent stage—no pathology
evade effects of response	mycobacteria—survive unharmed in granulomatous response designed to localize and destroy infection
depress host's response	HIV—destroys T cells malaria—depresses immune responsiveness
antigenic change	viruses, spirochetes, trypanosomes—all change target antigens so host response is ineffective
rapid replication	viruses, bacteria, protozoa—producing acute infections before recovery and immunity
survival in weakly responsive individuals	genetic heterogeneity in host population means some individuals respond weakly or to not at all, allowing organism to reproduce freely; examples in all groups

Fig. 8.7 Evasion strategies of parasites.

Changes in parasites create new problems for hosts

From what has been said above, it can be appreciated that there is no such thing as a static host–parasite relationship, and that concepts of unchanging 'pathogenicity' or 'harm-lessness' cannot be justified. Each relationship is an 'arms race', changes in one member being countered by changes in the other. Quite subtle changes in either can completely change the balance of the relationship, towards greater or lesser pathogenicity for example.

Perhaps the most important contemporary illustration of this situation is the dramatic and explosive appearance of HIV infections. This group of viruses was originally restricted to non-human primates, but changes in the virus have permitted extensive infections in humans. Of a different nature, but relevant to the general theme, is the acquisition of drug resistance in bacteria and protozoa (*Fig. 8.8*). Although the underlying genetic and metabolic changes do not by themselves influence pathogenicity, the expression of such changes in the face of intense and selective chemotherapy certainly does so.

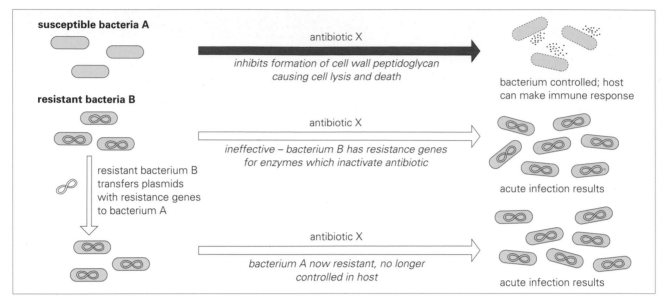

Fig. 8.8 Antibiotic resistance in bacteria. The activity of many antibiotics can be blocked by bacterial enzymes coded for by genes located on cytoplasmic DNA in plasmids. The ability of bacteria to transfer plasmids between individual organisms means that strains or species previously susceptible to an antibiotic can acquire the ability to produce such enzymes and so gain antibiotic resistance directly from resistant organisms. These newly resistant forms are then differentially selected under antibiotic treatment, the susceptible individuals being deleted from the population.

Host adaptations to overcome changes in parasites

Changes in the host can also alter the balance of a host–parasite relationship. A particularly dramatic example is the intense selection for resistant genotypes in rabbit populations exposed to the myxomatosis virus, which took place concurrently with selection for reduced pathogenicity in the virus itself (see Chapter 12). There are no exactly equivalent examples in humans, but in evolutionary time there have been major selective influences on populations prompting changes to permit survival in the face of life-threatening infections. A good example is the selective pressure exerted by *falciparum* malaria, which has been responsible for the persistence of many alleles associated with hemoglobinopathies (e.g. sickle cell hemoglobin). Although these abnormalities are detrimental to a varying degree, they persist because they are (or were) associated with resistance to malarial infection. Malaria has also changed the frequency of certain HLA antigens in areas where infection was severe.

Social and behavioral changes can be as important as genetic changes in altering host–parasite relations

Social and behavioral changes can alter host–parasite relations both positively and negatively *(Fig. 8.9)*. Although many bacterial infections of the intestine have declined in importance with changes in human lifestyle, there are other contemporary microbiologic problems in the developed world whose onset can be traced directly to sociologic, environmental and even medical change *(Fig. 8.9)*. A particularly good example is disease arising from domestication of pets (e.g. toxoplasmosis) because it illustrates that human freedom from some infections arises primarily because of lack of contact with the organisms and not from any innate resistance to the establishment of the infection itself. Diseases arising from contact with infected animals or animal products (zoonotic infections) constitute a constant threat that can be realized by behavioral or environmental changes that alter established patterns of human–animal contact.

SOCIAL AND BEHAVIORAL CHANGES AND INFECTIOUS DISEASES	
the causes	the results
altered environments (e.g. air conditioning)	water in cooling systems provides growth conditions for Legionella
changes in food production and food-handling practices	intensive husbandry under antibiotic protection leads to drug-resistant bacteria; deep-freeze, fast-food and inadequate cooking allow bacteria and toxins to enter body (e.g. *Listeria, Salmonella*)
routine use of antibiotics in medicine	emergence of antibiotic-resistant bacteria as hazards to hospitalized patients (e.g. methicillin-resistant *Staphylococcus aureus*)
routine use of immunosuppressive therapy	development of opportunistic infections in patients with reduced resistance (e.g. *Pseudomonas, Candida, Pneumocystis*)
altered sexual habits	promiscuity increases sexually transmitted diseases (e.g. gonorrhea, genital herpes, AIDS)
breakdown of filtration systems overuse of limited water supplies	transmission of animal infections leading to diarrheal and other infections (e.g. cryptosporidiosis, giardiasis, leptospirosis)
increase in ownership of pets, particularly exotic species	transmission of animal infections (e.g. *Chlamydia, Salmonella, Toxoplasma, Toxocara*)
increased frequency of journeys to tropical and subtropical countries	exposure to exotic organisms and vectors (e.g. malaria, viral encephalitides)

Fig. 8.9 Lifestyle changes and infectious diseases.

KEY FACTS

- The body is colonized by many organisms (the normal flora) which can be positively beneficial. They live on or within the body without causing disease, and play an important role in protecting the host from pathogenic microbes.

- The normal flora is predominantly made up of bacteria, but includes fungi and protozoa.

- Members of the normal flora can be harmful if they enter previously sterile parts of the body. They can be important causes of hospital-acquired infections.

- The usual relationship between the normal flora and the body is an example of beneficial symbiosis; parasitism (in the broad sense, covering all pathogenic microbes) is a harmful symbiosis.

- The biological context of host–parasite relationships, and the dynamics of the conflict between two species in this relationship, provide a basis for understanding the causes and control of infectious diseases.

- Changes in medical practice, in human behavior and, not least, in infectious organisms, are broadening the spectrum of organisms responsible for disease.

? QUESTIONS

1. Which of the following have representatives in the normal flora?
    A. *Candida*
    B. Streptococci
    C. Staphylococci
    D. *Bacteroides*
    E. All of these

2. The greatest number of bacteria forming the normal flora are found:
    A. In the mouth
    B. On the skin
    C. In the large intestine
    D. In the vagina
    E. In the nose

3. Which is not true of parasites?
    A. Their host provides their environment
    B. They rely on the host for their metabolic needs
    C. Their hosts control their development
    D. They always cause disease
    E. They have adaptations to evade immune responses

4. Factors relevant to altered patterns of infectious disease in modern society include:
    A. Increased travel
    B. Greater ownership of pets
    C. Antibiotic use
    D. Air conditioning
    E. All of these

FURTHER READING

Mims CA, Nash A, Stephen J. *Pathogenesis of Infectious Disease*, 5th edition. New York: Academic Press, 2001.

The adversaries—host defenses

2

9. The innate defenses of the body *71*

10. Adaptive responses provide a 'quantum leap' in effective defense *87*

11. The cellular basis of adaptive immune responses *99*

The innate defenses of the body

INTRODUCTION

In the preceding chapters, we have outlined some of the fundamental characteristics of the myriad types of micro- and macroparasites that may infect the body. We now turn to consider the ways in which the body seeks to defend itself against infection by these organisms.

The body has both 'innate' and 'adaptive' immune defenses

When an organism infects the body, the defense systems already in place may well be sufficient to prevent replication and spread of the infectious agent, thereby preventing development of disease. These established mechanisms are referred to as constituting the 'innate' immune system. However, should innate immunity be insufficient to parry the invasion by the infectious agent, the so-called 'adaptive' immune system then comes into action, although it takes time to reach its maximum efficiency *(Fig. 9.1)*. When it does take effect, it generally eliminates the infective organism, allowing recovery from disease.

The main feature distinguishing the adaptive response from the innate mechanism is that specific memory of infection is imprinted on the adaptive immune system, so that should there be a subsequent infection by the same agent, a particularly effective response comes into play with remarkable speed. It is worth emphasizing, however, that there is close synergy between the two systems, with the adaptive mechanism greatly improving the efficiency of the innate response.

The contrasts between these two systems are set out in *Figure 9.2*. On the one hand, the soluble factors such as lysozyme and complement, together with the phagocytic cells, contribute to the innate system, while on the other the lymphocyte-based mechanisms that produce antibody and T

COMPARISON OF INNATE AND ADAPTIVE IMMUNE SYSTEMS		
	innate immune system	adaptive immune system
major elements		
soluble factors	lysozyme, complement, acute phase proteins, e.g. C-reactive protein, interferon	antibody
cells	phagocytes natural killer cells	T lymphocytes
response to microbial infection		
first contact	+	++
second contact	+	++++
	non-specific no memory	specific memory
	resistance not improved by repeated contact	resistance improved by repeated contact

Fig. 9.2 Comparison of innate and adaptive immune systems. Innate immunity is sometimes referred to as 'natural', and adaptive as 'acquired'. There is considerable interaction between the two systems. 'Humoral' immunity due to soluble factors contrasts with immunity mediated by cells. Primary contact with antigen produces both adaptive and innate responses, but if the same antigen persists or is encountered a second time the specific adaptive response to that antigen is much enhanced.

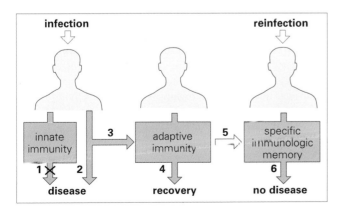

Fig. 9.1 Innate and adaptive immunity. An infectious agent first encounters elements of the innate immune system. These may be sufficient to prevent disease (1), but if not, disease may result (2). The adaptive immune system is then activated (3) to produce recovery (4) and a specific immunologic memory (5). Following reinfection with the same agent, no disease results (6) and the individual has acquired immunity to the infectious agent.

lymphocytes are the main elements of the adaptive immune system. Not only do these lymphocytes provide improved resistance by repeated contact with a given infectious agent, but the memory with which they become endowed shows very considerable specificity to that infection. For instance, infection with measles virus will induce a memory to that microorganism alone and not to another virus such as rubella.

DEFENSE AGAINST ENTRY INTO THE BODY

A variety of biochemical and physical barriers operate at the body surfaces

Before an infectious agent can penetrate the body, it must overcome biochemical and physical barriers that operate at the body surfaces. One of the most important of these is the skin, which is normally impermeable to the majority of infectious agents. Many bacteria fail to survive for long on the skin because of the direct inhibitory effects of lactic acid and fatty acids present in sweat and sebaceous secretions and the lower pH to which they give rise (Fig. 9.3). However, should there be skin loss, as can occur in burns for example, infection becomes a major problem.

The membranes lining the inner surfaces of the body secrete mucus, which acts as a protective barrier, inhibiting the adherence of bacteria to the epithelial cells, thereby preventing them from gaining access to the body. Microbial and other foreign particles trapped within this adhesive mucus may be removed by mechanical means such as ciliary action, coughing and sneezing. The flushing actions of tears, saliva and urine are other mechanical strategies that help to protect the epithelial surfaces. In addition, many of the secreted body fluids contain microbicidal factors: for example, the acid in gastric juice, spermine and zinc in semen, lactoperoxidase in milk, and lysozyme in tears, nasal secretions and saliva.

The phenomenon of microbial antagonism is associated with the normal bacterial flora of the body. These commensal organisms suppress the growth of many potentially pathogenic bacteria and fungi at superficial sites, first by virtue of their physical advantage of previous occupancy, especially on epithelial surfaces, second by competing for essential nutrients, or third by producing inhibitory substances such as acid or colicins. The latter are a class of bactericidins that bind to the negatively charged surface of susceptible bacteria and form a voltage-dependent channel in the membrane, which kills by destroying the cell's energy potential.

DEFENSES ONCE THE MICROORGANISM PENETRATES THE BODY

Despite the general effectiveness of the various barriers, microorganisms successfully penetrate the body on many occasions. When this occurs, two main defensive strategies come into play based on:

- the mechanism of phagocytosis, involving engulfment and killing of microorganisms by specialized cells, the 'professional phagocytes';
- the destructive effect of soluble chemical factors, such as bactericidal enzymes.

Two types of professional phagocyte

Perhaps because of the belief that professionals do a better job than amateurs, the cells that shoulder the main burden of our phagocytic defenses have been labeled 'professional phagocytes'. These consist of two major cell families, as originally defined by Elie Metchnikoff, the Russian zoologist (see panel):

- the large macrophages;
- the smaller polymorphonuclear granulocytes, which are generally referred to as polymorphs or neutrophils because their cytoplasmic granules do not stain with hematoxylin and eosin.

As a very crude generalization, it may be said that the polymorphs provide the major defense against pyogenic (pus-forming) bacteria, while the macrophages are thought to be at their best in combatting organisms capable of living within the cells of the host.

Macrophages are widespread throughout the tissues

Macrophages originate as bone marrow promonocytes, which develop into circulating blood monocytes (Fig. 9.5) and finally become the mature macrophages, which are widespread throughout the tissues and collectively termed the 'mononuclear phagocyte system' (Fig. 9.6). These macrophages are present throughout the connective tissue and are associated with the basement membrane of small blood vessels. They are particularly concentrated in the lung (alveolar macrophages), liver (Kupffer cells) and the lining of lymph node medullary sinuses and splenic sinusoids (Fig. 9.7) where they are well

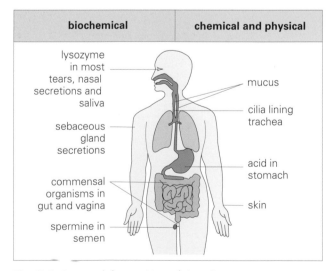

biochemical	chemical and physical

lysozyme in most tears, nasal secretions and saliva

sebaceous gland secretions

commensal organisms in gut and vagina

spermine in semen

mucus

cilia lining trachea

acid in stomach

skin

Fig. 9.3 Exterior defenses. Most of the infectious agents encountered by an individual are prevented from entering the body by a variety of biochemical and physical barriers. The body tolerates a variety of commensal organisms, which compete effectively with many potential pathogens.

LESSONS IN MICROBIOLOGY

Elie Metchnikoff (1845–1916)

This perceptive Russian zoologist can legitimately be regarded as the father of the concept of cellular immunity in which it is recognized that certain specialized cells mediate the defense against microbial infections. He was intrigued by the motile cells of transparent starfish larvae and made the critical observation that a few hours after introducing a rose thorn into the larvae the rose thorn became surrounded by the motile cells. He extended his investigations to mammalian leukocytes, showing their ability to engulf microorganisms, a process that he termed 'phagocytosis' (literally, eating by cells).

Because he found this process to be even more effective in animals recovering from an infection, he came to the conclusion that phagocytosis provided the main defense against infection. He defined the existence of two types of circulating phagocytes: the polymorphonuclear leukocyte, which he termed a 'microphage', and the larger 'macrophage'.

Although Metchnikoff held the somewhat polarized view that cellular immunity based upon phagocytosis provided the main, if not the only, defense mechanism against infectious microorganisms, we now know that the efficiency of the phagocytic system is enormously enhanced through cooperation with humoral factors, in particular antibody and complement.

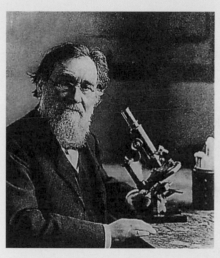

Fig. 9.4 Elie Metchnikoff (1845–1916). (Courtesy of the Wellcome Institute Library, London.)

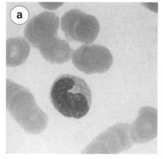 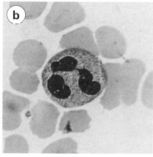

Fig. 9.5 Phagocytic cells. (a) Blood monocyte and (b) polymorphonuclear neutrophil, both derived from bone marrow stem cells. (Courtesy of PM Lydyard.)

placed to filter off foreign material *(Fig. 9.8)*. Other examples are the brain microglia, kidney mesangial cells, synovial A cells and osteoclasts in bone. In general, these are long-lived cells that depend upon mitochondria for their metabolic energy and show elements of rough-surfaced endoplasmic reticulum *(Fig. 9.9)* related to the formidable array of different secretory proteins that these cells generate.

Polymorphs possess a variety of enzyme-containing granules

The polymorph is the dominant white cell in the bloodstream and, like the macrophage, shares a common hemopoietic stem cell precursor with the other formed elements of the

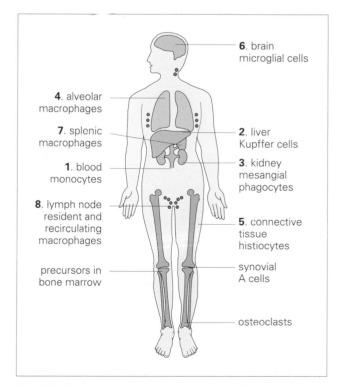

Fig. 9.6 The mononuclear phagocyte system. Tissue macrophages are derived from blood monocytes, which are manufactured in the bone marrow. (The numbers relate to those in *Figure 9.7*.)

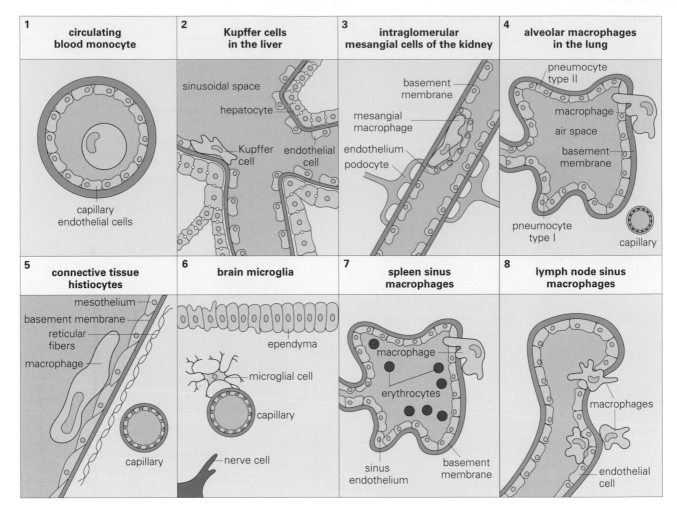

| 1 circulating blood monocyte | 2 Kupffer cells in the liver | 3 intraglomerular mesangial cells of the kidney | 4 alveolar macrophages in the lung |

Fig. 9.7 Cellular disposition of mononuclear phagocytes.

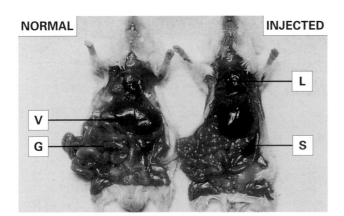

Fig. 9.8 Localization of intravenously injected particles in the mononuclear phagocyte system. (Right) A mouse was injected with fine carbon particles and killed five minutes later. Carbon accumulates in organs rich in mononuclear phagocytes: lungs (L), liver (V), spleen (S) and areas of the gut wall (G). (Left) Normal organ color shown in a control mouse. (Courtesy of PM Lydyard.)

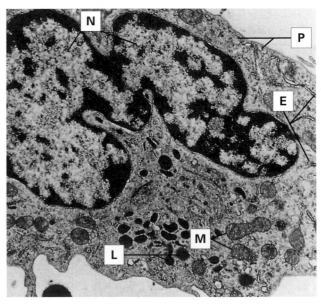

Fig. 9.9 Monocyte (×8000), with 'horseshoe' nucleus (N). Phagocytic and pinocytic vesicles (P), lysosomal granules (L), mitochondria (M) and isolated profiles of rough-surfaced endoplasmic reticulum (E) are evident. (Courtesy of B Nichols. Copyright Rockefeller University Press.)

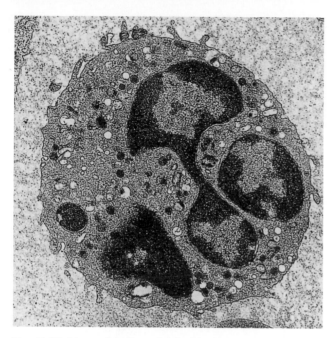

Fig. 9.10 Neutrophil. The multi-lobed nucleus and cytoplasmic granules are well displayed. (Courtesy of D McLaren.)

blood. It has no mitochondria, but uses its abundant cytoplasmic glycogen stores for its energy requirements; therefore, glycolysis enables these cells to function under anaerobic conditions, such as those in an inflammatory focus. The polymorph is a non-dividing, short-lived cell with a segmented nucleus; the cytoplasm is characterized by an array of granules, including:

- the primary azurophilic granule, which contains myeloperoxidase, some lysozyme and families of cationic proteins;
- the secondary 'specific' granules associated with lactoferrin and lysozyme;
- the tertiary granules typical of the conventional lysosome with acid hydrolases (Fig. 9.10).

Phagocytosis and killing

Phagocytes recognize pathogen-associated molecular patterns (PAMPs)

The first event in the uptake and digestion of a microorganism by the professional phagocyte involves the attachment of the microbe to the surface of the cell through the recognition of repeating molecular patterns, PAMPs, on the microbe by receptors on the phagocyte surface (Fig. 9.11). Generally speaking, these receptors bind to PAMPs composed of repeating carbohydrate motifs such as Gram-negative lipopolysaccharide, yeast cell wall mannans and mycobacterial glycolipids. Examples of intracellular PAMPs are the unmethylated guanosine–cytosine (CpG) sequences of bacterial DNA and double-stranded RNA from RNA viruses.

The phagocyte is activated through PAMP recognition

The attached microbe may then signal through the phagocyte receptors to initiate the ingestion phase by activating an actin–myosin contractile system, which sends arms of cytoplasm around the particle until it is completely enclosed

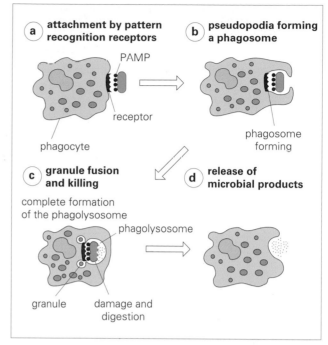

Fig. 9.11 Phagocytosis. (a) Phagocytes attach to microorganisms (blue icon) via their cell surface receptors which recognize pathogen-associated molecular patterns (PAMPs) such as lipopolysaccharide. (b) If the membrane now becomes activated by the attached infectious agent, the pathogen is taken into a phagosome by pseudopodia, which extend around it. (c) Once inside the cell, the various granules fuse with the phagosome to form a phagolysosome. (d) The infectious agent is then killed by a battery of microbicidal degradation mechanisms, and the microbial products are released.

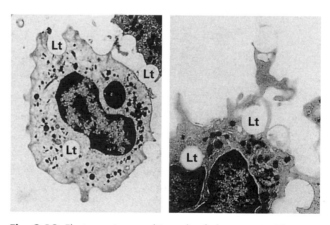

Fig. 9.12 Electron micrographic study of phagocytosis. These two micrographs show human phagocytes engulfing latex particles (Lt). (a) ×3000; (b) ×4500. (Courtesy of CHW Horne.)

within a vacuole (phagosome; Figs 9.11 and 9.12). Shortly afterwards, the cytoplasmic granules fuse with a phagosome and discharge their contents around the incarcerated microorganism.

The internalized micobe is the target for a fearsome array of killing mechanisms

As phagocytosis is initiated, the attached microbes also signal through one of a family of 'Toll-like' receptors (so called because of their homology with the Drosophila Toll component linked to embryonic differentiation), each of which engineers the defensive response to different types of infection. This leads to an NFκB mediated activation of a unique plasma membrane reduced nicotinamide adenine dinucleotide phosphate (NADPH) oxidase which reduces oxygen to a series of powerful microbicidal agents, namely superoxide anion, hydrogen peroxide, singlet oxygen and hydroxyl radicals (*Fig. 9.13*; see also Chapter 14). Subse-

quently, the peroxide, in association with myeloperoxidase, generates a potent halogenating system from halide ions, which is capable of killing both bacteria and viruses.

As superoxide anion is formed, the enzyme superoxide dismutase acts to convert it to molecular oxygen and hydrogen peroxide, but in the process consumes hydrogen ions. Therefore initially there is a small increase in pH, which facilitates the antibacterial function of the families of cationic proteins derived from the phagocytic granules. These

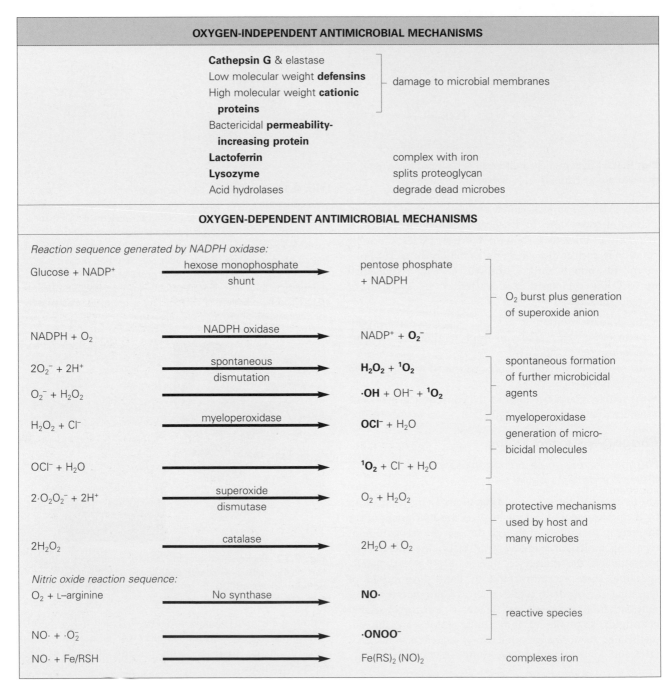

Fig. 9.13 Antimicrobial mechanisms in phagocytic vacuoles. Microbicidal species in bold letters. Fe/RSH, a complex of iron with a general sulfhydryl molecule; Fe(RS)$_2$, oxidised Fe/RSH; O$_2^-$, superoxide anion; ^{1}O$_2$, singlet (activated) oxygen; ·OH, hydroxyl free radical; NADPH, reduced nicotinamide adenine dinucleotide phosphate; NADP$^+$, oxidized NADPH; H$_2$O$_2$, hydrogen peroxide; OCl$^-$, hypochlorite anion; NO·, nitric oxide; ·ONOO$^-$, peroxynitrite radical.

molecules damage microbial membranes by the proteolytic action of cathepsin G and by direct adherence to the microbial surface. The defensins have an amphipathic structure which allows them to insert into microbial membranes to form destabilizing voltage-regulated ion channels. These antibiotic peptides reach extraordinarily high concentrations within the phagosome and act as disinfectants against a wide spectrum of bacteria, fungi and enveloped viruses. Other important factors are:

- lactoferrin, which complexes iron to deprive bacteria of essential growth elements;
- lysozyme, which splits the proteoglycan cell wall of bacteria;
- nitric oxide which can lead not only to iron seclusion but, together with its derivative, the peroxynitrite radical, can also be directly microbicidal.

The pH now falls so that the dead or dying microorganisms are extensively degraded by acid hydrolytic enzymes, and the degradation products released to the exterior.

Phagocytes are mobilized and targeted onto the microorganism by chemotaxis

Phagocytosis cannot occur unless the bacterium first attaches to the surface of the phagocyte, and clearly this cannot happen unless both have become physically close to each other. There is therefore a need for a mechanism that mobilizes phagocytes from afar and targets them onto the bacterium. Many bacteria produce chemical substances, such as formyl methionyl peptides, which directionally attract leukocytes, a process known as 'chemotaxis'. However, this is a relatively weak signaling system, and evolution has provided the body with a far more effective 'magnet' that uses a complex series of proteins collectively termed 'complement'.

Activation of the complement system

Complement resembles blood clotting, fibrinolysis and kinin formation in being a major triggered enzyme cascade system. Such systems are characterized by their ability to produce a rapid, highly amplified response to a trigger stimulus mediated by a cascade phenomenon in which the product of one reaction is the enzymic catalyst of the next. The most abundant and most central component is C3 (complement components are designated by the letter 'C' followed by a number), and the cleavage of this molecule is at the heart of all complement-mediated phenomena.

In normal plasma, C3 undergoes spontaneous activation at a very slow rate to generate the split product C3b. This is able to complex with another complement component, factor B, which is then acted upon by a normal plasma enzyme, factor D, to produce the C3-splitting enzyme C3bBb. This C3 convertase can then split new molecules of C3 to give C3a (a small fragment) and further C3b. This represents a positive feedback circuit with potential for runaway amplification; however, the overall process is restricted to a tick-over level by powerful regulatory mechanisms, which break the unstable soluble-phase C3 convertase into inactive cleavage products (*Fig. 9.14*).

In the presence of certain molecules, such as the carbohydrates on the surface of many bacteria, the C3

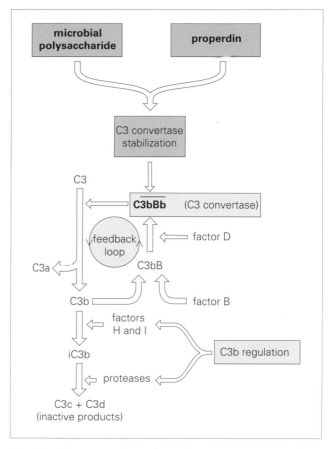

Fig. 9.14 Activation of complement by microorganisms. C3b is formed by the spontaneous breakdown of C3 complexes with factor B to form C3bB which is split by factor D to produce a C3 convertase C3bBb, capable of further cleaving C3. The convertase is heavily regulated by factors H and I but can be stabilized on the surface of microbes and properdin. The horizontal bar indicates an enzymically active complex. iC3b, inactive C3b.

convertase can become attached and stabilized against breakdown. Under these circumstances, there is active generation of new C3 convertase molecules, and what is known as the 'alternative' complement pathway can swing into full tempo (see Chapter 10).

Complement synergizes with phagocytic cells to produce an acute inflammatory response

Activation of the alternative complement pathway with the consequent splitting of very large numbers of C3 molecules has important consequences for the orchestration of an integrated antimicrobial defense strategy (*Fig. 9.15*). Large numbers of C3b produced in the immediate vicinity of the microbial membrane bind covalently to that surface and act as opsonins (molecules that make the particle they coat more susceptible to engulfment by phagocytic cells; see below). This C3b, together with the C3 convertase, acts on the next component in the sequence, C5, to produce a small fragment, C5a which, together with C3a, has a direct effect on mast cells to cause their degranulation. Consequently, mediators of vascular permeability and factors chemotactic for polymorphs are released. The nature of this degranulation process and of

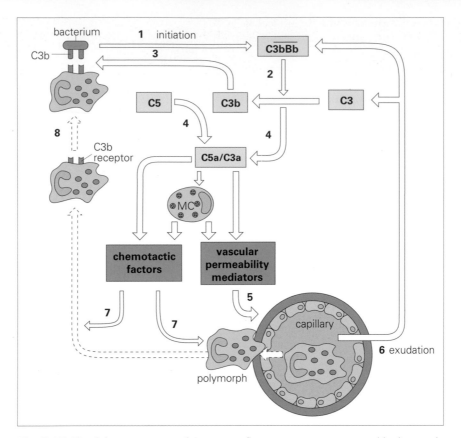

Fig. 9.15 The defensive strategy of the acute inflammatory reaction initiated by bacterial activation of the alternative complement pathway. Activation of the C3bBb C3 convertase by the bacterium (1) leads to the generation of C3b (2) (which binds to the bacterium (3)), C3a and C5a (4), which recruit mast cell (MC) mediators. These in turn cause capillary dilation (5), exudation of plasma proteins (6), and chemotactic attraction (7) and adherence of polymorphs to the C3b-coated bacterium (8). The polymorphs are then activated for the final kill.

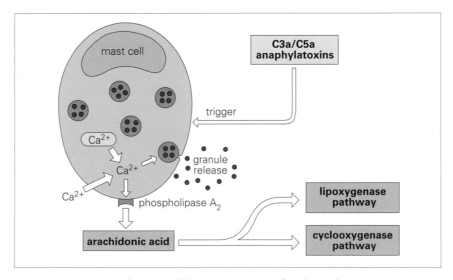

Fig. 9.16 Triggering of a mast cell leading to release of mediators by two major pathways: (1) granule release of pre-formed mediators, and (2) arachidonic acid produced by activation of phospholipase A_2 generating the lipoxygenase and cyclo-oxygenase subpathways. Intracellular calcium (Ca^{2+}) and cyclic adenosine monophosphate (cAMP) are central to the initiation of these events, but details are still unclear.

MAST CELL MEDIATORS		
	pre-formed	**effect**
granule release	histamine	vasodilation, increased capillary permeability, chemokinesis, bronchoconstriction
	heparin	anticoagulant
	tryptase	activates C3
	β-glucosaminidase	splits off glucosamine
	ECF	eosinophil chemotaxis
	NCF	neutrophil chemotaxis
	platelet activating factor	mediator release
	newly synthesized	**effect**
lipoxygenase pathway	leukotrienes C4 and D4 leukotriene B4	vasoactive, bronchoconstriction, chemotaxis and/or chemokinesis
cyclooxygenase pathway	prostaglandins, thromboxanes	affect bronchial muscle, platelet aggregation and vasodilation

Fig. 9.17 Mediators released by mast cell triggering. Chemotaxis refers to directed migration of granulocytes up the concentration gradient of the mediator, whereas chemokinesis describes randomly increased motility of these cells. (ECF, eosinophil chemotactic factor; NCF, neutrophil chemotactic factor.)

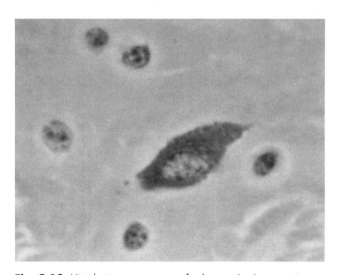

Fig. 9.18 Histologic appearance of a human (gut) connective tissue mast cell showing the dark blue cytoplasm with brownish granules. Alcian blue and safranin, ×600. (Courtesy of TSC Orr.)

the products to which it gives rise are shown in *Figures 9.16 and 9.17*; the circulating equivalent of the tissue mast cell *(Figs 9.18 and 9.19)*, the basophil, is shown in *Figure 9.20*.

The vascular permeability mediators increase the permeability of capillaries by modifying the intercellular forces between the endothelial cells of the vessel wall. This allows the exudation of fluid and plasma components, including more complement, to the site of the infection. These mediators *(Fig. 9.17)* also upregulate molecules such as intercellular adhesion molecule-1 (ICAM-1) and endothelial cell leukocyte adhesion molecule-1 (ELAM-1), which bind to specific complementary molecules on the polymorphs and encourage them to stick to the walls of the capillaries, a process termed 'margination'.

The chemotactic factors, on the other hand, provide a chemical gradient which attracts marginated polymorphonuclear leukocytes from their intravascular location, through the walls of the blood vessels, and eventually leads them to the site of the C3b-coated bacteria that initiated the whole activation process. Polymorphs have a well-defined receptor for C3b on their surface, and as a result the opsonized bacteria adhere very firmly to the surface of these newly arrived cells.

The processes of capillary dilation (erythema), exudation of plasma proteins and of fluid (edema) due to hydrostatic and osmotic pressure changes, and the accumulation of neutrophils, are collectively termed the 'acute inflammatory response', and result in a highly effective way of focusing phagocytic cells onto complement-coated microbial targets.

It also seems clear that the macrophage can be stimulated by certain bacterial toxins such as the lipopolysaccharides (LPS), by the action of C5a, and by the phagocytosis of C3b-coated bacteria, to secrete other potent mediators of acute inflammation, which reinforce the mast cell-directed pathway *(Fig. 9.21)*.

C9 molecules form the 'membrane attack complex', which is involved in cell lysis

We have already introduced the idea that following the activation of C3, the next component to be cleaved is C5; the larger C5b fragment that results becomes membrane bound. This subsequently binds components C6, C7 and C8, which

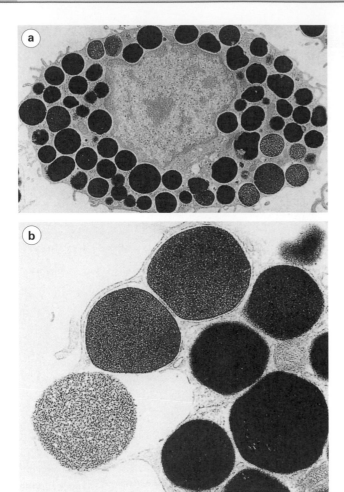

Fig. 9.19 Electron micrographs of rat peritoneal mast cells. These show (a) the undegranulated cell with its electron-dense granules ×6000 and (b) a granule in the process of exocytosis ×30 000. (Courtesy of TSC Orr.)

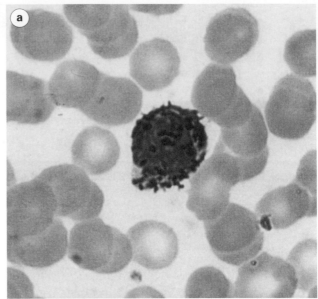

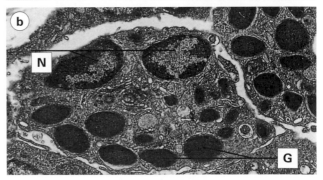

Fig. 9.20 Morphology of the basophil. (a) This blood smear shows a typical basophil with its deep violet–blue granules. Wright's stain, ×1500. (b) Electron micrograph showing the ultrastructure of the basophil. Basophils in guinea pig skin showing the nuclei (N) and characteristic randomly distributed granules (G). ×6000. (Courtesy of D McLaren.)

form a complex capable of inducing a critical conformational change in the terminal component C9. The unfolded C9 molecules become inserted into the lipid bilayer and polymerize to form an annular 'membrane attack complex' (MAC) *(Figs 9.22 and 9.23)*. This behaves as a transmembrane channel that is fully permeable to electrolytes and water; because of the high internal colloid osmotic pressure of cells, there is a net influx of sodium (Na^+), and this frequently leads to lysis.

Acute phase proteins

Certain proteins in the plasma, collectively termed 'acute phase proteins', increase in concentration in response to early 'alarm' mediators such as the cytokines interleukin-1 (IL-1), IL-6 and tumor necrosis factor (TNF), released as a result of infection or tissue injury. Many acute phase reactants such as mannose binding protein and C-reactive protein (CRP) increase dramatically during inflammation *(Fig. 9.24)*. Like the professional phagocytes, both use pattern recognition receptors to bind to molecular patterns on the pathogen (PAMPs), to generate defensive effector functions *(Fig. 9.25)*.

Other acute phase reactants show more moderate rises, usually less than five-fold *(Fig. 9.26)*. In general, these proteins are thought to have defensive roles.

Other extracellular antimicrobial factors

There are many microbicidal agents that operate at short range within phagocytic cells, but also appear in various body fluids in sufficient concentration to have direct inhibitory effects on infectious agents. For example, lysozyme is present in fluids such as tears and saliva in amounts capable of acting against the proteoglycan wall of susceptible bacteria. Similarly, lactoferrin may appear in the blood in sufficient concentration to complex iron and deprive bacteria of this important growth factor. Whether agents that normally act over a short range, such as reactive oxygen metabolites or TNF (a cytotoxic molecule produced by macrophages and other cell types), can reach concentrations in the body fluids that are adequate to allow them to act at a distance from the cell producing them, will be discussed in Chapter 14, particularly when considering the mechanisms by which the bloodborne forms of parasites such as malaria are attacked.

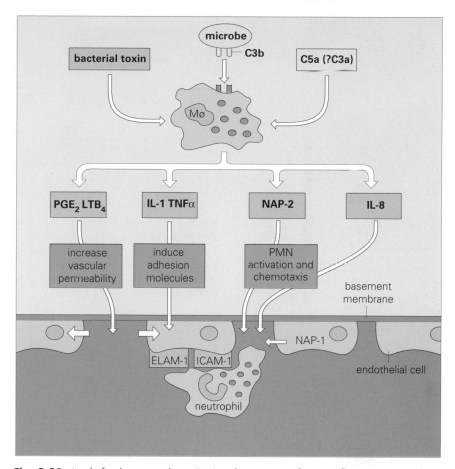

Fig. 9.21 A role for the macrophage (Mφ) in the initiation of acute inflammation. Stimulation induces macrophage secretion of mediators. Blood neutrophils stick to the adhesion molecules on the endothelial cell and use them to provide traction as they force their way between the cells, through the basement membrane (with the help of secreted elastase) and up the chemotactic gradient. During this process they become progressively activated by neutrophil activating peptide-2 (NAP-2). (PGE$_2$, prostaglandin E$_2$; LTB$_4$, leukotriene B$_4$; IL-1, interleukin-1; PMN, polymorphonuclear neutrophil; TNFα, tumor necrosis factor alpha; ELAM-1, endothelial cell leukocyte adhesion molecule-1; ICAM-1, intercellular adhesion molecule-1.)

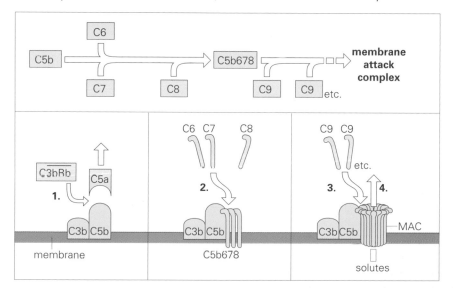

Fig. 9.22 Assembly of the C5b–9 membrane attack complex (MAC). (1) Recruitment of a further C3b into the C3bBb enzymic complex generates a C5 convertase which cleaves C5a from C5 and leaves the remaining C5b attached to the membrane. (2) Once C5b is membrane bound, C6 and C7 attach themselves to form the stable complex C5b67, which interacts with C8 to yield C5b678. (3) This unit has some effect in disrupting the membrane, but primarily causes the polymerization of C9 to form tubules traversing the membrane. The resulting tubule is referred to as a MAC. (4) Disruption of the membrane by this structure permits the free exchange of solutes, which are primarily responsible for cell lysis.

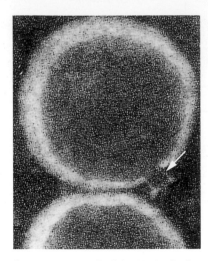

Fig. 9.23 Electron micrograph of the MAC. The funnel-shaped lesion (arrowed) is due to a human C5b–9 complex that has been reincorporated into lecithin liposomal membranes. ×234 000. (Courtesy of J Tranum-Jensen and S Bhakdi.)

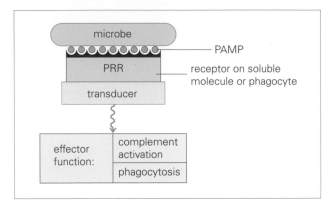

Fig. 9.25 A major defensive strategy in which soluble factors, such as CRP and mannose binding protein, and professional phagocytes use their pattern recognition receptors (PRR) to bind to the pathogen-associated molecular patterns (PAMPs) on the microbial surface and signal through their transducer structures to initiate appropriate effector functions.

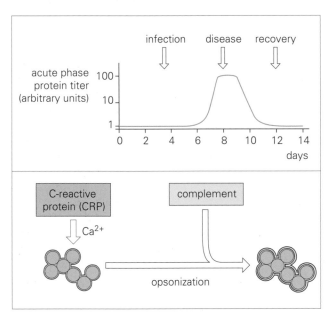

Fig. 9.24 Acute phase proteins, here exemplified by C-reactive protein (CRP), are serum proteins that increase rapidly in concentration (sometimes up to 100-fold) following infection (graph). They are important in innate immunity to infection. CRP recognizes and binds in a calcium (Ca^{2+}) dependent fashion to molecular groups found on a wide variety of bacteria and fungi. In particular, it uses its pattern recognition to bind the phosphocholine moiety of pneumococci. The CRP acts as an opsonin and activates complement with all the associated sequelae. Mannose binding protein reacts not only with mannose but several other sugars, enabling it to bind to a wide variety of Gram-negative and -positive bacteria, yeasts, viruses and parasites, subsequently activating the complement system and phagocytic cells.

Interferons are a family of broad spectrum antiviral molecules

Interferons (IFNs) are widespread throughout the animal kingdom and are discussed further in Chapter 14. They were first recognized by the phenomenon of viral interference, in

ACUTE PHASE PROTEINS PRODUCED IN RESPONSE TO INFECTION IN THE HUMAN	
acute phase reactant	**role**
dramatic increases in concentration:	
C-reactive protein	fixes complement, opsonizes
mannose binding protein	fixes complement, opsonizes
α_1 acid glycoprotein	transport protein
serum amyloid A protein	complexes chondroitin sulfate
moderate increases in concentration:	
α_1 proteinase inhibitors	inhibits bacterial proteases
α_1 anti-chymotrypsin	inhibits bacterial proteases
C3, C9, factor B	increase complement function
ceruloplasmin	O_2 scavenger
fibrinogen	coagulation
angiotensin	blood pressure
haptoglobin	binds hemoglobin
fibronectin	cell attachment

Fig. 9.26 Acute phase proteins produced in response to infection in the human. (Adapted from Stadnyk AW and Gauldie J. The acute phase protein response during parasitic infection. *Immunol Today* 1991; 7:A7–A12.)

which a cell infected with one virus is found to be resistant to superinfection by a second unrelated virus. Leukocytes produce many different alpha interferons (IFNα), while fibroblasts and probably all cell types synthesize IFNβ. A third type (IFNγ) is not a component of the innate immune system and will be discussed in Chapter 10 as a member of the important cytokine family.

When cells are infected by a virus, they synthesize and secrete IFNs, which bind to specific receptors on nearby uninfected cells. The bound IFN exerts its antiviral effect by

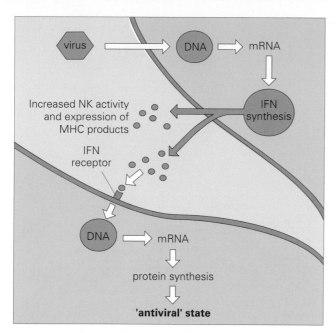

Fig. 9.27 The action of interferon (IFN). Virus infecting a cell induces the production of IFN. This is released and binds to IFN receptors on other cells. The IFN induces the production of antiviral proteins, which are activated if virus enters the second cell. (NK, natural killer; MHC, major histocompatibility complex.)

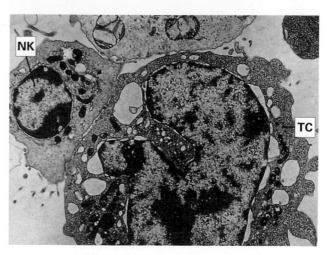

Fig. 9.28 Electron micrograph of an NK cell killing a tumor cell (TC). NK cells bind to and kill IgG antibody-coated (see *Fig. 10.15*), and even non-coated, tumor cells. It is essential for the membranes of the two cells to be closely apposed in order for the NK cell to deliver the 'kiss of death'. ×4500. (Courtesy of P Lydyard.)

facilitating the synthesis of two new enzymes, which interfere with the machinery used by the virus for its own replication. The mechanism of action of IFN is discussed more fully in Chapter 14; the net result is to set up a cordon of infection-resistant cells around the site of virus infection, so restraining its spread *(Fig. 9.27)*. IFN is highly effective in vivo, as supported by experiments in which mice injected with an antiserum to murine IFN were found to be killed by several hundred times less virus than was needed to kill the controls. It should be emphasized, however, that IFN seems to play a significant role in recovery from, rather than prevention of, viral infections.

Extracellular killing

Natural killer cells attach to virally infected cells, allowing them to be differentiated from normal cells

There is a widely held view that viruses represent fragments of the genome of multicellular organisms that have achieved the ability to exist in an extracellular state. The small number of genes present in the viral genome, however, do not include those required for viral replication. Accordingly, it is essential for viruses to penetrate the cells of an infected host in order to subvert the cells' replicative machinery towards viral replication. Clearly, it is in the interests of the host to try to kill such infected cells before the virus has had a chance to reproduce. Natural killer (NK) cells are cytotoxic cells that appear to have evolved to carry out just such a task. These are large granular lymphocytes (LGLs) *(Fig. 9.28)* that attach themselves by lectin-like receptors to structures, presumably glycoproteins, on the surface of virally infected cells and allow them to be differentiated from normal cells; activation of the NK cell results in the extracellular release of its granule

contents into the space between the target and effector cells. These contents include perforin molecules, which resemble C9 in many respects, especially in their ability to insert into the membrane of the target cell and polymerize to form annular transmembrane pores, like the MAC. This permits the entry of another granule protein, granzyme B, which leads to death of the target cell by apoptosis (programmed cell death), a process mediated by a cascade of proteolytic enzymes termed caspases, which terminates with the ultimate fragmentation of DNA by a Ca-dependent endonuclease *(Fig. 9.29)*.

Subsidiary mechanisms which can activate the caspase pathway include engagement of Fas on the target cell by the NK Fas ligand, and binding of tumor necrosis factor (TNF) released from the NK granules to surface receptors. TNF was first recognized as a product of activated macrophages known to be capable of killing certain other cells, particularly some tumor cells.

Yet a further mode of cytotoxicity can be turned on by the activated macrophage, involving the direct 'burning' of the surface of another cell by means of a stream of reactive oxygen intermediates, produced at the macrophage membrane by the respiratory oxygen burst, as discussed previously (see *Fig. 9.13*).

Eosinophils act against large parasites

It takes little imagination to realize that professional phagocytes are far too small to be capable of physically engulfing large parasites such as helminths. An alternative strategy, such as killing by an extracellular broadside of the type discussed above, would seem to be a more appropriate form of defense. Eosinophils appear to have evolved to fulfil this role. These polymorphonuclear relatives of the neutrophil have distinctive cytoplasmic granules, which stain strongly with acidic dyes *(Fig. 9.30)* and have a characteristic ultrastructural appearance. A major basic protein (MBP) has been identified

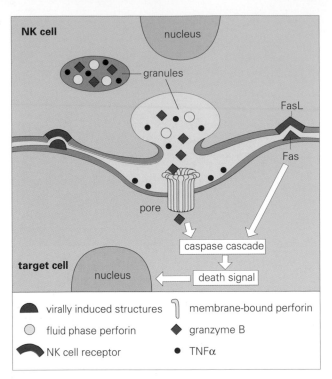

Fig. 9.29 Schematic model of lysis of virally infected target cell by a natural killer (NK) cell. As the NK cell receptors bind to the surface of the virally infected cell, there is exocytosis of granules and release of cytolytic mediators into the intercellular cleft. A calcium (Ca^{2+})-dependent conformational change in the perforin enables it to insert and polymerize within the membrane of the target cell to form a transmembrane pore, which allows entry of granzyme B into the target cell, where it causes programmed cell death (apoptosis). A back-up cytolytic system using engagement of the Fas receptor with its ligand (FasL), can also trigger apoptosis as can binding of granule-derived tumor necrosis factor alpha (TNFα) to its receptor.

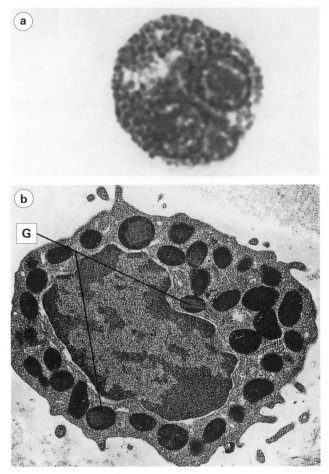

Fig. 9.30 The eosinophil granulocyte is capable of extracellular killing of parasites (e.g. worms) by releasing its granule contents. (a) Morphology of the eosinophil. This blood smear enriched for granulocytes shows an eosinophil with its multilobed nucleus and heavily-stained cytoplasmic granules. Leishman's stain. ×1800. (Courtesy of P Lydyard.) (b) Electron micrograph showing the ultrastructure of a guinea pig eosinophil. The mature eosinophil contains granules (G) with central crystalloids. ×8000. (Courtesy of D McLaren.)

in the core of the granule, while the matrix has been shown to contain an eosinophilic cationic protein, a peroxidase and a perforin-like molecule. Eosinophils have surface receptors for C3b and when activated generate copious amounts of active oxygen metabolites.

Many helminths can activate the alternative complement pathway but, although resistant to C9 attack, their coating with C3b allows adherence to the eosinophils through their C3b surface receptors. Once activated, the eosinophil launches its extracellular ammunition, which includes the release of major basic proteins and the cationic protein to damage the parasite membrane, with a possibility of a further 'chemical burn' from the oxygen metabolites and 'leaky pore' formation by the perforins.

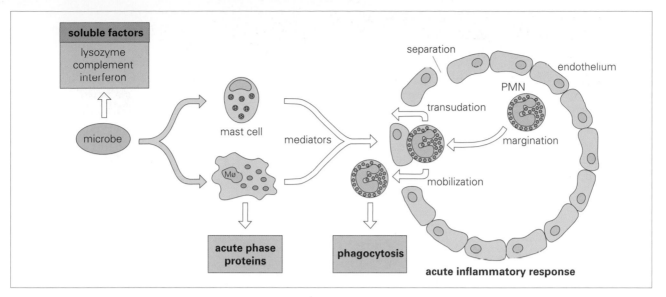

Fig. 9.31 Mobilization of defensive components of innate immunity. Microbes, either through complement activation or through direct effects on macrophages, release mediators which increase capillary permeability to allow transudation of plasma bactericidal molecules, and chemotactically attract plasma polymorphs from the bloodstream to the infection site. (PMN, polymorphonuclear neutrophil.)

 KEY FACTS

- The innate system of immune defense consists of a formidable barrier to entry and second-line defense by phagocytes and circulating soluble factors. Colonization of the body by normally non-pathogenic ('opportunistic') microorganisms occurs whenever there is a hereditary or acquired deficiency in any of these functions.

- The main phagocytic cells are polymorphonuclear neutrophils and macrophages. They adhere to the surface of the microbe by receptors which recognize pathogen-associated molecular patterns (PAMPs). This activates the engulfment process so that the organisms are taken inside the cell in a phagocytic vacuole which fuses with cytoplasmic granules. A formidable array of oxygen-dependent and oxygen-independent microbicidal mechanisms then comes into play.

- The complement system, a multicomponent triggered enzyme cascade, is used to attract phagocytic cells to the microbes and engulf them.

- The most abundant complement component, C3, is split by a convertase enzyme formed from its own cleavage product C3b and factor B and stabilized against breakdown caused by factors H and I through association with the microbial surface. As it is formed, C3b becomes covalently linked to the microorganism.

- The next most abundant component, C5, is activated to yield a small peptide, C5a, while residual C5b binds to the surface of the microorganism and assembles the terminal components C6–9 into a membrane attack complex (MAC), which is freely permeable to solutes and can lead to osmotic lysis. In addition, C5a is a potent chemotactic agent for polymorphs and greatly increases capillary permeability.

- C3a and C5a act on mast cells, causing the release of further mediators such as histamine, LTB_4 and $TNF\alpha$, with effects on capillary permeability and adhesiveness and neutrophil chemotaxis. They also activate neutrophils, which bind to the C3b-coated microbes by their surface C3b receptors and then ingest them.

- The influx of polymorphs and increase in vascular permeability constitute the potent antimicrobial acute inflammatory response.

- Inflammation can also be initiated by tissue macrophages, which subserve a similar role to that of the mast cell since signaling by bacterial toxins, C5a or by C3b-coated bacteria adhering to surface complement receptors on tissue macrophages causes the release of $TNF\alpha$, LTB_4, PGE_2, NCF and a neutrophil-activating peptide.

- Other humoral defenses include the acute phase proteins such as CRP, and the IFNs, which can block viral replication.

- Virally infected cells can be killed by NK cells.

KEY FACTS

- Extracellular killing can also be effected by C3b-bound eosinophils, which may be responsible for the failure of many large parasites to establish a foothold in potential hosts.

- It is probably true to say that engulfment and killing by phagocytic cells is the mechanism used to dispose of the majority of microbes, and the

mobilization and activation of these cells by orchestrated responses such as the acute inflammatory response *(Fig. 9.31)* is a key feature of innate immunity. However, not every organism is readily susceptible to phagocytosis or even to killing by complement or lysozyme, and this brings us to the role of the adaptive immune response, which is explored in Chapter 10.

QUESTIONS

1. Which of the following does *not* protect the external body surfaces:
   A. Skin
   B. Mucus
   C. Gastric acid
   D. Salivary amylase
   E. Gut microflora

2. The mononuclear phagocyte system includes:*
   A. Monocytes
   B. Kupffer cells
   C. Skin keratinocytes
   D. Lymph node medullary macrophages
   E. Endothelial cells

3. A polymorphonuclear neutrophil (PMN):*
   A. Generates reactive oxygen intermediates
   B. Is closely similar to a mast cell
   C. Contains microbicidal cytoplasmic granules
   D. Is a professional phagocytic cell
   E. Has granules which stain with eosin

4. C3b:
   A. Is chemotactic
   B. Is an anaphylatoxin
   C. Opsonizes bacteria
   D. Directly injures bacteria
   E. Is the precursor of C3

5. Natural killer (NK) cells:*
   A. Respond to interferon
   B. Contain perforin
   C. Contain granzymes
   D. Kill only by damaging the target cell outer membrane
   E. Resemble small lymphocytes

6. Antibacterial effects are shown by:*
   A. C-reactive protein
   B. Mannose binding protein
   C. Lysozyme
   D. Interferon
   E. Complement

*Question has more than one correct answer.

FURTHER READING

Aderem A, Underhill DM. Mechanisms of phagocytosis in macrophages. *Ann Rev Immunol* 1999; 17:593–623.

Alt F, Marrack P, eds. *Curr Opin Immunol* [appears bimonthly; issue no. 1 of each volume deals with 'Innate Immunity'].

Neth O, Jack DL, Dodds AW et al. Mannose-binding lectin binds to a range of clinically relevant microorganisms and promotes complement deposition. *Infect Immun* 2000; 68:688–93.

Roitt IM, Brostoff J, Male D. *Immunology,* 6th edition. London: Elsevier Science, 2002.

Ryan JC, Naper C, Hayashi S, Daws MR. Physiologic functions of activating natural killer (NK) complex-encoded receptors on NK cells. *Immunol Rev* 2001; 181:126–37.

Adaptive responses provide a 'quantum leap' in effective defense

INTRODUCTION

Infectious agents frequently find ways around the innate defenses

In Chapter 9, we discussed the many ways in which the primary or innate defenses of the body may counteract microbial infection. However, infectious agents frequently find ways around these defenses, as there is a huge number of different microorganisms surrounding us and they have a powerful ability to mutate. For example:

- The surface of some microbes fails to activate the alternative complement pathway.
- Other microbes can activate the alternative complement pathway, but do so at the end of flagella, so that the membrane attack complex builds up at a site distant from the body of the organism and therefore causes no damage.
- In other cases, microorganisms taken into the body of the macrophage develop subterfuges that prevent the development of the awesome battery of microbicidal mechanisms that the macrophage normally expresses (see Chapter 16).
- Cells infected with certain viruses may prove to be resistant to the cytotoxic action of natural killer cells, or the viruses may be only weak stimulators of interferon, so that cell-to-cell transmission of the virus proceeds unchecked.
- Yet another microbial subterfuge is the production of bacterial toxins that can kill the phagocyte if not neutralized.

Adaptive responses act against microorganisms that overcome the innate defenses

It is clear that the body needs to provide immune defenses that can be 'tailor-made' to each individual variant of the different species of microorganisms. Ideally, these should link the organism directly into the various killing mechanisms of the innate system. In this chapter, we shall see how evolution has achieved this by inserting specific recognition sites on antibody molecules and on certain lymphocytes. When an infectious agent enters the body, the lymphocytes respond to it and produce a reaction that is specific for that particular microorganism. Furthermore, the magnitude of this response increases with time, often to quite high levels, so that we speak of it as an 'adaptive' or 'acquired' response. We know that the body produces millions of different antibodies, which as a population are capable of recognizing virtually any pathogen that has arisen or might arise.

THE ROLE OF ANTIBODIES

The acute inflammatory response

Antibodies act as adaptors to focus acute inflammatory reactions

Antibodies are immunoglobulin molecules (*Figs 10.1 and 10.2*) which are synthesized by host B lymphocytes (so-called because they mature in the bone marrow; see *Fig. 11.2*) when they make contact with an infectious microbe, which acts as a foreign antigen (i.e. it generates antibodies). Each antibody has two identical recognition sites that are complementary in shape to the surface of the foreign antigen and which enable it to bind with varying degrees of strength to that antigen. The recognition site is hypervariable in that antibodies of different antigen specificities each has a unique amino acid sequence in this region. This hypervariability is confined to three loops on the heavy and three on the light peptide chains which make up the antibody molecule (*Fig. 10.1*) and are referred to as complementarity determining regions (CDRs) because they make complementary contact with the antigen. Thus, the amino acid sequences of these CDRs determine which antigen is recognized by a given antibody. Other sites on the antibody molecule are specialized for functions such as activating the complement system and inducing phagocytosis by macrophages and polymorphs (*Fig. 10.3*). Therefore, when a microbial antigen is coated with several of these adaptor antibody molecules, they induce complement fixation and phagocytosis, processes that the microbe may well have evolved to try and avoid. In this way, the reluctant microorganism becomes drawn into the innate defense mechanism of the acute inflammatory response. We will now examine the ways in which antibody can mediate these different phenomena.

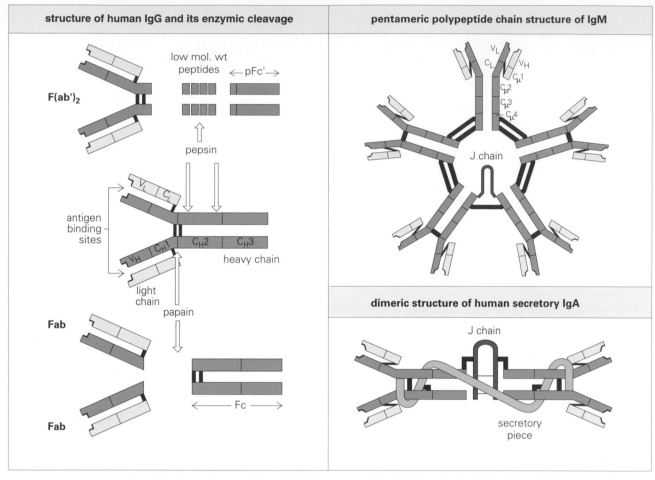

Fig. 10.1 The structure of immunoglobulins. The basic structure of immunoglobulins is a unit consisting of two identical light polypeptide chains and two identical heavy polypeptide chains linked together by disulfide bonds (black bars). Each chain is made up of individual globular domains. Different antibodies have different V_L and V_H domains, the highly variable regions of the light and heavy chains, respectively. This hypervariability is confined to three loops on the V_L and three on the V_H domains. These make up the antigen-binding site (highlighted in red in the figure). In contrast, the remaining domains (C_L, C_H1, etc.) are relatively constant in amino acid structure. Cleavage of human immunoglobulin G (IgG) by pepsin induces a divalent antigen-binding fragment, $F(ab')_2$ and a pFc' fragment composed of two terminal C_H3 domains. Papain produces two univalent antigen binding fragments, Fab, and an Fc portion containing the C_H2 and C_H3 heavy chain domains. Polymerization of the basic immunoglobulin units to form IgM and IgA is catalyzed by the J (joining) chain. The portion of the transporter (which transfers IgA across the mucosal cell to the lumen) which remains attached to the IgA is termed 'secretory piece'.

Antibody complexed with antigen activates complement through the 'classical' pathway

When antibody molecules bind an antigen, the resulting complex activates the first component of complement, C1, converting it into an esterase ($C\overline{1qrs}$). This initiates a second route of complement activation (*Fig. 10.4*) termed the 'classical' pathway, mainly because scientists discovered it before the 'alternative' pathway (see Chapter 9), although the evidence indicates that the alternative pathway is of greater antiquity in evolutionary terms. The activated first component splits off a small peptide from each of the succeeding components C4 and C2, the residual fragments forming a composite, the $C\overline{4b2b}$ complex. The $C\overline{4b2b}$ complex has the enzymatic ability or property of a C3 convertase. It has a similar function to the alternative pathway C3 convertase, $C\overline{3bBb}$, and the sequence of events following the splitting of

C3 is indistinguishable from that occurring in the alternative pathway. C3a and C5a anaphylatoxins are formed, and C3b binds to the surface of the microbe–antibody complex (*Fig. 10.5*; compare *Fig. 9.15*). Subsequently, the later components are assembled into a membrane attack complex (MAC) (see *Fig. 9.22*), which may help to kill the microorganism if it has been focused onto a vulnerable site.

The classical pathway can also be activated through the binding of acute phase proteins such as C-reactive protein and mannose binding protein (see below) to carbohydrates on microbial surfaces.

The acute inflammatory reaction can also be initiated by antibody bound to mast cells

A specialized antibody, immunoglobulin E (IgE), has a backbone site with a high affinity for specific receptors on the

BIOLOGICAL PROPERTIES OF MAJOR IMMUNOGLOBULIN CLASSES IN THE HUMAN					
designation	IgG	*IgA	IgM	IgD	IgE
major characteristics	most abundant internal Ig	protects external surfaces	very efficient against bacteremia	mainly lymphocyte receptor	initiates inflammation raised in parasitic infections causes allergy symptoms
antigen binding	++	++	++	++	++
complement fixation (classical)	++	—	+++	+	—
cross placenta	++	—	—	—	—
fix to homologous mast cells and basophils	—	—	—	—	++
binding to macrophages and polymorphs	+++	1	—	—	+

Fig. 10.2 Biologic properties of major immunoglobulin (Ig) classes in the human. (* Dimer in external secretion carries secretory piece; IgA dimer and IgM contain J chains.)

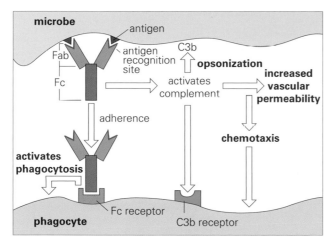

Fig. 10.3 The antibody adaptor molecule. Antibodies (anti-foreign bodies) are produced by host lymphocytes on contact with invading microbes, which act as antigens (i.e. generate antibodies). Each antibody *(Fig. 10.1)* has a recognition site (Fab) enabling it to bind antigen, and a backbone structure (Fc) capable of some secondary biologic action such as activating complement and phagocytosis. Thus in the present case, antibody bound to the microbe activates complement and initiates an acute inflammatory reaction (cf. *Fig. 9.15*). The C3b generated fixes to the microbe and, together with the antibody molecules, facilitates adherence to Fc and C3b receptors on the phagocyte and thence microbial ingestion.

surface of mast cells. When microbial antigen attaches to these cell-bound antibodies the surface receptors are cross-linked and transduce a signal to the interior of the cell. This signal leads to the release of mediators capable of increasing vascular permeability and inducing polymorph chemotaxis *(Fig. 10.6)*.

Activation of phagocytic cells

Antigen–antibody complexes activate phagocytic cells

Other sites on the Fc backbone of certain types of antibody molecule bind to specialized Fc receptors on the surface of phagocytic cells. If there is more than one antibody in the antigen–antibody complex, these receptors are cross-linked so inducing the cell to put out arms of cytoplasm, which enclose the complex in a phagocytic vacuole *(Fig. 10.7)*. Note also that there is a 'bonus effect' of multivalent binding of reversible ligand–receptor links; for example, the association constant for a complex binding through two antibody molecules to the phagocyte is the product rather than the sum of the individual association constants.

Blocking microbial reactions

Antibodies block microbial interactions by combining with one of the reacting molecules

For example, an antibody directed against the influenza hemagglutinin will prevent the virus from attaching to its specific receptor on a cell, making it unable to infect that cell *(Fig. 10.8)*. Likewise, antibodies to an essential transport molecule on a bacterial surface can prevent the uptake of that nutrient and cause a metabolic block. As a final example, an antibody to a bacterial toxin will prevent damage to the cells with which the toxin would otherwise interact.

THE ROLE OF T LYMPHOCYTES

Defense against intracellular organisms

Viruses and many different species of microorganisms can live within cells, where they are shielded from attack by antibody. The body has therefore evolved a defense system against such

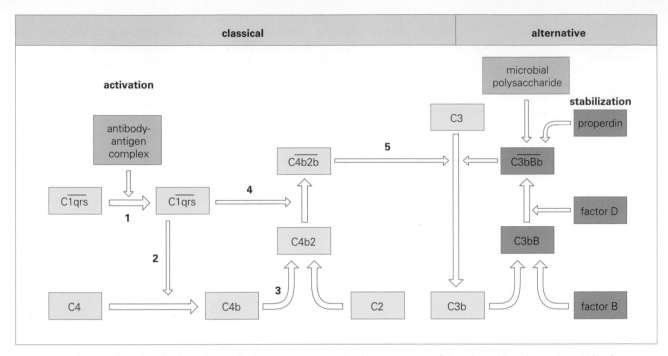

Fig. 10.4 The complex of antibody with microbial antigen activates the first component of the 'classical' pathway (step 1) leading to cleavage of C3 through the C4b2b C3 convertase (step 5). This contrasts with the activation of the 'alternative' pathway, which depends upon stabilization of the C3 convertase (C3bBb) on the microbial surface produced by the feedback loop (cf. *Fig. 9.14*). The classical pathway is in general antibody dependent, the alternative pathway is not. A bar (—) indicates an active complex.

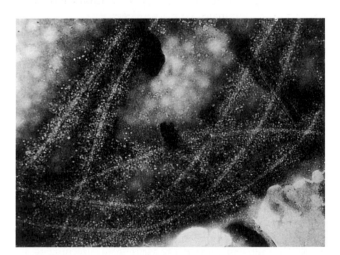

Fig. 10.5 Electron microscopy of C3-coated salmonella flagella. The flagella have been incubated with anti-flagellum antibody and complement. The electron-dense material extending 30 nm on either side of each flagellum is believed to be C3b. The interpretation of this is that complement fixation by antibody results in a heavy macromolecular coating of C3b on biologic membranes to which complement has been fixed. ×700 000. (Courtesy of A Feinstein and E Munn.)

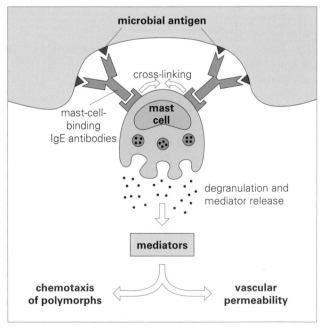

Fig. 10.6 Degranulation of mast cells by interaction of microbial antigen with specific antibodies of the IgE class, which bind to special receptors on the mast cell surface. The cross-linking of receptors caused by this interaction leads to the release of mediators, which induce an increase in vascular permeability and attract polymorphs—that is, they provoke an acute inflammatory reaction at the site of the microbial antigen.

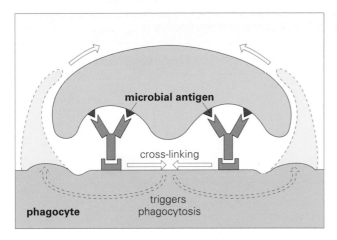

Fig. 10.7 The binding of a microbe to a phagocyte by more than one antibody cross-links the antibody receptors on the phagocyte surface and triggers phagocytosis of the microorganism which is engulfed by the extending cytoplasmic projections.

organisms based upon the T lymphocyte, so-called because it matures in the thymus gland.

T lymphocytes bind to peptide derived from intracellular organisms complexed with major histocompatibility complex

As microorganisms go through their various lifecycles they sometimes die within the cells they infect. The proteins derived from these dead organisms are fragmented by intracellular enzymes ('processing') and the peptides are incorporated into cytoplasmic vacuoles where they bind to a molecule of the major histocompatibility complex (MHC) *(Fig. 10.9)*. (MHC molecules were originally discovered because of their ability to bring about the most violent rejection of grafts interchanged between members of the same species. We now know that one of their important functions is to act as cellular surface markers. Class I MHC molecules are present on virtually every cell in the body and can therefore be used as a marker indicating an instance of 'cell'. Class II MHC molecules appear mainly on macrophages and B cells.)

A specialized T cell receptor (TCR) on the T lymphocyte surface *(Fig. 10.10)* is analogous to an antibody molecule in its ability to recognize foreign antigen. It resembles the immunoglobulin Fab portion in structure, with α and β chains instead of heavy and light chains, again with hypervariable loops to contact the antigen. However, unlike the antibody recognition site which interacts directly with a foreign antigen, the T cell surface receptor is specialized for binding to the complex of MHC molecule and peptide derived from the intracellular organism. Thus, not only is the MHC a molecular signal for 'cell', but the foreign peptide is a signal that the cell has an intracellular microbe. Therefore, when the TCR recognizes these two moieties together, the T lymphocyte must be binding to an infected cell of a type indicated by the class of the MHC *(Fig. 10.11)*. The T lymphocyte then becomes activated and, depending upon its particular characteristics, sets off an effector mechanism to deal with the intracellular microorganisms, as explained below.

T lymphocytes help macrophages kill intracellular parasites

The task of recognizing macrophages that have unwelcome guests, such as *Listeria* or tubercle bacilli living within them, falls mainly to a subset of lymphocytes called the TH1 T helper cells *(Fig. 10.11)*. When a specific TH1 cell combines with a complex of class II MHC molecule and microbial peptide on the surface of an infected macrophage, the T cell is triggered to release macrophage activating factors, notably interferon gamma (IFNγ) (see Chapter 9). This unleashes previously suppressed microbicidal mechanisms within the macrophage, so leading to the death of the intracellular parasites *(Fig. 10.12)*. In general, TH1 cells evoke a chronic inflammatory response dominated by macrophages.

T lymphocytes inhibit intracellular replication of viruses

Cells infected with virus express complexes consisting of class I MHC and a virally derived peptide on their surface. These are recognized by the specific receptors on cytotoxic T (Tc) cells *(Fig. 10.13)*, which are therefore led into close proximity to their virally infected target. The target cell is then killed by similar extracellular mechanisms to those described in Chapter 9. Since the virally derived peptides appear on the cell surface at a very early stage of infection, the Tc cells kill

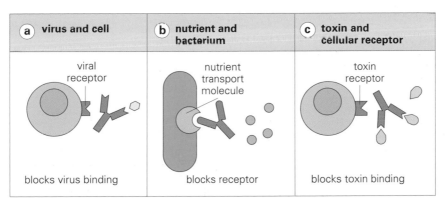

Fig. 10.8 Because of its size, antibody can block interactions between (a) a virus and a cell, (b) a nutrient and a bacterium and (c) a toxin and a cellular receptor.

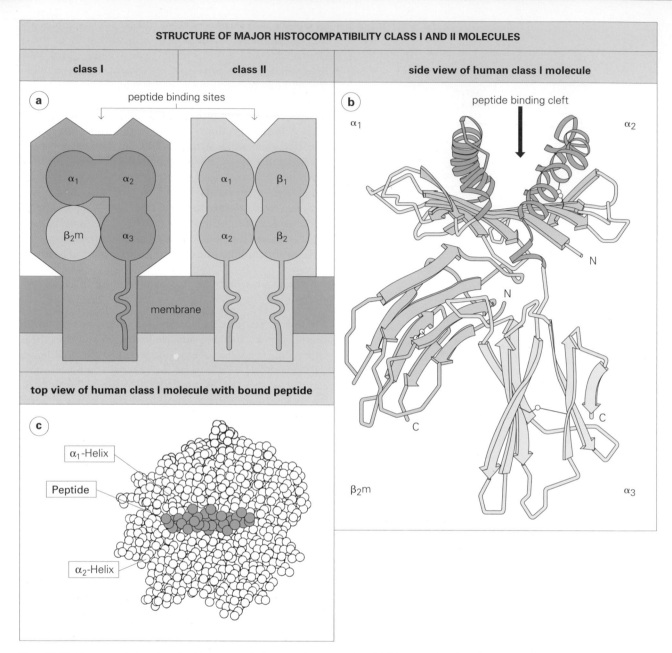

Fig. 10.9 Class I and class II major histocompatibility complex molecules. (a) Diagram showing domains and transmembrane segments; the α-helices and β-pleated sheets are viewed end-on. (b) Side view of human class I molecule (HLA-A2) based on X-ray crystallographic structure showing the cleft and the typical immunoglobulin folding of the α3 and β2-microglobulin (β2m) domains (four antiparallel β-strands on one face and three on the other). The strands making the β-pleated sheet are shown as thick gray arrows in the amino to carboxyl direction, α-helices are represented as helical ribbons. The inside facing surfaces of the two helices and the upper surface of the β-pleated sheet form a cleft which binds the peptide. (Adapted from PI Bjorkman et al., *Nature* 1987; 329:512, with permission.). (c) Top view of a peptide bound tightly within the MHC class I cleft, in this case peptide 309-317 from HIV-1 reverse transcriptase bound to HLA-A2. This is the 'view' seen by the combining site of the T cell receptor described below. (Based on DAA Vignali and JL Strominger, *The Immunologist* 1994; 2:112, with permission.)

the cell before the virus has had an opportunity to replicate significantly, and the host has won an important battle. The natural killer (NK) cell fulfils a similar function to that of the Tc cell, but because it lacks the specialized receptors for recognizing the particular viral peptide in association with class I MHC, its chances of binding strongly to the surface of the infected target cell are much less than those of the Tc cell.

However, it is of interest that both the Tc cell and the TH cell are capable of releasing IFNs, particularly IFNγ, which markedly improve the performance of the NK cell, so making a useful integrated system. An important additional responsibility of these IFNs is to render adjacent cells resistant to replication of viral particles, which gain entrance through intercellular transport mechanisms *(Fig. 10.14).*

EXTRACELLULAR ATTACK ON LARGE INFECTIOUS AGENTS

Defensive cells attack the antibody-coated surfaces of parasites

Where a parasite is demonstrably larger than a phagocytic cell, it is physically impossible for phagocytosis to occur. However, it is still possible for the defensive cells to deliver an extracellular attack on the surface of the parasite. This can occur through the phenomenon of 'antibody-dependent cellular cytotoxicity' (ADCC) in which effector cells bind through their surface receptors to antibody molecules coating the target cell *(Fig. 10.15)*. The result of this interaction is to induce activation of the effector cell and the release of materials to damage the parasite target. Major cell types that indulge in this type of activity are:

- macrophages;
- eosinophils;
- NK cells.

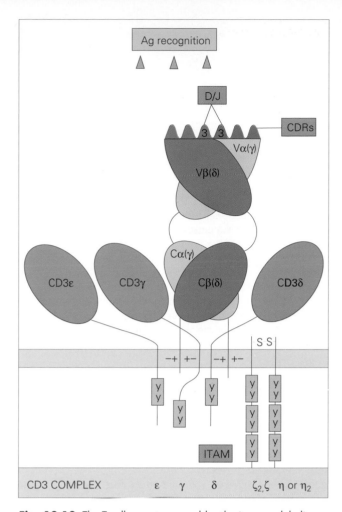

Fig. 10.10 The T cell receptor resembles the immunoglobulin Fab antigen-binding fragment in structure, with the highly variable (complementarity determining) regions (CDRs) making contact with the MHC–peptide antigen complex. This produces a signal which is transduced by the invariant CD3 complex composed of γ, δ, ε and ζ/η chains, through their cytoplasmic immune receptor tyrosine-based activation motifs (ITAM) which contact protein tyrosine kinases.

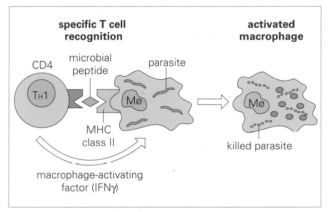

Fig. 10.12 T helper (TH1) cells trigger the killing of intracellular parasites within macrophages (MØ). Recognition of the infected macrophage by the TH1 cell TCR results in lymphocyte activation with release of IFNγ. This then activates the macrophage, which turns on its microbicidal mechanisms to kill the intracellular parasite.

| type | designation | target | | T cell | function |
		MHC class	cell type	ligand for MHC	
T helper	TH1	II	macrophage	CD4*	help macrophages to kill intracellular infection
T helper	TH2	II	B cells	CD4	help B cells to make antibody
cytotoxic T cell	Tc	I	most cells	CD8	kill virally infected cells before significant replication
*See page 102 and *Figure 11.6*.					

Fig. 10.11 Specialized subpopulations of T cells.

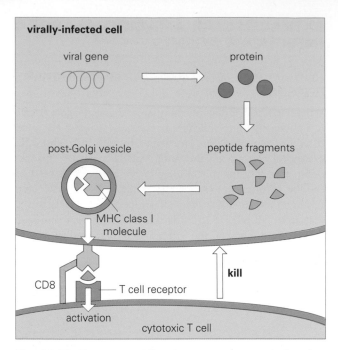

Fig. 10.13 The cytotoxic T lymphocytes are activated when their specific cell surface receptors recognize an infected cell by binding to a surface MHC class I molecule that is associated with a peptide fragment derived from a degraded intracellular viral protein.

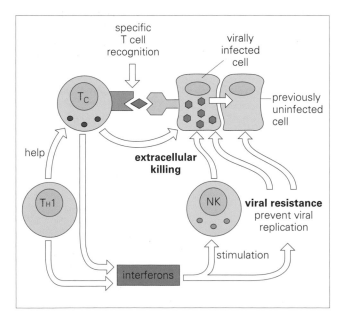

Fig. 10.14 Cytotoxic T (Tc) cells specifically recognize surface MHC class I plus peptide derived from degraded viral protein and kill the infected cells before the virus replicates. Natural killer (NK) cells can do the same, though far less effectively; however their activity is enhanced by interferons (IFNs) produced by Tc and TH1 cells. Local production of IFNs also prevents adjacent cells from becoming infected by intercellular viral transport.

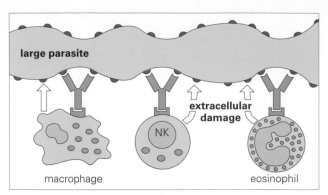

Fig. 10.15 Antibody-dependent cellular cytotoxicity. Different effector cells bind to the parasite surface through their receptor for antibody and damage the parasite target. Macrophages burn the target cell surface by a stream of reactive oxygen intermediates generated by the respiratory oxygen burst, NK cells induce apoptosis by perforin/granzyme, TNF and Fas/FasL mechanisms (see. p. 83) while eosinophils damage the target cell membrane by release of a major basic protein, a perforin-like molecule and copious reactive oxygen metabolites. The antibodies mostly belong to the IgG class (see *Figs 10.1 and 10.2*).

LOCAL DEFENSES AT MUCOSAL SURFACES

The immune mechanisms involving the acute inflammatory response and T-cell-mediated systems operate well within the milieu of the body. It is worth examining, however, the special nature of the defenses required to protect the body at the mucosal surfaces which face the exterior, for example in the lung and the gastrointestinal tract *(Fig. 10.16)*.

The first line of defense aims to prevent the microbe from adhering to the mucosal surface. Adhesion to the mucosal surface is a prerequisite for penetrating the body. To prevent this there is the innate mechanism of mucus production. In addition, a special antibody, IgA, is synthesized by the lymphoid aggregates, some of which are organized (adenoids, tonsil, Peyer's patches), while others are less organized (lamina propria, lung, urinogenital tract). Together these lymphoid aggregates constitute the mucosal-associated lymphoid tissue (MALT). The IgA is then actively transported by a carrier molecule into the lumen and is associated with the mucosal surface in a high concentration where it continues to bear a portion of the carrier called 'secretory piece' (see *Fig. 10.1*). When coated with such IgA antibodies, the adhesion of infectious agents to the mucosa is greatly diminished, but they can still be captured by local macrophages with surface receptors for IgA. Mast cells tend to cluster in the submucosal region and, should a microorganism break through the mucosal barrier, it could encounter a mast cell that has bound the specialized IgE antibody to its surface; on reaction with this surface antibody, the mast cell is triggered to release mediators of the acute inflammatory reaction. By increasing vascular permeability, these mediators will bring about the flooding of the site with plasma proteins, including other classes of antibody and complement, while chemotactic agents will attract polymorphonuclear leukocytes.

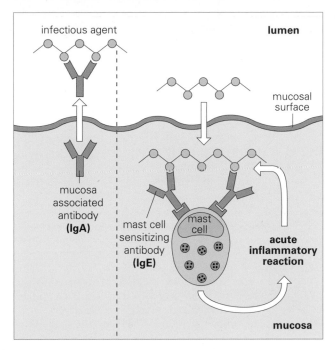

Fig. 10.16 Defense of body mucosal surfaces. A specialized antibody associated with the mucosal surface—secretory immunoglobulin A (IgA)—blocks adherence of the microbe to the mucosa and hence entry into the body. An infectious agent gaining entrance to the body will fire IgE-sensitized mast cells, which cluster beneath the surface and generate a protective local acute inflammatory response by attracting complement-fixing antibodies, complement and polymorphs from the blood.

Larger parasites, such as nematodes, within the lumen of the gut pose special problems

It is thought that antigens derived from the nematode may penetrate the submucosal space and activate T and B cells and degranulate sensitized mast cells. The latter will produce an acute inflammation at the mucosal surface and almost certainly lead to an outflow of antibody, complement and probably effectors of ADCC into the lumen. In the lumen, the antibody, complement and effectors of ADCC can then interact with the parasite and inflict metabolic damage. In the meantime, the interaction with sensitized TH cells will lead to the release of soluble factors termed cytokines, which include a mediator capable of stimulating the goblet cells lining the intestinal villi. The goblet cells then release their mucins into the lumen where they coat the damaged parasite and facilitate expulsion from the body *(Fig. 10.17).*

A subset of T cells bearing γδ receptors dominates the mucosal epithelium

In the human, T lymphocytes expressing αβ receptors represent the large majority of T cells in the blood, but a subset composed of γδ chains dominates the intestinal epithelium and skin. Unlike αβ T cells, the γδ subset can recognize antigen directly without the need for antigen processing. Heat shock proteins released from stressed or damaged cells are potent stimulators of γδ T cells as are low molecular weight phosphate-containing non-proteinaceous antigens such as isopentenyl pyrophosphate and alkylamines which occur in a wide range of pathogens. γδ T cells can also collaborate with mucosal epithelial cells expressing surface CD1 molecules (containing β_2 microglobulin but non-classical MHC-like chains) which have a hydrophobic cleft enabling them to present lipid and glycolipid microbial antigens such as lipoarabinomannan, the mycobacterial cell wall component.

KEY FACTS

- The evolution of the adaptive response has provided the body with a powerful series of mechanisms that extend and exploit the innate mechanisms of defense. Thus, this lymphocyte-mediated response greatly augments the innate defense against each particular infecting organism.

- In most cases, the effector mechanisms involve the innate systems of defense such as phagocytosis, complement activation and macrophage intracellular killing.

- Taking an overall view of the adaptive responses, humoral immunity mediated by antibody produced by B lymphocytes is effective in neutralizing bacterial toxins, and, by interacting with complement, mast cells and polymorphs,

produces the acute inflammatory reaction *(Fig. 10.18).* This response is especially effective against extracellular microbes, and the 'quantum leap' provided by antibody in the clearance of extracellular bacteria from the blood is clearly shown in the example in *Figure 10.19.* The IgE-mediated acute inflammatory response and secreted IgA defend the mucosal surfaces against extracellular infections.

- In contrast, the T cell-mediated response is directed to intracellular organisms. The receptor on the T cell recognizes an infected cell as a target by binding to the surface major histocompatibility complex (MHC) molecule, which is a marker for a cell, linked to a peptide derived by degradation of intracellular microbial protein.

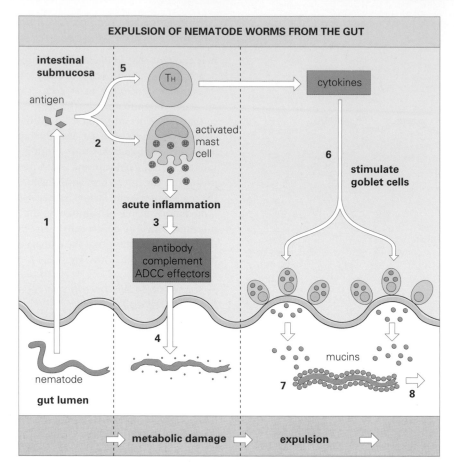

Fig. 10.17 Expulsion of nematode worms from the gut. Worm antigen (1) is thought to trigger an acute inflammatory reaction in the submucosa (2). This facilitates the recruitment of complement and possibly antibody-dependent cellular cytotoxicity (ADCC) effectors (3), which damage the parasite (4). Soluble factors (cytokines), released by antigen-specific triggering of T helper cells (5), stimulate the secretion of mucins by goblet cells (6), which coat the worm (7) and aid its expulsion (8).

- T cells are divided into T helper TH1, T helper TH2 and cytotoxic Tc cells. CD4 TH1 cells recognize class II MHC on macrophages and produce soluble factors (cytokines), firstly chemotactic factors and secondly IFNγ, which activate phagocytic cells to switch on their intracellular antimicrobial mechanisms. CD4 TH2 cells recognize class II MHC on B cells and help them to produce antibody. CD8 Tc cells recognize MHC class I on most cells and are effective against viruses, killing virally infected targets and preventing the spread of virus through the local production of interferons. Tc cells can also be divided into subsets expressing either TH1 or TH2 type cytokine patterns.

- *Figure 10.20* emphasizes the close interactions between innate and acquired mechanisms leading to defense against extracellular microorganisms on the one hand, and intracellular infections on the other. In keeping with these concepts, deficiencies in humoral immunity from whatever cause, predispose the individual to infection by extracellular organisms, whereas defects in T-cell-mediated responses are primarily associated with intracellular infections.

- The first contact with antigen evokes a response that leaves behind a memory of the encounter so that the subsequent response to a second contact with antigen is more powerful and evolves more rapidly than on the first occasion. The cellular bases for these phenomena are explained in Chapter 11. The production of memory by a primary interaction with antigen provides the basis for vaccination, where the first contact is with an avirulent form of the microorganism or its component antigens.

- The other point to stress at this stage is the specificity of memory—infection with measles, for example, produces a subsequent immunity to that virus, but does not afford protection against an unrelated virus such as mumps.

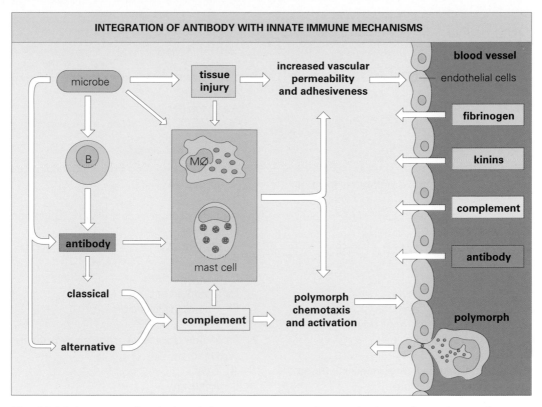

Fig. 10.18 Integration of antibody with the innate immune mechanisms, leading to the production of a protective acute inflammatory reaction. The activated endothelial cells allow exudation of soluble proteins from the circulation and express accessory molecules, which aid the binding of the polymorphs to the capillary wall and their subsequent escape into the infected site. (Mφ, macrophage.)

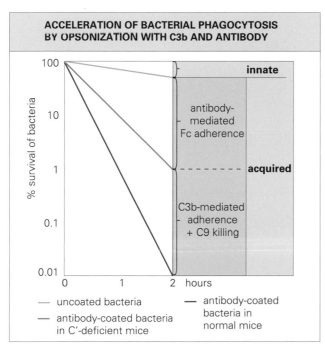

Fig. 10.19 The slow rate of phagocytosis of uncoated bacteria (innate immunity) is increased many times by acquired immunity through coating with antibody and then C3b (opsonization). Killing may also take place through the C5–9 terminal complement components. This is a hypothetical, but realistic situation; the natural proliferation of the bacteria has been ignored.

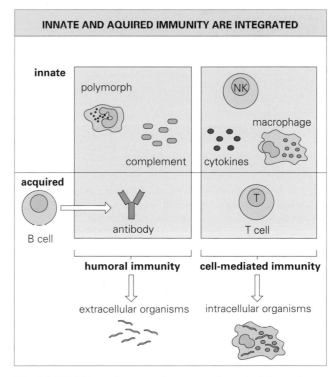

Fig. 10.20 The mechanisms of innate and acquired immunity are integrated to provide the basis for humoral and cell-mediated immunity. Deficiencies of humoral immunity predispose to infection with extracellular organisms, and deficiencies of T cell-mediated responses are associated primarily with intracellular infections.

QUESTIONS

1. Complement component C3 is cleaved by:*
A. C3b
B. C3bBb
C. Factor B
D. C1
E. C42

2. The classical and alternative pathways meet at complement component:
A. C4
B. C4b
C. Factor D
D. C5
E. C3

3. Plasma cells:*
A. Synthesize and secrete antibody
B. Are derived from T cells
C. Are derived from B cells
D. Secrete large amounts of gamma interferon
E. Have a high RNA content

4. A plasma cell secretes:
A. Antibody of similar specificity to that on the surface of the parent B cell
B. Antibody of two antigen specificities
C. The antigen it recognizes
D. Many different types of antibody
E. Lysozyme

---

* Question has more than one correct answer.

5. T cell surface receptors for antigen partly recognize:*
A. Cytokines
B. MHC
C. ADCC
D. Antibody
E. Peptides derived from intracellular processing of proteins

6. Clonal selection occurs when a B lymphocyte encounters:
A. Cytokines
B. Antigen
C. T lymphocytes
D. Complement
E. Chemotactic factors

7. Protection against microorganisms inside cells is provided by:
A. T cells
B. Antibody
C. C3b
D. C1
E. The membrane attack complex

8. Cells bearing MHC class I plus peptide are targets for specific:
A. B cells
B. Cytotoxic T cells
C. T_H1 cells
D. T_H2 cells
E. Interdigitating dendritic cells

FURTHER READING

Alt F, Marrack P, eds. *Curr Opin Immunol* [appears bimonthly; issue no. 4 of each volume deals with 'Immunity to Infection'].

Delves PJ, Roitt IM, eds. *Encyclopedia of Immunology*, 2nd edition. London: Academic Press, 1998. [contains articles on IgG, IgA, IgM, IgD and IgE and immunoglobulin function and domains.]

Griffiths GM. The cell biology of CTL killing. *Curr Opin Immunol* 1995; 7:343–8.

Roitt IM, Delves PJ. *Roitt's Essential Immunology*, 10th edition. Oxford: Blackwell Science, 2001.

The cellular basis of adaptive immune responses

INTRODUCTION

As we saw in the previous chapter, adaptive immune responses are generated by lymphocytes *(Fig. 11.1)* which are derived from stem cells differentiating within the primary lymphoid organs (bone marrow and thymus). From there they colonize the secondary lymphoid tissues where they mediate the immune responses to antigens *(Fig. 11.2)*. The lymph nodes are concerned with responses to antigens which are carried into them from the tissues, while the spleen is concerned primarily with antigens which reach it from the bloodstream *(Fig. 11.3)*. Communication between these tissues and the rest of the body is maintained by a pool of recirculating lymphocytes which pass from the blood into the lymph nodes, spleen and other tissues and back to the blood by the major lymphatic channels such as the thoracic duct *(Fig. 11.4)*. This traffic of lymphocytes between the tissues, the bloodstream and the lymph nodes enables antigen-sensitive cells to seek the antigen and to be recruited to sites at which a response is occurring. In addition, unencapsulated aggregates of lymphoid tissue termed 'mucosa-associated lymphoid tissue' or MALT, lie in the mucosal surface where they have the job of responding to antigens from the environment, particularly the heavy bacterial load in the intestine, by producing IgA antibodies for mucosal secretions. The lymphocytes which constitute the MALT system recirculate between these mucosal tissues using specialized homing receptors *(Fig. 11.5)*.

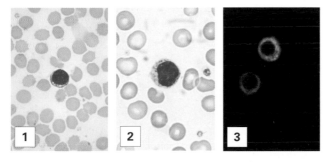

Fig. 11.1 Lymphocytes and plasma cells. (1) Small B and T lymphocytes have a round nucleus and a high nuclear:cytoplasmic ratio. (2) A large granular lymphocyte with a lower nuclear:cytoplasmic ratio, an indented nucleus and azurophilic cytoplasmic granules. Fewer than 5% of T helpers, and 30–50% of cytotoxic T cells, γδ T cells and natural killer (NK) cells have this morphology. (3) Antibody formed when B cells differentiate into plasma cells here stained with fluoresceinated anti-human IgM (green) and rhodaminated anti-human IgG (red) showing extensive intracytoplasmic staining. Note that plasma cells produce only one class of antibody as the distinct staining reveals. (1 and 2, stained with Giemsa, courtesy of A Stevens and J Lowe; 3, adapted from A Zucker-Franklin et al., *Atlas of Blood Cells: Function and Pathology*, 2nd edition, vol. 11, Milan: EE Ermes; Philadelphia: Lea and Febinger, 1988.)

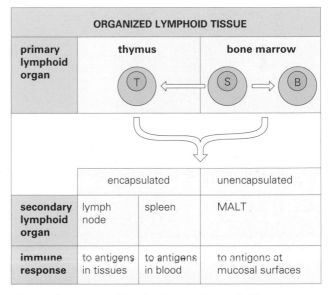

ORGANIZED LYMPHOID TISSUE			
primary lymphoid organ	**thymus**	**bone marrow**	
	T	S	B
		encapsulated	**unencapsulated**
secondary lymphoid organ	lymph node	spleen	MALT
immune response	to antigens in tissues	to antigens in blood	to antigens at mucosal surfaces

Fig. 11.2 Organized lymphoid tissue. Stem cells (S) arising in the bone marrow differentiate into immunocompetent B and T cells in the primary lymphoid organs. These cells then colonize the secondary lymphoid tissues where immune responses are organized. (MALT, mucosa-associated lymphoid tissue.)

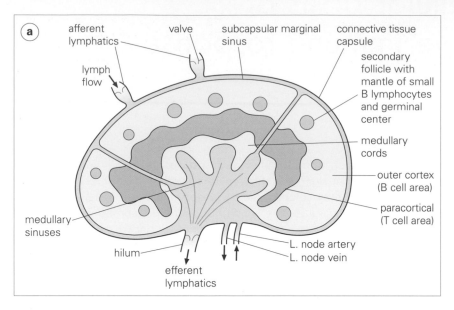

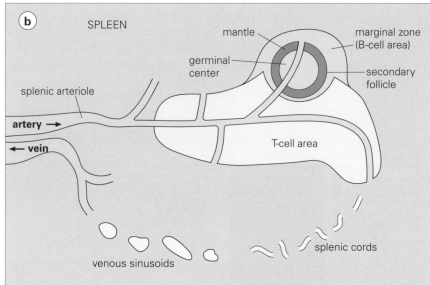

Fig. 11.3 The anatomy of a lymph node and the spleen. (a) Diagrammatic representation of section through a whole lymph node. The cortex is essentially a B cell region where differentiation within the germinal centers of secondary follicles to antibody-forming plasma cells and memory cells occurs. (b) Diagrammatic representation of spleen showing B and T cell areas. (Adapted from IM Roitt and PJ Delves, *Roitt's Essential Immunology*, 10th edition. Oxford: Blackwell Science, 2001.)

B AND T CELL RECEPTORS

B and T cells can be distinguished by their surface markers

As they differentiate into populations with differing functions, B and T cells acquire molecules on their surface that reflect these specializations. It is possible to produce homogeneous antibodies of a single specificity—termed 'monoclonal antibodies'—that can recognize such surface markers. When laboratories from all over the world compared the monoclonal antibodies they had raised, it was found that groups or clusters of monoclonal antibodies were each recognizing a common molecule on the surface of the lymphocyte. Each surface component so defined, was referred to as a 'CD' molecule *(Fig. 11.6)*, where CD refers to a 'cluster determinant'.

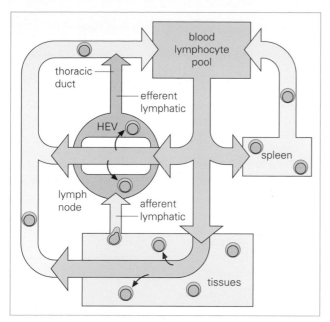

Fig. 11.4 The lymphocytes move through the circulation and enter the lymph nodes via the specialized endothelial cells of the postcapillary venules (HEVs). They leave through the efferent lymphatic vessels and pass through other nodes, finally entering the thoracic duct which empties into the circulation at the left subclavian vein (in humans). Lymphocytes enter the white pulp areas of the spleen in the marginal zones; they pass into the sinusoids of the red pulp and leave via the splenic vein. (Adapted from Roitt IM, Brostoff J, Male D. *Immunology*, 6th edition. London: Elsevier Science, 2002.)

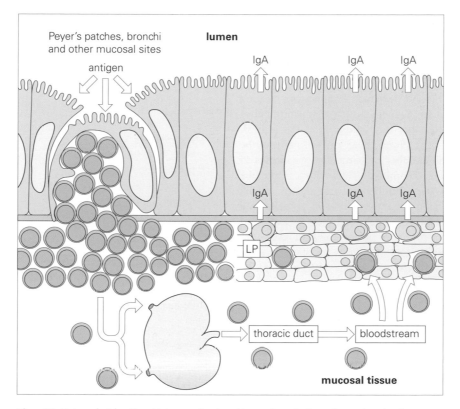

Fig. 11.5 Lymphoid cells which are stimulated by antigen in Peyer's patches (or the bronchi or another mucosal site) migrate via the regional lymph nodes and thoracic duct into the bloodstream and thence to the lamina propria (LP) of the gut or other mucosal surfaces which might be close to or distant from the site of priming. Thus lymphocytes stimulated at one mucosal surface may become distributed selectively throughout the MALT system. This is mediated through specific adhesion molecules on the lymphocytes and the mucosal high-walled endothelium of the postcapillary venules. (Same source as *Fig. 11.4*.)

Each lymphocyte expresses an antigen receptor of unique specificity on its surface

Among the surface markers on the B and T cells referred to above are the receptors on the plasma membrane which are used to identify foreign antigens. B cells possess surface immunoglobulin whereas the T cell receptor (TCR) on the surface of the T lymphocyte acts as an antigen recognition unit (see *Fig. 10.10*). We now know that despite the very large number of different components that could be combined together in multiple ways to give a diversity of surface receptors, each B lymphocyte rearranges its germline genes coding for these receptors so that it selects one and only one of the specificities for each receptor polypeptide chain. It then expresses that receptor molecule on its surface (*Fig. 11.7*). Once this occurs, the other genes coding for these antigen receptors in the lymphocyte are no longer used. In other words, following this genetic rearrangement process, the lymphocyte becomes committed to the synthesis and expression of a single receptor type. An analogous process occurs in the rearrangement of the αβ and γδ genes coding for the TCR. Just as for B cells, each T cell expresses one and only one specific combination of receptor peptides, and therefore shows a single specificity to which it is committed for the whole of its lifespan.

CLONAL EXPANSION OF LYMPHOCYTES

Antigen selects and clonally expands lymphocytes bearing complementary receptors. As there is such a large number of different possible specificities that lymphocytes can express, perhaps of the order of millions, there must of necessity be only a relatively small number of particular specificities to which lymphocytes are committed. Thus, when a microbe invades the body, the total number of lymphocytes initially committed to recognizing the antigens that go to make up a particular microbe is relatively small, and must be expanded to provide a sufficient number to protect the host. Evolution has provided a masterful solution to this problem. When a microbe enters the body, its component antigens combine with only those B lymphocytes whose surface receptors are complementary to the shape of these antigens. The B cells that bind the antigen become activated and proliferate clonally under the influence of soluble growth factors termed cytokines (see section on cytokines below) to form a large population of cells derived from the original (*Fig. 11.8*). The majority of these events occur within the lymphoid structure known as a germinal center (*Fig. 11.3*).

In the case of B cells, a large proportion of the clonally expanded lymphocytes become plasma cells (*Fig. 11.1*), dedicated to the synthesis and secretion of antibodies. Since these plasma cells are derived from a parent cell that is already committed to the production of only one specific antibody, the final product is identical to the molecule that was posted on the surface of the original antigen-recognizing cell. Or at least almost so, because somatic mutation of the lymphocytes within the germinal centers which are synthesizing this antibody, fine tunes the binding efficiency of the eventual product. The net result is that we have the production of large

SURFACE MARKERS ON B AND T CELLS			
function/identity	**CD designation**	**B cells**	**T cells**
antigen receptors			
Surface immunoglobulin	—	++	–
T cell αβ, γδ	—	–	++
TCR signal transducer	CD3	–	++
receptors for			
Leukocyte function antigen-3 (LFA-3)	CD2	–	++
MHC class II (T helpers)	CD4	–	++
MHC class I (cytotoxic T cells)	CD8	–	++
Complement (CR2)	CD21	++	–
Complement (CR1)	CD35	++	+
IgG (FcγIIR)	CDw32	++	–
IgE (FcεR)	CD23	+	–
Interleukin-2 (IL–2 α-chain)	CD25	act*	act*
MHC			
Class I	—	++	++
Class II	—	++	act*
other markers			
Differentiation marker	CD5	subset	++
Restricted leukocyte common antigen	CD45R	+	memory
*activated cells only			

Fig. 11.6 Surface markers on B and T cells. (IL, interleukin; MHC, major histocompatibility complex; TCR, T cell receptor; Fc, dimer of immunoglobulin heavy chain excluding the Fab V_H and C_H1 domains in *Fig. 10.1*.)

amounts of antibody which, like that on the surface of the parent cell, can combine with the invading antigen (*Fig. 11.8*).

A similar process of clonal selection and expansion occurs with T cells, producing a large number of T cell effectors with the same specificity as the original parent cell; some of these cells release cytokines, whereas others have cytotoxic functions so that they act as effectors of T-cell-mediated immunity. One difference between T and B cells is that the T cell receptors do not undergo further selection as a result of somatic mutation. Of crucial significance is the fact that in the case of both B and T cells, a fraction of the clonally expanded population differentiate into resting memory cells (*Fig. 11.8*). Thus, more cells are capable of recognizing the microbial

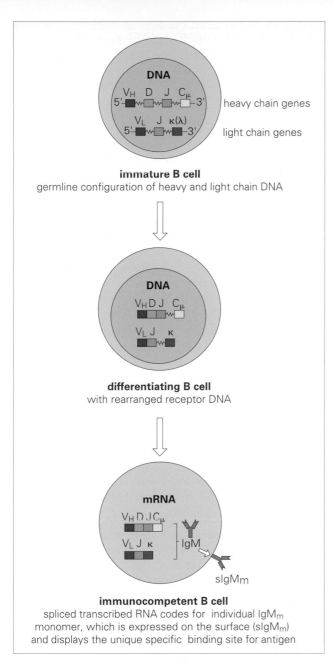

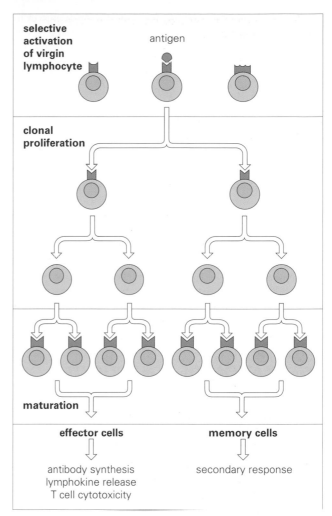

Fig. 11.7 Differentiation events leading to the expression of unique IgM monomer sIgM on the surface of an immunocompetent B lymphocyte. There are of the order of 50 germline V_H genes encoding the major portion of the variable region, with 25 minigenes encoding the D segment and 6 the J region. As the cell differentiates, V_H, D and J segments on one chromosome randomly fuse to generate lymphocytes with a very wide range of individual heavy chain variable domains. Variable region light chain domains are then formed by random V_L to J recombination. Finally, the variable and constant region genes respectively recombine to encode a single antibody molecule which is expressed on the mature B cell surface as an sIgM antigen receptor. When activated for antibody production, the transmembrane segment of IgM which normally holds the molecule on the surface is spliced out at the RNA stage and the soluble form of the IgM is secreted. Subsequently, heavy chain constant region gene switch can occur to generate the various immunoglobulin classes, IgG, IgA, etc. Leader sequences have been omitted for simplicity.

Fig. 11.8 Generation of a large population of effector and memory cells after primary contact of B or T cell with antigen. A fraction of the progeny of the original antigen-reactive lymphocytes become non-dividing memory cells, whereas the others become the effector cells of humoral or cell-mediated immunity. Memory cells require fewer cycles before they develop into effectors, thus shortening the reaction time for the secondary response.

antigen in any subsequent infection than in the initial virgin population that existed before the primary infection occurred.

THE ROLE OF MEMORY CELLS

Secondary immune responses are bigger and brisker than primary responses

In general, memory cells, as compared with naïve cells, are more readily stimulated by a given dose of antigen. This occurs because they have greater combining power, in the case of B cells through mutation and selection during the primary response, and for T cells, which do not undergo affinity maturation, through increased expression of accessory adhesion molecules, CD2, LFA-1, LFA-3 and intercellular adhesion molecule-1 (ICAM-1), which enable the lymphocyte to bind more strongly to the specialized cells which present antigen. These factors, combined with the increased number of lymphocytes specific for a given antigen present in the memory pool produced by the primary response, result in a much stronger antibody or T cell response on second contact with antigen. This provides the principle for vaccination (*Fig. 11.9*). The microbe or antigen to be used for vaccination is modified in such a way that it no longer produces disease or damage, but still retains the majority of its antigenic shapes. The primary response produced by the vaccination gives rise to a pool of memory cells, which can generate an abundant secondary response on subsequent contact with the antigen during a natural infection. Memory is usually long-lived, often extending over many years. There are many possible reasons for this: memory cells themselves may be innately long-lived or they may be sustained by gentle proliferation through subsequent contact with antigen present in reservoirs within the body or introduced by subclinical infection. An alternative mechanism in the case of T cells may be through stimulation by the cytokine IL-15 and in the case of B cells by anti-idiotypes (anti-antibodies produced in response to the combining region of the first antibody which may stimulate the memory B cells by 'tweaking' their surface receptors).

STIMULATION OF LYMPHOCYTES

T lymphocytes are activated by antigen presented on specialized cells

Naïve T cells are potently stimulated by interdigitating dendritic cells (IDC), which are specialized antigen-presenting cells (APCs). Immature IDCs in the tisues take up antigen which is then processed and presented on the surface as a peptide complexed with MHC class II. The IDC migrates to the T cell region of the draining lymph node where it stimulates several T lymphocytes with which it makes contact through recognition of the MHC–peptide complex by the specific T cell receptor and by accessory interaction of the B7 costimulator with surface CD28 (*Fig. 11.10*).

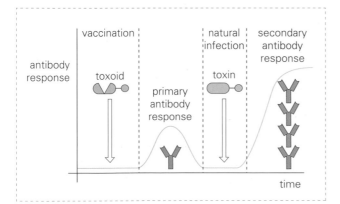

Fig. 11.9 Primary and secondary responses. The antibody response on the second contact with antigen is more rapid and more intense. Therefore, following vaccination with a benign form of the antigen (a chemically modified form of tetanus toxin in the example shown) to produce a primary response, subsequent contact with antigen in the form of a natural infection evokes the more efficient secondary response.

As noted above, primed T cells are more readily stimulated by antigen than naïve cells, and in this case macrophages can function as the antigen-presenting cell.

Some antigens stimulate B cells without the need for intervention by T lymphocytes

These so-called T-independent antigens are of two main types:

- Antigens of the first type contain molecular features that enable them to stimulate a wide variety of B cells independently of their specific antigen receptors; they are therefore referred to as 'polyclonal activators'. Those B cells carrying surface receptors that recognize epitopes on the polyclonal activator attract the molecule to their surfaces and are preferentially stimulated relative to the remainder of the B cell population (*Fig. 11.11*).
- The second type of T-independent antigen involves repeating determinants presented on the surface of specialized macrophages located within the marginal zone associated with splenic secondary follicles with germinal centers or within the lymph node subcapsular sinus (*Fig. 11.3a & b*), which can cross-link immunoglobulin receptors on the B cell and apparently stimulate the lymphocyte directly (*Fig. 11.11*).

One feature of both these types of T-independent antigen is that they give rise mainly to low affinity IgM rather than IgG antibody responses and rarely induce a memory response.

Antibody production frequently requires T cell help

The majority of antigens will stimulate B cells only if they have the assistance of T lymphocyte helper (TH) cells. The sequence of events is as follows:

- In stage 1, the antigen is processed by an antigen-presenting cell and primes a TH cell with a complementary receptor on its surface as described above.
- In stage 2, a B cell with surface receptors complementary to an epitope on the original antigen, captures the antigen on its receptor, internalizes it and, after processing, also presents a derived peptide on its surface in association with endogenous MHC class II molecules. This is the complex against which the TH cell was originally primed, and recognition of the processed antigen by the primed TH cell causes stimulation of the B cell, with subsequent activation, proliferation and maturation (*Fig. 11.12*).

It should be noted that although the TH cell recognizes a processed determinant of the antigen, the B cell is programmed to make only antibody with the same specificity as its surface receptor, and therefore the antibodies that finally result will be directed against the epitope on the antigen recognized by the B cell surface receptor.

CYTOKINES

Cytokines are soluble intercellular communication factors in the immune response

Interactions between the APC, the TH cell and the B cell are effected by the recognition of processed antigen in association with MHC class II molecules by the TCR, as indicated in *Figure*

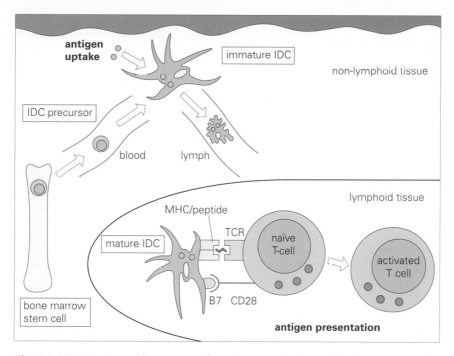

Fig. 11.10 Migration and maturation of interdigitating dendritic cells. The precursors of the IDCs are derived from bone marrow stem cells. They travel via the blood to non-lymphoid tissues. These immature IDCs, e.g. Langerhans' cells in skin, are specialized for antigen uptake. Subsequently they travel via the afferent lymphatics to take up residence within secondary lymphoid tissues, where they express high levels of MHC class II and costimulatory molecules such as B7. These cells are highly specialized for the activation of naïve T cells. (Reproduced with permission from IM Roitt and PJ Delves, *Roitt's Essential Immunology,* 10th edition. Oxford: Blackwell Science, 2001.)

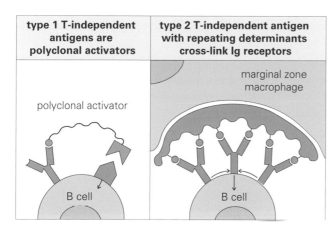

Fig. 11.11 B cell activation by T-independent antigens. The requirements for an antigen-presenting cell (APC) for type 2 antigens is still uncertain. (Ig, immunoglobulin.)

11.12. Following this recognition process, the cells act on each other by releasing soluble factors termed cytokines *(Fig. 11.13)*, which react with appropriate complementary surface receptors on the target cell. For example, in the activated T cell, the gene encoding the IL-2 receptor (IL-2R) is derepressed and the IL-2R molecule is expressed on the surface of the lymphocytes. A subpopulation of TH cells is also induced to synthesize IL-2, which acts as a growth factor for T cells by combining with the IL-2R, causing proliferation *(Fig. 11.8)*.

Cytokine production helps to define T helper subsets

Helper T cell clones can be divided into two main types with distinct cytokine secretion phenotypes *(Fig. 11.14)*. This makes biological sense in that TH1 cells producing cytokines such as IFNγ would be especially effective against intracellular infections with viruses and organisms which grow in macrophages, whereas TH2 cells are very good helpers for B cells and would seem to be adapted for defense against parasites which are vulnerable to IL-4-switched IgE, IL-5-induced eosinophilia and IL-3/4-stimulated mast cell proliferation. The skewing of phenotype towards the extreme TH1/TH2 patterns occurs during the immune response and is partly determined by the nature of the antigen stimulus. There is mutual antagonism between these two subsets in that IL-4 downregulates TH1 cells and IFNγ suppresses the activity of TH2 lymphocytes. Attention has been drawn to the existence of a TH3 subset also referred to as T regulatory-1 (Tr1) cells since they produce transforming growth factor beta (TGFβ) and IL-10 which can mediate immunosuppressive effects and have been implicated in the maintenance of self-tolerance (see *Fig. 11.17* below). *Figure 11.15* shows the broad sweep of

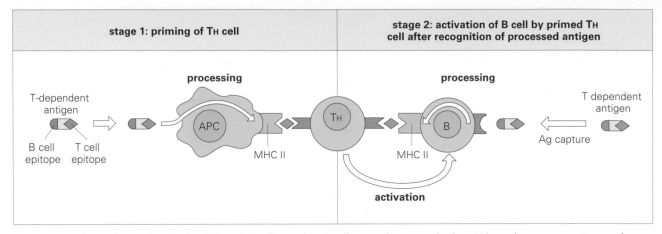

Fig. 11.12 The mechanism by which T helper (TH) cells stimulate B cells to synthesize antibody to T-dependent antigens. See text for a detailed description of the sequence of events. (Ag, antigen; APC, antigen-presenting cell; MHC, major histocompatability complex.)

the cytokine network and the involvement of many different cell types.

The recruitment of the different cells participating in the immune response to the optimal anatomical location, is mediated by a very large number of relatively low molecular weight chemoattractant cytokines, termed chemokines, which act through surface receptors on their target cell. These include: IL-8, which potently attracts neutrophils; macrophage chemotactic factor MCP-1; and RANTES, which attracts T, NK and dendritic cells plus monocytes, eosinophils and basophils to sites of inflammation.

REGULATORY MECHANISMS

Unlimited expansion of clones must be checked by regulatory mechanisms

Once lymphocyte clones are activated by antigen, they clearly cannot be allowed to go on dividing indefinitely, otherwise they would completely fill the body of the host. There are therefore several mechanisms regulating the expansion of these dividing lymphocytes.

One of the most important factors controlling the immune response is the concentration of antigen. There is of course a distinct evolutionary advantage in a system where the immune response is switched on by antigen and switched off when the antigen is no longer present. It is perhaps not surprising then that selective processes have guided the production of such a system in which the immune response is antigen-driven through the direct effect of antigen on the lymphocyte receptors. As the antigen is eliminated by metabolic catabolism and by clearance through the immune response, the stimulus to the immune system disappears.

Antibody itself has feedback potential

IgM produced early in the response has a positive feedback, stimulating the response in its fledgling stages. In contrast, IgG in sufficient concentrations produces negative feedback and acts to downregulate the immune response. We have already mentioned TH3 regulatory cells, which act to

downregulate both TH cells and B cells, whether through antigen-specific or idiotype-specific mechanisms. In the latter case, the epitopes on one lymphocyte receptor (idiotype) recognized by the receptor on another lymphocyte (the anti-idiotype) can form a network of interactions through which suppression may be mediated (Fig. 11.16).

TOLERANCE MECHANISMS

Tolerance mechanisms prevent immunologic self-reactivity

To avoid reaction against the body's own components, it is essential for the immune system to develop non-reactivity or 'tolerance' to self molecules. In essence, it is thought that cells that are autoreactive are either:

- eliminated by some form of clonal deletion;
- made anergic early in the life of the cell;
- sometimes silenced through T regulatory cells later in life (Fig. 11.17).

T cells are more readily tolerized than B cells at a given antigen concentration

There is extremely good evidence that self molecules in the thymus can lead to the deletion or 'anergy' of the specific T cell clone, although autoreactive T cells will survive if the concentration of MHC/self-peptide on the appropriate antigen-presenting cell is too low. B cells in contact with a relatively high concentration of self proteins are also subject to clonal deletion or anergy, but there is less need to tolerize other B cells in the sense that autoreactive B cells directed to thymus-dependent antigens will be unable to respond (helpless) if the corresponding TH cells to that molecule have been tolerized, be it through clonal deletion or suppression by T-regulators (Fig. 11.17).

Unresponsiveness will also result if self components cannot be seen or recognized by the immune system. This may occur because over a long period of time the repertoire has lost the genes giving rise to autoreactive receptors.

CYTOKINES: HORMONES OF THE IMMUNE SYSTEM		
factor	source	actions
IL-1 α/β	macrophages	inflammatory
IL-2	T cells	T and B cell proliferation
IL-3	T cells	pluripotent growth
IL-4	T cells	T and B proliferation, activation of macrophages
IL-5	T cells	eosinophil differentiation, B cell growth
IL-6	T cells	B cell differentiation
IL-7	T cells	B and T cell proliferation
IL-8	T cells	PMN activation
IL-9	T cells	mast cell growth
IL-10	T cell/B cell, macrophages	inhibition of TH1 cytokine production
IL-11	BM stromal cells	induction acute phase proteins
IL-12	Monocytes, Mφ	induction of TH1 cells
IL-13	T cells	inhibits mononuclear phagocyte inflammation: proliferation and differentiation B-cells
IL-15	Antigen-presenting cells	proliferation T-, NK and activated B-cells; maintenance T-memory cells
IL-16	CD8 T, CD4 (not preformed)	chemotaxis CD4 T cells and eosinophils
IL-17	T cells	proinflammatory; stimulates production of cytokines including TNFα, IL-1β, –6, –8, G-CSF
IL-18	macrophages, dendritic cells	induces IFNγ production by T; enhances NK cytotoxicity
IL-19	monocytes	modulates TH1 activity
IL-20	keratinocytes?	regulation of inflammatory responses to skin?
IL-21	TH cells	regulation hematopoiesis; NK differentiation; B activation; T costimulation
IL-22	T cells	inhibits IL-4 production by TH2
IL-23	dendritic cells	induces proliferation and IFNγ production by TH1; induces proliferation of memory cells
IFNα	multiple	antiviral
IFNβ	multiple	antiviral
IFNγ	T cells	antiviral, activation of macrophages, inhibition of T$_H$2 cells MHC induction
	NK cells	
TNFα	monocytes	cytotoxicity, cachexia, fever
lymphotoxin (TNFβ)	T cells	cytotoxicity, cachexia, fever
TGFβ	T cells/macrophages	inhibits activation of NK and T cells, macrophages; inhibits proliferation of B and T cells
GM-CSF	T cells	growth of granulocytes and monocytes
G-CSF	macrophages	growth of granulocytes
M-CSF	macrophages	growth of monocytes
Steel factor	BM stromal cells	stem cell division (c-kit ligand)

Fig. 11.13 Known cytokines and their actions. (BM, bone marrow; G-CSF, granulocyte colony stimulating factor; GM-CSF, granulocyte–macrophage colony stimulating factor; IFN, interferon; IL, interleukin; M-CSF, macrophage colony stimulating factor; NK, natural killer cell; PMN, polymorphonuclear lymphocyte; TGF, transforming growth factor; TNFα, tumor necrosis factor alpha.)

However, even if autoreactive T cells are present, they will not be activated if the self antigen (sAg) is anatomically secluded or is not presented in processed form in combination with MHC class II molecules in adequate concentrations. Therefore, they will also be unable to react with processed sAg presented on the surface of cells that do not express class II. Since most cells express class I molecules, it seems reasonable to assume that the cytotoxic T (Tc) cells capable of reacting against cells expressing processed intracellular components have been deleted, are helpless or are suppressed.

CYTOKINE PATTERNS OF T-CELL SUBSET CLONES		
	TH1	TH2
IFNγ		
IL-2		
Lymphotoxin (TNFβ)		
TNF (TNFα)		
GM-CSF		
IL-3		
IL-4		
IL-5		
IL-6		
IL-13		

☐ ++   ▨ +   ☐ negative   TH1/2, T-helper 1/2.

Fig. 11.14 Cytokine patterns of T cell clones define two subsets of helper cells: TH1 and TH2. IL-10 is not listed; although classed as a TH2 cytokine in the mouse, it is produced by TH1 and TH2 cells in the human. Similar cytokine patterns are seen in two subsets of CD8 Tc cells.

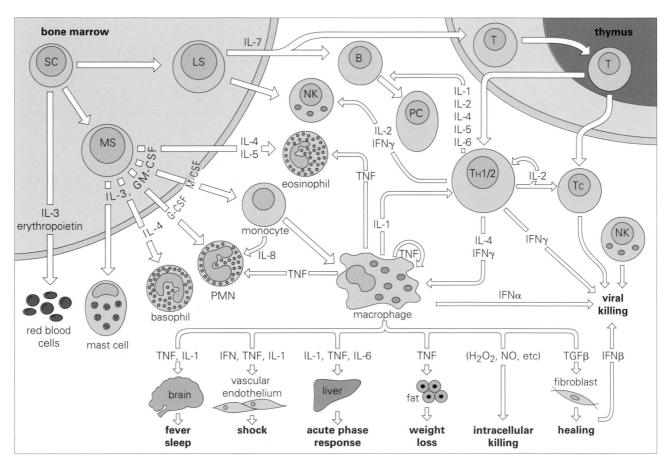

Fig. 11.15 Cellular interactions mediated by cytokines. T helper (TH) cells tend to skew into two major subsets: TH1, producing interleukin-2 (IL-2) and interferon-γ (IFNγ), which activate macrophage-mediated chronic inflammatory reactions; and TH2, producing IL-4, IL-5 and IL-6, which act to support B cell antibody responses. (G-CSF, granulocyte colony stimulating factor; GM-CSF, granulocyte–macrophage colony stimulating factor; H₂O₂, hydrogen peroxide; LS, lymphoid stem cell; M-CSF, macrophage colony stimulating factor; MS, myeloid stem cell; NK, natural killer cell; NO, nitric oxide; PC, plasma cell; PMN, polymorphonuclear lymphocyte; SC, stem cell; Tc, cytotoxic T cell; TGFβ, transforming growth factor beta; TNF, tumor necrosis factor) (Adapted from JHL Playfair, 2001.)

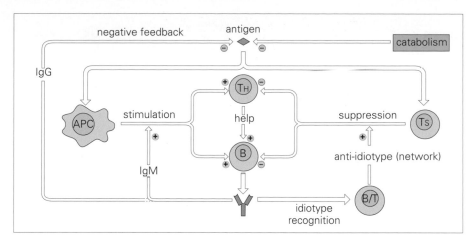

Fig. 11.16 Regulation of the immune response. T help for cell-mediated immunity is subject to similar regulation. The recruitment of B cells by anti-idiotype T helper (TH) cells and direct activation of anti-idiotype T suppressor (TS) cells by idiotype-positive TH cells have been omitted for the sake of clarity. (APC, antigen-presenting cell.)

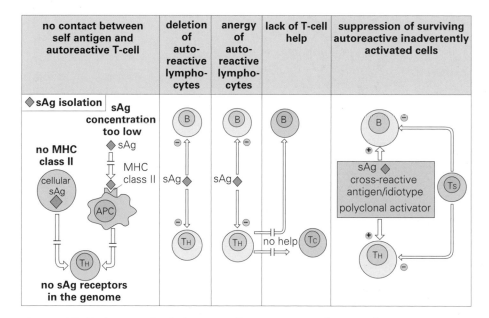

Fig. 11.17 Mechanisms of self-tolerance. Self antigens (sAg) will not stimulate autoreactive TH cells if they are anatomically isolated, or if there is too low a concentration of processed peptide–major histocompatibility complex class II (MHC II) molecules, or if there is no MHC II on the cell. Both B and T cells can be silenced by clonal deletion or made anergic (still living, but unresponsive) by contact with self antigen. Too low a concentration of presented sAg will fail to silence differentiating immature lymphocytes bearing the cognate receptors, leading to the survival of populations of autoreactive T and B cells. TH cells are the most readily tolerized population, and surviving autoreactive B cells and cytotoxic T (TC) cells cannot function without T cell help. Furthermore, inadvertent stimulation of surviving autoreactive cells may be checked by T suppressor (TS) cells probably of the TH3/Tr1 subset. Cells that are dead, unreactive or suppressed are shown in gray. (APC, antigen-presenting cell.) (Modified from IM Roitt and PJ Delves, 2001.)

KEY FACTS

- Each lymphocyte expresses either antibody or a TCR with a single specificity for antigen.

- A lymphocyte bearing a complementary antibody or TCR on its surface will bind antigen, be activated, proliferate to form a clone, and differentiate into antibody-forming cells or effectors of cell-mediated immunity, and also form a large pool of memory cells.

- Second contact with antigen stimulates the pool of memory cells to produce a larger and faster response than the primary reaction. Therefore, vaccination with a benign form of the antigen prepares the individual for an effective response on second contact with the antigen during a natural infection.

- Many antigens require T cell help before they can activate B cells, and the interactions are mediated by a variety of soluble cytokines.

- Unlimited expansion of clones is restricted by antigen concentration, antibody feedback, T cell suppression and apoptosis.

- Reactivity to self is prevented by a variety of tolerance mechanisms.

QUESTIONS

1. Immunological unresponsiveness to self antigens is called:
   A. Tolerance
   B. Tolerogen
   C. Memory
   D. Acquired immunity
   E. ADCC

2. Cytokines always act:
   A. By binding to specific receptors
   B. At long range
   C. Antagonistically with other cytokines
   D. Synergistically with other cytokines

3. Which of the following is characteristically produced by the TH2 CD4 cells which provide help for antibody production, but not by TH1 cells?
   A. IFNγ
   B. Lymphotoxin (TNFβ)
   C. GM-CSF
   D. IL-4
   E. IL-1

4. Negative feedback on adaptive B cell responses is mediated by:*
   A. Antigen-specific IgM
   B. Antigen-specific IgG
   C. Antigen neutralization
   D. Fcγ receptors on macrophages
   E. F(ab')$_2$ anti-μ

*Question has more than one correct answer.

FURTHER READING

Alt F, Marrack P, eds. *Curr Opin Immunol* [appears bimonthly; issues 1, 2 and 3 of each volume contain critical reviews].

Playfair JHL. *Immunology at a Glance*, 7th edition. Oxford: Blackwell Science, 2001.

Roitt IM, Delves PJ. *Roitt's Essential Immunology*, 10th edition. Oxford: Blackwell Science, 2001.

Roitt IM, Brostoff J, Male DK, eds. *Immunology*, 6th edition. London: Elsevier Science, 2002.

The conflicts

3

12. Background to the infectious diseases *113*

13. Entry, exit and transmission *123*

14. Immune defenses in action *143*

15. Spread and replication *157*

16. Parasite survival strategies and persistent infections *167*

17. Pathologic consequences of infection *183*

Microbes rapidly evolve characteristics that enable them to overcome the host's defenses

Microorganisms faced with the antimicrobial defenses of the host species have evolved and developed a variety of characteristics that enable them to bypass or overcome these defenses and carry out their obligatory steps (Fig 12.1). Infectious microorganisms evolve with extraordinary speed in comparison with their hosts. This is partly because they multiply much more rapidly, the generation time of an average bacterium being 1 hour or less compared with about 20 years for the human host. Rapid evolutionary change is also favored in bacteria that can hand over genes (carried on plasmids) directly to other bacteria, including unrelated bacteria. Antibiotic resistance genes, for instance, can thereby be transferred rapidly between species. This rapid rate of evolution ensures that microbes are always many steps ahead of the host's antimicrobial defenses. Indeed, if there are possible ways around the established defenses, microorganisms are likely to have discovered and taken advantage of them. Infectious microorganisms therefore owe their success to this ability to adapt and evolve, exploiting weak

HOST DEFENSES AND THE MICROBES' ANSWER

defense	microbial answer	mechanism	example
antimicrobial immune responses	infect glands or epithelial surfaces	virus has tropism for cells in glands or on surfaces	cytomegalovirus, rabies virus (salivary glands)
	relatively inaccessible to circulating antibody or immune cells		
	suppress immune responses	invade immune tissues	HIV, measles
	vary microbial antigens either in individually infected host, or during spread in host community	switch on different surface antigens	*Trypanosoma* spp., *Borrelia recurrentis*
		mutation, genetic recombination	influenza virus, streptococci, gonococci

Fig. 12.2 Host defenses and microbial evasion strategies: mechanical and other barriers. Microbes evolve fast and are generally one step ahead in this ancient conflict, but it must be remembered that the antimicrobial defenses themselves represent the host's answer to invading microbes. Although inflammation is not listed as a host defense in its own right, many of these defenses depend on local inflammation. Inflammation (Chapter 9) means an increased blood supply and the delivery of antibodies, complement, immune cells and phagocytes to the site of infection. In the days before antibiotics, people applied hot poultices to staphylococcal boils and abscesses so as to increase the amount of inflammation and hasten recovery. Microbes that interfere with the action of complement or with chemotaxis (staphylococci, streptococci, *Pseudomonas aeruginosa*, herpes simplex viruses) will thereby tend to reduce inflammation.

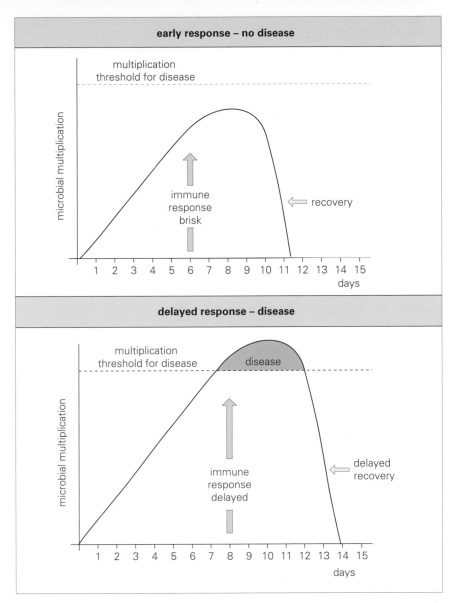

Fig. 12.3 Every infection is a race. Delays in mobilizing host adaptive defenses can lead to disease or death.

points in the host's defenses, as outlined in *Figures 12.2–12.4*. The host in turn has had to respond to such strategies by slowly improving defenses, adding extra features, and having multiple defense mechanisms with overlap and a good deal of duplication.

HOST–PARASITE RELATIONSHIPS

The speed with which host adaptive responses can be mobilized is crucial

Every infection is a race between the capacity of the microorganism to multiply, spread and cause disease and the ability of the host to control and finally terminate the infection *(Fig. 12.3)*. For instance, a 24-hour delay before an important host response comes into operation can give a decisive advantage to a rapidly growing microorganism. From the host's point of view, it may allow enough damage to cause disease. More importantly from the microbe's point of view, it

may give the microbe the opportunity to be shed from the body in larger amounts or for an extra day or two. A microbe that achieves this will be rapidly selected for in evolution.

Adaptation by both host and parasite leads to a more stable balanced relationship

The picture of conflict between host and parasite, usually and appropriately described in military terms, is central to an understanding of the biology of infectious disease. As with military conflicts, adaptation on both sides (see panel on myxomatosis) tends to lessen the damage and incidence of death in the host population, leading to a more stable and balanced relationship. The successful parasite gets what it can from the host without causing too much damage, and in general the more ancient the relationship the less the damage. Many microbial parasites, not only the normal flora (see Chapter 8), but also polioviruses, meningococci and

LESSONS IN MICROBIOLOGY

Myxomatosis

Myxomatosis provides a well-studied classic example of the evolution of an infectious disease unleashed on a highly susceptible population. Myxomavirus, which is spread mechanically by mosquitoes, normally infects South American rabbits (*Sylvilagus brasiliensis*), but they remain perfectly well, developing only a virus-rich skin swelling at the site of the mosquito bite. The same virus in the European rabbit (*Oryctolagus cuniculus*) causes a rapidly fatal disease.

Myxomavirus was successfully introduced into Australia in 1950 as an attempt to control the rapidly increasing rabbit population. Initially, more than 99% of infected rabbits died *(Fig. 12.4)*, but then two fundamental changes occurred:

- First, new, less lethal strains of virus appeared and replaced the original strain. This occurred because rabbits infected with these strains survived for longer and their virus was therefore more likely to be transmitted.
- Second, the rabbit population changed its character, as those that were genetically more susceptible to the infection were eliminated. In other words, the virus selected out the more resistant host, and the less lethal virus strain proved to be a more successful parasite. If the rabbit population had been eliminated, the virus

would also have died out, but the host–parasite relationship quite rapidly settled down to reach a state of better balanced pathogenicity. Australian rabbits now face a new threat, a calicivirus introduced from Europe which spreads by contact, and causes a lethal hemorrhagic disease.

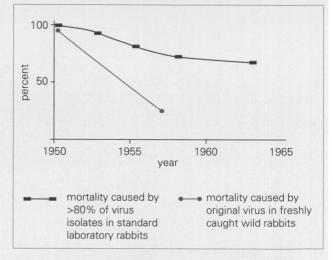

Fig. 12.4 Myxomatosis is the best-studied example of the appearance of a highly lethal microbe in a host population that gradually settles down to a state of more balanced pathogenicity. *Vibrio cholerae* has progressed in this direction, and perhaps HIV is destined to tread the same path.

---

pneumococci and others, live for the most part in peaceful coexistence with their human host.

Some microorganisms remain at body surfaces, perhaps spreading locally, but failing to invade deeper tissues. These include the common cold viruses, wart viruses, mycoplasmas and skin fungi. Often the disease is mild, but severe illness can occur when powerful toxins are produced and act either locally (cholera) or at distant sites (diphtheria).

Four types of infection can be distinguished

The four types of infecting microorganisms *(Fig. 12.5)* are:

- microorganisms with specific mechanisms for attaching to, or penetrating, the body surfaces of normal healthy hosts (most viruses and certain bacteria);
- microorganisms introduced into normal healthy hosts by biting arthropods (e.g. malaria, plague, typhus, yellow fever);
- microorganisms introduced into otherwise normal healthy hosts via skin wounds or animal bites (clostridia, rabies, *Pasteurella multocida*);
- microorganisms able to infect a normal healthy host only when surface or systemic defenses are impaired (see

Chapter 30)—as occurs with burns, insertion of foreign bodies (cannulas and catheters), urinary tract infections in men (stones, enlarged prostate, see Chapter 20), bacterial pneumonia following initial viral damage (post-influenza) or depressed immune responses (immunosuppressive drugs or diseases such as AIDS).

CAUSES OF INFECTIOUS DISEASES

More than one hundred microbes quite commonly cause infection

Humans are host to many different microorganisms. In addition to the scores of microbes that form the normal flora, there are more than one hundred that quite commonly cause infection, some of them remaining in the body for many years afterwards, and several hundred others that are responsible for less common infections. Against this rich background of parasitic activity, how do we prove that a certain microorganism is the culprit in a given disease? In some instances (anthrax, cholera, tetanus) the causative microorganism is identified and incriminated at an early stage, but in the case of glandular fever and viral hepatitis it is not so easy.

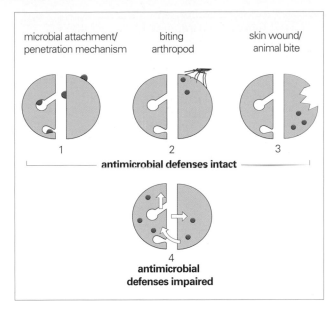

Fig. 12.5 Four types of microbial infection can be distinguished. (The diagrams show a schematic representation of the body surfaces of a host, similar to that in Figure 13.1.) Surface or systemic defenses of the host can be impaired in a variety of ways.

Koch's postulates to identify the microbial causes of specific diseases

In 1890, Robert Koch (see panel) set out as 'postulates' the following criteria he felt to be necessary for a microorganism to be accepted as the cause of a given disease:

- The microbe must be present in every case of the disease.
- The microbe must be isolated from the diseased host and grown in pure culture.
- The disease must be reproduced when a pure culture is introduced into a non-diseased susceptible host.
- The microbe must be recoverable from an experimentally infected host.

However, modifications were needed in order to include certain bacterial diseases and the new world of viral diseases. The microbe could not always be grown in the laboratory (*Treponema pallidum*, wart viruses), and for certain microbes—hepatitis B, Epstein–Barr virus (EBV)—there were (initially) no susceptible animal species. The criteria were modified therefore on several occasions to accommodate these problems and finally reformulated and brought up to date by AS Evans in 1976.

In the early days of microbiology, Koch's postulates brought a welcome clarity. The germ theory of disease causation had only recently been set out following Koch's

LESSONS IN MICROBIOLOGY

Robert Koch (1843–1910)

In 1876, while in general practice in Berlin, Robert Koch *(Fig. 12.6)* isolated the anthrax bacillus, and became the first to show a specific organism as the cause of a disease. In 1882 he discovered *Mycobacterium tuberculosis* as the cause of tuberculosis. He then went on to lead the 1883 expedition to Egypt and India, and discovered the cause of cholera: *Vibrio cholerae*.

Koch was the founder of the 'germ theory' of disease, which maintained that certain diseases were caused by a single species of microbe. In 1890, he set out his 'postulates' as ground rules (see text). New techniques were necessary to meet the exacting requirements of the postulates, and Koch became the first to grow bacteria in 'colonies', initially on potato slices and later, with his pupil Petri, on solid gelatin media.

Koch himself could not reproduce cholera in animals, however, and not all microbes could be cultivated. His neat rules therefore had to be modified. Nevertheless, he brought order and clarity to medicine—until then diseases were attributed to miasmas or mists, to punishments from the Gods or devils, or to unfortunate conjunctions of the stars and planets. However, there was resistance to his ideas. A distinguished Munich physician, Max Von

Petternkofer, believed that he had put paid to the new theory when he drank a pure culture of *V. cholerae* and suffered no more than mild diarrhea!

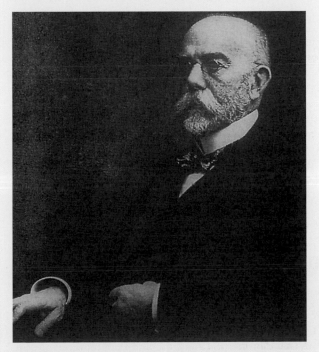

Fig. 12.6 Robert Koch (1843–1910).

classic studies on anthrax (1876) and tuberculosis (1882), and methods for isolating microbes in pure culture and identifying them were only just being developed.

Nowadays conclusions about causation are reached using enlightened common sense

Nowadays, with our vastly increased technology and understanding of infection, those attempts to make lists and apply rigid criteria may seem old fashioned. Perhaps we can now reach conclusions about causation using common sense. For instance, we recognize that diseases sometimes do not appear until many years after a specific infection (subacute sclerosing panencephalitis, Creutzfeldt–Jakob disease; see Chapter 24). Again, molecular genetic techniques may identify previously uncultivable causative organisms. The polymerase chain reaction was used to amplify and sequence small amounts of mRNA from the bowel of patients with Whipple's disease, a rare multisystem disorder. A unique 16s mRNA was identified, belonging to a previously uncharacterized, uncultivable bacterium *Tropheryma whippelii*. Nevertheless, gray areas remain, especially in diseases of possible or probable microbial etiology where the microbe does not act alone. Cofactors or genetic and immunologic factors in the host may play a vital part. Examples include:

- the cancers associated with viruses (hepatitis B, genital wart viruses, EBV);
- diseases of possible microbial origin where a number of different microbes may be involved (postviral fatigue syndrome, exacerbations of multiple sclerosis);
- diseases that might be infectious, but occur in only a very small proportion of genetically predisposed individuals (rheumatoid athritis, juvenile diabetes mellitus).

Possible problems in assigning disease etiology

Finally, there are two interesting possibilities that could give problems in assigning disease etiology, although neither has yet been shown to apply to human disease:

- First, in some infections the DNA of the causative virus is integrated into the genome of the host, and is transmitted vertically. It therefore behaves as a genetic attribute. This is known to occur, for instance, with mammary tumor virus in mice.
- Second, the causative microbe triggers off the disease process and then disappears completely from the body and is no longer detectable. This is known to be the case in the cerebellar hypoplasia occurring in hamsters and cats after intrauterine infection with parvovirus. There are no known examples in humans.

THE BIOLOGIC RESPONSE GRADIENT

It is uncommon for a microbe to cause exactly the same disease in all infected individuals

Hence a physician must be able to make a diagnosis when only some of the possible signs and symptoms are present. The exact clinical picture depends upon many variables such as infecting dose and route, age, sex, presence of other

FREQUENCY OF CLINICALLY APPARENT DISEASE	
infection	approximate % with clinically apparent disease*
*Pneumocystis jiroveci***	0
poliomyelitis (child)	0.1–1.0
Epstein–Barr virus (1–5 year old child)	1.0†
rubella	50
influenza (young adult)	60
whooping cough typhoid malaria anthrax	>90
gonorrhea (adult male) measles	99
rabies HIV (?)	100

*on primary infection **formerly *P. carinii*
†30–75% in young adults

Fig. 12.7 The likelihood of developing clinical disease often depends upon age and sex, as shown. When there is a lengthy incubation period the proportion with clinical disease may increase with time, from a few percent to (probably) 100% in the case of HIV.

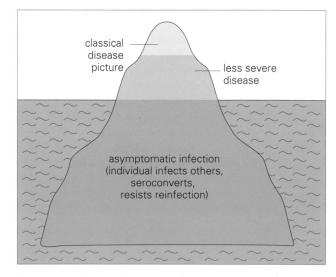

Fig. 12.8 The 'iceberg' concept of infectious disease.

microbes, nutritional status and genetic background. Infections such as measles or cholera give a fairly consistent disease picture, but others such as syphilis cause such a wide spectrum of pathology that Sir William Osler (1849–1919) stated that 'He who knows syphilis, knows medicine'.

There is great variation not only in the nature, but also in the severity of clinical disease. Many infections are asymptomatic in more than 90% of individuals, the clinically characterized illness applying to only an occasional unfortunate host *(Fig. 12.7)*. This illness can be mild or severe. Asymptomatically infected individuals are important because although they develop immunity and resistance to reinfection, they are not identified, move normally in the community and can infect others. Clearly there is little point in isolating a clinically infected patient when there is a high frequency of asymptomatically infected individuals in the community. This phenomenon can be represented as an iceberg *(Fig. 12.8)*.

KEY FACTS

- Faced with host defenses (see Chapters 9–10), the microbes (see Chapters 1–7) have developed mechanisms to bypass them, and in turn the host defenses have had to be modified, although slowly, in response.

- There is a conflict between the microbe and host, and every infectious disease is the result of this ancient conflict. Details of the host–microbe conflict are given in Chapters 9–17, an outline of diagnostic methods in Chapter 32, and a central account of infectious diseases according to the body systems involved in Chapters 18–30.

- Speed matters. Every infection is a race between microbial replication and spread and the mobilization of host responses.

- There are four types of infection depending upon whether host defenses are intact or impaired.

- It is sometimes difficult to incriminate a specific microbe as the cause of a disease.

- Microbes do not necessarily produce the same disease in all infected individuals. A biologic response gradient causes a spectrum that can range from an asymptomatic to a lethal infection.

FURTHER READING

Burnet FM, White DO. *The Natural History of Infectious Disease,* 4th edition. Cambridge: Cambridge University Press, 1972.
Falkow W. Koch's postulates applied to microbial pathogenicity. *Rev Infect Dis* 1988; 10.S274.

Mims CA, Nash A, Stephen J. *Mims' Pathogenesis of Infectious Disease,* 5th edition. London: Academic Press, 2001.
Smith GA. Virus strategies for evasion of the host response to infection. *Trends Microbiol* 1994; 2:81–8.

? QUESTIONS

1. How could you prove that a virus was the cause of diabetes mellitus?

2. Everyone dies after developing rabies, so how is this infection maintained in nature?

3. List the steps that a successful microbe must accomplish in the host. Which are the most important?

4. If a virus, for example myxomavirus, has gene products that interfere with immune responses or with the action of a cytokine, how could you show that this really mattered in the infected host?

5. Since every infection is a race, what is it that prevents all microbes from completing their infection within a few days?

6. Phagocytes have impressive antimicrobial powers, yet many microbes seem to multiply in them. Why is this?

Entry, exit and transmission

INTRODUCTION

Microorganisms must attach to, or penetrate, the host's body surfaces

The mammalian host can be considered as a series of body surfaces *(Fig. 13.1)*. To establish themselves on or in the host, microorganisms must either attach to, or penetrate, one of these body surfaces. The outer surface, covered by skin or fur, protects and isolates the body from the outside world, forming a dry, horny, relatively impermeable outer layer. Elsewhere, however, there has to be more intimate contact and exchange with the outside world. Therefore in the alimentary, respiratory and urinogenital tracts, where food is absorbed, gases exchanged and urine and sexual products released, the lining consists of one or more layers of living cells. In the eye, the skin is replaced by a transparent layer of living cells, the conjunctiva. Well-developed cleansing and defense mechanisms are present at all these body surfaces, and entry of microorganisms always has to occur in the face of these natural mechanisms. Successful microorganisms therefore possess efficient mechanisms for attaching to, and often traversing, these body surfaces.

Receptor molecules

There are often specific molecules on microbes that bind to receptor molecules on host cells, either at the body surface (viruses, bacteria) or in tissues (viruses). These receptor molecules, of which there may be more than one, are not, of course, present for the benefit of the virus or other infectious agent; they have specific functions in the life of the cell. Very occasionally the receptor molecule is present only in certain cells, which are then uniquely susceptible to infection. Examples include the CD4 molecule for HIV and the C3d receptor (CR_2) for Epstein–Barr virus. In these cases the presence of the receptor molecule determines virus tropism and accounts for the distinctive pattern of infection. Receptors are therefore critical determinants of cell susceptibility, not only at the body surface, but in all tissues. After binding to the susceptible cell, the microorganism can multiply at the surface (mycoplasma, *Bordetella pertussis*) or enter the cell and infect it (viruses, chlamydia; see Chapter 15).

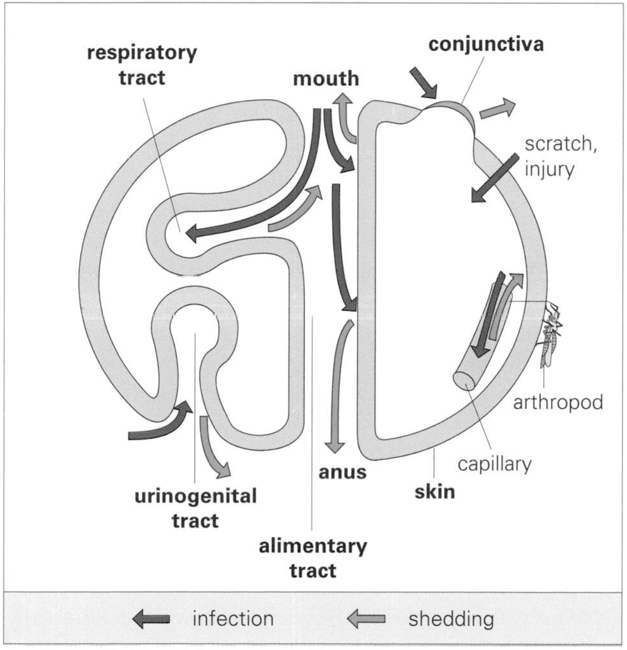

Exit from the body

Microorganisms must also exit from the body if they are to be transmitted to a fresh host. They are either shed in large numbers in secretions and excretions or are available in the blood for uptake, for example by blood-sucking arthropods or needles.

SITES OF ENTRY

Skin

Microorganisms gaining entry via the skin may cause a skin infection or infection elsewhere

Microorganisms which infect or enter the body via the skin are listed in *Figure 13.2*. On the skin, microorganisms other than residents of the normal flora (see Chapter 8) are soon inactivated, especially by fatty acids (skin pH is about 5.5), and probably by substances secreted by sebaceous and other glands, and certain peptides formed locally by keratinocytes protect against invasion by group A streptococci. Materials produced by the normal flora of the skin also protect against infection. Skin bacteria may enter hair follicles or sebaceous glands to cause styes and boils, or teat canals to cause staphylococcal mastitis.

Fig. 13.1 Body surfaces as sites of microbial infection and shedding.

MICROORGANISMS THAT INFECT VIA THE SKIN		
microorganism	**disease**	**comments**
arthropod-borne viruses	various fevers	150 distinct viruses, transmitted by bite of infected arthropod
rabies virus	rabies	bite from infected animals
wart viruses	warts	infection restricted to epidermis
staphylococci	boils, etc	commonest skin invaders
Rickettsia	typhus, spotted fevers	infestation with infected arthropod
leptospira	leptospirosis	contact with water containing infected animals' urine
streptococci	impetigo, erysipelas	concurrent pharyngeal infection in one-third of cases
Bacillus anthracis	cutaneous anthrax	systemic disease following local lesion at inoculation site
Treponema pallidum and *T. pertenue*	syphilis, yaws	warm, moist skin more susceptible
Yersinia pestis, Plasmodia	plague, malaria	bite from infected rodent flea or mosquito
Trichophyton spp. and other fungi	ringworm, athlete's foot	infection restricted to skin, nails, hair
Ankylostoma duodenale (or *Necator americanus*)	hookworm	silent entry of larvae through skin of e.g. foot
filarial nematodes	filariasis	bite from infected mosquito, midge, blood-sucking fly
Schistosoma spp.	schistosomiasis	larvae (cercariae) from infected snail penetrate skin during wading or bathing

Fig. 13.2 Microorganisms that infect via the skin. Some remain restricted to the skin (wart viruses, ringworm), whereas others enter the body after growth in the skin (syphilis) or after mechanical transfer across the skin (arthropod-borne infections, schistosomiasis).

Several types of fungi (the dermatophytes) infect the non-living keratinous structures (stratum corneum, hair, nails) produced by the skin. Infection is established as long as the parasites' rate of downward growth into the keratin exceeds the rate of shedding of the keratinous product. When the latter is very slow, as in the case of nails, the infection is more likely to become chronic.

Wounds, abrasions or burns are more common sites of infection. Even a small break in the skin can be a portal of entry if virulent microorganisms such as streptococci, leptospira or hepatitis B virus are present at the site. A few microbes, such as leptospira or the larvae of *Ankylostoma* and *Schistosoma*, are able to traverse the unbroken skin by their own activity.

Biting arthropods

Biting arthropods such as mosquitoes, ticks, fleas and sandflies (see Chapter 27) penetrate the skin during feeding and can thus introduce infectious agents or parasites into the body. The arthropod transmits the infection and is an essential part of the lifecycle of the microorganism. Sometimes the transmission is mechanical, the microorganism contaminating the mouth parts without multiplying in the arthropod. In most cases, however, the infectious agent multiplies in the arthropod and, as a result of millions of years of adaptation, causes little or no damage to that host. After an incubation period it appears in the saliva or feces and is transmitted during a blood feed. The mosquito for instance, injects saliva directly into host tissues as an anticoagulant, whereas the human body louse defecates as it feeds, and *Rickettsia rickettsii*, which is present in the feces, is introduced into the bite wound when the host scratches the affected area.

The conjunctiva

The conjunctiva can be regarded as a specialized area of skin. It is kept clean by the continuous flushing action of tears, aided every few seconds by the windscreen wiper action of the eyelids. Therefore the microorganisms that infect the normal conjunctiva (chlamydia, gonococci) must have efficient attachment mechanisms (see Chapter 25). Interference with local defenses due to decreased lacrimal gland secretion or conjunctival or eyelid damage allows even non-specialist microorganisms to establish themselves. Contaminated fingers often carry infectious material to the conjunctiva (e.g. trachoma).

Respiratory tract

Some microorganisms can overcome the respiratory tract's cleansing mechanisms

Air normally contains suspended particles, including smoke, dust and microorganisms. Efficient cleansing mechanisms (see Chapters 18 and 19) deal with these constantly inhaled particles. With about 500–1000 microorganisms per m^3 inside buildings, and a ventilation rate of 6 l/min at rest, as many as 10 000 microorganisms per day are introduced into the lungs. In the upper or lower respiratory tract, inhaled microorganisms, like other particles, will be entrapped in mucus, carried to the back of the throat by ciliary action, and swallowed. Those that invade the normal healthy respiratory tract have developed specific mechanisms to avoid this fate.

Interfering with cleansing mechanisms

The ideal strategy is to attach firmly to the surfaces of cells forming the mucociliary sheet. Specific molecules on the organism (often called adhesins) bind to receptor molecules on the susceptible cell *(Fig. 13.3)*. Examples of such respiratory infections are given in *Figure 13.4*.

Inhibiting ciliary activity is another way of interfering with cleansing mechanisms. This helps invading microorganisms establish themselves in the respiratory tract. *B. pertussis* for instance not only attaches to respiratory epithelial cells, but also interferes with ciliary activity, while other bacteria *(Fig. 13.5)* produce various ciliostatic substances of generally unknown nature.

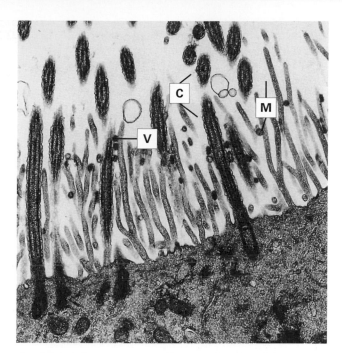

Fig. 13.3 Influenza virus attachment to ciliated epithelium. Influenza virus particles (V) attached to cilia (C) and microvilli (M). Electron micrograph of thin section from organ culture of guinea pig trachea one hour after addition of the virus. (Courtesy of RE Dourmashkin.)

Avoiding destruction by alveolar macrophages

Inhaled microorganisms reaching the alveoli encounter alveolar macrophages, which remove foreign particles and keep the air spaces clean. Most microorganisms are destroyed by these macrophages, but one or two pathogens have learnt

MICROBIAL ATTACHMENT IN THE RESPIRATORY TRACT			
microorganism	**disease**	**microbial adhesin**	**receptor on host cell**
influenza A virus	influenza	hemagglutinin	sialyloligosaccharides
rhinovirus	common cold	capsid protein	ICAM-1 (CD54)
coxsackie A viruses			integrin or ICAM-1
parainfluenza virus type 1, respiratory syncytial virus	respiratory illness	envelope protein	sialoglycolipids
Mycoplasma pneumoniae	atypical pneumonia	mycoplasmal molecule on 'foot'	neuraminic acid
Haemophilus influenzae *Strep. pneumoniae,* *Klebsiella pneumoniae*	respiratory disease	surface molecule	carbohydrate sequence in glycolipid
measles virus	measles	hemagglutinin	CD46

Fig. 13.4 Microbial attachment in the respiratory tract. ICAM-1, intercellular adhesion molecule-1; CD46, membrane cofactor protein involved in complement regulation; integrins, family of adhesion receptors (e.g. laminin receptor) expressed on many cell types.

INTERFERENCE WITH CILIARY ACTIVITY IN RESPIRATORY INFECTIONS		
cause	mechanisms	importance
infecting bacteria interfere with ciliary activity (*B. pertussis, H. influenzae, P. aeruginosa, M. pneumoniae*)	production of ciliostatic substance (tracheal cytotoxin from *B. pertussis*, at least 2 substances from *H. influenzae*, at least 7 from *P. aeruginosa*	++
viral infection	ciliated cell dysfunction or destruction by influenza, measles	+++
atmospheric pollution (automobiles, cigarette smoking, etc.)	acutely impaired mucociliary function	?+
inhalation of unhumidified air (indwelling tracheal tubes, general anesthesia)	acutely impaired mucociliary function	+
chronic bronchitis, cystic fibrosis	chronically impaired mucociliary function	+++

Fig. 13.5 Interference with ciliary activity in respiratory infections. Although microbes can actively interfere with ciliary activity (first item), a more general impairment of mucociliary function also acts as a predisposing cause of respiratory infection.

either to avoid phagocytosis or to avoid destruction after phagocytosis. Tubercle bacilli, for instance, survive in the macrophages, and respiratory tuberculosis is thought to be initiated in this way. Inhalation of as few as 5–10 bacilli is enough. The vital role of macrophages in antimicrobial defenses is dealt with more thoroughly in Chapter 14. Alveolar macrophages are damaged following inhalation of toxic asbestos particles and certain dusts, and this leads to increased susceptibility to respiratory tuberculosis.

Gastrointestinal tract

Some microorganisms can survive the intestine's defenses of acid, mucus and enzymes

Apart from the general flow of intestinal contents, there are no particular cleansing mechanisms in the intestinal tract, except insofar as diarrhea and vomiting can be included in this category. Under normal circumstances, multiplication of resident bacteria is counterbalanced by their continuous passage to the exterior with the rest of the intestinal contents. Ingestion of a small number of non-pathogenic bacteria, followed by growth in the lumen of the alimentary canal, produces only relatively small numbers within 12–18 hours, the normal intestinal transit time.

Infecting bacteria must attach themselves to the intestinal epithelium *(Fig. 13.6)* if they are to establish themselves and multiply in large numbers. They will then avoid being carried straight down the alimentary canal to be excreted with the rest of the intestinal contents. The concentration of micro-organisms in feces depends on the balance between the production and removal of bacteria in the intestine. *Vibrio cholerae (Figs 13.7, 13.8)* and the rotaviruses both establish specific binding to receptors on the surface of intestinal epithelial cells. For *V. cholerae*, establishment in surface mucus

may be sufficient for infection and pathogenicity. The fact that certain microbes infect mainly the large bowel (*Shigella* spp.) or small intestine (most salmonellae, rotaviruses) indicates the presence of specific receptor molecules on mucosal cells in these sections of the alimentary canal.

Infection sometimes involves more than mere adhesion to the lumenal surface of intestinal epithelial cells. *Shigella flexneri*, for example, can only enter these cells from the basal surface. Initial entry occurs after uptake by M cells, and the bacteria then invade local macrophages. This gives rise to an inflammatory response with an influx of polymorphs, which in turn causes some disruption of the epithelial barrier. Bacteria can now enter on a larger scale from the intestinal lumen and invade epithelial cells from below. The bacteria enhance their entry by exploiting the host's inflammatory response.

Crude mechanical devices for attachment

Crude mechanical devices are used for the attachment and entry of certain parasitic protozoans and worms. *Giardia lamblia*, for example, has specific molecules for adhesion to the microvilli of epithelial cells, but also has its own microvillar sucking disk. Hookworms attach to the intestinal mucosa by means of a large mouth capsule containing hooked teeth or cutting plates. Other worms (e.g. *Ascaris*) maintain their position by 'bracing' themselves against peristalsis, while tapeworms adhere closely to the mucus covering the intestinal wall, the anterior hooks and sucker playing a relatively minor role for the largest worms. A number of worms actively penetrate into the mucosa as adults (*Trichinella, Trichuris*) or traverse the gut wall to enter deeper tissues (e.g. the embryos of *Trichinella* released from the female worm and the larvae of *Echinococcus* hatched from ingested eggs).

MICROBIAL ATTACHMENT IN THE INTESTINAL TRACT			
microorganism	**disease**	**attachment site**	**mechanism**
poliovirus	poliomyelitis	intestinal epithelium	viral capsid protein reacts with specific receptor on cell (perhaps ICAM*)
rotavirus	diarrhea	intestinal epithelium	viral outer capsid protein binds to sialic-acid-containing oligosaccharide receptor on cell
Vibrio cholerae *Escherichia coli* (certain strains) *Salmonella typhi*	cholera diarrhea enteric fever	intestinal epithelium	specific bacterial molecule (adhesin)** binds to fucose/mannose receptor on cell
Shigella spp.	dysentery	colonic epithelium	Ipa molecule on bacteria binds to integrin on host cell***
Giardia lamblia	diarrhea	duodenal, jejunal epithelium	protozoa bind to mannose-6 phosphate on host cell; also have mechanical sucker
Entamoeba histolytica	dysentery	colonic epithelium	lectin on surface of amebae binds to asialofetuin on host cell
Ankylostoma duodenale	hookworm	intestinal epithelium	four hooks

*intracellular adhesion molecule; has important functions in inflammatory and 'social' life of cells; acts as receptor molecule for poliovirus on cells *in vitro*

**often on pili or fimbriae (e.g. up to 200 pili, each bearing adhesins, on *E. coli*)

***after attachment *Shigella* (and other pathogenic bacteria) induces epithelial cell to engulf it

Fig. 13.6 Microbial attachment in the intestinal tract.

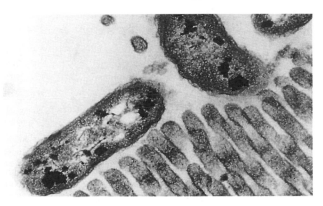

Fig. 13.7 Attachment of *Vibrio cholerae* to brush border of rabbit villus. Thin section electron micrograph, ×10 000. (Courtesy of ET Nelson.)

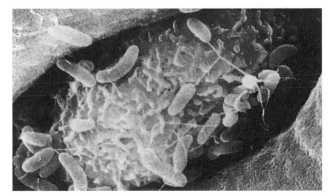

Fig. 13.8 Adherence of *Vibrio cholerae* to M cells in human ileal mucosa. (Courtesy of T Yamamoto.)

Mechanisms to counteract mucus, acids, enzymes and bile

Successful intestinal microbes must counteract or resist mucus, acids, enzymes and bile

Mucus protects epithelial cells, perhaps acting as a mechanical barrier to infection. It may contain molecules that bind to microbial adhesins, therefore blocking attachment to host cells. It also contains secretory IgA antibodies, which protect the immune individual against infection. Motile microorganisms (*V. cholerae*, salmonellae and certain strains of *Escherichia coli*) can propel themselves through the mucus layer and are therefore more likely to reach epithelial cells to make specific attachments; *V. cholerae* also produces a mucinase, which probably helps its passage through the mucus. Non-motile microorganisms, in contrast, rely on random and passive transport in the mucus layer.

MICROBIAL SUCCESS IN THE GASTROINTESTINAL TRACT		
property	**examples**	**consequence**
specific attachment to intestinal epithelium	poliovirus, rotavirus, *Vibrio cholerae*	microorganism avoids expulsion with other gut contents and can establish infection
motility	*V. cholerae*, certain *Escherichia coli* strains	bacteria travel through mucus and are more likely to reach susceptible cell
production of mucinase (neuraminidase)	*V. cholerae*	may assist transit through mucus
acid resistance	*Mycobacterium tuberculosis*	encourages intestinal tuberculosis (acid labile microorganisms depend on protection in food bolus or in diluting fluid) increased susceptibility in individuals with achlorhydria
	Helicobacter pylori	establish residence in stomach
	enteroviruses (hepatitis A, poliovirus, coxsackieviruses, echoviruses)	infection and shedding from gastrointestinal tract
bile resistance	*Salmonella*, *Shigella*, enteroviruses	intestinal pathogens
	Enterococcus faecalis, *E. coli*, *Proteus*, *Pseudomonas*	establish residence
resistance to proteolytic enzymes	reoviruses in mice	permits oral infection
anaerobic growth	*Bacteroides fragilis*	most common resident bacteria in anaerobic environment of colon

Fig. 13.9 Microbial properties that aid success in the gastrointestinal tract.

LESSONS IN MICROBIOLOGY

How to survive stomach acid—the neutralization strategy of *Helicobacter pylori*

This bacterium was discovered a mere 18 years ago, and was shown to be a human pathogen when two courageous doctors in Perth, Western Australia, drank a potion containing the bacteria and developed gastritis. The infection spreads from person to person by the oral–oral or fecal–oral route, and 150 years ago nearly all humans were infected as children. Today, in countries with improved hygiene, this is put off until later in life, until at the age of 50 more than half of the population have been infected. After being eaten, the bacteria attach by special adhesins to the stomach wall. Most microbes (e.g. *V. cholerae*) are soon killed at the low

pH encountered in the stomach. *H. pylori*, however, protects itself by releasing large amounts of urease, which acts on local urea to form a tiny cloud of ammonia round the invader. The attached bacteria cause inflammation, dyspepsia and occasionally a duodenal or gastric ulcer, so that treatment of these ulcers is by antibiotics rather than merely antacids. Ninety percent of duodenal ulcers are due to *H. pylori*, and the rest to aspirin or NSAIDs. The bacteria do not invade tissues, and they stay in the stomach for years, causing asymptomatic chronic gastritis. For unknown reasons some infected individuals develop stomach cancer. *H. pylori* was the third bacterium for which the entire genome was sequenced; several toxins have been characterized, but their exact role is still uncertain.

As might be expected, microorganisms that infect by the intestinal route are often capable of surviving in the presence of acid, proteolytic enzymes and bile. This also applies to microorganisms shed from the body by this route *(Fig. 13.9)*.

All organisms infecting by the intestinal route must run the gauntlet of acid in the stomach. *Helicobacter pylori* has evolved a specific defense (see panel). The fact that tubercle bacilli resist acid conditions favors the establishment of intestinal tuberculosis, but most bacteria are acid sensitive and prefer slightly alkaline conditions. For instance, volunteers who drank different doses of *V. cholerae* contained in 60 ml saline showed a 10 000-fold increase in susceptibility to cholera when 2 g of sodium bicarbonate was given with the bacteria. The minimum disease-producing dose was 10^8 bacteria without bicarbonate and 10^4 bacteria with bicarbonate. Similar experiments have been carried out in volunteers with *Salmonella typhi*, and the minimum infectious dose of 1000–10 000 bacteria was again significantly reduced by the ingestion of sodium bicarbonate.

When the infecting microorganism penetrates the intestinal epithelium (*Shigella*, *S. typhi*, hepatitis A and other enteroviruses) the final pathogenicity depends upon:

- subsequent multiplication and spread;
- toxin production;
- cell damage;
- inflammatory and immune responses.

Microbial exotoxin, endotoxin and protein absorption

Microbial exotoxins, endotoxins and proteins can be absorbed from the intestine on a small scale. Diarrhea generally promotes the uptake of protein, and absorption of protein also takes place more readily in the infant, which in some species needs to absorb antibodies from milk. As well as large molecules, particles the size of viruses can also be taken up from the intestinal lumen. This occurs in certain sites in particular, such as those where Peyer's patches occur. Peyer's patches are isolated collections of lymphoid tissue lying immediately below the intestinal epithelium, which in this region is highly specialized, consisting of so-called M cells (see *Fig. 13.8*). M cells take up particles and foreign proteins and deliver them to underlying immune cells with which they are intimately associated by cytoplasmic processes.

Urinogenital tract

Microorganisms gaining entry via the urinogenital tract can spread easily from one part of the tract to another

The urinogenital tract is a continuum, so microorganisms can spread easily from one part to another, and the distinction between vaginitis and urethritis, or between urethritis and cystitis, is not always easy or necessary (see Chapters 20 and 21).

Vaginal defenses

The vagina has no particular cleansing mechanisms, and repeated introductions of a contaminated, sometimes pathogen-bearing foreign object (the penis), makes the vagina particularly vulnerable to infection, forming the basis for sexually transmitted diseases (see Chapter 21). Nature has responded by providing additional defenses. During reproductive life, the vaginal epithelium contains glycogen due to the action of circulating estrogens, and certain lactobacilli colonize the vagina, metabolizing the glycogen to produce lactic acid. As a result the normal vaginal pH is about 5.0, which inhibits colonization by all except the lactobacilli and certain other streptococci and diphtheroids. Normal vaginal secretions contain up to 10^8/ml of these commensal bacteria. If other microorganisms are to colonize and invade they must either have specific mechanisms for attaching to vaginal or cervical mucosa or take advantage of minute local injuries during coitus (genital warts, syphilis) or impaired defenses (presence of tampons, estrogen imbalance). These are the microorganisms responsible for sexually transmitted diseases.

Urethral and bladder defenses

The regular flushing action of urine is a major urethral defense, and urine in the bladder is normally sterile.

The bladder is more than an inert receptacle, and in its wall there are intrinsic, but poorly understood, defense mechanisms. These include a protective layer of mucus and the ability to generate inflammatory responses and produce secretory antibodies and immune cells.

Mechanism of urinary tract invasion

The urinary tract is nearly always invaded from the exterior via the urethra, and an invading microorganism must first and foremost avoid being washed out during urination. Specialized attachment mechanisms have therefore been developed by successful invaders (e.g. gonococci, *Fig. 13.10*). A defined peptide on the bacterial pili binds to a carbohydrate polymer on the urethral cell, and the cell is then induced to engulf the bacterium. This is referred to as parasite-directed endocytosis and also occurs with chlamydia.

The foreskin is a handicap in genitourinary infections. This is because sexually transmitted pathogens often remain in the moist area beneath the foreskin after detumescence, giving them increased opportunity to invade. All sexually transmitted infections are commoner in uncircumcized males.

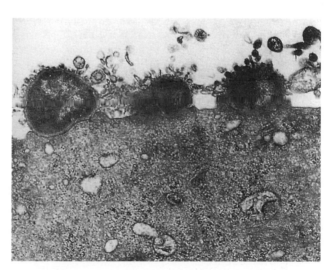

Fig. 13.10 Adherence of gonococci to the surface of a human urethral epithelial cell. (Courtesy of PJ Watt.)

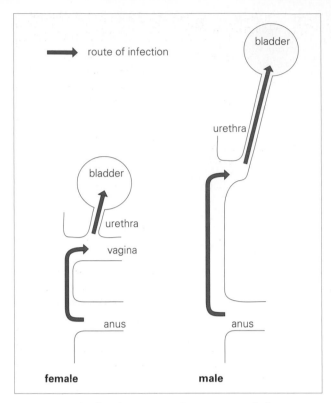

Fig. 13.11 The female urinogenital tract is particularly vulnerable to infection with fecal bacteria, mainly because the urethra is shorter and nearer to the anus.

Intestinal bacteria (mainly *E. coli*) are common invaders of the urinary tract, causing cystitis. Sexual anatomy is a major determinant of infection *(Fig. 13.11)*. Spread to the bladder is no easy task in the male, where the flaccid urethra is 20 cm long. Therefore urinary infections are rare in males unless organisms are introduced by catheters or when the flushing activity of urine is impaired (see Chapter 20). Things are different in females. Not only is the urethra much shorter (5 cm), but it is also very close to the anus *(Fig. 13.11)*, which is a constant source of intestinal bacteria. Urinary infections are about 14 times more common in women, and at least 20% of women have a symptomatic urinary tract infection at some time during their life. The invading bacteria often begin their invasion by colonizing the mucosa around the urethra and probably have special attachment mechanisms to cells in this area. Bacterial invasion is favored by the mechanical deformation of the urethra and surrounding region that occurs during sexual intercourse, which can lead to urethritis and cystitis. Bacteriuria is about 10 times more common in sexually active women than in nuns. The foreskin causes trouble again in urinary tract infection by fecal bacteria. These infections are commoner in uncircumcized infants because the prepuce may harbor fecal bacteria on its inner surface.

Oropharynx

Microorganisms can invade the oropharynx when mucosal resistance is reduced

Commensal microorganisms in the oropharynx are described in Chapter 18.

Oropharyngeal defenses

The flushing action of saliva provides a natural cleansing mechanism (about 1 liter/day is produced, needing 400 swallows), aided by masticatory and other movements of the tongue, cheek and lips. On the other hand, material borne backwards from the nasopharynx is firmly wiped against the pharynx by the tongue during swallowing and microbes therefore have an opportunity to enter the body at this site. Additional defenses include secretory IgA antibodies, antimicrobial substances such as lysozyme, the normal flora, and the antimicrobial activities of leukocytes present on mucosal surfaces and in saliva.

Mechanisms of oropharyngeal invasion

Attaching to mucosal or tooth surfaces is obligatory for both invading and resident microorganisms. For instance, different types of streptococci make specific attachments via lipoteichoic acid molecules on their pili to the buccal epithelium and tongue (resident *Streptococcus salivarius*), to teeth (resident *Strep. mutans*), or to pharyngeal epithelium (invading *Strep. pyogenes*).

Factors that reduce mucosal resistance allow commensal and other bacteria to invade, as in the cases of gum infections caused by vitamin C deficiency, or of *Candida* invasion (thrush) promoted by changed resident flora after broad spectrum antibiotics. When salivary flow is decreased for 3–4 hours, as between meals, there is a four-fold increase in the number of bacteria in saliva (see Chapter 18). In dehydrated patients salivary flow is greatly reduced and the mouth soon becomes overgrown with bacteria. As at all body surfaces, there is a shifting boundary between good behavior by residents and tissue invasion according to changes in host defenses.

EXIT AND TRANSMISSION

Microorganisms have a variety of mechanisms to ensure exit from the host and transmission

Successful microbes must leave the body and then be transmitted to fresh hosts. Highly pathogenic microbes (e.g. Ebola virus, *Legionella pneumophila*) will have little impact on host populations if their transmission from person to person is uncommon or ineffective. Nearly all microbes are shed from body surfaces, this being the route of exit to the outside world. Some, however, are extracted from inside the body by vectors, for example the blood-sucking arthropods that transmit yellow fever, malaria and filarial worms. *Figure 13.12* lists the types of infection and their role in the transmission of the microbe and provides a summary of the host defenses and the ways in which they are evaded. Transfer from one host to another forms the basis for the epidemiology of infectious disease (see Chapter 31).

Transmission depends upon three factors:

- the number of microorganisms shed;
- the microorganism's stability in the environment;
- the number of microorganisms required to infect a fresh host (the efficiency of the infection).

TYPES OF INFECTION AND THEIR ROLE IN TRANSMISSION				
type of infection	host defenses	microbial evasion mechanism	examples	value of evasion mechanism in transmission
respiratory tract	mucociliary clearance alveolar macrophage	adhere to epithelial cells, interfere with ciliary action replicate in alveolar macrophage	influenza virus, pertussis *Legionella*, tuberculosis	essential essential
intestinal tract	mucus, peristalsis acid, bile	adhere to epithelial cells resist acid, bile	rotavirus, *Salmonella* poliovirus	essential essential
liver	Kupffer cells and endothelial cells	localize in sinusoid, bypass Kupffer cells and endothelial cells	hepatitis viruses	essential: • microbe from liver → bile → gut (hepatitis A); • microbe from liver → blood (hepatitis B, yellow fever)
reproductive tract	flushing action of urine and sexual secretions, mucosal defenses	adhere to urethral/vaginal epithelial cells	gonococcus, *Chlamydia*	essential
urinary tract	flushing action of urine	adhere to urethral/epithelial cells reach urine from tubular epithelium	*Escherichia coli* polyomavirus	no value valuable
central nervous system	enclosed in bony 'box' of skull and vertebral column	reach CNS via nerves or blood vessels that enter skull or vertebral column	bacterial meningitis, viral encephalitis (e.g. rabies)	no value (except rabies)
skin, mucosa	layers of constantly shed cells (mucosa) dead keratinized cell layers (skin)	invade skin/mucosa from below infect basal epidermal layer infect via minor abrasions	varicella, measles papillomaviruses staphylococci, streptococci	essential essential valuable
		penetrate intact skin	schistosomiasis, ankylostomiasis, anthrax	essential
vascular system	skin	injection of microbe by biting vector, replication in blood cells or in vascular endothelial cells	malaria, yellow fever	essential

Fig. 13.12 Types of infection. For each type of host defense the successful microbe has an answer, which may or may not be important for transmission.

Number of microorganisms shed

Obviously the more virus particles, bacteria, protozoa and eggs that are shed, the greater the chance of reaching a fresh host. There are, however, many hazards. Most of the shed microorganisms die, and only an occasional one survives to perpetuate the species.

Stability in the environment

Microorganisms that resist drying spread more rapidly in the environment than those that are sensitive to drying (*Fig. 13.13*). Microorganisms also remain infectious for longer periods in the external environment when they are resistant to thermal inactivation. Certain microorganisms

MICROBIAL RESISTANCE TO DRYING AS A FACTOR IN TRANSMISSION		
stability on drying	examples	consequence
stable	tubercle bacilli staphylococci	spread more readily in air (dust, dried droplets)
	clostridial spores anthrax spores histoplasmal spores	spread readily from soil
unstable	Neisseria meningitidis streptococci Bordetella pertussis common cold viruses influenza virus measles	require close (respiratory) contact
	gonococci HIV Treponema pallidum	require close (sexual) contact
	polioviruses hepatitis A Vibrio cholerae leptospira	spread via water, food
	yellow fever virus malaria trypanosomes	spread via vectors (i.e. remain in a host)
	larvae/eggs of worms	need moist soil (except pinworms)

Fig. 13.13 Microbial resistance to drying as a factor in transmission. Microbes that are already dehydrated such as spores and artificially freeze-dried viruses are also more resistant to thermal inactivation. Spores can survive for years in soil.

have developed special forms (e.g. clostridial spores, amebic cysts) that enable them to resist drying, heat inactivation and chemical insults, and this testifies to the importance of stability in the environment. If still alive, microorganisms are more thermostable when they have dried. Drying directly from the frozen state (freeze-drying) can make them very resistant to environmental temperatures. The fact that spores and cysts are dehydrated accounts for much of their stability. Microorganisms that are sensitive to drying depend for their spread on close contact, vectors, or contamination of food and water for spread.

Number of microorganisms required to infect a fresh host

The efficiency of the infection varies greatly between microorganisms, and helps explain many aspects of transmission. For instance, volunteers ingesting 10 *Shigella dysenteriae*

bacteria (from other humans) will become infected, whereas as many as 10^6 *Salmonella* spp. (from animals) are needed to cause food poisoning. The route of infection also matters. A single tissue culture infectious dose of a human rhinovirus instilled into the nasal cavity causes a common cold, and although this dose contains many virus particles, about 200 such doses are needed when applied to the pharynx. As few as 10 gonococci can establish an infection in the urethra, but many thousand times this number are needed to infect the mucosa of the oropharynx or rectum.

Other factors affecting transmission

Genetic factors in microorganisms also influence transmission. Some strains of a given microorganism are therefore more readily transmitted than others, although the exact mechanism is often unclear. Transmission can vary independently of the ability to do damage and cause disease (pathogenicity or virulence).

Activities of the infected host may increase the efficiency of shedding and transmission. Coughing and sneezing are reflex activities that benefit the host by clearing foreign material from the upper and lower respiratory tract, but they also benefit the microorganism. Strains of microorganism that are more able to increase fluid secretions or irritate respiratory epithelium will induce more coughing and sneezing than those less able and will be transmitted more effectively. They will therefore be positively selected for. Similar arguments can be applied to the equivalent intestinal activity—diarrhea. Although diarrhea eliminates the infection more rapidly (prevention of diarrhea often prolongs intestinal infection), from the microbe's point of view it is a highly effective way of contaminating the environment and spreading to fresh hosts.

TYPES OF TRANSMISSION BETWEEN HUMANS

Microorganisms can be transmitted to humans by humans, vertebrates and biting arthropods. Transmission is most effective when it takes place directly from human to human. The commonest worldwide infections are spread by the respiratory, fecal–oral or venereal routes. A separate set of infections are acquired from animals, either directly from vertebrates (the zoonoses) or from biting arthropods. Infections acquired from other species are either not transmitted or transmit very poorly from human to human. Types of transmission are illustrated in *Figure 13.14*.

Transmission from the respiratory tract
Respiratory infections spread rapidly when people are crowded together indoors

An increase in nasal secretions with sneezing and coughing promotes effective shedding from the nasal cavity. In a sneeze *(Fig. 13.15)* up to 20 000 droplets are produced, and during a common cold, for instance, many of them will contain virus particles.

A smaller number of microorganisms (hundreds) are expelled from the mouth, throat, larynx and lungs during coughing (whooping cough, tuberculosis). Talking is a less important source of airborne particles, but does produce

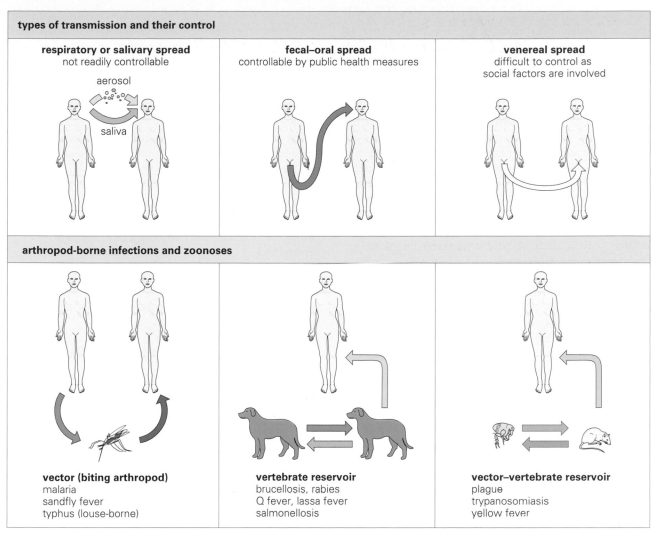

types of transmission and their control

respiratory or salivary spread
not readily controllable

aerosol

saliva

fecal–oral spread
controllable by public health measures

venereal spread
difficult to control as
social factors are involved

arthropod-borne infections and zoonoses

vector (biting arthropod)
malaria
sandfly fever
typhus (louse-borne)

vertebrate reservoir
brucellosis, rabies
Q fever, lassa fever
salmonellosis

vector–vertebrate reservoir
plague
trypanosomiasis
yellow fever

Fig. 13.14 Types of transmission and their control. Arthropod-borne infections and zoonoses can be controlled by controlling vectors or by controlling animal infection; there is virtually no person to person transmission of these infections.

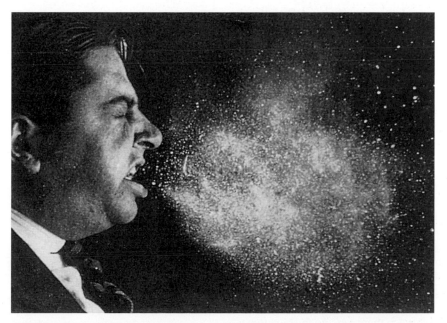

Fig. 13.15 Droplet dispersal following a violent sneeze. Most of the 20 000 particles seen are coming from the mouth. (Reprinted with permission from FR Moulton (ed.), *Aerobiology*, 1942. American Association for the Advancement of Science.)

them, especially when the consonants f, p, t and s are used. It is surely no accident that many of the most abusive words in the English language begin with these letters, so that a spray of droplets (possibly infectious) is delivered with the abuse!

The size of inhaled droplets determines their initial localization. The largest droplets fall to the ground after traveling approximately 4 m, and the rest settle according to size. Those 10 mm or so in diameter can be trapped on the nasal mucosa. The smallest (1–4 mm diameter) are kept suspended for an indefinite period by normal air movements, and it is particles of this size that are likely to pass the turbinate baffles in the nose and reach the lower respiratory tract.

When people are crowded together indoors, respiratory infections spread rapidly—for example the common cold in schools and offices and meningococcal infections in military recruits. This is perhaps why respiratory infections are common in winter. The air in ill-ventilated rooms is also more humid, favoring survival of suspended microorganisms such as streptococci and enveloped viruses. Air conditioning is another factor, as the dry air leads to impaired mucociliary activity. Respiratory spread is, in one sense, unique. Material from one person's respiratory tract can be taken up almost immediately into the respiratory tract of other individuals. This is in striking contrast to the material expelled from the gastrointestinal tract, and helps explain why respiratory infections spread so rapidly when people are indoors.

Handkerchiefs, hands and other objects can carry respiratory infection such as common cold viruses from one individual to another, although coughs and sneezes provide a more dramatic route. Transmission from the infected conjunctiva is referred to in Chapter 25.

The presence of receptors (*Fig. 13.4*) and local temperature as well as initial localization can determine which part of the respiratory tract is infected. For instance, it can be assumed that rhinoviruses arrive in the lower respiratory tract on a large scale, but fail to grow there because, like leprosy bacilli, they prefer the cooler temperature of the nasal mucosa.

Transmission from the gastrointestinal tract

Intestinal infection spreads easily if public health and hygiene are poor

The spread of an intestinal infection is assured if public health and hygiene are poor, the microbe appears in the feces in sufficient numbers and there are susceptible individuals in the vicinity. Diarrhea gives it an additional advantage, and the key role of diarrhea in transmission has been referred to above. During most of human history there has been a large scale recycling of fecal material back into the mouth, and this continues in developing countries. The attractiveness of the fecal–oral route for microorganisms and parasites is reflected in the great variety that are transmitted in this way.

Intestinal infections have been to some extent controlled in developed countries. The great public health reforms of the 19th century led to the introduction of adequate sewage disposal and a supply of purified water. For instance, in England two hundred years ago there were no flushing toilets and no sewage disposal and much of the drinking water was contaminated. Cholera and typhoid spread easily, and in

London the Thames became an open sewer. Nowadays, as in other cities, a complex underground disposal system separates sewage from drinking water. Intestinal infections are still transmitted in developed countries, but via food and fingers rather than by water and flies. Therefore, although each year in the UK there are dozens of cases of typhoid acquired on visits to developing countries, the infection is not transmitted to others.

The microorganisms that appear in feces usually multiply in the lumen or wall of the intestinal tract, but there are a few that are shed into bile. For instance, hepatitis A (enterovirus 72) enters bile after replicating in liver cells.

Transmission from the urinogenital tract

Urinogenital tract infections are often sexually transmitted

Urinary tract infections are common, but most are not spread via urine. Urine can contaminate food, drink and living space. Those infections that are spread by urine are listed in *Figure 13.16*.

Sexually transmitted diseases (STDs)

Microorganisms shed from the urinogenital tract are often transmitted as a result of mucosal contact with susceptible

HUMAN INFECTIONS TRANSMITTED VIA URINE		
infection	details	value in transmission
schistosomiasis	parasite eggs excreted in bladder	+++
typhoid	bacterial persistence in bladder scarred by schistosomiasis	+
polyomavirus infection	commonly excreted in urine in normal pregnancy	?
cytomegalovirus infection	commonly excreted in infected children	?
leptospirosis	infected rats and dogs excrete bacteria in urine	++
lassa fever (and South American hemorrhagic fevers)	persistently infected rodent excretes virus in urine	+++

Fig. 13.16 Human infections transmitted via urine. Schistosomiasis is the major infection transmitted in this way, the eggs undergoing development in snails before reinfecting humans. Viruses are shed in the urine after infecting tubular epithelial cells in the kidney.

individuals, typically as a result of sexual activity. If there is a discharge, organisms are carried over the epithelial surfaces and transmission is more likely. Some of the most successful sexually transmitted microorganisms (gonococci, chlamydia) therefore induce a discharge. Other microorganisms are transmitted effectively from mucosal sores (ulcers), for example *Treponema pallidum* and herpes simplex virus. The human papillomaviruses are transmitted from genital warts or from foci of infection in the cervix where the epithelium, although apparently normal, is dysplastic and contains infected cells (see Chapter 21).

The transmission of STDs is determined by social and sexual activity. Recent changes in the size of the human population and way of life have had a dramatic effect on the epidemiology of STDs. People now have an increased number of sexual partners because of increasing population density, increased movement of people, the decline of the idea that sexual activity is sinful and the knowledge that STDs are treatable and pregnancy is avoidable. In addition, the contraceptive pill has favored the spread of STDs by discouraging the use of mechanical barriers to conception. Condoms have been shown to reliably retain herpes simplex virus, HIV, chlamydia and gonococci in simulated coital tests of the syringe and plunger type (see Chapter 21).

STDs are, however, transmitted with far less speed and efficiency than respiratory or intestinal infections. Influenza can be transmitted to a multitude of others during one hour in a crowded room, or a rotavirus to a score of children during a morning at kindergarten, but STDs can only spread to each person by a separate sexual act. Promiscuity is therefore essential. Frequent sexual activity is not enough without promiscuity because stable partners can do no more than infect each other. The increased general level of promiscuity in society together with the huge numbers of sexual partners of certain individuals such as prostitutes has led to a dramatic rise in the incidence of STDs.

As almost all mucosal surfaces of the body can be involved in sexual activity, microorganisms have had increasing opportunity to infect new body sites. The meningococcus, a nasopharyngeal resident, has therefore sometimes been recovered from the cervix, the male urethra, and the anal canal, while occasionally gonococci and chlamydia infect the throat and anal canal. The possibilities are illustrated in all their complexity in *Figure 13.17*, apparently limited only by anatomic considerations. It is no surprise that genito-oro-anal contacts have sometimes allowed intestinal infections such as salmonella, giardia, hepatitis A, shigella, and pathogenic amebae to spread directly between individuals despite good sanitation and sewage disposal.

Semen as a source of infection

It might be expected that semen is involved in the transmission of infection, and this is the case in viral infections of animals such as blue tongue and foot and mouth disease. In humans, cytomegalovirus is often present in large quantities in semen, and the fact that it is also recoverable from the cervix suggests that it is sexually transmitted. Hepatitis B and HIV are also present in semen, and although the quantities are probably small, their presence plays a role in both homosexual and heterosexual transmission.

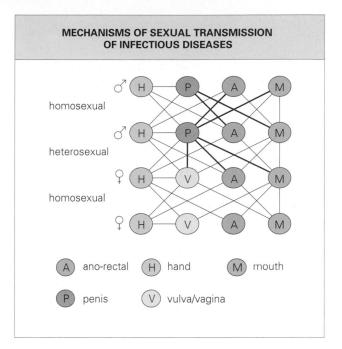

Fig. 13.17 The mechanisms of sexual transmission of infection. (Redrawn from Wilcox RR, The rectum as viewed by the venereologist. Br J Ven Dis 1981; 57:1–6.)

Perinatal transmission

The female genital tract can also be a source of infection for the newborn child (see Chapter 23). During passage down an infected birth canal, microorganisms can be wiped onto the conjunctiva of the infant or inhaled, leading to a variety of conditions such as conjunctivitis, pneumonia and bacterial meningitis.

Transmission from the oropharynx
Oropharyngeal infections are often spread in saliva

Saliva is often the vehicle of transmission. Microorganisms such as streptococci and tubercle bacilli reach saliva during upper and lower respiratory tract infections, while certain viruses infect the salivary glands and are transmitted in this way. Paramyxovirus, herpes simplex virus, cytomegalovirus and human herpesvirus type 6 are shed into saliva. In young children, fingers and other objects are regularly contaminated by saliva, and each of these infections is acquired by this route. Epstein–Barr virus is also shed into saliva, but is transmitted less effectively, perhaps because it is present only in cells or in small amounts. In developed countries people often escape infection during childhood, and become infected as adolescents or adults during the extensive salivary exchanges (mean 4.2 ml/h) that accompany deep kissing (see Chapter 18). Saliva from animals is the source of a few infections, and these are included in *Figure 13.18*.

Transmission from the skin
Skin can spread infection by shedding or direct contact

Dermatophytes (fungi such as those that cause ringworm) are shed from skin and also from hair and nails, the exact source

HUMAN INFECTIONS TRANSMITTED VIA SALIVA	
microorganism	**comments**
herpes simplex, paramyxovirus	infection generally during childhood
cytomegalovirus, Epstein–Barr virus	adolescent/adult infection is common
rabies virus	shed in saliva of infected dogs, wolves, jackals, vampire bats, etc.
Pasteurella multocida	bacteria in upper respiratory tract of dogs, cats, etc. appears in saliva and is transmitted via bites, scratches
Streptobacillus moniliformis	present in rat saliva and infects man (rat bite fever)

Fig. 13.18 Human infections transmitted via saliva.

depending on the type of fungus (see Chapter 26). Skin is also an important source of certain other bacteria and viruses, as outlined in *Figure 13.19*.

Shedding to the environment

The normal individual sheds desquamated skin scales into the environment at a rate of about 5×10^8/day, the rate depending upon physical activities such as exercise, dressing and undressing. The fine white dust that collects on indoor surfaces, especially in hospital wards, consists largely of skin scales. Staphylococci are present, and different individuals show great variation in staphylococcal shedding, but the reasons are unknown.

Transmission by direct contact or by contaminated fingers is much more common than following release into the environment, and microorganisms transmitted in this way include potentially pathogenic staphylococci and human papillomaviruses.

Transmission in milk

Milk is produced by a skin gland. Microorganisms are rarely shed into human milk, and examples include HIV, cytomegalovirus and human T cell lymphotropic virus 1 (HTLV1), but milk from cows, goats and sheep can be important

INFECTIONS TRANSMITTED FROM THE SKIN		
microorganism	**disease**	**comments**
staphylococci	boils, carbuncles, etc, neonatal skin sepsis	pathogenicity varies, skin lesions or nose picking are common sources of infection
Treponema pallidum	syphilis	mucosal surfaces more infectious than skin
Treponema pertenue	yaws	regular transmission from skin lesions
Streptococcus pyogenes	impetigo	vesicular (epidermal) lesions crusting over, common in children in hot, humid climates
Staphylococcus aureus	impetigo	less common; bullous lesions, especially in newborn
dermatophytes	skin ringworm	different species infect skin, hair, nails
herpes simplex virus	herpes simplex, cold sore	up to 10^6 infectious units per ml of vesicle fluid
varicella-zoster virus	varicella, zoster	vesicular skin lesions occur but transmission is usually respiratory*
coxsackievirus A16	hand, foot and mouth disease	vesicular skin lesions but transmission fecal and respiratory
papillomaviruses	warts	many types**
Leishmania tropica	cutaneous leishmaniasis	skin sores are infectious
Sarcoptes scabei	scabies	eggs from burrows transmitted by hand (also sexually)

Fig. 13.19 Human infections transmitted from the skin. (*Except in zoster, where a localized skin eruption occurs and the respiratory tract is generally unaffected. **Generally direct contact, but plantar warts are commonly spread following contamination of floors.)

HUMAN INFECTIONS TRANSMITTED VIA MILK		
microorganism	type of milk	importance in transmission
mumps virus	human	–
cytomegalovirus	human	–
HIV	human	+
HTLV1	human	+
Brucella	cow, goat, sheep	++
Mycobacterium bovis	cow	++
Coxiella burnetii (Q fever rickettsia)	cow	+
Campylobacter jejuni	cow	++
Salmonella spp. Listeria monocytogenes Staphylococcus spp. Streptocuccus pyogenes Yersinia enterocolitica	cow	+

Fig. 13.20 Human infections transmitted via milk. Human milk is rarely a significant source of infection. All microbes listed are destroyed by pasteurization.

sources of infection (*Fig. 13.20*). Other bacteria can be introduced into milk after collection.

Transmission from blood

Blood can spread infection via arthropods or needles

Blood is often the vehicle of transmission. Microorganisms and parasites spread by blood-sucking arthropods (see below) are effectively shed into the blood. Infectious agents present in blood (hepatitis viruses, HIV) are also transmissible by needles, either in transfused blood or when contaminated needles are used for injections or intravenous drug misuse. Intravenous drug misuse is a well-known factor in the spread of these infections. In addition at least 12 000 million injections are given each year, worldwide, about one in ten of them for vaccines. Unfortunately in parts of the developing world, disposable syringes tend to be used more than once without being properly sterilized in between ('If it still works, use it again'). To prevent this the World Health Organization (WHO) is encouraging the use of new types of syringe in which, for instance, the plunger cannot be withdrawn once it has been pushed in.

TRANSPLACENTAL TRANSMISSION OF INFECTION	
microorganism	effect
rubella virus, cytomegalovirus	placental lesion, abortion, stillbirth, malformation
HIV	childhood AIDS
hepatitis B virus	antigen carriage in infant, but most of these infections are perinatal or postnatal
Treponema pallidum	stillbirth, congenital syphilis with malformation
Listeria monocytogenes	meningoencephalitis
Toxoplasma gondii	stillbirth, CNS disease

Fig. 13.21 Human infections transmitted via the placenta.

Blood is also the source of infection in transplacental transmission and this generally involves initial infection of the placenta (see Chapter 23).

Vertical and horizontal transmission

Vertical transmission takes place between parents and their offspring

When transmission is direct from parents to offspring via for example sperm, ovum, placenta (*Fig. 13.21*), milk or blood, it is referred to as vertical. This is because it can be represented as a vertical flow down a page (*Fig. 13.22*) just like a family pedigree. Other infections, in contrast, are said to be horizontally transmitted, with an individual infecting unrelated individuals by contact, respiratory or fecal–oral spread. Vertically transmitted infections can be subdivided as shown in *Figure 13.23*. Strictly speaking, these infections are able to maintain themselves in the species without spreading horizontally as long as they do not affect the viability of the host. Various retroviruses are known to maintain themselves vertically in animals (e.g. mammary tumor virus in milk, sperm and ovum of mice), but this does not appear to be important in humans, except possibly for HTLV1, where milk transfer seems to be important. There are, however, many retrovirus sequences present in the normal human genome. These DNA sequences are too incomplete to produce infectious virus particles, but can be regarded as amazingly successful parasites. They presumably do no harm and survive within the human species, watched over, conserved and replicated as part of our genetic constitution.

TRANSMISSION FROM ANIMALS

Humans and animals share a common susceptibility to certain pathogens

Humans live in daily contact, directly or indirectly, with a wide variety of other animal species, both vertebrate and

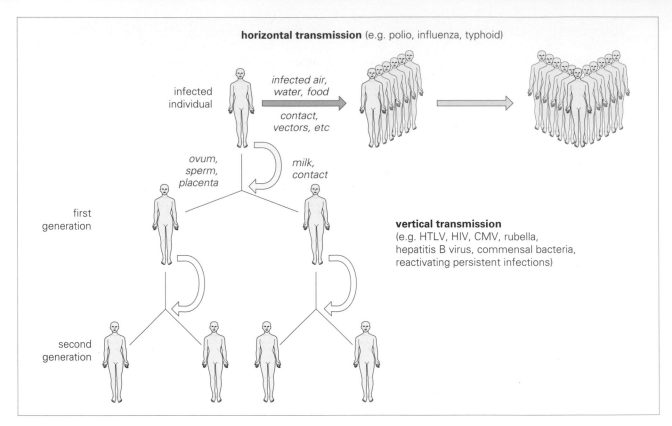

horizontal transmission (e.g. polio, influenza, typhoid)

infected individual

infected air, water, food

contact, vectors, etc

ovum, sperm, placenta

milk, contact

first generation

vertical transmission
(e.g. HTLV, HIV, CMV, rubella, hepatitis B virus, commensal bacteria, reactivating persistent infections)

second generation

Fig. 13.22 Vertical and horizontal transmission by infection. Most infections are transmitted horizontally, as might be expected in crowded human populations. Vertical transmission becomes more important in small isolated communities (see Chapter 17). (CMV, cytomegalovirus; HTLV, human T cell lymphotropic virus.)

TYPES OF VERTICAL TRANSMISSION		
type	**route**	**examples**
prenatal	placenta	rubella cytomegalovirus syphilis toxoplasmosis
perinatal	infected birth canal	gonococcal/ chlamydial conjunctivitis hepatitis B
postnatal	milk or direct contact	cytomegalovirus hepatitis B HIV, HTLV1
germline	viral DNA sequences in human genome	many retroviruses

Fig. 13.23 Types of vertical transmission. (HTLV, human T cell lymphotropic virus.)

invertebrate, not only sharing a common environment, but also a common susceptibility to certain pathogens. The degree to which animal contacts transmit infection depends upon the type of environment (urban/rural, tropical/temperate, hygienic/insanitary) and on the nature of the contact. Close contact is made with vertebrate animals used for food or as pets, and with invertebrate animals adapted to live or feed on the human body. Less intimate contact is made with many other species, which nevertheless may transmit pathogens equally well. For convenience, animal-transmitted infections can be divided into two categories:

• those involving arthropod and other invertebrate vectors;
• those transmitted directly from vertebrates (zoonoses).

More detailed accounts of these infections are given in Chapters 27 and 28.

Invertebrate vectors

Insects, ticks and mites—the bloodsuckers—are the most important vectors spreading infection

By far the most important vectors of disease belong to these three groups of arthropods. Many species are capable of transmitting infection, and a wide range of organisms is transmitted *(Fig. 13.24).* In the past, insects have been responsible for some of the most devastating epidemic diseases, for example fleas and plague and lice and typhus. Even today one of the world's most important infectious diseases, malaria, is transmitted by the *Anopheles* mosquito. The distribution and epidemiology of these infections are determined by the climatic conditions that allow the vectors to breed and the organism to complete its development in their bodies. Some diseases are therefore purely tropical and subtropical, for example malaria, sleeping sickness and yellow

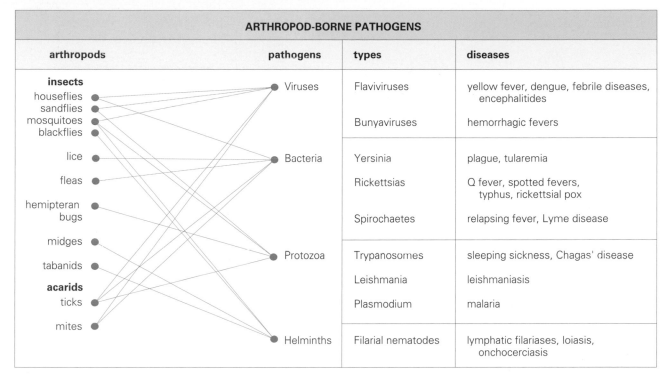

ARTHROPOD-BORNE PATHOGENS			
arthropods	pathogens	types	diseases
insects	Viruses	Flaviviruses	yellow fever, dengue, febrile diseases, encephalitides
houseflies			
sandflies		Bunyaviruses	hemorrhagic fevers
mosquitoes			
blackflies			
lice	Bacteria	Yersinia	plague, tularemia
fleas		Rickettsias	Q fever, spotted fevers, typhus, rickettsial pox
hemipteran bugs		Spirochaetes	relapsing fever, Lyme disease
midges	Protozoa	Trypanosomes	sleeping sickness, Chagas' disease
tabanids		Leishmania	leishmaniasis
acarids		Plasmodium	malaria
ticks			
mites	Helminths	Filarial nematodes	lymphatic filariases, loiasis, onchocerciasis

Fig. 13.24 Arthropod-borne pathogens. Mosquitoes are a major source of infection. Note that, with the exception of pneumonic plague, none is transmitted from human to human.

fever, while others are much more widespread, for example plague and typhus.

Passive carriage

Insects may carry pathogens passively on their mouth parts, on their bodies, or within their intestines. Transfer onto food or onto the host occurs directly as a result of the insect feeding, regurgitating or defecating. Many important diseases, such as trachoma, can be transmitted in this way by common species such as houseflies and cockroaches.

Blood-feeding species have mouthparts adapted for penetrating skin in order to reach blood vessels or to create small pools of blood (*Fig. 13.25*). The ability to feed in this way provides access to organisms in the skin or blood. The mouthparts can act as a contaminated hypodermic needle, carrying infection between individuals.

Biologic transmission

This is much more common, the blood-sucking vector acting as a necessary host for the multiplication and development of the pathogen. Almost all of the important infections (listed in *Fig. 13.24*) are transmitted in this way. The pathogen is reintroduced into the human host, after a period of time, at the next blood meal. Transmission can be by direct injection, usually in the vector's saliva (malaria, yellow fever), or by contamination from feces or regurgitated blood deposited at the time of feeding (typhus, plague).

Other invertebrate vectors spread infection either passively or by acting as an intermediate host

Many invertebrates used for food convey pathogens (*Fig. 13.26*). Perhaps the most familiar are the shellfish

Fig. 13.25 Female *Anopheles* mosquito feeding. (Courtesy of CJ Webb.)

(molluscs and crustacea) associated with food poisoning and acute gastroenteritis. These aquatic animals accumulate viruses and bacteria in their bodies, taking them in from contaminated waste, and transferring them passively. In other cases the relationship between the pathogen and the invertebrate is much closer. Many parasites, especially worms, must undergo part of their development in the invertebrate before being able to infect a human. Humans are infected when they eat the invertebrate (intermediate) host. Dietary habits are therefore important in infection.

Aquatic molluscs (snails) are necessary intermediate hosts for schistosomes—the blood flukes. They become infected by larval stages, which hatch from eggs passed into water in the urine or feces of infected people. After a period of

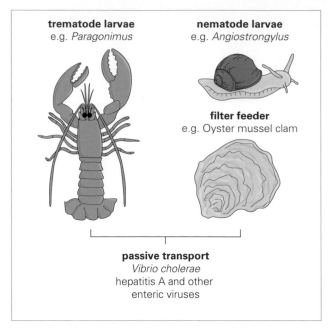

Fig. 13.26 Microorganisms transmitted via invertebrates used for food. Filter-feeding molluscs living in estuaries near sewage outlets are a common source of infection.

development and multiplication large numbers of infective stages (cercariae) escape from the snails. These can rapidly penetrate through human skin, initiating the infection that will result in adult flukes occupying visceral blood vessels (see Chapter 30).

Transmission from vertebrates

Many pathogens are transmitted directly to humans from vertebrate animals

Strictly, the term zoonoses can apply to any infection transmitted to humans from infected animals, whether this is direct (by contact or eating) or indirect (via an invertebrate vector). Here, however, zoonoses are used to describe infections of vertebrate animals that can be transmitted directly. Many pathogens are transmitted in this way *(Fig. 13.27)* by a variety of different routes including contact, inhalation, bites, scratches, contamination of food or water, and ingestion as food.

The epidemiology of zoonoses depends upon the frequency and the nature of contact between the vertebrate and the human hosts. Some are localized geographically, being dependent for example upon local food preferences. Where these involve eating uncooked animal products such as fish or amphibia, a variety of parasites (especially tapeworms and nematodes) can be acquired. Others are associated with occupation, for example if this involves contact with raw animal products (butchers in the case of toxoplasmosis and Q fever) or frequent contact with domestic stock (farm workers in the case of brucellosis and dermatophyte fungi). In urban areas, zoonoses are most likely to be acquired by eating or drinking infected animal products or by contact with dogs, cats and other domestic pets.

ZOONOSES—HUMAN INFECTIONS TRANSMITTED FROM VERTEBRATES		
pathogens	vertebrate vector	diseases
viruses		
arenaviruses	mammals	Lassa fever, lymphocytic choriomeningitis, Bolivian hemorrhagic fever
poxviruses	mammals	cowpox, orf
rhabdoviruses	mammals	rabies
bacteria		
Bacillus anthracis	mammals	anthrax
Brucella	mammals	brucella
Chlamydia	birds	psittacosis
Leptospira	mammals	leptospirosis (Weil's disease)
Listeria	mammals	listeriosis
Salmonella	birds, mammals	salmonellosis
Mycobacterium tuberculosis	mammals	tuberculosis
fungi		
Cryptococcus	birds	meningitis
dermatophytes	mammals	ringworm
protozoa		
Cryptosporidium	mammals	cryptosporidiosis
Giardia	mammals	giardiasis
Toxoplasma	mammals	toxoplasmosis
helminths		
Ancylostoma	mammals	hookworm disease
Echinococcus	mammals	hydatid disease
Taenia	mammals	tapeworms
Toxocara	mammals	toxocariasis (visceral larval migrans)
Trichinella	mammals	trichinellosis

Fig. 13.27 Human infections transmitted directly from vertebrates (birds and mammals).

Domestic pets or pests?

Dogs and cats are the commonest domestic pets, and both are reservoirs of infection for their owners *(Fig. 13.28)*. The pathogens concerned are spread by contact, bites and scratches, by vectors, and by contamination with fecal material. Major infections transmitted in these ways include:

- toxocariasis from dogs;
- toxoplasmosis from cat.

Both are almost universal in their distribution.

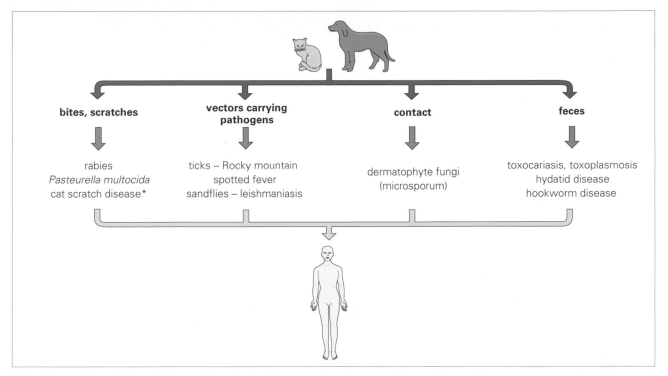

Fig. 13.28 Man's best friends? Zoonoses transmitted from dogs and cats. (*A benign infection, with skin lesions and lymphadenopathy, shown to be due to a recently discovered bacterium, *Afipia catei*.)

Humans may acquire hydatid disease from tapeworm eggs passed in dog feces where dogs are used for herding domestic animals and have access to infected carcasses. In rural areas of many countries this has been, or remains, an important infection.

Many species of birds are kept as pets and some can pass on serious infections to those in contact with them. Contact is usually through inhalation of infected particulate material. Perhaps the most important of these is psittacosis caused by *Chlamydophila* (formerly *Chlamydia*) *psittaci*, which despite the common name 'parrot fever' can be acquired from many avian species.

The recent trend in developed countries towards keeping unusual or exotic pets (especially reptiles, exotic birds and mammals) raises new risks of zoonotic infection. Many reptiles, for example, pass human-infective *Salmonella* spp. in their droppings. Exotic birds and mammals can carry a range of viruses that could be transmitted under the correct conditions. Diagnosis of infections under these circumstances can be difficult if the physician does not know of the existence of such pets.

KEY FACTS

- To establish infection in the host, microbes must attach to, or pass across, body surfaces.

- Many microbes have developed chemical or mechanical mechanisms to attach themselves to the surface of the respiratory, urinogenital or alimentary tracts. In the skin they generally depend upon entry via small wounds or arthropod bites.

- Microbes must exit from the body after replication in order to be transmitted to fresh hosts. This also takes place across body surfaces.

- Efficient shedding of microbes from the skin or respiratory, urinogenital or alimentary tracts, or delivery into the blood or dermal tissues for uptake during arthropod feeding, are vital stages in their lifecycles.

- Many human infections come from animals, either directly (zoonoses) or indirectly (via blood-sucking arthropods), and the incidence of these infections depends upon exposure to infected animals or arthropods.

? QUESTIONS

1. Place the following types of transmission in order according to the speed with which the infection generally spreads in the community: sexual, fecal–oral, respiratory, zoonotic.

2. Why are so many arthropod-borne infections and zoonoses not transmitted directly from human to human?

3. Would you expect urine to be an effective vehicle for transmitting an infection? If not, why not?

4. Could you transmit a respiratory infection to others if you did not cough or sneeze?

5. List the routes and the tissues or the cells involved in vertical transmission.

6. Is there anything to stop a microbe, transmitted by the sexual route, that attaches to and infects urethral epithelial cells, from doing the same to respiratory epithelial cells?

FURTHER READING

Cohen MS, Sparling PF. Mucosal infection with *Neisseria gonorrhoeae*. *J Clin Investig* 1992; 89:1699–1705.

Falkow S. Bacterial entry into eukaryotic cells. *Cell* 1991; 65:1099–1102.

Haywood AM. Virus receptors: binding, adhesion, strengthening and changes in viral structure. *Virology* 1994; 68:1–5.

Mims CA. The transmission of infection. *Rev Med Microbiol* 1995; 6:217–27.

Mims CA, Nash A, Stephen J. *Mims' Pathogenesis of Infectious Disease*, 5th edition. London: Academic Press, 2001.

Simonsen L, Kane A, Lloyd J et al. Unsafe injections in the developing world and transmission of blood-borne pathogens: a review. *Bull WHO* 1999; 77:789–800.

Warren KS. The control of helminths; non-replicating infectious agents of man. *Am Rev Publ Health* 1981; 2:101–16.

INTRODUCTION

The barrier effects of the skin and mucous membranes and their adjuncts such as cilia have already been referred to (see Chapter 9). We now turn to the back-up mechanisms called rapidly into play when an organism has penetrated these barriers—namely, complement, the phagocytic and cytotoxic cells, and a variety of cytotoxic molecules. While they lack the dramatic specificity and memory of adaptive (i.e. lymphocyte-based) immune mechanisms, these natural defenses are vital to survival—particularly in invertebrates, where they are the only defense against infection (adaptive responses only evolved with the earliest vertebrates).

In addition to these non-specific mechanisms, the immune system enables the specific recognition of antigens by T and B cells as part of adaptive immunity. Broadly speaking, antibodies are particularly important in combatting infection by extracellular microbes, particularly pyogenic bacteria, while T cell immunity is required to control intracellular infections with bacteria, viruses, fungi or protozoa. Their value is illustrated by the generally disastrous results of defects in T and/or B cells, or their products, discussed in more detail in Chapter 30. This chapter gives examples of how these different types of immunity contribute to the body's defenses against microbes.

Antimicrobial peptides protect the skin against invading bacteria

A number of proteins that are expressed at epithelial surfaces, and by polymorphonuclear leukocytes (PMNs), can have a direct antibacterial effect. These include β-defensins, dermicidins and cathelicidins. Dermicidin is made by sweat glands and secreted into sweat; it is active against *Escherichia coli*, *Staphylococcus aureus* and *Candida albicans*. Mice whose PMNs and keratinocytes are unable to make cathelicidin become susceptible to infection with group A streptococcus.

Lysozyme is one of the most abundant antimicrobial proteins in the lung. Genetically engineered transgenic mice that had two to four times more lysozyme than control mice in their bronchoalveolar lavage were shown to be much better at killing group B streptococci. The transgenic mice were also more resistant to infection by *Pseudomonas aeruginosa* (*Fig. 14.1*).

COMPLEMENT

The alternative pathway of complement activation is part of the early defense system

The basic biology of the complement system and its role in inducing the inflammatory response and promoting chemotaxis, phagocytosis and vascular permeability have been described in Chapter 9. Here we are concerned with its ability to directly damage microorganisms as part of the early response to infection. Contrary to what might be expected from the dramatic lysis of many kinds of bacteria in the test tube, the action of complement in vivo is restricted mainly to the neisseria. Patients deficient in C5, C6, C7, C8 or C9 are unable to eliminate gonococci and meningococci, with the increased risk of developing septicemia or becoming a carrier.

It should be emphasized that only the alternative pathway of complement activation or the mannan-binding lectin pathway form part of this natural 'early defense' system. Activation through the classical pathway occurs only after an antibody response has been made. It is not surprising to learn,

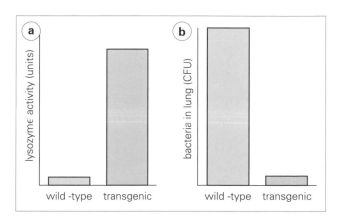

Fig. 14.1 Transgenic mice making greater amounts of lysozyme are more resistant to infection with *Pseudomonas aeruginosa*. (a) The transgenic mice made 18-fold more lysozyme than the wild-type control mice. (b) The transgenic mice showed much greater killing of *Pseudomonas aeruginosa* in the lungs following intratracheal infection than the wild-type mice. (Redrawn from from Akinbi et al. *J Immunol* 2000; 165:5760).

therefore, that the alternative pathway appears to have evolved first.

ACUTE PHASE PROTEINS AND PATTERN RECOGNITION RECEPTORS

C-reactive protein is an antibacterial agent produced by liver cells in response to cytokines

Among the acute phase proteins produced in the course of most inflammatory reactions, C-reactive protein (CRP) is particularly interesting in being an antibacterial agent, albeit of very restricted range. CRP is a pentameric β-globulin, somewhat resembling a miniature version of IgM (molecular weight 130 000 compared with 900 000 for IgM). It reacts with phosphorylcholine in the wall of some streptococci and subsequently activates both complement and phagocytosis. CRP is produced by liver cells in response to cytokines, particularly interleukin-6 (IL-6, see Chapter 11), and levels can rise as much as 1000-fold in 24 hours—a much more rapid response than that of antibody (see Chapter 9). Therefore, CRP levels are often used to monitor inflammation, for example in rheumatic diseases. Most of the other acute phase proteins are produced in increased amounts early in infection and have not just antimicrobial activity but can act as opsonins, antiproteases, play an immunomodulatory role or be involved in the fibrinolytic or anticoagulant pathways. For example, many of the complement components are acute phase proteins. Those with a role in protection against infection are also termed pattern recognition receptors, such as mannose-binding lectin. Some acute phase proteins such as lipopolysaccharide binding protein may reduce pathology by binding toxic bacterial products such as lipopolysaccharide.

Macrophages can recognize bacteria as foreign using Toll-like receptors

Another family of surface receptors, called Toll-like receptors, on macrophages and other cells, bind conserved microbial molecules such as lipopolysaccharide (LPS) (endotoxin), bacterial DNA, double-stranded RNA or bacterial flagellin. Pattern recognition receptors recognize these repeated structures (pathogen-associated molecular patterns, see Chapter 9) and this leads to release of pro-inflammatory cytokines such as tumor necrosis factor alpha (TNFα), IL-1 and IL-6. Signaling through the Toll-like receptors also leads to the increased expression of major histocompatibility complex (MHC) molecules and of co-stimulatory molecules, thus enhancing antigen presentation and usually leading to the activation of T helper 1 (TH1) cells.

Collectins

Collectins are proteins that bind to carbohydrate molecules expressed on bacterial and viral surfaces. This results in cell recruitment, activation of the alternative complement cascade, and macrophage activation. One of the collectins, surfactant protein A, has been shown to play a role in the innate defense of the lung against infection with group B streptococci. Mice deficient in surfactant protein A were much more susceptible to infection, developing greater pulmonary infiltration and dissemination of bacteria to the spleen, compared with those able to produce the collectin.

Mannan-binding lectin (MBL) is another collectin found in serum. Binding of MBL to carbohydrates containing mannose on microorganisms leads to complement activation, through the mannan-binding lectin pathway. Many individuals have low serum concentrations of MBL due to mutations in the *MBL* gene or its promoter. A recent study of children with malignancies showed that MBL deficiency increased the duration of infections.

FEVER

A raised temperature almost invariably accompanies infection (see Chapter 29). In many cases the cause can be traced to the release of cytokines such as IL-1 or IL-6, which play important roles in both immunity and pathology (see Chapter 11). However, the interesting question as to whether the raised temperature itself is of benefit to the host remains unsettled.

It is probably unwise to generalize about the benefit or otherwise of fever

Several microorganisms have been shown to be susceptible to high temperature. This was the basis for the 'fever therapy' of syphilis by deliberate infection with blood-stage malaria, and the malaria parasite itself may also be damaged by high temperatures, though it is obviously not totally eliminated. In general, however, one would predict that successful parasites were those that were adapted to survive episodes of fever; indeed the 'stress' or 'heat-shock' proteins produced by both mammalian and microbial cells in response to stress of many kinds, including heat, are thought to be part of their protective strategy. On the other hand, several host immune mechanisms might also be expected to be more active at higher temperatures: examples are complement activation, lymphocyte proliferation and the synthesis of proteins such as antibody and cytokines.

NATURAL KILLER CELLS

Natural killer cells are a rapid but non-specific means of controlling viral and other intracellular infections

Natural killer (NK) cells provide an early source of cytokines and chemokines during infection, until there is time for the activation and expansion of antigen-specific T cells. NK cells can provide an important source of interferon-gamma (IFNγ) during the first few days of infection (*Fig. 14.2*). NK cell cytokine production can be induced by monokines such as IL-12 and IL-18 that are in turn induced by macrophages in response to LPS or other microbial components. NK cells can also act as cytotoxic effector cells, lysing host cells infected with viruses and some bacteria, as they make both cytotoxic granules and perforin. They recognize their targets by means of a series of activating and inhibitory receptors that are not antigen-specific. The inhibitory receptors recognize the complex of MHC class I and self peptide; if both this inhibitory receptor and another NK-cell-activating receptor

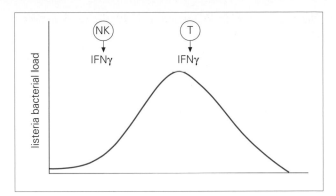

Fig. 14.2 In many intracellular infections, such as with *Listeria*, a source of IFNγ is needed to activate macrophages and induce bacterial killing, but it takes several days for antigen-specific T cells to become activated and proliferate. NK cells can provide a source of IFNγ until the adaptive T cell response can take over. In the period between NK cell and T cell production of IFNγ, some IFNγ may also be produced by other T cell subpopulations, including γδ T cells and NK T cells.

are engaged, the NK cell will not be activated. However if there is insufficient MHC class I on the surface, the inhibitory receptor is not engaged and the NK cell is activated to kill the target cell. This is an effective strategy as some viruses inhibit MHC class I expression on the cells they infect. NK cells are therefore a more rapid but less specific means of controlling viral and other intracellular infections. Their importance is highlighted by the ability of mice lacking both T and B cells (severe combined immunodeficiency, SCID) to control some virus infections.

PHAGOCYTOSIS

Phagocytes engulf, kill and digest would-be parasites

Perhaps the greatest danger to the would-be parasite is to be recognized by a phagocytic cell, engulfed, killed and digested *(Fig. 14.3)*. A description of the various stages of phagocytosis is given in Chapter 9. Phagocytes (principally macrophages) are normally found in the tissues where invading micro-organisms are more likely to be encountered. In addition, phagocytes present in the blood (principally the PMNs) can be rapidly recruited into the tissues when and where required. Only about 1% of the normal adult bone marrow reserve of 3×10^{12} PMNs is present in the blood at any one time, representing a turnover of about 10^{11} PMNs per day. Most macrophages remain within the tissues, and well under 1% are present in the blood as monocytes. PMNs are short lived, but macrophages can live for many years (see below).

Intracellular killing by phagocytes

Phagocytes kill organisms using either an oxidative or a non-oxidative mechanism

The mechanisms by which phagocytes kill the organisms they ingest are traditionally divided into oxidative and non-oxidative, depending upon whether the cell consumes oxygen in the process. Respiration in PMNs is non-mitochondrial

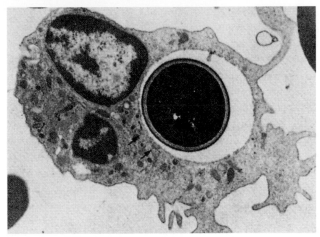

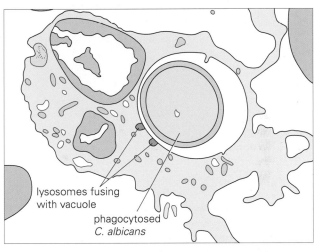

lysosomes fusing with vacuole

phagocytosed *C. albicans*

Fig. 14.3 Electron micrograph and diagrammatic representation of neutrophil containing phagocytosed *Candida albicans*. ×7000. (Courtesy of H Valdimarsson.)

and anaerobic, and the burst of oxygen consumption, the so-called 'respiratory burst' *(Fig. 14.4)*, that accompanies phagocytosis represents the generation of microbicidal reactive oxygen intermediates (ROIs).

Oxidative killing

Oxidative killing involves the use of ROIs

The importance of ROIs in bacterial killing was revealed by the discovery that PMNs from patients with chronic granulomatous disease (CGD) did not consume oxygen after phagocytosing staphylococci. Patients with CGD have one of three kinds of genetic defect in a PMN membrane enzyme system involving nicotinamide adenine dinucleotide phosphate (NADPH) oxidase. The normal activity of this system is the progressive reduction of atmospheric oxygen to water with the production of ROIs such as the superoxide ion, hydrogen peroxide and free hydroxyl radicals, all of which can be extremely toxic to microorganisms *(Fig. 14.5)*.

CGD patients are unable to kill staphylococci and certain other bacteria and fungi, which consequently cause deep chronic abscesses. They can, however, deal with catalase-negative bacteria such as pneumococci because these produce, and do not destroy, their own hydrogen peroxide in sufficient

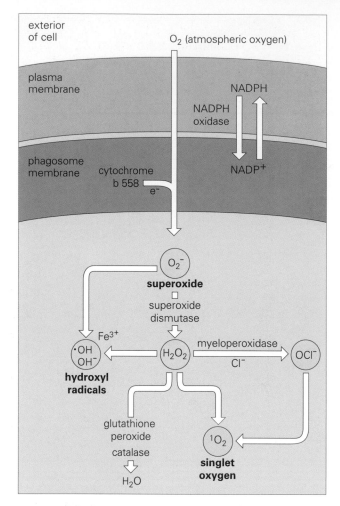

Fig. 14.4 The principal molecules involved in the respiratory burst. Oxygen is progressively reduced by the addition of electrons (e⁻). (NADPH, nicotinamide adenine dinucleotide phosphate.)

The way in which ROIs actually kill microorganisms is controversial

ROIs can damage cell membranes (lipid peroxidation), DNA and proteins (including vital enzymes), but in some cases it may be the altered pH that accompanies the generation of ROIs that does the damage. Killing of some bacteria and fungi (e.g. *Escherichia coli*, *Candida*) occurs only at an acid pH, while killing of others (e.g. staphylococci) occurs at an alkaline pH. There may also be a need for protease activity (e.g. cathepsins, elastase), with enzyme solubilization occurring as a result of the influx of H^+ and K^+ into the phagocytic vesicle.

Cytotoxic lipids prolong the activity of ROIs

As already mentioned, one of the targets of the toxic ROIs is lipid in cell membranes. ROIs are normally extremely short lived (fractions of a second), but their toxicity can be greatly prolonged by interaction with serum lipoproteins to form lipid peroxides. Lipid peroxides are stable for hours and can pass on the oxidative damage to cell membranes, both of the parasite (e.g. malaria-infected red cell) and of the host (e.g. vascular endothelium). The cytotoxic activity of normal serum to some blood trypanosomes has been traced to the high density lipoproteins, and in cotton rats to a macroglobulin.

Non-oxidative killing

Non-oxidative killing involves the use of the phagocyte's cytotoxic granules

Oxygen is not always available for killing microorganisms; indeed some bacteria grow best in anaerobic conditions (e.g. the *Clostridia* of gas gangrene), and oxygen would in any case

---

SOME ORGANISMS KILLED BY REACTIVE OXYGEN AND NITROGEN SPECIES		
bacteria	**fungi**	**protozoa**
Staphylococcus aureus	*Candida albicans*	*Plasmodium*
Escherichia coli	*Aspergillus*	*Leishmania* (nitric oxide)
Serratia marcescens		

Fig. 14.5 Organisms killed by reactive oxygen species.

PMN AND EOSINOPHIL GRANULE CONTENTS		
PMN		**eosinophil**
primary (azurophil)	**specific (heterophil)**	
myeloperoxidase	lysozyme	peroxidase
acid hydrolases	lactoferrin	cationic proteins
cathepsins G, B, D	alkaline phosphatase	ECP
defensins	NADPH oxidase	MBP
BPI	collagenase	neurotoxin
cationic proteins	histaminase	lysophospholipase
lysozyme		

Fig. 14.6 Contents of polymorphonuclear leukocyte (PMN) and eosinophil granules. (BPI, bactericidal permeability increasing protein; ECP, eosinophil cationic protein; MBP, major basic protein; NADPH, nicotinamide adenine dinucleotide phosphate).

---

amounts to interact with the cell myeloperoxidase, producing the highly toxic hypochlorous acid. The defective PMNs from CGD patients can be readily identified in vitro by their failure to reduce the yellow dye nitroblue tetrazolium to a blue compound (the 'NBT test', see Chapter 32).

be in short supply in a deep tissue abscess. Phagocytic cells therefore contain a number of other cytotoxic molecules. The best studied are the proteins in the various PMN granules *(Fig. 14.6)*, which act on the contents of the phagosome as the granules fuse with it. Note that the transient fall in pH accompanying the respiratory burst enhances the activity of the cationic microbicidal proteins and defensins.

Another phagocytic cell, the eosinophil, is particularly rich in cytotoxic granules *(Fig. 14.6)*. The highly cationic (i.e. basic) contents of these granules give them their characteristic acidophilic staining pattern. Five distinct eosinophil cationic proteins are known and seem to be particularly toxic to parasitic worms, at least in vitro. Because of the enormous difference in size between parasitic worms and eosinophils, this type of damage is limited to the outer surfaces of the parasite. The eosinophilia typical of worm infections is presumably an attempt to cope with these large and almost indestructible parasites. Both the production and level of activity of eosinophils is regulated by T cells and macrophages and mediated by cytokines such as interleukin 5 (IL-5) and tumor necrosis factor (TNF).

Monocytes and macrophages also contain cytotoxic granules. Unlike PMNs *(Fig. 14.7)*, macrophages contain little or no myeloperoxidase, but secrete large amounts of lysozyme. Lysozyme is an antibacterial molecule maintained at a concentration of about 30 mg/ml in serum, though this concentration can increase to as high as 800 mg/ml in rare cases of monocytic leukemia. Macrophages are extremely sensitive to activation by bacterial products (e.g. LPS) and T cell products, e.g. IFNγ. Activated macrophages have a greatly enhanced ability to kill both intracellular and extracellular targets.

Nitric oxide

A major secreted product of the activated macrophage is nitric oxide (NO), one of the reactive nitrogen intermediates (RNIs) generated during the conversion of arginine to citrulline by arginase. NO is strongly cytotoxic to a variety of cell types, and RNIs are generated in large amounts during infections (e.g. leishmaniasis, malaria). Arginase can also cause damage by leading to a deprivation of arginine, which is an essential amino acid for some viruses (e.g. herpes simplex) and parasites (e.g. the liver fluke *Schistosoma*).

CYTOKINES

Cytokines contribute to both infection control and infection pathology

Early studies with supernatants from cultures of lymphocytes and macrophages revealed a family of non-antigen-specific molecules with diverse activities, that were involved in cell-to-cell communication. These are now collectively known as 'cytokines'. They play many crucial roles in protection against infectious diseases. The way in which these molecules acquired their sometimes rather misleading names, and the bewildering overlap of function between molecules of quite different structure, are described in detail in Chapter 11.

Cytokines are of importance in infectious disease for two contrasting reasons:

POLYMORPHONUCLEAR LEUKOCYTES AND MACROPHAGES COMPARED		
	PMN	**macrophage**
site of production	bone marrow	bone marrow
duration in marrow	14 days	54 hours
duration in blood	7–10 hours	20–40 hours (monocyte)
average life span	4 days	months–years
numbers in blood	$(2.5$–$7.5) \times 10^9/l$	$(0.2$–$0.8) \times 10^9/l$
marrow reserve	10 × blood	–
numbers in tissues	(transient)	100 × blood
principal killing mechanisms	oxidative non-oxidative	oxidative nitric oxide cytokines
activated by	TNFα, IFNγ, GM-CSF, microbial products	TNFα, IFNγ, GM-CSF, microbial products (e.g. LPS)
important deficiencies	CGD myeloperoxidase chemotactic Chediak–Higashi	lipid storage diseases
major secretory products	lysozyme	over 80, including: lysozyme, cytokines (TNFα, IL-1), complement factors

Fig. 14.7 The major phagocytic cells—PMNs and macrophages—differ in a number of important respects. (CGD, chronic granulomatous disease; GM-CSF, granulocyte–macrophage colony-stimulating factor; IFN, interferon; IL, interleukin; LPS, lipopolysaccharide; TNFα, tumor necrosis factor alpha.)

- They can contribute to the control of infection.
- They can contribute to the development of pathology.

The latter harmful aspect—of which TNF in septic shock is a good example—is discussed in Chapter 12. The beneficial effects can be direct or more often indirect via the induction of some other antimicrobial process.

HUMAN INTERFERONS			
	IFNα	**IFNβ**	**IFNγ**
alternative name	'leukocyte' IFN	'fibroblast' IFN	'immune' IFN
principal source	all cells	all cells	T lymphocytes (NK cells)
inducing agent	viral infection (or dsRNA)	viral infection (or dsRNA)	antigen (or mitogen)
number of species	22*	1	1
chromosomal location of gene(s)	9	9	12
antiviral activity	+++	+++	+
immunoregulatory activity:			
macrophage action	–	–	++
MHC I upregulation	+	+	+
MHC II upregulation	–	–	+
*each species coded by a different gene			

Fig. 14.8 Human interferons (IFNs). (dsRNA, double stranded ribonucleic acid; MHC, major histocompatibility complex.)

Interferons

The best-established antimicrobial cytokines are the interferons (IFNs) *(Fig. 14.8)*. The name is derived from the demonstration in 1957 that virus-infected cells secreted a molecule that interfered with viral replication in bystander cells. IFN of all three types (α, β and γ) interact with specific receptors on most cells, one for α and β and another for γ, following which they induce an antiviral state via the generation of at least two types of enzyme: a protein kinase and a 2′,5′-oligoadenylate synthetase. Both of these enzymes result in the inhibition of viral RNA translation and therefore of protein synthesis *(Fig. 14.9)*.

IFNα and IFNβ constitute a major part of the early response to viruses

IFNα and IFNβ are produced rapidly within 24 hours of infection, and constitute a major part of the early response to viruses. IFNγ is mainly a T cell product and is therefore produced later, although, as discussed above, an early IFNγ response may be mounted by NK cells.

IFNs can also inhibit virus assembly at a later stage (e.g. retroviruses), while many of the other effects of IFN contribute to the antiviral state, for example the enhancement of cellular MHC expression and the activation of NK cells and macrophages *(Fig. 14.10)*. Unlike cytotoxic T cells, IFN normally inhibits viruses without damaging the host cell.

Although best known for their antiviral activity, IFNs have recently been shown to be induced by, and active against, infections with a wide range of organisms, including rickettsia, mycobacteria and several protozoa. The role of IFNγ is discussed further under T cells, below. Some intracellular organisms (e.g. *Leishmania*) can counteract the effect of IFNγ on MHC expression, thereby facilitating their own survival.

In animal experiments, treatment with antibodies to IFNα greatly increases susceptibility to viral infection; conversely, treatment with IFNα has proved useful for some human virus infections, notably chronic hepatitis B (see Chapter 22).

Other cytokines

TNFα production can be good or bad

A striking example of a potentially useful role for TNF in infection is the inhibition of the proliferation of B lymphocytes by Epstein–Barr virus (EBV). EBV infection in people with malaria can lead to Burkitt's lymphoma, a monoclonal tumor of B cells, and TNF levels have been shown to be raised in malaria. However, TNF is also thought to contribute to the pathology of malaria as well as to that due to bacterial endotoxins (see Chapter 12). This illustrates the often confusing role that cytokines play in infectious diseases of all kinds—'enough is enough' and 'too much is dangerous' seem to be the rules for these powerful molecules. Paradoxically, TNF concentration is raised in HIV infection and has been found to enhance the replication of HIV in T cells—a 'positive feedback' with worrying potential. The role of T-cell-derived cytokines such as IFNγ in immunity to infection is discussed below.

ANTIBODY-MEDIATED IMMUNITY

The key property of the antibody molecule is to bind specifically to antigens on the foreign microbe. In many cases this is followed by secondary binding to other cells or molecules of the immune system (e.g. phagocytes, complement). These

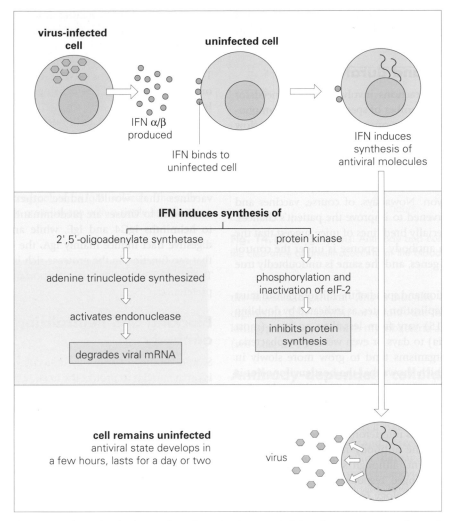

Fig. 14.9 The molecular basis of interferon (IFN) action. (eIF-2, eukaryotic initiation factor 2.

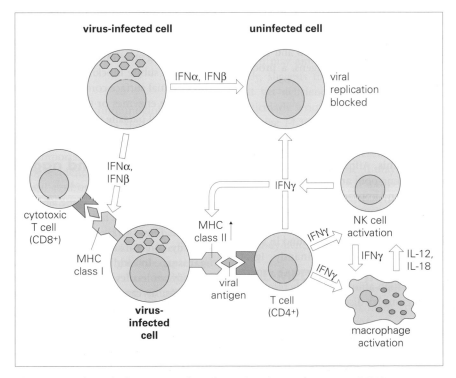

Fig. 14.10 The multiple activities of interferons (IFNs) in viral immunity. (MHC, major histocompatability complex; NK, natural killer.)

ANTIBODY AND CMI IN RESISTANCE TO SYSTEMIC INFECTIONS		
type of resistance	antibody	CMI
recovery from primary infection	yellow fever polioviruses coxsackie viruses	poxviruses: e.g. ectromelia (mice), vaccinia (man) herpes-type viruses: herpes simplex varicella-zoster cytomegalovirus
	streptococci staphylococci *Neisseria meningitidis* *Haemophilus influenzae*	LCM virus (mice) measles tuberculosis leprosy typhoid
	Candida spp. *Giardia lamblia* ?malaria	systemic fungal infections ?chronic mucocutaneous candidiasis
resistance to re-infection	nearly all viruses including measles most bacteria	tuberculosis leprosy
resistance to reactivation of latent infection	?herpes simplex	varicella-zoster cytomegalovirus tuberculosis *Pneumocystis jiroveci**

Fig. 14.14 Antibody and cell-mediated immunity (CMI) in resistance to systemic infections. Either antibody or CMI is known to be the major factor in these examples. But in many other infections there is no information, and sometimes both types of immunity are important. (*formerly *P. carinii*.)

MHC molecule that is recognized by its T cell receptor. Some examples of the importance of antibody and cell-mediated immunity in resistance to systemic infections are given in *Figure 14.14*.

T cell immunity correlates with control of bacterial growth in leprosy

In leprosy, there is a spectrum of disease, ranging from the paucibacillary tuberculoid forms to the multibacillary lepromatous disease. T cell immunity, as measured by lymphocyte proliferation, secretion of TH1 cytokines such as IFNγ, or delayed type hypersensitivity skin testing, is found in response to the antigens of *M. leprae* in patients with tuberculoid leprosy, but lost in patients with lepromatous

leprosy. The value of T cell stimulation leading to macrophage activation and bacterial killing is clearly illustrated by experiments in which lepromatous leprosy patients' skin lesions were injected with IFNγ. This resulted in an influx of T cells and macrophages into the skin lesions, and a reduction in the number of bacteria. Another good example of the protective role of IFNγ and TH1 immunity is seen in animal models of *Leishmania* infection: i.e. some mouse strains such as C57BL/6 are resistant to disease, controlling the infection and making a good TH1 cytokine response, whereas others such as BALB/c are susceptible, fail to make IFNγ and cannot control parasite growth (see *Fig. 14.16*).

The protective effects of making IFNγ, which then binds to its specific receptor on macrophages and induces macrophage activation and the production of antimicrobial molecules, are illustrated very clearly by the consequences of a failure in IFNγ synthesis or of binding to its receptor. Mice in which the gene for IFNγ has been inactivated ('knocked-out') become very susceptible to intracellular infections. Recently, individuals with mutations in the genes for the IFNγ receptor have been indentified. Such individuals are susceptible to infections with mycobacteria, or to disseminated infections following BCG vaccination (*Fig. 14.17*).

Some bacteria evade protective TH1 responses by inducing antigen-specific regulatory T cells. *Bordetella pertussis* infection induces regulatory T cells specific for its filamentous hemagglutinin and pertactin. These regulatory T cells produce IL-10 which then suppresses TH1 immunity.

Is a positive delayed type hypersensitivity skin test an indicator of immunity?

The most widely used test of T cell immunity in man is the delayed type hypersensivity (DTH) skin test, in which induration induced by the intradermal injection of antigen is measured 2–3 days later. Such tests can be used to screen for T cell anergy—for example by using candidin, as most individuals will have been exposed to *Candida*. The most widely used skin test is the Mantoux skin test using antigens from *M. tuberculosis*. However, although production of the TH1 cytokine IFNγ correlates with the skin test response (see *Fig. 14.18*), this test is neither diagnostic nor a correlate of immunity. Unfortunately, many of the antigens in the purified protein derivative of *M. tuberculosis* used as the antigen in this test are cross-reactive with those in other mycobacteria, including BCG and non-tuberculous environmental myco-bacteria. This means that skin test positivity may be found in BCG-vaccinated subjects, and in people not exposed to *M. tuberculosis* itself. In addition, some of those with a large skin test response are at increased risk of developing tuberculosis, showing that strong T cell responses can be induced during disease progression.

Cytotoxic T lymphocytes kill by inducing 'leaks' in the target cell

The well-known cytotoxic T lymphocyte (CTL) is unusual in that both antigen-specific recognition and killing of the target are carried out by the same cell. The recognition step, involving an antigenic fragment that becomes associated with a class I MHC molecule, is discussed in Chapter 10, and

THERAPEUTIC ROLE OF CYTOKINES IN INFECTION

organism	cytokine	comments
Viruses		
hepatitis C	IFNα	usually given with ribavirin
hepatitis B	IFNγ	used if mutants develop during long-term therapy with lamivudine
HIV	IFNα, IL-2	given intermittently
Bacteria		
M. tuberculosis	IFNγ	aerosolized treatment given on trial basis to patients with multi-drug-resistant TB
M. leprae	IFNγ, IL-2	bacterial numbers reduced if injected directly into skin lesions in trials
general	IFNγ	given prophylactically to patients with chronic granulomatous disease to prevent bacterial infections
Fungi		
systemic mycoses	GM-CSF, M-CSF	treatment of neutropenic patients with myelogenous leukemia or after bone marrow transplantation
aspergillosis	IFNγ	given to patients with chronic granulomatous disease

Fig. 14.15 Examples of the therapeutic use of cytokines in infectious diseases in humans. Other cytokine treatments are currently under investigation. (GM-CSF, granulocyte–macrophage colony stimulating factor; IFN, interferon; IL, interleukin; M-CSF, macrophage colony stimulating factor.)

PROTECTIVE INFLUENCE OF IFNγ IN LEISHMANIA INFECTION

mouse strain	phenotype	production of IFNγ	IL-4
C57BL/6	resistant	+	–
BALB/c	susceptible	–	+

Fig. 14.16 Cytokine production in the spleens of mice infected with *Leishmania major*. The resistant phenotype (C57BL/6 mice) was associated with the production of the TH1 cytokine IFNγ, whereas the susceptible phenotype was associated with the production of the TH2 cytokine IL-4. (From Heinzel et al. *J Exp Med* 1989; 169:59, with permission.)

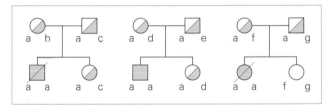

Fig. 14.17 Genetic mutations in the IFNγ receptor cause susceptibility to mycobacterial infections. Three Maltese families had children who were susceptible to atypical mycobacterial infection (solid symbols), two of whom died (slashed symbols). Individuals with carrier status are shown with half-filled symbols. All of the affected children were homozygous for the disease locus a on chromosome 6q22–q23, with a point mutation in the gene for the IFNγ receptor. This mutation introduces a stop codon resulting in a non-functional trucated protein. (From Newport et al. *N Engl J Med* 1996; 335:1941–9, with permission. Copyright Massachusetts Medical Society.)

displays the high degree of specificity characteristic of adaptive responses. The killing mechanism, however, is relatively non-specific. It appears to involve the induction of 'leaks' in the target cell by the insertion of perforin, a 66 kDa molecule that is structurally and functionally similar to the terminal complement component C9 (80 kDa; *Fig. 14.19*). Other molecules, including granzymes and cytokines such as TNFα may also be involved, and their effects may be either direct or indirect. Target cell death may be due to:

- leakage;
- induction of apoptosis—a 'suicide' program built into all cells and induced by Fas/FasL interactions, granzymes and TNFα.

These mechanisms are thought to operate principally against virus-infected cells, but some cells infected with other intracellular parasites, including mycobacteria (e.g. *M. leprae* in Schwann cells) and even protozoa (e.g. *Theileria parva* in lymphocytes) may also be susceptible. Most cytotoxic T cells are CD8-positive, recognizing MHC class-I-restricted peptide epitopes, but cytotoxicity can also be mediated by CD4 T cells and by γδ T cells. Surprisingly, it now seems that CD8 T cells are activated in some bacterial infections such as tuberculosis where the microbe remains within the phagosome and does not escape into the cytoplasm. This may result from a process

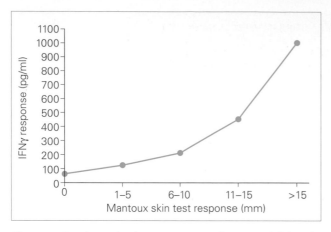

Fig. 14.18 Relationship between IFNγ production and delayed type hypersensitivity response. IFNγ responses to *M. tuberculosis* purified protein derivative were measured in vitro in healthy young adults. Skin test responses to the same antigen were measured by induration in the Mantoux skin test. (From Black et al. *Int J Tuberc Lung Dis* 2001; 5:664–72.)

called cross-priming, where bacterial antigens taken up by a dendritic cell are processed not only for MHC class II but also for MHC class I presentation. The lysis of an infected target cell may not always kill the intracellular microbe, but its release from its hideaway may lead to phagocytosis and subsequent killing by a more highly activated macrophage (*Fig. 14.20*).

Another interesting recent finding is that not all CD8 T cells can act as effector cytotoxic T cells. More human CD8 T cells express the granule protease granzyme A than the pre-formed effector molecule perforin. In HIV infection, two-thirds of the CD8 T cells express granzymes but only one-third express perforin. This may explain why virus-infected cells escape killing by antigen-specific CD8 T cells in HIV infection.

A summary of cytotoxic molecules made by cells involved in both natural and adaptive immunity is given in *Figure 14.21*.

RECOVERY FROM INFECTION

The everyday concept of an infectious disease is one where the patient is ill for a period of days to months and then recovers. In some cases he is subsequently immune to the disease. In such circumstances one can be fairly certain that adaptive (lymphocyte-based) mechanisms have been at work, since: (1) the existence of disease symptoms implies that natural defense mechanisms, which act rapidly, did not succeed in eliminating the parasite; (2) a period of days or weeks is typical of the time that adaptive immune mechanisms take to reach maximal levels; and (3) subsequent immunity is a sign of the immunological memory exclusive to lymphocytes, whose ability to specifically recognize antigens, to proliferate into clones, and to survive as memory cells, allows the host to progressively adapt to the infectious organisms in the environment. Thus, the older individuals are, the better they are adapted to the environment—until old age begins to weaken the immune system itself.

In the early stages of an infection, however, adaptive immunity can appear somewhat clumsy and ineffective. Since the lymphocytes are programmed to recognize the shapes of antigenic epitopes, they cannot distinguish virulent from harmless parasites, nor can they 'know' which type of immune response will be most effective. Thus, it is likely that the majority of responses in any individual infection will be irrelevant to recovery, and the demonstration of antibody, cytokines or cytotoxic cells is no proof that they are doing anything useful. Often one mechanism is responsible for recovery and another for resistance to re-infection (e.g. cytotoxic cells and interferon in recovery from measles, antibody in prevention of a second attack). In many infections, notably

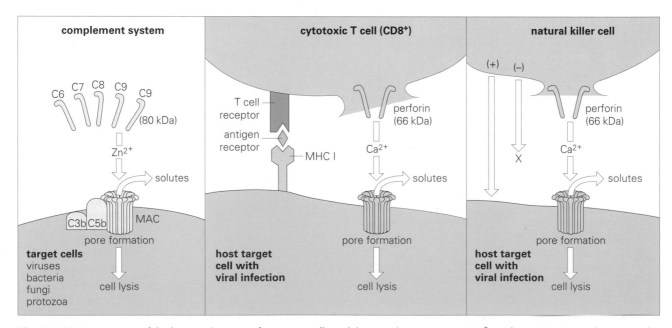

Fig. 14.19 Comparison of the lytic mechanisms of cytotoxic cells and the complement system. (Ca²⁺, calcium; MAC, membrane attack complex; MHC, major histocompatability complex; Zn²⁺, zinc.)

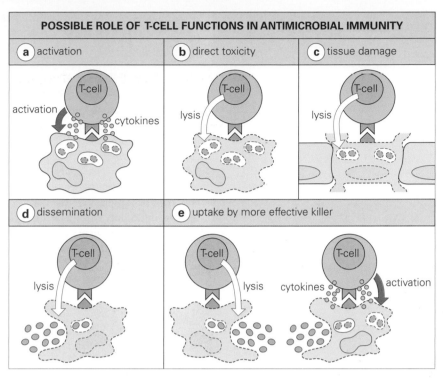

Fig. 14.20 Possible roles for T cells in immunity to intracellular microbes. (a) The T cell activates intracellular killing mechanisms by secretion of cytokines such as IFNγ, e.g. in a macrophage. (b) The T cell directly kills cell and parasite. (c) The T cell destroys vital tissue in the process of killing the parasite. (d) By lysing cells the T cell allows still-living parasites to disseminate. (e) Parasites released in this way may be phagocytosed by a more effective host cell. (Redrawn from Kaufman SH. *Rev Infect Dis* 1989; 11(Suppl 2):S448–54.

those by protozoa or helminths, there is still controversy as to which of the numerous responses that can be detected are useful, harmful or neutral. This distinction can only be made by repeated and patient observation and correlation, aided by study of deficiency syndromes if they occur and by animal experiments where good models exist.

The reason for an individual's failure to recover from an infection can also be hard to pinpoint. If the infection is one from which most people recover (e.g. measles), or from which they do not suffer at all (e.g. pneumocystis), an immuno-deficiency should be considered (see Chapter 30). Infections that are rapidly fatal in normal individuals (e.g. Lassa fever) are frequently those to which the evolving human immune system has not been exposed, since they are normally maintained in animals and only accidentally infect man (see Zoonoses, Chapter 28). But if the infection normally runs a prolonged course without either being eliminated or killing the host, the parasite can be considered to be successful, and this success will be due to one or more survival strategies. These are the subject of Chapter 16.

KEY FACTS

- Protection against infectious organisms that penetrate the outer barriers of the skin and mucous membranes is mediated by a variety of early defense mechanisms, which constitute innate immunity.
- These early defense mechanisms occur more rapidly but are less specific than the adaptive mechanisms based on lymphocyte responses.
- Important early defense mechanisms include the acute phase response, the complement system, IFNs, phagocytic cells and NK cells. Together these act as a first line of defense during the initial hours or days of infection.

- Adaptive immunity, mediated by antibody and T cells, is responsible for recovery from infection in many cases, although these mechanisms take days to weeks to reach peak efficiency.
- Sometimes, as in the common viral infections, cell-mediated immunity is responsible for recovery from infection, and antibody for the maintenance of immunity.
- Failure to recover from infection may be due to some deficiency of host immunity or to successful evasion strategies used by the microorganism.

CYTOTOXIC MOLECULES		
host component		**effective against**
major cell source	**molecule**	
liver cells macrophage	complement C1–3 complement C5–9	bacteria, fungi *Neisseria* streptococci
macrophage, neutrophil, eosinophils	reactive oxygen intermediates (plus peroxidase)	bacteria, fungi, malaria
macrophage	lysozyme interferon (α,β) tumor necrosis factor reactive nitrogen intermediates	Gram-positive bacteria viruses viruses, bacteria, malaria leishmania, malaria
neutrophil	defensins cathepsins lactoferrin	bacteria, fungi bacteria, fungi bacteria, yeasts
eosinophil	cationic proteins	schistosome worms
T lymphocyte	cytokines perforins granzymes	viruses, some bacteria, fungi, protozoa
natural killer cell	perforins granzymes	viruses
liver, fat	high density lipoprotein low density lipoprotein (oxidized)	trypanosomes malaria
kidney	urea	bacteria

Fig. 14.21 Some important cytotoxic molecules that operate against infectious organisms.

QUESTIONS

1. Macrophages can kill parasites using:*
   A. Reactive oxygen intermediates
   B. Major basic protein
   C. Cytotoxic lipid peroxides
   D. Antibodies
   E. Nitric oxide

2. Interferons act as antiviral agents by:*
   A. Damaging the host cell
   B. Inhibiting virus assembly
   C. Inhibiting viral RNA translation
   D. Preventing viral invasion

3. Antibodies can enhance immunity to infection by:*
   A. Opsonizing the parasite for subsequent phagocytosis
   B. Causing direct lysis of the parasite
   C. Inducing phagocyte activation directly
   D. Blocking microbial entry into the host cell
   E. Inducing antibody-dependent cellular cytotoxicity

4. Immunity to an intracellular pathogen such as *M. tuberculosis* requires:*
   A. Antigen-specific T cells
   B. Production of cytokines such as IFNγ
   C. Mediators produced by eosinophils
   D. IgE antibodies

*Question has more than one correct answer.

FURTHER READING

Alt F, Marrack P, eds. *Curr Opin Immunol* [appears bimonthly; issue no. 4 of each volume deals with 'Immunity to infection'].
Roitt IM, Brostoff J, Male D. *Immunology*, 6th edition. London: Elsevier Science, 2002.

INTRODUCTION

An infection may be a surface infection or a systemic infection

Many successful microorganisms multiply in epithelial cells at the site of entry on the body surface, but fail to spread to deeper structures or through the body. Local spread takes place readily on a fluid-covered mucosal surface, often aided by ciliary action, and large-scale movements of fluid spread the infection to more distant areas on the surface. This is obvious in the gastrointestinal tract. In the upper respiratory tract, high 'winds' (coughing, sneezing) can splatter infectious agents onto new areas of mucosa, or into the openings of sinuses or the middle ear, while the gentler downward trickle of mucus during sleep may seed an infectious agent into the lower respiratory tract. As a result, large areas of the body surface can be involved within a few days, with shedding to the exterior. There is not enough time for a primary immune response to be generated, and therefore non-adaptive responses—interferon, natural killer cells—are more important in controlling the infection. These surface infections therefore show a 'hit-and-run' pattern.

In contrast, other microorganisms spread systemically through the body via lymph or blood. They often undergo a complex or stepwise invasion of various tissues before reaching the final site of replication and shedding to the exterior (e.g. measles, typhoid). Surface and systemic infections and their consequences are compared in *Figure 15.1*.

FEATURES OF SURFACE AND SYSTEMIC INFECTIONS

A variety of factors determine whether an infection is a surface or a systemic infection

What prevents surface infections from spreading more deeply? Why do the microbes that cause systemic infections leave the relatively safe haven of the body surface to spread through the body, where they will bear the full onslaught of host defenses? These are important questions. For instance, what are the factors that persuade meningococci residing harmlessly on the nasal mucosa to invade deeper tissues, reach the blood and meninges, and cause meningitis (see Chapter 24)? The answer is not known.

Temperature is one factor that can restrict microbes to body surfaces. Rhinovirus infections, for instance, are restricted to the upper respiratory tract because they are temperature sensitive, replicating efficiently at 33°C, but not at the temperatures encountered in the lower respiratory tract (37°C). *Mycobacterium leprae* is also temperature sensitive, which accounts for its replication being more or less limited to nasal mucosa, skin and superficial nerves.

The site of budding is a factor that can restrict viruses to body surfaces. Influenza and parainfluenza viruses invade surface epithelial cells of the lung, but are liberated by budding from the free (external) surface of the epithelial cell, not from the basal layer from where they could spread to deeper tissues (*Fig. 15.2*).

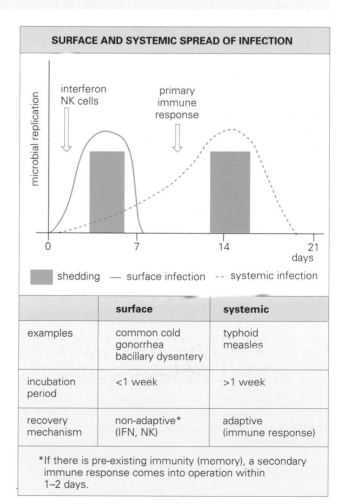

SURFACE AND SYSTEMIC SPREAD OF INFECTION

	surface	systemic
examples	common cold gonorrhea bacillary dysentery	typhoid measles
incubation period	<1 week	>1 week
recovery mechanism	non-adaptive* (IFN, NK)	adaptive (immune response)

*If there is pre-existing immunity (memory), a secondary immune response comes into operation within 1–2 days.

Fig. 15.1 Surface and systemic infections. (IFN, interferon; NK, natural killer.)

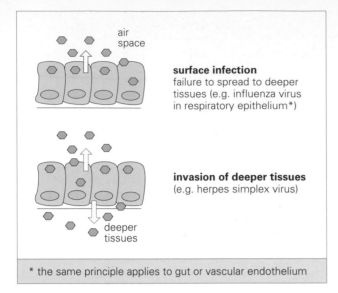

Fig. 15.2 Topography of virus release from epithelial surfaces can determine the pattern of infection.

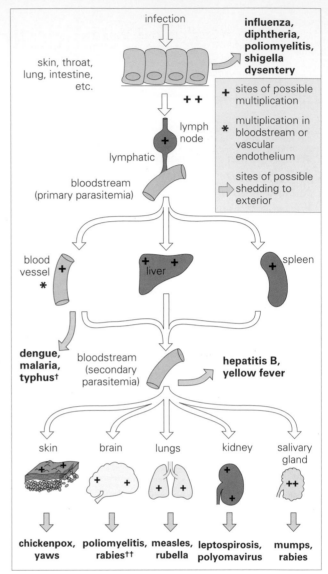

Fig. 15.3 The spread of infection throughout the body. Bone marrow and muscle are possible sources for secondary parasitemia in addition to blood vessels, liver and spleen. †In dengue, malaria and typhus, multiplication occurs in blood cells or vascular endothelium. ††Poliovirus invades from the blood but is not shed from the brain, whereas rabies invades and later translocates from the brain via peripheral nerves.

Many microorganisms are obliged to spread systemically because they fail to spread and multiply at the site of initial infection, the body surface. In the case of measles or typhoid, there is, for unknown reasons, next to no replication at the site of initial respiratory or intestinal infection. Only after spreading through the body systemically are large numbers of microorganisms delivered back to the same surfaces, where they multiply and are shed to the exterior. Other microorganisms need to spread systemically because they have committed themselves to infection by one route while major replication and shedding occurs at a different site. The microbe must reach the replication site, and there is then no need for extensive replication at the site of initial infection. For instance, mumps and hepatitis A viruses infect via the respiratory and alimentary routes, respectively, but must spread through the body to invade and multiply in salivary glands (mumps) and liver (hepatitis A).

In systemic infections there is a stepwise invasion of different tissues of the body

This stepwise invasion is illustrated in *Figure 15.3*, and such infections include measles *(Fig. 15.4)* and typhoid *(Fig. 15.5)*. Although the final sites of multiplication may be essential for microbial shedding and transmission (e.g. measles), they are sometimes completely unnecessary from this point of view (e.g. meningococcal meningitis, paralytic poliomyelitis). These microbes are not shed to the exterior after multiplying in the meninges or spinal cord.

For the microbe, systemic spread is fraught with obstacles, and a major encounter with immune and other defenses is inevitable. Microorganisms have therefore been forced to develop strategies for bypassing or countering these defenses (see Chapter 16).

Rapid replication is essential for surface infections

The rate of replication of the infecting microorganism is of central importance, and doubling times vary from 20 minutes

to several days *(Fig. 15.6)*. Hit-and-run (surface) infections need to replicate rapidly, whereas a microorganism that divides every few days (e.g. *Mycobacterium tuberculosis*) is likely to cause a slowly evolving disease with a long incubation period. Microorganisms nearly always multiply faster in vitro than they do in the intact host, as might be expected if host defenses are performing a useful function. In the host, microorganisms are phagocytosed and killed and the supply of nutrients may be limited. The net increase in numbers is slower than in laboratory cultures where microbes are not only free from attack by host defenses, but also every effort has been made to supply them with optimal nutrients, susceptible cells, and so on.

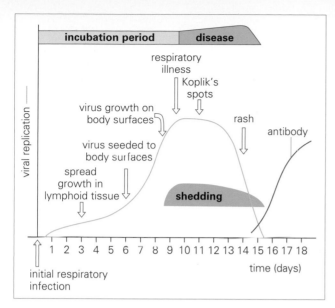

Fig. 15.4 The pathogenesis of measles. Virus invades body surfaces via blood vessels, reaches surface epithelium first in the respiratory tract where there are only 1–2 layers of epithelial cells and then in mucosae (Koplik's spots) and finally in the skin (rash).

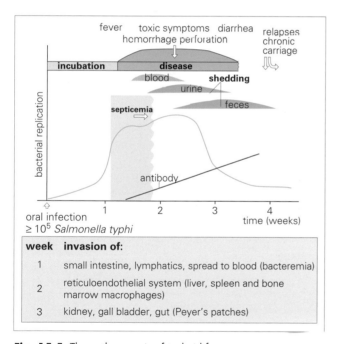

week	invasion of:
1	small intestine, lymphatics, spread to blood (bacteremia)
2	reticuloendothelial system (liver, spleen and bone marrow macrophages)
3	kidney, gall bladder, gut (Peyer's patches)

Fig. 15.5 The pathogenesis of typhoid fever.

MECHANISMS OF SPREAD THROUGH THE BODY

Spread to lymph and blood

Invading microbes encounter a variety of defenses on entering the body

After traversing the epithelium and its basement membrane at the body surface, invading microbes face the following defences:

REPLICATION RATES OF MICROORGANISMS		
microorganism	situation	mean doubling time
most viruses	in cell*	< 1 h
many bacteria, e.g. *Escherichia coli, staphylococci*	in vitro	20–30 min
Salmonella typhimurium	in vitro in vivo	30 min 5–12 h
Mycobacterium tuberculosis	in vitro in vivo	24 h many days
Mycobacterium leprae[†]	in vivo	2 weeks
Treponema pallidum[†]	in vivo	30 h
Plasmodium falciparum	in vitro/in vivo (erythrocyte or hepatic cell)	8 h

*but some viruses show greatly delayed replication or delayed spread from cell to cell
[†]cannot be cultivated in vitro

Fig. 15.6 Replication rates of different microorganisms.

- tissue fluids containing antimicrobial substances (antibody, complement);
- local macrophages (histiocytes). Subcutaneous and submucosal macrophages are a threat to microbial survival;
- the physical barrier of local tissue structure. Local tissues consist of various cells in a hydrated gel matrix; although viruses can spread by stepwise invasion of cells, invasion is more difficult for bacteria, and those that spread effectively sometimes possess special spreading factors (e.g. streptococcal hyaluronidase);
- the lymphatic system. The rich network of the lymphatic system soon conveys microorganisms to the battery of phagocytic and immunologic defenses awaiting them in the local lymph node (*Fig. 15.7*). Macrophages, strategically placed in the marginal and other lymph sinuses, constitute an efficient filtering system for lymph.

The infection may be halted at any stage, but by multiplying locally or in lymph nodes and by evading phagocytosis the microorganism can ultimately reach the bloodstream. Therefore, a minor injury to the skin, followed by a red streak (inflamed lymphatic) and a tender, swollen local lymph node are classic signs of streptococcal invasion. Most bacteria cause a great deal of inflammation when they invade in this way. In the early stages lymph flow increases, but eventually if there is

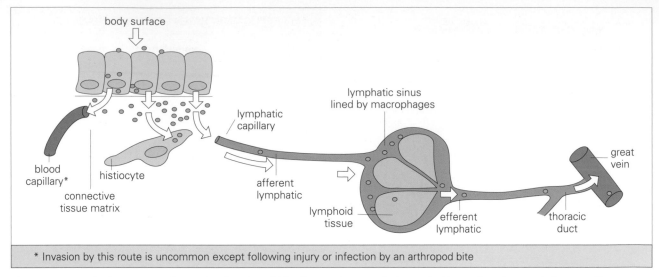

* Invasion by this route is uncommon except following injury or infection by an arthropod bite

Fig. 15.7 Microbial invasion and spread to lymph and blood. Microbes (or other particles) beneath surface epithelium readily enter local lymphatics.

enough inflammation and tissue damage in the node itself, the flow of the lymph may cease. In contrast, viruses and other intracellular microorganisms often invade lymph and blood silently and asymptomatically during the incubation period; this is facilitated when they infect monocytes or lymphocytes without initially damaging them.

Spread from blood

The fate of microorganisms in the blood depends upon whether they are free or associated with circulating cells

Viruses or small numbers of bacteria can enter the blood without causing a general body disturbance. For instance transient bacteremias are fairly common in normal individuals (e.g. they may occur after defecation or brushing teeth), but the bacteria are usually filtered out and destroyed in macrophages lining the liver and spleen sinusoids. Under certain circumstances the same bacteria have a chance to localize in less well-defended sites, such as congenitally abnormal heart valves in the case of viridans streptococci causing infective endocarditis, or in the ends of growing bones in the case of *Staphylococus aureus* osteomyelitis.

If microorganisms are free in the blood they are exposed to body defenses such as antibodies and phagocytes. However, if they are associated with circulating cells, these cells can protect them from host defenses and carry them around the body. For example, many viruses, such as Epstein–Barr virus (EBV) and rubella, and intracellular bacteria (*Listeria, Brucella*) are present in lymphocytes or monocytes and, if not damaged or destroyed, these 'carrying cells' protect and transport them. Malaria infects erythrocytes, and a few viruses infect platelets.

On entering the blood, microorganisms are exposed to macrophages of the reticuloendothelial system (see Chapter 9). Here in the sinusoids, where blood flows slowly, they are often phagocytosed and destroyed. But certain microorganisms survive and multiply in these cells (*Salmonella*

typhi, Leishmania donovani, yellow fever virus). The microorganism may then:

- spread to adjacent hepatic cells in the liver (hepatitis viruses), or splenic lymphoid tissues (measles virus);
- re-invade the blood (*S. typhi*, hepatitis viruses).

Each circulating microorganism invades characteristic target organs and tissues

If uptake by reticuloendothelial macrophages is not complete within a short time, or if large numbers of microorganisms are present in the blood, there is an opportunity for localization elsewhere in the vascular system. Why each circulating microorganism invades characteristic target organs and tissues *(Fig. 15.8)* is not completely understood, but may be due to:

- specific receptors for the microorganism, leading to localization on the vascular endothelium of certain target organs;
- random localization in organs throughout the body, only some of them being suitable for subsequent colonization and replication;
- accumulation of circulating microbes in sites where there is local inflammation, because of the slower flow and sticky endothelium in inflamed vessels.

After localization and organ invasion, the replicating microbe is shed from the body if the organ has a surface with access to the outside world *(Fig. 15.3)*. It may also be shed back into the bloodstream, either directly or via the lymphatic system.

Spread via nerves

Certain viruses spread via peripheral nerves from peripheral parts of the body to the central nervous system and vice versa

Tetanus toxin reaches the central nervous system (CNS) by this route. Rabies, herpes simplex virus (HSV) and varicella-zoster virus (VZV) travel in axons (see Chapters 13 and 24)

CIRCULATING MICROBES THAT INVADE ORGANS VIA SMALL BLOOD VESSELS		
microbe	disease	principal organs invaded*
viruses		
hepatitis B	hepatitis B	liver
rubella	congenital rubella	placenta (fetus)
varicella-zoster virus	chickenpox	skin, respiratory tract
polio	poliomyelitis	brain, spinal cord
mumps	mumps	parotid, mammary glands
bacteria		
Rickettsia rickettsi	Rocky Mountain spotted fever	skin
Treponema pallidum	secondary syphilis	skin, mucosae
Neisseria meningitidis	meningitis	meninges
protozoa		
Trypanosoma cruzi	Chagas' disease	heart, skeletal muscle
Plasmodium spp.	malaria	liver
helminths		
Schistosoma spp. (larvae)	schistosomiasis	veins of bladder, bowel
Ascaris lumbricoides (larvae)	ascariasis	lung
Ancylostoma duodenale (larvae)	hookworm	lung
*in liver, sinusoids; elsewhere, capillaries, venules		

Fig. 15.8 Circulating micoorganisms that invade organs via small blood vessels.

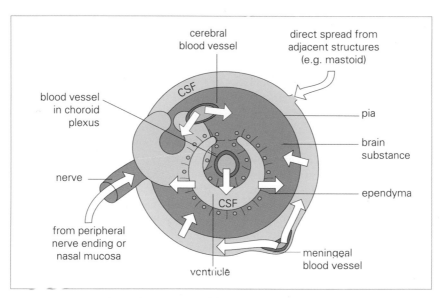

Fig. 15.9 Routes of microbial invasion of the central nervous system. (CSF, cerebrospinal fluid.)

and although the rate is slow, being accounted for by axonal flow (up to 10 mm/hour), this movement is important in the pathogenesis of these infections. Rabies not only reaches the CNS largely by peripheral nerves, but takes the same route from the CNS when it invades the salivary glands. Few, if any, host defenses are in a position to control this type of viral spread once nerves are invaded. Routes of invasion of the CNS are illustrated in *Figure 15.9*.

An uncommon route of spread to the CNS is via olfactory nerves with axons terminating on olfactory mucosa. For instance, certain free-living amebae (e.g. *Naegleria* spp.) found in sludge at the bottom of freshwater pools may take this route and cause meningoencephalitis in swimmers (see Chapter 24). Viruses and bacteria in the nasopharynx (e.g. meningococci, poliovirus) generally spread to the CNS via the blood.

Spread via cerebrospinal fluid

Once microorganisms have crossed the blood–cerebrospinal barrier they spread rapidly in the cerebrospinal fluid spaces

Such microorganisms can then invade neural tissues (echoviruses, mumps virus) as well as multiply locally (*Neisseria meningitidis*, *Haemophilus influenzae*, *Streptococcus pneumoniae*) and possibly infect ependymal and meningeal cells.

Spread via other routes

Rapid spread from one visceral organ to another can take place via the pleural or peritoneal cavity

Both the pleural and peritoneal cavities are lined by macrophages, as if in expectation of such invasion, and the peritoneal cavity contains an antimicrobial armory, consisting of the omentum (the 'abdominal policeman'), and many lymphocytes, macrophages and mast cells. Injury or disease in an abdominal organ provides a source of infection for peritonitis, as do chest wounds or lung infections for pleurisy.

GENETIC DETERMINANTS OF SPREAD AND REPLICATION

The pathogenicity of a microorganism is determined by the interplay of a variety of factors

These factors are referred to in Chapters 12 and 16. A distinction is sometimes made between pathogenicity and virulence: virulence implies a quantitative measure of pathogenicity. For instance, it can be expressed as the number of organisms necessary to cause death in 50% of individuals: lethal dose 50 (LD50). Nearly all pathogenicity factors are controlled by host and microbial genes. It has long been known that there are host genetic influences on susceptibility to infectious disease, and that mutations in microorganisms affect their pathogenicity. Within the past 15 years some of these genetic factors have been revealed by the application of molecular genetics techniques, and as a result it is increasingly possible to identify the specific gene products involved. Progress has also been made, though with greater difficulty, in understanding the mode of action of these gene products.

Genetic determinants in the host

The ability of a microorganism to infect and cause disease in a given host is influenced by the genetic constitution of the host

At a relatively gross level, some human pathogens either do not infect other species or infect only closely related primates (e.g. measles, trachoma, typhoid, hepatitis B, warts), whereas others infect a very wide range of hosts (rabies, anthrax). Also, within a given host species, there are genetic determinants of susceptibility. The best examples are found in animals, but there are examples for human disease (see below).

One example at the molecular level is the sickle cell gene and susceptibility to malaria. Malaria merozoites (see Chapter 27) parasitize red blood cells and metabolize hemoglobin, freeing heme and using globin as a source of amino acids. The sickle cell gene causes a substitution of the amino acid valine

for glutamic acid at one point in the β-polypeptide chain of the hemoglobin molecule. The new hemoglobin (hemoglobin S) becomes insoluble when reduced, and precipitates inside the red cell envelope, distorting the cell into the shape of a sickle. In homozygous individuals there are two of these genes and the individual has the disease sickle cell anemia, because their red cells are so fragile they sickle under normal circumstances. But in the heterozygote (sickle cell trait) the gene is less harmful, and provides resistance to severe forms of falciparum malaria, which ensures its selection in endemic malarial regions. The gene would be eliminated from populations after 10–20 generations unless it conferred some advantage. Restriction endonuclease analyses of the gene in Indian and West African populations have revealed that it arose independently in these malarious countries. Homozygotes, however, show increasing susceptibility to other infections, particularly *Strep. pneumoniae*, as a result of splenic dysfunction following repeated splenic infarcts.

Susceptibility often operates at the level of the immune response

A poor immune response to a given infection can lead to increased susceptibility to disease, whereas an immune response that is too vigorous may lead to immunopathologic disease (see Chapter 17). Of particular importance are the major histocompatibility complex (MHC) genes on chromosome 6, coding for MHC class II (HLA DP, DQ, DR) antigens and controlling specific immune responses (see Chapters 10 and 11). For example, susceptibility to leprosy (see Chapter 26) is strongly influenced by MHC class II genes. People with the HLA DR3 antigen are more susceptible to tuberculoid leprosy, whereas those with HLA DQ1 are more susceptible to lepromatous leprosy.

Studies of identical twins (see panel) provide evidence that genetic determinants affect susceptibility to tuberculosis. The present day European population shows considerable resistance to this disease. During the great epidemics of pulmonary tuberculosis in Europe in the 17th, 18th and 19th centuries, genetically susceptible individuals were weeded out. In 1850 mortality rates in Boston, New York, London, Paris and Berlin were over 500/100 000, but with improvements in living conditions these fell to 180/100 000 by 1900, and they have fallen even more since then. However, previously unexposed populations, especially in Africa and the Pacific Islands, show much greater susceptibility to respiratory tuberculosis. In the Plains Indians living in the Qu'Appelle Valley reservation in Saskatchewan, Canada, in 1886, tuberculosis spread through the body to infect glands, bones, joints and meninges, giving a death rate of 9000/100 000.

Genetic determinants in the microbe

Virulence is likely to be coded for by more than one microbial gene

Virulence is determined by numerous factors such as adhesion, penetration into cells, antiphagocytic activity, production of toxins and interaction with the immune system. Consequently, different genes and gene products are probably involved at different stages in pathogenesis.

LESSONS IN MICROBIOLOGY

Genetically determined susceptibility to infection

There are several classic examples of susceptibility to infectious disease determined by unidentified but presumably genetic factors in the human host.

The Lubeck disaster due to vaccination with virulent tubercle bacilli

In Lubeck, Germany, in 1926, living virulent tubercle bacilli instead of attenuated (vaccine) bacilli were inadvertently given to 249 babies. There were 76 deaths, but the rest, who developed only minor lesions, survived and were alive and well 12 years later. Each received the same inoculum, and it seems likely that the differences in outcome were largely due to genetic factors in the host.

A military misfortune due to contamination of yellow fever vaccine with hepatitis B virus

In 1942, more than 45 000 US military personnel were vaccinated against yellow fever, but were inadvertently injected at the same time with hepatitis B virus present as a contaminant in the human serum used to stabilize the vaccine. There were 914 clinical cases of hepatitis, of which 580 were mild, 301 moderate and 33 severe. Even with a given batch of vaccine the incubation period varied in the range 10–20 weeks. Serologic tests were not then available, so the number of subclinical infections is unknown. In this case both physiologic and genetic influences on susceptibility may have played a part.

Identical twins are affected similarly by respiratory tuberculosis

A study of tuberculosis in twins when at least one twin had the disease, showed that, for identical twins, the other twin was affected in 87% of cases. With non-identical twins the equivalent figure was only 26%. In addition, the identical twins had a similar type of clinical disease.

ATTENUATION OF PATHOGENS IN VITRO		
pathogen	passage	attenuated (live) product
Mycobacterium bovis	10 years of repeated passage in glycerin–bile–potato medium	bacille Calmette–Guérin (BCG) vaccine
rubella virus	27 passages in human diploid cells	rubella vaccine (Wistar RA 27/3)

Fig. 15.10 Examples of attenuation of pathogens following repeated passage in vitro.

often due to acquisition or loss of genetic elements such as integrons, pathogenicity islands, transposons and plasmids (see Chapters 2 and 33).

Changes in the virulence of a microorganism take place during artificial culture in the laboratory. For instance, in the classical procedure for obtaining a live vaccine (see Chapter 34), a microorganism is repeatedly grown (passaged) in vitro, and this generally leads to reduced pathogenicity in the host. The new strain is then referred to as 'attenuated' (Fig. 15.10).

Our understanding of the genetic basis for microbial pathogenicity had advanced rapidly in recent years due to DNA cloning and genetic manipulation techniques. For instance, by introducing or deleting/inactivating genome segments, the virulence genes can be identified. Examples are shown in *Figure 15.11*. Rapid advances in genomics are also making major contributions to our understanding of virulence genes and conditions affecting their expression. For many viruses the entire genome has been sequenced, thus allowing the assignment of functions to specific loci.

OTHER FACTORS AFFECTING SPREAD AND REPLICATION

Various other factors have an influence on susceptibility to infectious disease (Fig. 15.12). In most cases it is not known whether this involves differences in microbial spread and replication or differences in host immune and inflammatory reponses. Infections in hosts with immunologic and other defects are described in Chapter 33.

The brain can influence immune responses

When stress (a loosely used word) is associated with malnutrition or crowding it may be difficult to disentangle the separate influences of these various factors on susceptibility to infection, as in the case of tuberculosis. The brain can, however, influence immune responses, acting via the hypothalamus, pituitary and adrenal cortex. It has long been known that glucocorticoids, which have powerful actions on immune cells, are needed for resistance to infection and trauma. A shortage of glucocorticoids, as in Addison's disease, or an excess, as with steroid therapy, results in increased

Under natural circumstances microorganisms are constantly undergoing genetic change, such as mutations. The single-stranded RNA viruses in particular show very high mutation rates. Mutations affecting surface antigens undergo rapid selection in the host under immune pressure (antibody, cell-mediated immunity), as in the case of the rapidly evolving M proteins of streptococci, and the capsid proteins of picornaviruses. In addition, genetic changes in bacteria are

THE MOLECULAR BASIS OF MICROBIAL PATHOGENICITY		
microorganism	**gene or gene product**	**effect on virulence**
Streptococcus pyogenes	M protein; 60 mm long coiled coil extending from bacterial cell wall with N terminal hypervariable domain	antiphagocytic role; inhibits opsonization; exact mechanism unknown
	amino acid sequence overlap with host components (myosin, tropomyosin, keratin, etc.)	autoimmune complication
Yersinia enterocolitica	invasion (inv) gene codes for 92 kDa protein on bacterial surface	required for uptake of bacteria into epithelial cells and macrophages of Peyer's patches
Shigella spp.	ipa B (invasion plasmid antigen B) gene	mediates lysis of vacuolar membrane and escape of bacteria into cytoplasm of colonic epithelial cells*
Leishmania donovani	Arg–Gly–Asp sequence of gp63 surface protein	binds to C3b receptor on macrophage and thereby infects this cell
Neisseria gonorrhoeae	genes for proteins of pili (fimbriae) and for certain outer membrane proteins	proteins mediate attachment to mucosal cells, independent control of each gene makes *N. gonorrhoeae* the 'master chameleon', altering its surface antigens to evade host immune responses
herpes simplex virus type I	gene for envelope glycoprotein C (gC)	gC acts as receptor for C3b, blocking the classical pathway and enabling virus or virus-infected cell to resist lysis by complement plus antibody

*Shigellae enter gut wall via M cells in Peyer's patches, then invade colonic epithelial cells from basolateral surfaces. In this, as in other bacterial infections, invasiveness depends upon coordinated expression of many different genes.

Fig. 15.11 Examples of the molecular basis of microbial pathogenicity.

susceptibility to infection *(Fig. 15.12)*. In addition, the brain, the endocrine and the immune systems often use the same molecular messengers—cytokines, peptide hormones, neurotransmitters. Neural cells, for instance, have receptors for interferons and for interleukins—IL-1, IL-2, IL-3, IL-6—and thymic lymphocytes can produce prolactin and growth hormone. Immune–neuroendocrine cross-talk now has molecular respectability and provides an acceptable basis for the influence of the brain on immunity and infectious disease.

HOST FACTORS INFLUENCING SUSCEPTIBILITY TO INFECTIOUS DISEASE			
factor	example	alteration in susceptibility	mechanism
pregnancy	hepatitis viruses	more lethal outcome	?increased metabolic burden for liver in pregnancy
	urinary infections	pyelonephritis more common	reduced peristalsis in ureter
malnutrition	measles	more severe; more lethal	vitamin A deficiency; depressed CMI
age	respiratory syncytial virus	more severe; more lethal in infant	small diameter of airways
	mumps, chickenpox, Epstein–Barr virus infection	more severe in adult	?increased immunopathology
atmospheric pollution	raised sulfur dioxide levels	excess acute respiratory disease	?interference with mucociliary defenses
	silicosis	increased susceptibility to tuberculosis	?damage to lung macrophages
foreign bodies	necrotic bone fragments	chronic osteomyelitis more common	antimicrobial defenses less effective in necrotic tissue
	necrotic tissue	increased susceptibility to *Clostridium perfringens*	anaerobic necrotic tissues favor bacterial growth
stress, hormones	glucocorticoid production: *decreased* (Addison's disease)	increased susceptibility to infection	hypersensitivity to inflammatory/immune responses?
	increased (steroid therapy)	increased susceptibility to infection	reduction in protective immune/inflammatory responses

Fig. 15.12 Host factors influencing susceptibility to infectious disease. (CMI, cell-mediated immunity.)

KEY FACTS

- Infections restricted to the body surfaces (e.g. common cold, shigella dysentery) have shorter incubation periods than systemic infections (e.g. measles, typhoid), and adaptive (immune) host responses tend to be less important.

- Microbes with a slow growth rate (e.g. *M. tuberculosis*) tend to cause diseases which evolve slowly.

- Spread through the body takes place primarily via lymph and blood. The fate of circulating microbes depends upon whether they are free or present in circulating blood cells.

- Uptake by reticuloendothelial cells in liver and spleen focuses infection into these organs, but specific localization in the vascular bed of other organs (e.g. mumps virus in salivary glands, meningococci in meninges) is not understood.

- Viruses can spread in either direction along nerve axons, and this is important in the pathogenesis of recurrent herpes simplex virus infection, zoster and rabies.

- Pathogenicity and virulence are strongly influenced by genetic factors in the host (e.g. tuberculosis in identical twins) and by genetic factors in the microbe (e.g sickle cell trait in falciparum malaria).

QUESTIONS

1. What are the routes by which microbes can reach (a) the salivary glands and (b) the liver?

2. Is invasion of the CNS ever of any value from the microbe's point of view?

3. Give examples of microbes that (a) travel free in the plasma and (b) travel in association with blood cells. What are the consequences in each case?

4. Why can tuberculosis and leprosy bacilli not cause rapid 'hit-and-run' infections?

5. Give an example of a change in a single human gene that causes an important change in susceptibility to an infectious disease.

 FURTHER READING

Alonzo de Velasco E, Verheul AF, Verhoef J, Snippe H. Streptococcus pneumoniae: virulence factors, pathogenesis and vaccines. *Microbiol Rev* 1995; 59:591–603.

Griffin JW, Watson DF. Axonal transport in neurologic disease. *Ann Neurol* 1988; 23:3–13.

Mims CA, Nash A, Stephen J. *Mims' Pathogenesis of Infectious Disease*, 5th edition. London: Academic Press, 2001.

Savino W, Dardenne M. Immune–neuroendocrine interactions. *Immunol Today* 1995; 16:318–22.

Townsend GC, Scheld WM. In vitro models of the blood–brain barrier to study bacterial meningitis. *Trends Microbiol* 1995; 3:441–5.

Parasite survival strategies and persistent infections

INTRODUCTION

Most common infectious organisms have developed 'answers' to host defenses

So far we have concentrated on the battery of mechanisms available to the host, both natural and adaptive, to keep out and destroy the parasite. Powerful as these are, they are obviously not 100% effective, otherwise healthy people would never have infections. In fact, most of the common infectious organisms described in this book have developed 'answers' to host defenses because their ability to survive as human parasites has depended upon this. They successfully infect humans and are of concern to the physician precisely because they have developed strategies for evading or actively interfering with host defenses.

Strategies to evade natural non-adaptive defenses such as the phagocyte

These include the following.

- *Killing or avoiding being killed by phagocytes.* Successful parasites have evolved numerous ingenious antiphagocytic devices. Antiphagocytic devices *(Fig. 16.1)* range from killing or inhibiting the phagocyte itself, via more subtle ways of eluding contact, to protection against intracellular death allowing the microorganism to survive within the phagocyte—a very serious challenge to the host.
- *Interfering with ciliary action* (see *Fig. 13.5*).
- *Interfering with complement's alternative pathway.* For instance *(Fig. 16.2)*, the insertion of the C567 complex is prevented by the long side chains of the cell wall polysaccharides of smooth strains of *Salmonellae* and by the capsules of staphylococci, which, unlike the cell wall, do not activate complement. Certain bacteria, for example streptococci and campylobacter, actively inhibit complement activation, while a covering of non-complement fixing antibody, for example IgA, is yet another way of avoiding lysis. Anti-complement activity is also a feature of several protozoan and helminthic infections, for example infections with *Leishmania* and the hydatid worm *Echinococcus granulosus*.
- *Producing iron binding molecules.* Nearly all bacteria need iron, but the host's iron-binding proteins such as trans-ferrin limit the availability of this element. Accordingly, certain bacteria (e.g. *Neisseria*) produce their own powerful iron-binding proteins to circumvent the shortage.
- *Blocking interferons.* Host cells respond to double-stranded DNA (dsRNA) from infecting microbes (including all viruses), by forming interferons alpha and beta. These are produced rapidly, within 24 hours, after infection and are part of the non-adaptive response. Certain viruses are either poor inducers of interferons (hepatitis B) or produce molecules that block the action of interferons in cells (hepatitis B, HIV, adenoviruses, Epstein–Barr virus, vaccinia

virus). Interferon gamma (IFNγ), an essential part of the adaptive response, is also affected.

Strategies to evade adaptive defenses

Strategies to evade adaptive defenses are more sophisticated than those for evading innate defenses

The success of microbes in evading or interfering with adaptive (immune) defenses is discussed in this chapter. The strategies involved are more sophisticated than those for evading innate defenses, because lymphocytes are programmed so that their cell receptors can recognize virtually any shape (B cells) or amino acid sequence (T cells), provided it is not identical to self; for example:

- The polysaccharide capsules of bacteria prevent non-immune contact between phagocytes and the bacterial cell wall, but are quickly recognized as foreign by B cell surface receptors (immunoglobulin), leading to the formation of antibody with consequent opsonization and phagocytosis of the bacteria.
- Many microorganisms such as bacteria and fungi can resist intracellular destruction by macrophages, but their peptides are presented in association with major histocompatability complex (MHC) molecules on the macrophage surface, and their presence is detected by T cells. A new set of cytotoxic and other immune mechanisms is then brought into action.

In both these examples the lymphocytes are behaving like a highly specialized and sharply observant secret police force in contrast to the everyday activities of the more pedestrian macrophages.

PARASITE SURVIVAL STRATEGIES

Parasite survival strategies can take as many forms as there are parasites, but they can be usefully classified according to the immune component that is evaded and the means selected to

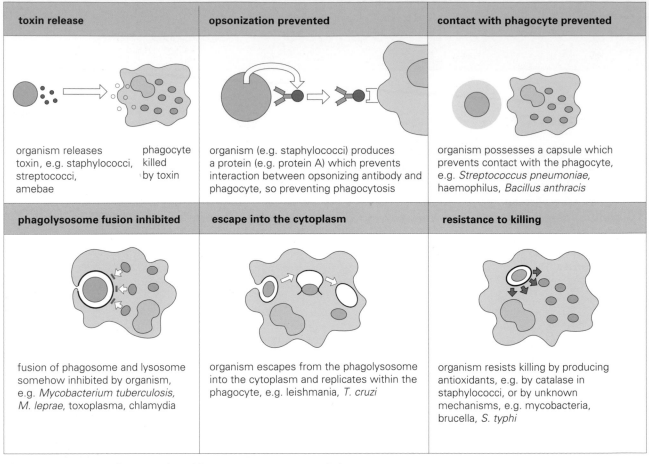

toxin release	opsonization prevented	contact with phagocyte prevented
organism releases toxin, e.g. staphylococci, streptococci, amebae — phagocyte killed by toxin	organism (e.g. staphylococci) produces a protein (e.g. protein A) which prevents interaction between opsonizing antibody and phagocyte, so preventing phagocytosis	organism possesses a capsule which prevents contact with the phagocyte, e.g. *Streptococcus pneumoniae*, haemophilus, *Bacillus anthracis*
phagolysosome fusion inhibited	**escape into the cytoplasm**	**resistance to killing**
fusion of phagosome and lysosome somehow inhibited by organism, e.g. *Mycobacterium tuberculosis*, *M. leprae*, toxoplasma, chlamydia	organism escapes from the phagolysosome into the cytoplasm and replicates within the phagocyte, e.g. leishmania, *T. cruzi*	organism resists killing by producing antioxidants, e.g. by catalase in staphylococci, or by unknown mechanisms, e.g. mycobacteria, brucella, *S. typhi*

Fig. 16.1 Various mechanisms adopted by microorganisms to avoid phagocytosis.

do this (see Chapter 12). As a result, the microbe is able to undergo what are often quite lengthy periods of growth and spread during the incubation period before being shed and transmitted to the next host, as occurs in hepatitis B and tuberculosis. Shedding of the microbe for just a few extra days after clinical recovery gives more extensive transmission in the community, and this is a worthwhile result for the microbe.

Some microbes are able to persist in the host

Certain microbes are able to remain (persist) in the host for many years, often for life. From the microbe's point of view, persistence is worthwhile only if shedding occurs during the persistence. Persistent microbes fall into two categories:

- those that are shed more or less continuously, such as the Epstein–Barr virus (EBV) into saliva, hepatitis B virus into blood, and eggs into feces in various helminth infections;
- those that are shed intermittently, such as herpes simplex virus (HSV), polyomaviruses, typhoid bacilli, tubercle bacilli and malaria parasites.

Viruses are particularly good at thwarting immune defenses

Viruses are able to thwart immune defenses for a number of reasons:

- Their invasion of tissues and cells is often 'silent'. Unlike most bacteria, they do not form toxins, and as long as they

do not cause extensive cell destruction there is no sign of illness until the onset of immune and inflammatory responses, sometimes several weeks after infection as occurs in hepatitis B virus and EBV infections.
- Viruses such as rubella virus, wart viruses, hepatitis B virus and EBV can infect cells for long periods without adverse effects on cell viability.

Virus latency is a type of persistence and is based on an intimate molecular relationship with the infected cell. The viral genome continues to be present in the host without producing antigens or infectious material, and only does so very occasionally, when the virus reactivates (becomes patent).

Strategies for evading host defenses cause a rapid 'hit-and-run' infection

One evasion strategy for microorganisms is to cause a rapid 'hit-and-run' infection. The microbe invades, multiplies and is shed within a few days, before adaptive immune defenses have had time to come into action. Infections of the body surfaces (rhinoviruses, rotaviruses) come into this category. Otherwise, the principal strategies employed by parasites to elude the lymphocyte (as discussed in the following pages) are:

- concealment of antigens;
- antigenic variation;
- immunosuppression.

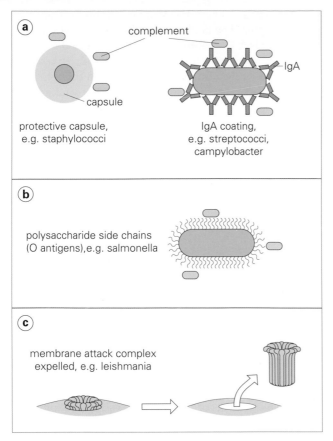

Fig. 16.2 Three ways by which microorganisms can avoid damage by complement: (a) failure to trigger complement; (b) protection of the membrane from attack; (c) expulsion of the membrane attack complex C5–9.

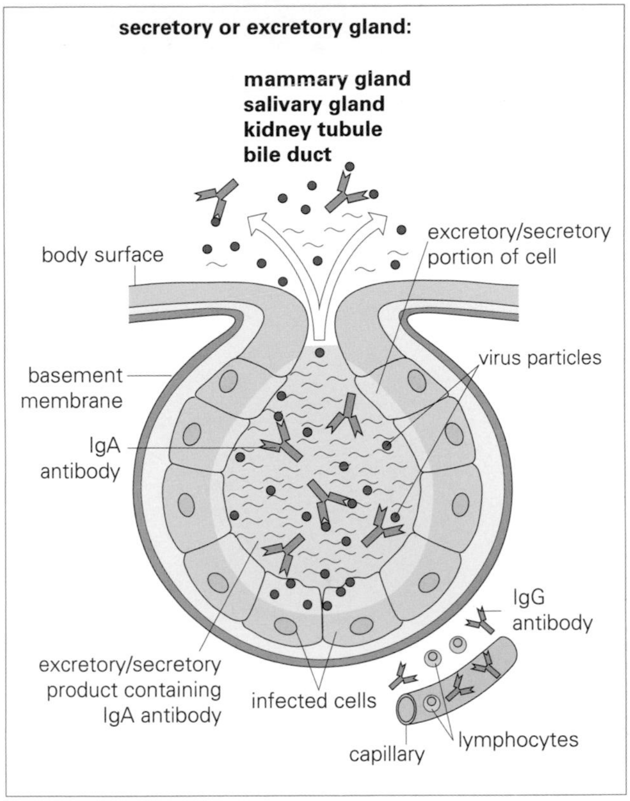

Fig. 16.3 Viral infection of cell surfaces facing the external world. Infection of the surface epithelium of, for instance, a secretory or excretory gland allows direct shedding of the virus to the exterior, as well as avoidance of host immune defenses.

Concealment of antigens

A spy in a foreign country can conceal his presence from the police by hiding, by never venturing out of doors, or by adopting the disguise of a native. Parasites have the same choice. Places to hide include the interior of host cells (though the MHC molecules act as 'informers' for this compartment, picking up and transporting microbial peptides to the cell surface where they will be recognized) and particular sites in the body where lymphocytes do not normally circulate ('privileged sites', the equivalent of 'no-go' areas).

Remaining inside cells without their antigens being displayed on the surface prevents recognition

If a microbe can remain inside cells without allowing its antigens to be displayed on the cell surface, it will remain unrecognized ('incognito') as far as immune defenses are concerned. Even if specific antibody and T cell responses have been induced the microbe inside such a cell is unaffected. Persistent latent viruses such as HSV in sensory neurones behave in this way. During reactivation, of course, re-exposure and boosting of immune defenses is inevitable.

Other strategies are possible. Several viruses (HIV in macrophages, coronaviruses) display their proteins 'secretly' on the walls of intracellular vacuoles instead of at the cell surface, and bud into these vacuoles. Adenoviruses have taken more active steps to avoid antigen display. One of the adenoviral proteins (E19) combines with class I MHC molecules and prevents their passage to the cell surface so that infected cells are not recognized by cytotoxic T cells.

Colonizing privileged sites keeps the microbe out of reach of circulating lymphocytes

The vast numbers of microbes that colonize the skin and the intestinal lumen, together with those that are shed directly into external secretions, are effectively out of reach of circulating lymphocytes. They are exposed to secretory antibodies, which although able to bind to the microbe (e.g. influenza virus) and render it less infectious, are generally unable to kill the microbe or control its replication in or on the epithelial surface *(Figs 16.3, 16.4)*. A local inflammatory response, however, can enhance host defenses.

Within the body it is more difficult to avoid lymphocytes and antibodies, but certain sites are safer than others. These include the central nervous system, joints, testes and placenta. Here lymphocyte circulation is less intense, and access of antibodies and complement is more restricted. However, as soon as inflammatory responses are induced, then lymphocytes, monocytes and antibodies are rapidly delivered and the site loses its privilege.

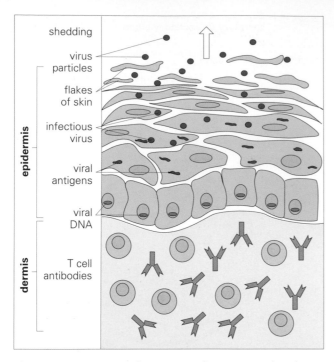

Fig. 16.4 Wart virus replication in epidermis—a privileged site? Cell differentiation such as keratinization controls virus replication, and as a result virus matures when it is physically removed from immune defenses.

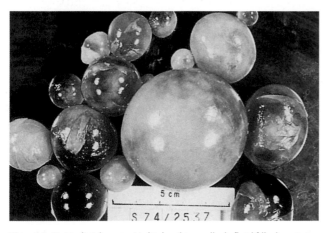

Fig. 16.5 Hydatid cysts. Multiple, thin-walled, fluid-filled cysts in a surgical specimen. The lung is a common site. (Courtesy of JA Innes.)

Additional privileged sites can be created by the infectious organism itself. A good example is the hydatid cyst that develops in liver, lung or brain around growing colonies of the tapeworm *Echinococcus granulosus* (Fig. 16.5) inside which the worms can survive even though the blood of the host contains protective levels of antibody.

Perhaps the most highly privileged site of all is host DNA, and this is occupied by the retroviruses. Retroviral RNA is transcribed by the reverse transcriptase into DNA as a necessary part of the replicative cycle, and this then becomes integrated into the DNA of the host cell (see Chapter 21). Once integrated, and as long as there is no cell damage and

viral products are not expressed on the cell surface where they can be recognized by immune defenses, the virus enjoys total anonymity. This is what makes complete cure and complete removal of virus from a patient infected with HIV such a daunting task. The intragenomic site becomes even more privileged if the egg or sperm is infected. The viral genome will then be present in all embryonic cells and transferred from one generation to another as if it were the host's own DNA. Luckily this does not happen with HIV or with human T cell lymphotropic virus (HTLV) 1 and 2. However, the 'endogenous' retroviruses of humans present in profusion as DNA sequences in our genome, but not expressed as antigens, come into this category. They are part of our inheritance. This surely represents the ultimate, the final logical step in parasitism, at the borderline between infection and heredity.

Mimicry sounds like a useful strategy, but does not prevent the host from making an antimicrobial response

If the microbe can in some way avoid inducing an immune response, this can be regarded as a 'concealment' of its antigens. One method is by mimicking host antigens, as such self antigens are not recognized as foreign (Fig. 16.6). Numerous examples are known of parasite-derived molecules that resemble those of the host (Fig. 16.7). In the case of viral proteins, mimicry based on amino acid sequence homology (sharing of 8–10 consecutive amino acids) is seen to be common when computer comparisons are made between viral and host proteins. Perhaps the most celebrated example, however, is the cross-reaction between group A beta-hemolytic streptococci and human myocardium. This cross-reaction underlies the development of rheumatic heart disease, following repeated streptococcal infection because of antibody made against the cross-reacting determinant meromyosin (see Fig. 16.6). The fact that the host makes such autoantibodies shows that in this case mimicry does not protect the bacteria. The conclusion is that, although mimicry sounds like a useful strategy for microbes and occurs quite frequently, it is probably an accident rather than a sinister microbial strategy. It does not prevent the host from making an antimicrobial and autoimmune response.

Microbes can conceal themselves by taking up host molecules to cover their surface

This is illustrated in *Figure 16.7*. A superb example of this is the blood fluke *Schistosoma*, which acquires a complete surface coat of host blood group glycolipids, MHC antigens and immunoglobulin molecules from the plasma. Such a worm must indeed be virtually invisible even to a lymphocyte. For unknown reasons, however, this strategy is essentially restricted to worms.

The uptake of immunoglobulin molecules by the microbe seems to be a more widespread phenomenon. A number of viruses and bacteria produce Fc receptors, which are displayed on their surface and bind immunoglobulin molecules of all specificities in an immunologically useless upside-down position (*Fig. 16.8*, and see below). This prevents the access of specific antibodies or T cells to the microbe or the infected cell.

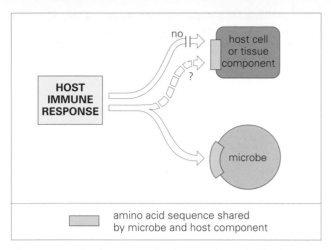

Fig. 16.6 Molecular mimicry by the microbe probably does not restrain the immune response, but host cells and tissue can then be subject to immune damage, for example rheumatic heart disease following streptococcal infection is caused by antibodies reacting with meromyosin, the cross-reacting determinant.

Tolerization

Tolerizing the host prevents the induction of an immune response

An alternative strategy for the microbe is to avoid inducing an immune response or to induce a poor response. There are four possible methods:

- infection during early embryonic life;
- the production of large quantities of the microbial antigen or of antigen–antibody complexes;
- exploiting 'gaps' in the host's immune repertoire;
- upsetting the balance between antibody and cell-mediated immune responses—between T helper cell (TH) 1 and 2 responses.

Infection during early embryonic life

Before development of the immune system, a time when antigens present are regarded as 'self', infection could possibly result in immune tolerance. However, in the case of intra-uterine infection with cytomegalovirus (CMV), rubella virus and syphilis, the fetus does eventually produce IgM antibody, which is detectable in umbilical cord blood. But cell-mediated responses are more seriously impaired. Children with congenital CMV or rubella fail to develop lymphoproliferative responses to CMV or rubella antigens and consequently take years to clear the virus from the body (see Chapter 23). In some cases infection in the neonatal period is more likely to result in tolerance than infection in later life. Therefore, neonatal infection with hepatitis B virus frequently results in permanent carriage of the virus, though the mechanism is unknown.

Production of large quantities of microbial antigen or antigen–antibody complexes

Large quantities of microbial antigen or antigen–antibody complexes circulating in the body can cause immune tolerance to that antigen. Anergy, as evidenced by normal antibody but depressed cell-mediated immune responses

MIMICRY AND UPTAKE OF HOST ANTIGENS		
microbe's strategy	parasite	corresponding host antigen
mimicry	Epstein–Barr virus streptococci	human fetal thymus* cardiac muscle (meromyosin)
	klebsiella	HLA-B27**
	Mycobacterium tuberculosis	65 kDa heat shock protein
	Neisseria meningitidis	embryonic brain
	treponema	cardiolipin†
	Mycoplasma pneumoniae	erythrocytes††
	plasmodia	thymosin-α₁
	Trypanosoma cruzi	heart, nerve
	schistosoma	glutathione transferase
antigen uptake	cytomegalovirus	β₂-microglobulin
	schistosoma	glycolipids, HLA, Ig, etc.
	filarial nematodes	albumin

*also cross-reacts with erythrocytes of certain species and is the basis for the Paul Bunnell (heterophil antibody) test
**possible basis for ankylosing spondylitis
†basis for Wassermann-type antibody test for syphilis
††basis for cold agglutinin test

Fig. 16.7 Some examples of mimicry or uptake of host antigens by parasites. (HLA, human leukocyte antigen; Ig, immunoglobulin.)

to the invading microbe, is seen in disseminated coccidioido-mycosis and cryptococcosis, and in visceral and diffuse cutaneous leishmaniasis, in each case associated with large amounts of microbial antigen in the circulation.

Exploiting 'gaps' in the host's immune repertoire

There are likely to be certain peptides to which the host makes a poor immune response, based on the nature of the host's MHC class II molecules. These represent genetically determined 'gaps' in the host's immune repertoire, and microbes, as they evolve, might be be expected to match these peptides. In other words, microbes may be constantly 'probing' the immune repertoire of the host, seeking out weaknesses. There is no proof that this occurs, but it is conceivable, for instance, that the great susceptibility of African people to tuberculosis is due to a genetically determined, poor cell-mediated immune response to key *M. tuberculosis* antigens. Europeans show greater resistance because of the 'weeding out' of genetically susceptible individuals over hundreds of years. It has been estimated that 30% of all adult deaths in Europe in the 19th century were due to tuberculosis.

Upsetting the balance between antibody and TH1 and TH2 responses

Resistance to infection often depends upon a suitable balance between antibody and TH1 and TH2 responses (see Chapter

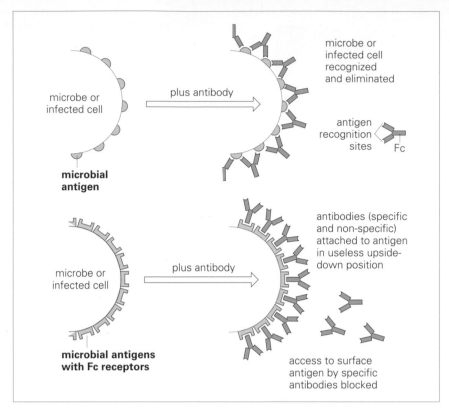

Fig. 16.8 The production of Fc receptors is of some benefit to microbes, for example staphylococci, streptococci, herpes simplex virus, varicella-zoster virus and cytomegalovirus.

10). Good defense against tuberculosis and herpesviruses needs cell-mediated immunity, whereas antibody is required for good defense against polioviruses or *Streptococcus pneumoniae.* In active tuberculosis, T cells making IL-4 can be detected, with a reduction in the beneficial TH1 cytokine response. By inducing an ineffective type of response a microbe can promote its own survival. Some bacteria evade protective TH1 responses by inducing antigen-specific regulatory T cells. *Bordetella pertussis* infection induces regulatory T cells specific for its filamentous hemagglutinin and pertactin. These regulatory T cells produce IL-10, and thus suppress TH1 immunity to two vital bacterial components which help the bacteria attach to host cells.

ANTIGENIC VARIATION

Reverting to the metaphor of a spy in foreign territory, there is another way to confuse the enemy—by repeated changes in appearance. The African trypanosome, the causative organism of sleeping sickness, does this, and so do a wide range of viruses, bacteria and protozoa. Antigenic variation can occur:

- during the course of infection in a given individual;
- during spread of the microbe through the host community (Fig. 16.9).

As a strategy for evading host immune responses, antigenic variation depends upon variation occurring in antigens whose recognition is involved in protection. Antigenic variation is common as the microbe passes through the host community and it tends to be more important in longer-lived hosts, such

as humans in whom microbial survival is favored by multiple re-infections during the lifetime of a given individual. Also it is more common in infections limited to respiratory or intestinal epithelium where the incubation period is less than 1 week and the microbe can commonly infect, multiply and be shed from the body before a significant secondary immune response is generated. During systemic infections (e.g. measles, mumps, typhoid) the incubation period is longer and secondary responses have more opportunity to come into action and control an infection by an antigenic variant. Accordingly, antigenic variation is not an important feature of these systemic infections.

At the molecular level there are three main mechanisms for antigenic variation:

- mutation;
- recombination;
- gene switching.

The best known example of mutation is the influenza virus

As the influenza virus spreads through the community there are repeated mutations in the genes coding for hemagglutinin and neuraminidase (see Chapter 19), causing small antigenic changes that are sufficient to reduce the effectiveness of B and T cell memory built up in response to earlier infections. This is called 'antigenic drift'. Human rhinoviruses and enteroviruses are evolving rapidly and show a similar drift. Antigenic drift could account for the wealth of antigenic types of staphylococci, streptococci and pneumococci. During polio-

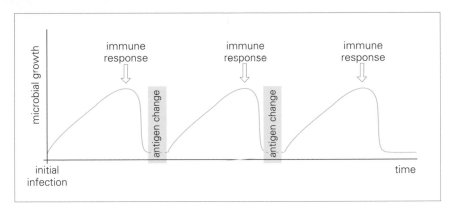

Fig. 16.9 Antigenic variation as a microbial strategy. The change in antigens may take place in the originally infected individual, enabling the microbe to undergo renewed growth (e.g. trypanosomiasis), or it may take place as the microbe passes through the host population, enabling it to reinfect a given individual (e.g. influenza).

DEPRESSED IMMUNE RESPONSES CAUSED BY MICROBIAL INFECTIONS			
parasite		**feature of immunosuppression**	**mechanism**
viruses	HIV	↓Ab ↓CMI long lasting	↓CD4+ T cells immunosuppressive molecule (gp41) ↓ antigen presentation by infected APC polyclonal activation of B cells
	Epstein–Barr virus	↓CMI temporary	includes polyclonal activation of infected B cells*
	measles	↓CMI temporary**	differentiation blocked in infected T and B cells
	cytomegalovirus	↓CMI temporary	unknown; very occasional infection of mononuclear cells
	varicella-zoster virus mumps	↓CMI temporary	infection of T cells
bacteria	*M. leprae* (lepromatous leprosy)	↓CMI	polyclonal activation of B cells induction of suppressor T cells
protozoa	*Trypanosoma* *Plasmodia* *Toxoplasma* *Leishmania*	↓Ab ↓CMI	?
Ab, antibody; CMI, cell-mediated immunity; APC, antigen-presenting cell			

Fig. 16.10 Depressed immune responses in microbial infections. In most cases the mechanisms are unclear, but possible important factors are listed. For HIV, the depressed responses are seen later, after initial neutralizing antibody and cytotoxic cell responses. There are at least nine possible mechanisms involved in HIV immunosuppression, but decreased numbers of CD4+ T cells is probably the most important.
*Also, the BCRF1 gene of the virus codes for an IL-10-like molecule that enhances antibody rather than protective CMI responses.
**Patients with a positive tuberculin skin test become temporarily negative during measles infection. Measles also stops macrophages producing IL-12, a molecule needed for the TH1-type (protective) immune response.

virus epidemics, mutations occur at the rate of about two base substitutions per week, some of them involving the main antigenic sites on the virus. HIV (see Chapter 21) undergoes antigenic drift, but in this case it occurs during infection of a given individual, which helps to explain the difficulties experienced by the immune system in controlling this infection. Mutations affecting the epitopes recognized by cytotoxic T (Tc) cells are the source of 'escape mutants'.

The classic example of recombination involves influenza A virus

More extensive and sudden alterations in antigens can take place by the exchange of genetic material between two different microbes. The classic example is genetic 'shift' in influenza A virus, in which human and avian virus strains recombine (see Chapter 19). As a result, a completely new strain of influenza A virus suddenly emerges, brandishing a hemagglutinin or neuraminidase of avian origin. This new virus, not previously experienced by the present population, gives rise to an influenza pandemic.

Gene switching was first demonstrated in African trypanosomes

Gene switching represents the most dramatic form of antigenic variation and was first demonstrated in the African trypanosomes, *Trypanosoma gambiense* and *T. rhodesiense* (see Chapter 27). These organisms carry genes for about one thousand quite distinct surface molecules known as variant-specific glycoproteins, which cover almost the entire surface and are immunodominant. The trypanosome can switch from the use of one gene to another, much as a B cell does with the immunoglobulin heavy chain constant genes. The effect on the host is a sequence of unrelated infections at approximately weekly intervals. This enables the trypanosome to persist while the immune system is constantly trying to catch up with it. The main stimulus for each gene switch is possibly the antibody response itself, but the exact

mechanism is not clear. About 10% of the trypanosome genome consists of surface coat genes, but this is a worthwhile investment for the parasite.

Gene switching is thought to result in the relapsing persistent course of certain infections

Gene switching is also thought to be responsible for the relapsing persistent course of certain other infections, including that by *Borrelia recurrentis* (relapsing fever) and brucellosis. It is also important in gonorrhea, not because of antigenic variation, but because changes in bacterial properties are desirable at different stages of the infection. For instance, attachment to urethral epithelium is vital early in infection by *Neisseria gonorrhoeae*, but attachment to phagocytes is less desirable. Hence there is a switching of genes coding for the pilin and outer membrane proteins that mediate attachment. However, gonococci also show great antigenic variation as they circulate through the host community, and this is achieved by genetic rearrangements and recombinations in the repertoire of pilin genes.

IMMUNOSUPPRESSION

Many virus infections cause a general temporary immunosuppression

A large variety of microorganisms cause immunosuppression in the infected host. As a subversive strategy this makes sense, but the extent to which the microbe benefits is often

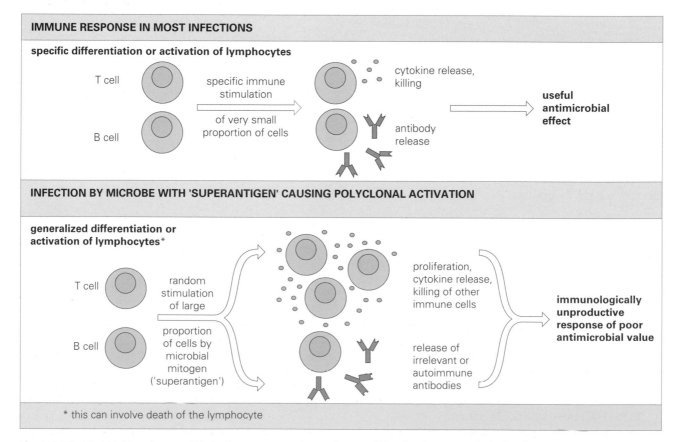

Fig. 16.11 Microbial interference with the immune system by production of T or B cell mitogens (polyclonal activators).

debatable. The host shows a depressed immune response to antigens of the infecting microbe (antigen-specific suppression) or, more commonly, both to antigens of the infecting microbe and unrelated antigens. HIV is one of the most spectacular, but by no means the only microbe that interferes with the immune system in this way, as the death of CD4 T cells results in a disastrous loss of T cell function *(Fig. 16.10)*. The mechanism is generally not understood, but it often involves invasion of the immune system by the microbe—in other words 'to evade, invade'.

Clearly it would benefit the microbe if most responses to its own but not to other antigens were suppressed, but this is uncommon. However, a general immunosuppression, as long as it is temporary, might give the microbe enough time to grow, spread and be shed before being eliminated. This is what happens in many virus infections. A lasting general immunosuppression would be detrimental to the microbe because susceptibility to other infections would cause unnecessary damage to the host species. From this point of view HIV has certainly overstepped the mark.

Different microbes have different immunosuppressive effects

Immunosuppression by microbes often involves actual infection of immune cells:

* T cells (HIV, measles);
* B cells (EBV);
* macrophages (HIV, leishmania);
* dendritic cells (HIV).

This may result in impaired cell function, such as blocking of cell division, blocking of release of interleukin 2 (IL-2) or other cytokines, or in cell death.

Additional immunosuppressive actions taken by microbes include the release of immunosuppressive molecules. For instance, the gp41 polypeptide formed by HIV acts as an 'immunologic anesthetic', temporarily blocking T cell function. Other microbes (poxviruses, herpesviruses, *T. cruzi*) release molecules that interfere with the action of complement or with immunologically important cytokines such as IL-2, IFNs (see above) or tumor necrosis factor (TNF).

Certain microbe toxins are immunomodulators

A particularly dramatic form of immune interference is practiced by the staphylococci. Many strains liberate exotoxins (staphylococcal enterotoxin, epidermolytic toxin and toxic shock syndrome toxin) that are responsible for disease. At first sight, producing these toxins seems to be of no advantage to the staphylococci, but it is now recognized that they have extremely powerful immunomodulatory actions—they are the most potent T cell mitogens known, and act at picomolar concentrations. They function as 'superantigens' and, after binding to class II MHC molecules on antigen-presenting cells, act as polyclonal activators of T cells (see *Fig. 16.11*.). A large proportion (2–20%) of all T cells respond by dividing and releasing cytokines; only 0.001–0.01% are capable of doing this in response to a regular antigen.

It would be logical to presume that these toxins, which are coded for by plasmids, were acquired by the parasite to upset immune responses and therefore to help in the eternal battle with host defenses. As if to confirm this, it has been found that similar molecules are produced by certain streptococci and mycoplasmas.

Possible mechanisms by which the staphylococcal toxins may interfere with immune defenses include:

* excessive local liberation of cytokines by activated cells, upsetting the delicate balance of immune regulation;
* killing of T cells or other immune cells;
* diversion of T cells of all specificities into immunologically unproductive activity by polyclonal activation (see *Fig. 16.11*).

Less dramatic polyclonal activation is seen in many other infections. Microbes may cause polyclonal activation of B cells as well as T cells, for example in EBV and HIV infections, and this can be interpreted as an 'immunodiversion' by the infecting microbe, or in the case of EBV as production of a supply of B cells in which the virus can grow. One consequence is that a range of 'irrelevant', sometimes autoimmune, antibodies are formed (e.g. heterophil antibodies in EBV infection).

Successful microbes often interfere with signaling between immune cells, with cytotoxic T cell recognition or with host apoptotic responses

Many microbes interfere with host molecules such as cytokines, chemokines, MHC, apoptotic and complement receptors, all of which are essential components of host defence. Many DNA viruses code for fake molecules or fake cell receptors for the host molecules, and this disrupts the antimicrobial response. Herpes simplex virus (HSV) produces a molecule, gC (glycoprotein C), that functions as a receptor for C3b. It is present on the virus particle and on the infected cell and interferes with complement activation, protecting both the virus and the infected cell from destruction by antibody and complement.

EB virus produces a homologue of IL-10, which favors a humoral rather than the more protective CMI response induced by IL-12. Virulent strains of *Mycobacterium tuberculosis* induce IL-10 production by infected macrophages, which again favors the infecting microbe. Furthermore, *M. tuberculosis*, as well as other intracellular organisms (*Leishmania major, Histoplasma capsulatum*) inhibit IL-12 production by the infected macrophages. T cells are therefore not activated by IL-12 to form IFNγ, and the immune response is again pushed away from the protective TH1 pattern.

Adenoviruses and herpesviruses reduce MHC class I expression on infected cells, so that cytotoxic T cells fail to recognize such cells. Other viruses (rotaviruses, adenoviruses) interfere with the production or action of interferons.

A strategy useful for one microbe is not necessarily good for others. For example, a local cell infected with a virus can commit suicide by undergoing apoptosis, a useful defense if it takes place before virus replication is complete. Accordingly, certain viruses (HSV, EBV, HIV) code for proteins that interfere with apoptosis, permitting long-term infection of the cell. Other viruses, however, such as measles, induce apoptosis, as do certain bacteria (*Shigella flexneri, Salmonella*) after encountering macrophages, enabling them to escape destruction. It may be useful to induce apoptosis in one cell but not in another. Thus, HIV inhibits apoptosis in the infected immune cell, but induces apoptosis in neighboring uninfected cells

Some microbes interfere with the local expression of the immune response in tissues

Some microbes do not interfere with the development of an immune response, but actively interfere with its expression in tissues. For instance *N. gonorrhoeae*, *Strep. pneumoniae* and many strains of *Haemophilus influenzae* liberate a protease that cleaves human IgA antibody. These bacteria are residents or invaders of mucosae where IgA antibodies operate, and the ability to produce such an enzyme seems unlikely to be mere coincidence.

An equally worthwhile local interference practiced by so many different infectious agents that it is likely to be significant, is the production by the microbe of Fc receptor molecules (see *Fig. 16.8*). The best-known example is protein A, a cell wall protein excreted from virulent staphylococci that inhibits the phagocytosis of antibody-coated bacteria, as shown in *Figure 16.8*. Certain herpesviruses (HSV, varicella-zoster virus (VZV), CMV) code for molecules that act as Fc receptors for IgG, and streptococci produce an Fc receptor for IgA.

PERSISTENT INFECTIONS					
	microorganism	site of persistence	infectiousness of persistent microorganism	consequence	shedding of microorganism to exterior
viruses	herpes simplex	dorsal root ganglia	–	activation, cold sore	+
		salivary glands	+	none known	+
	varicella-zoster	dorsal root ganglia	–	activation, zoster	+
	cytomegalovirus	lymphoid tissue	–	activation ± disease	+
	Epstein–Barr virus	lymphoid tissue	–	lymphoid tumor	–
		epithelium	–	nasopharyngeal carcinoma	–
		salivary glands	+	none known	+
	hepatitis B	liver (virus shed into blood)	+	chronic hepatitis: liver cancer	+
	adenoviruses	lymphoid tissue	–	none known	+
	polyomaviruses BK and JC (man)	kidney	–	activation (pregnancy, immunosuppression)	+
	T cell leukemia viruses	lymphoid and other tissues	±	late leukemia, neurologic disease	–
	paramyxovirus	brain	±	subacute sclerosing panencephalitis	–
	HIV	lymphocytes, macrophages	+	chronic disease	+
chlamydia	trachoma	conjunctiva	+	chronic disease and blindness	?
rickettsia	*Rickettsia prowazeki*	lymph node	?	activation	+
bacteria	*Salmonella typhi*	gall bladder urinary tract	+	intermittent shedding in urine, feces	+
	Mycobacterium tuberculosis	lung or lymph node (macrophages?)	?	activation, tuberculosis in middle aged	+
	Treponema pallidum	disseminated	±	chronic disease	–
protozoa	*Plasmodium vivax*	liver	?	activation, clinical malaria	+
	Toxoplasma gondii	lymphoid tissue, muscle, brain	±	activation, neurologic disease	–
	Trypanosoma cruzi	blood, macrophages	±	chronic disease	–

Fig. 16.12 Examples of persistent infections in humans. Shedding to the exterior takes place either directly, for example via skin lesions, saliva or urine, or indirectly via the blood (hepatitis B, malaria).

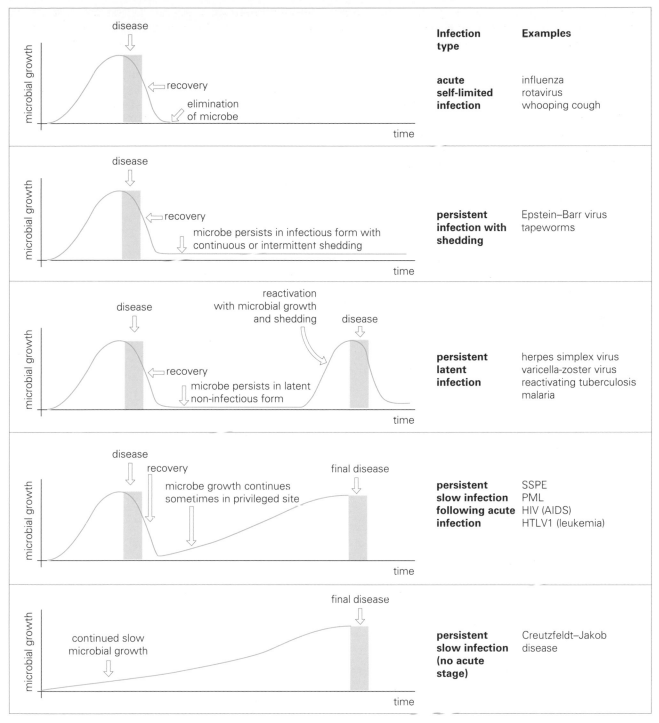

Fig. 16.13 Patterns of acute and persistent infections. For some microbes (e.g. CMV, tuberculosis) the distinction between persistence in infectious form and true latency is not clear. (HTLV1, human T cell leukemia virus 1; PML, progressive multifocal leukencephalopathy; SSPE, subacute sclerosing panencephalitis.)

Other examples include the production by *Pseudomonas* of an elastase that inactivates the C3b and C5a components of complement and hence tends to inhibit opsonic and other host defense functions of complement.

Unfortunately, although the above phenomena look convincingly like microbial adaptations for upsetting host defenses, it is not always easy to prove that this is the case.

PERSISTENT INFECTIONS

Persistent infections represent a failure of host defenses

One way of looking at persistent infections (*Fig. 16.12*) is to regard them as failures of host defenses. Host defenses are

LESSONS IN MICROBIOLOGY

Persistence is of survival value for the microbe

Persistence without any further shedding as occurs in subacute sclerosing panencephalitis and progressive multifocal leukencephalopathy (see Chapter 24) is of no survival value, but there are obvious advantages if the microbe is also shed, either continuously or intermittently. This is especially true when the host species consists of small isolated groups of individuals *(Fig. 16.14)*. Measles, for instance, is not normally a persistent infection. It only infects humans, does not survive for long outside the body and has nowhere else to go (i.e. there is no animal reservoir). Without a continued supply of fresh susceptible humans the virus could not maintain itself and would become extinct. There has to be, at all times, someone acutely infected with measles. From studies of island communities it is clear that you need a minimum of about 500 000 humans to maintain measles without reintroduction from outside. In paleolithic times, when humans lived in small, isolated groups, measles could not have existed in its present form.

In contrast, persistent and latent infections are admirably adapted for survival under these circumstances. VZV can maintain itself in a community of less than 1000 individuals. Children get chickenpox, the virus persists in latent form in sensory neurones, and later in life the virus reactivates to cause shingles. By this time a new generation of susceptible individuals has appeared and the shingles vesicles provide a fresh source of virus.

Serologic studies show that the viral infections prevalent in small, completely isolated Indian communities in the Amazon basin are persistent or latent (e.g. due to adenoviruses, polyomaviruses, papillomaviruses, herpesviruses) rather than non-persistent (e.g. due to influenza, measles, poliovirus). The same principles apply to non-viral infections.

Those present in small communities are either persistent/latent (typhoid, respiratory tuberculosis) or have an animal reservoir for maintenence of the microbe.

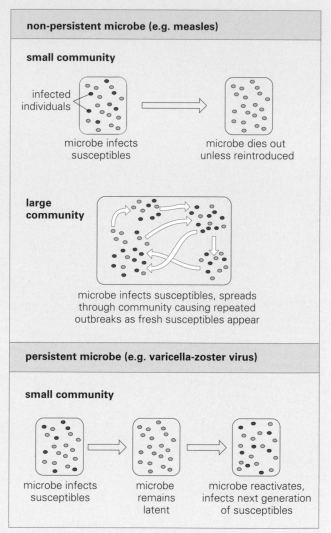

Fig. 16.14 Persistence is a microbial survival strategy.

designed to control microbial growth and spread and to eliminate the microbe from the body. The microbe may persist:

- in a flagrantly defiant infectious form, as with hepatitis B in the blood or the schistosome in the blood vessels of the alimentary tract or bladder;
- in a form with low or partial infectivity, for instance adenoviruses in the tonsils and adenoids;
- in a completely non-infectious form, often without producing any microbial antigens. Latent virus infections

are classic examples of this type of persistence. In the case of HSV, viral DNA persists for many years, probably for life, in sensory neurones in the dorsal root ganglia.

The molecular basis for viral latency has still not been elucidated. It involves special adaptations by the virus to the state of latency—in the case of HSV and VZV there is a very limited transcription of viral RNA in infected neurones, known as 'latency-associated transcripts'. The viral genome is not integrated with host DNA, and instead of being linear it is circular, and exists in free episomal form.

REACTIVATION OF PERSISTENT INFECTIONS		
circumstance	infectious agent	site of shedding
old age	varicella-zoster virus	skin vesicles
	tuberculosis	saliva
pregnancy	polyomaviruses (BK, JC)	urine
	cytomegalovirus	cervix
	herpes simplex virus 2	cervix
	Epstein–Barr virus	saliva
leukemias, lymphomas (e.g. Hodgkin's disease)	varicella-zoster virus	skin vesicles
	polyomavirus (JC)	CNS (PML)*
post-transplant immuno-suppression	herpes simplex virus	skin/mucosal lesions
	varicella-zoster virus	skin vesicles
	wart viruses	skin
	cytomegalovirus	viremia, pneumonitis*
	Epstein–Barr virus	saliva
	hepatitis B	blood
HIV infection	Pneumocystis jiroveci**	lung*
	Toxoplasma gondii	CNS*
	varicella-zoster virus	skin vesicles
	herpes simplex virus	skin/mucosal lesions
	Mycobacterium tuberculosis	lung
	polyomavirus (JC)	CNS (PML)*
* no shedding from these sites ** formerly P. carinii		

Fig. 16.15 Reactivation of persistent infections. (PML, progressive multifocal leukencephalopathy.)

Latent infections can become patent

Latent infections are so-called because they can become patent. This is where they become of immense medical interest, and the legacy of latent herpesvirus infections in man is described in Chapter 26. Different patterns of persistent infections are illustrated in *Figure 16.13*, and they are important for four main reasons:

- They can be reactivated.
- They are sometimes associated with chronic disease, as in the case of chronic hepatitis B infections, subacute sclerosing panencephalitis following measles, and AIDS.
- They are sometimes associated with cancers, such as hepatocellular carcinoma with hepatitis B virus, and

KEY FACTS

- Many successful parasites have adopted strategies for evading immune responses. These enable them to stay in the body long enough to complete their business of infection and shedding to fresh hosts. Some parasites persist indefinitely in the body.
- Mechanisms of immune evasion include:
  - concealing parasite antigens from the host (staying inside host cells, infecting 'privileged sites');
  - changing parasite antigen, either in the infected individual (trypanosomiasis) or during spread through the host population (influenza);
  - direct action on immune cells (e.g. HIV on CD4+ T cells) or on immune signaling systems (e.g. production of fake cytokine molecules);
  - local interference with immune defenses (production of IgA proteases, Fc receptors).
- During persistent infections the microbe may continue to multiply and be able to infect others (HIV, hepatitis B).
- Alternatively, during persistent infections the microbe enters into a latent state and later in life reactivates with renewed multiplication and the ability to infect others (herpesviruses).

Burkitt's lymphoma and nasopharyngeal carcinoma with EBV.
- From the microbial viewpoint, they enable the infectious agent to persist in the host community (see panel).

Reactivation

Reactivation is clinically important in immunosuppressed individuals

Reactivation occurs in immunocompromised patients, and is of major clinical importance in those immunosuppressed as a result of chronic disease or infection (AIDS), tumors (leukemias, lymphomas), or in those immunosuppressed by the physician following transplantation *(Fig. 16.15)*. Reactivation also occurs during naturally occurring periods of immunocompromise, the most important of these being pregnancy and old age. From the microbe's point of view, latency is an adaptation that allows reactivation with renewed growth and shedding of the infectious agent during these naturally occurring periods.

Features of reactivation in herpesvirus infections are described in Chapters 21 and 26. We still know very little about reactivation mechanisms at the molecular level, as might be expected in view of our ignorance about the latent

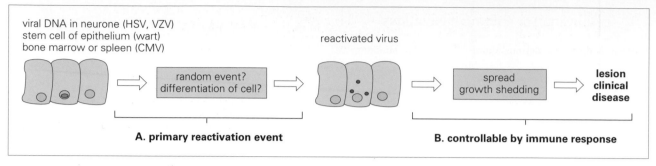

Fig. 16.16 Two stages in reactivation of latent viruses. (CMV, cytomegalovirus.)

state itself. Latency is often thought of as a period when the microbe is in deep sleep. However, recent experiments suggest it may be a more active state. For example, *M. tuberculosis* needs to make certain proteins to keep itself patent. Other products – called resuscitation promoting factors – may be needed to wake up a latent microbe.

It is useful to distinguish two stages in reactivation

The first event (stage A) in reactivation *(Fig. 16.16)*, the resumption of viral activity in the latently infected cell, is the most mysterious stage. In the case of HSV, this can be triggered by sensory stimuli arriving in the neurone (from skin areas responding to sunlight) and also by certain fevers (i.e. during other infections) or by hormonal influences. Little more than this is known!

The second event (stage B) involves the spread and replication of the reactivated virus. HSV must travel down the sensory axon to the skin or mucosal surface, infect and spread in subepithelial tissues and then in the epithelium, finally forming a virus-rich vesicle (more than one million infectious

units/ml of vesicle fluid). All this takes at least 3–4 days. Stage B is less mysterious than stage A and can be controlled by the immune system. Therefore, cold sores may be associated with poor lymphocyte responses to HSV antigens, and zoster with declining cell-mediated responses (specifically to VZV antigens) in old people.

Stage A probably occurs more frequently than stage B, because immune defenses often arrest the process during stage B before final production of the lesion. Hence as many as 10–20% of HSV reactivation episodes are thought to be 'non-lesional' with burning, tingling and itching at the site, but no signs of a cold sore. Also, zoster may involve no more than the sensory prodrome associated with virus reactivation and replication in sensory neurones; skin lesions are prevented by host defenses.

Reactivation of EBV and CMV with appearance of the virus in saliva (EBV) or blood (CMV) is generally asymptomatic. In immunologically deficient individuals, however, reactivation may progress to cause clinical disease: either hepatitis and pneumonitis in the case of CMV or the rarer hairy tongue leukoplakia due to EBV (see Chapter 30).

? QUESTIONS

1. Could molecular mimicry be a mere biologic accident? If it were, would you expect it to be more common with short (4–5) than with long (7–8) amino acid sequences?

2. Why should antigenic variation involve especially the outer (surface) molecules of a parasite?

3. Based on your understanding of herpesvirus latency:
   (a) Could you catch shingles after contact with a case of chickenpox?
   (b) Could you develop a cold sore a few weeks after contact with a patient with a cold sore?

4. Under what circumstances might a wart virus in the epidermis be exposed to immune defenses?

FURTHER READING

Alcami A, Koszinowski UH. Viral mechanisms of immune evasion. *Trends Microbiol* 2000; 8:410–18.

Fitzpatrick DR, Bielefeldt-Ohmann H. Mechanisms of herpes virus immuno-evasion. *Microb Pathogen* 1991; 10:253–259.

Garcia-Blanco MA, Cullen BR. Molecular basis of latency in pathogenic human viruses. *Science* 1991; 254:815–20.

Lower R, Lower J, Kurth R. The viruses in all of us: characteristics and biologic significance of human retrovirus sequences. *Proc Natl Acad Sci USA* 1996; 93:5177–84.

Maizels RM, Bundy DAP, Selkirk ME et al. Immunologic modulation and evasion by helminth parasites in human populations. *Nature* 1993; 365:797–805.

Mocarski ES. Immunomodulation by cytomegaloviruses: manipulative strategies beyond evasion. *Trends Microbiol* 2002; 10:332–9.

Nau GJ, Richmond JF, Schlesinger A et al. Human macrophage activation programs induced by bacterial pathogens. *Proc Natl Acad Sci USA* 2002; 99:1503–8.

INTRODUCTION

Symptoms of infections are produced by the microorganisms or by the host's immune responses

Symptoms that appear rapidly after the acquisition of an infection are usually due to the direct action of the invading microbe or its secretions. Thus a virus in a cell may cause metabolic 'shut-down' or lyse the cell. Bacteria, however, provoke most of their acute effects by releasing toxins, but may also cause distress by inducing inflammation. The inflammatory response is, of course, an important component of host protection, vascular permeability being vital for the rapid mobilization of cells such as neutrophils, and serum components such as complement and antibody. Inflammation is therefore intrinsically a healthy sign, and it is interesting that some virulent bacteria (e.g. staphylococci) can to some extent inhibit the inflammatory response.

Often, however, pathologic changes are secondary to the activation of immunologic mechanisms that are normally thought of as protective. These may involve the natural or the adaptive immune system or, more usually, both (Fig. 17.1). Tissue damage resulting from adaptive immune responses is usually referred to as 'immunopathology' and is quite common in infectious diseases, particularly those that are chronic and persistent. The immunologic basis of these mechanisms of tissue damage is described in Chapter 11.

Certain viruses can cause permanent malignant change in cells. Examples include HTLV1 and 2 (lymphomas, leukemias), Epstein–Barr virus (nasopharyngeal carcinoma and Burkitt's lymphoma), genital papilloma viruses (cervical cancer), and hepatitis B virus (liver cancer). Cofactors may be involved.

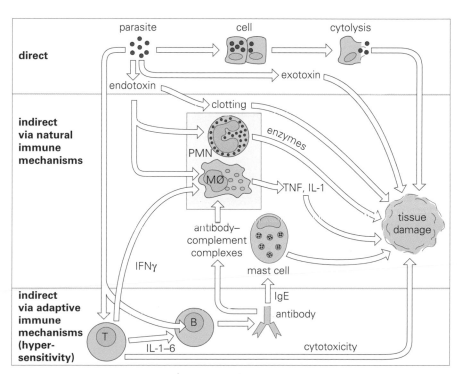

Fig. 17.1 Pathologic effects of infection: a general scheme. Infectious parasitic organisms can cause disease directly (top) or indirectly via overactivation of various immune mechanisms, either natural (center) or adaptive (bottom). (IFN, interferon; IL, interleukin; Mφ, macrophage; PMN, polymorphonuclear leukocyte, TNF, tumor necrosis factor.)

PATHOLOGY CAUSED DIRECTLY BY THE MICROORGANISM

Direct effects may result from cell rupture, organ blockage or pressure effects

Organisms that multiply in cells and subsequently spread usually do so by rupturing the cell. Many viruses and some intracellular bacteria and protozoa behave in this way (Fig. 17.2). It is important to realize that many others do not. For example, viruses or bacteria may remain latent (e.g. herpes simplex virus and varicella-zoster virus in nerve ganglia, and *Mycobacterium tuberculosis* in macrophages), and many viruses can bud from a cell without disrupting it. The type of cell infected may also have an influence on survival of the organism, thus HIV lyses T cells, but persists in macrophages. Other direct effects include:

- blockage of major hollow viscera by worms;
- blockage of lung alveoli by dense growth of, for example, *Pneumocystis*;
- mechanical effects of large cysts (e.g. hydatid).

Exotoxins are a common cause of serious tissue damage, especially in bacterial infection

The parasite may actively secrete 'exotoxins' (Fig. 17.3). In some cases these are clearly part of its strategy for entry, spread or defense against the host, but sometimes they seem to be of little or no benefit to the parasite.

Most exotoxins are proteins and are often coded not by the bacterial DNA, but in plasmids (e.g. *Escherichia coli*) or phages (e.g. botulism, diphtheria, scarlet fever). In some cases they consist of two or more subunits, one of which is required for binding and entry to the cell while the other switches on or inhibits some cellular function.

Powerful toxins are generally secreted from extracellular microbes. Microbes that multiply in cells cannot afford to cause serious damage at too early a stage, and such toxins therefore tend to be less prominent in intracellular infections due to *Mycobacteria*, *Chlamydia*, or *Mycoplasma*. For example, leprosy patients with lepromatous disease have huge bacterial loads for many years without any toxicity. Although many toxins can kill host cells, lower concentrations may be important by causing dysfunction in immune or phagocytic cells. For example, concentrations of streptolysin well below the cell-killing level will inhibit leukocyte chemotaxis, and the staphylococcal enterotoxin and epidermolytic toxins also have immunomodulatory activity at exceedingly low (nanogram to picogram) levels.

Inactivation of toxins without altering antigenicity results in successful vaccines

Toxins can often be inactivated (e.g. by formaldehyde) without altering their antigenicity, and the resulting toxoids are among the most successful of all vaccines (see Chapter 34), the classic examples being diphtheria and tetanus toxoids. Toxins are generally more highly conserved in their structure

ORGANISMS THAT DIRECTLY DAMAGE TISSUE		
organism	cell or tissue damaged	mechanism
viruses poliovirus rhinovirus HIV coxsackievirus rotavirus	neurones URT mucosa CD4, T cells, macrophages, pancreatic β cells, heart enterocytes	cytopathic
bacteria *Streptococcus mutans* mycobacteria	teeth macrophages	acid production damaged macrophage releases cytokines
fungi *Histoplasma*	macrophages	damaged macrophage releases cytokines
protozoa *Plasmodium*	erythrocytes	damaged erythrocyte removed
helminths *Ascaris* *Echinococcus*	intestinal occlusion biliary occlusion hydatid cyst	mechanical mechanical, inflammation pressure effects

Fig. 17.2 Many organisms directly damage or destroy the tissues they infect. This is especially common with cytopathic viruses. (URT, upper respiratory tract.)

EXOTOXINS OF IMPORTANCE IN DISEASE

organism	exotoxin	tissue damaged	action	disease
bacteria				
Clostridium tetani	tetanospasmin	neurones	spastic paralysis	tetanus
Clostridium perfringens	α-toxin	erythrocytes, platelets, leukocytes, endothelium	cell lysis	gas gangrene
Clostridium botulinum	neurotoxin	nerve–muscle junction	flaccid paralysis	botulism
Corynebacterium diphtheriae	diphtheria toxin	throat, heart, peripheral nerve	inhibits protein synthesis	diphtheria
Shigella dysenteriae	enterotoxin	intestinal mucosa	—	dysentery
Escherichia coli	enterotoxin	intestinal epithelium	fluid loss from	gastroenteritis
Vibrio cholerae	enterotoxin		intestinal cells	cholera
Staphylococcus aureus	α-toxin	red and white cells	hemolysis	abscesses
	hemolysin	(via cytokines)	hemolysis	
	leucocidin	leukocytes	destroys leukocytes	
	enterotoxin	intestinal cells	induces vomiting diarrhea	food poisoning
	TSST1	—	release of cytotoxins	toxic shock syndrome
	epidermolytic	epidermis	—	scalded skin syndrome
Streptococcus pyogenes	streptolysin O and S	red and white cells	hemolysis	hemolysis pyogenic lesion
	erythrogenic	skin capillaries	skin rash	scarlet fever
Bacillus anthracis	cytotoxin	lung	pulmonary edema	anthrax
Bordetella pertussis	pertussis toxin	trachea	kills epithelium	whooping cough
Legionella pneumophila	numerous	neutrophils	cell lysis	Legionnaires' disease
Listeria monocytogenes	hemolysin	leukocytes, monocytes	cell lysis	listeriosis
Pseudomonas aeruginosa	exotoxin A	cells	cell lysis	various infections
fungi				
Aspergillus fumigatus	aflatoxin	liver	carcinogenic	?liver damage/cancer*
protozoa				
Entamoeba histolytica	enterotoxin	colonic epithelium	cell lysis	amebic dysentery

Fig. 17.3 Important exotoxins in disease. Many bacteria and a few other organisms damage host tissues by secreting exotoxins. Some bacterial exotoxins are among the most powerful toxins known. Vaccination, by inducing antibody, is often very effective in protection. (TSST1, toxic shock syndrome toxin.)* In turkeys and pigs from *A. fumigatus*-contaminated ground nuts but not so far in humans.

than the surface antigens of the organism secreting them. This allows for more effective cross-immunity and explains, for example, why scarlet fever (caused by streptococcal erythrotoxin) usually occurs only once, while streptococcal infections recur almost indefinitely.

An interesting offshoot of the two subunit structure of toxins is that by changing the specificity of the part responsible for attachment, the specificity of the toxin for a particular cell type can be changed. An example is the plant toxin ricin—the A subunit can be attached to a monoclonal antibody to make it a specific poison for tumor cells. The same strategy could obviously be used against parasites if desired.

Mode of action of toxins and consequences

These can be be considered under five headings (*Fig. 17.4*).

Bacteria may produce enzymes to promote their survival or spread

A number of bacteria release enzymes that break down the tissues or the intercellular substances of the host, allowing the infection to spread freely. Among these enzymes are hyaluronidase, collagenase, DNase and streptokinase. Some staphylococci release a coagulase, which deposits a protective

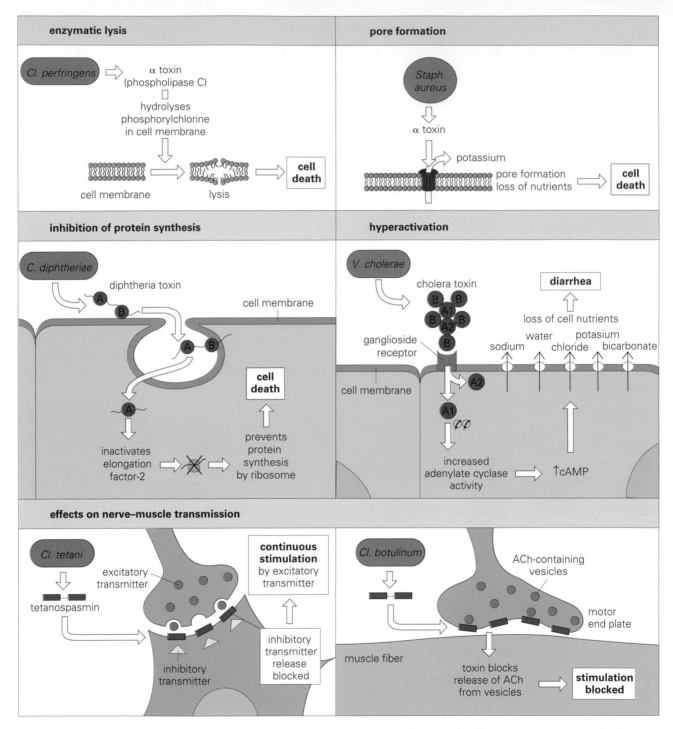

Fig. 17.4 The mode of action of some exotoxins. Bacterial toxins act in a variety of ways. Often the toxin is a two-chain molecule, one chain being concerned with entry into cells while the other has inhibitory activity against some vital function. (ACh, acetylcholine; cAMP, cyclic adenosine monophosphate; C., *Corynebacterium*; Cl., *Clostridium*; Staph., *Staphylococcus*; V., *Vibrio*.)

layer of fibrin onto and around the cells, thus localizing them.

Toxins may damage or destroy cells and are then known as hemolysins

Cell membranes can be damaged enzymatically by lecithinases or phospholipases, or by insertion of pore-forming molecules, which destroy the integrity of the cell. The collective term for such toxins is 'hemolysins',

although many cells other than red blood cells can be affected. Both staphylococci and streptococci produce pore-forming toxins; pseudomonads release enzymatic hemolysins.

Toxins may enter cells and actively alter some of the metabolic machinery

Characteristically these toxin molecules have two subunits. The A subunit is the active component, while the B subunit is a binding component needed to interact with receptors on the cell membrane. When binding occurs, the A subunit, or the whole toxin–receptor complex, is taken into the cell by endocytosis, and the A subunit becomes activated. Two well-studied toxins of this type are those of diphtheria (see Chapter 18) and cholera.

Diphtheria toxin blocks protein synthesis

Diphtheria toxin is synthesized as a single polypeptide (from bacteriophage *n* genes) and binds by the B subunit to target cells (*Fig. 17.4*). The polypeptide is partially cleaved and then the entire toxin–receptor complex is internalized. The A subunit then splits off and passes into the cytosol, where it inactivates the transfer of amino acids from transfer RNA to the polypeptide chain during translation of mRNA by ribosomes. It does this by catalyzing attachment of adenosine diphosphate (ADP) ribose to the elongation protein (ADP ribosylation), effectively blocking protein synthesis.

Cholera toxin results in massive loss of water from intestinal epithelial cells

Cholera toxin is released as a complex of five B subunits surrounding the A subunit. The latter is cleaved into two fragments—A1 and A2—held by disulfide bonds. The B subunits bind to ganglioside receptors on intestinal epithelial cells, leading to internalization of the A subunits, which then separate from one another (*Fig. 17.4*). The A1 portion then ADP-ribosylates one of the regulatory molecules involved in the production of cyclic adenosine monophosphate (cAMP). As a result the molecule is unable to turn off production. The increased levels of cAMP in the cell change the sodium/chloride flux across the cell membrane, resulting in a massive outflow of water and electrolytes from the cell and causing the profuse diarrhea of cholera. The exotoxins of *Escherichia coli* and salmonella have similar actions, as does pertussis toxin.

Tetanus and botulinum toxins are among the most potent affecting nerve impulses

One gram of botulinum toxin is sufficient to kill 10 million people! Tetanus and botulinum toxins have the characteristic A + B structure, the B subunit binding to ganglioside receptors on nerve cells. The internalized A subunit of tetanus is carried by axonal transport from the point of production to the central nervous system (CNS), where it interferes with synaptic transmission in inhibitory neurones by blocking neurotransmitter release. This allows the excitatory transmitter to continuously stimulate the motor neurones, causing spastic paralysis. Botulinum toxin enters the body via the intestine, escaping digestion and crossing the gut wall. The toxin affects peripheral nerve endings at the neuromuscular junction, blocking presynaptic release of acetylcholine. This prevents muscle contraction, causing flaccid paralysis.

Diarrhea

Diarrhea is an almost invariable result of intestinal infections

Diarrhea is one of the major causes of death in children worldwide (see Chapter 22). It can be considered as:

- a means for the host to rid itself rapidly of the infectious organism;
- a means for the infection to spread to other hosts.

Diarrhea is a feature of a wide range of organisms, but in only a few cases is the exact mechanism understood. While toxins are often the cause (cholera, shigella), microbial invasion and damage to epithelial cells may also be important. The pathophysiology, with changes in electron transport or loss of enterocytes, has been elucidated in some cases. Many of the organisms causing diarrhea can be 'picked up' from food, but the term 'food poisoning' is usually reserved for those cases where toxins are already present in the food rather than being generated during the growth of organisms in the intestine. As would be expected, 'food poisoning' causes symptoms earlier—that is, hours after exposure rather than days (*Fig. 17.5*).

PATHOLOGIC ACTIVATION OF NATURAL IMMUNE MECHANISMS

Overactivity can damage host tissues

The very potent natural immune mechanisms discussed in Chapter 14 have in-built safety as far as specificity is

INFECTIOUS CAUSES OF DIARRHEA		
food poisoning (due to pre-formed toxin in food)		
	onset	source
Staphylococcus aureus	1–6 hours	cream, meat, poultry
Clostridium perfringens	8–20 hours	reheated meat
Clostridium botulinum	12–36 hours	canned food
Bacillus cereus	1–20 hours	reheated foods
intestinal infections		
	onset	source
rotavirus	2–5 days	contact (fecal–oral)
salmonella	1–2 days	eggs
shigella	1–4 days	fecal–oral
campylobacter	1–4 days	poultry, domestic animals
Vibrio cholerae	2 days	fecal–oral
Escherichia coli	1–4 days	traveller's diarrhea
Yersinia enterocolitica	days–weeks	pets (e.g. dogs)
Giardia lamblia	1–2 weeks	contaminated water
Entamoeba histolytica	days–weeks	
Cryptosporidium	days–weeks	fecal–oral, opportunistic (e.g. in AIDS)
Isopora belli		

Fig. 17.5 Infectious causes of diarrhea. Worldwide, infectious diarrhea is the major cause of infant mortality.

concerned. They have had to evolve in the constant presence of the host's 'self' antigens, to which they do not therefore respond. However, they are not so well controlled quantitatively, and there are many cases when overactivity not only damages an invading parasite, but also damages innocent host tissues. The expression of natural immunity often causes a certain amount of inflammation—and this can be severe, with tissue damage. Complement, polymorphs and tumor necrosis factor (TNF) play important roles.

Microbial endotoxin activates the immune system and induces cytokines, causing a bewildering variety of biologic effects *(Fig. 17.6)*. At the clinical level, it can be responsible for septic shock.

Endotoxins are typically lipopolysaccharides

'Endotoxins' of bacteria and other microorganisms have a deceptively similar name to exotoxins, but are profoundly different in their significance. Unlike exotoxins, these are integral parts of the microbial cell wall and are normally released only when the cell dies. Endotoxins are particularly characteristic of Gram-negative bacteria. A typical lipopolysaccharide (LPS) endotoxin is composed of:

- a lipid portion (lipid A) inserted into the cell wall, responsible for much of the toxic activity;
- a conserved core polysaccharide;
- the highly variable O-polysaccharide, responsible for the serologic diversity which is a feature of organisms such as salmonellae and shigellae.

LPSs stimulate an extraordinary range of host responses—or perhaps one should say a wide range of responses have evolved to respond to LPSs. In the words of Lewis Thomas 'when we sense lipopolysaccharide, we are likely to turn on

every defence at our disposal' *(Fig. 17.6)*. Evidently the body needs to be aware of invading Gram-negative bacteria at the earliest possible stage.

Clinically, the most important effects of LPS are:

- fever;
- vascular collapse (or shock).

As mentioned in Chapter 14, fever may benefit host or parasite or both, and is currently considered to be mainly due to the action of two cytokines—interleukin 1 (IL-1) and tumor necrosis factor (TNF)—on the hypothalamus. Both these cytokines are produced by macrophages in response to LPS (and to analogous molecules from other organisms, see below).

Endotoxin shock is usually associated with systemic spread of organisms

The commonest example of endotoxin (or 'septic') shock is septicemia with Gram-negative bacteria such as *E. coli* or *Neisseria meningitidis*. However, many other organisms also release molecules that stimulate TNFα and/or IL-1 production *(Fig. 17.7)* and therefore function in part like LPS, although they are more or less unrelated in structure. In the 'toxic shock syndrome' of young women with staphylococcal infections of the genital tract, toxic shock syndrome toxin (TSST1) is the mediator, yet it is a superantigen, activating a large proportion of all T cells (up to 1 in 5, see Chapter 16). Perhaps the enormous numbers of activated T cells produce enough cytokines to cause the toxic effect.

Septic shock, however, is a complex phenomenon, and other bacterial components, such as peptidoglycans, may also play a part. In streptococcal infections the culprits are pyrogenic (erythrogenic) exotoxins released by the bacteria.

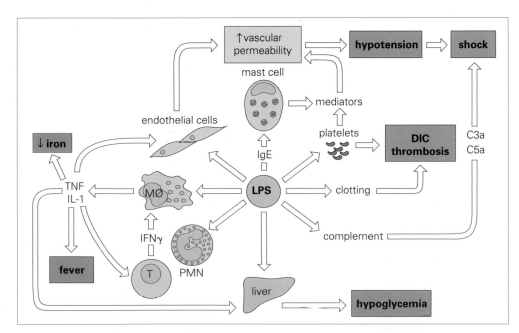

Fig. 17.6 The many activities of bacterial endotoxin. Lipopolysaccharide (LPS) activates almost every immune mechanism as well as the clotting pathway and as a result LPS is one of the most powerful immune stimuli known. (DIC, disseminated intravascular coagulation; IFN, interferon; IL, interleukin; Mφ, macrophage; PMN, polymorphonuclear leukocyte; TNF, tumor necrosis factor.)

IMPORTANT ENDOTOXINS AND FUNCTIONALLY RELATED MOLECULES		
organisms	toxin	cytokines induced
bacteria		
Gram-negative		
Salmonella		
Shigella	LPS	TNF, IL-1
Escherichia coli		
Neisseria		
meningitidis		
Gram-positive		
Staphylococcus aureus	TSST1	TNF
mycobacteria	lipoarabinomannan	TNF
Bordetella pertussis	endotoxin	TNF
fungi		
yeasts	zymosan	TNF
protozoa		
Plasmodium	phospholipids (exoantigens)	TNF

Fig. 17.7 Important endotoxins and functionally related molecules. Most endotoxins are lipopolysaccharides (LPS) and exert their main effects by stimulating cytokine release. (IL, interleukin; TNF, tumor necrosis factor; TSST1, toxic shock syndrome toxin.)

The involvement of cytokines in the pathogenesis of shock is by no means a purely academic concern, because it suggests the possibility of treatment by antagonists of a small number of cytokines (e.g. by monoclonal antibodies or inhibitors) rather than by antibodies to the toxins themselves, which are of enormous antigenic diversity. This idea is discussed further in Chapter 33.

The cytokine most closely linked to disease at present is TNF

Raised concentrations of TNFα in the serum have been shown to correlate with severity in patients with meningococcal septicemia and with *Plasmodium falciparum* malaria. However, animal experiments indicate that in such cases TNFα probably synergizes with other cytokines such as IL-1 and interferon-gamma (IFNγ) to produce its full effects. In meningococcal disease, TNFα levels in blood and cerebrospinal fluid (CSF) can change independently, the former being raised in septicemia and the latter in meningitis; it therefore appears that the production and/or effects of TNFα can be restricted to a particular body compartment.

Complement is involved in several tissue-damaging reactions

The activation of complement is a vital part of immunity to many bacteria, viruses and protozoa (see Chapter 14).

Complement can, however, be involved in tissue-damaging reactions, for example immune complex disease, which also involves antibody and, usually, polymorphonuclear leukocytes (PMNs). Complement also plays an important role in the acute inflammatory response by generating the chemotactic factors C3a and C5a (see Chapter 9).

Direct activation of complement by LPS may contribute to the shock induced by toxic amounts of this endotoxin in which the levels of complement components (e.g. C3) drop profoundly; this response appears to involve both the classical and the alternative pathways, which are activated by the lipid and polysaccharide components, respectively. C3a and C5a are produced in large amounts, and there is frequently a severe decrease in the number of PMNs because of aggregation of these cells, adherence to vessel walls, and their activation to release toxic molecules, both oxidative and non-oxidative. When this occurs in the pulmonary capillaries, severe pulmonary edema may result—the 'adult respiratory distress syndrome' (ARDS).

Disseminated intravascular coagulation is a rare but serious feature of bacterial septicemia

Disseminated intravascular coagulation (DIC) can be a feature of bacterial (e.g. meningococcal) septicemia, but is also seen in some virus infections such as Ebola fever (Chapter 28). The relative contributions of immune complexes, platelets, and direct activation of the clotting pathway via the effect of LPS on Hageman factor, remain controversial. For example, the hemorrhagic phenomena of yellow fever are probably secondary to coagulation defects due to the extensive liver damage, whereas in dengue ('hemorrhagic') fever it has been suggested that there is immune complex deposition in blood vessels. However, in all these hemorrhagic syndromes the role of cytokines such as TNF also needs to be considered.

Mast cell degranulation in response to LPS is usually secondary to IgE antibody formation

Some insect venoms, however, may be able to activate mast cells directly, and reactions of this kind are called 'anaphylactoid'.

PATHOLOGIC CONSEQUENCES OF THE IMMUNE RESPONSE

Overreaction of the immune system is known as 'hypersensitivity'

Adaptive immune responses are vital to defense against infection, as witnessed by the increased susceptibility to infectious disease of immunodeficient patients (see Chapter 30). The antimicrobial effects of lymphocyte responses act mainly by specifically focusing or enhancing non-specific effector mechanisms (see Chapter 10). This may, however, also enhance the pathologic effects outlined above. The tissue-damaging effects of hypersensitivity are referred to as 'immunopathologic'. Coombs and Gell classified hypersensitivity into four types in 1958, based on the immunologic mechanism underlying the tissue damaging reaction.

Each of the four main types of hypersensitivity can be of microbial or non-microbial origin

Hypersensitivity of microbial origin includes some of the most serious of these responses *(Fig. 17.8)*. Organisms of many sorts can be involved, but one common feature is that the infection is prolonged, with continuous or repeated antigenic stimulation.

Type I hypersensitivity

Allergic reactions are a feature of worm infections

The most dramatic allergic (type I) reaction is that following the rupture of a hydatid cyst. Slow leakage of worm antigens ensures that the patient's mast cells are sensitized with specific IgE, and the massive flood of antigens on rupture may cause acute fatal anaphylaxis, with vascular collapse and pulmonary edema. Even the small amount of antigen used in diagnostic skin tests can have this effect, although this is rare.

Another worm associated with high levels of IgE is *Ascaris*, but here the pathologic consequences are mainly respiratory, with eosinophilic infiltrates and asthmatic episodes corresponding to passage of the parasite through the lung. The itching rashes characteristic of helminth infections when the worms die in the skin are probably also of this type, an example being 'swimmer's itch' due to animal or avian schistosomes.

Why allergic reactions are such a feature of worm infections is not really clear, but they may be due to some feature of the antigens; in addition, it has been suggested that IgE plays a role in protection against worms. One would hope so, as in all other respects this class of antibody appears to be nothing but a nuisance.

Type II hypersensitivity

Type II reactions are mediated by antibodies to the infectious organism or autoantibodies

Strictly speaking, type II reactions are mediated by antibody (usually IgG) leading to cytotoxicity, either extracellular or intracellular (e.g. after phagocytosis). Antibody binds to the cell and, if complement is activated, the cell is lysed. Cytotoxicity by T cells is considered under type IV reactions. An important distinction can be made between antibodies to the (foreign) infectious organism and autoantibodies; the former kill host cells because they display foreign antigens, whereas the latter bind to unaltered host antigens, and both types of response occur in infectious disease *(Fig. 17.8)*. In the latter case, of course, the interesting question is why autoantibodies should be formed during infection, and several mechanisms have been postulated for this. However the whole question of autoimmunity remains highly controversial.

In blood-stage malaria, microbial antigens attach themselves to host cells

It has been shown that the hemolytic anemia of blood-stage malaria is due not to autoantibody as previously thought, but to antibodies to parasite-derived antigen that have been picked up by red cells. In some cases it may be the antigen–antibody complex that binds to the cell. A similar reaction can occur following quinine treatment of *Plasmodium falciparum* malaria—blackwater fever.

Antimyocardial antibody of group A β-hemolytic streptococcal infection is the classic autoantibody triggered by infection

This reaction is due to the presence of the same cross-reacting carbohydrate antigen on the bacterium and the myocardium. However, as more protein sequences are obtained and compared, numerous other similar examples have come to light, and it is possible that cross-reaction between microbial and human antigens may underlie a number of diseases of currently unknown origin. Whether this mimicry of host antigens has any survival value to the microbe is discussed in Chapter 16.

Type III hypersensitivity

Immune complexes cause disease when they become lodged in tissues or blood vessels

The formation of immune complexes can lead to phagocytosis and removal of antigen, but also to complement activation. Complications occur when the complexes escape removal by the phagocytes of the reticuloendothelial system and become lodged in the tissues or blood vessels, attracting complement and neutrophils. Release of lysosomal enzymes then results in local damage, which is particularly serious in small blood vessels, especially in the renal glomeruli. Immune complex disease is a major cause of both acute and chronic glomerulonephritis, and the majority of cases are probably the result of infection. There is also an important group in which autoantigen–autoantibody complexes are responsible (e.g. DNA–anti-DNA in systemic lupus erythematosus), but even these may ultimately be the consequence of a viral infection.

Like most other immunopathologic conditions, immune complex deposition is usually a feature of chronic infection (e.g. malaria). However, a persistent antigenic stimulus is not the only prerequisite, indicated by the fact that the most serious form of malarial nephropathy is found in *Plasmodium malariae* (quartan) malaria, which progresses despite successful treatment of the infection, while the nephropathy of *P. falciparum* (malignant tertian) malaria typically recovers after the infection has been cured. Predisposing factors may include a poor antibody response (in terms of amount or affinity), a particular tendency of the antigen itself to bind to vascular endothelium, or inhibition of the normal function of phagocytes or complement in removing circulating complexes.

Acute glomerulonephritis occurs as a serious complication of streptococcal infection (Chapter 18) and is at least partly due to localization in glomeruli of immune complexes containing streptococcal antigens (see *Fig. 17.10*). Polymorph infiltration and alterations in the basement membrane cause leakage of albumin, even red cells, in the urine. The glomerulonephritis appears a few weeks after the infection has been terminated. When complexes are deposited over a long period (malarial nephropathy) the mesangial cell intrusions and fusion of foot processes cause a more irreversible impairment of glomerular function (chronic glomerulonephritis).

HYPERSENSITIVITY OF MICROBIAL ORIGIN

Coombs and Gell classification	principal mechanism	examples

type I (allergic/anaphylactic)	IgE, mast cells	helminths
		  Ascaris
		  hydatid (ruptured cyst)
		? viral skin rash
		? upper respiratory tract
		  viral infections

type II (cytotoxic)	IgG to surface
	complement
	cytotoxic cells
		virus infected cells
		malaria infected erythrocytes
		autoantibodies in:
		  Mycoplasma
		  streptococci
		  Trypanosoma cruzi

type III (immune complex-mediated)	immune complexes
	complement
	PMN
		in tissues:
		  allergic alveolitis
		  actinomycosis
		in blood vessels:
		  glomerulonephritis
		  malaria
		  streptococci
		  hepatitis B
		  syphilis

type IV (cell-mediated)	T lymphocytes
	cytokines
	macrophages (and other
	  non-specific cells)
		granuloma
		  tuberculosis
		  leprosy (tuberculoid)
		  schistosomiasis (eggs)
		  Histoplasma
		mononuclear infiltration
		  ± cell damage in many
		  virus infections (i.e. tissue delayed-type
		  hypersensitivity responses) with CD4, CD8, cytokines
		  and macrophages playing roles
		viral rashes

autoimmunity	cross-reaction with host polyclonal B cell activation	streptococcal myocarditis African trypanosomiasis

Fig. 17.8 Hypersensitivity of microbial origin. All four classic types of hypersensitivity can be induced by infectious organisms, types II and III being the most commonly encountered. Note that some mechanisms mediating hypersensitivity also take part in protective immunity. (PMN, polymorphonuclear leukocyte.)

Occupational diseases associated with inhalation of fungi are the classic examples of immune complex deposition in the tissues

Immune complex deposition in the tissues, made famous by the work of Arthus on antigens injected into the skin of animals with pre-existing antibody (mainly IgG), manifests as a combination of thrombosis in small blood vessels and necrosis in the tissues due to PMN degranulation *(Fig. 17.9)*. Perhaps the best-studied examples are the occupational diseases associated with inhalation of fungi (e.g. farmer's

lung, pigeon-fancier's disease, maple bark stripper's disease) in which chronic inflammation of the lung can lead to a state of destruction and fibrosis known as 'extrinsic allergic alveolitis', an unfortunate name since classical (IgE-mediated) allergy does not seem to be involved.

Another well-known model of immune complex disease is serum sickness

Serum sickness follows repeated injections of foreign protein, leading to circulating complexes, which deposit in the kidneys

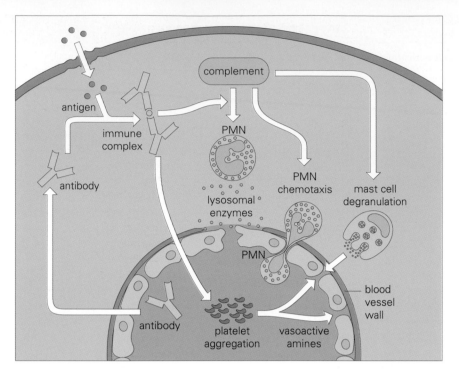

Fig. 17.9 The Arthus reaction. Microbial antigens that enter the tissues (e.g. fungal particles in the lung) encounter antibody and form immune complexes. These activate complement and initiate chemotaxis of polymorphonuclear leukocytes (PMNs), and degranulation of these and tissue mast cells. The resulting inflammatory response is further potentiated by damage induced by PMN-derived lysosomal enzymes.

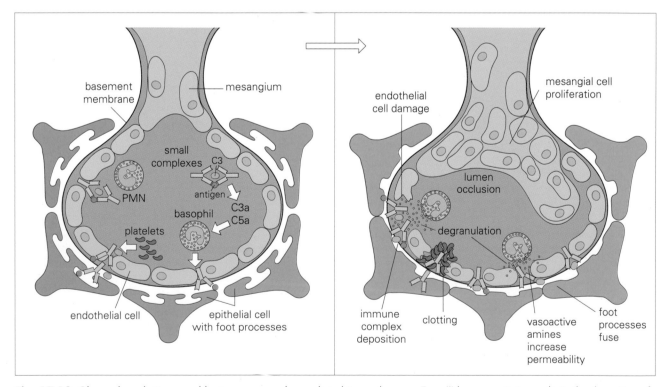

Fig. 17.10 Glomerulonephritis caused by immune complex-mediated tissue damage. Type III hypersensitivity results in the deposition of immune complexes in the bloodvessel walls, particularly at sites of high pressure, filtration or turbulence such as the kidney. (PMN, polymorphonuclear leukocyte.)

CELL-MEDIATED RESPONSES			
immune cells or molecules	protective effect against	pathologic effect	skin test
cytotoxic T cells (CD8)	virus infections _Theileria_ ? mycobacteria	local tissue loss	–
basophils T cells	?	inflammation	24 h (Jones-Mote)
T cells macrophages cytokines giant cells epithelioid cells eosinophils	intracellular organisms viruses bacteria fungi protozoa worms	mononuclear cell infiltration granuloma fibrosis calcification (>14 days)	delayed/tuberculin type (>2 days)

Fig. 17.11 Cell-mediated immunity in protection and disease. The nomenclature of cell-mediated immune responses is complicated. Although often described in terms of skin tests, their real significance is related to protective and/or pathologic reactions in the tissues.

(Fig. 17.10), skin and joints. This was common in the pre-antibiotic days of passive serotherapy for infectious disease (see Chapter 35). It is also a possible complication of treatment with monoclonal (usually murine) antibody, which is an increasingly attractive approach to many conditions, and this is one of the reasons why determined efforts are being made to produce monoclonal antibodies in which as much of the molecule as possible is humanized.

Type IV hypersensitivity

Cell-mediated immune responses invariably cause some tissue destruction, which may be permanent

Despite the examples of antibody-mediated tissue damage discussed above, the antibody response generally achieves its purpose in eliminating invading organisms without any trace of damage to the host. Cell-mediated (type IV) responses are not quite so sure-footed, in that the activation of both T cells and macrophages invariably causes some tissue destruction, which may be reparable if not too prolonged, but can also lead to fibrosis and even calcification with serious permanent loss of tissue.

Confusion has occurred due to the use of a number of terms to describe and subdivide type IV responses. Some reflect actual pathologic conditions while others describe the results of diagnostic skin tests, and none corresponds exactly to the processes by which cell-mediated immunity protects against infection _(Fig. 17.11)_.

From the medical viewpoint granuloma formation is the most important type IV response

The cell-mediated response to microbial antigen is responsible for granuloma formation and plays a major role in diseases such as tuberculosis, tuberculoid leprosy, lymphogranuloma inguinale, and in _Toxocara_ infection. The complex involvement of the cytokine network in type IV responses poses certain paradoxes. For example, the tendency

of some granulomas to undergo necrosis (e.g. caseation in tuberculosis) whereas others do not (e.g. leprosy, sarcoidosis) may be explained in terms of the different pattern of cytokines involved. TNF, often in association with some microbial products, is especially likely to cause necrosis through its effects on vascular endothelium, which probably accounts for much of its antitumor activity.

The clinical features of schistosomiasis are produced by cell-mediated immunity

The price paid for protective cell-mediated immunity is particularly well illustrated by the helminth disease schistosomiasis. _Schistosoma mansoni_ (the blood fluke) lays eggs in the mesenteric venous system, some of which become lodged in small portal vessels in the liver. Strong cell-mediated reactions to secreted enzymes lead to granulomatous reactions around each egg, resulting in egg destruction and sparing of liver parenchyma from the toxic effects of the egg enzymes. However, the coalescent calcified granulomas ultimately cause portal cirrhosis, with portal hypertension, esophageal varices and hematemesis (see Chapter 22).

The rather unexpected effect of malnutrition in reducing the incidence and severity of certain diseases (e.g. typhus, malaria) may be attributable to a reduction in immuno-pathology, though in the majority of diseases (e.g. measles, meningococcal infection, tuberculosis) the reverse is true. Indeed, poor nutrition is regarded as a major factor predisposing to the greater severity of many common infections in tropical countries.

SKIN RASHES

A variety of skin rashes have an immunologic origin

The ways in which infections can affect the skin are detailed in Chapter 26, but here it should be mentioned that some

SKIN RASHES AND THEIR IMMUNOLOGIC BASIS			
organism	**disease**	**character**	**pathogenic basis**
viruses			
measles	measles	maculopapular rash	T cells; immune complex; allergy
rubella	German measles	maculopapular rash	T cells; immune complex; allergy
varicella-zoster	chickenpox/zoster	vesicular rash	viral cytopathic
hepatitis B	hepatitis B	urticarial	immune complexes
bacteria			
Streptococcus pyogenes	scarlet fever	erythematous rash	erythrogenic toxin
Treponema pallidum	syphilis	disseminated infectious rash in secondary stage	immune complexes
Treponema pertenue	yaws	disseminated infectious rash in secondary stage	
Salmonella typhi	typhoid, enteric fever	sparse rose spots	immune complexes
Neisseria meningitidis	meningitis, spotted fever	petechial or maculopapular lesions	immune complexes
Mycobacterium leprae	tuberculoid leprosy	blotchy skin lesions	T cells, macrophages
Rickettsia prowazeki and others	typhus	maculopapular or hemorrhagic rash	thrombosis
fungi			
dermatophytes	dermatophytoid or allergic rash	–	immune complexes? hypersensitivity to fungal antigens
Blastomyces dermatitidis	blastomycosis	papule or pustule developing into granuloma	T cells
protozoa			
Leishmania tropica	cutaneous leishmaniasis	papules ulcerating to form crusted infectious sores	T cells, macrophages

Fig. 17.12 Many skin rashes represent immunologic reactions occurring in the skin. It is suspected that several skin diseases of unknown origin are in fact caused by viruses, either directly or indirectly.

rashes are considered to be immunologically mediated. For example the characteristic skin rash of measles is absent in children with T cell deficiency (e.g. thymic aplasia or DiGeorge syndrome), who instead develop a fatal systemic infection, indicating that the skin lesions are T cell mediated and represent some form of successful cell-mediated immunity. In contrast, if children with T cell deficiency are vaccinated with live vaccinia virus they develop an inexorable spreading skin lesion, which is clearly a direct and not an immunopathologic effect.

Figure 17.12 lists the more common skin conditions of immunologic origin in which an infectious organism is thought to be involved. Further details can be found in Chapter 26.

VIRUSES AND CANCER

A variety of RNA and DNA viruses can cause permanent malignant changes within cells *(Fig. 17.13)*. Such malignant transformation by these 'tumor viruses' has been extensively studied. An account of proviruses and oncogenes (genes causing malignancy) is included in Chapter 3. However, only a small number of human cancers have been shown to be associated with such tumor viruses *(Fig. 17.14)*.

Human T cell lymphotropic viruses (HTLVs) are associated with certain lymphomas and leukemias

HTLV1 and HTLV2 are retroviruses that have no oncogenes (see Chapter 3). Their proviral DNA is detectable in the cellular DNA of certain malignant lymphomas and leukemias. HTLV1 is known to cause adult T cell leukemia and lymphoma, particularly in Southern Japan, the Caribbean islands and West Africa. Less is known about the geographic distribution of HTLV2, which can be isolated from hairy T cell leukemia. The carcinogenic nature of HTLV1 is not due to activation of a cellular oncogene, but is due to the *tat* gene product enhancing transcription of host genes involved in cell division. These infections are described in more detail in Chapter 26.

Epstein–Barr virus (EBV) is associated with nasopharyngeal carcinoma

EBV is closely linked with the development of nasopharyngeal carcinoma (NPC) (see Chapter 18), which is common in Southern China and other parts of Asia (12–30 cases/100 000 people/year), less common in parts of North Africa, and rare elsewhere in the world. The reason for this restricted geographic distribution is unknown. There is no convincing

MALIGNANT TRANSFORMATION	
changes	details
morphology	loss of shape; rounding decreased adhesion to surface

growth, contact	loss of contact inhibition of
	  growth and movement
	increased ability to grow
	  from a single cell
	increased ability to
	  grow in suspension
	capacity for continued growth
	  (immortalization)

cellular properties	DNA synthesis induced chromosomal changes appearance of new antigens (viral or cellular in origin)
biochemical properties	loss of fibronectin reduced cAMP

Fig. 17.13 Malignant transformation. These changes occur when tumor viruses cause transformation of cultured cells. Many of these changes are obviously relevant for tumor production in vivo. (cAMP, cyclic adenosine monophosphate.)

evidence for specific carcinogenic EBV strains, but these effects could be due to the presence locally of cocarcinogens such as nitrosamines in salted fish. EBV DNA can be demonstrated in the cancer cells, but the precise mechanism for tumorigenicity is unknown; cellular oncogenes have not been implicated.

People at high risk of developing NPC show high IgA titers to EBV capsid antigen a year or more before clinical symptoms appear.

EBV is associated with Burkitt's lymphoma

Burkitt's lymphoma, a tumor of immature B cells, occurs in parts of East Africa (e.g. Uganda) and in Papua New Guinea in 6–14-year-old children, especially boys. EBV DNA is present in the tumor cells, but most of the many copies of the EBV gene are not integrated into the host cell DNA. The tumor is probably caused by the action of EBV on B cells, causing them to proliferate and making activation of cellular oncogenes more likely. The cellular oncogene c-myc is translocated from chromosome 8 to the immunoglobulin heavy chain locus on chromosome 14, where it is expressed. As a result of this, the B cell may be prevented from entering the resting stage. There is also downregulation of adhesion and human leukocyte antigen (HLA) molecules, so that the EBV-containing cells, which are normally subject to immune control, develop into tumor cells. The Burkitt's lymphoma cells also show other chromosomal abnormalities, but their role in tumorigenesis is unclear.

The fact that EBV is a common worldwide infection, whereas Burkitt's lymphoma, like NPC, is strikingly localized geographically, points once again to the involvement of local cofactors, perhaps chemical or infectious cocarcinogens.

HIV does not appear to be associated with non-endemic Burkitt's lymphoma nor with the lymphomas seen in immunosuppressed (e.g. post-renal-transplant) patients. It may, however, be involved in HIV-associated lymphomas. About 3% of patients with AIDS develop non-Hodgkin's lymphomas, 20% of these occurring in the brain. However, there is no good evidence to suggest that Hodgkin's lymphomas are of EBV origin.

VIRUSES AND HUMAN CANCER				
viruses	cancer	strength of association	viral genome in cancer cells	cofactor
Epstein–Barr virus	Burkitt's lymphoma nasopharyngeal carcinoma Hodgkin's disease	++ ++ –	+ + –	malaria nitrosamines –
human papillomavirus	cervical cancer skin cancer	++ +/–	+ +	?cigarettes ?HSV2 ?UV light
hepatitis B virus hepatitis C virus	liver cancer liver cancer	++ ++	+ –	?aflatoxin ?hepatocyte regeneration
HTLV1	T cell leukemia	++	+	–
HSV2	cervical cancer	+/–	+/–	–

Fig. 17.14 Viruses and human cancer. Many viruses transform cells in culture, but only a few are important in human cancer. The associations are strongly supported by studies of naturally occurring or experimentally induced cancers in animals. (HTLV, human T cell lymphotropic virus; HSV, herpes simplex virus; UV, ultraviolet.)

Certain human papillomavirus infections are associated with cervical cancer

There are clear associations between the development of cervical cancer and infection with certain of the 77 distinct genotypes of human papillomavirus (HPV; see Chapters 3, 21 and 26). They account for more than 80% of cervical cancers. Penile, vulval and rectal cancers are also associated with these types of HPV. Those at high risk include types 16 and 18, and those with low risk types 6 and 11. The latter cause cervical lesions, but have a lower risk of progression to malignancy.

In most primary and metastatic cancer cells, the HPV genomes are present in integrated form (i.e. within the host genome), and certain viral genes *(E6, E7)* are transcribed and translated. Integration occurs at different chromosomal locations and the *E6* and *E7* open reading frames seem to be involved in transformation of epithelial cells and in maintenance of the transformed state, probably by binding to and inactivating tumor-suppressing cellular proteins concerned with regulation of the cell cycle. Cervical cancer is an uncommon sequel to infection with these strains of HPV, and cocarcinogens such as cigarette smoke and herpes simplex virus (HSV) have been implicated.

HPV infection is associated with squamous cell carcinoma of the skin

It is possible that ultraviolet light acts as a cocarcinogen, as is known to be the case with papillomaviruses and skin cancers in sheep and cattle. People with the rare autosomal recessive disease epidermodysplasia verruciformis are infected with 10–20 different but less common types of HPV, and 35% of patients develop multiple squamous cell carcinomas of the skin. Of these tumors 90% contain HPV5 or HPV8 DNA.

HPVs may also play a role in the genesis of the skin cancers that appear in immunosuppressed patients (e.g. renal transplant recipients), and cutaneous warts are common in these patients. However, there is no evidence that skin cancers in healthy individuals are associated with HPV infection.

Hepatitis B and hepatitis C viruses are major causes of hepatocellular carcinoma

Integrated hepatitis B virus (HBV) sequences are found in the tumor cells of hepatocellular carcinoma (HCC). The exact mechanism is unclear, but insertion of HBV sequences may activate cellular oncogenes (e.g. of the *myc* family) or alter cell growth control by transcriptional transactivation.

HCC is more common in certain parts of the world (e.g. west Africa), and this may be due to the presence of cocarcinogens (e.g. aflatoxin). However, the closely related hepadnavirus of woodchucks (see panel) causes the same tumor in these animals in the apparent absence of cocarcinogens. Perhaps HBV-associated HCC in humans is a sequel to the continuous hepatocyte regeneration that occurs during persistent carriage of HBV.

The mechanism by which hepatitis C virus (HCV) causes HCC is considered to be indirect, as HCV sequences are not integrated into tumor cells. It is thought that the persistent hepatocyte damage and inflammation in HCV carriers results in HCC. Once cirrhosis is established, there is a 1–4% risk of HCC.

Several DNA viruses can transform cells in which they are unable to replicate

In addition, the viral genome is sometimes integrated into the host cell genome. Extensive studies have been carried out with the conclusion that despite high oncogenicity in vitro and in laboratory animals, these viruses do not seem to be important in human cancer. For instance:

- Human adenoviruses transform cells in culture and cause sarcomas experimentally in hamsters. About 10% of the adenovirus genome integrates, and the T antigen is expressed. However, adenoviruses are not associated with human cancer.
- Polyomavirus (Latin: *poly*, many; *oma*, tumors), a mouse papovavirus, and simian vacuolating virus 40 (SV40), a monkey papovavirus, both cause tumors in experimentally

LESSONS IN MICROBIOLOGY

The many faces of hepatitis B

Classic epidemiologic studies on hepatitis B virus in Taiwan showed two things. First, 90% of those infected in infancy became carriers, as did 23% of those infected at 1–3 years, but only 3% of those infected as university students. Second, among 3454 carriers of HBsAg there were 184 cases of hepatocellular carcinoma, whereas there were only 10 cases among 19 253 non-carriers. Eighty percent of all liver cancers are due to hepatitis B.

Worldwide there are about 350 million carriers of this virus and therefore, with liver cancer causing up to 2 million deaths each year, hepatitis B virus is second only to tobacco as a human carcinogen.

The mechanism of carcinogenesis is not clear. Nearly all human cancers show chromosomal integration of the virus, but there is great variation in integration site and in the number of copies of the viral genome.

Very similar viruses infect woodchucks, ground squirrels and Pekin ducks. In Northwest USA, 30% of woodchucks are carriers and most develop liver cancer in later life. In this host the virus infects not only liver cells but also lymphoid cells in the spleen, peripheral blood and thymus, and pancreatic acinar cells and bile duct epithelium.

inoculated hamsters. The viral DNA is integrated into tumor cells, and T antigens are expressed. Are these viruses, or their human equivalents (BK and JC viruses), linked with human cancers? An incident occurred about 30 years ago when thousands of children were accidentally inoculated with SV40 virus present in certain batches of poliovirus vaccine. The formalin inactivation procedure had failed to kill the SV40 virus present in the monkey kidney cells in which the polio vaccine had been grown. There was, however, no consequent increase in tumor incidence in the SV40-infected individuals. Nevertheless, evidence is accumulating that JC, BK and SV40 viruses are associated with certain cancers of the brain, with certain lymphomas and with other tumors.

Kaposi's sarcoma is probably caused by a virus

Kaposi's sarcoma is 300-times more common among patients with AIDS than among other immunosuppressed groups, but is seen almost entirely in those who acquired HIV by sexual contact. Human Herpes Virus 8 (HHV8) appears to be sexually transmitted and is present in the tumors

Bacteria associated with cancer

The association between *Helicobacter pylori* and stomach and duodenal cancer is referred to in Chapter 22, but the mechanism is not known.

KEY FACTS

- Tissue damage or disease can be caused by infectious organisms in several ways.

- Infectious organisms may destroy cells directly (e.g. cytopathic viruses), release toxins that destroy cells or their cellular function (e.g. staphylococcus or tetanus toxins), overstimulate normal defense systems (e.g. LPS) or stimulate excessive or prolonged adaptive responses.

- Such effects of infectious organisms on defense systems may be antibody- or T-cell-mediated and are collectively known as 'hypersensitivity reactions' or 'immunopathology'.

- Some viruses have been shown to be involved in the initiation of tumors, with the viral genome being found in the cancer cells. The restricted geographic distribution of some of these tumors may be due to the local presence of cocarcinogens.

? QUESTIONS

1. Distinguish between exotoxins and endotoxins.

2. What is 'septic shock' and how might it be prevented?

3. What is an immune complex and how can it cause disease?

4. Which types of skin rash have an immunologic origin?

5. Which viruses are suspected of causing cancer?

FURTHER READING

Bosch FX, Manos MM, Munoz N et al. Prevalence of human papillomavirus in cervical cancer; a worldwide perspective. *J Natl Cancer Inst* 1995; 87:796–802.

Collier LH, ed. *Topley and Wilson's Microbiology and Microbial Infections*, 9th edition, Vol 1: Virology; Ch 12: Oncogenicity, pp 211–34. London: Edward Arnold, 1998.

Hacker J, Blum-Oehler G, Muhldorfer I, Tschape H. Pathogenicity islands of virulent bacteria: structure, function and impact on microbial evolution. *Mol Microbiol* 1997; 23:1089–97.

Mims CA, Nash A, Stephen J. *Mims' Pathogenesis of Infectious Disease*, 5th edition. London: Academic Press, 2001.

Rees AJ, Andres GA, Peters DK, eds. Symposium on pathogenetic mechanisms in nephritis. *Kidney Int* 1989; 35:921–1033.

Sriskandan S, Cohen J. The pathogenesis of septic shock. *J Infect* 1995; 30:201–6.

Stephen J. Pathogenesis of infectious diarrhoea: mini-review. *Canadian J Gastroenterol* 2001; 15:669–83.

Clinical manifestation and diagnosis of infections by body system

4

18. Upper respiratory tract infections   *201*

19. Lower respiratory tract infections   *217*

20. Urinary tract infections   *241*

21. Sexually transmitted diseases   *251*

22. Gastrointestinal tract infections   *277*

23. Obstetric and perinatal infections   *313*

24. Central nervous system infections   *323*

25. Infections of the eye   *343*

26. Infections of the skin, soft tissue, muscle and associated systems   *349*

27. Vector-borne infections   *383*

28. Multisystem zoonoses   *401*

29. Fever of unknown origin   *413*

30. Infections in the compromised host   *423*

THE CLINICAL MANIFESTATIONS OF INFECTION

As there are at least 150 different infectious diseases to describe, a system of classification is essential. In Chapters 18–26, infections are classified according to the body system primarily involved at the clinical level. For example, rhinoviruses specifically cause infection of the upper respiratory tract, and bacillary or amebic dysentery are gastrointestinal tract infections. Other infections characteristically cause damage predominantly to one part of the body, although other parts may be affected. Thus, tuberculosis is considered in Chapter 19 (lower respiratory tract infections) and typhoid in Chapter 22 (gastrointestinal tract infections), these being the sites primarily affected. Again, when microbes are transmitted as a result of certain states or activities, they can be grouped together with others acquired in the same way, even though more than one system may be involved. Hence syphilis and AIDS are dealt with in Chapter 21 (sexually transmitted diseases) and rubella in Chapter 23 (obstetric and perinatal infections).

The systems approach is useful because it includes infections caused by a wide variety of microbes on the basis of the clinical syndrome produced. As with any system of classification, however, there are gray areas and overlaps. Referral to the Appendix, where definitive accounts of the most important infectious organisms are given, will help clarify any ambiguities.

Chapters 27 and 28 deal with those infections that cannot be readily pigeon-holed into systems. These include multisystem infections (i.e. infections that are not obviously localized to any one system of the body). Many multisystem infections are also multihost in that they can be transmitted:

• from person to person by an intermediate vector (usually an arthropod), their distribution depending upon climate, ecology and the presence of adequate numbers of the required arthropod (see Chapter 27);
• directly to humans from other vertebrates, in which case they are known as 'zoonoses' (see Chapter 28), with distributions ranging from highly restricted (Rocky Mountain spotted fever, Lassa fever) to widespread (Q fever, leptospirosis).
  Finally, there are two further disease groupings, founded on clinical presentation:
• those presenting as 'fevers of unknown origin' (see Chapter 29);
• those seen in the compromised host (see Chapter 30).

The latter category has become increasingly important because of the large number of patients whose defenses are impaired as a result of disease (cystic fibrosis, diabetes mellitus), infection (AIDS), immunosuppressive therapy (transplant patients) or other causes (e.g. burns, catheters).

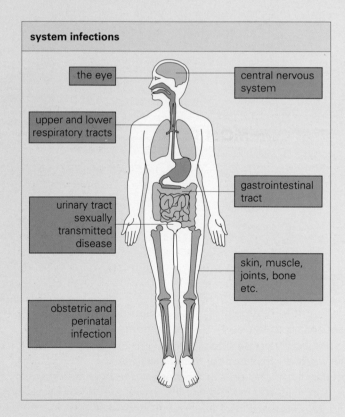

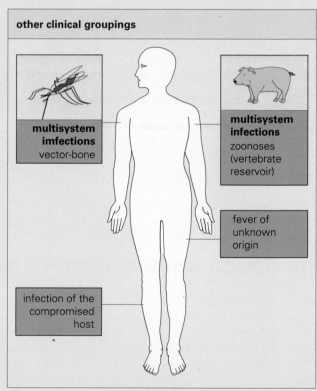

INTRODUCTION

The mucociliary system and the flushing action of saliva are defenses against upper respiratory tract infection

The air we inhale contains millions of suspended particles, including microorganisms. Nearly all these microorganisms are harmless, except in the vicinity of infected individuals where the air may contain large numbers of pathogenic microorganisms. Efficient cleansing mechanisms (see Chapters 9 and 13) are therefore vital components of the body's defense against infection of both the upper and lower respiratory tract. Infection takes place against the background of these natural defense mechanisms, and it is then appropriate to ask why the defenses have failed. For the upper respiratory tract, the mucociliary system is important in the nasopharynx, and the flushing action of saliva in the oropharynx.

As on other surfaces of the body (see Chapter 8), a variety of microorganisms live harmlessly in the upper respiratory tract and oropharynx *(Fig. 18.1)*; they colonize the nose, mouth, throat and teeth and are well adapted to life in these sites. Normally they are well-behaved guests, not invading tissues and not causing disease. However, as in other parts of the body, resident microorganisms can cause trouble when host resistance is weakened.

The upper and lower respiratory tracts form a continuum for infectious agents

We distinguish between upper and lower respiratory tract infections, but the respiratory tract from the nose to the alveoli is a continuum as far as infectious agents are concerned *(Fig. 18.2)*. There may, however, be a preferred 'focus' of infection (e.g. nasopharynx for coronaviruses and rhinoviruses); but parainfluenza viruses, for instance, can infect the nasopharynx to give rise to a cold, as well as the larynx and trachea (croup or laryngotracheitis), and occasionally the bronchi and bronchioles (bronchitis, bronchiolitis or pneumonia).

Two useful generalizations can be made about upper and lower respiratory tract infections

These are that:

- Many microorganisms are restricted to the surface epithelium, but others spread to other parts of the body, before returning to the respiratory tract, oropharynx, salivary glands *(Fig. 18.3)*.
- Two groups of microbes can be distinguished: 'professional' and 'secondary' invaders.

Professional invaders are those that successfully infect the normally healthy respiratory tract *(Fig. 18.4)*. They generally possess specific properties that enable them to evade local host defenses, such as the attachment mechanisms of respiratory viruses *(Fig. 18.5)* and the other devices shown in *Figure 18.4*. Secondary invaders only cause disease when host defenses are already impaired *(Fig. 18.4)*.

THE COMMON COLD

Rhinoviruses and coronaviruses together cause more than 50% of colds

Viruses are the commonest invaders of the nasopharynx, and a great variety of types *(Fig. 18.5)* are responsible for the common cold. They induce a flow of virus-rich fluid from the nasopharynx, and when the sneezing reflex is triggered, large numbers of virus particles are discharged into the air. Transmission is therefore by aerosol and also by virus-contaminated hands (see Chapter 13). Most of these viruses possess surface molecules that bind them firmly to host cells or to cilia or microvilli protruding from these cells. As a result, they are not washed away in secretions and are able to initiate infection in the normally healthy individual. Virus progeny from the first infected cell then spread to neighboring cells and via surface secretions to new sites on the mucosal surface. After a few days, damage to epithelial cells and the secretion of fluid containing inflammatory mediators such as bradykinin lead to common cold-type symptoms *(Fig. 18.6)*.

Common cold virus infections are diagnosed by clinical appearance

In view of the large variety of viruses and because common colds are generally mild and self-limiting with no systemic spread, laboratory tests are not worthwhile. Diagnosis becomes important when the lower respiratory tract is involved, as for instance with influenza viruses or in children with respiratory syncytial virus (RSV) infection. The antigens of these viruses can be detected in exfoliated cells in the

NORMAL FLORA OF THE RESPIRATORY TRACT	
type of resident*	**microorganism**
common residents (>50% of normal people)	oral streptococci *Neisseria* spp., *Branhamella* corynebacteria *Bacteroides* anaerobic cocci (*Veillonella*) fusiform bacteria** *Candida albicans*** *Streptococcus mutans* *Haemophilus influenzae*
occasional residents (<10% of normal people)	*Streptococcus pyogenes* *Streptococcus pneumoniae* *Neisseria meningitidis*
uncommon residents (<1% normal people)	*Corynebacterium diphtheriae* *Klebsiella pneumoniae* *Pseudomonas* ⌐ especially after *Escherichia coli* ∟ antibiotic *C. albicans* ⌐ treatment
residents in latent state in tissues:[†] lung lymph nodes etc. sensory neurone/ glands connected to mucosae	*Pneumocystis jiroveci*[††] *Mycobacterium tuberculosis* cytomegalovirus (CMV) herpes simplex virus Epstein–Barr virus

*all except tissue residents are present in the oronasopharynx or on teeth
**present in mouth; also *Entamoeba gingivalis*, *Trichomonas tenax*, micrococci, *Actinomyces* spp.
***all except *M. tuberculosis* are present in most humans
[††]formerly *P. carinii*

Fig. 18.1 The normal flora of the respiratory tract.

nasopharyngeal aspirates from children (see *Fig. 19.4*), and a rise in virus-specific antibodies will confirm the diagnosis, which is generally retrospective. Virus isolation is tedious and can be difficult, but is usually carried out for public health purposes by central laboratories when, for instance, there is a new pandemic strain of influenza virus. Reference laboratories are now using molecular methods to detect and then sequence influenza viruses for typing purposes and check that the vaccine strains are a good match with the circulating strains.

Treatment of the common cold is symptomatic

It is often said that a common cold will resolve in 48 hours if vigorous treatment with anticongestants, analgesics and antibiotics is undertaken, while untreated it will take two days! There are no worthwhile vaccines for the common cold viruses, and treatment is for the most part symptomatic. There are, however, influenza virus vaccines.

PHARYNGITIS AND TONSILLITIS

About 70% of acute sore throats are caused by viruses

Microorganisms that cause acute pharyngitis are listed in *Figure 18.7*. Common cold and other upper respiratory tract viruses inevitably encounter the submucosal lymphoid tissues that form a defensive ring around the oropharynx (*Fig. 18.2*). The throat becomes sore (pharyngitis) either because the overlying mucosa is infected or because of inflammatory and immune responses in the lymphoid tissues themselves. Adenoviruses are common causes, often infecting the conjunctiva as well as the pharynx to cause pharyngoconjunctival fever. Epstein–Barr virus (EBV) and cytomegalovirus (CMV) multiply locally in the pharynx (*Fig. 18.8*), and herpes simplex virus (HSV) and certain coxsackie A viruses multiply in the oral mucosa to produce a painful local lesion or ulcer. Certain enteroviruses (e.g. coxsackie A16) can cause additional vesicles on the hands and feet and in the mouth (hand, foot and mouth disease, *Fig. 18.9*).

Cytomegalovirus infection

CMV can be transmitted by saliva, urine, blood, semen and cervical secretions

CMV is the largest human herpesvirus (*Fig. 18.10*), and there is only one serotype. As with animal CMVs it is species specific; humans are the natural hosts, and animal CMVs do not infect humans. The name refers to the multinucleated cells, which together with the intranuclear inclusions, are characteristic responses to infection with this virus. CMV was originally called 'salivary gland' virus and is transmitted by saliva and other secretions.

Urine is an additional source of infection in children, and in infected pregnant women the virus can spread via the blood to the placenta and fetus. Semen and cervical secretions may also contain virus, and it can therefore be spread by sexual contact. It is often present in milk in small quantities, but this is of doubtful significance in transmission. CMV can also be transmitted by blood transfusions and organ transplants.

CMV infection is often asymptomatic, but can reactivate and cause disease when cell-mediated immunity (CMI) defenses are impaired

After clinically silent infection in the upper respiratory tract, CMV spreads locally to lymphoid tissues and then systemically in circulating lymphocytes and monocytes to involve lymph nodes and the spleen. The infection then localizes in epithelial cells in salivary glands and kidney tubules, and in cervix, testes and epididymis, from where the virus is shed to the outside world (*Fig. 18.11*).

Infected cells may be multinucleated or bear intranuclear inclusions, but pathologic changes are minor and infection is generally asymptomatic. In young adults, a glandular fever

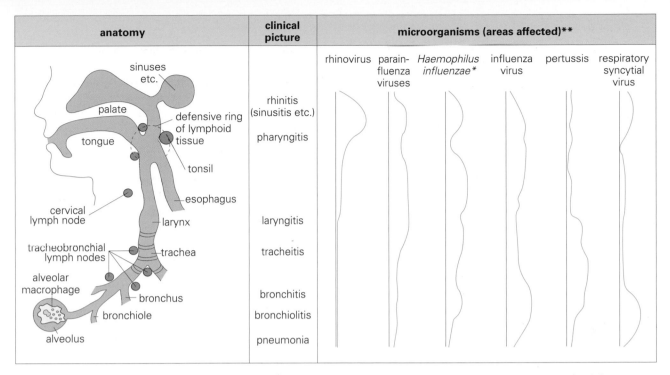

Fig. 18.2 The respiratory tract as a continuum. (*Asymptomatic nasopharyngeal colonization is common. **Magnitude of rhinitis, laryngitis, etc. shown by area between black and blue lines.)

TWO TYPES OF RESPIRATORY INFECTION		
type	**examples**	**consequences**
restricted to surface	common cold viruses influenza streptococci in throat chlamydia (conjunctivitis) diphtheria pertussis *Candida albicans* (thrush)	local spread local (mucosal) defenses important adaptive (immune) response sometimes too late to be important in recovery short incubation period (days)

spread through body	measles, mumps, rubella
	EBV, CMV
	Chlamydophila psittaci
	Q fever
	cryptococcosis
		little or no lesion at entry site
		microbe spreads through body, returns to surface for
		   final multiplication and shedding, e.g. salivary gland
		   (mumps, CMV, EBV), respiratory tract (measles)
		adaptive immune response important in recovery
		longer incubation period (weeks)

Fig. 18.3 After entry via the respiratory tract, microbes either stay on the surface epithelium or spread through the body. (*formerly *Chlamydia psittaci*; CMV, cytomegalovirus; EBV, Epstein–Barr virus.)

type illness can occur, but without heterophil antibodies which are found in most individuals with EBV infection, exceptions being children under 14 years of age. There is fever and lethargy, and abnormal lymphocytes and mononucleosis in blood smears. The virus inhibits T cell responses, and there is a temporary reduction in their immune reactivity to other antigens.

Although specific antibodies and CMI responses are generated, these fail to clear the virus (see Chapter 16), which often continues to be shed in saliva and urine for many

months. The infection is, however, eventually controlled by CMI mechanisms, although infected cells remain in the body throughout life and can be a source of reactivation and disease when CMI defenses are impaired.

CMV owes its success in our species to its ability to evade immune defenses. For instance, it presents a poor target for cytotoxic T (Tc) cells by interfering with the transport of major histocompatibility complex (MHC) class I molecules to the cell surface (see Chapter 10), and it induces Fc receptors on infected cells (see Chapter 16).

RESPIRATORY INVADERS—PROFESSIONAL OR SECONDARY		
type	**requirement**	**examples**
professional invaders (infect healthy respiratory tract)	adhesion to normal mucosa (in spite of mucociliary system)	respiratory viruses (influenza, rhinoviruses) *Streptococcus pyogenes* (throat) *Strep. pneumoniae* *Mycoplasma pneumoniae* chlamydia (psittacosis, chlamydial conjunctivitis and pneumonia, trachoma)
	ability to interfere with cilia	*Bordetella pertussis, M. pneumoniae, Strep. pneumoniae* (pneumolysin)
	ability to resist destruction in alveolar macrophage ability to damage local (mucosal, submucocal) tissues	*Legionella, Mycobacterium tuberculosis* *Corynebacterium diphtheriae* (toxin), *Strep. pneumoniae* (pneumolysin)
secondary invaders (infect when host defenses impaired)	initial infection and damage by respiratory virus (e.g. influenza virus)	*Staphylococcus aureus; Strep. pneumoniae*, pneumonia complicating influenza
	local defenses impaired (e.g. cystic fibrosis) chronic bronchitis, local foreign body or tumor depressed immune responses (e.g. AIDS, neoplastic disease) depressed resistance (e.g. elderly, alcoholism, renal or hepatic disease)	*Staph. aureus, Pseudomonas* *Haemophilus influenzae, Strep. pneumoniae* *Pneumocystis jiroveci*, cytomegalovirus, *M. tuberculosis* *Strep. pneumoniae, Staph. aureus*, *H. influenzae*

Fig. 18.4 The two types of respiratory invader.

CMV infection can cause fetal malformations and pneumonia in immunodeficient patients

In the natural host, the human infant or child, CMV causes no illness, and in general it causes a mild illness in adults. Two circumstances, however, interfere with this harmonious host–parasite balance:

• Primary infection during pregnancy allows spread of virus from the blood to the placenta and then to the fetus, resulting in congenital abnormalities as described in Chapter 23. Reactivation of infection during pregnancy also occurs and leads to fetal infection, but rarely to congenital abnormalities. However, CMV is second only to Down's syndrome as a cause of mental retardation in babies.

• In immunodeficient patients such as bone marrow or solid organ transplant recipients and rarely in AIDS patients (see Chapter 30), CMV infection causes an interstitial pneumonia with infiltrating infected mononuclear cells. Other sites affected include the CNS, with focal cerebral 'micronodular' lesions with infected mononuclear cells, together with a variety of other complications, including retinitis. In addition, the gastrointestinal tract may be involved, with a colitis and hepatitis.

Clinical diagnosis of primary infection is rarely possible, because it is so commonly asymptomatic. However, in symptomatic immunocompetent individuals, CMV IgM detection is used to make the diagnosis. CMV antigen or CMV DNA detection methods are used on bronchoalveolar fluid to make the diagnosis in individuals with CMV pneumonitis.

Multinucleated cells or cells with prominent intranuclear inclusions may be seen in lung biopsy material. CMV IgM and IgG serology is available but is unlikely to be of diagnostic help in immunosuppressed patients. The management of post-transplant recipients involves CMV DNA monitoring of whole blood or plasma samples and pre-emptive therapy on detecting CMV viremia (see Chapter 30).

Antiviral treatment of CMV retinitis and pneumonia

While ganciclovir or foscarnet is often an effective treatment, aciclovir is ineffective. As CMV pneumonitis is considered to be an immunopathological disease, CMV specific or human normal immunoglobulin is given in addition to the antiviral agent to potentially block the response to pneumocytes expressing the target antigens.

There is no vaccine, but trials of live and inactivated vaccines have been carried out. Contact between congenitally infected children and susceptible pregnant women should be avoided. Blood for transfusion of newborns, and solid organ and bone marrow transplants, should preferably come from CMV antibody negative donors.

Epstein–Barr virus infection

EBV is transmitted in saliva

EBV, like CMV, is species specific. EBV is structurally and morphologically identical to other herpesviruses (see Chapter 3), but is antigenically distinct. A major antigen is the viral

VIRUSES CAUSING COMMON COLDS

virus	types involved	attachment mechanism	disease
rhinoviruses (>100 types)*	several at any given time in the community	capsid protein binds to ICAM-1 type molecule on cell**	common cold
coxsackie virus A (24 types)†	especially A21	capsid protein binds to ICAM-1 type molecule on cell**	common cold; also oropharyngeal vesicles (herpangina) and hand, foot and mouth disease (A16)
influenza viruses	several	hemagglutinin binds to neuraminic acid-containing glycoprotein on cell	may also invade lower respiratory tract
parainfluenza virus (4 types)	1, 2, 3, 4	viral envelope protein binds to glycoside on cell	may also invade larynx
respiratory syncytial virus	(2 types)	G protein on virus attaches to receptor on cell	may also invade lower respiratory tract
coronaviruses (several types)	all	viral envelope protein binds to glycoprotein receptors on cell	common cold; severe acute respiratory syndrome
adenovirus (41 types)	5–10 types	penton fiber binds to cell receptor	mainly pharyngitis; also conjunctivitis, bronchitis
echovirus (34 types)	4, 9, 11, 20, 25	—	common cold

*a given type shows little or no neutralization by antibody against other types

**ICAM-1: intercellular adhesion molecule expressed on a wide variety of normal cells, member of immunoglobulin superfamily, coded on chromosome 19

†Coxsackie virus A9 binds to vitronectin, an integrin protein; types 1 and 8 bind to very-late-activating antigen-2 (an integrin) and 6, 7, 12, 21 to decay-accelerating factor (CD55) on cell.

Fig. 18.5 Common cold viruses and their mechanisms of attachment.

capsid antigen (VCA) used in diagnostic tests. Other useful antigens diagnostically are the early antigens (EA) which are produced before viral DNA synthesis, and the EBV-associated nuclear antigens (EBNA), which are located in the nucleus of the infected cells. Humans are the natural hosts.

EBV is transmitted by the exchange of saliva, for instance during kissing, and is a ubiquitous infection. In developing countries, infection probably occurs via close contact in early childhood and is subclinical. In developed countries infection occurs in two peaks at 1 to 6 years and 14 to 20 years of age, and in most cases causes illness.

The clinical features of EBV infection are immunologically mediated

Clinical and immunologic events in EBV infection are illustrated in *Figure 18.12*. EBV replicates in B lymphocytes, after making a specific attachment to the C3d receptor (CD21) on these cells, and also in certain epithelial cells. The pathogenesis of the disease and the clinical features can be accounted for on this basis. Virus is shed in saliva from infected epithelial cells and possibly lymphocytes in salivary glands, and from the oropharynx, with clinically silent spread to B lymphocytes in local lymphoid tissues and elsewhere in the body (lymph nodes, spleen).

T lymphocytes respond immunologically to the infected B cells (outnumbering the latter by about 50 to 1) and appear in peripheral blood as 'atypical lymphocytes' (*Fig. 18.13*). Much of the disease is attributable to an immunologic civil war, as specifically activated T cells respond to the infected B cells. In the naturally infected infant or small child these immune responses are weak and there is generally no clinical disease. Older children, however, become unwell, and young adults especially develop infectious mononucleosis or glandular fever 4–7 weeks after initial infection. This is characterized by fever, sore throat (see *Fig. 18.8*), often with petechiae on the hard palate, lymphadenopathy and splenomegaly, with anorexia and lethargy as prominent features. Hepatitis may occur, with mild elevations of hepatocellular enzymes in 90% of cases and jaundice in 9%. Splenic rupture may occur.

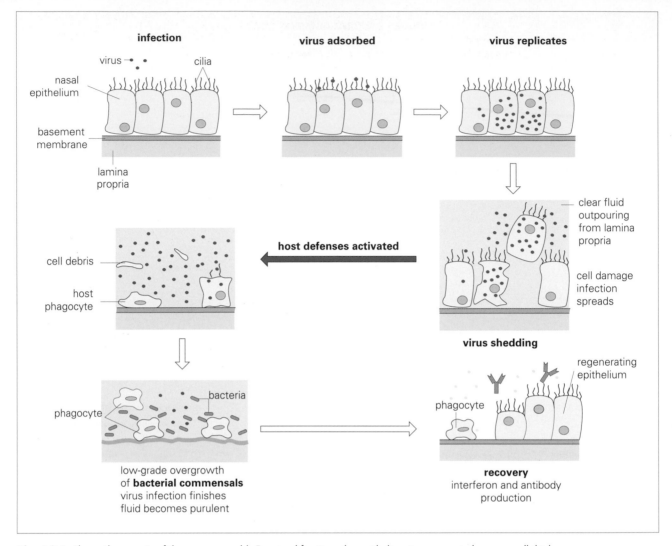

Fig. 18.6 The pathogenesis of the common cold. For simplification, the epithelium is represented as one cell thick.

Less than 1% of cases develop neurologic complications, including aseptic meningitis and encephalitis, nearly always with complete recovery.

The symptoms are presumably due to the action of cytokines released during the intense immunologic activity. The infected B cells are stimulated to differentiate and produce antibodies; this polyclonal activation of B cells is responsible for the production of heterophil antibodies (reacting with erythrocytes of sheep or horses) and a variety of autoantibodies. Spontaneous recovery usually occurs in 2–3 weeks, but the symptoms may persist for a few months. The virus remains as a latent infection in spite of antibody and CMI responses, and saliva often remains infectious for months after clinical recovery.

The autoantibodies produced in response to EBV infection include IgM antibodies to erythrocytes (cold agglutinins), which are present in most cases. About 1% of cases develop an autoimmune hemolytic anemia, which subsides within 1–2 months.

A 'hairy tongue' condition caused by EBV replication in squamous epithelial cells in the tongue occurs in immuno-deficient patients.

EBV remains latent in a small proportion of B lymphocytes

EBV is well equipped to evade immune defenses (see Chapter 16). It acts against complement and interferon, and produces a fake interleukin 10 (IL-10) molecule that interferes with the action of the host's own IL-10 (an important immuno-regulatory cytokine). EBV also prevents apoptosis (lysis) of infected cells, and the boldness of its strategy has enabled it to take up permanent residence within the immune system.

EBV DNA is present in episomal form in a small pro-portion of B lymphocytes, and a few copies may be integrated into the cell genome. Later in life, immunodeficiency can lead to reactivation of infection so that EBV reappears in the saliva, usually with no clinical symptoms; this occurs in more than 50% of renal transplant patients.

Laboratory tests for diagnosing infectious mononucleosis should include viral capsid antigen IgM detection

Infectious mononucleosis is diagnosed clinically by the characteristic syndrome and the appearance of the throat. Laboratory diagnosis is by:

CAUSE OF ACUTE PHARYNGITIS		
organisms	examples	comments
viruses	rhinoviruses, coronaviruses	a mild symptom in the common cold
	adenoviruses (types 3, 4, 7, 14, 21)	pharyngoconjunctival fever
	parainfluenza viruses	more severe than common cold
	influenza viruses, cytomegalovirus	not always present
	coxsackie A and other enteroviruses	small vesicles (herpangina)
	Epstein–Barr virus	occurs in 70–90% of glandular fever patients
	herpes simplex virus type 1	can be severe, with palatal vesicles or ulcers
bacteria	*Streptococcus pyogenes*	causes 10–20% of cases of acute pharyngitis; sudden onset; mostly in 5-10-year-old children
	Neisseria gonorrhoeae	often asymptomatic; usually via orogenital contact
	Corynebacterium diphtheriae	pharyngitis often mild, but toxic illness can be severe
	Haemophilius influenzae	epiglottitis
	Borrelia vincenti plus fusiform bacilli	Vincent's angina; commonest in adolescents and adults

Fig. 18.7 Microorganisms that cause acute pharyngitis.

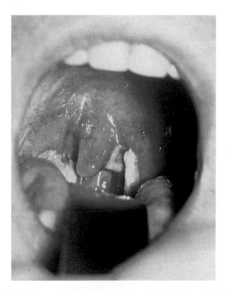

Fig. 18.8 Infectious mononucleosis caused by Epstein–Barr virus. The tonsils and uvula are swollen and covered in white exudate. There are petechiae on the soft palate. (Courtesy of JA Innes.)

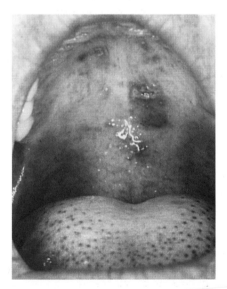

Fig. 18.9 Ulcers on the hard palate and tongue in hand, foot and mouth disease due to coxsackie A virus. (Courtesy of JA Innes.)

- Demonstrating atypical lymphocytes, comprising up to 30% of nucleated cells, in a blood smear. A number of viral infections cause an atypical lymphocytosis, therefore this is not specific to EBV.
- Demonstrating heterophil antibodies to horse (or sheep) erythrocytes in the 'monospot' test. These are present in 90% of cases, but less commonly in infected children. Titers fall during recovery and disappear by 6 months, so previous infection is not detected.
- Demonstrating EBV-specific antibody. Detection of VCA IgM indicates current infection. VCA IgG and EBNA IgG are markers of previous exposure.
- Demonstrating EBV DNA by DNA hybridization or the polymerase chain reaction.

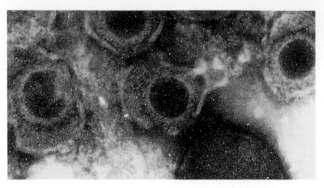

Fig. 18.10 Electron micrograph of cytomegalovirus particles. This is the largest human herpes virus, with a diameter of 150–200 nm, and a dense DNA core. (Courtesy of DK Banerjee.)

Treatment of EBV infection is limited

At present no antiviral agent has been shown to have a clinical benefit, although high doses of aciclovir have an effect in vitro. There is no licensed vaccine, but vaccine preparations have been tested in animal models using various viral envelope glycoproteins.

Cancers associated with EBV

EBV is closely associated with Burkitt's lymphoma in African children

Burkitt's lymphoma *(Fig. 18.14)* is virtually restricted to parts of Africa and Papua New Guinea, so it is clear that EBV alone is not enough to cause the lymphoma. The most likely co-carcinogen is malaria, which acts by weakening T cell control of EBV infection and perhaps by causing polyclonal activation of B cells, the increased turnover rendering them more susceptible to neoplastic transformation.

EBV is closely associated with other B cell lymphomas in immunodeficient patients

For example, B cell lymphomas occur in 1–10% of solid organ transplant recipients, especially children, when primary EBV infection occurs post-transplantation. EBV DNA and RNA transcripts are found in the tumor cells, which also show a translocation of the c-*myc* oncogene on chromosome 8 to the immunoglobulin heavy chain locus on chromosome 14 (see Chapter 17).

EBV infection is also closely associated with nasopharyngeal carcinoma

Nasopharyngeal carcinoma (NPC) is a very common cancer in China and southeast Asia. EBV DNA is detectable in the tumor cells, and a cocarcinogen, possibly ingested nitros-amines from preserved fish, is likely. Host genetic factors controlling human leukocyte antigens (HLA) and immune responses may confer susceptibility to NPC.

Bacterial infections

Bacteria responsible for pharyngitis include:

- *Strep. pyogenes* (group A β-hemolytic, *Fig. 18.15*), the commonest and most important to diagnose because it can lead to complications (see below), but can be readily treated with penicillin;
- *Corynebacterium diphtheriae*;
- *Haemophilus influenzae* (type B), which occasionally causes severe epiglottitis with obstruction of the airways, especially in young children;
- *Borrelia vincenti* together with certain fusiform bacilli, which can cause throat or gingival ulcers;
- *Neisseria gonorrhoeae*.

Each of these types of bacteria attach to the mucosal surface, sometimes invading local tissues.

CYTOMEGALOVIRUS (CMV) INFECTION		
site of infection	result	comment
salivary glands	salivary transmission	importance of kissing and contaminated hands
tubular epithelium of kidney	virus in urine	probable role in transmission
cervix, testis/epididymis	sexual transmission	up to 10^7 infectious doses/ml of semen in an acutely infected male
lymphocytes, macrophages	virus spread through body via infected cells mononucleosis may occur immunosuppressive effect	probable site of persistent infection
placenta, fetus	congenital abnormalities	greatest damage in fetus after primary maternal infection rather than reactivation

Fig. 18.11 The effects of cytomegalovirus (CMV) infection. CMV is a 'well behaved' parasite, causing little or no damage to the host unless it infects the fetus or placenta to cause congenital abnormalities or it reactivates following depressed cell-mediated immunity (post-transplant, AIDS) to cause viremia, fever, hepatitis or pneumonia.

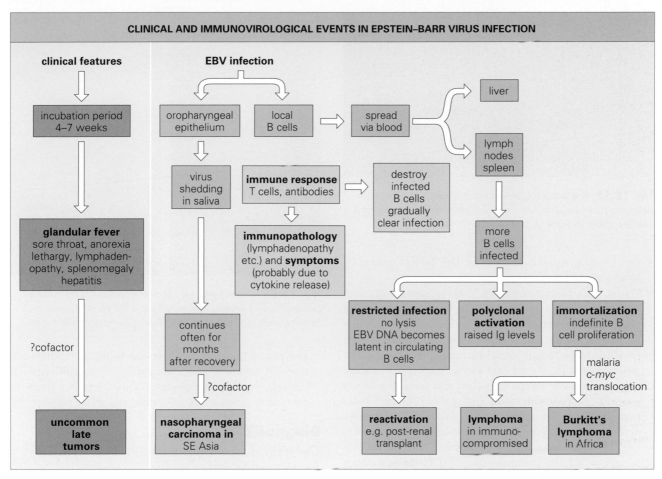

CLINICAL AND IMMUNOVIROLOGICAL EVENTS IN EPSTEIN–BARR VIRUS INFECTION

Fig. 18.12 Clinical and immunovirologic events in Epstein–Barr virus (EBV) infection in adolescents or adults. A milder, often subclinical infection occurs in children.

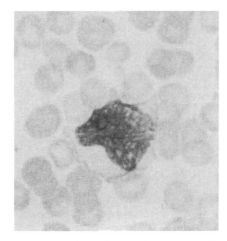

Fig. 18.13 An atypical lymphocyte characteristic of Epstein–Barr virus infection.

Complications of Strep. pyogenes *infection*

Complications of Strep. pyogenes *throat infection include quinsy, scarlet fever, rheumatic fever, rheumatic heart disease and glomerulonephritis*

These complications are important enough to be listed separately, although most are uncommon in developed countries where there is good access to medical care and

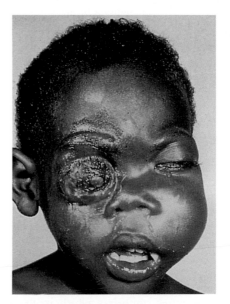

Fig. 18.14 Burkitt's lymphoma affecting the maxilla and eye in an African child. (Courtesy of DH Wright.)

probably less exposure to streptococci. The complications include:

• Peritonsillar abscess ('quinsy'), an uncommon complica-tion of untreated streptococcal sore throat.

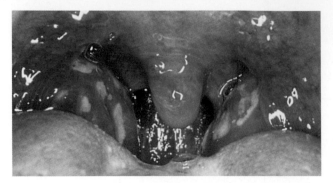

Fig. 18.15 Streptococcal tonsillitis due to group A β-hemolytic *Streptococcus pyogenes* with intense erythema of the tonsils and a creamy-yellow exudate. (Courtesy of JA Innes.)

- Otitis media, sinusitis, mastoiditis (see below), caused by local spread of *Strep. pyogenes*.
- Scarlet fever. Certain strains of *Strep. pyogenes* produce an erythrogenic toxin coded for by a lysogenic phage. The toxin spreads through the body and localizes in the skin to induce a punctate erythematous rash (scarlet fever; *Fig. 18.16*). The tongue is initially furred, but later red. The rash begins as facial erythema and then spreads to involve most of the body except the palms and soles. The face is generally flushed with circumoral pallor. The rash fades over the course of a week and is followed by extensive desquamation. The skin lesions themselves are not serious, but they signal infection by a potentially harmful streptococcus, which in pre-antibiotic days could sometimes spread through the body to cause cellulitis and septicemia.
- Rheumatic fever. This is an indirect complication. Antibodies formed to antigens in the streptococcal cell wall cross-react with the sarcolemma of human heart, and with tissues elsewhere. Granulomas are formed in the heart (Aschoff's nodules), and 2–4 weeks after the sore throat the patient (usually a child) develops myocarditis or pericarditis, which may be associated with subcutaneous nodules, polyarthritis and, rarely, chorea. Chorea is a disease of the central nervous system resulting from antistreptococcal antibodies reacting with neurones.
- Rheumatic heart disease. Repeated attacks of *Strep. pyogenes* with different M types (see Appendix) can lead to damage to the heart valves. Certain children have a genetic predisposition to this immune-mediated disease. If a primary attack is accompanied by rising or high antistreptolysin O (ASO) antibody levels (see Appendix), future attacks must be prevented by penicillin prophylaxis throughout childhood. In many developing countries, rheumatic heart disease is the commonest type of heart disease.
- Acute glomerulonephritis. Antibodies to streptococcal components combine with these components to form circulating immune complexes, which are then deposited in glomeruli, together, probably, with autoantibodies to glomerular components. Here, the complement and coagulation systems are activated, resulting in local inflammation. Blood appears in the urine (red cells, protein) and there are signs of an acute nephritis syndrome (edema, hypertension) 1–2 weeks after the sore throat. ASO antibodies are usually elevated. Only four to five of the 65

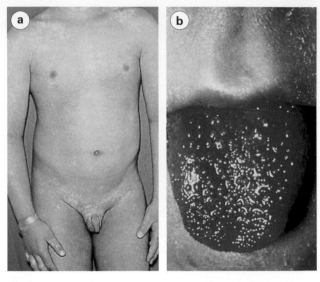

Fig. 18.16 Scarlet fever. (a) Punctate erythema is followed by peeling for 2–3 weeks. (b) The tongue is furred at first and then becomes raw with prominent papillae. (Courtesy of WE Farrar.)

M types of *Strep. pyogenes* give rise to this condition, and repeated infection with different 'nephritogenic' types is unlikely. Penicillin prophylaxis is therefore not given. In contrast to rheumatic fever, second attacks are rare.

Diagnosis

Generally a laboratory diagnosis is not necessary for pharyngitis and tonsillitis

There are many possible viral causes of pharyngitis and tonsillitis, and the clinical condition is generally not serious enough to seek laboratory help. EBV or CMV infection is diagnosed by the presence of lymphocytosis and atypical lymphocytes, but EBV is distinguished from CMV by detecting heterophil antibodies using the Paul-Bunnell or monospot test and VCA IgM, whereas CMV diagnosis is made by detecting CMV IgM. HSV is readily isolated in the laboratory, but clinical diagnosis is usually adequate. Bacteria are identified by culturing throat swabs (see Chapter 32). It is especially important to diagnose *Strep. pyogenes* infection because of the possible complications (see above) and because, unlike *Strep. pneumoniae*, it remains susceptible to penicillin. Using a latex antigen test a rapid diagnosis can be made directly from a throat swab, but this is not widely used, and bacterial culture is the gold standard. Resistance to erythromycin and tetracycline, however, is increasing. Although during the winter months up to 16% of schoolchildren carry group A streptococci in the throat without symptoms, treatment is recommended.

PAROTITIS

Mumps virus is spread by intimate contact and infects the salivary glands

There is only one serotype of this single-stranded RNA paramyxovirus. It spreads by airborne droplets, salivary secretions and possibly urine. Close contact is necessary—either at school, as the peak incidence is at 5–14 years of age, or in crowded adult communities such as prisons, garrisons and ships.

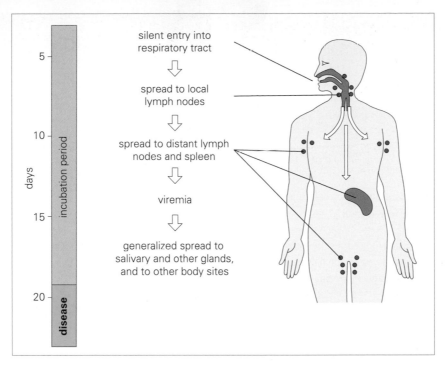

Fig. 18.17 The pathogenesis of mumps. Understanding the pathogenesis of this infection helps to explain the disease picture, sites of shedding and the complications that can arise, but little is known about the events that occur during the first week of infection.

After entry into the body—the primary site of replication is the epithelium of the upper respiratory tract or eye—the virus spreads systemically, undergoing a lengthy period of growth in lymphoid tissues (lymphocytes and monocytes) and reticuloendothelial cells. After approximately 7-10 days the virus re-enters the blood and localizes in salivary and other glands and body sites including the central nervous system, testis, pancreas and ovary (Fig. 18.17). Infected cells lining the ducts degenerate and finally, after an incubation period of 18–21 days, the inflammation, with lymphocyte infiltration and often edema, results in disease. After a prodromal period of malaise and anorexia lasting 1–2 days, the parotid gland becomes painful, tender and swollen, and is sometimes accompanied by submandibular gland involvement (Fig. 18.18). This is the classic sign of mumps although it is present only in 30–40% of infections. However, other tissues in the body may be invaded, with clinical consequences such as inflammation of the testis and pancreas, resulting respectively in orchitis and pancreatitis (Fig. 18.19). CMI as well as antibody responses appear, and the patient usually recovers within one week. There is life-long resistance to reinfection.

Mumps is diagnosed on the basis of parotitis

Laboratory diagnosis is made:

- by isolating virus in cell culture or detecting viral RNA in saliva, cerebrospinal fluid (CSF) or urine;
- by detecting mumps-specific IgM antibody.

Treatment and prevention

There is no specific treatment, but mumps is prevented by using the attenuated live virus vaccine, which is safe and

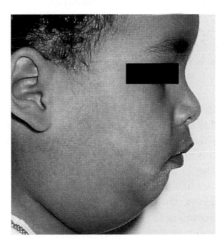

Fig. 18.18 Enlarged submandibular glands in a child with mumps. (Courtesy of JA Innes.)

effective. This is usually given in combination with measles and rubella vaccines (MMR vaccine).

Combined MMR has been a controversial issue in the UK after autism and bowel disorders were reported as associated with immunization. However, a series of epidemiological studies showed no association with immunization.

OTITIS AND SINUSITIS

Otitis and sinusitis can be caused by many viruses and a range of secondary bacterial invaders

Many viruses are capable of invading the air spaces associated with the upper respiratory tract (sinuses, middle ear,

PATHOGENESIS OF MUMPS		
site of growth	**result**	**comment**
salivary glands	inflammation, parotitis virus shed in saliva (from 3 days before to 6 days after symptoms)	often absent; can be unilateral
meninges	meningitis ⎤ ⎥ up to 7 days after parotitis	common (in about 10% cases)
brain	encephalitis ⎦	less common; complete recovery is the rule, deafness is a rare complication
kidney	virus present in urine	no clinical consequences
testis, ovary	epididymo-orchitis; rigid tunica albuginea around testis makes orchitis more painful and more damaging in male	common in adults (20% in adult males); often unilateral; not a significant cause of sterility
pancreas	pancreatitis	rare complication (possible role in juvenile diabetes mellitus)
mammary gland	virus detectable in milk; mastitis in 10% post-pubertal females	–
thyroid	thyroiditis	rare
myocardium	myocarditis	rare
joints	arthritis	rare

Fig. 18.19 Clinical consequences of mumps virus invasion of different body tissues.

mastoid). Mumps virus or respiratory syncytial virus (RSV) for instance, can cause vestibulitis or deafness, which is generally temporary. The range of secondary bacterial invaders is the same as for other upper respiratory tract infections—that is, *Strep. pneumoniae* and *H. influenzae* and sometimes anaerobes such as *Bacteroides fragilis*. Brain abscess is a major complication (see Chapter 24). Blockage of the eustachian (auditory) tube or the opening of sinuses, caused by allergic swelling of the mucosa, prevents mucociliary clearance of infection, and the local accumulation of inflammatory bacterial products causes further swelling and blockage.

Acute otitis media

Common causes of acute otitis media are viruses, Strep. pneumoniae *and* H. influenzae

This condition is extremely common in infants and small children, partly because the eustachian (auditory) tube is open more widely at this age. A study in Boston showed that 83% of 3-year-olds had had at least one episode, and 46% had had three or more episodes since birth. At least 50% of the attacks are viral in origin (especially RSV), and the bacterial invaders are nasopharyngeal residents, most commonly *Strep. pneumoniae* or *H. influenzae,* and sometimes *Strep. pyogenes* or *Staph. aureus*. There may be general symptoms, and acute otitis media should be considered in

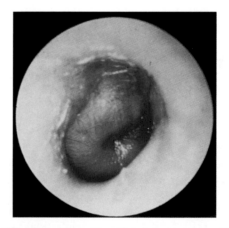

Fig. 18.20 Acute otitis media with bulging ear drum. (Courtesy of M Chaput de Saintonge.)

any child with unexplained fever, diarrhea or vomiting. The ear drum shows dilated vessels with bulging of the drum at a later stage *(Fig. 18.20)*. Fluid often persists in the middle ear for weeks or months ('glue ear') regardless of therapy, and contributes to impaired hearing and learning difficulties in infants and small children.

If acute attacks are inadequately treated there may be continued infection with a chronic discharge through a perforated drum and impaired hearing. This is 'chronic suppurative otitis media'.

Otitis externa

Causes of otitis externa are Staph. aureus, Candida albicans and Gram-negative opportunists

Infections of the outer ear can cause irritation and pain, and must be distinguished from otitis media. In contrast to the middle ear, the external canal has a bacterial flora similar to that of the skin (staphylococci, corynebacteria and, to a lesser extent, propionibacteria), and the pathogens responsible for otitis media are rarely found in otitis externa. The warm moist environment favors *Staph. aureus, Candida albicans* and Gram-negative opportunists such as *Proteus* and *Pseudomonas aeruginosa*.

Ear drops containing polymyxin or other antibiotics are usually an effective treatment.

Acute sinusitis

The etiology and pathogenesis of acute sinusitis are similar to those of otitis media. Clinical features include facial pain and localized tenderness. It may be possible to identify the causative bacteria by microscopy and culture of pus aspirated from the sinus, but sinus puncture is not often carried out. In addition, as is the case for otitis media, the patient can be treated empirically with ampicillin or amoxicillin, or with the newer oral cephalosporins (e.g. cefixime) to deal with beta-lactamase-producing organisms.

ACUTE EPIGLOTTITIS

Acute epiglottitis is generally due to H. influenzae *capsular type B infection*

Acute epiglottitis is most often seen in young children. For unknown reasons, *H. influenzae* capsular type B spreads from the nasopharynx to the epiglottis, causing severe inflammation and edema. There is usually a bacteremia.

Acute epiglottitis is an emergency and necessitates intubation and treatment with antibiotics

Acute epiglottitis is characterized by difficulty in breathing because of respiratory obstruction and, until the airway has been secured (intubation), extreme care must be taken when examining the throat in case the swollen epiglottis is sucked into the edematous airway and causes total obstruction. Treatment is begun immediately with antibiotics effective against *H. influenzae* (cefotaxime, chloramphenicol). The clinical diagnosis is confirmed by isolating bacteria from the blood and possibly the epiglottis. The *H. influenzae* type B (Hib) vaccine greatly reduces the frequency of this and other infections due to *H. influenzae* type B.

Respiratory obstruction due to diphtheria (see below) is rare in developed countries, but the characteristic false membrane and local swelling can extend from the pharynx to involve the uvula.

ORAL CAVITY INFECTIONS

Saliva flushes the mouth and contains a variety of antibacterial substances

The oral cavity is continuous with the pharynx, but is dealt with separately because of the presence of teeth, which are subject to a particular set of microbiologic problems. The normal mouth contains commensal microorganisms, some of which are, to a large extent restricted to the mouth (Fig. 18.1). Most of them make specific attachments to teeth or mucosal surfaces and are shed into the saliva as they multiply. The liter or so of saliva secreted each day mechanically flushes the mouth. It also contains secretory antibodies, polymorphs, desquamated mucosal cells and antibacterial substances such as lysozyme and lactoperoxidase. When salivary flow is decreased for a few hours, as between meals, there is a four-fold increase in the number of bacteria in saliva, and in dehydrated patients or in severe illnesses such as typhoid or pneumonia, the mouth becomes foul because of microbial overgrowth.

Oral candidiasis

Changes in the oral flora produced by broad spectrum antibiotics and impaired immunity predispose to thrush

The presence of commensal bacteria in the mouth makes it difficult for invading microorganisms to become established, but changes in oral flora upset this balance. For instance, prolonged administration of broad spectrum antibiotics allows the normally harmless *C. albicans* to flourish, penetrating the epithelium with its pseudomycelia, and causing thrush. Oral thrush (candidiasis, *Fig. 18.21*) is also seen when immunity is impaired, as in HIV infection and malignancy, and occasionally in newborn infants and the elderly. It sometimes spreads to involve the esophagus. The diagnosis is readily confirmed by Gram stain and culture of scraped material, which shows large Gram-positive budding yeasts.

Topical antifungal agents (e.g. nystatin or clotrimazole) or oral fluconazole (see Chapter 33) are effective treatments for thrush, together with attention to any predisposing factors.

Another example of the shifting boundary between harmless coexistence and tissue invasion by resident microbes is seen with vitamin C deficiency, which reduces mucosal resistance and allows residents to cause gum infections.

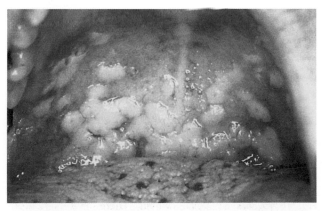

Fig. 18.21 Oral candidiasis. (Courtesy of JA Innes.)

Caries

In the USA and western Europe 80–90% of people are colonized by Streptococcus mutans, *which causes dental caries*

The microorganisms specifically adapted for life on teeth form a film called dental plaque on the tooth surface. This is a complex mass containing about 10^9 bacteria/g embedded in a polysaccharide matrix *(Fig. 18.22)*. The film, visible as a red layer when a dye such as erythrocin is taken into the mouth, is largely removed by thorough brushing, but re-establishes itself within a few hours. The clean teeth become covered with salivary glycoproteins to which certain streptococci (especially *Strep. mutans* and *Strep. sobrinus*) become attached and multiply. In the USA and western Europe, 80–90% of people are colonized by *Strep. mutans. Strep. mutans* itself synthesizes glucan (a sticky high molecular weight polysaccharide) from sucrose and this forms a matrix between these streptococci. Certain other bacteria, including anaerobic filamentous fusobacteria and actinomycetes, are also present. When the teeth are not cleaned for several days, plaque becomes thicker and more extensive—a tangled forest of microorganisms.

The bacteria in plaque use dietary sugar and form lactic acid, which decalcifies the tooth locally. Proteolytic enzymes from the bacteria help to break down other components of the enamel to give rise to a painful cavity in the tooth (caries). Infection may then spread into the pulp of the tooth to form a pulp or root abscess, and from here to the maxillary or mandibular spaces.

The pH in an active caries lesion may be as low as 4.0
Therefore caries usually develops in crevices on the tooth when suitable bacteria *(Strep. mutans)* are in the plaque and there is a regular supply of sucrose. It may legitimately be regarded as an infectious disease—one of the most prevalent infectious diseases in developed countries due to closely placed bacteria-coated teeth and a sugary, often fluoride-deficient, diet.

Periodontal disease

Actinomyces viscosus, Actinobacillus *and* Bacteroides *spp. are commonly involved in periodontal disease*

A space (the gingival crevice) readily forms between the gums and tooth margin, and it may be considered as an oral backwater. It contains polymorphs, complement, IgG and IgM antibodies, and easily becomes infected. Gingival crevices normally contain an average of 2.7×10^{11} microbes/g, and 75% of them are anaerobes. Bacteria such as *Actinomyces viscosus, Actinobacillus* and *Bacteroides* spp. are commonly involved. In periodontal disease, the space enlarges to become a 'pocket', with local inflammation, an increasing number of polymorphs and a serum exudate. The inflamed gum bleeds readily and later recedes, while the multiplying bacteria cause halitosis. Finally, the structures supporting the teeth are affected, with reabsorption of ligaments and weakening of bone, causing the teeth to loosen. Periodontal disease with gingivitis is almost universal, although its severity varies greatly. It is a major cause of tooth loss in adults.

LARYNGITIS AND TRACHEITIS

Parainfluenza viruses are common causes of laryngitis

Viral infections of the upper respiratory tract may spread downwards to involve the larynx and the trachea. Usually the cause is a parainfluenza virus, but sometimes it is RSV, influenza virus or an adenovirus. Diphtheria (see below) may involve the larynx or trachea.

In adults, laryngeal infection (laryngitis) and tracheitis cause hoarseness and a burning retrosternal pain on breathing in and out. The larynx and trachea have non-expandable rings of cartilage in the wall, and are easily obstructed in children because of their narrowness. Swelling of the mucous membrane may lead to croup, which consists of a dry cough and inspiratory stridor ('crowing'). Difficulty with respiration may lead to hospital admission.

Bacteria such as group A streptococci, *H. influenzae* and *Staph. aureus* are less common causes of laryngitis and rachitis.

DIPHTHERIA

Diphtheria is caused by toxin-producing strains of C. diphtheriae *and can cause life-threatening respiratory obstruction*

Diphtheria is now rare in developed countries due to widespread immunization with toxoid (see Chapter 34), but it is still common in developing countries. Non-toxigenic strains occur in the normal pharynx, but bacteria producing the extracellular toxin (exotoxin; see Chapter 2) must be present to cause disease. They can colonize the pharynx (especially the tonsillar regions), the larynx, the nose and occasionally the genital tract, and in the tropics or in indigent people with poor skin hygiene, the skin.

Adhesion mechanisms are not understood, but the bacteria multiply locally without invading deeper tissues or spreading through the body. The toxin destroys epithelial cells

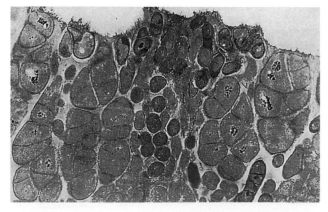

Fig. 18.22 Dental plaque on the deep surface of a child's tooth. ×20 000. (e, enamel.) (Courtesy of HN Newman.)

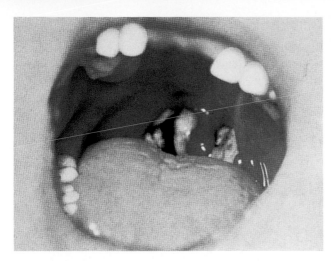

Fig. 18.23 Pharyngeal diphtheria. Characteristic diphtheria 'false membrane' in a child, with local inflammation. (Courtesy of Norman Begg.)

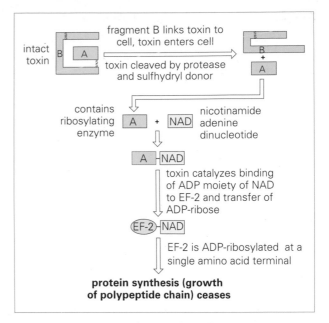

Fig. 18.24 Mechanism of action of diphtheria toxin. (ADP, adenosine diphosphate; EF-2, elongation factor-2.)

LESSONS IN MICROBIOLOGY

Diphtheria toxin

The genes encoding toxin production are carried by a temperate bacteriophage which, during the lysogenic phase, is integrated into the bacterial chromosome. The toxin is synthesized as a single polypeptide (molecular weight 62 000; 535 amino acids) consisting of:

- fragment B (binding) at the carboxy terminal end, which attaches the toxin to the host cells (or to any eukaryotic cell);
- fragment A (active) at the amino terminal end, which is the toxic fragment.

Toxic fragment A is only formed by protease cleavage and reduction of disulfide bonds after uptake of the toxin into the cell. Fragment A inactivates elongation factor-2 (EF-2) by adenosine diphosphate (ADP) ribosylation and thereby inhibits protein synthesis (Fig. 18.24). Prokaryotic and mitochondrial protein synthesis are not affected because a different EF is involved. A single bacterium can produce 5000 toxin molecules per hour and the toxic fragment is so stable within the cell that a single molecule can kill a cell. For unknown reasons myocardial and peripheral nerve cells are particularly susceptible.

and polymorphs, and an ulcer forms which is covered with a necrotic exudate forming a 'false membrane'. This soon becomes dark and malodorous, and bleeding occurs on attempting to remove it. There is extensive inflammation and swelling (Fig. 18.23) and the cervical lymph nodes may be enlarged to give a 'bull neck' appearance.

Nasopharyngeal diphtheria is the most severe form of the disease. When the larynx is involved, it can result in life-threatening respiratory obstruction. Anterior nasal diphtheria is a mild form of the disease if it occurs on its own, because the toxin is less well absorbed from this site, and a nasal discharge may be the main symptom. The patient will, however, be highly infectious.

Diphtheria toxin can cause fatal heart failure and a polyneuritis

The toxin (see panel and Fig. 18.24) is absorbed into the lymphatics and blood, and has several effects:

- Constitutional upset, with fever, pallor, exhaustion.
- Myocarditis, usually within the first two weeks. Electrocardiographic changes are common and cardiac failure can occur. If this is not lethal, complete recovery is usual.
- Polyneuritis, which may occur after the onset of illness, due to demyelination. It may, for instance, affect the ninth cranial nerve, resulting in paralysis of the soft palate and regurgitation of fluids.

Diphtheria is managed by immediate treatment with antitoxin and antibiotic

Diphtheria is a life-threatening disease, and clinical diagnosis is a matter of urgency. As soon as the diagnosis is suspected clinically the patient is isolated to reduce the risk of the toxigenic strain spreading to other susceptible individuals, and treatment is begun with antitoxin. The antitoxin is produced in horses, and tests for hypersensitivity to horse serum should be carried out. Penicillin or erythromycin is given as an adjunct. Laryngeal diphtheria may require tracheotomy.

The diagnosis is confirmed in the laboratory by isolation and identification of the organism (see Appendix and Chapter 32) and demonstrating toxin production by a gel-diffusion precipitin reaction (Elek test).

Contacts may need chemoprophylaxis or immunization

Contacts of diphtheria patients should be tested for carriage of toxigenic *C. diphtheriae* and if necessary be given chemoprophylaxis or immunization. Toxigenic bacteria may be carried and transmitted by asymptomatic convalescents or by apparently healthy individuals.

Diphtheria is prevented by immunization

Diphtheria has almost disappeared from developed countries as a result of the immunization of children with a safe effective toxoid vaccine (see Chapter 34). However, the disease re-appears when immunization is neglected. In 1990, epidemics began in the Russian Federation, and by 1994 all 15 of the Newly Independent States were involved. Worldwide, there are still 100 000 cases and up to 8000 deaths per year.

KEY FACTS

- The respiratory tract from the nose to alveoli is a continuum, and any given microbe can cause disease in more than one segment.

- Some respiratory infections are restricted to the surface epithelium (influenza, diphtheria, pertussis), while others spread throughout the body (measles, rubella, mumps, CMV, EBV).

- 'Professional' invaders infect the healthy respiratory tract (e.g. common cold viruses, influenza viruses, mumps, CMV, EBV, *M. tuberculosis*), whereas 'secondary' invaders cause disease when host defenses are impaired (e.g. *Staph. aureus, Pneumocystis jiroveci, Pseudomonas*).

- Common diseases of the teeth and neighboring structures—caries, periodontal disease—are of microbial etiology.

- Diphtheria is a life-threatening disease caused by a biochemically defined bacterial toxin, and is completely preventable by vaccination.

QUESTIONS

An 18-month-old girl presents to the accident and emergency department in the early hours of the morning having woken up screaming with a fever. Her parents are unable to console her. She has a 3-day history of cold and snuffles. On examination she is flushed and irritable and her ear drums are bright red and bulging.

1. What is the diagnosis?

2. What are the most likely pathogens?

3. How would you treat her?

4. What are the possible complications of this condition?

FURTHER READING

Efstratiou A, George RC. Microbiology and epidemiology of diphtheria. *Rev Med Microbiol* 1996; 7:31–42.

Fischetti VA. Streptococcal M protein: molecular design and biological behaviour. *Clin Microb Rev* 1989; 2:285–314.

Henderson FW, Collier AM, Sanyal MA et al. A longitudinal study of respiratory viruses and bacteria in the etiology of acute otitis media with effusion. *N Engl J Med* 1982; 366:1377–83.

McMillan JA, Sandstrom C, Weiner LB et al. Viral and bacterial organisms associated with acute pharyngitis in a school-aged population. *J Pediatr* 1986; 109:747–52.

Shaw JH. Causes and control of dental caries. *N Engl J Med* 1987; 317:996.

Turner RB, Hendley JO, Gwaltney JM. Shedding of infected ciliated epithelial cells in rhinovirus colds. *J Infect Dis* 1982; 145:849–53.

Lower respiratory tract infections

INTRODUCTION

Although the respiratory tract is continuous from the nose to the alveoli, it is convenient to distinguish between infections of the upper and lower respiratory tract, even though the same microorganisms might be implicated in infections of both. Infections of the upper respiratory tract and associated structures are the subject of Chapter 18. Here, we discuss infections of the lower respiratory tract. These infections tend to be more severe than infections of the upper respiratory tract, and the choice of appropriate antimicrobial therapy is important and may be life saving.

Lower respiratory tract infections can be broadly divided into acute and chronic

Among the acute infections, four major syndromes can be identified:

- acute bronchitis;
- acute exacerbations of chronic bronchitis;
- acute bronchiolitis;
- pneumonia.

Influenza is a specific infection that if severe may proceed to bronchitis or pneumonia. Whooping cough will be considered in this chapter as a serious and acute infection of the lower respiratory tract.

The latter part of this chapter deals with chronic infections, including:

- specific infections such as tuberculosis and aspergillosis;
- conditions such as lung abscesses and empyema;
- infections in cystic fibrosis patients.

ACUTE INFECTIONS

Whooping cough

Whooping cough is caused by the bacterium Bordetella pertussis

Whooping cough or pertussis is a severe disease of childhood. *Bordetella pertussis* is confined to humans and is spread from person to person by airborne droplets. The organisms attach to, and multiply in, the ciliated respiratory mucosa, but do not invade deeper structures. Surface components such as filamentous hemagglutinin and fimbrial agglutinogens play an important role in specific attachment to respiratory epithelium.

B. pertussis infection is associated with the production of a variety of toxic factors

Some of these toxic factors affect inflammatory processes, while others damage ciliary epithelium. They are:

- Pertussis toxin, which resembles diphtheria and other toxins (see Chapters 17 and 18) in being a subunit toxin with an active (A) unit and a binding (B) unit. The A unit is an adenosine diphosphate (ADP)–ribosyl transferase, which catalyzes the transfer of ADP–ribose from nicotinamide adenine dinucleotide (NAD) to host cell proteins. The functional consequence of this is a disruption of signal transduction to the affected cell, but the toxin probably has other effects on the cell surface as well.
- Adenylate cyclase toxin, which is a single peptide that can enter host cells and cause them to increase their cyclic adenosine monophosphate (cAMP) to supraphysiologic levels. In neutrophils this results in an inhibition of defense functions such as chemotaxis, phagocytosis and bactericidal killing. This toxin may also be responsible for the hemolytic properties of *B. pertussis*.
- Tracheal cytotoxin, which is a cell wall component derived from the peptidoglycan of *B. pertussis* that specifically kills tracheal epithelial cells (see Chapter 2).
- Endotoxin, which differs from the classic endotoxin of other Gram-negative rods, but has functional similarities and may play a role in the pathogenesis of infection.

B. pertussis infection is characterized by paroxysms of coughs followed by a 'whoop'. After an incubation period of 1–3 weeks, *B. pertussis* infection is manifest first as a catarrhal illness with little to distinguish it from other upper respiratory tract infections. This is followed up to 1 week later by a dry non-productive cough, which becomes paroxysmal. A paroxysm is characterized by a series of short coughs producing copious mucus, followed by a 'whoop', which is a characteristic sound produced by an inspiratory gasp of air. Despite the severity of the cough, the symptoms are confined to the respiratory tract, and lobar or segmental collapse of the lungs can occur *(Fig. 19.1)*.

Complications include central nervous system (CNS) anoxia, exhaustion and secondary pneumonia due to invasion of the damaged respiratory tract by other pathogens.

The early clinical picture is non-specific, and the true diagnosis may not be suspected until the paroxysmal phase. The organisms can be isolated on suitable media from throat swabs or on 'cough plates' (see Chapter 32 and Appendix), but they are fastidious and do not survive well outside the host's environment.

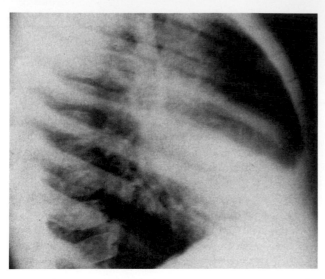

Fig. 19.1 Chest radiograph showing patchy consolidation and collapse of the right middle lobe in whooping cough. (Courtesy of JA Innes.)

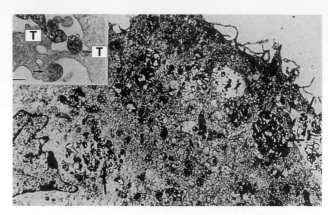

Fig. 19.2 Opsonized *Mycoplasma pneumoniae* cells (arrowed) phagocytosed by an alveolar macrophage (bar, 2 μm). The insert shows *M. pneumoniae* cells adhering with the tip organelle (T) to macrophage surfaces. (Reproduced from E Jacobs, 1991; with permission from Churchill Livingstone Medical Journals.)

Whooping cough is managed with supportive care and erythromycin

Supportive care is of prime importance. Infants are at greatest risk of complications, and admission to hospital should be considered for children under 1 year of age. For specific antibacterial treatment to be effective it must penetrate the respiratory mucosa and inhibit or kill the infecting organism. Erythromycin is the drug of choice. Although the treatment is often not begun until the disease is recognized in the paroxysmal phase, it does appear to reduce its severity and duration. It also reduces the risk of organisms in the throat, thereby helping to reduce the infectivity of the patient, and helps to reduce the risk of secondary infections.

Erythromycin prophylaxis of close contacts of active cases is helpful in controlling the spread of infection.

Whooping cough can be prevented by active immunization

For many years a whole cell vaccine comprising a killed suspension of *B. pertussis* cells has been used. It is usually combined with purified diphtheria and tetanus toxoids and administered as 'DPT' or 'triple' vaccine. The efficacy of pertussis vaccine is generally high, but variable, and recent years have seen major concerns about side effects. These take the form of:

- fever, malaise and pain at the site of administration, which may occur in up to 20% of infants and are not serious;
- convulsions, thought to be associated with the vaccine in about 0.5% of vaccinees;
- encephalopathy and permanent neurologic sequelae associated with vaccination, with an estimated rate of 1 in 100 000 vaccinations (< 0.001%).

Concern about side effects led to a marked fall in uptake of the vaccine and subsequently to a marked increase in the incidence of whooping cough (see Chapter 31). Efforts are now concentrated on the production of subunit vaccines containing only the 'protective' antigens. The difficulty has been in identifying these antigens, but combinations of inactivated pertussis toxin and filamentous hemagglutinin appear to be promising, and such vaccines are already in use in Japan and some other countries.

Acute bronchitis

Acute bronchitis is an inflammatory condition of the tracheobronchial tree, usually due to infection

Causative agents include rhinoviruses and coronaviruses, which are also found infecting the upper respiratory tract, and lower tract pathogens such as influenza virus, adenoviruses and *Mycoplasma pneumoniae*. Secondary bacterial infection with *Streptococcus pneumoniae* and *Haemophilus influenzae* may also play a role in pathogenesis. The degree of damage to the respiratory epithelium varies with the infecting agent:

- With influenza virus infection it may be extensive and leave the host prone to secondary bacterial invasion (post-influenza pneumonia; see below).
- With *Mycoplasma pneumoniae* infection, specific attachment of the organism to receptors on the bronchial mucosal epithelium *(Fig. 19.2)* and the release of toxic substances by the organism results in sloughing of affected cells.

A cough is the most prominent presentation, and treatment is largely symptomatic. The value of antibiotics is uncertain, but they are usually recommended.

Acute exacerbations of chronic bronchitis

Infection is only one component of chronic bronchitis

Chronic bronchitis is a condition characterized by cough and excessive mucus secretion in the tracheobronchial tree that are not attributable to specific diseases such as bronchiectasis, asthma or tuberculosis. Infection appears to be only one component of the syndrome, the others being cigarette smoking and inhalation of dust or fumes from the workplace. Bacterial infection does not appear to initiate the disease, but is probably significant in perpetuating it and in producing the characteristic acute exacerbations. *Strep. pneumoniae* and unencapsulated strains of *H. influenzae* are the organisms most frequently isolated, but interpretation of the significance of their presence in sputum is difficult because they are also commonly found in the normal throat flora and can therefore contaminate expectorated sputum. Other bacteria such as *Staphylococcus aureus* and *Mycoplasma pneumoniae* are less commonly associated with infection and exacerbation. Viruses are frequent causes of acute infection.

Antibiotic therapy may be helpful in the treatment of acute exacerbations, although its efficacy is difficult to assess.

Bronchiolitis

75% of bronchiolitis infections are caused by respiratory syncytial virus

Bronchiolitis is a disease restricted to childhood, and usually to children under 2 years of age. The bronchioles of a young child have such a fine bore that if their lining cells are swollen by inflammation the passage of air to and from the alveoli can be severely restricted. Infection results in necrosis of the epithelial cells lining the bronchioles and leads to peribronchial infiltration, which may spread into the lung fields to give an interstitial pneumonia (see below). As many as 75% of these infections are caused by respiratory syncytial virus (RSV) and most of the remaining 25% are also of viral etiology, although *M. pneumoniae* is implicated occasionally.

Respiratory syncytial virus infection

RSV is the most important cause of bronchiolitis and pneumonia in infants

RSV is a typical paramyxovirus, and two major strains have been identified: group A and group B. Its surface spikes bear G protein (not hemagglutinin or neuraminidase) for attachment to the cell, and fusion (F) protein. The latter initiates viral entry by fusing the viral envelope to the cell membrane, and also fuses host cells to form syncytia.

RSV infection is transmitted by droplets and to some extent by hands. Outbreaks occur each winter (*Fig. 19.3*), and during the RSV season infection can spread in hospitals as well as in the community. Nearly all individuals have been infected by 2 years of age. About 1 in every 100 infants with RSV bronchiolitis or pneumonia requires admission to hospital.

RSV infection can be particularly severe in young infants

After inhalation, the virus establishes infection in the nasopharynx and lower respiratory tract. Clinical illness appears after an incubation period of 4–5 days. The illness can be particularly severe in young infants, with peak mortality at 3 months of age, the virus invading the lower respiratory tract by direct surface spread to cause bronchiolitis or pneumonia. Young infants develop a cough, rapid respiratory rate and cyanosis. In young children and adults, however, the virus is restricted to the upper respiratory tract, causing a less severe common cold-type illness. Otitis media is quite common. Secondary bacterial infection is rare.

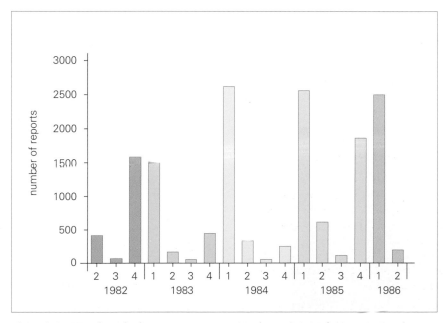

Fig. 19.3 Acute bronchiolitis in respiratory syncytial virus (RSV) infection. Seasonal variation is evident in quarterly reports of RSV infection in England and Wales. (Redrawn from Communicable Disease Surveillance Centre.)

The manifestations of RSV infection appear to have an immunopathologic basis

Maternal antibodies in the infant react with virus antigens, perhaps with the liberation of histamine and other mediators from the host's cells. In early trials a killed vaccine was used and, during subsequent natural RSV infection, the vaccinees had more frequent and severe lower respiratory tract disease compared with unimmunized children, supporting an immune-mediated pathogenesis.

Neutralizing antibodies are formed, at lower levels in younger infants, but cell-mediated immunity (CMI) is needed to terminate the infection. The virus continues to be shed from the lungs of children lacking CMI for many months. Apparently healthy children may continue to show depressed pulmonary function or wheeze even 1–2 years after apparent recovery.

Recurrent infections are common, but are less severe. The reason for recurrence, which is also a feature of parainfluenza virus infection, is unknown.

RSV-specific antigens are detectable in smears of exfoliated cells, and ribavirin is indicated for severe disease

RSV-specific antigens are detectable by immunofluorescence (*Fig. 19.4*) or enzyme-linked immunosorbent assay (ELISA) methods (see Chapter 32) in smears of exfoliated cells obtained by nasopharyngeal lavage. Virus isolation is less commonly useful, and success depends on inoculating respiratory secretions as soon as possible into cell cultures. Polymerase chain reaction (PCR) detection of viral RNA is also helpful.

The antiviral agent ribavirin, used as an aerosol, has occasionally been used successfully for severe disease. At present there is no vaccine.

Hantavirus pulmonary disease

Sin Nombre virus, a hantavirus present in wild rodents, caused severe pulmonary disease in 1993 when it infected people in south-west USA. Viral invasion of the pulmonary capillary endothelium led to fluid outpouring into the lungs, and at least 26 deaths were reported.

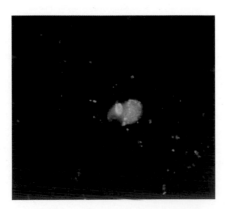

Fig. 19.4 Immunofluorescent preparation from the nasopharynx showing respiratory syncytial virus-infected cells (bright green). (Courtesy of H Stern.)

Pneumonia

Pneumonia has long been known as 'the old man's friend' as it is the most common cause of infection-related death in the USA and Europe. It is caused by a wide range of microorganisms giving rise to indistinguishable symptoms. The challenge lies not in the clinical diagnosis of pneumonia—except perhaps in children, in whom it may be more difficult to diagnose—but in the laboratory identification of the microbial cause (see Appendix). In the absence of such identification, the choice of antimicrobial therapy may not be optimal.

Microorganisms reach the lungs by inhalation, aspiration or via the blood

Microorganisms gain access to the lower respiratory tract by inhalation of aerosolized material or by aspiration of the normal flora of the upper respiratory tract. The size of inhaled particles is important in determining how far they travel down the respiratory tract; only those less than about 5 µm diameter reach the alveoli. Less frequently, the lungs become seeded with organisms as a result of spread via the blood from other infected sites. Healthy individuals are susceptible to infection by a range of pathogens possessing adhesins, which allow the pathogens to attach specifically to the respiratory epithelium. In addition, people with impaired defenses, for example if immunocompromised, with preceding viral damage, or with cystic fibrosis, may develop infections with organisms that do not cause infections in health. An example is *Pneumocystis jiroveci*, an important cause of pneumonia in people with AIDS.

The respiratory tract has a limited number of ways in which it can respond to infection

The host's response can be defined by the pathologic and radiologic findings, but the terms can be confusing because they are applied differently in different situations. However, four descriptive terms are in common use (*Fig. 19.5*):

- Lobar pneumonia refers to involvement of a distinct region of the lung. The polymorph exudate formed in response to infection, clots in the alveoli and renders them solid. Infection may spread to adjacent alveoli until constrained by anatomic barriers between segments or lobes of the lung. Thus one lobe may show complete consolidation.
- Bronchopneumonia refers to a more diffuse patchy consolidation, which may spread throughout the lung as a result of the original pathologic process in the small airways.
- Interstitial pneumonia involves invasion of the lung interstitium and is particularly characteristic of viral infections of the lungs.
- Lung abscess, sometimes referred to as necrotizing pneumonia, is a condition in which there is cavitation and destruction of the lung parenchyma.

The outcomes common to all these conditions are respiratory distress resulting from the interference with air exchange in the lungs, and systemic effects as a result of infection in any part of the body.

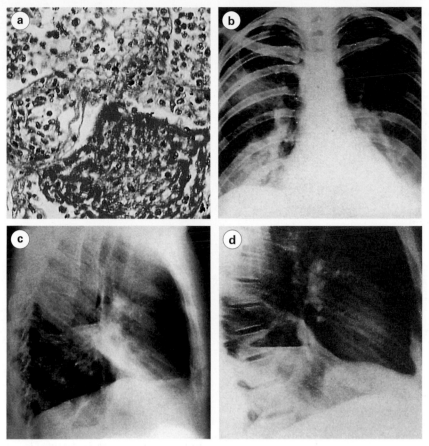

Fig. 19.5 Four types of pneumonia. (a) Pneumococcal lobar pneumonia, showing consolidated alveoli filled with neutrophils and fibrin. (Hematoxylin and eosin stain) (Courtesy of ID Starke and ME Hodson.) (b) Mycoplasma bronchopneumonia, with patchy consolidation in several areas of both lungs. (Courtesy of JA Innes.) (c) Interstitial pneumonia due to influenza virus. (Courtesy of ID Starke and ME Hodson.) (d) Lung abscess, showing an abscess cavity in the lower lobe of the right lung. (Courtesy of JA Innes.)

CAUSES OF PNEUMONIA RELATED TO AGE	
children	**adults**
mainly viral (e.g. respiratory syncytial virus, parainfluenza) or bacterial secondary to viral respiratory infection (e.g. after measles)	bacterial causes more common than viral
neonates may develop interstitial pneumonitis caused by *Chlamydia trachomatis* acquired from the mother at birth	etiology varies with age, underlying disease, occupational and geographic risk factors

Fig. 19.6 Pneumonia in children is more often viral in origin or bacterial secondary to a viral respiratory infection. In adults, bacterial pneumonia is more common.

A wide range of microorganisms can cause pneumonia

Age is an important determinant *(Fig. 19.6):*

- Most childhood pneumonia is caused either by viruses or by bacteria invading the respiratory tract secondary to viral infection, e.g. after measles infection. Neonates born to mothers with genital *Chlamydia trachomatis* infection may develop a chlamydial interstitial pneumonitis (see Chapter 21) resulting from colonization of the respiratory tract during birth.
- In the absence of an underlying disorder such as cystic fibrosis, pneumonia is unusual in older children. Children and young adults with cystic fibrosis are very prone to lower respiratory tract infection, caused characteristically by *Staph. aureus, H. influenzae* and *Pseudomonas aeruginosa.*
- The cause of pneumonia in adults depends upon a number of risk factors such as age, underlying disease and exposure to pathogens through occupation, travel, or contact with animals.

Pneumonia acquired in hospital tends to be caused by a different spectrum of organisms, particularly Gram-negative

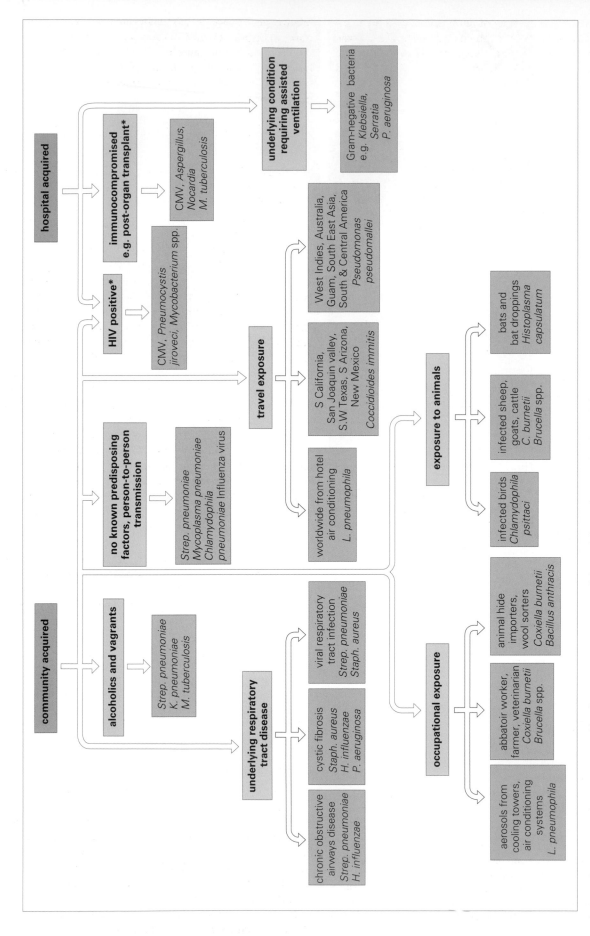

Fig. 19.7 Many pathogens are capable of causing pneumonia in adults, and the etiology is related to risk factors such as the exposure to pathogens through occupation, travel and contact with animals. The elderly are more likely to be infected and tend to have a more severe illness than young adults. (*These infections are often reactivating endogenous infections rather than community or hospital acquired.) (C., Coxiella; CMV, cytomegalovirus; H., Haemophilus; K., Klebsiella; L., Legionella; M., Mycobacterium; P., Pseudomonas; Staph., Staphylococcus; Strep., Streptococcus.)

bacteria. The causative agents of adult pneumonia are summarized in *Figure 19.7*. Although clinical and epidemiologic clues help to suggest the likely cause, microbiologic investigations are essential to confirm the diagnosis and ensure optimal antimicrobial therapy.

It is often difficult to distinguish between bacterial and viral pneumonias clinically

Viral pneumonias show a characteristic interstitial pneumonia on chest radiography more often than bacterial pneumonias *(Fig. 19.5c)*, and for the sake of clarity are described separately below. Infections with RSV have been described earlier in this chapter, and opportunist pathogens, such as *P. jiroveci*, associated specifically with pneumonia in the immunocompromised are described in Chapter 30.

Bacterial pneumonia

Strep. pneumoniae *is the classic bacterial cause of acute community-acquired pneumonia*

In the past, 50–90% of pneumonias were caused by *Strep. pneumoniae* (the 'pneumococcus'), but in recent years the

COMMON CAUSES OF PNEUMONIA IN COMMUNITY-BASED STUDIES IN THREE COUNTRIES

pathogen	percentage* of cases for which a pathogen was identified		
	Sweden	Denmark	Canada
Streptococcus pneumoniae	66	26	11
Legionella pneumophila	4	30	5
Mycoplasma Chlamydia	9	8	10
Haemophilus influenzae	13	32	8
Moraxella catarrhalis	3	0	1
Staphylococcus aureus	0	7	6
viral cause (not specified)	15	13	21

*note that more than one possible cause was isolated from some patients, therefore accounting for totals greater than 100%

Fig. 19.8 Despite the numerous possible pathogens, the vast majority of infections are caused by just a few. *Streptococcus pneumoniae* is the classic cause of lobar pneumonia, but its incidence has been declining in recent years in comparison with the incidence of the so-called atypical causes of pneumonia such as *Mycoplasma* and *Legionella*. (Data from TJ Marrie et al., 1987 and SS Pedersen, 1989.)

relative importance of this pathogen has decreased and it now causes only 25–60% of cases *(Fig. 19.8)*. *H. influenzae* is estimated to be the cause of 5–15% of cases, but the true incidence is difficult to determine because this organism frequently colonizes the upper respiratory tract of bronchitic patients (see above).

A variety of bacteria cause primary atypical pneumonia

When penicillin, an effective antibiotic treatment for pneumococcal infection, became widely available, a significant proportion of cases of pneumonia failed to respond to this treatment and were labeled 'primary atypical pneumonia'. 'Primary' refers to pneumonia occurring as a new event, not secondary to influenza for example, and 'atypical' to the facts that *Strep. pneumoniae* is not isolated from sputum from such patients, the symptoms are often general as well as respiratory, and the pneumonia fails to respond to penicillin or ampicillin. The causes of atypical pneumonia include *M. pneumoniae*, *Chlamydophila* (formerly *Chlamydia*) *pneumoniae* and *Chlamydophila* (formerly *Chlamydia*) *psittaci*, *Legionella pneumophila* and *Coxiella burnetii*. The relative importance of these pathogens varies in different studies *(Fig. 19.8)*. Infection with *C. pneumoniae* is common. About 50% of adults have antibodies, and in the USA it causes up to 300 000 cases of pneumonia each year in adults. *Mycoplasma pneumoniae* and *C. pneumoniae* appear to be solely human pathogens, whereas *C. psittaci* and *Coxiella burnetii* are acquired from infected animals, and *Legionella pneumophila* is acquired from contaminated environmental sources *(Fig. 19.7)*.

Moraxella catarrhalis (previously *Branhamella catarrhalis*) is increasingly recognized as a cause of pneumonia, particularly in patients with carcinoma of the lung or other underlying lung disease. Other etiologic agents of pneumonia associated with particular underlying diseases, occupations or exposure to animals and travel are summarized in *Figure 19.7* and described in other chapters. It is important to note that a causative organism is not isolated in as many as 35% of lower respiratory tract infections.

Patients with pneumonia usually present feeling unwell and with a fever

Signs and symptoms of a chest infection include:

- chest pain, which may be pleuritic;
- a cough, which may produce sputum;
- shortness of breath;
- difficulty and pain on breathing.

Some infections result in symptoms confined mainly to the chest, whereas others such as Legionnaires' disease caused by *L. pneumophila* have a much wider systemic involvement, and the patient may present with mental confusion, diarrhea and evidence of renal or liver dysfunction. However, the distinction between localized and systemic symptoms is not usually reliable enough for an accurate diagnosis.

Chest examination may reveal abnormal crackling sounds, called 'rales', and evidence of consolidation, even before changes become evident on radiography.

Patients with pneumonia usually have shadows in one or more areas of the lung

The chest radiograph is an important adjunct to the clinical diagnosis. Patients with pneumonia usually have shadows indicating consolidation (see above for descriptions of lobar, broncho- and interstitial pneumonia). However, careful interpretation is required to differentiate between infection and non-infective processes such as tumors.

Pneumonia is the most common cause of death from infection in the elderly

It is also an important cause of death in the young and previously healthy. Complications of infection include spread of the infecting organisms:

- directly to extrapulmonary sites such as the pleural space, giving rise to empyema (see below);
- indirectly via the blood to other parts of the body.

For example, the majority of patients with pneumococcal pneumonia have positive blood cultures, and pneumococcal meningitis not infrequently follows pneumonia in the elderly.

Sputum samples are best collected in the morning and before breakfast

Microscopic examination and culture of expectorated sputum remain the mainstays of respiratory bacteriology, despite doubts about the value of these procedures. Collection of sputum is non-invasive, but more invasive techniques, such as transtracheal aspiration, bronchoscopy and bronchoalveolar lavage, and open lung biopsy, may yield more useful results.

Sputum samples are best collected in the morning because sputum tends to accumulate while the patient is lying in bed, and before breakfast to reduce contamination by food particles and bacteria from food. It is important that the specimen submitted for examination is truly sputum and not simply saliva. A physiotherapist can be of great assistance to ill patients who may be unable to cough unaided.

The usual laboratory procedures on sputum specimens from patients with pneumonia are Gram stain and culture

Examination of the Gram-stained sputum (see Chapter 32) can give a presumptive diagnosis within minutes if the film reveals a host response in the form of abundant polymorphs and the putative pathogen, e.g. Gram-positive diplococci characteristic of *Strep. pneumoniae* (Fig. 19.9). The presence of organisms in the absence of polymorphs is suggestive of contamination of the specimen rather than infection, but it is important to remember that immunocompromised patients may not be able to mount a polymorph leukocyte response. Also remember that the causative agents of atypical pneumonia, with the exception of *L. pneumophila* (Fig. 19.10), will not be seen in Gram-stained smears.

Standard culture techniques will allow the growth of the bacterial pathogens such as *Strep. pneumoniae*, *Staph. aureus*, *H. influenzae*, and *Klebsiella pneumoniae* and other non-fastidious Gram-negative rods. Special media or conditions are required for the causative agents of atypical pneumonia, including *L. pneumophila* (Fig. 19.10, see Appendix).

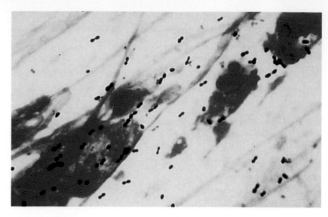

Fig. 19.9 Gram-stained smears of sputum can help the physician make a rapid diagnosis if, like this, they contain abundant Gram-positive diplococci characteristic of pneumococci, as well as polymorphs. However, many of the important causes of pneumonia will not be stained by Gram's stain.

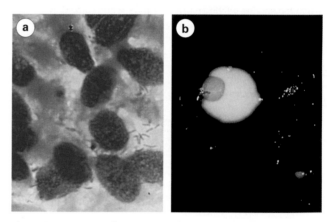

Fig. 19.10 *Legionella pneumophila*. (a) Gram stain of a bronchial biopsy specimen in a patient with fulminant Legionnaires' disease. (Courtesy of S Fisher-Hoch.) (b) Culture plate showing white colonies on buffered charcoal yeast extract medium. (Courtesy of I Farrell.)

Rapid non-cultural techniques have been applied successfully to the diagnosis of pneumococcal pneumonia. Detection of pneumococcal antigen by agglutination of antibody-coated latex particles (see Chapter 32) can be used with both sputum and urine specimens, as antigen is excreted in the urine. Use of this technique means the result is available within 1 hour of receipt of the specimen, but antibiotic susceptibility tests cannot be performed unless the organisms are isolated.

Microbiologic diagnosis of atypical pneumonia is usually confirmed by serology

As mentioned above, several important causes of pneumonia will not be revealed in Gram-stained sputum smears and cannot be grown on simple routine culture media. For these reasons the diagnosis is usually confirmed by serologic tests rather than by culture. In some infections, IgM, antigen or genome detection are being used to make the diagnosis at an early stage. A single high titer of specific antibodies, or preferably demonstration of a rising titer between the acute

SEROLOGIC DIAGNOSIS OF 'ATYPICAL' PNEUMONIA	
pathogen	test
Mycoplasma pneumoniae	complement fixation test (CFT) IgM by latex agglutination or ELISA
Legionella pneumophila	urinary antigen test or rapid microagglutination test
Chlamydophila pneumoniae Chlamydophila psittaci	microimmunofluorescence or ELISA using species-specific antigens
Coxiella burnetii	CFT (phase I and phase II antigens)

Fig. 19.11 Several of the bacterial causes of pneumonia are difficult to grow in the laboratory, so examination of the patient's serum for specific antibodies is the usual method of diagnosis. It is always better to demonstrate a rising titer between acute and convalescent phase sera than to rely on a single sample. (ELISA, enzyme-linked immunosorbent assay.)

and convalescent phase of the disease, is required; therefore serologic diagnosis is often retrospective. The important serologic tests are shown in *Figure 19.11*.

Pneumonia is treated with appropriate antimicrobial therapy

Once the cause of the pneumonia has been identified, selection of the appropriate antimicrobial therapy is relatively straightforward *(Fig. 19.12)*, though there is increasing incidence of penicillin and ampicillin resistance in pneumococci in some countries.

The choice of treatment is more difficult when sputum is not produced or does not reveal the pathogen. It is therefore important to take a full history and use invasive diagnostic techniques if appropriate to help establish the cause.

Prevention of pneumonia involves measures to minimize exposure, and pneumococcal immunization post-splenectomy and for those with sickle cell disease

Respiratory infections are usually transmitted by airborne droplets, so person-to-person spread is virtually impossible to prevent, although less crowding and better ventilation help to reduce the chances of acquiring infection. Infections acquired from sources other than humans may be more amenable to prevention—for example by avoiding contact with sick animals (Q fever) or birds (psittacosis). The contamination of cooling systems and hot water supplies by legionellae has been the subject of intense study, and regulations are now in force in the UK and elsewhere to provide guidance for maintenance engineers.

Immunization is available for a few respiratory pathogens. A pneumococcal vaccine incorporating the polysaccharide capsular antigens of the most common types of *Strep. pneumoniae* is recommended for those at particular risk, e.g. post-splenectomy or individuals with sickle cell disease who are unable to deal effectively with capsulate organisms.

Viral pneumonia

Viruses can invade the lung from the bloodstream as well as directly from the respiratory tract

Many viruses cause pneumonia *(Fig. 19.13)* and, as with viral infections of the upper respiratory tract, generally accomplish infection in the face of normal host defenses. Perfectly healthy individuals are susceptible, and most of these viruses have surface molecules that attach specifically to the respiratory epithelium. RSV can cause pneumonia in infants and is described earlier in this chapter.

Even when viruses of this group do not themselves cause pneumonia they may damage respiratory defenses, laying the ground for secondary bacterial pneumonia. Sometimes the virus fails to spread significantly to air spaces, but remains in interstitial tissues to cause interstitial pneumonitis. An example is cytomegalovirus (CMV) pneumonitis in immuno-deficient patients such as bone marrow transplant recipients.

Parainfluenza virus infection

As with RSV, parainfluenza viruses are most likely to cause lower respiratory tract disease, croup and pneumonia, in children.

There are four types of parainfluenza viruses with differing clinical effects

The surface spikes of parainfluenza viruses are composed of hemagglutinin plus neuraminidase on one type of spike and fusion proteins on another. The four types of virus have different antigens. After infection by respiratory droplets these viruses spread locally on respiratory epithelium.

Parainfluenza viruses 1–3 cause pharyngitis, croup, otitis media, bronchiolitis and pneumonia. Croup is seen in children under 5 years of age, and consists of acute laryngo-tracheobronchitis with a harsh cough and hoarseness. Parainfluenza virus 4 is less common and generally causes a common-cold-type illness.

Virus-specific antigens can often be detected in cells from respiratory washings, and the virus can be isolated. Ribavirin is an effective antiviral but there is no vaccine.

Adenovirus infection

Adenoviruses cause about 5% of acute respiratory tract illness overall

There are 41 antigenic types of adenovirus, some of which cause upper respiratory tract infections such as pharyngo-conjunctival fever and sore throat (see Chapter 18) and lower respiratory tract infections. Adenovirus respiratory tract infections generally cause non-specific symptoms in children under 5 years of age. As maternal antibody wanes, lower respiratory tract illnesses become more frequent, especially with adenovirus 7.

Types 3, 4 and 7 have caused outbreaks of respiratory illness ranging from pharyngitis to atypical pneumonia in

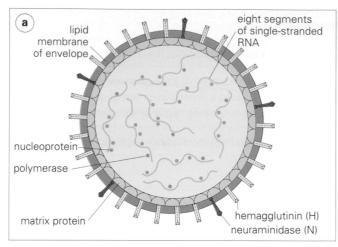

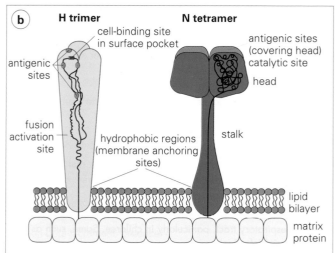

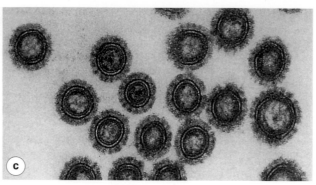

Fig. 19.14 The influenza A virus particle (a), with detail enlarged (b) to show surface hemagglutinin (H) and neuraminidase (N). Each particle has approximately 500 H spikes, which bind to the host cell and fuse the viral envelope to the cell's plasma membrane to initiate infection, and approximately 100 N spikes, which release the virus from the cell surface. Nucleoprotein and polymerase proteins are closely associated with RNA segments to form ribonucleoprotein (RNP). The N tetramer is propeller-shaped as viewed from the end. Detail of only one unit of H trimer and N tetramer is shown. The three-dimensional structure is known from X-ray crystallographic analysis. Electron micrograph (c) shows sectioned influenza virus particles. ×300 000. (Courtesy of D Hockley.)

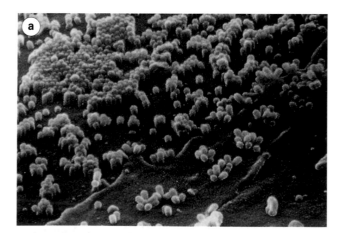

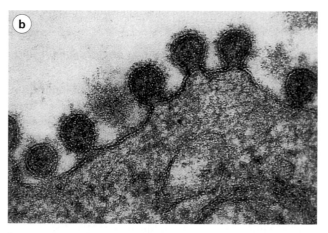

Fig. 19.15 Influenza virus budding from the surface of an infected cell. (a) Scanning electron micrograph. ×27 000. (b) In section. ×350 000. (Courtesy of D Hockley.)

1957 and 1968 by the less severe Asian and Hong Kong influenza pandemics, respectively. In 1976, there was a swine influenza scare in Fort Dix, USA, and in 1997, 18 people in Hong Kong became ill from an avian influenza A virus, H5N1. Six of the infected people subsequently died. The outbreak ceased after public health authorities ordered the slaughter of all live chickens in Hong Kong. Five human infections were reported in 1999 in Hong Kong and South China with another avian strain, influenza A, H9N2. There was neither evidence of wider spread nor human-to-human transmission with either strain.

Epidemics and pandemics are due to the appearance of new strains of viruses so that a given individual is regularly re-infected with different strains. This is in contrast to viruses that undergo

PANDEMIC HUMAN INFLUENZA VIRUSES				
type	subtype*	year	clinical severity	prototype virus
A	H3N2 (?)	1889	moderate	designation based on serologic studies, viruses not isolated
	H1N1 (swine)	1918	severe	
	H2N2 (Asian)	1957	severe	A/Japan/57/H2N2
	H3N2 (Hong Kong)**	1968	moderate	A/Hong Kong/68/H3N2
	H1N1	1977	mild	A/USSR/77
B	none	1940	moderate	B/Lee/40
C	none	1947	very mild	C/Taylor/47
*antigenic shift in influenza A virus is shown by the appearance of novel combination of H and N antigens				
**amino acid and base sequence analysis suggests that recombination between H3N8 (from ducks) and H2N2 gave rise to H3N2				

Fig. 19.16 Human influenza viruses. Novel strains of virus arising in one continent spread rapidly to other continents, causing outbreaks during appropriate times of the year (winter months in temperate climates). There is a World Health Organization global surveillance system for influenza involving more than 100 laboratories in 79 different countries. New strains affecting humans include H5N1, an avian strain which caused 18 infections in humans in Hong Kong in 1997, and H9N2, an avian strain which caused 5 in infections in humans in Hong Kong and South China.

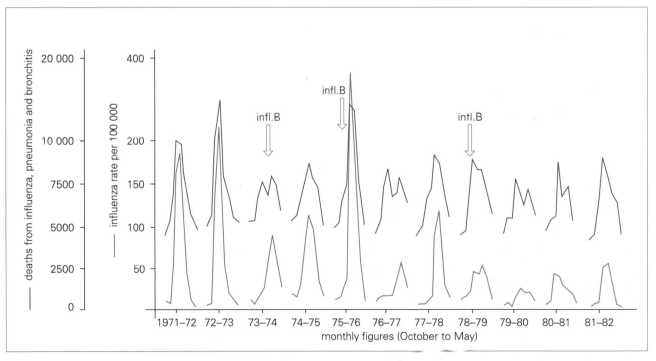

Fig. 19.17 Outbreaks of influenza within a community are reflected by a general increase in deaths from acute respiratory disease. Notifications of new cases of clinical influenza are paralleled by an increase in deaths attributed to influenza, pneumonia and bronchitis. Monthly figures from October to May for England and Wales (1971–83) are shown. The peaks are due to the spread of different strains of influenza A (H3N2 and H1N1) and influenza B (arrows) viruses in the community. (Data from the Office of Population, Censuses and Surveys.)

minimal antigenic variation (monotypic viruses) such as measles or mumps, for which one infection confers life-long immunity.

Transmission of influenza is by droplet inhalation

Influenza occurs throughout the world. Except in the tropics, the infection is almost entirely restricted to the coldest months of the year. This is largely because, during cold weather, people spend more time inside buildings with limited air space, which favors transmission, and perhaps also because of decreased host resistance. Influenza activity within a community is reflected not only in the numbers of people becoming ill and consulting doctors, but also in excess mortality due to acute respiratory disease, such as pneumonia, which particularly affects the elderly (*Fig. 19.17*).

The initial symptoms of influenza are due to direct viral damage and associated inflammatory responses. The virus enters the respiratory tract in droplets and attaches to sialic acid receptors on epithelial cells via the H glycoprotein of the virus envelope. Fewer virus particles are needed to infect the lower respiratory tract than the upper respiratory tract. Just 1–3 days after infection the cytokines liberated from damaged cells and from infiltrating leukocytes cause symptoms such as chills, malaise, fever and muscular aches. There are also respiratory symptoms such as a runny nose and cough. Most people feel better within 1 week. The direct viral damage and associated inflammatory responses can be severe enough to cause bronchitis and interstitial pneumonia.

Influenzal damage to the respiratory epithelium predisposes to secondary bacterial infection

Secondary bacterial invaders include staphylococci, pneumococci and *H. influenzae*. Life-threatening influenza is often due to secondary bacterial infection, especially with *Staph. aureus*, the viral infection being brought under control by antibody and cell-mediated immune responses to the infecting virus. Interferon probably plays a part during the early stages of the infection. Although antiviral antibodies may not be detected within the serum for 1–2 weeks, they are produced at an earlier stage, but are complexed with viral antigens in the respiratory tract.

Mortality due to secondary bacterial pneumonia is higher in apparently healthy individuals over 60 years of age and in those with impaired resistance due to, for example, chronic cardiorespiratory disease or renal disease. Pregnant women are also more vulnerable.

Rarely, influenza causes CNS complications

CNS complications include encephalomyelitis and polyneuritis. These appear to be indirect immunopathologic complications rather then due to CNS invasion by the virus. Guillain–Barré syndrome, a polyneuropathy with proximal, distal or generalized motor weakness, occurred as a significant but rare (1/100 000) sequel to the widespread vaccination of citizens in the USA with inactivated H3N2 influenza virus in 1976. However, subsequent vaccines have not been associated with this syndrome.

During influenza epidemics a diagnosis can generally be made clinically

Influenza-infected cells are seen after fluorescent antibody or immunoperoxidase staining of cells obtained from nasal aspirates. PCR detection of influenza viral RNA can also be carried out, together with sequence analysis for typing purposes. A rise in specific antibodies can be detected by hemagglutination inhibition, complement fixation test or ELISA (see Chapter 32) in paired serum samples taken within a few days of illness and 7–10 days later. The virus can also be isolated from throat washings taken within 1–2 days of onset after inoculation into eggs or into certain cell cultures. This takes several days and is more important for public health authorities following infection with new virus strains rather than for diagnosis in individual patients.

Vaccines and antiviral agents can be used to prevent influenza

The aim of immunization is to help prevent infection, and those at risk of complications from influenza infection should be offered vaccine before the 'flu season'.

Influenza virus vaccines in regular use are:

- those consisting of egg-grown virus, which are then purified, formalin-inactivated and extracted with ether;
- the less reactogenic purified H and N antigens prepared from virus that has been disrupted ('split') by lipid solvents.

Influenza A (H3N2 and H1N1 strains) and influenza B are included in the vaccine. The exact virus strains are reviewed annually in relation to the viruses circulating the previous year. The vaccines are given by parenteral injection, and provide protection against disease in up to 70% of individuals for about one year. Vaccination of individuals at high risk, especially those over 65 years of age and those with chronic cardiopulmonary disease, is recommended. It might be expected that the respiratory route would be a better way of inducing respiratory immunity, and trials with live attenuated virus vaccines administered intranasally are in progress.

Rimantadine or amantadine inhibit the replication of influenza A viruses compared with the neuraminidase inhibitors, zanamivir and oseltamivir, which act on both influenza A and B. These antivirals can reduce the severity of the infection, but only if given within 1–2 days of disease onset. They have also been shown to be effective when used for prophylaxis.

SARS-associated coronavirus infection

An outbreak of severe respiratory disease with no identifiable cause was reported from Guangdong Province in the People's Republic of China in November 2002. The agent spread to mainly parts of east and southeast Asia, as well as Toronto in Canada, and was eventually reported in 30 countries. The World Health Organization (WHO) issued a global health alert in March 2003 concerning Severe Acute Respiratory Syndrome (SARS). The main symptoms were high fever >38° C, cough, shortness of breath or difficulty in breathing. Chest X-rays consistent with pneumonia were also seen. Close contact with someone infected with the SARS agent was the highest risk of the infection spreading from person to person and occurred mostly in family members and hospital staff caring for SARS patients. The incubation period was generally between two and seven days, with a 10 day maximum.

The SARS associated coronavirus (SARS CoV), a new member of the coronavirus family, was identified by virus isolation in cell culture and electron microscopy in conjunction with molecular methods. Diagnostic methods included PCR detection and serology. The rapid identification of the SARS associated coronavirus, implementation of infection control on a scale not seen previously involving face masks, checking for fever in the community and at airports which resulted in rapid isolation on detecting symptom onset, international scientific networking, and immediate availability of data set a global standard for investigation of disease outbreaks.

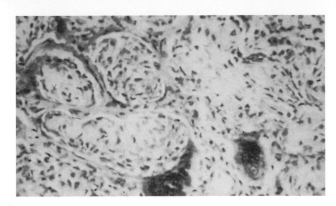

Fig. 19.18 Lung biopsy in measles pneumonia showing inflammatory cell infiltrate, proliferation of the alveolar lining cells and large, darkly staining, multinucleate giant cells. (Hematoxylin and eosin stain.) (Courtesy of ID Starke and ME Hodson.)

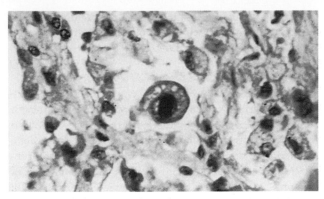

Fig. 19.19 Owl's eye inclusion body in cytomegalovirus infection. Large numbers of virus particles accumulate in the nucleus of the enlarged infected cell to produce a single dense inclusion. (Hematoxylin and eosin stain.) (Courtesy of ID Starke and ME Hodson.)

By July 2003, just slightly more than four months since the virus began moving between countries via international air travel, WHO reported that all known chains of person-to-person transmission of the SARS virus had been broken. The largest outbreaks occurred in mainland China, with 5327 cases and 348 deaths, and Hong Kong, where 1755 cases and 298 deaths were reported.

Measles

Secondary bacterial pneumonia is a frequent complication of measles in developing countries

Measles is dealt with in detail as a multisystem infection in Chapter 26. It is mentioned here because:

- It can cause 'giant cell' pneumonia in those with impaired immune responses.
- The virus replicates in the lower respiratory tract and, under certain circumstances, causes sufficient damage to lead to secondary bacterial pneumonia.

Secondary bacterial pneumonia is now uncommon in developed countries, but is a frequent complication among children in developing countries, and measles remains a major cause of death in childhood. Depressed immune responsiveness, inadequate vaccination programs, malnutrition (especially vitamin A) and poor medical care to deal with complications, tip the host–parasite balance markedly in favor of the virus.

After an incubation period of 10–14 days, there is fever, a runny nose, conjunctivitis and cough. Koplik's spots and then the characteristic rash appear 1–2 days later. The virus replicates in the epithelium of the nasopharynx, middle ear and lung, interfering with host defenses and enabling bacteria such as pneumococci, staphylococci and meningococci to establish infection. Pneumonia generally results in those with measles being admitted to hospital, but otitis media is also common. Virus replication continues unchecked in children with severely impaired cell-mediated immune responses, giving rise to a giant cell pneumonia, which is a rare and

usually fatal manifestation (Fig. 19.18). Other complications are referred to in Chapter 26, and the neurologic complications in Chapter 24.

Measles is diagnosed clinically, but when the incidence is low, detection of specific IgM responses, measles virus isolation, and measles viral RNA detection can be helpful.

Antibiotics are needed for secondary bacterial complications of measles, but the disease can be prevented by immunization

If severe, ribavirin treatment is available, but antibiotics are needed for bacterial complications. Children with severe measles generally have very low levels of serum retinol; recovery is hastened and death is made less likely when they are given 400 000 IU vitamin A.

Measles is prevented by a highly effective, live, attenuated vaccine, given with mumps and rubella vaccines (MMR, see Chapter 34). Since immunization began, the number of cases has declined by 70%. In the USA, after a rise to nearly 30 000 cases in 1990, the number has fallen to 488 (47 of them imported) in 1996. It was planned to eliminate the disease in the Americas by the year 2000, and the WHO are hoping for global eradication by 2010–15. Before the vaccine was available in the 1960s, there were 135 million cases and 7–8 million deaths each year worldwide. Measles is still a killer, but deaths had already been reduced to one million a year by 1996.

CMV infection

CMV infection can cause an interstitial pneumonia in immunocompromised patients

As discussed in Chapter 18, the virus does not normally replicate on respiratory epithelium or cause respiratory illness; but in immunocompromised patients, in particular bone marrow transplant recipients, it can give rise to an interstitial pneumonia. CMV DNA can be detected and quantified, the virus can be isolated and characteristic inclusions demonstrated in lung tissue (Fig. 19.19).

CHRONIC INFECTIONS

Tuberculosis

Tuberculosis is one of the most serious infectious diseases of the developing world

Tuberculosis kills about three million people and infects almost nine million others every year wherever poverty, malnutrition and poor housing prevail. It affects the apparently healthy as well as being a serious disease of the immunocompromised, as has become particularly obvious in patients with AIDS. Tuberculosis is primarily a disease of the lungs, but may spread to other sites or proceed to a

MYCOBACTERIA ASSOCIATED WITH HUMAN DISEASE	
species	**clinical disease**
*slow growers	
M. tuberculosis	tuberculosis
M. bovis	bovine tuberculosis
M. leprae	leprosy
M. avium ⎤ **	disseminated infection in AIDS
M. intracellulare ⎦	patients
M. kansasii	lung infections
M. marinum	skin infections and deeper infections (e.g. arthritis, osteomyelitis) associated with aquatic activity
M. scrofulaceum	cervical adenitis in children
M. simiae	lung, bone and kidney infections
M. szulgai	lung, skin and bone infections
M. ulcerans	skin infections
M. xenopi	lung infections
M. paratuberculosis	? association with Crohn's disease
*rapid growers	
M. fortuitum	opportunist infections with
M. chelonae	introduction of organisms into deep subcutaneous tissues; usually associated with trauma or invasive procedures

*slow growers require >7 days for visible growth from a dilute inoculum; rapid growers require <7 days for visible growth from a dilute inoculum

***M. avium* complex; recent studies show that the two species are distinct. Of the *M. avium* complex, serotypes 1–6 and 8–11 are assigned to *M. avium*, serotypes 7, 12–17, 19, 20 and 25 assigned to *M. intracellulare*

Fig. 19.20 Many species of mycobacteria are associated with occasional disease, but the major pathogens of the genus are *M. tuberculosis, M. bovis. and M. leprae.*

generalized infection ('miliary' tuberculosis). It is also referred to in Chapters 20, 24 and 26.

Tuberculosis is caused by Mycobacterium tuberculosis

Other species of mycobacteria—so-called atypical mycobacteria, mycobacteria other than tuberculosis (MOTT) or non-tuberculous mycobacteria (NTM)—also cause infection in the lungs *(Fig. 19.20).*

Infection is acquired by inhalation of *M. tuberculosis* in aerosols and dust. Airborne transmission of tuberculosis is efficient because infected people cough up enormous numbers of mycobacteria, projecting them into the environment, where their waxy outer coat (see Chapter 2) allows them to withstand drying and therefore survive for long periods of time in air and house dust.

The pathogenesis of tuberculosis depends upon the history of previous exposure to the organism

In primary infection (i.e. infection in individuals encountering *M. tuberculosis* for the first time), the organisms are engulfed by the alveolar macrophages in which they can both survive and multiply. Non-resident macrophages are attracted to the site, ingest the mycobacteria and carry them via the lymphatics to the local hilar lymph nodes. In the lymph nodes the immune response, predominantly a CMI response, is stimulated. The CMI response is detectable 4–6 weeks after infection by introducing purified protein derivative (PPD) of *M. tuberculosis* into the skin. A positive result is shown by local induration and erythema, 48–72 hours later.

The CMI response helps to curb further spread of M. tuberculosis

However, some *M. tuberculosis* organisms may have already escaped to set up foci of infection in other body sites. Sensitized T cells release lymphokines that activate macrophages and increase their ability to destroy the mycobacteria. The body reacts to contain the organisms within 'tubercles', which are small granulomas consisting of epithelioid cells and giant cells *(Fig. 19.21).* The lung lesion plus the enlarged lymph

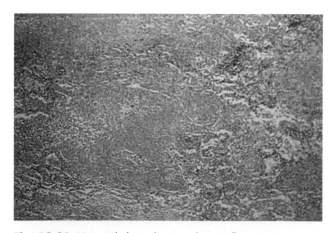

Fig. 19.21 Histopathology showing dense inflammatory infiltration, granuloma formation and caseous necrosis in pulmonary tuberculosis. (Courtesy of R Bryan.)

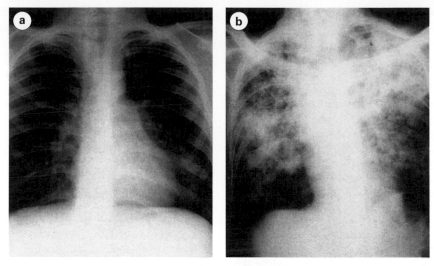

Fig. 19.22 Chest radiographs of (a) primary tuberculosis, showing the Ghon focus in the lower left lung, and (b) post-primary pulmonary tuberculosis showing advanced disease. (Courtesy of JA Innes.)

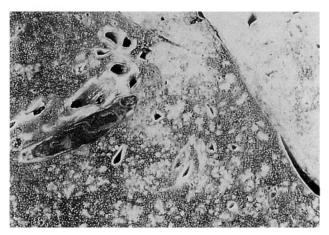

Fig. 19.23 Miliary tuberculosis. Gross specimen of lung showing the cut surface covered with white nodules, which are the miliary foci of tuberculosis. (Courtesy of JA Innes.)

nodes is often called the Ghon or primary complex. After a time the material within the granulomas becomes necrotic and caseous or cheesy in appearance.

The tubercles may heal spontaneously, become fibrotic or calcified, and persist as such for a lifetime in people who are otherwise healthy. They will show up on a chest radiograph as radio-opaque nodules *(Fig. 19.22)*. However, in a small percentage of people with primary infection, and particularly in the immunocompromised, the mycobacteria are not contained within the tubercles, but invade the bloodstream and cause disseminated disease ('miliary' tuberculosis, *Fig. 19.23*).

Secondary tuberculosis is due to reactivation of dormant mycobacteria, and is usually a consequence of impaired immune function resulting from some other cause such as malnutrition, infection (e.g. AIDS), chemotherapy for treatment of malignancy, or corticosteroids for the treatment of inflammatory diseases.

Tuberculosis illustrates the dual role of the immune response in infectious disease

On the one hand, the CMI response controls the infection and, when it is inadequate, the infection disseminates or reactivates. On the other hand, nearly all the pathology and disease is a consequence of this CMI response, as *M. tuberculosis* causes little or no direct or toxin-mediated damage.

Reactivation occurs most commonly in the apex of the lungs. This site is more highly oxygenated than elsewhere, allowing the mycobacteria to multiply more rapidly to produce caseous necrotic lesions, which spill over into other sites in the lung, and from where organisms spread to more distant sites in the body.

Primary tuberculosis is often asymptomatic

In contrast to pneumonia, which is usually an acute infection, the onset of tuberculosis is insidious, the infection proceeding for some time before the patient becomes sufficiently ill to seek medical attention. Primary tuberculosis is usually mild and asymptomatic and in 90% of cases does not proceed further. However, clinical disease develops in the remaining 10%.

Mycobacteria have the ability to colonize almost any site in the body. The clinical manifestations are variable: fatigue, weight loss, weakness and fever are all associated with tuberculosis. Infection in the lungs characteristically causes a chronic productive cough, and the sputum may be blood-stained as a result of tissue destruction. Necrosis may erode blood vessels, which can rupture and cause death through hemorrhage.

Complications of M. tuberculosis infection arise from local spread or dissemination

The organism may disseminate via the lymphatics and bloodstream to other parts of the body. This usually occurs at the time of primary infection, and in this way chronic foci are established, which may proceed to necrosis and destruction in, for example, the kidney. Alternatively, spread may be by extension to a neighboring part of the lung, for instance when a tubercle erodes into a bronchus and discharges its contents, or into the pleural cavity, resulting in a pleural effusion.

Although the number of cases of pulmonary tuberculosis has been declining in developed countries since the beginning of the 20th century, hastened by the advent of specific chemotherapy, the incidence of extrapulmonary tuberculosis has stayed roughly constant for many years and therefore makes up a greater proportion of the tuberculosis caseload in developed countries than in developing countries.

The Ziehl–Neelsen stain of sputum can provide a diagnosis of tuberculosis within 1 hour, whereas culture can take 6 weeks

A diagnosis of tuberculosis is suggested by the clinical signs and symptoms referred to above, supported by characteristic changes on chest radiography (Fig. 19.22) and positive skin test reactivity in the tuberculin (Mantoux) test. These tests are confirmed by microscopic demonstration of acid-fast rods and culture of *M. tuberculosis*. Microscopic examination of a smear of sputum stained by Ziehl–Neelsen's method or by auramine (see Chapter 32 and Appendix) often reveals acid-fast rods (Fig. 19.24). This result can be obtained within 1 hour of receipt of the specimen in the laboratory. This is important because *M. tuberculosis* can take up to 6 weeks to grow in culture (although radiometric methods may reduce the time required for detection, see Appendix) and therefore confirmation of the diagnosis is necessarily delayed. Rapid non-culture tests to detect mycobacteria—for example using the polymerase chain reaction (PCR, see Chapter 32)—are becoming increasingly available. Further tests are required to identify the mycobacterial species and to establish susceptibility to antituberculous drugs.

Specific antituberculous drugs and prolonged therapy are needed to treat tuberculosis

Mycobacteria are innately resistant to most antibacterial agents, and specific antituberculous drugs have to be used; these are reviewed in Chapter 33. The key features of treatment are the use of:

- combination therapy—usually three drugs (e.g. isoniazid, rifampicin, ethambutol) to prevent emergence of resistance;
- prolonged therapy—minimum 6 months—which is necessary to eradicate these slow-growing intracellular organisms.

The number of strains resistant to the first-line antituberculous drugs has increased and has stimulated health agencies to monitor treatment more carefully (e.g. DOTS—directly observed treatment, short-course) and rekindled research interest in finding new agents.

Tuberculosis is prevented by improved social conditions, immunization and chemoprophylaxis

The steady decline in incidence of tuberculosis since the beginning of the 20th century, and before specific preventive measures were available, underlines the importance of improvements in social conditions in the prevention of this and many other infectious diseases. However, recent years have seen an increase in the number of cases associated with AIDS; in some countries in the developing world, HIV infection and AIDS are threatening to overwhelm tuberculosis control programs. An estimated one-third of AIDS-related deaths in 1995 were thought to be due to tuberculosis.

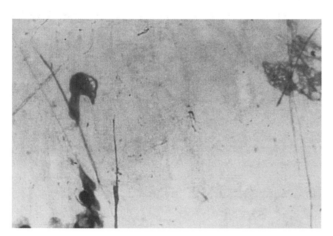

Fig. 19.24 Pulmonary tuberculosis. Sputum preparation showing pink-stained, acid-fast tubercle bacilli. (Ziehl–Neelsen stain.) (Courtesy of JA Innes.)

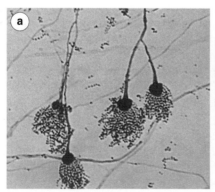
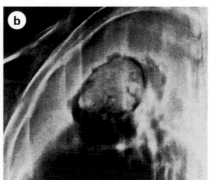
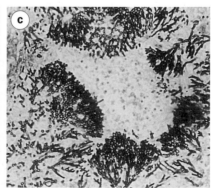

Fig. 19.25 *Aspergillus fumigatus*. (a) Lactophenol cotton blue stained preparation showing the characteristic conidiophores. (b) Aspergilloma. Tomogram showing fungus ball contained within the lung cavity, outlined by air space. (Courtesy of JA Innes.) (c) Invasive aspergillosis. Histologic section showing fungal hyphae invading the lung parenchyma and blood vessels. (Grocott stain.) (Courtesy of C Kibbler.)

Immunization with a live attenuated vaccine, the so-called BCG (bacille Calmette-Guérin) vaccine, has been used effectively in situations where tuberculosis is prevalent. Immunization, which confers positive skin test reactivity, does not prevent infection, but it allows the body to react quickly to limit proliferation of the organisms. In areas where there is a low prevalence of disease, immunization has been largely replaced by chemoprophylaxis.

Prophylaxis with isoniazid for 1 year is recommended for people who have had close contact with a case of tuberculosis. It is also advocated for individuals who show recent conversion to skin test positivity, when it is essentially early treatment of subclinical infection rather than prophylaxis.

Fungal infections

Disease associated with fungal infection is most commonly seen in patients with defective immunity, either as a consequence of immune suppressive treatment or of concomitant disease. A number of species can cause opportunistic infections, and two are of particular importance: *Aspergillus fumigatus* and *Pneumocystis jiroveci*.

Aspergillus fumigatus

Aspergillus fumigatus *can cause allergic bronchopulmonary aspergillosis, aspergilloma or disseminated aspergillosis*

The genus *Aspergillus* contains many species and these are ubiquitous in the environment. They do not form part of the normal flora. Their spores are regularly inhaled without harmful consequences, but some species, notably *A. fumigatus*, are able to cause a range of diseases, including:

- Allergic bronchopulmonary aspergillosis, which is, as its name suggests, an allergic response to the presence of *Aspergillus* antigen in the lungs and occurs in patients with asthma.
- Aspergilloma in patients with pre-existing lung cavities or chronic pulmonary disorders. *Aspergillus* colonizes a cavity and grows to produce a fungal ball, a mass of entangled hyphae—the aspergilloma (Fig. 19.25). The fungi do not invade the lung tissue, but the presence of a large aspergilloma can cause respiratory problems.
- Disseminated disease in the immunosuppressed patient when the fungus invades from the lungs.

  Treatment of invasive aspergillosis is very difficult due to the limited number and toxic nature of antifungal agents active against *Aspergillus* (see Chapter 33) and the lack of functional host defenses.

Pneumocystis jiroveci *(formerly P. carinii)*

Pneumocystis *pneumonia is an important opportunistic infection in AIDS*

P. jiroveci is an atypical fungus, commonly found in normal humans and in rodents. Infection spreads by droplet transmission. Disease occurs in debilitated and immune-deficient individuals. Before the advent of highly active antiretroviral therapy (HAART), a high proportion of AIDS patients develop pneumocystis pneumonia, and this can be fatal.

Pneumocystis occurs as a trophic form, up to 5 µm diameter, as sporocysts and spore cases. Spores are released when these

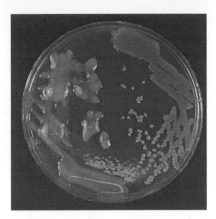

Fig. 19.26 *Pseudomonas aeruginosa* isolated from the sputum of patients with cystic fibrosis characteristically grows in a very mucoid colonial form, shown here on the left of the picture, with the normal colonial form on the right for comparison.

cases rupture. Disease is associated with an interstitial pneumonitis, with plasma cell infiltration. Infections of sites other than the lung have also been reported.

Cystic fibrosis

Cystic fibrosis is the most common lethal inherited disorder among Caucasians, with an incidence of approximately 1 in 2500 live births. The disease is characterized by pancreatic insufficiency, abnormal sweat electrolyte concentrations and production of very viscid bronchial secretions. The latter tend to lead to stasis in the lungs and this predisposes to infection.

P. aeruginosa *colonizes the lungs of almost all 15–20-year-olds with cystic fibrosis*

The respiratory mucosa of individuals with cystic fibrosis presents a different environment for potential pathogens to that found in healthy individuals without cystic fibrosis, and the common infecting organisms and the nature of infections differ from other lung infections. These invaders include:

- *Staph. aureus*, which causes respiratory distress and lung damage, but can be well controlled by specific anti-staphylococcal chemotherapy;
- *Pseudomonas aeruginosa*, which is the pathogen of paramount importance (see below);
- in recent years *P. cepacia*, another member of the genus *Pseudomonas*, which has become an increasing problem;
- *H. influenzae*, typically non-encapsulated strains, which may be found in association with *Staph. aureus* and *P. aeruginosa*; their pathogenic significance is unclear, but they appear to contribute to respiratory exacerbations.

P. aeruginosa infection is uncommon in those under 5 years of age, but colonizes the lungs of almost all patients aged 15–20 years, often encouraged by its intrinsic resistance to antistaphylococcal agents. Early in the course of infection, normal colony types are grown from sputum cultures, but as infection progresses the organism changes to a highly mucoid form, almost mimicking the mucoid secretions of the patient (Fig. 19.26). These mucoid forms are thought to grow in microcolonies in the lung, but most of the lung damage is

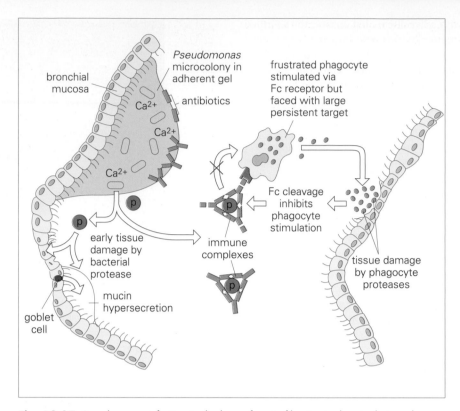

Fig. 19.27 *Pseudomonas* infection in the lung of cystic fibrotics is chronic, but rarely invasive beyond the bronchial mucosa. The organisms are thought to grow in microcolonies embedded in a calcium (Ca^{2+})-dependent mucoid alginate gel, which contains DNA and tracheobronchial mucin, and attaches to the bronchial mucosa. This protects the organisms from the host defenses and provides a physical and electrolyte barrier to antibiotics. Much of the damage to tissue is thought to be due to the slow release of bacterial proteases (which disrupt the mucosa and cause mucin hypersecretion), immunopathologic mechanisms exacerbated by the size, antigenicity and persistence of the alginate matrix, and the indirect action of immune complexes associated with *Pseudomonas* antigens (P). Tissue damage is also caused by phagocyte proteases. Intermittent exacerbations can be explained by the cleavage of the Fc of immune complexes by these proteases and consequent inhibition of further phagocyte stimulation. (Redrawn from Govan and Glass, 1990.)

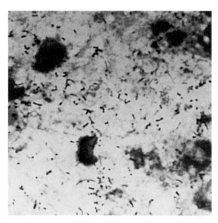

Fig. 19.28 Gram-stain of pus from a lung abscess showing Gram-positive cocci and both Gram-negative and Gram-positive rods. (Courtesy of JR Cantey.)

due to immunologic responses to the organisms and to the alginate, which forms the mucoid material *(Fig. 19.27)*. *P. aeruginosa* rarely invades beyond the lung even in the most severely infected individuals.

Although specific antibacterial chemotherapy can reduce the symptoms of infection and improve the quality of life, infections, particularly with *P. aeruginosa* and *P. cepacia*, are impossible to eradicate and are frequently a cause of death. Heart–lung transplantation is a successful alternative treatment for some patients.

Lung abscess

Lung abscesses usually contain a mixture of bacteria including anaerobes

This is a suppurative infection of the lung, sometimes referred to as 'necrotizing pneumonia'. The most common predisposing cause is aspiration of respiratory or gastric secretions as a result of altered consciousness. The infection is therefore endogenous in origin and cultures often reveal a mixture of bacteria, with anaerobes such as *Bacteroides* and *Fusobacterium* playing an important role *(Fig. 19.28)*.

Patients with lung abscesses may be ill for at least 2 weeks before presentation and usually produce large amounts of sputum, which, if foul smelling, gives a strong hint of the presence of anaerobes and often suggests the diagnosis. Most diagnoses are made from chest radiographs *(Fig. 19.5d)* and the cause confirmed by microbiologic investigation.

Treatment of lung abscess should include an anti-anaerobic drug and last 2–4 months

Because of the likely presence of anaerobes, a suitable anti-anaerobic agent such as metronidazole should be part of the treatment regimen, and treatment may be needed for 2–4 months to prevent relapse. If diagnosis and treatment are delayed, infection may spread to the pleural space, giving rise to empyema (see below).

Pleural effusion and empyema

Up to 50% of patients with pneumonia have a pleural effusion

Pleural effusions arise in a variety of different diseases. Sometimes the organisms infecting the lung spread to the pleural space and give rise to a purulent exudate or 'empyema'.

Pleural effusions can be demonstrated radiologically, but detection of empyema can be difficult, particularly in a patient with extensive pneumonia.

Aspiration of pleural fluid provides material for microbiologic examination, and *Staph. aureus*, Gram-negative rods and anaerobes are commonly involved.

Treatment should be directed at drainage of pus, eradication of infection and expansion of the lung.

PARASITIC INFECTIONS

A variety of parasites localize to the lung or involve the lung at some stage in their development

Such parasites include:

- Nematodes such as *Ascaris* and the hookworms (see Chapters 6 and 22), which migrate through the lungs as they move to the small intestine, breaking out of the capillaries around the alveoli to enter the bronchioles. The damage caused by this process, and the development of inflammatory responses, can lead to a transient pneumonitis.
- Schistosome larvae, which may cause mild respiratory symptoms as they migrate through the lungs (see Chapters 6 and 22).
- The microfilariae of filarial nematodes such as *Wuchereria* or *Brugia*, which appear in the peripheral circulation with a regular diurnal or nocturnal periodicity, their appearance coinciding with the time at which the vector blood-sucking insects are likely to feed. Outside these periods the larvae

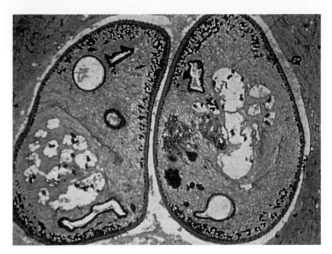

Fig. 19.29 Two adult *Paragonimus* contained within a fibrous cyst in the lung. (Courtesy of H Zaiman.)

become sequestered in the capillaries of the lung. Under certain conditions, as yet undefined, and in certain individuals, the presence of the larvae triggers a condition known as 'tropical pulmonary eosinophilia' (TPE or Weingarten's syndrome). This is characterized by cough, respiratory distress and marked eosinophilia; microfilariae are usually absent from the blood.

- *Ascaris* and *Strongyloides* infections, which may also trigger a pulmonary eosinophilia, although the condition is distinct from TPE.
- *Echinococcus granulosus* infection, which leads to the development of hydatid cysts in a proportion (20–30%) of cases due to localization of the larvae of the tapeworm in the lungs (see Chapters 6 and 22). These cysts may reach a considerable size, causing respiratory distress, largely as a consequence of the mechanical pressure exerted on lung tissue.
- *Entamoeba histolytica* infection, which may rarely involve the lung.
- *Paragonimus westermani*, the oriental lung fluke, which is the most important example of one of the very few adult parasites that live in the lung. Infection is acquired by eating crustaceans containing the infective metacercariae. These migrate from the intestine across the body cavity and penetrate into the lungs. The adults develop within fibrous cysts, which connect with the bronchi to provide an exit for the eggs *(Fig. 19.29)*. Infections cause chest pain and difficulty in breathing, and can cause bronchopneumonia when large numbers of parasites are present. Praziquantel is an efficient anthelmintic for this infection.

KEY FACTS

- Although continuous from nose to alveoli, the respiratory tract is divided into 'upper' and 'lower' from the viewpoint of infection.

- Infections in the lower respiratory tract are spread by the airborne route (except parasites), are acute or chronic, tend to be severe and may be fatal without correct treatment. They are caused by a wide range of organisms—usually bacteria or viruses, but also fungi and parasites.

- Bronchitis, an inflammatory condition of the tracheobronchial tree, is usually chronic with acute exacerbations associated with infection by viruses and bacteria. The disease is characterized by cough and excessive mucus production, and the diagnosis is clinical. Antibiotics are often given, but their efficacy is uncertain.

- Bronchiolitis, usually caused by RSV, is acute and severe in young children. RSV causes outbreaks in the community and in hospitals. The disease has an immunopathologic basis, and specific treatment (ribavirin) may be considered. No vaccine is available.

- Pneumonia is caused by a variety of pathogens depending upon the patients' age, previous or underlying disease, and occupational and geographic factors. Correct microbiologic diagnosis is essential to optimize therapy. Mortality from pneumonia remains significant.

- *B. pertussis* colonizes the ciliated respiratory epithelium causing the specifically human infection whooping cough. Pertussis toxin and other toxic factors are important for virulence. Diagnosis is clinical, alerted by the characteristic paroxysmal cough. Supportive care is paramount; antibiotics play a peripheral role. Prevention by immunization is effective, and new safer vaccines are becoming available.

- Influenza viruses cause endemic, epidemic and pandemic infections as a result of the capacity of the virus for antigenic drift and shift. The disease is acute in onset and can be clinically severe. Viral damage to the respiratory mucosa predisposes to secondary bacterial pneumonia. Antiviral agents are available, but of limited efficacy. Immunization is important, but needs to be kept up to date due to the frequent antigenic changes in the circulating virus.

- Tuberculosis, a major killer, is becoming more common because of its association with AIDS. Infection is usually chronic. Primary infection with *M. tuberculosis* results in a localized pulmonary lesion, while secondary disease arises from reactivation as a result of an impairment of immune function. Clinical diagnosis is supported by demonstrating the acid-fast *M. tuberculosis* in sputum. Effective treatment is available, but long courses of drug combinations are essential. Chemoprophylaxis and BCG immunoprophylaxis are important in prevention.

- *A. fumigatus* causes disease in the lung ranging from invasive disease in the immunocompromised to allergic conditions in the otherwise healthy. Effective treatment is difficult because of the limited number of active antifungals and lack of host defenses.

- Cystic fibrosis is an inherited disease that predisposes to a particular pattern of lung disease characterized by infection with *P. aeruginosa*. Infection can be controlled by antibacterials, but rarely eradicated.

- Various species of parasites pass through or localize in the lungs at some stage in their lifecycle. Damage is limited unless the parasite load is high, and is usually immunopathologic in nature.

QUESTIONS

A 30-year-old man presents with a 10-day history of tiredness, headache, fever and dry cough. He smokes 20 cigarettes a day, his past medical history is unremarkable, and there is nothing else of note on systems review. Relevant findings on examination include a temperature of 38°C, dyspnea and a skin rash consistent with erythema multiforme. Auscultation of his chest reveals a few scattered crepitations and is otherwise unremarkable. The results of investigations are: hemoglobin 10 g/dl; white cell count $6 \times 10^9/l$; erythrocyte sedimentation rate 45 mm/h; urea and electrolytes normal; chest radiograph, patchy shadowing.

1. What is the differential diagnosis?

2. Which questions particularly relevant to the differential diagnosis have not been asked?

3. What further investigations would you perform?

4. The results of some of these investigations are: *Mycoplasma* particle agglutination test titer 1024; *Mycoplasma* CFT acute serum titer 160; *Mycoplasma* CFT convalescent serum titer 2560; cold agglutinins, positive. What is the diagnosis?

5. How would you treat this patient?

FURTHER READING

Alonzo de Velasco E, Verheul AF, Verhoef J, Snipple H. Streptococcus pneumoniae: virulence factors, pathogenesis, and vaccines. *Microbiol Rev* 1995; 59:591–603.

Couch RB, Kasel JA, Glezen WP et al. Influenza: Its control in persons and populations. *J Infect Dis* 1986; 153:431–47.

Department of Health and Welsh Office. The control of legionellae in health care premises. London: HMSO, 1988.

Govan JRW, Glass S. The microbiology and therapy of cystic fibrosis lung infections. *Rev Med Microbiol* 1990; 1:19–28.

Hutchinson DN. Nosocomial legionellosis. *Rev Med Microbiol* 1990; 1:108–15.

Jacobs E. Mycoplasma pneumoniae virulence factors and the immune response. *Rev Med Microbiol* 1991; 2:83–90.

Kawaoka Y, Webster RG. Molecular mechanisms of acquisition of virulence in influenza virus in nature. *Microb Pathogenesis* 1988; 5:311–18.

La Via WV, Marks MI, Stutman HR. Respiratory syncytial virus puzzles. Clinical features, pathophysiology, treatment and prevention. *J Pediatr* 1992; 121:503–10.

Marrie TJ, Grayston JT, Wang P, Kuo C-C. Pneumonia associated with the TWAR strain of Chlamydia. *Ann Intern Med* 1987; 106:507–11.

Moser MR, Bender TR, Marelolis NS et al. An outbreak of influenza aboard a commercial airliner. *Am J Epidemiol* 1979; 110:1–7.

Pedersen SS. Clinical efficacy of ciprofloxacin in lower respiratory tract infections. *Scand J Infect Dis* 1989; Suppl.60:89–97.

Sudre P, ten Dam G, Kochi A. Tuberculosis: a global overview of the situation today. *Bull WHO* 1992; 70:149–59.

Webster RG, Bean WJ, Gorman OT et al. Evolution and ecology of influenza viruses. *Microbiol Rev* 1992; 56:152–79.

Van den Hoogen BG, de Jong JC, Groen J et al. A newly discovered human pneumovirus isolated from young children with respiratory tract disease. *Nat Med* 2001; 7:719–24.

- The human polyomaviruses, JC and BK, enter the body via the respiratory tract, spread through the body and infect epithelial cells in the kidney tubules and ureter, where they establish latency with persistence of the viral genome. About 35% of kidneys from healthy individuals contain polyomavirus DNA sequences. However, during normal pregnancy the viruses may reactivate asymptomatically, with the appearance of large amounts of virus in the urine. Reactivation also occurs in immunocompromised patients (see Chapter 30) and may lead to hemorrhagic cystitis.
- High titers of cytomegalovirus (CMV) and rubella may be shed asymptomatically in the urine of congenitally infected infants (see Chapter 23).
- In contrast to asymptomatic shedding, some serotypes of adenovirus have been implicated as a cause of hemorrhagic cystitis.
- The rodent-borne hantavirus responsible for Korean hemorrhagic fever, infects capillary blood vessels in the kidney and can cause a renal syndrome with proteinuria.
- Finally, a number of other viruses can infect the kidneys, including mumps and HIV.

Urine samples may be investigated by electron microscopy, virus isolation, and genome detection methods.

Very few parasites cause UTIs

Other causes of UTI include:

- The fungi *Candida* spp. and *Histoplasma capsulatum*.
- The protozoan *Trichomonas vaginalis* (see Chapter 21),

which can cause urethritis in both males and females, but is most often considered as a cause of vaginitis.
- Infections with *Schistosoma haematobium* (see Chapter 27), which result in inflammation of the bladder and commonly hematuria. The eggs penetrate the bladder wall, and in severe infections large granulomatous reactions can occur and the eggs may become calcified. Bladder cancer is associated with chronic infections, although the mechanism is uncertain. Obstruction of the ureter as a result of egg-induced inflammatory changes can also lead to hydronephrosis.

PATHOGENESIS

A variety of mechanical factors predispose to UTI

Anything that disrupts normal urine flow or complete emptying of the bladder or facilitates access of organisms to the bladder will predispose an individual to infection (*Fig. 20.2*). The shorter female urethra is a less effective deterrent to infection than the male urethra (see Chapter 13). Sexual intercourse facilitates the movement of organisms up the urethra, particularly in females, so the incidence of UTI is higher among sexually active women than among celibate women. Preceding bacterial colonization of the periurethral area of the vagina is perhaps important (see below).

In male infants, UTIs are more common in the uncircumcised, and this is associated with colonization of the inside of the prepuce and urethra with fecal organisms.

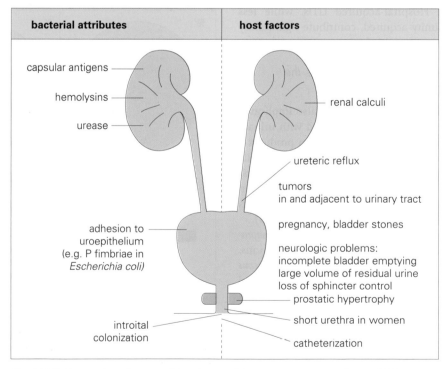

Fig. 20.2 Bacterial attributes and host factors favoring urinary tract infection (UTI). Abnormalities of the urinary tract tend to predispose to infection. Bacterial adherence factors have been studied in detail, but relatively little is known about other bacterial virulence factors in UTI.

Pregnancy, prostatic hypertrophy, renal calculi, tumors and strictures are the main causes of obstruction to complete bladder emptying

When there is a residual urine of more than 2–3 ml, infection is more likely. Infection, superimposed on urinary tract obstruction, may lead to ascent of infection to the kidney and rapid destruction of renal tissue.

Loss of neurologic control of the bladder and sphincters (e.g. in spina bifida, paraplegia or multiple sclerosis), and the resultant large residual volume of urine in the bladder, causes a functional obstruction to urine flow, and such patients are particularly prone to recurrent infections.

Vesicoureteral reflux (reflux of urine from the bladder cavity up the ureters, sometimes into the renal pelvis or parenchyma) is common in children with anatomic abnormalities of the urinary tract and may predispose to ascending infection and kidney damage. Reflux may also occur in association with infection in children without underlying abnormalities, but tends to disappear with age.

Despite reports that pyelonephritis (infection of the kidney) is a common finding in people with diabetes mellitus at postmortem, clinical surveys have failed to produce convincing evidence that there is a significant difference in the prevalence of UTI between people of the same age with and without diabetes mellitus. However, people with diabetes mellitus may have more severe UTIs, and if diabetic neuropathy interferes with normal bladder function, persistent UTIs are common.

Catheterization is a major predisposing factor for UTI

During insertion of the catheter, bacteria may be carried directly into the bladder and, while in situ, the catheter facilitates bacterial access to the bladder either via the lumen of the catheter or by tracking up between the outside of the catheter and the urethral wall *(Fig. 20.3)*. The catheter disrupts the normal bladder's protective function action and allows bacteria to get a foothold. Thus, duration of catheterization is directly associated with increased probability of infection (i.e. risk of UTI increases by about 3–5% each day of catheterization).

A variety of virulence factors are present in the causative organisms

The conflict between host and parasite in the urinary tract has been discussed in Chapter 13. Most urinary tract pathogens originate in the fecal flora, but only the aerobic and facultative species such as *E. coli* possess the attributes required to colonize and infect the urinary tract. The ability to cause infection of the urinary tract is limited to certain serogroups of *E. coli* such as O (somantic) serotypes (e.g. O1, O2, O4, O6, O7 and O75) and K (capsular) serotypes (e.g. K1, K2, K3, K5, K12 and K13). These serotypes differ from those associated with gastrointestinal tract infection (see Chapter 22), which has led to use of the term 'uropathogenic *E. coli*' (UPEC). The success of these strains is attributable to a variety of genes in chromosomal pathogenicity islands (Chapter 2) which are not found in fecal *E. coli*. For example, UPEC typically contain genes associated with colonization of the periurethral areas. For example, specific fimbriae (pili) enable adherence to urethral and bladder epithelium. Studies with other species of urinary tract pathogens have confirmed the presence of similar adhesins for uroepithelial cells *(Fig. 20.4)*.

Other features of *E. coli* which appear to assist in the localization of organisms in the kidney and in renal damage include:

- The capsular acid polysaccharide (K) antigens are associated with the ability to cause pyelonephritis and are known to enable *E. coli* strains to resist host defenses by inhibiting phagocytosis.

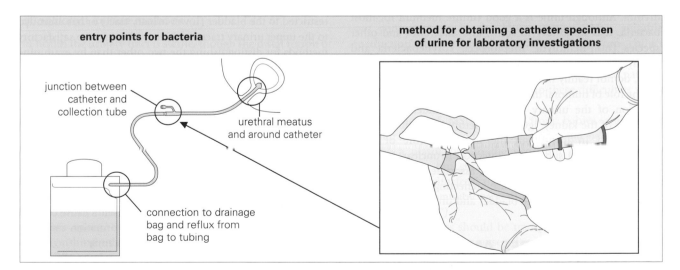

entry points for bacteria

junction between catheter and collection tube

urethral meatus and around catheter

connection to drainage bag and reflux from bag to tubing

method for obtaining a catheter specimen of urine for laboratory investigations

Fig. 20.3 The urinary catheter. Catheterization is an important predisposing factor for infection. Bacteria can be pushed into the bladder as the catheter is inserted and, while the catheter is in place, bacteria reach the bladder by tracking up between the outside of the catheter and the urethra. Contamination of the catheter drainage system by bacteria from other sources can also result in infection. Specimens of bladder urine for laboratory investigations can be collected from catheterized patients as shown. The second port (above) is for putting fluids into the bladder. Urine from the drainage bag should not be tested because it may have been standing for several hours.

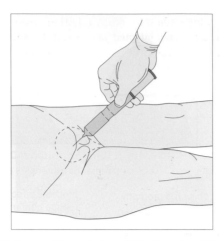

Fig. 20.7 Suprapubic aspiration of bladder urine. Urine samples can be collected directly from the bladder by insertion of a needle. This method is useful in young children from whom it is difficult to obtain uncontaminated midstream urine specimens.

For patients with a catheter, a catheter specimen of urine is used for microbiologic examination

Patients should not be catheterized simply to obtain a urine sample. Urine is obtained from patients who have a catheter in situ by withdrawing a sample with a syringe and needle from the catheter tube as shown in *Figure 20.3*. Urine that has been standing in the catheter drainage bag for hours is unsuitable for testing because the organisms may have multiplied to give much greater numbers than those present in the patient.

Special urine samples are required to detect M. tuberculosis and Schistosoma haematobium

These include:

- three early morning urine samples on consecutive days for *M. tuberculosis*; these do not require the same precautions during collection as an MSU sample, because the culture technique prohibits the growth of organisms other than mycobacteria;
- the last few milliliters of a morning urine sample collected after exercise for detection of *S. haematobium*.

Laboratory investigations

Urine specimens should be examined macroscopically and microscopically and should be cultured by quantitative or semiquantitative methods, as summarized in Chapter 32.

Microscopic examination of urine allows a rapid preliminary report

Bacteria may be seen on microscopy when present in the specimen in large numbers. However, they are not necessarily indicative of infection, but may indicate that the specimen has been poorly collected or left at room temperature for a prolonged period of time.

The presence of red and white blood cells, although abnormal, is not necessarily indicative of UTI. Hematuria may be present in association with:

- infection of the urinary tract and elsewhere (e.g. bacterial endocarditis);
- renal trauma;
- calculi;
- urinary tract carcinomas;
- clotting disorders;
- thrombocytopenia.

Occasionally, red blood cells may contaminate urine specimens of menstruating women.

White blood cells are present in the urine in very small numbers (e.g. < 10/ml) in health; a count of over 10/ml is considered abnormal, but is not always associated with bacteriuria. Sterile pyuria is an important finding and may reflect:

- concurrent antibiotic therapy;
- other diseases such as neoplasms or urinary calculi;
- infection with organisms not detected by routine urine culture methods (see Appendix).

Renal tubular cells, seen in the urine of aspirin-misusers, may be confused with white blood cells. Urinary casts are also indicative of renal tubular damage.

A laboratory diagnosis of significant bacteriuria requires quantification of the bacteria

Culture media and methods are outlined in the Appendix. Conventional methods produce results within 18–24 hours, but rapid methods (e.g. based on bioluminescence, turbidimetry, leukocyte esterase/nitrate reductase test, etc.) are also available. In some laboratories, direct antibiotic susceptibility tests are set up on detecting abnormal numbers of white blood cells or bacteria on microscopy so that both culture and susceptibility results are available within 24 hours.

Interpretation of the significance of bacterial culture results depends upon a variety of factors

These factors relate to:

- collection—specimen collection must be carried out properly;
- storage—the urine must be cultured within 1 hour of collection or held at 4°C for not more than 18 hours before culture;
- antibiotic treatment—in a patient receiving antibiotics, smaller numbers of organisms may be significant and may represent an emerging resistant population; simple laboratory methods are available to detect antibacterial substances;
- fluid intake—the patient may be taking more or less fluid than usual, and this will clearly influence the quantitative result;
- the specimen—the quantitative guidelines are valid for MSU specimens; they do not apply to catheter specimens, suprapubic aspirates or nephrostomy samples.

TREATMENT

Uncomplicated UTI is treated with an oral antibacterial as a single dose or for 3 days

Uncomplicated UTI (cystitis) generally resolves spontaneously within 4 weeks in up to 40% of patients; however, treatment with antibacterial agents reduces symptoms and insures bacterial eradication. Oral antimicrobial chemotherapy is generally as either a single dose or for 3 days, depending upon the drug. The commonly prescribed agents are shown in *Figure 20.8*. The choice of agent should be based on the results of susceptibility tests. However, for uncomplicated UTIs in patients in the community, therapy is often 'best guess', at least until laboratory results are available. This requires a knowledge of the likely pathogens and their antibiotic susceptibility patterns in the locality. Follow-up cultures should be carried out after treatment has been completed (at least 2 days later) to confirm eradication of the infecting organism. In addition to antibacterial therapy, the patient should be advised to drink large volumes of fluid to help the normal flushing out process.

Children and pregnant women with asymptomatic bacteriuria should be treated with antibacterials and followed up to check for eradication of the infection. Instrumentation of the urinary tract should be delayed in patients with significant bacteriuria until appropriate treatment has rendered the urine sterile.

Complicated UTI (pyelonephritis) should be treated with a systemic antibacterial agent

The organism should be known to be susceptible to the antibacterial, and systemic treatment should continue until the signs and symptoms subside. It can then be replaced by oral therapy. The usual length of treatment is at least 10 days, but longer treatment may be necessary to sterilize the kidney.

Hospital-acquired infections or recurrent infections, particularly in catheterized patients, may be caused by antibiotic-resistant organisms, and the agent of choice will depend upon the antibacterial susceptibility pattern. If possible, the catheter should be removed, as eradication of infection is extremely difficult to achieve in catheterized patients and some would advocate treatment only when the patient complains of symptoms or before invasive procedures. Guidelines for catheter care and for the prevention of catheter-associated UTIs are shown in *Figure 20.9*.

COMMON ORAL ANTIBACTERIALS FOR URINARY TRACT INFECTIONS		
antibacterial	**class of agent***	**comments**
ampicillin amoxicillin	beta-lactam beta-lactam	note that >50% of Gram-negative rods causing UTI are beta-lactamase producers and are therefore resistant
co-amoxiclav	beta-lactam + beta-lactamase inhibitor	active against most Gram-negative rods, resistant to ampicillin by virtue of beta-lactamase production
cefalexin cefuroxime	beta-lactam beta-lactam	relatively beta-lactamase stable, therefore wider spectrum than ampicillin, increasing antimicrobial resistance
trimethoprim	antimetabolite/nucleic-acid synthesis inhibitor	incidence of resistant strains increasing
co-trimoxazole	combination of trimethoprim with sulfamethoxazole (also antimetabolite nucleic-acid synthesis inhibitor)	may be useful in 'blind' treatment but more toxic than trimethoprim alone; resistance also an issue
nitrofurantoin	urinary antiseptic	for uncomplicated UTI only; not active in alkaline pH (therefore not useful for *Proteus* infections)
nalidixic acid	quinolone	for uncomplicated UTI; Gram-negative infections only; not active against Gram-positive
ciprofloxacin levofloxacin	quinolone	very broad spectrum; not highly active against enterococci

Fig. 20.8 Oral antibacterials for urinary tract infections (UTIs). Several different classes of antibacterial are available in oral formulations and suitable for treatment of UTI. Nitrofurantoin and nalidixic acid are useful only for lower UTIs as they do not achieve adequate serum and tissue concentrations to treat upper UTIs. Newer generation quinolones are available (Chapter 33.).

INTRODUCTION

Sexually transmitted infections usually cause diseases

In some instances, sexually transmitted infections (STIs) may not result in overt disease symptoms, such as in the early stages of HIV infection and asymptomatic gonorrhea in females. This is particularly troublesome since asymptomatic or unreported sexually transmitted diseases (STDs) are generally untreated, thus facilitating further cycles of infection and spread. While STDs are of major medical importance throughout the world, HIV infection/AIDS has had the greatest global impact, affecting an estimated 42 million adults by 2003. In addition to HIV, new cases of other STDs occur globally with alarming frequency (hundreds of millions of new cases) each year.

The incidence of most STDs is increasing

This is typified by the situation in England, Wales and Northern Ireland where, between 1995 and 2000, the number of new STD reports from genitourinary medicine clinics more than tripled. A similar situation exists in other countries, including the USA. The reasons for this increase include:

- increasing density and mobility of human populations;
- the difficulty of engineering changes in human sexual behavior;
- the absence of vaccines for almost all STIs

The last two factors may change. There is already evidence of changes in male homosexual behavior, leading to decreased transmission of some STDs in this group, and eventually there will be vaccines for certain infections—herpes simplex, gonorrhea, HIV.

The emergence of HIV infection and AIDS has overshadowed other STDs and has had an immense impact as a new and highly lethal infectious disease. Measuring plasma HIV-1 RNA load and CD4 counts or percentage have become the mainstay in management of HIV infection with regard to monitoring disease progress and response to antiretroviral therapy in resource rich countries.

The 'top ten' STDs are listed in *Figure 21.1* while those that are less common are listed in *Figure 21.2*; *Figure 21.3* gives examples of the strategies used by the microorganisms to overcome host defenses.

STDS AND SEXUAL BEHAVIOR

The general principles of entry, exit and transmission of the microorganisms that cause STDs are set out in Chapter 13.

The spread of STDs is inextricably linked with sexual behavior

There are therefore many more opportunities for controlling STIs than, for instance, respiratory infections. Infected but asymptomatic individuals play an important role, and important determinants are promiscuity and sexual practices involving contact between different orifices and mucosal surfaces (see Chapter 13).

- Transmission between heterosexuals or male homosexuals can take place following oral or anal intercourse. The gonococcus, for instance, causes pharyngitis and proctitis, although it infects stratified squamous epithelium less readily than columnar epithelium.
- Condom usage is another major determinant. Condoms have been shown to retain gonococci, herpes simplex virus (HSV), HIV and chlamydia in simulated coital tests of the syringe and plunger type (even when the 'infected' plunger was left in place for an extra 8 hours!).

Further discussion of the control of STDs is included in Chapter 31.

Various host factors influence the risk of acquiring an STD

It is not surprising that the type of sexual activity is important or that genital lesions or ulcers increase the risk of acquiring infections such as HIV. Other factors are less well understood, such as the numerous observations that uncircumcised men have a higher risk of infection.

STDs do not necessarily occur singly, and the possibility of multiple infection must always be borne in mind. For instance, syphilis can accompany gonorrhea, and there is evidence that genital herpes may be reactivated during an attack of gonorrhea.

SYPHILIS

Syphilis is caused by the spirochete Treponema pallidum *and is less common than other STDs*

Treponema pallidum (see Appendix), is closely related to the treponemes that cause the non-venereal infections of pinta

THE TOP TEN SEXUALLY TRANSMITTED DISEASES

organism	disease	comment	treatment
papillomaviruses (types 6 & 11 associated with visible genital warts)	genital warts, dysplasias	the commonest of all STDs, associated with cancer of cervix, penis, etc.	podophyllin, cryotherapy
Chlamydia trachomatis (D–K serotypes)	non-specific urethritis	increasing incidence	doxycycline, azithromycin
C. trachomatis (L1, L2, L3 serotypes)	lymphogranuloma venereum	mainly tropical countries	doxycycline, tetracycline, erythromycin
Candida albicans	vaginal thrush, balanitis	very common; predisposing factors	nystatin, fluconazole
Trichomonas vaginalis	vaginitis, urethritis	very common	metronidazole
herpes simplex virus types 1 and 2	genital herpes	increasing; problem of latency and reactivation	aciclovir, valaciclovir, famciclovir
Neisseria gonorrhoeae	gonorrhea	decreasing incidence in developed countries	ceftriaxone, ciprofloxacin
HIV	AIDS	incidence increasing worldwide	nucleoside, nucleotide and non-nucleoside reverse transcriptase inhibitors, fusion inhibitors; protease inhibitors
Treponema pallidum	syphilis	decreasing incidence in developed countries	penicillin
hepatitis B virus	hepatitis	300 million carriers worldwide	lamivudine, adefovir, interferon alpha
Haemophilus ducreyi	chancroid	mainly tropical	erythromycin, ceftriaxone

Fig. 21.1 The 'top ten' sexually transmitted diseases (STDs).

OTHER SEXUALLY TRANSMITTED DISEASES

organism	disease	comment	treatment
Calymmatobacterium granulomatis	granuloma inguinale	tropical	tetracycline, co-trimoxazole
Sarcoptes scabiei	genital scabies	common	permethrin cream
Phthirus pubis	pediculosis pubis	common	permethrin cream
Mycoplasma Ureaplasma (T strains)	non-specific urethritis	less important than chlamydia	tetracycline, erythromycin
Gardnerella vaginalis	vaginitis	acts together with anaerobes	metronidazole

Fig. 21.2 Other sexually transmitted diseases. No vaccines available.

STRATEGIES ADOPTED BY SEXUALLY TRANSMITTED MICROORGANISMS TO COMBAT HOST DEFENSES

host defenses	microbial strategies	examples
integrity of mucosal surface	specific attachment mechanism	gonococcus or chlamydia to urethral epithelium
urine flow (for urethral infection)	specific attachment; induce own uptake and transport across urethral epithelial surface in phagocytic vacuole	gonococcus
	infection of urethral epithelial or subepithelial cells	herpes simplex virus (HSV), chlamydia
phagocytes (especially polymorphs)	induce negligible inflammation	*Treponema pallidum*; mechanism unclear, perhaps poorly activates alternative complement pathway due to sialic acid coating
	resist phagocytosis	gonococcus (capsule) *T. pallidum* (absorbed fibronectin)
complement	C3d receptor on microbe binds C3b/d and reduces C3b/d-mediated polymorph phagocytosis	*Candida albicans*
inflammation	induce strong inflammatory response, yet evade consequences	gonococcus, *C. albicans*, HSV, chlamydia
antibodies (especially IgA)	produce IgA protease	gonococcus
cell-mediated immune response (T cells, lymphokines, natural killer cells, etc.)	antigenic variation; allows re-infection of a given individual wth an antigenic variant	gonococcus, chlamydia, papillomaviruses (not HSV or *T. pallidum*)
	antigenic variation within a given individual	HIV
	poorly understood factors cause ineffective cell-mediated immune response	*T. pallidum*, HIV

Fig. 21.3 Strategies adopted by sexually transmitted microorganisms to combat host defenses.

SPIRAL ORGANISMS OF MEDICAL IMPORTANCE

family	genus	species	subspecies	disease
Spirochaetaceae	*Treponema*	*pallidum*	*pallidum*	syphilis
		pallidum	*pertenue*	yaws
		carateum	–	pinta
	Borrelia	*recurrentis*	–	relapsing fever
		burgdorferi	–	Lyme disease
Leptospiraceae	*Leptospira*	interrogans	(serovar) *icterohaemorrhagiae*	leptospirosis (Weil's disease)

Fig. 21.4 Spiral organisms of medical importance.

and yaws *(Figs 21.4 and 21.5)*. T. pallidum has a worldwide distribution, and syphilis remains a problem (it is the third most frequent bacterial STD in the USA), especially in developing countries, due to the serious sequelae and the risk of congenital infection.

T. pallidum enters the body through minute abrasions on the skin or mucous membranes. Transmission of T. pallidum requires close personal contact because the organism does not survive well outside the body and is very sensitive to drying, heat and disinfectants. Horizontal spread (see Chapter 13) occurs through sexual contact, and vertical spread via transplacental infection of the fetus (see Chapter 23).

Local multiplication leads to plasma cell, polymorph and macrophage infiltration, with later endarteritis. The bacteria multiply very slowly, and the average incubation period is 3 weeks.

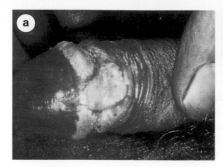 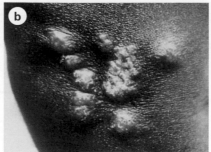 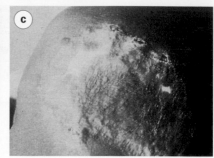

Fig. 21.5 (a) Typical penile chancre of primary syphilis. (Courtesy of RD Catterall.) Yaws (b) and pinta (c) are endemic in tropical and subtropical countries and are spread by direct contact. (Courtesy of PJ Cooper and G Griffin.)

Classically, T. pallidum *infection is divided into three stages*

The three classical stages of syphilis are primary, secondary and tertiary syphilis (*Fig. 21.6*). However, not all patients go through all three stages; a substantial proportion remains permanently free of disease after suffering the primary or secondary stages of infection. The lesion of primary syphylis is illustrated in *Fig. 21.5*. The secondary stage may be followed by a latent period of some 3–30 years, after which the disease may recur—the tertiary stage. Unlike most bacterial pathogens, *T. pallidum* can survive in the body for many years despite a vigorous immune response. It has been suggested that the healthy treponeme evades recognition and elimination by the host by maintaining a cell surface rich in lipid. This layer is antigenically unreactive and the antigens are only uncovered in dead and dying organisms when the host is then able to respond. Tissue damage is mostly due to the host response.

Despite many years of effort, *T. pallidum* still cannot be cultivated in the laboratory in artificial media. It has therefore been difficult to study possible virulence factors at a molecular level, although genes have been cloned in *Escherichia coli* and major proteins have been characterized.

An infected woman can transmit T. pallidum *to her baby in utero*

Congenital syphilis is acquired after the first three months of pregnancy. The disease may manifest as:

- serious infection resulting in intrauterine death;
- congenital abnormalities, which may be obvious at birth;
- silent infection, which may not be apparent until about 2 years of age (facial and tooth deformities).

Laboratory diagnosis of syphilis

As *T. pallidum* cannot be grown in vitro, laboratory diagnosis hinges on microscopy and serology.

Microscopy

Exudate from the primary chancre should be examined by either:

- dark-field microscopy immediately after collection;
- ultraviolet (UV) microscopy after staining with fluorescein-labeled anti-treponemal antibodies.

The organisms have tightly wound, slender coils with pointed ends and are sluggishly motile in unstained preparations. *T. pallidum* is very thin (about 0.2 μm diameter, compared with *E. coli*, which is about 1 μm) and cannot be seen in Gram-stained preparations. Silver impregnation stains can be used to demonstrate the organisms in biopsy material.

Serology

Serologic tests for syphilis are the mainstay of diagnosis. They are divided into non-specific and specific tests for the detection of antibodies in patients' serum.

Non-specific tests (non-treponemal tests) for syphilis are the VDRL and RPR tests

The term non-specific is used because the antigens are not treponemal in origin, but are from extracts of normal mammalian tissues. Cardiolipin, from beef heart, allows the detection of anti-lipid IgG and IgM formed in the patient in response to lipoidal material released from cells damaged by the infection, as well as to lipids in the surface of *T. pallidum*. The two tests in common use today are:

- the Venereal Disease Research Laboratory (VDRL) test;
- the rapid plasma reagin (RPR) test.

Both are available in kit form.

Non-specific tests show up as positive within 4–6 weeks of infection (or 1–2 weeks after the primary chancre appears) and decline in positivity in tertiary syphilis or after effective antibiotic treatment of primary or secondary disease. Therefore, these tests are useful for screening. However, they are non-specific and may give positive results in conditions other than syphilis (biologic false positives, *Fig. 21.7*). All positive results should therefore be confirmed by a specific test. However, treatment (e.g. especially during the primary and secondary stages) tends to result in seroreversion to these tests. Thus, with confirmed disease (see below), these tests can provide at least an indication of therapeutic efficacy.

Commonly used specific tests for syphilis are the treponemal antibody test, FTA-ABS test and the MHA-TP

These tests use recombinant proteins or treponemal antigens extracted from *T. pallidum*. Tests in common use include:

- enzyme-linked immunosorbent assays which detect IgM and IgG;

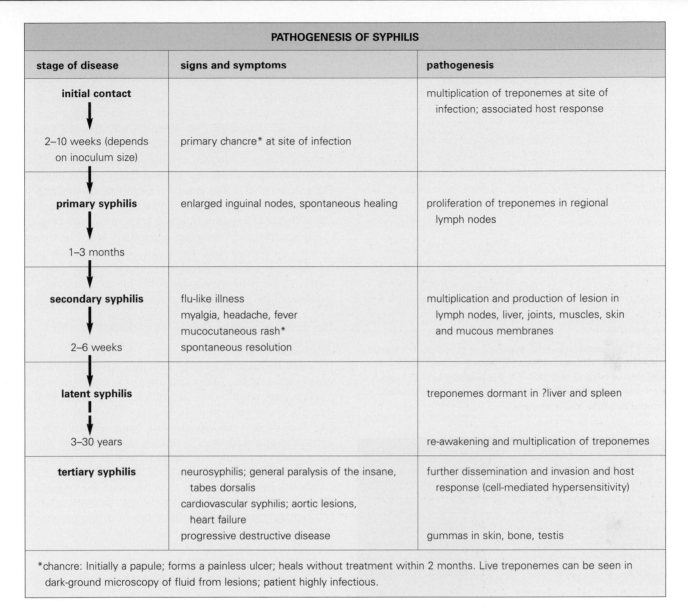

	PATHOGENESIS OF SYPHILIS	
stage of disease	**signs and symptoms**	**pathogenesis**
initial contact 2–10 weeks (depends on inoculum size)	primary chancre* at site of infection	multiplication of treponemes at site of infection; associated host response
primary syphilis 1–3 months	enlarged inguinal nodes, spontaneous healing	proliferation of treponemes in regional lymph nodes
secondary syphilis 2–6 weeks	flu-like illness myalgia, headache, fever mucocutaneous rash* spontaneous resolution	multiplication and production of lesion in lymph nodes, liver, joints, muscles, skin and mucous membranes
latent syphilis 3–30 years		treponemes dormant in ?liver and spleen re-awakening and multiplication of treponemes
tertiary syphilis	neurosyphilis; general paralysis of the insane, tabes dorsalis cardiovascular syphilis; aortic lesions, heart failure progressive destructive disease	further dissemination and invasion and host response (cell-mediated hypersensitivity) gummas in skin, bone, testis
*chancre: Initially a papule; forms a painless ulcer; heals without treatment within 2 months. Live treponemes can be seen in dark-ground microscopy of fluid from lesions; patient highly infectious.		

Fig. 21.6 The pathogenesis of syphilis. A feature of *Treponema pallidum* infection is its chronic nature, which seems to involve a delicately balanced relationship between pathogen and host.

- the fluorescent treponemal antibody absorption (FTA-ABS, *Fig. 21.8*) test in which the patient's serum is first absorbed with non-pathogenic treponemes to remove cross-reacting antibodies before reaction with *T. pallidum* antigens;
- the microhemagglutination assay for *T. pallidum* (MHA-TP).

These tests should be used to confirm that a positive result with a non-specific test is truly due to syphilis. Also, because they become positive earlier in the course of the disease, they can be used for confirmation when the clinical picture is strongly indicative of syphilis. They tend to remain positive for many years and may be the only positive test in patients with late syphilis. However, they remain positive after appropriate antibiotic treatment and cannot therefore be used as indicators of therapeutic response. They can also give false positive reactions *(Fig. 21.7)*.

Confirmation of a diagnosis of syphilis depends upon several serologic tests

Positive serologic test results for babies born to infected mothers may represent passive transfer of maternal antibody or the baby's own response to infection. These two possibilities can be distinguished by testing for IgM and retesting at 6 months of age, by which time maternal antibody levels have waned. Antibody titers remain elevated in babies with congenital syphilis.

At present several serologic tests are needed to confirm a diagnosis of syphilis. None of these tests distinguishes syphilis from the non-sexually transmitted treponematoses, yaws and pinta. Western blot assays using whole *T. pallidum* cells as antigen appear to have excellent potential as a specific confirmatory test in the future.

FALSE POSITIVES IN SYPHILIS SEROLOGY	
test	**conditions associated with false positive results**
non-specific (non-treponemal) VDRL RPR	viral infection, collagen vascular disease, acute febrile disease, post-immunization, pregnancy, leprosy, malaria
specific (treponemal) FTA-ABS MHA-TP	diseases associated with increased or abnormal globulins, lupus erythematosus, skin diseases, antinuclear antibodies, drug misuse, pregnancy

Fig. 21.7 Serologic tests for syphilis and conditions associated with false-positive results. (FTA-ABS, fluorescent treponemal antibody absorption test; MHA-TP, microhemagglutination assay for *T. pallidum*; RPR, rapid plasma reagin test; VDRL, Venereal Disease Research Laboratory test.)

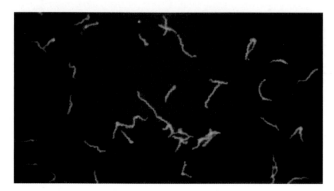

Fig. 21.8 The fluorescent treponemal antibody absorption test for syphilis. Antibody in the patient's serum binds to bacteria and is visualized by a fluorescent dye.

Treatment

Penicillin is the drug of choice for treating people with syphilis and their contacts

Penicillin is very active against *T. pallidum* (*Fig. 21.1*). For patients who are allergic to penicillin, treatment with tetracycline or doxycycline should be given. Only penicillin therapy reliably treats the fetus when administered to a pregnant mother.

Prevention of secondary and tertiary disease depends upon early diagnosis and adequate treatment. Contact tracing with screening and treatment is also important. Several STDs may be present in one patient concurrently, and patients with other STDs should be screened for syphilis.

Congenital syphilis is completely preventable if women are screened serologically early in pregnancy (less than 3 months) and those who are positive are treated with penicillin.

GONORRHEA

Gonorrhea is caused by the Gram-negative coccus Neisseria gonorrhoeae (the 'gonococcus')

This bacterium is a human pathogen and does not cause natural infection in other animals. Therefore its reservoir is human and transmission is direct, usually through sexual contact, from person to person. The organism is sensitive to drying and does not survive well outside the human host, so intimate contact is required for transmission. It is thought that a woman has a 50% chance of becoming infected after a single sexual intercourse with an infected man, while a man has a 20% chance of acquiring infection from an infected woman.

Asymptomatically infected individuals (almost always women, see below) form the major reservoir of infection. Infection may also be transmitted vertically from an infected mother to her baby during childbirth. Infection in babies is usually manifest as ophthalmia neonatorum (see Chapter 23).

The gonococcus has special mechanisms to attach itself to mucosal cells

The usual site of entry of gonococci into the body is via the vagina or the urethral mucosa of the penis, but other sexual practices may result in the deposition of organisms in the throat or on the rectal mucosa. Special adhesive mechanisms (*Fig. 21.9*) prevent the bacteria from being washed away by urine or vaginal discharges. Following attachment, the gonococci rapidly multiply and spread through the cervix in women, and up the urethra in men. Spread is facilitated by various virulence factors (*Fig. 21.9*), although the organisms do not possess flagella and are non-motile. Production of an IgA protease helps to protect them from the host's secretory antibodies.

Host damage in gonorrhea results from gonococcal-induced inflammatory responses

The gonococci invade non-ciliated epithelial cells, which internalize the bacteria and allow them to multiply within intracellular vacuoles, protected from phagocytes and antibodies. These vacuoles move down through the cell and fuse with the basement membrane, discharging their bacterial contents into the subepithelial connective tissues. *Neisseria gonorrhoeae* does not produce a recognized exotoxin. Damage to the host results from inflammatory responses elicited by the organism. Persistent untreated infection can result in chronic inflammation and fibrosis.

Infection is usually localized, but in some cases bacteria isolates (e.g. resistant to the bactericidal action of serum, etc.) can invade the bloodstream and so spread to other parts of the body.

Gonorrhea is initially asymptomatic in many women, but can later cause infertility

Symptoms develop within 2–7 days of infection and are characterized:

- in the male by urethral discharge (*Fig. 21.10*) and pain on passing urine (dysuria);
- in the female by vaginal discharge.

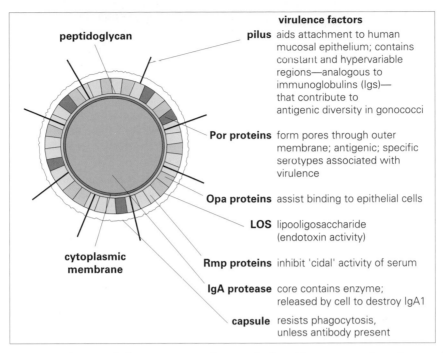

Fig. 21.9 The spread of *Neisseria gonorrhoeae* is facilitated by various virulence factors. Changes in the surface structure of the gonococcus render the organism avirulent.

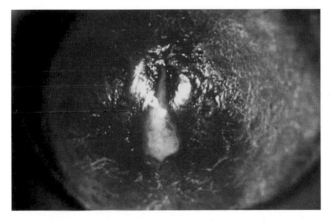

Fig. 21.10 Gonococcal urethritis. Typical purulent meatal discharge with inflammation of the glans. (Courtesy of J Clay.)

At least 50% of all infected women have only mild symptoms or are completely asymptomatic. They do not therefore seek treatment and will continue to infect others. Asymptomatic infection, however, is not the usual course of events in men. Women may not be alerted to their infection unless or until complications arise such as:

- pelvic inflammatory disease (PID);
- chronic pelvic pain;
- infertility resulting from damage to the fallopian tubes.

Ophthalmia neonatorum is characterized by a sticky discharge (see *Fig. 23.10*).

Gonococcal infection of the throat may result in a sore throat (see Chapter 18), and infection of the rectum also results in a purulent discharge.

In men, local complications of urethral infection are rare *(Fig. 21.11)*. Invasive gonococcal disease is much more

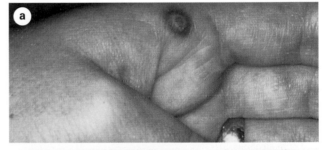

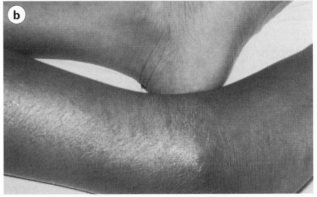

Fig. 21.11 Local and systemic complications of gonococcal infection. (a) Skin lesions start as erythematous papules, which often become pustular and hemorrhagic with necrotic centers. (Courtesy of JS Bingham.) (b) Septic arthritis of the ankle with marked erythema and swelling of the ankle and leg. (Courtesy of TF Sellers, Jr.)

common in infected women than in men, but prompt treatment is important in containing local infection. The common occurrence of asymptomatic infection in women is an important factor in the occurence of complications (i.e. the infection is unrecognized and untreated). In 10–20% of

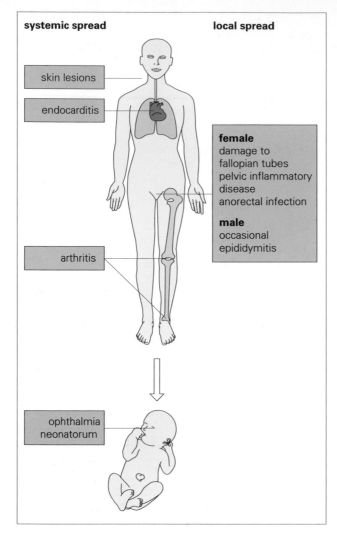

systemic spread | local spread

skin lesions

endocarditis

female
damage to
fallopian tubes
pelvic inflammatory
disease
anorectal infection

male
occasional
epididymitis

arthritis

ophthalmia
neonatorum

Fig. 21.12 Local and systemic spread of gonococcal infection and complications.

untreated women, infection spreads up the genital tract to cause pelvic inflammatory disease (PID) and damage to the fallopian tubes.

Disseminated infection occurs in 1–3% of women, but is less common in men (see above and *Fig. 21.12*). It is a function not only of the strain of gonococcus (see above), but also host factors (e.g. about 5% of people with disseminated infection have deficiencies in the late-acting components of complement [C5–C8]).

A diagnosis of gonorrhea is made from microscopy and culture of appropriate specimens

Urethral and vaginal discharges and other specimens where indicated are used for microscopy and culture. Although a purulent discharge is characteristic of local gonococcal infection, it is not possible to distinguish reliably between gonococcal discharge and that caused by other pathogens such as *Chlamydia trachomatis* on clinical examination.

With experience, the finding of Gram-negative intracellular diplococci in a smear of urethral discharge from a symptomatic male patient is a highly sensitive and specific test for the diagnosis of gonorrhea.

Culture is essential in the investigation of infection in women and asymptomatic men, and for specimens taken from sites other than the urethra. Specimens from symptomatic men should also be cultured:

- to confirm the identity of the isolate; misinterpretation of microscopy or culture results can cause severe distress and may result in litigation;
- to perform antibiotic susceptibility tests (see Chapter 32);
- to aid in the distinction between treatment failure and re-infection.

Because of the organism's sensitivity to drying, cultures should be made on warmed selective (i.e. modified Thayer Martin) and non-selective (chocolate blood agar) medium to insure recovery. Inoculation into appropriate transport medium is required if transfer to the laboratory will be delayed (no more than 48 hours). Blood cultures should be collected if disseminated disease is suspected, and joint aspirates may yield positive cultures.

Serologic tests are unsatisfactory. Recently, commercial kits with probes specific for both *N. gonorrhoeae* and *Chlamydia* DNA have become available, providing reliable results within about 2–4 hours.

Antibacterials used to treat gonorrhea are ceftriaxone and fluoroquinolones such as ciprofloxacin, but resistance is increasing

The antibacterial agents of choice are shown in *Figure 21.1*. Penicillinase-producing *N. gonorrhoeae* were first observed in 1976 with increasing resistance that has severely compromised the effective treatment of gonorrhea in many parts of the world, especially Southeast Asia. Resistance to fluoroquinolones is also on the increase. Since patients with gonorrhea may also be infected with chlamydia (see below) treatment regimens often include a combination of agents targeting both organisms (e.g. ceftriaxone and doxycycline, respectively). Early treatment of a significant proportion of sexually promiscuous patients achieves a striking reduction in the duration of infectiousness and transmission rates. Prophylactic use of antibacterials has no effect in preventing sexually-acquired gonorrhea, but the application of antibacterial eye drops to babies born to mothers with gonorrhea or suspected gonorrhea is effective. Infection can be prevented by the use of condoms.

Follow-up of patients and contact tracing are vital to control the spread of gonorrhea. At present, effective vaccines are not available, but the possibility of using some of the pilus proteins or other outer membrane components of the gonococcal cell as antigens is under investigation. However, immunization may prevent symptomatic disease without preventing infection, and the dangers of asymptomatic infection have been discussed above.

Repeated infections can occur with strains of bacteria with different pilin proteins.

CHLAMYDIAL INFECTION

C. trachomatis serotypes D–K cause sexually transmitted genital infections

The chlamydiae are very small bacteria that are obligate intracellular parasites. They have a more complicated lifecycle

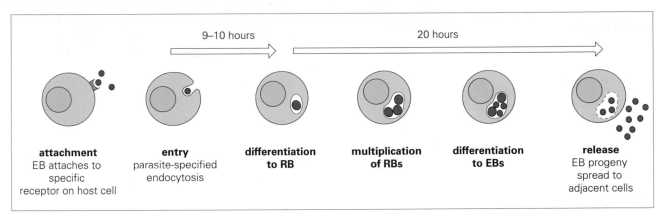

Fig. 21.13 The lifecycle of *Chlamydia*. (EB, elementary body; RB, reticulate body.)

MEDICALLY IMPORTANT SPECIES OF CHLAMYDIACEAE			
species	serotype	natural host	disease in humans
Chlamydia trachomatis	A,B,C	humans	trachoma
	D–K	humans	cervicitis urethritis proctitis conjunctivitis pneumonia (in neonates)
	L1,L2,L3	humans	lymphogranuloma venereum
Chlamydophila psittaci	?	birds and non-human mammals	pneumonia
Chlamydophila pneumoniae	?	humans	acute respiratory disease

Fig. 21.14 Medically important chlamydiaceae. *Chlamydia trachomatis* is the species associated with sexually transmitted disease.

CHLAMYDIA TRACHOMATIS: CLINICAL SYNDROMES AND THEIR COMPLICATIONS		
infection in	clinical syndromes	complications
men	urethritis epididymitis proctitis conjunctivitis	systemic spread Reiter's syndrome*
women	urethritis cervicitis bartholinitis salpingitis conjunctivitis	ectopic pregnancy infertility systemic spread: perihepatitis arthritis dermatitis
neonates	conjunctivitis	interstitial pneumonitis

*Urethritis, conjunctivitis, polyarthritis, mucocutaneous lesions

Fig. 21.15 Clinical syndromes and complications caused by *C. trachomatis*, serotypes D–K.

than free-living bacteria because they can exist in different forms:

- The elementary body (EB) is adapted for extracellular survival and for initiation of infection.
- The reticulate body (RB) is adapted for intracellular multiplication *(Fig. 21.13)*.

Traditionally, three species of *Chlamydia* were recognized: *C. trachomatis*, *C. psittaci* and *C. pneumoniae*. However the latter two have now been moved to a new genus, *Chlamydophila (Fig. 21.14)*. *Chlamydophila psittaci* and *Chlamydophila pneumoniae* infect the respiratory tract and have been discussed in Chapter 19. The species *Chlaymdia trachomatis* can be subdivided into different serotypes (also known as serovars)

and these have been shown to be linked characteristically with different infections:

- Serotypes A, B and C are the causes of the serious eye infection trachoma (see Chapter 25).
- Serotypes D–K are the cause of genital infection and associated ocular and respiratory infections *(Fig. 21.15)*.
- Serotypes L1, L2 and L3 cause the systemic disease lymphogranuloma venereum (LGV) (see below).

C. trachomatis serotypes D–K have a worldwide distribution whereas the distribution of LGV serotypes is more restricted.

The majority of infections are genital and are acquired during sexual intercourse. Asymptomatic infection is common, especially in women. Ocular infections in adults are probably acquired by autoinoculation from infected genitalia or by ocular–genital contact. Ocular infections in neonates are acquired during passage through an infected maternal birth canal, and the infant is also at risk of developing *C. trachomatis* pneumonia (see Chapter 19).

Chlamydiae enter the host through minute abrasions in the mucosal surface

They bind to specific receptors on the host cells and enter the cells by 'parasite-induced' endocytosis (see Chapter 13). Once inside the cell, fusion of the chlamydia-containing vesicle with lysozomes is inhibited by an unknown mechanism and the EB begins its developmental cycle *(Fig. 21.13)*. Within 9–10 hours of cell invasion the EBs differentiate into metabolically active RBs, which divide by binary fission and produce fresh EB progeny. These are then released into the extracellular environment within a further 20 hours.

The clinical effects of C. trachomatis *infection appear to result from cell destruction and the host's inflammatory response*

The released EBs invade adjacent cells or cells distant from the site of infection if carried in lymph or blood.

Growth of *C. trachomatis* serotypes D–K seems to be restricted to columnar and transitional epithelial cells, but serotypes L1, L2 and L3 cause systemic disease (LGV). The site of infection determines the nature of clinical disease *(Fig. 21.15)*. Genital tract infection with serotypes D–K is locally asymptomatic in most women, but usually symptomatic in men.

Laboratory tests are essential to diagnose chlamydial urethritis and cervicitis

Chlamydial urethritis and cervicitis cannot be reliably distinguished from other causes of these conditions on clinical grounds alone. The methods traditionally available include cell culture and direct antigen detection.

Most infected patients develop antibodies, but serology is unreliable for diagnostic purposes. As chlamydiae are obligate intracellular parasites, isolation must be performed in cell cultures. The specimen is suspended in fluid and centrifuged on to a monolayer of tissue culture (McCoy) cells pretreated with cycloheximide, which enhances the uptake of chlamydiae. After 48–72 hours, *C. trachomatis* forms characteristic cytoplasmic inclusions, which stain with iodine because they contain glycogen *(Fig. 21.16)* or can be visualized with immunofluorescent stains.

C. trachomatis *can be detected directly on microscopy using the direct fluorescent antibody test*

C. trachomatis can be detected directly in smears of clinical specimens made on microscope slides stained with fluorescein conjugated monoclonal antibodies and viewed by UV microscopy—the direct fluorescent antibody (DFA) test. The EBs stain as bright yellow-green dots *(Fig. 21.17)*. Results can be obtained within a few hours. Compared with culture, this method is extremely specific, but often not sensitive enough for asymptomatic infections. Chlamydial antigens can also be detected in specimens using an enzyme-linked immunosorbent assay (ELISA), but this test also suffers from reduced sensitivity in asymptomatic patients.

A variety of nucleic acid-based tests are now commercially available for chlamydial detection

Recently developed nucleic acid probe and amplification-based tests are capable of directly detecting *C. trachomatis* in specimens from infected individuals (e.g. cervix, urethra, urine, etc.). As mentioned previously, these commercially available kits can provide rapid (2–4 hours) and specific detection of both *N. gonorrhoeae* and *Chlamydia* DNA, which is important since patients are often coinfected with both organisms. These quick and accurate molecular approaches are used increasingly as the preferred test for the detection of these organisms.

Chlamydial infection is treated or prevented with doxycycline or tetracycline

It is important to remember that chlamydiae are not susceptible to the beta-lactam antibiotics, which are important for the treatment of gonorrhea and syphilis. It is recommended

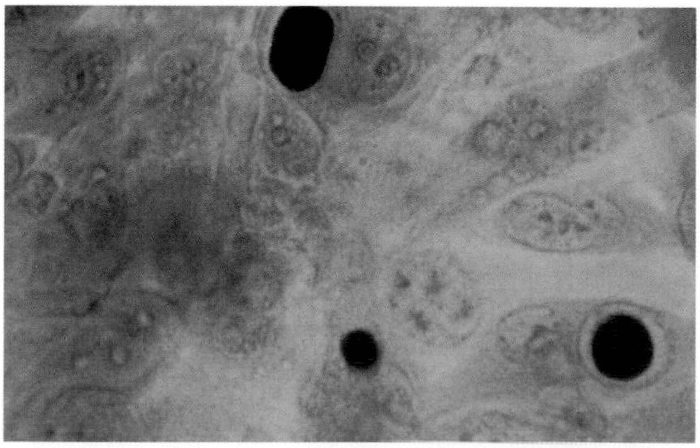

Fig. 21.16 Chlamydial inclusion bodies stained dark brown with iodine.

Fig. 21.17 Direct fluorescent antibody test for *Chlamydia trachomatis*. Elementary bodies can be seen as bright yellow-green dots under the ultraviolet microscope. (Courtesy of JD Treharne.)

that patients receiving treatment for gonorrhea also be treated with doxycycline for possible concurrent chlamydial infection *(Fig. 21.1)*. In addition, patients with clinically diagnosed chlamydial genital infections, their sexual contacts and babies born to infected mothers should be treated. Erythromycin should be used for babies.

Prevention depends upon recognizing the importance of asymptomatic infections. Early diagnosis and treatment of cases and of their sexual partners is important in order to avoid complications and reduce opportunities for transmission. Remember that STDs are not mutually exclusive, and patients may have concurrent infections with quite different pathogens.

OTHER CAUSES OF INGUINAL LYMPHADENOPATHY

Genital infections are common causes of inguinal lymphadenopathy (swelling of lymph nodes in the groin) among sexually active people. Syphilis and gonorrhea have been discussed above. Lymphogranuloma venereum (LGV), chancroid and donovanosis are more common in tropical and subtropical countries than in Europe and the USA but may be imported by travellers who have acquired the disease through sexual contact in these areas.

Lymphogranuloma venereum (LGV)

LGV is caused by C. trachomatis *serotypes L1, L2 and L3*

LGV is a serious disease especially common in Africa, Asia and South America. It occurs sporadically in Europe, Australia and North America, particularly among homosexual males. The prevalence appears to be higher among males than females, probably because symptomatic infection is more common in men.

LGV is a systemic infection involving lymphoid tissue and is treated with tetracycline or doxycycline

The clinical picture can be contrasted with the more restricted infection seen with *C. trachomatis* serotypes D–K (see above). The primary lesion is an ulcerating papule at the site of inoculation (after an incubation period of 1–4 weeks) and may be accompanied by fever, headache and myalgia. The lesion heals rapidly, but the chlamydiae proceed to infect the draining lymph nodes, causing characteristic inguinal buboes *(Fig. 21.18)*, which gradually enlarge. Chlamydiae may disseminate from the lymph nodes via the lymphatics to the tissues of the rectum to cause proctitis. Other systemic complications include fever, hepatitis, pneumonitis and meningo-encephalitis. The infection may resolve untreated, but:

- Abscesses may form in lymph nodes, which suppurate and discharge through the skin.
- Chronic granulomatous reactions in lymphatics and neighboring tissues can eventually give rise to fistula in ano or genital elephantiasis.

Cell culture methods are available (see above), but the chlamydial isolation rate is reported to be low (24–30%). Classically, the 'Frei' skin test was used in diagnosis. This involves intradermal injection of the LGV antigen, but it is unreliable, lacking sensitivity in early disease and lacking specificity because the Frei antigen is only genus specific. As discussed above, nucleic acid-based tests are also available. Treatment with tetracycline or doxycycline *(Fig. 21.1)* is recommended. Pregnant women and children under 9 years of age should be treated with erythromycin.

Chancroid (soft chancre)

Chancroid is caused by Haemophilus ducreyi *and is characterized by painful genital ulcers*

Infection by the Gram-negative bacterium *Haemophilus ducreyi* is manifest as painful non-indurated genital ulcers and local lymphadenitis *(Fig. 21.19)*. Note the difference between this and the chancre of primary syphilis, which is painless, but the ulcers may be confused with those of genital herpes, though they are usually larger and have a more ragged appearance. While the disease is endemic in some areas of the USA, cases generally tend to occur in distinct outbreaks. However, in Africa and Asia chancroid is the commonest cause of genital ulcers. Epidemiologic information is important because the diagnosis is usually clinical as the organism is difficult to grow

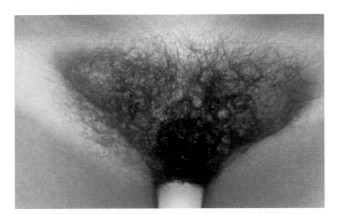

Fig. 21.18 Lymphogranuloma venereum. Bilateral enlargement of inguinal glands. (Courtesy of JS Bingham.)

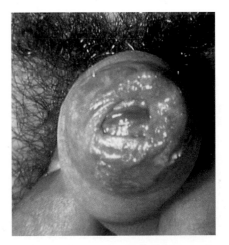

Fig. 21.19 Chancroid. Several irregular ulcers on the prepuce. (Courtesy of L Parish.)

in the laboratory. Chancroid may also be confused with donovanosis (see below).

Chancroid is diagnosed by microscopy and culture and treated with erythromycin, ceftriaxone or co-trimoxazole

Gram-stained smears of aspirates from the ulcer margin or enlarged lymph node characteristically show large numbers of short Gram-negative rods and chains, often described as having a 'school of fish' appearance, within or outside polymorphs. Aspirates should be cultured on a rich medium (GC agar with 1–2% hemoglobin, 5% fetal bovine serum, 10% CVA, and vancomycin [3 μg/ml]) at 33°C in 5–10% carbon dioxide. *H. ducreyi* will not tolerate higher temperatures. Growth is slow, and it may take 2–9 days for colonies to appear. Treatment with a macrolide (e.g. erythromycin or azithromycin) or ceftriaxone *(Fig. 21.1)* is generally recommended.

Donovanosis

Donovanosis is caused by Calymmatobacterium granulomatis *and is characterized by genital nodules and ulcers*

Donovanosis (granuloma inguinale or granuloma venereum) is rare in temperate climates, but common in tropical and subtropical regions such as the Caribbean, New Guinea, India and central Australia. The infection is characterized by nodules, almost always on the genitalia, which erode to form granulomatous ulcers that bleed readily on contact. The infection may extend and the ulcers may become secondarily infected. The pathogen is a Gram-negative rod, traditionally called *Calymmatobacterium granulomatis (Fig. 21.2)*. Genomic analysis has recently placed this organism into the genus *Klebsiella*, however most literature continues to use the *C. granulomatis* designation. The bacteria invade and multiply within mononuclear cells and are liberated when the cells rupture.

Donovanosis is diagnosed by microscopy and treated with tetracycline

The diagnosis of donovanosis is made by examining a smear from the lesion stained with Wright's or Giemsa stain. 'Donovan bodies' appear as clusters of blue- or black-stained organisms in the cytoplasm of mononuclear cells. Treatment with tetracyclines or co-trimoxazole is recommended *(Fig. 21.2)*.

MYCOPLASMAS AND NON-GONOCOCCAL URETHRITIS

Mycoplasma hominis, genitalium, *and* Ureaplasma urealyticum *may be causes of genital tract infection*

Although *Mycoplasma pneumoniae* has a proven role in the causation of pneumonia (see Chapter 19), the role of *M. hominis*, *M. genitalium*, and *Ureaplasma urealyticum* (which metabolizes urea; also called 'T strains') in STDs is less certain. These organisms frequently colonize the genital tracts of healthy sexually active men and women. They are less common in sexually inactive populations, which supports the view that they may be sexually transmitted. It is difficult to prove that they cause infection of the genital tract, but

M. genitalium may cause non-gonococcal urethritis, *M. hominis* may cause PID, postabortal and postpartum fevers, and pyelonephritis. *U. urealyticum* has also been associated with nongonococcal urethritis and prostatitis.

M. hominis, *M. genitalium*, and *U. urealyticum* are treated with either tetracyclines or erythromycin (some *Ureaplasmas* are tetracycline resistant) which is also the treatment for chlamydial infections.

OTHER CAUSES OF VAGINITIS AND URETHRITIS

Candida infection

Candida albicans *causes a range of genital tract diseases, which are treated with oral or topical antifungals*

These vary from mild superficial, localized infections in an otherwise healthy individual to disseminated often fatal infections in the immunocompromised. This yeast is a normal inhabitant of the female vagina, but in some women and in circumstances which are not clearly understood, the candidal load increases and causes an intensely irritant vaginitis with a cheesy vaginal discharge. This may be accompanied by urethritis and dysuria and may present as a urinary tract infection (see Chapter 20). The diagnosis can be confirmed by microscopy and culture of the discharge *(Fig. 21.20)*.

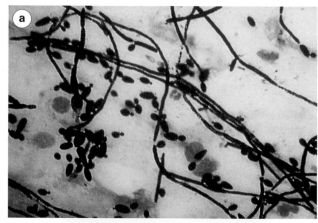

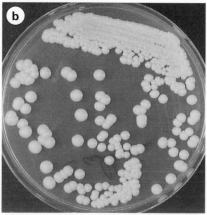

Fig. 21.20 *Candida albicans.* (a) Light microscopic appearance and (b) culture of vaginal discharge.

Treatment with an oral antifungal such as fluconazole or a topical preparation such as nystatin is recommended, but recurrence is frequent in a small proportion of women. Balanitis (inflammation of the glans penis) is seen in approximately 10% of male partners of females with vulvovaginal candidiasis, but urethritis is uncommon in men and is rarely symptomatic.

Trichomonas infection

Trichomonas vaginalis *is a protozoan parasite and causes vaginitis with copious discharge*

Trichomonas vaginalis inhabits:

- the vagina in women;
- the urethra (and sometimes the prostate) in men.

It is transmitted during sexual intercourse. In women, heavy infections cause vaginitis with a characteristic copious foul-smelling discharge. There is an associated increase in the vaginal pH. The infection should be distinguished from bacterial vaginosis (see below) by microscopic examination of the discharge, which shows actively motile trophozoites (*Fig. 21.21*).

Metronidazole is recommended for symptomatic T. vaginalis *infections*

In men, *Trichomonas vaginalis* is rarely symptomatic, but sometimes causes a mild urethritis; however, regular sexual partners of symptomatic women should be treated to prevent re-infection.

Bacterial vaginosis

Bacterial vaginosis is associated with Gardnerella vaginalis *plus anaerobic infection and a fishy-smelling vaginal discharge*

This non-specific vaginitis is a syndrome in women characterized by at least three of the following signs and symptoms:

- excessive malodorous vaginal discharge;
- vaginal pH greater than 4.5;
- presence of clue cells (vaginal epithelial cells coated with bacteria, *Fig. 21.22*).
- a fishy amine-like odor.

There is a significant increase in the numbers of *G. vaginalis* in the vaginal flora and a concomitant increase in the numbers of obligate anaerobes such as *Bacteroides* (*Fig. 21.2*).

G. vaginalis is consistently found in association with vaginosis, but is also found in 20–40% of healthy women. It is generally present in the urethra of male partners of women with vaginosis, indicating that it can be sexually transmitted. *G. vaginalis* has also been isolated from blood cultures from women with postpartum fever.

G. vaginalis has had a chequered taxonomic history, being first classified as a haemophilus, then as a corynebacterium, reflecting the fact that it tends to be Gram-variable (sometimes appearing Gram-negative, sometimes Gram-positive). It grows in the laboratory on human blood agar in a moist atmosphere enriched with carbon dioxide. The organism is

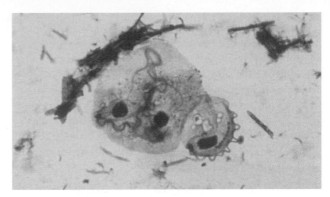

Fig. 21.21 Motile trophozoites in vaginal discharge in *T. vaginalis* infection. (Giemsa stain.) (Courtesy of R Muller.)

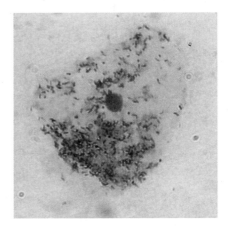

Fig. 21.22 Clue cells in bacterial vaginosis.

treated with oral metronidazole. Species of the genus *Mobiluncus* appear to be related to *G. vaginalis* and have also been implicated in vaginosis.

The pathogenesis of bacterial vaginosis is still unclear, but appears to be related to factors that disrupt the normal acidity of the vagina and the equilibrium between the different constituents of the normal vaginal flora. Whether any of these or other unknown factors are sexually transmissible is unclear.

GENITAL HERPES

Herpes simplex virus (HSV)-2 is the most common cause of genital herpes, but HSV-1 is being detected more frequently

HSV is a ubiquitous infection of humans worldwide. HSV-1 is generally transmitted via saliva causing primary oropharyngeal infection in children, and cold sores occur after virus reactivation. However, a separate virus strain, HSV-2, has emerged as a result of independent transmission by the venereal route. HSV-2 shows biologic and antigenic differences from the original HSV-1 strain, but special laboratory techniques are needed to distinguish them. There is little cross-immunity. Although originally recovered from separate sites, orogenital sexual practices have become prevalent enough to obscure the topographic difference between the strains, so that HSV-1 and HSV-2 can be recovered from oral and genital sites.

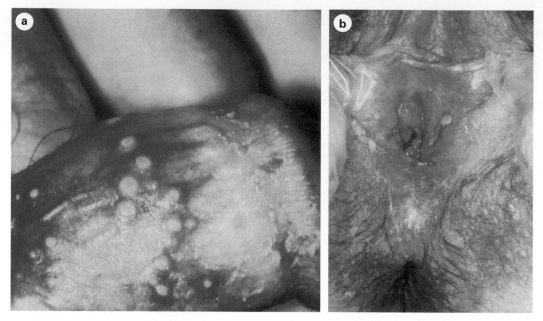

Fig. 21.23 Genital herpes. Vesicles (a) on the penis and (b) in the perianal area and vulva. Those on the labia minora and fourchette have ruptured to reveal characteristic herpetic erosions. (Courtesy of JS Bingham.)

Genital herpes is characterized by ulcerating vesicles that can take up to 2 weeks to heal

The primary genital lesion on the penis or vulva is seen 3–7 days after infection. It consists of vesicles that soon break down to form painful shallow ulcers *(Fig. 21.23)*. Local lymph nodes are swollen, and there may be constitutional symptoms including fever, headache and malaise. Occasionally the lesions are on the urethra, causing dysuria or pain on micturition. Healing takes up to 2 weeks, but the virus in the lesion travels up sensory nerve endings to establish latent infection in dorsal root ganglion neurones (see Chapter 24). From this site it can reactivate, travel down nerves to the same area, and cause recurrent lesions ('genital cold sores').

Aseptic meningitis or encephalitis occurs in adults as a rare complication, and spread of infection from mother to infant at the time of delivery can give rise to neonatal disseminated herpes or encephalitis.

Genital herpes is generally diagnosed from the clinical appearance, and aciclovir can be used for treatment

HSV can be isolated from vesicle fluid or ulcer swabs and the isolate typed by immunofluorescence using type-specific monoclonal antibodies. Recurrent genital infection is more frequent with HSV-2, therefore typing is of help in determining the prognosis. The cytopathic effect is characteristic and is generally seen within 1–2 days post-inoculation, with ballooning degenerating cells and multinucleate giant cells. HSV DNA detection methods which include type differentiation may be used which have a much greater sensitivity than virus isolation. A number of antivirals, including oral aciclovir, valaciclovir and famciclovir can be used for treatment of severe or early lesions, and aciclovir may need to

be given intravenously if there are systemic complications. Recurrent attacks are troublesome, and treatment options include starting an antiviral when prodromal symptoms occur or alternatively taking 6–12 months low-dose aciclovir or one of the alternative agents to stop or at least reduce the frequency of recurrences.

HUMAN PAPILLOMAVIRUS INFECTION

There are over 70 distinct types of human papillomaviruses, all infecting skin or mucosal surfaces, and the DNA of each showing less than 50% cross-hybridization with that of others. These are evidently ancient viral associates of man that have evolved extensively, and many of the different types are adapted to specific regions of the body.

Many papillomavirus types are transmitted sexually and cause genital warts

Warts (condylomata acuminata) appear on the penis, vulva and perianal regions *(Fig. 21.24)* after an incubation period of 1–6 months (see Chapter 26). They may not regress for many months and can be treated with podophyllin. The lesion on the cervix is a flat area of dysplasia visible by colposcopy as a white plaque *(Fig. 21.25)* after the local application of 5% acetic acid. Because of their association with cervical cancer, especially types 16 and 18, cervical lesions are best removed by laser or loop excision.

HUMAN IMMUNODEFICIENCY VIRUS

HIV is a retrovirus *(Fig. 21.26)*, so-called because this single-stranded RNA virus contains a *pol* gene that codes for a reverse transcriptase (Latin: *retro*, backwards).

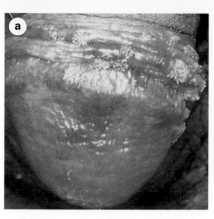 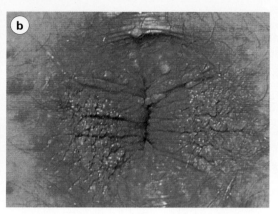 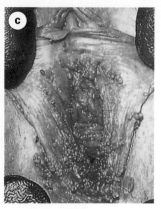

Fig. 21.24 Genital warts. (a) Warts on the penis are usually multiple, and on the shaft are often flat and keratinized. (b) Warts in the perianal area often extend into the anal canal. (c) Warts in the vulvoperineal area can enlarge dramatically and extend into the vagina. (Courtesy of JS Bingham.)

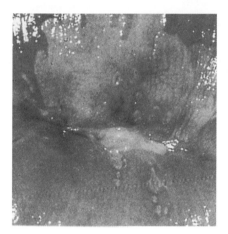

Fig. 21.25 Cervical dysplasia caused by papillomavirus should be removed by laser. (Courtesy of A Goodman.)

AIDS was first recognized in 1981 in the USA

In 1981, the Communicable Disease Center, Atlanta, USA noted an increase in requests to use pentamidine for *Pneumocystis carinii* (now classified as *P. jiroveci*) infection in previously well individuals who also suffered severe infections by other normally harmless microorganisms. These included *C. albicans* esophagitis, mucocutaneous HSV, toxoplasma CNS infection or pneumonia, and cryptosporidial enteritis; Kaposi's sarcoma was also often present. Patients had evidence of impaired immune function, as shown by skin test anergies, and depletion of CD4-positive T helper (TH) lymphocytes. This immunodeficiency syndrome appearing in an individual without a known cause such as treatment with immunosuppressive drugs was referred to as 'acquired immune deficiency syndrome' (AIDS). An internationally agreed definition of AIDS soon followed. Epidemics subsequently occurred in San Francisco, New York and other cities in the USA, and in the UK and Europe a few years later.

HIV, the causative virus of AIDS, was isolated from blood lymphocytes in 1983

It was recognized as belonging to the lentivirus (slow virus) group of retroviruses and related to similar agents in monkeys

HUMAN RETROVIRUSES	
virus	**comment**
HTLV1	endemic in West Indies and SW Japan; transmission via blood, human milk; can cause adult T cell leukemia, and HTLV1-associated myelopathy, also known as tropical spastic paraparesis
HTLV2	uncommon, sporadic occurrence; transmission via blood; can cause hairy T cell leukemia and neurological disease
HIV-1, HIV-2	transmission via blood, sexual intercourse; responsible for AIDS, HIV-2 West African in origin, closely related to HIV-1 but antigenically distinct
human foamy virus	causes foamy vacuolation in infected cells; little is known of its occurrence or pathogenic potential
human placental virus(es)	detected in placental tissue by electron microscopy and by presence of reverse transcriptase
human genome viruses	nucleic acid sequences representing endogenous retroviruses are common in the vertebrate genome, often in well-defined genetic loci; acquired during evolutionary history; not expressed as infectious virus; function unknown; perhaps should be regarded as mere parasitic DNA

Fig. 21.26 Human retroviruses. Human T cell lymphotropic virus (HTLV)1, HTLV2, HIV-1 and HIV-2 have been cultivated in human T cells in vitro. The human placental and genome viruses are not known as infectious agents. Retroviruses are also common in cats (FAIDS), monkeys (MAIDS), mice (mouse leukemia), and other vertebrates. (ARC, AIDS-related complex.)

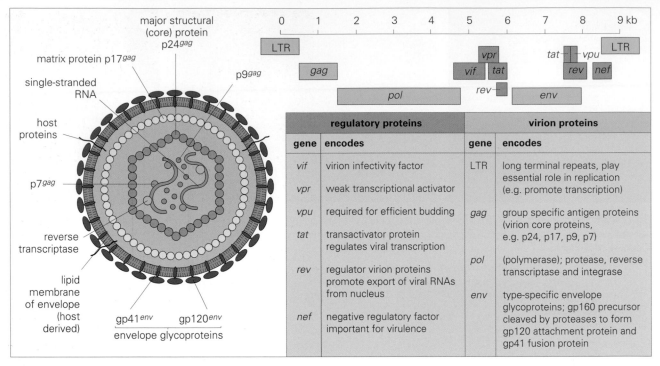

Fig. 21.27 The structure and genetic map of HIV. The *rev* and *tat* genes are divided into non-contiguous pieces and the gene segments spliced together in the RNA transcript. Occasional host proteins such as major histocompatibility complex (MHC) molecules are present in the envelope. (p) is protein and (gp) is glycoprotein. About 10^9 HIV-1 particles are produced each day at the peak of infection, and this, together with the low fidelity of reverse transcriptase, means that new virus variants are always appearing. Mutations are seen especially in *env* and *nef* genes. Any one patient contains many variants, and drug resistant and immune resistant mutants emerge. There are also macrophage-tropic and T cell-tropic populations of virus and syncytium-inducing and non-syncytium-inducing populations, with effects on disease progression. By genetic analysis HIV-1 strains are subdivided into group M (most HIV-1 isolates), which contains at least 10 subtypes (A–J) differing in geographic distribution, and groups N and O (African). The degree of cross-immunity between these strains is not clear.

and to visnavirus in sheep and goats. The structure of the viral particle and its genome are illustrated in *Figure 21.27* and its replication mechanism in *Figures 21.28* and *21.29*.

Virus replication is regulated by at least six genes. The replication cycle is often halted after integration of the provirus so that the infection remains latent in the cell. The *tat* and *rev* genes function as transactivating factors, and can increase production of viral RNAs and proteins when latently infected cells are:

- stimulated to differentiate (e.g. TH cells by antigen);
- stimulated by infection with certain other viruses such as HSV or cytomegalovirus (CMV).

HIV infection probably started in Africa in the 1950s, and 42 million people worldwide were infected by 2002

The molecular biologic evidence (in terms of nucleic acid sequence) indicates that both HIV-1 and the closely related HIV-2 seen in West Africa probably arose from closely related primate viruses. HIV-1 is separated into three groups, namely M (main), N (new) and O (outlier). The M group comprises the HIV-1 subtypes A to J, with the N and O groups focused in western central Africa. The geographical prevalence of the subtypes differs, with subtype B being most common in North America and Europe, and the non-B strains such as A and C being found more frequently in Africa. However, with increasing travel the subtype distribution is changing and,

together with the potential for mixed or superinfections, i.e. an HIV infected individual becoming infected with another strain, and viral recombination events, other subtypes are being seen such as the circulating recombinant forms (CRF). These may be important in having different rates of disease progression.

HIV-1 may have been present in humans in central Africa for many years, but in the late 1970s it began to spread rapidly *(Fig. 21.30)*, possibly with changed biologic properties as a result of increased transmission following major socio-economic upheavals and migrations of people from central to east Africa. Female prostitutes and male soldiers and workers travelling around the country played a major part. The disease soon appeared in Haiti and the USA, followed by Europe and Australasia.

In the late 1980s, HIV began to appear in Asian countries, beginning with Thailand, and by 1995 explosive spread was based on heterosexual transmission, with high infection rates in female sex workers and transmission among users of injected drugs in Asia.

Worldwide by the end of 2002 about 42 million adults and children will have been infected with HIV including:

- 29.4 million in sub-Saharan Africa;
- 7.2 million in Asia and the Pacific;
- 1.2 million in eastern Europe and Central Asia;
- 1 million in North America;
- 0.65 million in western Europe.

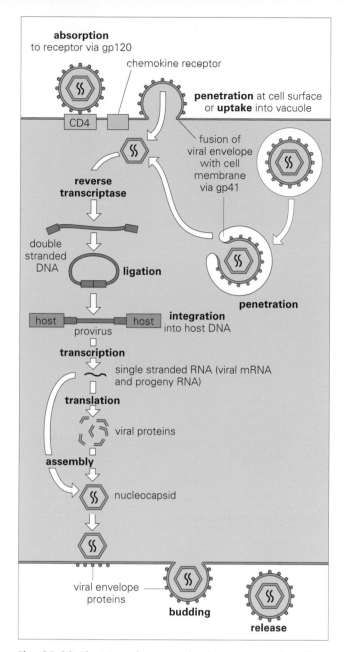

Fig. 21.28 The HIV replication cycle. The virus enters the cell either by fusion with the cell membrane at the cell surface or via uptake into a vacuole and release within the cell.

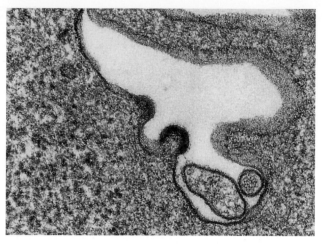

Fig. 21.29 Electron micrograph showing HIV budding from the cell surface before release. (Courtesy of D Hockley.)

molecule acts as a high affinity binding site for the viral gp120 envelope glycoprotein. Productive replication and cell destruction does not occur until the Tн cell is activated. Tн cell activation is greatly enhanced not only in attempts to respond to HIV antigens, but also as a result of the secondary microbial infections seen in patients. Monocytes and macrophages, Langerhans' cells and follicular dendritic cells also express the CD4 molecule and are infected, but are not generally destroyed, potentially acting as a reservoir for infection. Langerhans' cells, for example dendritic cells in the skin and genital mucosa, may be the first cells infected. Later in the disease there is a remarkable disruption of histologic pattern in lymphoid follicles as a result of the breakdown of follicular dendritic cells.

HIV-1 enters host cells by binding the viral gp120 to the CD4 receptor and a chemokine coreceptor on the host cell surface. The CCR5 beta-chemokine receptor is important in establishing the infection. Those people with CCR5 gene deletions are resistant to infection. On the other hand, disease progression has been associated with HIV variants using the CXCR4 alpha-chemokine receptor. Cell susceptibility to infection is therefore affected by the levels of these chemokine coreceptors; for example, their expression may be upregulated by opportunistic infections.

Five million people were newly infected in 2002, and 3.1 million died as a result of HIV infection that year. During this time the epidemic grew and was expected to continue at a high rate in China and India, with an estimated 1 million and 4 million infected individuals, respectively. It has been estimated that between 2002 and 2010 an additional 45 million people will become infected in 126 low and middle income countries; more than 40% will be from Asia and the Pacific regions.

HIV mainly infects cells bearing the CD4 cell surface antigen and also requires chemokine coreceptors

CD4-receptor-bearing cells include Tн cells, monocytes, dendritic cells and microglia (*Figs 21.31, 21.32*). The CD4

At first the immune system fights back against HIV infection, but then begins to fail

During the first few months virus-specific CD8-positive T cells are formed and reduce the viremia which is referred to as the HIV load. This is followed by the appearance of neutralizing antibodies. Even so, up to 10^{10} infectious virus particles and up to 10^{9} infected lymphocytes are produced daily. Then the immune system begins to suffer gradual damage, and the number of circulating CD4-positive T cells steadily falls and the HIV load rises. Nearly all infected CD4-positive T cells are in lymph nodes. The cell-mediated immune responses to viral antigens, as judged by lymphoproliferation, weaken, whereas responses to other antigens are normal. Perhaps the virus initially engineers a specific suppression of protective responses to itself. Eventually the patient loses the battle to replace lost T cells, and the number falls more rapidly. Skin

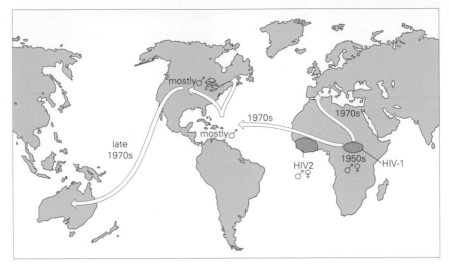

Fig. 21.30 Early spread of HIV infection (now worldwide). HIV-1 may have been present in central Africa for many years before increased migration and socioeconomic upheaval caused it to begin spreading in the late 1970s. Outside Africa, most infections occurred in men.

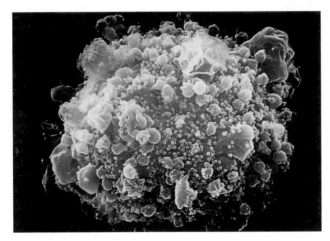

Fig. 21.31 Scanning electron micrograph of an HIV-infected TH cell. ×20 000. (Courtesy of D Hockley.)

test delayed type hypersensitivity (DTH) responses are absent, natural killer (NK) cell and cytotoxic T (Tc) cell activity is reduced, and there are various other immunologic abnormalities, including polyclonal activation of B cells. Functional changes in T lymphocytes—reduced responses to mitogens, reduced interleukin 2 (IL-2) and interferon-gamma (IFNγ) production—are also seen. As AIDS develops, responses to HIV and unrelated antigens are further depressed. The immune system has lost control. Plasma HIV-1 RNA load measurements have been shown to predict clinical outcome and are used in clinical management to help determine disease stage and progression as well as antiretroviral therapy response.

The exact mechanism of the immunosuppression in HIV infection is still unclear

The following factors need to be considered:

- TH cells directly killed by virus;
- TH cells induced to commit suicide (apoptosis, programmed cell death) by virus;

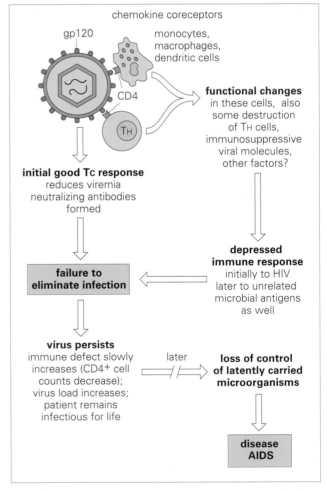

Fig. 21.32 The pathogenesis of AIDS. Although CD4 is the first receptor, there is secondary binding of the virus to chemokine receptors (not shown) on host cells, and this increases the efficiency of infection. Genetic defects in chemokine receptors may account for the failure of certain sex workers in Africa to become infected despite repeated exposure to HIV. (Tc, cytotoxic T cell; TH, T helper lymphocyte.)

- TH cells made vulnerable to immune attack by Tc cells;
- T cell replenishment impaired by damage to the thymus and lymph nodes and by infection of stem cells;
- defects in antigen presentation associated with infection of dendritic cells;
- immunosuppressive virus-coded molecules (gp120, gp41).

The host response is further handicapped by the high rate of viral evolution assisted by the lack of a reverse transcriptase proofreading function. The virus exists as a quasispecies, in other words the infection comprises a number of hetero-geneous strains. Some of the variants show resistance to currently circulating Tcs (i.e. are immune escape variants). Others show increased pathogenicity.

Before the advent of highly active antiretroviral therapy the immunosuppression was permanent, the patient remained infectious, the virus persisted in the body and death was due to opportunist infections and tumors.

HIV-2 appears to be transmitted less easily than HIV-1, probably because the viral load is lower, and the progression to AIDS is slower. HIV-2 is endemic in west Africa, and has spread to Portugal and parts of India.

Routes of transmission

In developed countries, homosexual men have so far been the group most vulnerable to HIV infection and AIDS, especially the passive partner in anal intercourse. Infection is transmitted primarily from male to male and from male to female *(Fig. 21.33)*, although not very efficiently compared with other STDs. Transmission from female to male, however, is a common and well-established feature of HIV in Africa and Asia. In randomly selected rural communities in parts of central and east Africa, up to 40% of the population is infected with HIV, mostly young adults.

Heterosexual transmission has not so far been as important in resource rich as in resource poor countries

One explanation for the greater heterosexual spread in developing countries is that other STIs are more common, causing ulcers and discharges, which are sources of infected lymphocytes and monocytes. Genital ulcers are associated with a four-fold increase in the risk of infection. Also, viral strains from Asia and sub-Saharan Africa have been shown to infect Langerhans' cells in genital mucosa more easily than do other strains. It is not clear whether HIV can infect males by the urethra or whether pre-existing genital skin breaks are necessary. As with other STDs, uncircumcised males are more likely to be infected.

HIV can also be transmitted vertically from infected mother to offspring, but the infant is not infected in 55–85% of pregnancies, the upper limit being associated with avoiding breastfeeding. Overall, the infant is infected in about 20% of pregnancies in utero and intrapartum. The transmission rate peri- and postnatally is around 11–16%, the higher end of the range depends on whether the child has been breastfed for up to 24 months. In resource rich countries, antenatal HIV screening, offering antiretroviral drugs during pregnancy and cesarean section delivery, avoiding breastfeeding, and giving antiretroviral drugs to the newborn infant have reduced the risk of HIV transmission to the child. In resource poor countries it has been shown that giving one dose of one antiretroviral drug to both mother and child reduced HIV transmission by 47%.

By the end of 2002, there were 3.2 million children under 15 years of age living with HIV or AIDS, 800 000 of whom were newly infected that year.

As infection in Africa does not generally occur until after the onset of sexual maturity, it is probable that arthropod transmission does not occur.

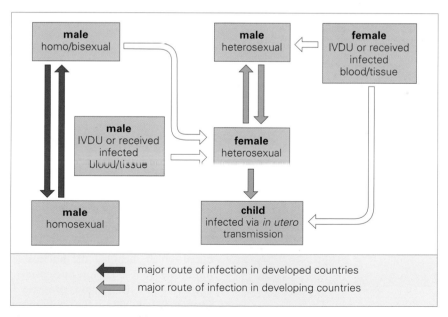

Fig. 21.33 Major routes of transmission of HIV. Although the heterosexual route of transmission has so far been well established only in developing countries, there is evidence that this route is becoming more important in the developed countries. (IVDU, intravenous drug user.)

Hemophiliacs who have received contaminated blood products have also been infected, though less commonly, as well as injecting drug users. As with other bloodborne virus infections, using contaminated needles can lead to infection, i.e. in tattooing, body piercing and acupuncture.

Finally, healthcare workers are at risk of HIV infection after sustaining needlestick or mucous membrane splash injuries involving an HIV-infected source. The risk of infection is approximately 1 in 400 and is dependent on a number of factors, including depth of the injury and amount of blood to which the recipient has been exposed. Wearing protective clothing such as gloves and goggles is part of universal precautions to avoid exposure.

Development of disease

Primary HIV infection may be accompanied by a mild mononucleosis-type illness

Signs and symptoms of the mild mononucleosis-type illness associated with HIV infection include fever, malaise and lymphadenopathy (Fig. 21.34). A maculopapular rash may

also occur. Antibody responses can be detected in a few weeks, and Tc cells are formed. The acute infection and rapid, widespread viral dissemination is followed by a chronic asymptomatic stage. Viral replication is reduced in line with the immune response, and the individual usually remains well. The duration of this stage is dependent on a number of factors including the viral phenotype, host immune response and use of antiretroviral therapy. Infected cells are, however, still present, and at a later stage the infected individual may develop weight loss, fever, persistent lymphadenopathy, oral candidiasis and diarrhea. Further viral replication takes place until finally, some years after initial infection, full-blown AIDS develops (Fig. 21.34).

Progression to AIDS

Viral invasion of the CNS, with self-limiting aseptic meningoencephalitis as the most common neurological picture, occurs in early infection.

A progressive HIV-associated encephalopathy is seen in individuals with AIDS and is characterized by multiple small nodules of inflammatory cells; most of the infected cells appear to be microglia or infiltrating macrophages. These cells express the CD4 antigen, and it has been suggested that infected monocytes carry the virus into the brain, but the picture is complicated by the various persistent infections that are activated and give rise to their own CNS pathology. These include infections by HSV, varicella-zoster virus (VZV), *Toxoplasma gondii*, JC virus (progressive multifocal leukoencephalopathy, PML) and *Cryptococcus neoformans*.

HIV exercises complex control over its own replication (Fig. 21.28). Replication is also affected by responses to other infections, which act as antigenic stimuli, and some of them directly as transactivating agents.

Some patients, especially in Africa, develop a wasting disease ('slim' disease), possibly due to unknown intestinal infections or infestations, and perhaps also to the direct effects of the virus infecting cells of the intestinal wall.

AIDS, symptomatic disease, consists of a large spectrum of microbial diseases acquired or reactivated as a result of the underlying immunosuppression due to HIV (Figs 21.35 and 21.36). The disease picture of AIDS is therefore an indirect result of infection with HIV.

Before the advent of antiretroviral therapy, one study in New York reported a mortality rate of 80% 5 years after the onset of the disease, and the average survival time after hospital admission was 242 days.

Treatment

Antiretroviral therapy results in a dramatic improvement in disease prognosis

In the 1990s, a range of antiretroviral therapies was introduced which included the nucleoside reverse transcriptase inhibitors (NRTIs), non-nucleoside reverse transcriptase inhibitors (NNRTIs) and protease inhibitors (PIs) (see Chapter 33). In 2003, a fusion inhibitor was added to the list. A study of monotherapy with AZT, an NRTI, was terminated prematurely after showing a significant clinical benefit in symptomatic individuals. The Concorde study revealed that monotherapy gave no benefit in treating asymptomatic

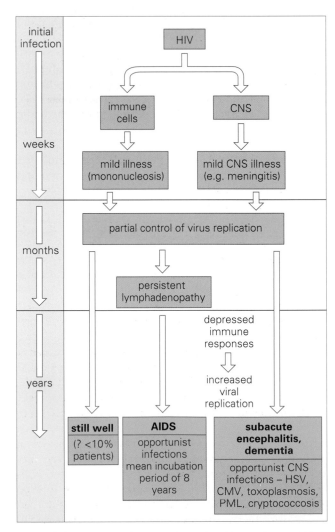

Fig. 21.34 The clinical features and progression of untreated HIV infection. (CMV, cytomegalovirus; CNS, central nervous system; HSV, herpes simplex virus; PML, progressive multifocal leukoencephalopathy.)

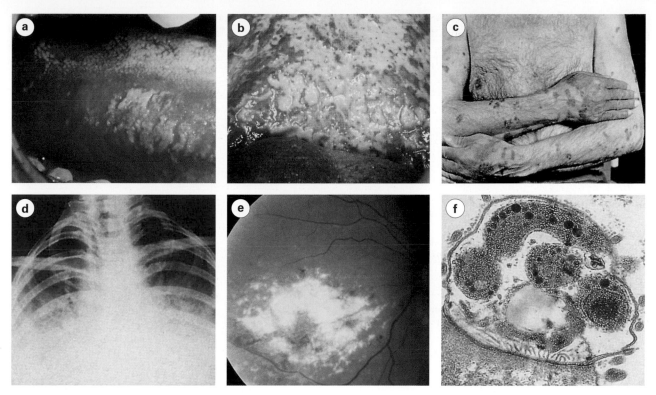

Fig. 21.35 Opportunist infections and tumors associated with HIV infection. (a) Hairy leukoplakia—raised white lesions of oral mucosa, predominently along the lateral aspect of the tongue, due to Epstein–Barr virus infection. (Courtesy of HP Holley.) (b) Extensive oral candidiasis. (Courtesy of WE Farrar.) (c) Kaposi's sarcoma—brown pigmented lesions on the upper extremities. (Courtesy of E Sahn.) (d) *Pneumocystis* pneumonia, with extensive infiltrates in both lungs. (Courtesy of JA Innes.) (e) Cytomegalovirus retinitis showing scattered exudates and hemorrhages, with sheathing of vessels. (Courtesy of CJ Ellis.) (f) Cryptosporidiosis—electron micrograph showing mature schizont with several merozoites attached to intestinal epithelium. (Courtesy of WE Farrar.)

individuals, but the Delta study, reported in 1996, demonstrated considerable advantages in treatment with two NRTIs. Subsequently, the NNRTI and PI classes of drugs were introduced, the latter having a different site of action. In combination with two NRTIs, the NNRTI or PI drugs have had a dramatic effect on progression to AIDS and led to the term highly active antiretroviral therapy (HAART). One drawback has been a number of important side effects of the drugs, including mitochondrial toxicity and altered fat distribution known as lipodystrophy. Treatment compliance with certain drugs is a problem because of the side effects and the number and frequency of pills taken each day. This is important, as missing any doses can lead to the development of drug resistance, thus limiting treatment options. Improved monitoring using plasma HIV load measurements and CD4 counts and percentages has shown the success of HAART, with rapid falls in plasma HIV load and rises in CD4 cells seen after initiating therapy. HIV is found in various compartments of the body including the CSF and genital tract. Antiretroviral drugs may not penetrate these sites, resulting in a high viral load detectable in semen despite suppression of the plasma HIV load. As a result, the incidence of AIDS and AIDS-related death in the UK has fallen by more than 40% since 1996.

Nucleoside reverse transcriptase inhibitor and fusion inhibitor classes of drugs are in use, and other antiretroviral drugs are being developed. In addition, other HIV targets are under investigation, as are immunotherapeutic approaches.

Development of antiretroviral resistance and cross-resistance is a feature

Plasma HIV-1 RNA load is a good indicator of viral replication, and failure of antiretroviral therapy is seen by a rise in viral load. It is estimated that up to 50% of those receiving HAART will fail annually. Antiretroviral resistance testing and therapeutic drug monitoring are part of clinical management. Drug resistance testing may be carried out when the plasma HIV-1 load is not suppressed whilst on antiretroviral therapy. Specific mutations in the reverse transcriptase and protease regions of plasma virus, associated with reduced susceptibility to one or more antiretroviral drugs, have been identified by nucleic acid sequencing, known as genotypic analysis. More than 15 drugs are licensed for HIV treatment, and some drug resistance mutations confer resistance to more than one drug of the same class, whereas others appear unique to specific drugs. There is also increasing evidence of transmission of drug-resistant HIV. The prevalence of drug-resistant viruses in newly infected individuals ranges from 5% to 20%, depending on factors such as whether the individual was infected by someone failing on antiretroviral therapy, this being less likely in those infected in resource poor regions. It may be useful to carry out baseline resistance testing in specific situations before starting treatment, as infection with a drug-resistant virus may affect the efficacy of subsequent therapy.

OPPORTUNIST INFECTIONS AND TUMORS IN AIDS	
viruses	disseminated CMV (including retina, brain, peripheral nervous system, gastrointestinal tract) HSV (lungs, gastrointestinal tract, CNS, skin) JC virus (brain – PML) EBV (hairy leukoplakia, primary cerebral lymphoma)
bacteria*	mycobacteria (e.g. *Mycoplasma avium*, *M. tuberculosis* – disseminated, extrapulmonary) *Salmonella* (recurrent, disseminated) septicemia
protozoa	*Toxoplasma gondii* (disseminated, including CNS) *Cryptosporidium* (chronic diarrhea) *Isospora* (with diarrhea, persisting more than one month)
fungi	*Pneumocystis jiroveci* (pneumonia) *Candida albicans* (esophagitis, lung infection) *Cryptococcus neoformans* (CNS) histoplasmosis (disseminated, extrapulmonary) *Coccidioides* (disseminated, extrapulmonary)
tumors	Kaposi's sarcoma** B cell lymphoma (e.g. in brain, some are EBV induced)
other	wasting disease (cause unknown) HIV encephalopathy

*also pyogenic bacteria (e.g. *Haemophilus*, *Streptococcus*, *Pneumococcus*) causing septicemia, pneumonia, meningitis, osteomyelitis, arthritis, abscesses etc.; multiple or recurrent infections, especially in children

**associated with HHV8, an independently-transmitted agent; 300-times as frequent in AIDS as in other immunodeficiencies

Fig. 21.36 Opportunist infections and tumors in AIDS. AIDS is defined as the presence of antibodies to HIV plus one of the conditions in this table. (CMV, cytomegalovirus; CNS, central nervous system; EBV, Epstein–Barr virus; HSV, herpes simplex virus; PML, progressive multifocal leukoencephalopathy.)

Treatment of AIDS involves prophylaxis and treatment of opportunist infections as well as using antiretrovirals

Depending on the CD4 count, prophylaxis is given for specific opportunistic infections such as *Pneumocystis jiroveci* and *Cryptococcus neoformans*. When opportunist infections are diagnosed, they are treated appropriately, for example co-trimoxazole or pentamidine with or without steroids for *P. jiroveci*, ganciclovir for CMV, and fluconazole or amphotericin for *C. neoformans* infection.

Laboratory tests

Laboratory tests for HIV infection involve both serological and molecular analysis

AIDS is a clinical definition; in the presence of antibodies to HIV, any of the conditions listed in *Figure 21.36*, regardless of the presence of other causes of immunodeficiency, indicate AIDS. The range and complexity of tests used for HIV-1 and -2 antibody screening, diagnosis of infection, and monitoring disease progression and response to therapy have increased dramatically.

Viral replication occurs during the incubation period, during which time the viral genome and, briefly, viral p24 antigen but not the host's antibody response, may be detected. HIV-1 and -2 diagnostic tests can be divided into antibody detection, combined antibody and antigen detection, antigen detection, and genome detection. The last can be divided into qualitative HIV-1 proviral DNA and quantitative HIV-1 RNA detection. In addition, antiretroviral drug resistance assays are becoming part of standard management.

Initially, an HIV-1 and -2 antibody or combination assay which includes antibody and p24 antigen is carried out (see Chapter 32). The latter have been developed to reduce the diagnostic window period. Assay reactivity is confirmed using an alternative HIV test format on the original unseparated sample stored in the laboratory. This is to ensure that a specimen separation error has not occurred. HIV type differentiation may be carried out using an immunoblot, where the antigens are coated on nitrocellulose strips. A positive result is confirmed on a further blood sample, to ensure that the original sample had not been mislabeled at collection.

If it is difficult to make a diagnosis because the sample is reactive in the tests but gives an indeterminate result, or the patient may have a seroconversion illness and the screening tests are negative, HIV-1 RNA or proviral DNA tests may be carried out on plasma and whole blood samples, respectively.

Part of monitoring HIV-1-infected individuals on or off antiretroviral therapy involves measuring the plasma HIV-1 RNA load, which can be quantified using several commercial assays using different methods. The main assay formats are based on reverse transcription polymerase chain reaction (RT-PCR), branched DNA signal amplification, and RNA transcription isothermal amplification.

In addition, part of the laboratory portfolio involves antiretroviral resistance genotypic analysis by automated DNA sequencing. This is a specialized test which is costly, and the interpretation of the results may be complicated.

Diagnosis of HIV infection in newborn infants is a problem. If IgG antibodies are present they are presumably of maternal origin, but commercial tests for virus-specific IgM and IgA antibodies, which would signify in-utero infection (see Chapter 23), are not yet available. Reference laboratories may have these in-house tests as part of their test portfolio. Samples from infants are tested at various time intervals up to 12–24 months for p24 antigen, HIV-1 RNA and/or HIV-1 proviral DNA, and HIV antibody to assess their HIV status.

Measures to control spread

Many developed countries have taken measures to reduce the spread of HIV

In developed countries, unlike in Africa and Asia, most cases so far have been in male homosexuals (*Fig. 21.37*), though the picture is changing. Blood donor HIV screening programs, in addition to other bloodborne viruses, are carried out, and those at risk of infection are discouraged from volunteering. Heat treatment of Factor VIII is carried out as a further precaution before this product is used to treat hemophiliac patients. HIV has a delicate outer envelope and is highly susceptible to heat and chemical agents. HIV is inactivated under pasteurization conditions and also by hypochlorites, even at concentrations as low as 1 in 10 000 ppm; 2.5% glutaraldehyde and ethyl alcohol are also effective against the virus.

The main effort in the prevention of HIV infection concerns mass public education programs. These involve inducements to change sexual behavior, particularly a reduction in promiscuous behavior, and the use of barrier contraceptives such as condoms. In resource rich countries the initial signs that male homosexuals were controlling the spread of STDs by altering sexual behavior seem to have reversed. The problem of transmission between injecting drug users is being tackled in some areas by measures that were originally controversial, such as the free distribution of clean needles and syringes.

The importance of reducing transmission rates is discussed in Chapter 31. The biggest risk for the future in developed countries is that heterosexual transmission becomes more common, following the African and Asian pattern. Unfortunately, the determinants of heterosexual transmission are not understood, but the means for prevention are nevertheless clear—condoms and decreased promiscuity. So far it has proved difficult to induce changes in sexual behavior of heterosexuals by means of public health educational programs via the media. If these changes in heterosexual behavior can take place, a dramatic reduction in the incidence of all STDs would be assured.

Vaccination

The prospects for a successful vaccine against HIV infection are limited, but there is hope

The prospects are limited partly because of viral antigenic variation as well as the slow neutralizing antibody response to HIV infection. Intensive work is in progress, and various subunit envelope glycoproteins, whole virus vaccines, and virus vectors to carry HIV antigens are being developed and tested. Trials are being carried out in animal (monkey) models and also preliminary trials in humans. Good virus-specific responses are probably needed. The danger of inducing antibodies that enhance infectivity has been noted. Enhancing antibodies are known to be important in the hemorrhagic shock syndrome caused by dengue virus. They combine with the virus without neutralizing it, and the complex then attaches to the Fc receptor present on monocytes, which ingest the complex and thus become infected. In other words, the antibody not only fails to protect, but is responsible for carrying the virus into the susceptible cell! The fact that there is a successful killed virus vaccine for a feline retrovirus (feline leukemia), and that a similar vaccine protects monkeys from simian AIDS does, however, give some hope for the development of an HIV vaccine.

To prevent sexual transmission, mucosal immunity is needed, and this is likely to come from a mucosally administered vaccine. Peptide vaccines at present seem less likely because of the general problem of immunogenicity (e.g. carrier proteins, adjuvants, see Chapter 34) and because numerous T cell epitopes would have to be included in view of the extensive class II major histocompatibility complex (MHC) antigen variations in human populations.

OPPORTUNIST STDs

Opportunist STDs include salmonellae, shigellae, hepatitis A, Giardia lamblia *and* Entamoeba histolytica *infections*

Although STDs are classically transmitted during heterosexual intercourse they can also be transmitted whenever two mucosal surfaces are brought together. Anal intercourse allows the transfer of microorganisms from penis to rectal mucosa or to anal and perianal regions. Gonococcal or papillomavirus lesions, for instance, may occur in any of these sites. A few microorganisms (hepatitis B, HIV) are transmitted more often across rectal mucosa. If there is oral–anal contact, a variety of intestinal pathogens are given the opportunity to spread as STDs and can then be regarded as 'opportunistic STDs'. These include salmonellae, shigellae, hepatitis A virus, *Giardia lamblia* and *Entamoeba histolytica* (see Chapter 22). They are less common nowadays, but *Entamoeba histolytica* was the major pathogen in the so-called 'gay bowel syndrome'. Together with chronic infections such as CMV and cryptosporidiosis, they contribute to intestinal symptoms and diarrhea in AIDS patients.

Infection route	Inner London				Outer London				Rest of England				Total by exposure*
	1989 or earlier	1990–94	1995–99	2000–02	1989 or earlier	1990–94	1995–99	2000–02	1989 or earlier	1990–94	1995–99	2000–02	
Sex between men	1968	3320	1719	221	50	195	163	34	650	1521	1060	283	11186
Sex between men and women	96	596	866	348	17	181	254	161	66	373	510	396	3864
Injecting drug use	46	202	133	20	1	10	15	3	29	137	130	22	748
IDU & sex between men	52	95	59	5	0	6	3	0	10	30	27	8	295
Blood factor	68	64	17	4	0	0	0	1	157	222	64	3	600
Blood/tissue transfer	16	20	16	3	2	4	2	0	21	26	18	6	141
Mother to infant	1	28	15	0	2	33	34	7	10	26	37	36	426
Other	1	5	4	0	1	0	1	0	1	5	5	0	23
Undetermined	10	22	14	10	3	6	5	2	12	31	29	22	171
Total	2258	4352	2843	611	76	435	477	208	956	2371	1880	776	17454

Fig. 21.37 Total numbers of AIDS cases reported in England by period of AIDS diagnosis, up to end of September 2002. More than twice as many people are infected (HIV-seropositive) and infectious. *Includes 211 cases where local authority of AIDS report is not recorded. (IDU, intravenous drug use.) (Data courtesy of PHLS Communicable Disease Surveillance Centre, London.)

Hepatitis B virus is often transmitted sexually

The virus and its surface antigen, HBsAg, are detectable in semen, saliva and vaginal secretions. Titers in blood are higher and, like HIV, transmission is more likely when genital areas are ulcerated or contaminated with blood (e.g. menstrual blood). Hepatitis B transmission among male homosexuals parallels the transmission of HIV, with passive anal intercourse as a high risk factor. Hepatitis D transmission is similar to that of hepatitis B. Hepatitis C is less commonly transmitted sexually; less than 5% of long-term sexual partners are infected.

ARTHROPOD INFESTATIONS

Infection with the pubic or crab louse causes itching and is treated with permethrin cream

The 'crab louse', *Phthirus pubis*, is distinct from the other human lice, *Pediculus humanus corporis* and *Pediculus humanus*

capitis. The crab louse is well adapted for life in the genital region, clinging tightly to the pubic hairs (see Chapter 6). Occasionally hairs on the eyebrows or in the axilla are colonized. It takes up to 10 blood feeds a day and this causes itching at the site of the bites. Eggs called 'nits' are seen attached to the pubic hairs, and the characteristic lice, up to 2 mm long, are visible (often at the base of a hair) under a hand lens or by microscopy. Infestation is common; for example there are more than 10 000 cases/year in the UK.

Treatment is by the application of 1% permethrin cream to all affected hair sites.

Genital scabies is also treated with permethrin cream or lindane

Sarcoptes scabiei (see Chapter 26) may cause local lesions on the genitalia, and can be spread as an STD. Patients may have evidence of scabies elsewhere on the body, with burrows between the fingers or toes. Genital scabies is treated with 5% permethrin cream.

 KEY FACTS

- Microorganisms transmitted by the sexual route in humans include representatives from all groups apart from the rickettsiae and helminths.

- STDs are becoming more widespread in the community rather than remaining confined to high risk groups.

- Genital herpes, warts and chlamydial urethritis are by far the most common of all the STDs, but HIV infection has had a major impact, eclipsing all the other well-known STDs because it is usually eventually lethal.

- Except for hepatitis A and B there are no vaccines for these infections, but antimicrobial chemotherapy is often available.

- At present, the best method of control is prevention.

- Transmission depends upon human behavior, which is notoriously difficult to influence.

- Long intervals between the onset of infectiousness and disease increase the chances of transmission.

 QUESTIONS

A 24-year-old art critic presents with a fever, dry cough and shortness of breath for 10 days, which have been getting worse. She seems very anxious, but otherwise nothing can be found either in the medical history or on physical examination. A blood sample is collected for an atypical pneumonia screen and her doctor gives her amoxycillin and erythromycin. Five days later she feels much worse and calls her doctor, who arranges for her admission to hospital. The results of the blood tests taken after she had been ill for 10 days are as follows; hemoglobin 13g/dl; white cell count 2.3×10^9/l; *Mycoplasma* latex agglutination test < 8; complement fixation test for antibodies to chlamydia group < 40, influenza A and B < 40, adenoviruses

< 40, *Mycoplasma pneumoniae* < 40, *Coxiella burnetii* < 40.

The patient later admits to weight loss and night sweats, and says that she has been worried because four years ago she had intimate contact over a few months with a boyfriend who was later diagnosed as HIV-1 seropositive. On examination the relevant findings are a temperature of 37.8° C, dyspnea, and tachypnea. There are no other findings in the respiratory system. A chest radiograph shows bilateral shadowing and a ground-glass appearance, sparing the upper zones. After appropriate counselling she consents to an HIV antibody screening test.

QUESTIONS

1. What is the most likely diagnosis?

2. What further investigations would you perform?

3. How would you manage her?

4. She improves over the next two weeks. What is her prognosis and how would you follow her up?

FURTHER READING

Hansfield H. *Color Atlas and Synopsis of Sexually Transmitted Diseases.* New York: McGraw-Hill, 2001.

Hirsch MS, Brun-Vezinet F, D'Aquila RT et al. Antiretroviral drug resistance testing in adult HIV-1 infection: recommendations of an International AIDS Society-USA Panel. *JAMA* 2000; 283(18):2417–26.

Ho DD, Neumann AU, Perelson AS et al. Rapid turnover of plasma virions and CD4 lymphocytes in HIV-1 infection. *Nature* 1995; 373:123–6.

Holmes K. *Sexually Transmitted Diseases.* New York: McGraw-Hill, 1998.

Lawn SD, Butera ST, Folks TM. Contribution of immune activation to the pathogenesis and transmission of human immunodeficiency virus type 1 infection. *Clin Microbiol Rev* 2001; 14:753–77.

Mellors JW, Rinaldo CR, Gupta P et al. Prognosis of HIV-1 infection predicted by the quantity of virus in plasma. *Science* 1996; 272:1167–70.

Shafer RW. Genotypic testing for human immunodeficiency virus type 1 infection drug resistance. *Clin Microbiol Rev* 2002; 15:247–77.

UNAIDS http://www.unaids.org

Wilfert CM. Prevention of mother-to-child transmission of HIV-1. *Antiviral Therapy* 2001; 6:161–77.

INTRODUCTION

Ingested pathogens may cause disease confined to the gut or involving other parts of the body

Ingestion of pathogens can cause many different infections. These may be confined to the gastrointestinal tract or initiated in the gut before spreading to other parts of the body. In this chapter we consider the important bacterial causes of diarrheal disease and summarize the other bacterial causes of food-associated infection and food poisoning. Viral and parasitic causes of diarrheal disease are discussed, as well as infections acquired via the gastrointestinal tract and causing disease in other body systems, including typhoid and paratyphoid fevers, listeriosis and some forms of viral hepatitis. For clarity, all types of viral hepatitis are included in this chapter. Infections of the liver can also result in liver abscesses, and several parasitic infections cause liver disease. Peritonitis and intra-abdominal abscesses can arise from seeding of the abdominal cavity by organisms from the gastrointestinal tract. Several different terms are used to describe infections of the gastrointestinal tract; those in common use are shown in *Figure 22.1*.

A wide range of microbial pathogens is capable of infecting the gastrointestinal tract, and the important bacterial and viral pathogens are listed in *Figure 22.2*. They are acquired by the fecal–oral route, from fecally contaminated food, fluids or fingers.

For an infection to occur, the pathogen must be ingested in sufficient numbers or possess attributes to elude the host defenses of the upper gastrointestinal tract and reach the intestine (*Fig. 22.3;* see also Chapter 13). Here they remain localized and cause disease as a result of multiplication and/or toxin production, or they may invade through the intestinal mucosa to reach the lymphatics or the bloodstream (*Fig. 22.4*). The damaging effects resulting from infection of the gastrointestinal tract are summarized in *Figure 22.5*.

Food-associated infection versus food poisoning

Infection associated with consumption of contaminated food is often termed 'food poisoning', but 'food-associated infection' is a better term. True food poisoning occurs after consumption of food containing toxins, which may be chemical (e.g. heavy metals) or bacterial in origin (e.g. from *Clostridium botulinum* or *Staphylococcus aureus*). The bacteria multiply and produce toxin within contaminated food. The organisms may be destroyed during food preparation, but the toxin is unaffected, consumed and acts within hours. In food-associated infections, the food may simply act as a vehicle for the pathogen (e.g. *Campylobacter*) or provide conditions in which the pathogen can multiply to produce numbers large enough to cause disease (e.g. *Salmonella*).

DIARRHEAL DISEASES CAUSED BY BACTERIAL OR VIRAL INFECTION

Diarrhea is the most common outcome of gastrointestinal tract infection

Infections of the gastrointestinal tract range in their effects from a mild self-limiting attack of 'the runs' to severe, sometimes fatal, diarrhea. There may be associated vomiting, fever and malaise. Diarrhea is the result of an increase in fluid and electrolyte loss into the gut lumen, leading to the production of unformed or liquid feces and can be thought of as the method by which the host forcibly expels the pathogen (and in doing so, aids its dissemination). However, diarrhea also occurs in many non-infectious conditions, and an infectious cause should not be assumed.

In the developing world, diarrheal disease is a major cause of mortality in children

In the developing world, diarrheal disease is a major cause of morbidity and mortality, particularly in young children. In the developed world it remains a very common complaint, but is usually mild and self-limiting except in the very young, the elderly and immunocompromised patients. Most of the pathogens listed in *Figure 22.2* are found throughout the world, but some such as *Vibrio cholerae*, have a more limited geographic distribution. However, such infections can be acquired by travelers to these areas and imported into their home countries.

Many cases of diarrheal disease are not diagnosed, either because they are mild and self-limiting and the patient does not seek medical attention, or because medical and laboratory

TERMS USED TO DESCRIBE GASTROINTESTINAL TRACT INFECTIONS

gastroenteritis

a syndrome characterized by gastrointestinal symptoms including nausea, vomiting, diarrhea and abdominal discomfort

diarrhea

abnormal fecal discharge characterized by frequent and/or fluid stool; usually resulting from disease of the small intestine and involving increased fluid and electrolyte loss

dysentery

an inflammatory disorder of the gastrointestinal tract often associated with blood and pus in the feces and accompanied by symptoms of pain, fever, abdominal cramps; usually resulting from disease of the large intestine

enterocolitis

inflammation involving the mucosa of both the small and large intestine

Fig. 22.1 As well as many colloquial expressions, several different clinical terms are used to describe infections of the gastrointestinal tract. Diarrhea without blood and pus is usually the result of enterotoxin production, whereas the presence of blood and/or pus cells in the feces indicates an invasive infection with mucosal destruction.

IMPORTANT BACTERIAL AND VIRAL PATHOGENS OF THE GASTROINTESTINAL TRACT

pathogen	animal reservoir	foodborne	waterborne
Bacteria			
Escherichia coli	+?	+(EHEC)	+(ETEC)
Salmonella	+	+++	+
Campylobacter	+	+++	+
Vibrio cholerae	–	+	+++
Shigella	–	+	–
Clostridium perfringens	+	+++	–
Bacillus cereus	–	++	–
Vibrio para-haemolyticus	–	++	–
Yersinia enterocolitica	+	+	–
Viruses			
rotavirus	–	–	–
noroviruses (previously known as SRSV or Norwalk-like viruses)	–	++	+

Fig. 22.2 Many different pathogens cause infections of the gastrointestinal tract. Some are found in both humans and animals while others are strictly human parasites. This difference has important implications for control and prevention. (EHEC, enterohemorrhagic (verotoxin-producing) *Escherichia coli*; ETEC, enterotoxigenic *E. coli*; SRSV, small round structured viruses.)

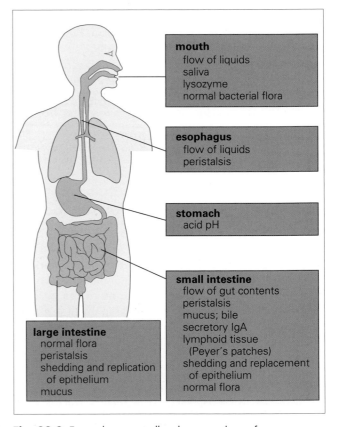

mouth
flow of liquids
saliva
lysozyme
normal bacterial flora

esophagus
flow of liquids
peristalsis

stomach
acid pH

small intestine
flow of gut contents
peristalsis
mucus; bile
secretory IgA
lymphoid tissue
(Peyer's patches)
shedding and replacement
of epithelium
normal flora

large intestine
normal flora
peristalsis
shedding and replication
of epithelium
mucus

Fig. 22.3 Every day we swallow large numbers of microorganisms. Because of the body's defense mechanisms, however, they rarely succeed in surviving the passage to the intestine in sufficient numbers to cause infection.

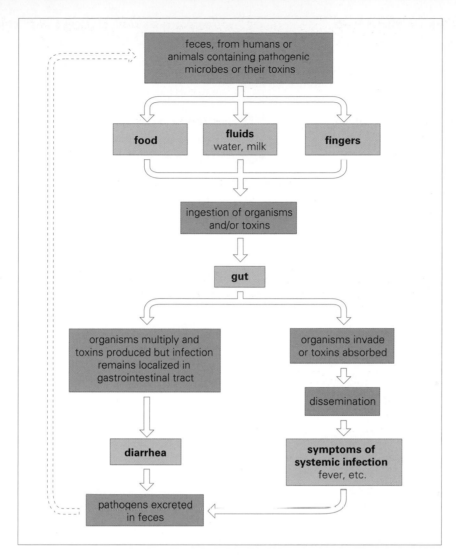

Fig. 22.4 Infections of the gastrointestinal tract can be grouped into those that remain localized in the gut and those that invade beyond the gut to cause infection in other sites in the body. In order to spread to a new host, pathogens are excreted in large numbers in the feces and must survive in the environment for long enough to infect another person directly or indirectly through contaminated food or fluids.

DAMAGE RESULTING FROM INFECTION OF THE GASTROINTESTINAL TRACT
pharmacologic action of bacterial toxins, local or distant to site of infection, e.g. cholera, staphylococcal food poisoning
local inflammation in response to superficial microbial invasion, e.g. shigellosis, amebiasis
deep invasion to blood or lymphatics; dissemination to other body sites, e.g. hepatitis A, enteric fevers
perforation of mucosal epithelium after infection, surgery or accidental trauma, e.g. peritonitis, intra-abdominal abscesses

Fig. 22.5 Infection of the gastrointestinal tract can cause damage locally or at distant sites.

facilities are unavailable, particularly in developing countries. It is generally impossible to distinguish on clinical grounds between infections caused by the different pathogens. However, information about the patient's recent food and travel history, and macroscopic and microscopic examination of the feces for blood and pus can provide helpful clues. A precise diagnosis can only be achieved by laboratory investigations. This is especially important in outbreaks, because of the need to instigate appropriate epidemiologic investigations and control measures.

Bacterial causes of diarrhea
Escherichia coli

This is one of the most versatile of all bacterial pathogens. Some strains are important members of the normal gut flora in man and animals (see Chapter 2), whereas others possess virulence factors that enable them to cause infections in the intestinal tract or at other sites, particularly the urinary tract (see Chapter 20). Strains that cause diarrheal disease do so by several distinct pathogenic mechanisms and differ in their epidemiology *(Fig. 22.6)*.

There are six distinct groups of E. coli with different pathogenetic mechanisms

Initially, all diarrhea-associated *Escherichia coli* were termed enteropathogenic *E. coli* (EPEC). However, greater insight into mechanisms of pathogenicity has led to specific group designations: enteropathogenic *E. coli* (EPEC), enterotoxigenic *E. coli* (ETEC), enterohemorrhagic *E. coli* (EHEC), enteroinvasive *E. coli* (EIEC), enteroaggregative *E. coli* (EAEC), and diffuse-aggregative *E. coli* (DAEC).

CHARACTERISTICS OF ESCHERICHIA COLI STRAINS CAUSING GASTROINTESTINAL INFECTIONS		
pathogenic group	**epidemiology**	**laboratory diagnosis***
enteropathogenic *E. coli* (EPEC)	EPEC strains belong to particular O serotypes cause sporadic cases and outbreaks of infection in babies and young children importance in adults less clear	isolate organisms from feces determine serotype of several colonies with polyvalent antisera for known EPEC types *adhesion to tissue culture cells can be demonstrated by a fluorescence actin staining test* *DNA-based assays for detection of attachment (virulence) factors*
enterotoxigenic *E. coli* (ETEC)	most important bacterial cause of diarrhea in children in developing countries most common cause of traveler's diarrhea water contaminated by human or animal sewage may be important in spread	isolate organisms from feces tests commercially available for immunologic detection of toxins from culture supernatants *gene probes specific for LT and ST genes available for detection of ETEC in feces and in food and water samples*
enterohemorrhagic (verotoxin-producing) *E. coli* (EHEC)	serotype O157 most important EHEC in human infections outbreaks and sporadic cases occur worldwide food and unpasteurized milk important in spread may cause hemolytic–uremic syndrome (HUS)	isolate organisms from feces proportion of EHEC in fecal sample may be very low (often <1% of *E. coli* colonies) usually sorbitol non-fermenters *Shiga toxin production and associated genes detected by biological, immunological and nucleic-acid-based assays*
enteroinvasive *E. coli* (EIEC)	important cause of diarrhea in areas of poor hygiene infections usually foodborne; no evidence of animal or environmental reservoir	isolate organisms from feces *test for enteroinvasive potential in tissue culture cells or nucleic-acid-based assys for invasion-associated genes*
enteroaggregative *E. coli* (EAEC) diffuse-aggregative *E. coli* (DAEC)	characteristic attachment to tissue culture cells cause diarrhea in children in developing countries role of toxins uncertain	*tissue culture assays for aggregative or diffuse adherence*

Fig. 22.6 *Escherichia coli* is a major cause of gastrointestinal infection, particularly in developing countries and in travelers. There is a range of pathogenic mechanisms within the species, resulting in more or less invasive disease. *Specialized tests are given in italics. (LT, heat-labile enterotoxin; ST, heat-stable enterotoxin.)

Enteropathogenic E. coli *(EPEC) do not appear to make any toxins*

They do produce bundle-forming pili (Bfp), intimin (an adhesin) and an associated protein (translocated intimin receptor, Tir). These virulence factors allow bacterial attachment to epithelial cells of the small intestine, leading to disruption of the microvillus (an 'attaching–effacing' mechanism of action; *Figs 22.6 and 22.7*) leading to diarrhea (see *Fig. 22.12*).

Enterotoxigenic E. coli *(ETEC) possess colonization factors (fimbrial adhesins)*

These bind the bacteria to specific receptors on the cell membrane of the small intestine (*Figs 22.6 and 22.8*). These organisms produce powerful plasmid-associated enterotoxins which are characterized as being either heat labile (LT) or heat stable (ST):

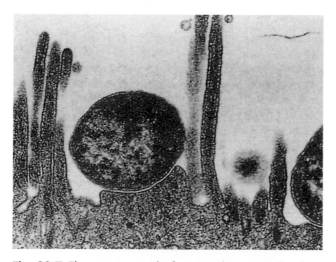

Fig. 22.7 Electron micrograph of enteropathogenic *Escherichia coli* adhering to the brush border of intestinal mucosal cells with localized destruction of microvilli. (Courtesy of S Knutton.)

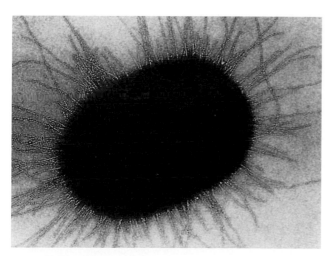

Fig. 22.8 Electron micrograph of enterotoxin *Escherichia coli*, showing pili necessary for adherence to mucosal epithelial cells. (Courtesy of S Knutton.)

- Heat-labile enterotoxin LT-I is very similar in structure and mode of action to cholera toxin produced by *V. cholerae*, and infections with strains producing LT-I can mimic cholera, particularly in young and malnourished children (see *Fig. 22.12*).
- Other ETEC strains produce heat-stable enterotoxins (STs) in addition to or instead of LT. STs have a similar but distinct mode of action to that of LT. ST_A activates guanylate cyclase activity, causing an increase in cyclic guanosine monophosphate, which results in increased fluid secretion. Immunoassays are commercially available for the identification of ETEC (*Fig. 22.6*).

Enterohemorrhagic E. coli *(EHEC) isolates produce a verotoxin*

The verotoxin (i.e. toxic to tissue cultures of 'vero'cells) is essentially identical to Shiga (*Shigella*) toxin. After attachment to the mucosa of the large intestine (by the 'attaching–effacing' mechanism also seen in EPEC) the produced toxin has a direct effect on intestinal epithelium, resulting in diarrhea (see *Fig. 22.12*). EHEC cause hemorrhagic colitis (HC) and hemolytic–uremic syndrome (HUS). In HC there is destruction of the mucosa and consequent hemorrhage; this may be followed by HUS. Verotoxin receptors have been identified on renal epithelium and may account for the kidney involvement. While there are many serotypes of EHEC, the most common one in the USA is O157:H7.

Enteroinvasive E. coli *(EIEC) attach specifically to the mucosa of the large intestine*

Utilizing plasmid-associated genes, they invade the cells by endocytosis. Inside the cell they lyse the endocytic vacuole, multiply and spread to adjacent cells, causing tissue destruction, inflammation, necrosis and ulceration, resulting in blood and mucus in stools (*Figs 22.6 and 22.12*).

Enteroaggregative E. coli *(EAEC) derive their name from their characteristic attachment pattern to tissue culture cells*

The pattern is an aggregative or 'stacked brick' formation. These organisms act in the small intestine to cause persistent diarrhea especially in children in developing countries. Their aggregative adherence ability is due to plasmid-associated fimbriae. EAEC also produce heat-labile toxins (an enterotoxin and a toxin related to *E. coli* hemolysin) but their role in diarrheal disease is uncertain.

Diffuse-aggregative E. coli *(DAEC) produce an alpha hemolysin and cytotoxic necrotizing factor 1*

They are also known as diffuse-adherent or cell-detaching *E. coli*. Their role in diarrheal disease, especially in young children, is incompletely understood and somewhat controversial, with some studies reporting no association.

EPEC and ETEC are the most important contributors to global incidence of diarrhea, while EHEC is more important in developed countries

The diarrhea produced by *E. coli* varies from mild to severe, depending upon the strain and the underlying health of the host. ETEC diarrhea in children in developing countries may be clinically indistinguishable from cholera. EIEC and EHEC strains both cause bloody diarrhea (see *Fig. 22.12*). Following EHEC infection, HUS is characterized by acute renal failure *(Fig. 22.9)*, anemia and thrombocytopenia, and there may be neurologic complications. HUS is the most common cause of acute renal failure in children in the UK and USA.

Specific tests are needed to identify strains of pathogenic E. coli

Because *E. coli* is a member of the normal gastrointestinal flora, specific tests are required to identify strains that may be responsible for diarrheal disease. These are summarized in *Figure 22.6*. Infections are more common in children and are also often travel-associated, and these factors should be considered when samples are received in the laboratory. It is important to note that specialized tests beyond routine stool cultures are required to identify specific diarrhea-associated *E. coli* types. Such tests are not ordinarily performed with uncomplicated diarrhea, which is usually self-limiting. However, concern regarding EHEC (e.g. bloody diarrhea) has led most laboratories in developed countries to screen for *E. coli* O157:H7.

Antibacterial therapy is not indicated for E. coli diarrhea

Specific antibacterial therapy is not indicated. Fluid replacement may be necessary, especially in young children. Treatment of HUS is urgent and may involve dialysis.

Provision of a clean water supply and adequate systems for sewage disposal are fundamental to the prevention of diarrheal disease. Food and unpasteurized milk can be important vehicles of infection, especially for EIEC and EHEC, but there is no evidence of an animal or environmental reservoir.

Salmonella

Salmonellae are the most common cause of food-associated diarrhea in many developed countries

However, in some countries (e.g. the USA and UK) they have been relegated to second place by *Campylobacter*. Like *E. coli*, the salmonellae belong to the family Enterobacteriaceae. Historically, salmonella nomenclature has been somewhat confusing, with more than two thousand serotypes defined on the basis of differences in the cell wall (O) and flagellar (H) antigens (Kauffmann–White scheme). However, more recent DNA hybridization studies indicate that there are only two species, the most important of which, for human infection, is *Salmonella enterica*. To simplify discussion and comparison, past convention has been to replace this species name with the serotype designation. While technically incorrect (the serotype is not a species) this practice is helpful when discussing interrelationships between different isolates, as for example in epidemiologic analysis when tracing the source of an outbreak. This convention is thus followed here [see Appendix] to maintain continuity with other scientific literature.

All salmonellae except for *Salmonella typhi* and *S. paratyphi* are found in animals as well as humans. There is a large animal reservoir of infection, which is transmitted to man via contaminated food, especially poultry and dairy products *(Fig. 22.10)*. Waterborne infection is less frequent. Salmonella infection is also transmitted from person to person, and secondary spread can therefore occur, for example within a family after one member has become infected after consuming contaminated food.

Salmonellae are almost always acquired orally in food or drink that is contaminated

Diarrhea is produced as a result of invasion by the salmonellae of epithelial cells in the terminal portion of the small intestine *(Fig. 22.11)*. Initial entry is probably through uptake by M cells (the 'antigenic samplers' of the bowel)

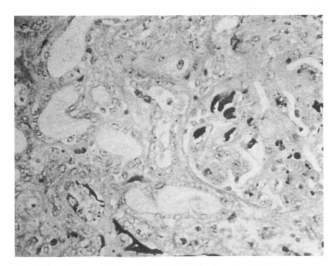

Fig. 22.9 Verotoxin-producing *Escherichia coli* infection, showing fibrin 'thrombi' in glomerular capillaries in hemolytic–uremic syndrome. (Weigert stain.) (Courtesy of HR Powell.)

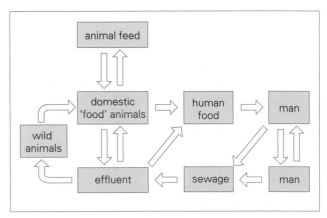

Fig. 22.10 The recycling of salmonellae. With the exception of *Salmonella typhi*, salmonellae are widely distributed in animals, providing a constant source of infection for man. Excretion of large numbers of salmonellae from infected individuals and carriers allows the organisms to be 'recycled'.

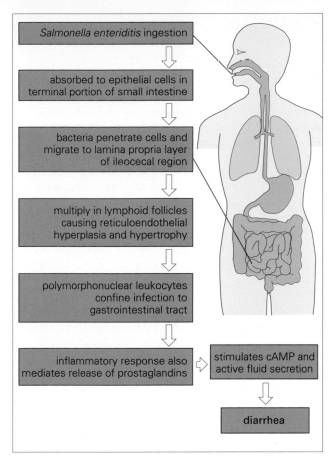

Fig. 22.11 The passage of salmonellae through the body. The vast majority of salmonellae cause infection localized to the gastrointestinal tract and do not invade beyond the gut mucosa. (cAMP, cyclic adenosine monophosphate.)

with subsequent spread to epithelial cells. A similar route of invasion occurs in *Shigella*, *Yersinia* and reovirus infections. The bacteria migrate to the lamina propria layer of the ileocecal region, where their multiplication stimulates an inflammatory response, which both confines the infection to the gastrointestinal tract and mediates the release of prostaglandins. These in turn activate cyclic adenosine monophosphate (cAMP) and fluid secretion, resulting in diarrhea.

Species of *Salmonella* that normally cause diarrhea (e.g. *S. enteritidis*, *S. choleraesuis*) may become invasive in patients with particular predispositions (e.g. children and patients with cancer or sickle cell anemia). The organisms are not contained within the gastrointestinal tract, but invade the body to cause septicemia; consequently, many organs become seeded with salmonellae, sometimes leading to osteomyelitis, pneumonia or meningitis.

In the vast majority of cases, *Salmonella* spp. cause an acute but self-limiting diarrhea, though in the young and the elderly the symptoms may be more severe. Vomiting is also common with enterocolitis, while fever is usually a sign of invasive disease *(Fig. 22.12)*. *S. typhi* and *S. paratyphi* invade the body from the gastrointestinal tract to cause systemic illness and are discussed in a later section.

Salmonella diarrhea can be diagnosed by culture on selective media

The methods for culturing fecal specimens on selective media are summarized in the Appendix. The organisms are not fastidious and can usually be isolated within 24 hours, although small numbers may require enrichment in selenite broth before culture. Preliminary identification can be made rapidly, but the complete result, including serotype, takes at least 48 hours.

Fluid and electrolyte replacement may be needed for salmonella diarrhea

Diarrhea is usually self-limiting and resolves without treatment. Fluid and electrolyte replacement may be required, particularly in the very young and the elderly. Unless there is evidence of invasion and septicemia, antibiotics should be positively discouraged because they do not reduce the symptoms or shorten the illness, and may prolong excretion of salmonellae in the feces. There is some evidence that symptomatic treatment with drugs that reduce diarrhea has the same adverse effect.

Salmonellae may be excreted in the feces for several weeks after a salmonella infection

Figure 22.10 illustrates the problems associated with the prevention of salmonella infections. The large animal reservoir makes it impossible to eliminate the organisms, and preventive measures must therefore be aimed at 'breaking the chain' between animal and man, and from person to person. Such measures include:

- maintaining adequate standards of public health (clean drinking water and proper sewage disposal);
- education programs on hygienic food preparation.

Following an episode of salmonella diarrhea, an individual can continue to carry and excrete organisms in the feces for several weeks. Although in the absence of symptoms the organisms will not be dispersed so liberally into the environment, thorough handwashing before food handling is essential. People employed as food handlers are excluded from work until three specimens of feces have failed to grow salmonella.

Campylobacter

Campylobacters *are among the commonest causes of diarrhea*

Campylobacter spp. are curved or S-shaped Gram-negative rods *(Fig. 22.13)*. They have long been known to cause diarrheal disease in animals, but are also one of the most common causes of diarrhea in humans. The delay in recognizing the importance of these organisms was due to their cultural requirements, which differ from those of the enterobacteria as they are microaerophilic and thermophilic (growing well at 42°C); they do not therefore grow on the media used for isolating *E. coli* and salmonellae. Several species of the genus *Campylobacter* are associated with human disease, but *Campylobacter jejuni* is by far the most common. *Helicobacter pylori*, previously classified as *Campylobacter pylori*, is an important cause of gastritis and gastric ulcers (see below).

CLINICAL FEATURES OF BACTERIAL DIARRHEAL DISEASE						
pathogen	incubation period	duration	symptoms			
			diarrhea	vomiting	abdominal cramps	fever
Salmonella	6h–2 days	48h–7 days	watery	+	+	+
Campylobacter	2–11 days	3 days–3 weeks	bloody	–	+	+
Shigella	1–4 days	2–3 days	bloody	–	+	+
Vibrio cholerae	2–3 days	up to 7 days	watery	+	+	–
Vibrio parahaemolyticus	8h–2 days	3 days	watery	+	+	+
Clostridium perfringens	8h–1 day	12h–1 day	watery	–	+	–
Bacillus cereus diarrheal emetic	8h–12h 15 min–4h	12h–1 day 12h–2 days	watery watery	– +	+ +	– –
Yersinia enterocolitica	4–7 days	1–2 weeks	bloody	–	+	+
enteropathogenic Escherichia coli (EPEC)	1–2 days	weeks	watery	+	+	+
enterotoxigenic Escherichia coli (ETEC)	1–7 days	2–6 days	watery	+	+	–
enterohemorrhagic Escherichia coli (EHEC)	3–4 days	5–10 days	bloody	+	+	–
enteroinvasive Escherichia coli (EIEC)	1–3 days	7–10 days	bloody	+	+	+

Fig. 22.12 The clinical features of bacterial diarrhea infection. It is difficult, if not impossible, to determine the likely cause of a diarrheal illness on the basis of clinical features alone, and laboratory investigations are essential to identify the pathogen.

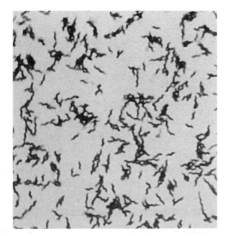

Fig. 22.13 *Campylobacter jejuni* infection. Gram stain showing Gram-negative, S-shaped bacilli. (Courtesy of I Farrell.)

As with salmonellae, there is a large animal reservoir of campylobacter in cattle, sheep, rodents, poultry and wild birds. Infections are acquired by consumption of contaminated food, especially poultry, milk or water. Recent studies have shown an association between infection and consumption of milk from bottles with tops that have been pecked by wild birds. Household pets such as dogs and cats can become infected and provide a source for human infection, particularly for young children. Person to person spread by the fecal–oral route is rare, as is transmission from food handlers.

Campylobacter *diarrhea is clinically similar to that caused by other bacteria such as salmonella and shigella*

The gross pathology and histologic appearances of ulceration and inflamed bleeding mucosal surfaces in the jejunum, ileum and colon (*Fig. 22.14*) are compatible with invasion of

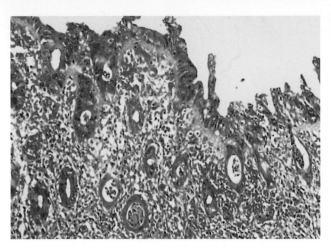

Fig. 22.14 Inflammatory enteritis caused by *Campylobacter jejuni*, involving the entire mucosa, with flattened atrophic villi, necrotic debris in the crypts and thickening of the basement membrane. (Cresyl-fast violet stain.) (Courtesy of J Newman.)

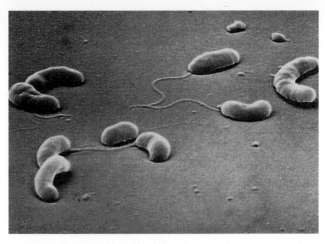

Fig. 22.15 Scanning electron micrograph of *Vibrio cholerae* showing comma-shaped rods with a single polar flagellum. ×13 000. (Courtesy of DK Banerjee.)

the bacteria, but the production of cytotoxins by *C. jejuni* has also been demonstrated. Invasion and bacteremia are not uncommon, particularly in neonates and debilitated adults.

The clinical presentation is similar to that of diarrhea caused by salmonellae and shigella, although the disease may have a longer incubation period and a longer duration. The key features are summarized in *Figure 22.12*.

Cultures for campylobacter *should be set up routinely in every investigation of a diarrheal illness*

The methods are described in the Appendix, but it is important to note that the media and conditions for growth differ from those required for the enterobacteria. Growth is often somewhat slow compared with that of the enterobacteria, but a presumptive identification should be available within 48 hours of culture.

Erythromycin is used for severe campylobacter *diarrhea*

Erythromycin is the antibiotic of choice for cases of diarrheal disease that are severe enough to warrant treatment. Invasive infections may require treatment with an additional antibiotic (e.g. quinolone, aminoglycoside, etc.).

The preventive measures for salmonella infections described above are equally applicable to the prevention of campylobacter infections, but there are no requirements for the screening of food handlers because contamination of food by this route is very uncommon.

Cholera

Cholera is an acute infection of the gastrointestinal tract caused by the comma-shaped Gram-negative bacterium *V. cholerae (Fig. 22.15)*. The disease has a long history characterized by epidemics and pandemics. The last cases of cholera acquired in the UK were in the 19th century following the introduction of the bacterium by sailors arriving from Europe, and in 1849 Snow published his historic essay *On the Mode of Communication of Cholera*.

Cholera flourishes in communities with inadequate clean drinking water and sewage disposal

The 1990s have witnessed the seventh pandemic of cholera spreading into Latin America. The disease remains endemic in southeast Asia and parts of Africa and South America. Unlike salmonellae and campylobacter, *V. cholerae* is a free-living inhabitant of fresh water, but causes infection only in humans. Asymptomatic human carriers are believed to be a major reservoir. The disease is spread via contaminated food; shellfish grown in fresh and estuarine waters have also been implicated. Direct person to person spread is thought to be uncommon. Therefore cholera continues to flourish in communities where there is absent or unreliable provision of clean drinking water and sewage disposal. Cases still occur in developed countries (e.g. the Gulf Coast of Louisiana and Texas in the United States), but high standards of hygiene mean that secondary spread should not occur.

V. cholerae *serotypes are based on somatic (O) antigens*

Serotype O1 is the most important and is further divided into two biotypes: classical and El Tor *(Fig. 22.16)*. The El Tor biotype, named after the quarantine camp where it was first isolated from pilgrims returning from Mecca, differs from classical *V. cholerae* in several ways. In particular it causes only a mild diarrhea and has a higher ratio of carriers to cases than classical cholera; carriage is also more prolonged, and the organisms survive better in the environment. The El Tor biotype, which was responsible for the seventh pandemic, has now spread throughout the world and has largely displaced the classical biotype.

In 1992 a new non-O1 strain (O139) arose in south India and spread rapidly. It is able to infect O1-immune individuals and cause epidemics, and has been proclaimed as the eighth pandemic strain of cholera. *V. cholerae* O139 appears to have originated from the El Tor O1 biotype when the latter acquired a new O (capsular) antigen by horizontal gene transfer from a non-O1 strain. This provided the recipient

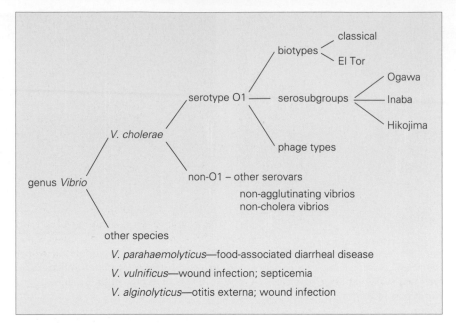

Fig. 22.16 *Vibrio cholerae* serotype O1, the cause of cholera, can be subdivided into different biotypes with different epidemiologic features, and into serosubgroups and phage types for the purposes of investigating outbreaks of infection. Although *V. cholerae* is the most important pathogen of the genus, other species can also cause infections of both the gastrointestinal tract and other sites.

strain with a selective advantage in a region where a large part of the population is immune to O1 strains.

Other species of *Vibrio* cause a variety of infections in man (*Fig. 22.16*). *V. parahaemolyticus* is another cause of diarrheal disease, but this is usually much less severe than cholera (see below).

The symptoms of cholera are caused by an enterotoxin

The symptoms of cholera are entirely due to the production of an enterotoxin in the gastrointestinal tract (see Chapter 17). However, the organism requires additional virulence factors to enable it to survive the host defenses and adhere to the intestinal mucosa. These are illustrated in *Figure 22.17* (see also Chapter 13).

The clinical features of cholera are summarized in *Figure 22.12*. The severe watery non-bloody diarrhea is known as rice water stool because of its appearance (*Fig. 22.18*) and can result in the loss of one liter of fluid every hour. It is this fluid loss and the consequent electrolyte imbalance that results in marked dehydration, metabolic acidosis (loss of bicarbonate), hypokalemia (potassium loss) and hypovolemic shock resulting in cardiac failure. Untreated, the mortality from cholera is 40–60%; rapidly instituted fluid and electrolyte replacement reduces the mortality to less than 1%.

Culture is necessary to diagnose sporadic or imported cases of cholera and carriers

In countries where cholera is prevalent, diagnosis is based on clinical grounds, and laboratory confirmation is rarely sought. It is worth remembering that ETEC infection can resemble

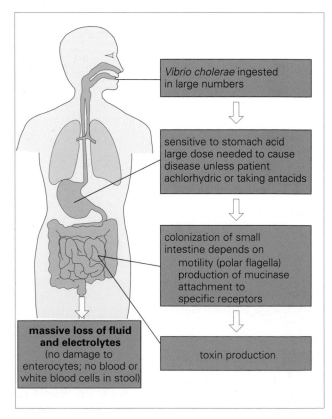

Fig. 22.17 The production of an enterotoxin is central to the pathogenesis of cholera, but the organisms must possess other virulence factors to allow them to reach the small intestine and to adhere to the mucosal cells.

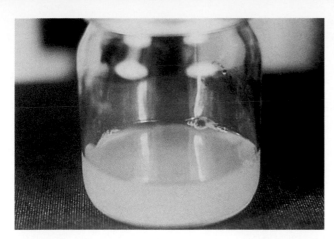

Fig. 22.18 Rice water stool in cholera. (Courtesy of AM Geddes.)

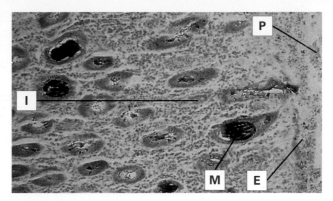

Fig. 22.19 Shigellosis. Histology of the colon showing disrupted epithelium covered by pseudomembrane and interstitial infiltration. Mucin glands have discharged their contents and the goblet cells are empty. (Colloidal iron stain.) (E, epithelium; I, interstitial infiltration; M, mucin in glands; P, pseudomembrane.) (Courtesy of RH Gilman.)

cholera in its severity—but, for both diseases, fluid and electrolyte replacement are of paramount importance. The methods are given in the Appendix.

Prompt rehydration with fluids and electrolytes is central to the treatment of cholera

Oral or intravenous rehydration may be used. Antibiotics are not necessary, but tetracycline may be given, as some evidence indicates that this reduces the time of excretion of *V. cholerae* thereby reducing the risk of transmission. There have, however, been reports of tetracycline-resistant *V. cholerae* in some areas.

As with other diarrheal disease, a clean drinking water supply and adequate sewage disposal are fundamental to the prevention of cholera. As there is no animal reservoir, it should in theory be possible to eliminate the disease. However, carriage in humans, albeit for only a few weeks, occurs in 1–20% of previously infected patients, making eradication difficult to achieve.

Killed whole-cell cholera vaccine is no longer recommended by the WHO

A killed whole-cell vaccine is available and is given parenterally, but is effective in only about 50% of those vaccinated, with protection lasting for only 3–6 months. It is no longer recommended by the World Health Organization (WHO) for travelers to cholera-endemic areas, although it may be required in certain countries. Oral vaccines (not available in the USA) appear to provide somewhat better protection.

Shigellosis

Symptoms of Shigella infection range from mild to severe depending upon the infecting species

Shigellosis is also known as bacillary dysentery (in contrast to amebic dysentery; see below) because in its more severe form it is characterized by an invasive infection of the mucosa of the large intestine causing inflammation and resulting in the presence of pus and blood in the diarrheal stool. However, symptoms range from mild to severe depending upon the species of *Shigella* involved and on the underlying state of health of the host. There are four species:

- *Shigella sonnei* causes most infections at the mild end of the spectrum.
- *Shigella flexneri* and *S. boydii* usually produce more severe disease.
- *Shigella dysenteriae* is the most serious.

Shigellosis is primarily a pediatric disease. When associated with severe malnutrition it may precipitate complications such as the protein deficiency syndrome 'kwashiorkor'. Like *V. cholerae*, shigellae are human pathogens without an animal reservoir, but unlike the vibrios, they are not found in the environment, being spread from person to person by the fecal–oral route and less frequently by contaminated food and water. Shigellae appear to be able to initiate infection from a small infective dose (10–100 organisms) and therefore spread is easy in situations where sanitation or personal hygiene may be poor (e.g. refugee camps, nurseries, day care centers and institutions for the handicapped).

Shigella diarrhea is usually watery at first, but later contains mucus and blood

Shigellae attach to, and invade, the mucosal epithelium of the distal ileum and colon, causing inflammation and ulceration *(Fig. 22.19)*. However, they rarely invade through the gut wall to the bloodstream. *S. dysenteriae* produce a (Shiga) toxin similar to that associated with enterohemorrrhagic *E. coli* (EHEC; see above), which can cause damage to the intestinal epithelium and glomerular endothelial cells, the latter leading to kidney failure (hemolytic–uremic syndrome, HUS; see above).

The main features of shigella infection are summarized in *Figure 22.12*. Diarrhea is usually watery at first, but later contains mucus and blood. Lower abdominal cramps can be severe. The disease is usually self-limiting, but dehydration can occur, especially in the young and elderly. Complications can be associated with malnutrition (see above).

Antibiotics should only be given for severe shigella diarrhea

Rehydration may be indicated. Antibiotics, especially those decreasing intestinal motility, should not be given except in severe cases. Plasmid-mediated resistance is common, and antibiotic susceptibility tests should be performed on shigella isolates if treatment is required.

Education in personal hygiene and proper sewage disposal are important. Cases may continue to excrete shigellae for a few weeks, but longer-term carriage is unusual; therefore with adequate public health measures and no animal reservoir, the disease is potentially eradicable.

Other bacterial causes of diarrheal disease

The pathogens described in the previous sections are the major bacterial causes of diarrheal disease. Salmonella and campylobacter infections and some types of *E. coli* infections are most often food-associated, whereas cholera is more often waterborne and shigellosis is usually spread by direct fecal–oral contact. Other bacterial pathogens that cause food-associated infection or food poisoning are described below.

V. parahaemolyticus *and* Yersinia enterocolitica *are foodborne Gram-negative causes of diarrhea*

V. parahaemolyticus is a halophilic (salt-loving) vibrio that contaminates seafood and fish. If these foods are consumed uncooked, diarrheal disease can result. The mechanism of pathogenesis is still unclear. Most strains associated with infection are hemolytic due to production of a heat-stable cytotoxin and have been shown to invade intestinal cells (in contrast to *V. cholerae,* which is non-invasive and cholera toxin, which is not cytotoxic).

The clinical features of infection are summarized in *Figure 22.12.* The methods used for the laboratory diagnosis of *V. parahaemolyticus* infection are given in the Appendix (e.g. special media for cultivation, etc.). Prevention of infection depends upon cooking fish and seafood properly.

Yersinia enterocolitica is a member of the *Enterobacteriaceae* and is a cause of food-associated infection especially among infants and particularly in colder parts of the world. The reason for this geographic distribution is unknown, but it has been speculated that it is because the organism prefers to grow at temperatures of 22–25°C. *Y. enterocolitica* is found in a variety of animal hosts including rodents, rabbits, pigs, sheep, cattle, horses and domestic pets. Transmission to humans from household dogs has been reported. The organism survives and multiplies, albeit more slowly, at refrigeration temperatures (4°C) and has been implicated in outbreaks of infection associated with contaminated milk as well as other foods.

The mechanism of pathogenesis is unknown, but the clinical features of the disease result from invasion of the terminal ileum, necrosis in Peyer's patches and an associated inflammation of the mesenteric lymph nodes *(Fig. 22.20).* The presentation, with enterocolitis and often mesenteric adenitis, can easily be confused with acute appendicitis, particularly in children. The clinical features are summarized in *Figure 22.12.* The laboratory diagnosis is outlined in the Appendix. As with *V. parahaemolyticus,* an indication of a suspicion of yersinia infection is useful so that the laboratory staff can process the specimen appropriately.

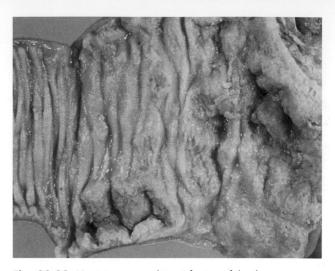

Fig. 22.20 *Yersinia enterocolitica* infection of the ileum, showing superficial necrosis of the mucosa and ulceration. (Courtesy of J Newman.)

Clostridium perfringens *and* Bacillus cereus *are spore-forming Gram-positive causes of diarrhea*

The Gram-negative organisms described in the previous sections invade the intestinal mucosa or produce enterotoxins, which cause diarrhea. None of these organisms produces spores. Two Gram-positive species are important causes of diarrheal disease, particularly in association with spore-contaminated food. These are *Clostridium perfringens* and *Bacillus cereus.*

Cl. perfringens is associated with diarrheal diseases in different circumstances, and the pathogenesis is summarized in *Figure 22.21:*

- Enterotoxin-producing strains are a common cause of food-associated infection.
- Much more rarely, β-toxin-producing strains produce an acute necrotizing disease of the small intestine, accompanied by abdominal pain and diarrhea. This form occurs after the consumption of contaminated meat by people who are unaccustomed to a high protein diet and do not have sufficient intestinal trypsin to destroy the toxin. It is traditionally associated with the orgiastic pig feasts enjoyed by the natives of New Guinea, but also occurred in people released from prisoner of war camps.

The clinical features of the common type of infection are shown in *Figure 22.12.* The laboratory investigation of suspected *Cl. perfringens* infection is outlined in the Appendix. The organism is an anaerobe and grows readily on routine laboratory media. Enterotoxin production can be demonstrated by a latex agglutination method.

Antibacterial treatment of *Cl. perfringens* diarrhea is rarely required. Prevention depends on thorough reheating of food before serving, or preferably avoiding cooking food too long before consumption.

Cl. perfringens is also an important cause of wound and soft tissue infections, as described in Chapter 26.

Bacillus cereus spores and vegetative cells contaminate many foods, and food-associated infection takes one of two forms:

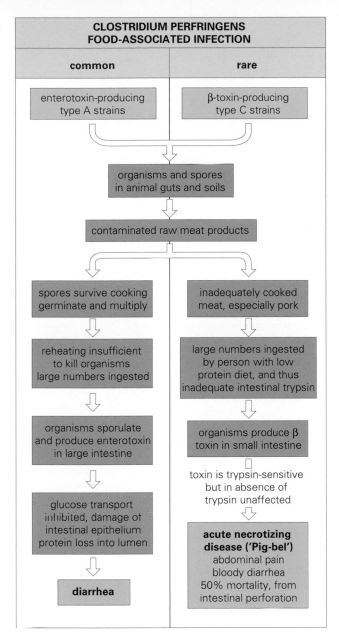

Fig. 22.21 *Clostridium perfringens* is linked with two forms of food-associated infection. The common, enterotoxin-mediated infection (left) is usually acquired by eating meat or poultry that has been cooked enough to kill vegetative cells, but not spores. As the food cools, the spores germinate. If reheating before consumption is inadequate (as it often is in mass catering outlets), large numbers of organisms are ingested. The rare form associated with β-toxin-producing strains (right) causes a severe necrotizing disease.

- diarrhea resulting from the production of enterotoxin in the gut;
- vomiting due to the ingestion of enterotoxin in food.

Two different toxins are involved, as illustrated in *Figure 22.22*. The clinical features of the infections are summarized in *Figure 22.12*. Laboratory confirmation of the diagnosis requires specific media as described in the Appendix. The emetic type of disease may be difficult to assign to *B. cereus* unless the incriminated food is cultured.

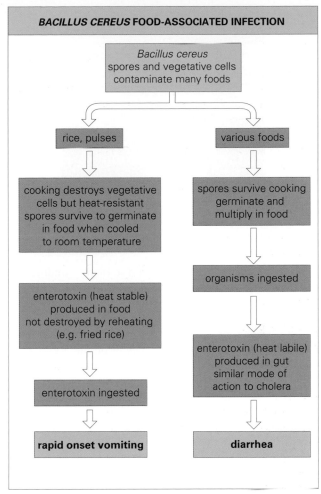

Fig. 22.22 *Bacillus cereus* can cause two different forms of food-associated infection. Both involve toxins.

As with *Cl. perfringens*, prevention of *B. cereus* food-associated infection depends upon proper cooking and rapid consumption of food. Specific antibacterial treatment is not indicated.

Antibiotic-associated diarrhea— *Clostridium difficile*

Treatment with broad spectrum antibiotics can be complicated by Cl. difficile *diarrhea*

All the infections described so far arise from the ingestion of organisms or their toxins. However, diarrhea can also arise from disruption of the normal gut flora. Even in the early days of antibiotic use it was recognized that these agents affected the normal flora of the body as well as attacking the pathogens. For example, orally administered tetracycline disrupts the normal gut flora, and patients sometimes become recolonized not with the usual facultative Gram-negative anaerobes but with *Staphylococcus aureus*, causing enterocolitis, or with yeasts such as *Candida*. Soon after clindamycin was introduced for therapeutic use, it was found to be associated with a severe diarrhea in which the colonic mucosa became covered with a characteristic fibrinous pseudomembrane (pseudomembranous colitis; *Fig. 22.23*).

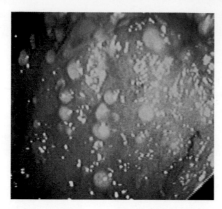

Fig. 22.23 Antibiotic-associated colitis due to *Clostridium difficile*. Sigmoidoscopic view showing multiple pseudomembranous lesions. (Courtesy of J Cunningham.)

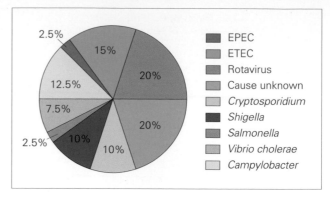

Fig. 22.24 Diarrheal disease is a major cause of illness and death in children in developing countries. This illustration shows the proportion of infections caused by different pathogens. Note that in as many as 20% of infections a cause is not identified, but many of these are likely to be viral. (Data from the WHO.) (EPEC, enteropathogenic *Escherichia coli*; ETEC, enterotoxigenic *E. coli*.)

However, clindamycin is not the cause of the condition; it merely inhibits the normal gut flora and allows *Cl. difficile* to multiply. This organism is commonly found in the gut of children and to a lesser extent in adults, but can also be acquired from other patients in hospital by cross-infection. In common with other clostridia, *Cl. difficile* produces exotoxins, two of which have been characterized: one is a cytotoxin and the other an enterotoxin, and both appear to play a role in producing diarrhea.

Although initially associated with clindamycin, *Cl. difficile* diarrhea has since been shown to follow therapy with many other broad spectrum antibiotics; hence the term antibiotic-associated diarrhea or colitis. The infection is often severe and may require treatment with the anti-anaerobic agent metronidazole, or with oral vancomycin. However, the recent emergence of vancomycin-resistant enterococci, probably originating in the gut flora, has led to the recommendation that oral vancomycin be avoided wherever possible (see Chapter 33).

Viral diarrhea

Over three million infants die of gastroenteritis each year, and viruses are the commonest cause

Non-bacterial gastroenteritis and diarrhea are usually caused by viruses. Infection is seen in all parts of the world, especially in infants and young children (*Fig. 22.24*). Its impact is staggering—in parts of Asia, Africa and Latin America more than three million infants die of gastroenteritis each year, and children may have a total of 60 days of diarrhea in each year. It has a major effect on nutritional status and growth. In the USA about 200 000 children less than 5 years of age are hospitalized each year because of infectious gastroenteritis.

Although viruses appear to be the commonest causes of gastroenteritis in infants and young children, viral gastroenteritis is not distinguishable clinically from other types of gastroenteritis. The viruses are specific to humans, and infection follows the general rules for fecal–oral transmission. Oral transmission of non-bacterial gastroenteritis was first demonstrated experimentally in 1945, but it was not until 1972 that viral particles were identified in feces by electron microscopy. It has been difficult or impossible to cultivate most of these viruses in cell culture.

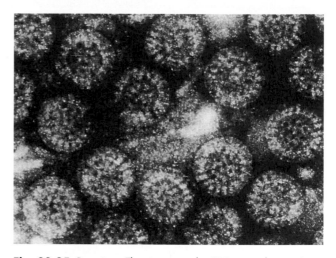

Fig. 22.25 Rotavirus. The virus particles (65 nm in diameter) have a well-defined outer margin and capsules radiating from an inner core to give the particle a wheel-like (hence 'rota') appearance. (Courtesy of JE Banatvala.)

Rotaviruses

These are morphologically characteristic viruses (*Fig. 22.25*), with a genome consisting of 11 separate segments of double-stranded RNA. Different rotaviruses infect the young of many mammals, including children, kittens, puppies, calves, foals and piglets, but it is thought that viruses from one host species occasionally cross-infect another. There are at least two human serotypes.

Replicating rotavirus causes diarrhea by damaging transport mechanisms in the gut

The incubation period is 1 to 2 days. After virus replication in intestinal epithelial cells there is an acute onset of vomiting, which is sometimes projectile, and diarrhea which lasts from 4 to 7 days. The replicating virus damages transport mechanisms in the gut, and loss of water, salt and glucose causes diarrhea (*Fig. 22.26*). Infected cells in the intestine are destroyed, resulting in villous atrophy. The villi, long finger-

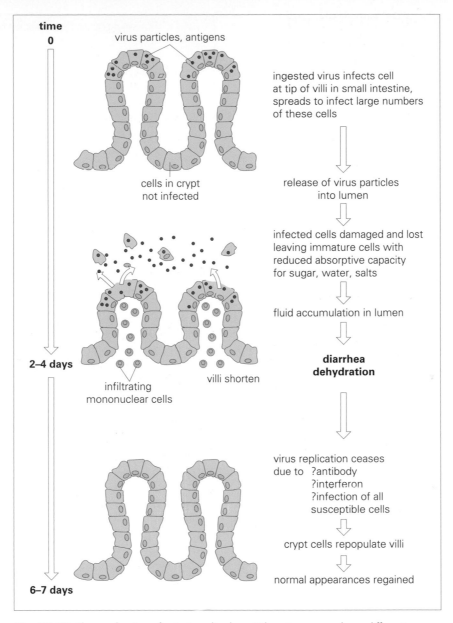

time 0

virus particles, antigens

ingested virus infects cell at tip of villi in small intestine, spreads to infect large numbers of these cells

cells in crypt not infected

release of virus particles into lumen

infected cells damaged and lost leaving immature cells with reduced absorptive capacity for sugar, water, salts

fluid accumulation in lumen

2–4 days

infiltrating mononuclear cells

villi shorten

diarrhea dehydration

virus replication ceases due to ?antibody
?interferon
?infection of all susceptible cells

crypt cells repopulate villi

normal appearances regained

6–7 days

Fig. 22.26 The mechanism of rotavirus diarrhea. Other viruses may have different mechanisms.

like projections, become flattened resulting in the loss of both the surface area for absorption and the digestive enzymes, and raised osmotic pressure in the gut lumen causes diarrhea. There is no inflammation or loss of blood. Exceedingly large numbers of virus particles, 10^{10}–10^{11}/g, appear in the feces. For unknown reasons, respiratory symptoms such as cough and coryza are quite common. The disease is more severe in infants in developing countries.

Infection is commonest in children under 2 years of age, and most frequent in the cooler months of the year. IgA antibodies in colostrum give protection during the first 6 months of life. Outbreaks are sometimes seen in nurseries. Older children are less susceptible to infection, nearly all of them having developed antibodies, but occasional infections occur in adults.

Rotaviruses are well-adapted intestinal infectious agents. As few as 10 ingested particles can cause infection, and by generating a diarrhea laden with enormous quantities of infectious particles these organisms have ensured their continued transmission and survival.

Rotavirus particles can be seen in fecal samples by electron microscopy

Laboratory diagnosis is generally not available in developing countries or necessary in developed countries, but during the acute stages the characteristic 65 nm particles can be seen in fecal samples by electron microscopy. They show cubic symmetry and an outer capsid coat arranged like the spokes of a wheel (*Fig. 22.25*). Viral antigen can be detected in feces by enzyme-linked immunosorbent assay (ELISA) (see Chapter 32).

Fluid and salt replacement can be life-saving in rotavirus diarrhea

Dehydration occurs readily in infants, and fluid and salt replacement orally or intravenously can be life-saving. There are no antiviral agents available, but a variety of live attenuated oral vaccines have undergone successful trials.

Other viruses

Other viruses causing diarrhea in humans include caliciviruses, astroviruses, adenoviruses and coronaviruses

Caliciviruses are 27 nm diameter, single-stranded RNA viruses that may cause 'winter vomiting disease'. They include the noroviruses, previously known as the small round structured viruses (SRSV) or Norwalk-like viruses (NLV). They have not yet been cultivated in vitro and cause gastroenteritis when fed to adult volunteers. One of the first identified outbreaks was in a school in Norwalk, Ohio in 1969. Infection is common in older children and adults. These viruses are highly infectious, spread rapidly and nosocomial infection is common. In 25–50% of cases there may be chills, headache, myalgia or fever as well as nausea, abdominal pain, vomiting and diarrhea, but recovery occurs within 24 to 48 hours. Laboratory diagnosis, important in outbreaks and for epidemiologic studies, is usually by electron microscopy or ELISA, and genome detection methods have improved the detection sensitivity. Viruses in this group are often implicated in diarrhea related to food or waterborne surfaces occurring after eating sewage-contaminated shellfish such as cockles or mussels.

Astroviruses are 28 nm single-stranded RNA viruses of which five serotypes are known and have characteristic five- or six-pointed star patterns. Most infections occur in childhood and are mild. Adenoviruses are unenveloped, 70–80 nm double-stranded DNA viruses of which types 40 and 41 are associated with gastroenteritis. Types 40 and 41 can only be grown in specialized cell culture lines. They are second to rotaviruses as a cause of acute diarrhea in young children in temperate climates. Coronaviruses have an uncertain role.

Although outbreaks of gastroenteritis often have a viral etiology it may be difficult to be sure about the exact role of a given virus when it is identified in feces, as there are a number of viruses that replicate in the gastrointestinal tract which are not associated with acute diarrheal illnesss.

FOOD POISONING

In this chapter the term 'food poisoning' is restricted to the diseases caused by toxins elaborated by contaminating bacteria in food before it is consumed (see above). The emetic toxin of *B. cereus* fits this definition, as do the diseases associated with the consumption of *Staph. aureus* enterotoxin and *Cl. botulinum* toxin.

Staphylococcus aureus

Eight different enterotoxins are produced by different strains of Staph. aureus

At least eight serologically distinct enterotoxins are produced by strains of *Staph. aureus*, the best understood of which are

STAPHYLOCOCCAL ENTEROTOXINS		
enterotoxin		
A	most commonly associated with food poisoning	
B	associated with staphylococcal enterocolitis (rare)	
C	rare	
D	second most common, alone or in combination with A	associated with contaminated milk products
E	rare	
TSST-1	toxic shock syndrome toxin, not food-associated	

Fig. 22.27 *Staphylococcus aureus* produces at least eight immunogically distinct enterotoxins, the most important of which are listed here. Strains may produce one or more of the toxins simultaneously. Enterotoxin A is by far the most common in food-associated disease.

enterotoxins A–E (*Fig. 22.27*). All are heat stable and resistant to destruction by enzymes in the stomach and small intestine. Their mechanism of action is incompletely understood; however, similar to the TSST-1 toxin of toxic shock syndrome (see Chapter 26), they generally behave as superantigens (see Chapter 16) binding to major histocompatibility complex (MHC) class II molecules, which results in T cell stimulation. Their effect on the central nervous system results in severe vomiting within 3–6 hours of consumption. Diarrhea is not a feature, and recovery within 24 hours is usual.

Up to 50% of *Staph. aureus* strains produce enterotoxin, and food (especially processed meats) is contaminated by human carriers. The bacteria grow at room temperature and release toxin. Subsequent heating may kill the organisms, but the toxin is stable. Often there are no viable organisms detectable in the food consumed, but enterotoxin can be detected by a latex agglutination test.

Botulism

Exotoxins produced by Cl. botulinum cause botulism

Botulism is a rare but serious disease caused by the exotoxin of *Cl. botulinum*. The organism is widespread in the environment, and spores can be isolated readily from soil samples and from various animals including fish. Seven serologically distinct toxins have been identified, but only four—A, B, E, and less frequently F—are associated with human disease. While not destroyed by digestive enzymes, the toxins are inactivated after 30 minutes at 80°C. The toxins are ingested in food (often canned or reheated) or produced in the gut after ingestion of the organism; they are absorbed from the gut into the bloodstream and then reach their site of action, the peripheral nerve synapses. The action of the toxin is to block neurotransmission (see Chapter 17).

Infant botulism is the most common form of botulism

There are three forms of botulism:

- foodborne botulism;
- infant botulism;
- wound botulism.

In foodborne botulism, toxin is elaborated by organisms in food, which is then ingested. In infant and wound botulism, the organisms are respectively ingested or implanted in a wound, and multiply and elaborate toxin in vivo. Infant botulism has been associated with feeding babies honey contaminated with *Cl. botulinum* spores.

The clinical disease is the same in all three forms and is characterized by flaccid paralysis leading to progressive muscle weakness and respiratory arrest. Intensive supportive treatment is urgently required, and complete recovery may take many months. Improvements in supportive care have reduced the mortality from around 70% to approximately 10%, but the disease, although rare, remains life-threatening. In addition, since botulinum toxin is one of the most potent biological toxins known to man, there is concern regarding its potential use as an agent of biowarfare.

Laboratory diagnosis of botulism involves injecting fecal and food samples into mice

Laboratory diagnosis depends largely upon demonstrating the presence of toxin by injecting samples of feces and food (if available) into mice that have been protected with botulinum antitoxin or left unprotected. Culture of feces or wound exudate for *Cl. botulinum* should also be performed. Because of bioterrorism concerns, current efforts are aimed at finding less time-consuming approaches to toxin detection, including polymerase chain reaction (PCR)-based assays for toxin sequences and ELISA (see Chapter 32) tests for functional toxin activity.

Polyvalent antitoxin is recommended as an adjunct to intensive supportive therapy for botulism

Since botulinum toxins are antigenic, they can be inactivated and used to produce antitoxin in animals. When botulism is suspected, antitoxin should be promptly administered along with supportive care, which may include mechanical ventilation (due to difficulty in breathing) and intravenous and nasogastric nutritional support (due to difficulty in swallowing). Antibiotics are generally used only for treatment of secondary infections.

It is not practicable to prevent food becoming contaminated with botulinum spores, so prevention of disease depends upon preventing the germination of spores in food by:

- maintaining food at an acid pH;
- storing food at less than 4°C;
- destroying toxin in food by heating for 30 minutes at 80°C.

HELICOBACTER PYLORI AND GASTRIC ULCER DISEASE

Helicobacter pylori is associated with most duodenal and gastric ulcers

It is now well established that the Gram-negative spiral bacterium *H. pylori* is associated with over 90% of duodenal ulcers and 70–80% of gastric ulcers (*Fig. 22.28*). *H. pylori* does not appear to play a role in gastroesophageal reflux disease (GERD) or non-ulcer dyspepsia, most commonly presenting with persistent or recurrent pain in the upper abdomen in the

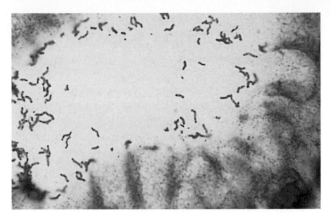

Fig. 22.28 *Helicobacter pylori* gastritis. Silver stain showing numerous spiral-shaped organisms adhering to the mucosal surface. (Courtesy of AM Geddes.)

absence of structural evidence of disease. Diagnosis is usually made on the basis of histologic examination of biopsy specimens, although the non-invasive urea breath test (*H. pylori* produces large amounts of urease) is the most rapid means of detecting the organism's presence. *H. pylori* can be cultured in the laboratory, but is difficult to grow.

The mechanism of pathogenicity is still being elucidated but involves a number of virulence factors including a cytotoxin, acid-inhibiting protein, adhesins, urease (which aids survival in the acidic environment) and other factors which disrupt the gastric mucosa. Eradication of *H. pylori* to promote the remission and healing of ulcers requires combination therapy such as a proton pump inhibitor and two antibiotics such as clarithromycin and amoxicillin (see Chapter 33). However, studies suggesting that *H. pylori* may actually provide protection from some esophageal and gastric cancers has led to active discussion regarding whether the organism should be eliminated from asymptomatic patients. The interrelationship between *H. pylori* and gastric disease is thus complex and remains to be further clarified.

PARASITES AND THE GASTROINTESTINAL TRACT

Many species of protozoan and worm parasites live in the gastrointestinal tract, infecting some 3.5 billions worldwide. Only a few are a frequent cause of serious pathology (*Fig. 22.29*) and these will form the focus of this part of the chapter.

Transmission of intestinal parasites is maintained by the release of lifecycle stages in feces

The different lifecycle stages include cysts, eggs and larvae. In most cases new infections depend either directly or indirectly upon contact with fecally derived material, infection rates therefore reflecting standards of hygiene and levels of sanitation. In general, the stages of protozoan parasites passed in feces are either already infective or become infective within a short time. These parasites are therefore usually acquired by swallowing infective stages in fecally contaminated food or water. Worm parasites, with two major exceptions (pinworm

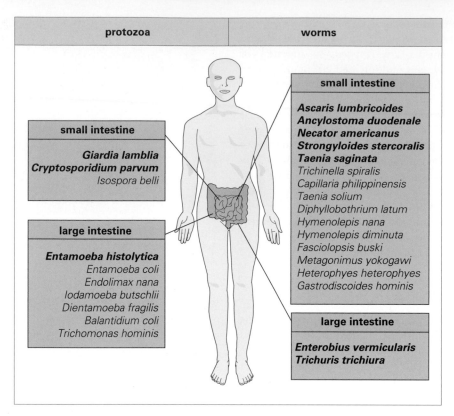

| protozoa | worms |

small intestine

Giardia lamblia
Cryptosporidium parvum
Isospora belli

large intestine

Entamoeba histolytica
Entamoeba coli
Endolimax nana
Iodamoeba butschlii
Dientamoeba fragilis
Balantidium coli
Trichomonas hominis

small intestine

Ascaris lumbricoides
Ancylostoma duodenale
Necator americanus
Strongyloides stercoralis
Taenia saginata
Trichinella spiralis
Capillaria philippinensis
Taenia solium
Diphyllobothrium latum
Hymenolepis nana
Hymenolepis diminuta
Fasciolopsis buski
Metagonimus yokogawi
Heterophyes heterophyes
Gastrodiscoides hominis

large intestine

Enterobius vermicularis
Trichuris trichiura

Fig. 22.29 Gastrointestinal parasites of man. The majority of these infections are found in developing countries, but all species also occur in the developed world and some have recently come to prominence because of their association with AIDS. The most important parasite species are highlighted in bold type.

and the dwarf tapeworm), produce eggs or larvae that require a period of development outside the host before they become infective. Transmission routes are more complex here:

- Some species are acquired through food or water contaminated with infective eggs or larvae, or are picked up directly via contaminated fingers.
- Some have larvae that can actively penetrate through the skin, migrating eventually to the intestine.
- Others are acquired by eating animals or animal products containing infective stages.

The symptoms of intestinal infection range from very mild, through acute or chronic diarrheal conditions associated with parasite-related inflammation, to life-threatening diseases caused by spread of the parasites into other organs of the body. Most infections fall into the first of these categories; indeed, in many parts of the world, intestinal parasitism is accepted as a normal condition of life.

Protozoan infections

Three species are of particular importance:

- *Entamoeba histolytica;*
- *Giardia lamblia;*
- *Cryptosporidium parvum.*

All three can give rise to diarrheal illnesses, but the organisms have distinctive features that allow a differential diagnosis to be made quite easily *(Fig. 22.30)*. Other more recently identified intestinal protozoans of concern, particularly in immune-suppressed patients, include *Cyclospora cayetanensis*, *Isospora belli* and the microsporidians.

Entamoeba histolytica

Entamoeba histolytica *infection is particularly common in subtropical and tropical countries*

For many years it was considered that infections with *E. histolytica* could be asymptomatic or pathogenic, with dysentery a key symptom when the amebae invaded the mucosa. A recent advance has been the discovery that two species are involved: *E. histolytica* being invasive and *E. dispar* being non-invasive. *E. histolytica* occurs worldwide, but is most often found in subtropical and tropical countries, where the prevalence may exceed 50%. The trophozoite stages of the amebae live in the large intestine on the mucosal surface. Reproduction of these stages is by simple binary fission, and there is periodic formation of resistant encysted forms, which pass out of the body. These cysts can survive in the external environment and act as the infective stages. Infection occurs when food or drink is contaminated either by infected food handlers or as a result of inadequate sanitation. Transmission can also take place as a result of anal sexual activity. The cysts pass intact through the stomach when swallowed and excyst in the small intestine, each giving rise to eight progeny. These adhere to the epithelial cells and damage them by phagocytosis and cytolysis. They can invade the mucosa and feed on host tissues including red blood cells, giving rise to amebic colitis.

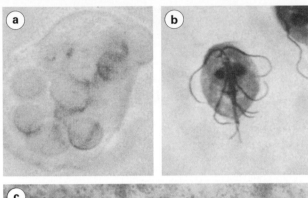

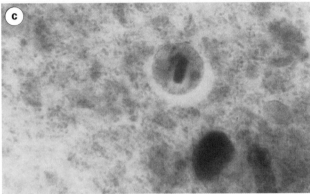

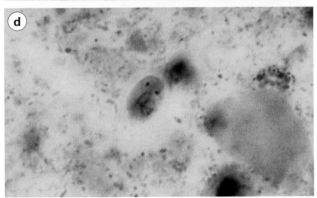

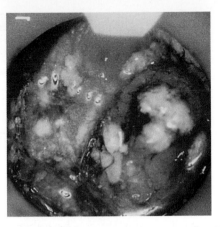

Fig. 22.31 Amebic colitis. Sigmoidoscopic view showing deep ulcers and overlying purulent exudate. (Courtesy of RH Gilman.)

FEATURES OF BACILLARY AND AMEBIC DYSENTERY		
	bacillary	**amebic**
organism	shigella	entameba
polymorphs and macrophages in stool	many	few
eosinophils and Charcot–Leydon crystals in stool	few or absent	often present
organisms in stool	many	few
blood and mucus in stool	yes	yes

Fig. 22.32 Features of bacillary and amebic dysentery.

Fig. 22.30 Protozoan infections of the gastrointestinal tract. (a) *Entamoeba histolytica*. Trophozoite found in the acute stage of the disease, which often contains ingested red blood cells. (b) *Giardia lamblia* trophozoite associated with acute infection in man. (Courtesy of DK Banerjee.) (c) Cyst of *E. histolytica*, with only one of the four nuclei visible. The broad chromatid bar is a semicrystalline aggregation of ribosomes. Hematoxylin and eosin stain. (d) Oval cyst of *G. lamblia* showing two of the four nuclei. Iron hematoxylin stain. (Courtesy of R Muller and JR Baker.)

E. histolytica *infection may cause mild diarrhea or severe dysentery*

Infections with *E. dispar* are asymptomatic. Invasion of the mucosa by *E. histolytica* may produce small localized superficial ulcers or involve the entire colonic mucosa with the formation of deep confluent ulcers *(Fig. 22.31)*. The former causes a mild diarrhea, whereas more severe invasion leads to 'amebic dysentery', which is characterized by mucus, pus and blood in the stools. Dysenteries of amebic and bacillary origin can be distinguished by a number of features *(Fig. 22.32)*.

Complications include perforation of the intestine, leading to peritonitis, and extraintestinal invasion. Trophozoites can spread via the blood to the liver, with the formation of an abscess, and may secondarily extend to the lung and other organs. Rarely, abscesses spread directly and involve the overlying skin.

E. histolytica *infection can be diagnosed in symptomatic patients from the presence of characteristic four-nucleate cysts in the stool*

These cysts may be infrequent in light infections, and repeated stool examination is necessary. Care must be taken to differentiate *E. histolytica* from other non-pathogenic species that might be present *(Fig. 22.33)*. Trophozoites can be found in cases of dysentery (when the stools are loose and wet), but they are fragile and deteriorate rapidly; specimens should therefore be preserved before examination. ELISA tests are available, as is a triage panel assay that can distinguish between *E. histolytica/E. dispar*, *Cryptosporidium parvum* and *Giardia lamblia*. Differentiation of *histolytica* and *dispar* requires immunological tests or PCR.

Entamoeba histolytica	Entamoeba coli	Endolimax nana	Iodamoeba bütschlii	red blood cell

Fig. 22.33 Characterisics of cysts (size and number of nuclei) are used to differentiate pathogenic from non-pathogenic protozoa. A red blood cell is shown for comparison.

Acute *E. histolytica* infection can be treated with metronidazole

Recovery from infection is usual, and there is some immunity to re-infection. Treatment may fail to clear the infection completely and the passage of infective cysts can continue. Metronidazole is useful against both the intestinal and extraintestinal sites of infection, but if the latter become secondarily infected with bacteria, additional antibiotics and drainage are necessary. Prevention of amebiasis in the community requires the same approaches to hygiene and sanitation as those adopted for bacterial infections of the intestine.

Giardia lamblia

Giardia was the first intestinal microorganism to be observed under a microscope. It was discovered by Anton van Leeuwenhoek in 1681, using the microscope he had invented to examine specimens of his own stool. It has a global distribution and at the present time is the most commonly diagnosed intestinal parasite in the USA.

Like *Entamoeba*, *Giardia* has only two lifecycle stages

The two lifecycle stages are the flagellate (four pairs of flagella) binucleate trophozoite and the resistant four-nucleate cyst. The trophozoites live in the upper portion of the small intestine, adhering closely to the brush border of the epithelial cells by specialized attachment regions (*Fig. 22.34*). They divide by binary fission and can occur in such numbers that they cover large areas of the mucosal surface. Cyst formation occurs at regular intervals, each cyst being formed as one trophozoite rounds up and produces a resistant wall. Cysts pass out in the stools and can survive for several weeks under optimum conditions. Infection occurs when the cysts are swallowed, usually as a result of drinking contaminated water. The minimum infective dose is very small: 10–25 cysts. Epidemics of giardiasis have occurred when public drinking supplies have become contaminated, but smaller outbreaks have been traced to drinking from rivers and streams that have been contaminated by wild animals. The genus *Giardia* is widely distributed in mammals, and there is suggestive evidence for cross-infection between certain animal hosts (e.g. beaver) and humans. Much of this is circumstantial, but case reports provide more direct evidence. Recent data suggest that *Giardia* may also be transmitted sexually.

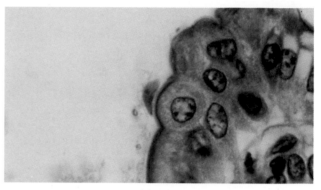

Fig. 22.34 Trophozoite of *Giardia lamblia* attached to the mucosal surface of the small intestine. (Iron hematoxylin stain.) (Courtesy of R Muller and JR Baker.)

Mild *Giardia* infections are asymptomatic, more severe infections cause diarrhea

The diarrhea may be:

- self-limiting, with 7–10 days being the usual course;
- chronic, and develop into a serious condition, particularly in patients with deficient or compromised immunologic defenses.

It is thought to arise from inflammatory responses triggered by the damaged epithelial cells and from interference with normal absorptive processes. Characteristically the stools are loose, foul-smelling and often fatty.

Diagnosis of *Giardia* infection is based on identifying cysts or trophozoites in the stool

Repeated examination is necessary in light infections, when concentration techniques improve the chances of finding cysts. Duodenal intubation or the use of recoverable swallowed capsules and threads may aid in obtaining trophozoites directly from the intestine. ELISA tests are available with good specificity.

Giardia infection can be treated with a variety of drugs

These include mepacrine hydrochloride, metronidazole and tinidazole, but none is completely successful. Community measures for prevention include the usual concerns with hygiene and sanitation, and improved treatment of drinking water supplies (largely filtration and chlorination) where these are suspected as a source. Care in drinking from potentially contaminated natural waters is also indicated.

Cryptosporidium parvum

Cryptosporidium parvum *is widely distributed in many animals*

Awareness of *Cryptosporidium parvum* as an important cause of diarrhea in humans was established during the early years of the AIDS epidemic, although similar parasites were known to be widely distributed in many animals. There are two major genotypes, one associated with human infection, one primarily with animals (including cattle), but cross-infection to humans does occur. The parasite has a complex lifecycle, going through both asexual and sexual phases of development in the same host. Transmission requires ingestion of a minimum of 10 or so of the resistant oocyst stage (4–5 mm diameter) in fecally contaminated material *(Fig. 22.35)*. In the small intestine the cyst releases infective sporozoites, which invade the epithelial cells, remaining closely associated with the apical plasma membrane. Here they form schizonts, which divide to release merozoites, and these then re-invade further epithelial cells. Eventually a sexual phase occurs and oocysts are released. Transmission probably occurs most often via drinking water contaminated by oocysts, either from other humans or from animals. In 1993, *C. parvum* caused a massive outbreak of watery diarrhea affecting 403 000 people in Milwaukee, USA. It was transmitted through the public water supply and probably originated from cattle.

C. parvum *diarrhea ranges from moderate to severe*

Symptoms of infection with *C. parvum* range from a moderate diarrhea to a more severe profuse diarrhea that is self-limiting in immunocompetent individuals (lasting 15–40 days), but can become chronic in immunocompromised patients. Cryptosporidiosis is a common infection in people with AIDS. In individuals with CD4+ T cell counts < 100/mm^3 diarrhea is prolonged, may become irreversible, and can be life-threatening.

Routine fecal examinations are inadequate for diagnosing C. parvum *diarrhea*

Concentration techniques and special staining (e.g. modified Ziehl–Neelsen stain) are necessary to recover and identify the

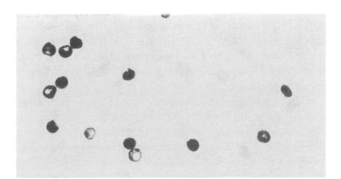

Fig. 22.35 *Cryptosporidium* oocysts in fecal specimen. (Courtesy of S Tzipori.)

oocysts. Direct immunofluorescence and ELISA tests can be used, and PCR is being developed.

Only immunocompromised patients need treatment for C. parvum *diarrhea*

Antiviral treatments improve the diarrhea in AIDS patients. The macrolide spiramycin has been used with limited success. Paromomycin and azithromycin reduced oocyst output but did not clear infection. Public health measures are similar to those outlined for controlling giardiasis, although *Cryptosporidium* is more resistant to chlorination.

Cyclospora, Isospora *and* Microsporidians

Cyclospora cayetanensis, identified in 1994, is now recognized as a cause of traveler's diarrhea. It can also be acquired from contaminated imported food; for example, Guatemalan raspberries were thought to be the cause of an outbreak in the USA in 1997. Birds may act as an important source of infection. Diarrhea can be prolonged and is severe in immune-suppressed individuals. Trimethoprim–sulfamethoxazole (co-trimoxazole) is effective. *Isospora belli*, like *Cyclospora* and *Cryptosporidium*, is a coccidian parasite, whose lifecycle stages take place in epithelial cells of the mucosa. AIDS patients may show particularly severe symptoms, persistent diarrhea causing weight loss and even death. Infections with microsporidia (an unusual group) have also become recognized as a cause of diarrhea in AIDS and other immune-suppressed patients. *Enterozoon bieneusi* is the commonest cause, although *Encephalitozoon intestinalis* also occurs. Transmission appears to be direct. Albendazole and metronidazole have been used successfully to treat infections.

'Minor' intestinal protozoans

The human intestine may harbour a large number of protozoa, many of which appear to be quite harmless *(Fig. 22.29)*. Some have a questionable role in disease—these include *Balantidium coli*, *Blastocystis hominis*, *Dientamoeba fragilis*, *Sarcocystis hominis*.

Worm infections

The most important intestinal worms clinically are the nematodes known as 'soil-transmitted helminths'

Soil-transmitted helminths fall into two distinct groups:

- *Ascaris lumbricoides* (large roundworm) and *Trichuris trichiura* (whipworm), in which infection occurs by swallowing the infective eggs;
- *Ancylostoma duodenale* and *Necator americanus* (hookworms) and *Strongyloides stercoralis*, which infect by active skin penetration by infective larvae, that then undertake a systemic migration through the lungs to the intestine.

With the exception of *Trichuris* (large intestine), all inhabit the small bowel.

The pinworm or threadworm *Enterobius vermicularis* is perhaps the commonest intestinal nematode in developed countries and is the least pathogenic. The females of this species, which live in the large bowel, release infective eggs onto the perianal skin. This causes itching, and transmission usually occurs directly from contaminated fingers, but the eggs are also light enough to be carried in dust.

The soil-transmitted helminths are commonest in the warmer developing countries. About one quarter of the world's population carry these worms, children being the most heavily infected section of the population. Transmission is favored where there is inadequate disposal of feces, contamination of water supplies, use of feces (night-soil) as fertilizer, or low standards of hygiene (see below). Vast numbers of eggs are released by each female (tens of thousands by *Trichuris* and *Ancylostoma* and hundreds of thousands by *Ascaris*).

Lifecycle and transmission

Female Ascaris and Trichuris *lay thick-shelled eggs in the intestine, which are expelled with feces and hatch after being swallowed by another host*

The thick-shelled eggs of *Ascaris* and *Trichuris* are shown in *Figure 22.36*. The eggs require incubation for several days at optimum conditions (warm temperature, high humidity) for the infective larvae to develop. Once this occurs, the eggs remain infective for many weeks or months, depending upon the local microclimate. After being swallowed the eggs hatch in the intestine, releasing the larvae. Those of *Ascaris* penetrate the gut wall and are carried in the blood through the liver to the lungs, climbing up the bronchi and trachea before being swallowed and once again reaching the intestine. The adult worms live freely in the gut lumen, feeding on intestinal contents. In contrast *Trichuris* larvae remain within the large bowel, penetrating into the epithelial cell layer, where they remain as they mature.

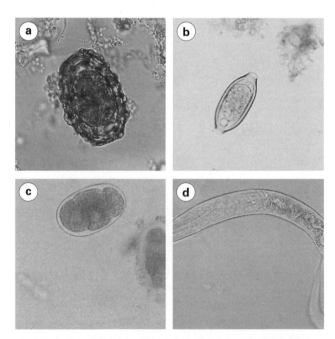

Fig. 22.36 Eggs and larvae of intestinal nematodes passed in feces. (a) Egg of *Ascaris* (fertile). (b) Egg of *Trichuris*. (c) Egg of hookworm. The ovum continues to divide in the fecal sample and may be at the 16- or 32-cell stage by the time the sample is examined. (d) Larva of *Strongyloides stercoralis*. (Courtesy of JH Cross.)

Adult female hookworms lay thin-shelled eggs that hatch in the feces shortly after leaving the host

A hookworm egg is shown in *Figure 22.36*. The larvae of these hookworms (*A. duodenale* and *N. americanus*) feed on bacteria until infective, and then migrate away from the fecal mass. Infection takes place when larvae come into contact with unprotected skin (or additionally, in the case of *Ancylostoma*, are swallowed). They penetrate the skin, migrate via the blood to the lungs, climb the trachea and are swallowed. Adult worms attach by their enlarged mouths to the intestinal mucosa, ingest a plug of tissue, rupture capillaries and suck blood.

The adult female Strongyloides *lays eggs that hatch in the intestine*

The lifecycle of *Strongyloides* is similar to that of hookworms, but shows some important differences. The adult worm exists as a parthenogenetic female that lays eggs into the mucosa. These eggs hatch in the intestine and the released larvae usually pass out in the feces (*Fig. 22.36*). Development outside the host can follow the hookworm pattern, with the direct production of skin-penetrating larvae or may be diverted into the production of a complete free-living generation, which then produces infective larvae. Under certain conditions, and particularly when the host is immunocompromised, *Strongyloides* larvae can reinvade before they are voided in the feces. This process of autoinfection can give rise to the severe clinical condition known as 'disseminated strongyloidiasis'. All soil-transmitted helminths are relatively long-lived (several months to years), but authenticated cases show that *Strongyloides* infections can persist for more than 30 years, presumably through continuous internal autoinfection.

Clinical features

In most individuals, worm infections produce chronic mild intestinal discomfort rather than severe diarrhea or other conditions. Infections may lead to hypersensitivity responses and can also reduce responses to vaccination. Each parasite has a number of characteristic pathologic conditions linked with it.

Large numbers of adult Ascaris *worms can cause intestinal obstruction*

The migration of *Ascaris* larvae through the lungs can cause severe respiratory distress (pneumonitis), and this stage is often associated with pronounced eosinophilia. Intestinal stages of infection can cause abdominal pain, nausea and digestive disturbances. In children with a suboptimal nutritional intake these disturbances can contribute to clinical malnutrition. Large numbers of adult worms can cause a physical blockage in the intestine, and this may also occur as worms die following chemotherapy. Intestinal worms tend to migrate out of the intestine, often up the bile duct, causing cholangitis. Perforation of the intestinal wall can also occur. Worms have occasionally been reported in unusual locations, including the orbit of the eye and the (male) urethra. *Ascaris* is highly allergenic, and infections often give rise to symptoms of hypersensitivity which may persist for many years after the infection has been cleared.

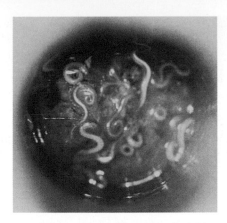

Fig. 22.37 Trichuriasis in a healthy, infected, child. Proctoscopic view showing numerous adult *Trichuris trichiura* attached to the intestinal mucosa. (Courtesy of RH Gilman.)

Moderate to severe Trichuris *infection can cause a chronic diarrhea*

As with all intestinal worms, children are the members of the community most heavily infected with *Trichuris*. Although usually regarded as of little clinical significance, recent research has shown that moderate to heavy infections in children can cause a chronic diarrhea *(Fig. 22.37)*, reflected in impaired nutrition and retarded growth. Occasionally, heavy infections lead to prolapse of the rectum.

Hookworm disease can result in an iron-deficiency anemia

Invasion of hookworm larvae through the skin and lungs can cause a dermatitis and pneumonitis, respectively. The blood-feeding activities of the intestinal worms can lead to an iron-deficiency anemia if the diet is inadequate. Heavy infections cause a marked debility and growth retardation.

Strongyloidiasis can be fatal in immunosuppressed people

Heavy intestinal infection with *Strongyloidiasis* causes a persistent and profuse diarrhea with dehydration and electrolyte imbalance. Profound mucosal changes can also lead to a malabsorption syndrome, which is sometimes confused with tropical sprue. People with diseases that suppress immune function, such as AIDS and cancer, or who are being treated with immunosuppressant drugs, are susceptible to the development of disseminated strongyloidiasis. Invasion of the body by many thousands of autoinfective larvae can be fatal.

The commonest sign of pinworm (threadworm) infection is anal pruritus. Occasionally this is accompanied by mild diarrhea. Migrating worms sometimes invade the appendix and have been linked with appendicitis. Invasion of the vagina has been reported in female children.

Laboratory diagnosis

All five of the soil-transmitted species can be diagnosed by finding eggs or larvae in the fresh stool, and direct smears or concentration techniques can be used. Immunodiagnosis of

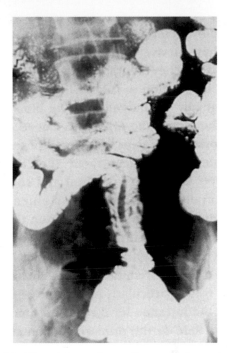

Fig. 22.38 Filling defect in the small intestine due to the presence of *Ascaris*, seen on a radiograph after a barium meal. (Courtesy of W Peters.)

intestinal parasites is still at an early stage. Infections with *Ascaris*, hookworms and *Strongyloides* are often accompanied by a marked blood eosinophilia. Although this is not diagnostic, it is a strong indicator of worm infection.

The eggs of Ascaris, Trichuris *and hookworms are characteristic*

These eggs are shown in *Figure 22.36* and are easily recognizable. Identification of the species of hookworm requires culture of the stool to allow the eggs to hatch and the larvae to mature into the infective third stage. The presence of adult *Ascaris* can sometimes be confirmed directly by radiography *(Fig. 22.38)*.

The presence of larvae in fresh stools is diagnostic of *Strongyloides* infection.

Pinworm infection is diagnosed by finding eggs on perianal skin

Although adult pinworms sometimes appear in the stools, the eggs are seldom seen because they are laid directly onto the perianal skin *(Fig. 22.39)*. They can be found by wiping this area with a piece of clear adhesive tape (the 'Scotch tape' test) and examining the tape under the microscope.

Treatment and prevention

A variety of anthelmintic drugs is available for treating intestinal nematodes. Piperazine has been used with great success against *Ascaris*, hookworms and pinworm, though many more recent drugs (albendazole, mebendazole, levamisole, pyrantel) can also be used and are also effective against trichuriasis and strongyloidiasis (especially albendazole and levamisole). At the community level, prevention can be

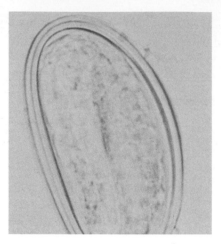

Fig. 22.39 Egg of *Enterobius* on perianal skin. (Courtesy of JH Cross.)

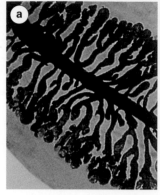

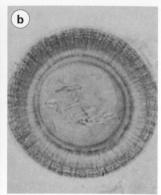

Fig. 22.40 *Taenia saginata*. (a) Gravid proglottids stained with India ink to show numerous side branches. (b) Egg containing six-hooked (hexacanth) larva. (Courtesy of R Muller and JR Baker.)

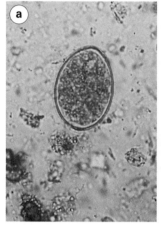

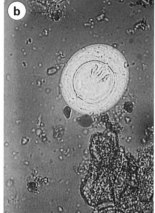

Fig. 22.41 Eggs of (a) *Diphyllobothrium latum* and (b) *Hymenolepis nana*. (Courtesy of R Muller and JR Baker.)

achieved through improved hygiene and sanitation, making sure that fecal material is disposed of properly.

Other intestinal worms

Many other worm species can infect the intestine, but most are uncommon in developed countries

Of the human tapeworms:

- The beef tapeworm *Taenia saginata*, transmitted through infected beef, is the most widely distributed. However, infection is usually asymptomatic, apart from the nausea felt on passing the large segments! Diagnosis involves finding these segments or the characteristic eggs in the stool *(Fig. 22.40)*.
- *Diphyllobothrium latum*, the broadfish tapeworm, is widely distributed geographically, but infection is restricted to individuals eating raw or undercooked fish carrying the infective larvae. The eggs of this species have a terminal 'lid' and are the diagnostic stage in the stool *(Fig. 22.41)*.
- *Hymenolepis nana*, the dwarf tapeworm, occurs primarily in children, infection occurring directly by swallowing eggs *(Fig. 22.41)*. This worm has the ability to undergo autoinfection within the host's intestine, so that a large number of worms can build up rapidly, leading to diarrhea and some abdominal discomfort.

All these tapeworms can be removed by praziquantel or niclosamide.

Intestinal symptoms (predominantly diarrhea and abdominal pain) are also associated with infections by the nematode *Trichinella spiralis*, which is better known clinically for the pathology caused by the bloodborne muscle phase (see Chapters 26 and 28). Infection with the two species of schistosome associated with mesenteric blood vessels (*Schistosoma japonicum* and *S. mansoni*) can also cause symptoms of intestinal disease. As the eggs pass through the intestinal wall they cause marked inflammatory responses, granulomatous lesions form, and diarrhea may occur in the early acute phase. Heavy chronic *S. mansoni* infection is associated with inflammatory polyps in the colon, while severe involvement of the small bowel is more common with *S. japonicum*.

SYSTEMIC INFECTION INITIATED IN THE GASTROINTESTINAL TRACT

We opened this chapter by noting that infections acquired by the ingestion of pathogens could remain localized in the gastrointestinal tract or could disseminate to other organs and body systems. Important examples of disseminated infection are the enteric fevers and viral hepatitis types A and E. Listeriosis also appears to be acquired via the gastrointestinal tract. For the sake of clarity and convenience, other types of viral hepatitis will also be discussed in this chapter.

Enteric fevers: typhoid and paratyphoid

The term 'enteric fever' was introduced in the last century in an attempt to clarify the distinction between typhus (see Chapter 27) and typhoid. For many years these two diseases had been confused, as the common root of their names suggests (typhus, a fever with delirium; typhoid, resembling typhus), but even before the causative agents were isolated (typhoid caused by *S. typhi* and typhus caused by *Rickettsia* spp.), it was pointed out that it was 'just as impossible to confuse the intestinal lesions of typhoid with the pathologic findings of typhus as it was to confuse the eruptions of measles with the pustules of smallpox'. In fact, enteric fevers can be caused by *S. typhi* and three additional salmonella species, but the name 'typhoid' has stuck.

S. typhi, *and paratyphi types* S. paratyphi A, S. schottmuelleri *(previously named* S. paratyphi B), *and* S. hirshfeldii *(previously named* S. paratyphi C) *cause enteric fevers*

These species of *Salmonella* are restricted to humans and do not have a reservoir in animals. Therefore, spread of the infection is from person to person, usually through contaminated food or water. After infection, people can carry the organism for months or years, providing a continuing source from which others may become infected. Typhoid Mary, a cook in New York City in the early 1900s, is one such example. She was a long-term carrier who succeeded in initiating at least 10 outbreaks of the disease.

The salmonellae multiply within, and are transported around, the body in macrophages

After ingestion, the salmonellae that survive the antibacterial defenses of the stomach and small intestine penetrate the gut mucosa through the Peyer's patches, probably in the jejunum or distal ileum *(Fig. 22.42)*. Once through the mucosal barrier, the bacteria reach the intestinal lymph nodes, where they survive and multiply within macrophages (see *Fig. 15.5*). They are transported in the macrophages to the mesenteric lymph nodes and thence to the thoracic duct and are eventually discharged into the bloodstream. Circulating in the blood, the organisms can seed many organs, most importantly in areas where cells of the reticuloendothelial system are concentrated (i.e. the spleen, bone marrow, liver and Peyer's patches). In the liver they multiply in Kupffer cells. From the reticuloendothelial system the bacteria reinvade the blood to reach other organs (e.g. kidney). The gallbladder is infected either from the blood or from the liver via the biliary tract, the bacterium being particularly resistant to bile. As a result *S. typhi* enters the intestine for a second time in much larger numbers than on the primary encounter and causes a strong inflammatory response in Peyer's patches, leading to ulceration, with the danger of intestinal perforation.

Rose spots on the upper abdomen are characteristic, but absent in up to half of patients with enteric fever

After an incubation period of 10–14 days (range 7–21 days), the disease has an insidious onset with non-specific symptoms of fever and malaise accompanied by aches and respiratory symptoms, and may resemble a flu-like illness (see Chapter 15). Diarrhea may be present, but constipation is just as likely. At this stage the patient often presents with a fever of unknown origin (FUO; see Chapter 29). In the absence of treatment the fever increases and the patient becomes acutely ill. Rose spots—erythematous maculopapular lesions that blanch on pressure *(Fig. 22.43)*—are characteristic on the upper abdomen, but may be absent in up to half of patients. They are transient and disappear within hours to days. Without treatment, an uncomplicated infection lasts 4–6 weeks.

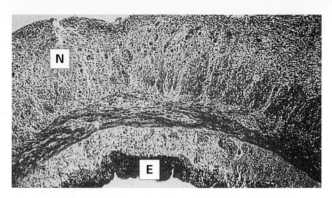

Fig. 22.42 Typhoid. Section of ileum showing a typhoid ulcer with a transmural inflammatory reaction, focal areas of necrosis (N) and a fibrinous exudate (E) on the serosal surface. (Hematoxylin and eosin stain.) (Courtesy of MSR Hutt.)

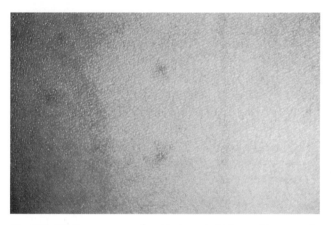

Fig. 22.43 Rose spots on the skin in typhoid fever. (Courtesy of WE Farrar.)

Before antibiotics, 12–16% of patients with enteric fever died, usually of complications

The complications can be classified into:

- those secondary to the local gastrointestinal lesions (e.g. hemorrhage and perforation; *Fig. 22.44*);
- those associated with toxemia (e.g. myocarditis, hepatic and bone marrow damage);
- those secondary to a prolonged serious illness;
- those resulting from multiplication of the organisms in other sites, causing meningitis, osteomyelitis or endocarditis.

Before antibiotics became available, 12–16% of patients died, usually of complications occurring in the third or fourth week of the disease. Relapse after an initial recovery was also common.

1–3% of patients with enteric fever become chronic carriers

Patients usually continue to excrete *S. typhi* in the feces for several weeks after recovery, and 1–3% become chronic carriers, which is defined as *S. typhi* excretion in feces or urine for 1 year after infection. Chronic carriage is more common in women, in older patients and in those with underlying disease of the gallbladder (e.g. stones) or urinary bladder (e.g. schistosomiasis).

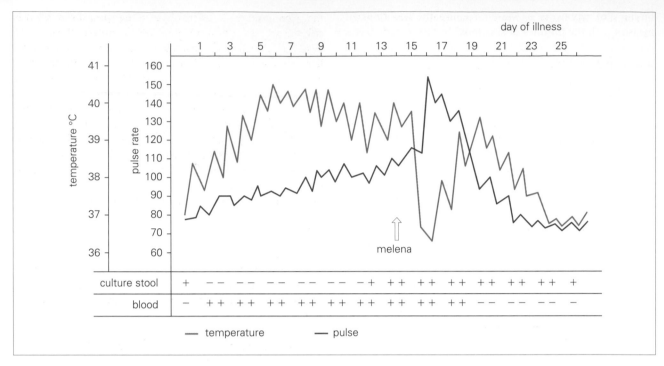

Fig. 22.44 The clinical course of typhoid fever. Chart of temperature, pulse rate and bacteriologic findings in a patient whose illness was complicated by massive hemorrhage. (Courtesy of HL DuPont.)

Diagnosis of enteric fever depends upon isolating S. typhi or paratyphi types using selective media

Diagnosis cannot be made on clinical grounds alone, although the presence of rose spots in a febrile patient is highly suggestive. Samples of blood, feces and urine should be cultured on selective media. An antibody response to infection can be detected by an agglutination test (Widal test), but non-specific cross-reaction with other enterobacteria may also cause an increase in H and O antibody levels. Interpretation of the results is complicated and depends upon a knowledge of the normal antibody titers in the population and whether the patient has been vaccinated. A demonstration of a rising titer between acute and convalescent phase sera is more useful than examination of a single sample. At best the results confirm the microbiologic diagnosis, at worst they are misleading.

Antibiotic treatment should be commenced as soon as enteric fever is diagnosed

Ciprofloxacin or ceftriaxone followed by cefixime have been effectively used in antimicrobial chemotherapy, which should continue for at least 1 week after the patient's temperature has returned to normal. Some antibiotics appear active in vitro, but do not achieve a clinical cure, presumably because they do not reach the bacteria in their intracellular location. Isolates of *S. typhi* resistant to a variety of antimicrobial agents have been reported.

Prevention of enteric fever involves public health measures, treating carriers and vaccination

Breaking the chain of spread of infection from person to person depends upon good personal hygiene, adequate sewage disposal and a clean water supply. These conditions exist in the developed world, where outbreaks of enteric fever are rare but still occur.

Typhoid carriers are a public health concern and should be excluded from employment involving food handling. Every effort should be made to eradicate carriage by antibiotic treatment, and if this is unsuccessful, removal of the gallbladder (the most common site of carriage) should be considered.

A single-dose injectable vaccine (Typhim Vi) which contains capsular polysaccharide antigen and an oral, live-attenuated, vaccine (strain Ty21a) are available and recommended for travelers to developing countries. However, with both vaccines protection is complete in only 50–80% of recipients.

Listeriosis

Listeria infection is associated with pregnancy and reduced immunity

Listeria monocytogenes is a Gram-positive coccobacillus that is widespread among animals and in the environment. It is becoming increasingly recognized as a foodborne pathogen, associated particularly with uncooked foods such as paté, contaminated milk, soft cheeses and coleslaw. Studies of cases involving unpasteurized milk suggest that fewer than one thousand organisms may cause disease, and the ability of the organism to multiply, albeit slowly, at refrigeration temperatures allows an infective dose to accumulate in goods stored in this way. Even then, the population at risk appears to primarily be:

- pregnant women, with the possibility of infection of the baby in the uterus or during birth;
- immunocompromised people;
- cancer patients (especially those with leukemia).

The disease usually presents as meningitis (see Chapter 24).

Viral hepatitis

An alphabetical litany of viruses directly target the liver, from hepatitis A to E

Hepatitis means inflammation and damage to the liver, and has differing etiologies including non-infectious multi-systemic conditions and drug toxicity as well as infectious agents. The latter include viruses and less commonly bacteria (e.g. *Leptospira* spp.), and other microorganisms. There is a broad spectrum of clinical illness ranging from asymptomatic, symptomatic with malaise, anorexia, nausea, abdominal pain and jaundice, to acute life-threatening liver failure, which is rare. Jaundice is a clinical term for the yellow tinge to the skin, sclera and mucous membranes. This is a result of liver cell damage which means that the liver cannot transport bilirubin into the bile, causing increased bilirubin levels in the body fluids. More than half of the liver must be damaged or destroyed before liver function fails. Regeneration of liver cells is rapid, but fibrous repair, especially when infection persists, can lead to permanent damage called cirrhosis. Cirrhosis results in a small, shrunken liver with poor function.

At least six different viruses are referred to as hepatitis viruses (*Fig. 22.45*), and generally they cannot be distinguished clinically. However, hepatitis A and E viruses are transmitted by the fecal–oral route and do not result in a carrier state; both infections resolve. In contrast, hepatitis B, D (delta), and C are transmitted by similar routes involving blood-contaminated equipment, although sexual transmission of hepatitis B is much more common than in hepatitis C, and all can lead to chronic carriage. Some agents have been reported

that were thought to be involved in the spectrum of what is referred to as non-A-to-E hepatitis. However, there is no evidence that the GB, hepatitis G and TT viruses infect the liver directly, the liver being affected as a bystander. Other viruses also cause hepatitis as part of a disease syndrome and are dealt with in other chapters. Dramatic elevations of serum aminotransferase concentration (alanine aminotransferase, ALT; aspartate aminotransferase, AST) are characteristic of acute viral hepatitis. Specific laboratory tests for hepatitis A, B, D, C and E viruses have been available for some years. With the exception of hepatitis A and B there are no licensed vaccines, and specific antiviral treatments with and without immunomodulators are available for hepatitis B and C.

Hepatitis A

This disease is caused by a single-stranded unenveloped RNA virus referred to as hepatitis A virus (HAV) and has been reclassified into its own genus *Hepatovirus* in the *Picornaviridae* family. There is only one serotype, and the virus is endemic worldwide.

HAV is transmitted by the fecal–oral route

Virus is excreted in large amounts in feces (10^8 infectious doses/g) and spreads from person to person by close contact (hands), by intimate contact (anal intercourse) or by contamination of food or water. The incubation period between infection and illness is 3–5 weeks, with a mean of 4 weeks; virus is present in feces 1–2 weeks before symptoms appear and during the first week (sometimes also the second and third week) of the illness. Person to person transmission can lead to outbreaks in places such as schools and camps, and viral contamination of water or food is a common source

VIRAL HEPATITIS					
virus	virus classification	type of virus	mode of infection	incubation period	other comments
hepatitis A (HAV)	Hepatovirus	ssRNA	fecal–oral	2–4 weeks	no carrier state
hepatitis B (HBV)	Hepadnavirus	dsDNA	blood-borne, sexual	6 weeks–6 months	carriage associated with liver cancer
hepatitis C (HCV)	Flavivirus	ssRNA	blood-borne,	2 months	carriage associated with liver cancer
hepatitis D (HDV)	Deltavirus	ssRNA	from blood	2–12 weeks	needs concurrent hepatitis B virus infection
hepatitis E (HEV)	Calicivirus	ssRNA	fecal–oral	6–8 weeks	common in Far East, no carrier state
yellow fever	Flavivirus	ssRNA	mosquito	3–6 days	no person-to-person spread, no carrier state

Fig. 22.45 The main viruses causing hepatitis in humans. Other viruses causing hepatitis include Epstein–Barr virus (mild hepatitis in 15% of infected adults and adolescents), cytomegalovirus and rarely herpes simplex virus, while intrauterine infection with rubella or cytomegalovirus causes hepatitis in the newborn. (ds, double-stranded; ss, single-stranded.)

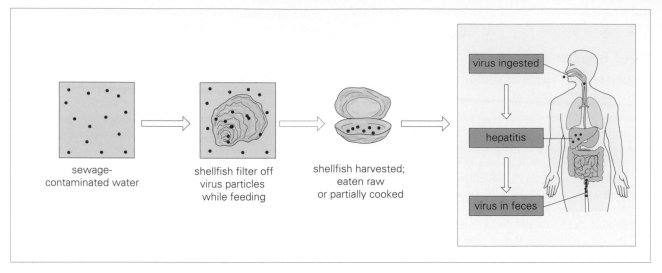

Fig. 22.46 Contamination of shellfish by hepatitis A virus (HAV) can lead to human infection.

of infection *(Fig. 22.46)*. In developing countries up to 90% of children have been infected by 5 years of age, whereas in developed countries up to 20% of young adults have been infected. The latter figure used to be higher but is mostly a result of improved sanitation and less overcrowding.

Clinically, hepatitis A is milder in young children than in older children and adults

After infection, the virus enters the blood from unknown sites in the gastrointestinal tract, where it may replicate. It then infects liver cells, passing into the biliary tract to reach the intestine and appears in feces *(Fig. 22.47)*. Relatively small amounts of virus enter the blood at this stage. Events during the rather lengthy incubation period are poorly understood, but liver cells are damaged, possibly by a direct viral action. Common clinical manifestations are fever, anorexia, nausea and vomiting; jaundice is more common in adults. The illness generally has a more sudden onset than hepatitis B. The best laboratory method for diagnosis is to detect HAV-specific IgM antibody in serum.

Pooled human normal immunoglobulin contains antibody to HAV and will prevent or attenuate infection if given as pre- or post-exposure prophylaxis. There is no antiviral therapy, but an effective formaldehyde-inactivated vaccine is now available which should be offered to a number of groups at particular risk of infection. These include travelers to HAV endemic countries, sewage workers, child daycare center staff, institutional care workers, male homosexuals, and individuals with chronic liver disease. The vaccine could also replace the immunoglobulin preparation in the post-exposure setting.

 ### Hepatitis E

Hepatitis E virus (HEV) spreads by the fecal–oral route

This disease, also known as enteric non-A–non-B hepatitis, is caused by a small single-stranded RNA virus, and shares similarities with the caliciviruses. The virus is excreted in feces and spreads by the fecal–oral route. Although uncommon in developed countries, it occurs as a waterborne infection in

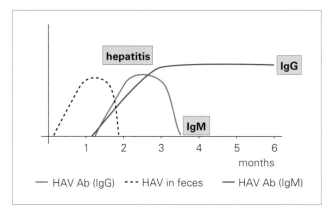

Fig. 22.47 The clinical and virologic course of HAV. (Ab, antibody.)

India and may be responsible for 50% of cases of sporadic hepatitis in developing countries. HEV has been identified in a variety of animals, and it is thought that they might be a reservoir for infection. Hepatitis E may therefore be another example of a zoonotic infection. The incubation period is 6–8 weeks. The disease is generally mild, but is severe in pregnant women, with a high mortality, up to 20% during the third trimester, due to fulminant hepatitis. The virus is eliminated from the body on recovery and there are no carriers. The diagnosis is made using serological tests to detect HEV-specific IgM. There is no vaccine.

Hepatitis B

This disease is caused by hepatitis B virus (HBV), a hepadna (hepatitis DNA) virus (see Appendix and panel) containing a partially double-stranded circular DNA genome and three important antigens: HB surface antigen, HB core antigen and HBe antigen *(Figs 22.48 and 22.49)*. HBe antigen is a soluble component secreted by the virus core, is expressed on the hepatocyte surface, and is targeted by the host immune system. Infection with a given strain of HBV confers resistance to all strains, but antigenic variation occurs. The four serological subtypes (adw, adr, ayw and ayr) have been superseded

LESSONS IN MICROBIOLOGY

Hepatitis A

In August 1988 the Florida Department of Health and Rehabilitation Services traced 61 people who had suffered serologically confirmed infection with HAV. These individuals resided in five different states, but 59 of them had eaten raw oysters from the same growing areas in Bay County coastal waters. The oysters had been gathered illegally from outside the approved harvesting areas and were contaminated with HAV. The mean incubation period of the disease was 29 days (range 16–48 days). Probable sources of fecal contamination near the oyster beds included boats with inappropriate sewage disposal systems and discharge from a local sewage treatment plant that contained a high concentration of fecal coliforms.

Hepadnaviruses

Hepadnaviruses are also found in woodchucks, ground squirrels and Pekin ducks. In each case the infection persists in the body, with HBsAg-like particles in the blood and chronic hepatitis and liver cancer as sequelae. These viruses often infect non-hepatic cells. In northeast USA for instance, 30% of woodchucks carry their own type of hepadnavirus and most develop liver cancer by later life. The virus replicates not only in liver cells, but also in lymphoid cells in the spleen, peripheral blood and thymus and in pancreatic acinar cells and bile duct epithelium.

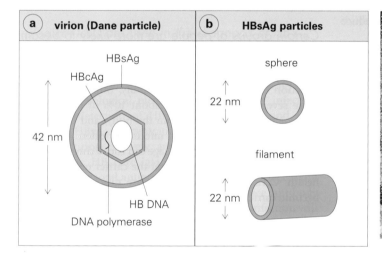

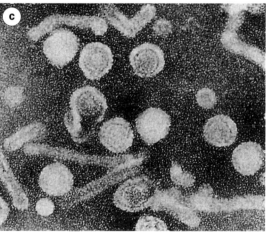

Fig. 22.48 During acute infection and in some carriers there are 10^6–10^7 infectious (Dane) particles/ml of serum (a), and as many as 10^{12} HB surface antigen (HBsAg) particles/ml (b). (c) Electron micrograph showing Dane particles and HBsAg particles. (Courtesy of JD Almeida.)

by the genetic classification in which the genotypes A to F have been determined. These may influence the clinical outcome of infection, response to antiviral treatment, and are useful in epidemiologic studies.

HB surface antigen can be found in blood and other body fluids

HBV can be transmitted by various routes, including:

- sexual intercourse;
- vertically from mother to child (intrauterine, peri- and postnatal infection; see Chapter 23);
- via blood and blood products, blood contaminated needles and equipment which may be used by injecting drug users;

- in association with tattooing, bodypiercing and acupuncture, again due to reusing needles which may be contaminated by blood.

Transmission has been reported in healthcare settings such as hemodialysis units because of contaminated hemodialysis equipment. This has been reduced dramatically since the introduction of regular HB surface antigen (HBsAg) monitoring of patients and disposable dialysis cartridges. In addition, incidents have been reported involving HBV transmission from hepatitis B carrier healthcare workers (HCWs) to their patients while carrying out exposure-prone procedures, such as cardiothoracic surgery, due to intraoperative needle-stick injuries resulting in blood-to-blood contact. Hepatitis B immunization and HBsAg screening of HCWs, and HBV DNA

QUESTIONS

A 24-year-old astrologer with a history of intravenous drug misuse sees his doctor because he has felt tired and unwell for the past few weeks. He has noticed that his urine is very dark, he feels nauseated, and does not feel like eating, and he has developed right-sided abdominal discomfort. A friend thinks that he looks 'yellow'. On examination he is tattooed, has yellow sclerae, and is tender in the right upper quadrant of his abdomen. His liver is enlarged, firm and smooth. The results of investigations, including the liver function tests are: AST, 1200 IU/l; ALT, 1000 IU/l; ALP, 100 IU/l; bilirubin, 60 mmol/l.

1. What is the most likely diagnosis and what is the differential diagnosis of a viral hepatitis in this setting?

2. What investigations would you perform?

3. How would you manage this man?

4. What other factors are important regarding the control of infection?

An 11-month-old baby girl is admitted to the pediatric unit with a 2-day history of fever, vomiting and copious watery diarrhea. She was a full-term normal delivery and has two siblings, one of whom had a mild diarrheal illness that cleared up 4 days earlier.

On examination she is unwell, mildly dehydrated, and febrile with a temperature of 38°C. Her abdomen is soft, and there are no other findings of note.

1. What would be your immediate management of this baby?

2. What viral causes of diarrhea are most likely?

3. How would a viral infection be diagnosed?

4. What is the natural course of the infection?

FURTHER READING

Blaser MJ, Ravdin JI, Guerrant RL et al. *Infections of the Gastrointestinal Tract.* Baltimore: Lippincott Williams and Wilkins, 1995.

Farthing MJ, Wakelin D, Keusch GT. *Enteric Infection: Intestinal Helminths*, vol. 2. London: Chapman and Hall, 1995.

Lauer G, Walker BD. Hepatitis C virus infection. *N Engl J Med* 2001; 345:41–52.

Mahoney FJ. Update on diagnosis, management, and prevention of hepatitis B virus infection. *Clin Microbiol Rev* 1999; 12:351–66.

Paradise LJ, Friedman H, Bendinelli M. *Enteric Infections and Immunity.* Dordrecht: Kluwer Academic, 1996.

Surawica CF, Owen R. *Gastrointestinal and Hepatic Infections.* Philadelphia: WB Saunders, 1995.

INTRODUCTION

During pregnancy a novel set of potentially susceptible tissues appear, including the fetus, the placenta and the lactating mammary glands. The placenta acts as an effective barrier, protecting the fetus from most circulating microorganisms, and the fetal membranes shield the fetus from microorganisms in the genital tract. Perforation of the amniotic sac, for instance, at a late stage of pregnancy, often results in fetal infection.

During pregnancy certain infections in the mother can be more severe than usual (malaria, hepatitis) or reactivate (HSV, CMV, polyomaviruses), and after delivery the raw uterine tissue is susceptible to streptococcal and other pathogens, causing puerperal sepsis.

The fetus, once infected via the placenta, is highly susceptible, but may survive certain pathogens and develop congenital abnormalities (rubella, CMV, *Toxoplasma gondii*, *Treponema pallidum*). Bacteria from the vagina (e.g. group B streptococci) can cause neonatal septicemia, meningitis and death, and a birth canal infected with *Neisseria gonorrhoeae* or *Chlamydia trachomatis* inoculates the infant to cause neonatal conjunctivitis. Maternal genital HSV infection can cause more serious neonatal disease and is probably underreported.

Maternal HIV infection often causes abortion, prematurity and low birth weight, and up to 40% of infants are infected in resource poor countries or where maternal infection is undiagnosed, about a third in utero and two thirds perinatally from maternal blood or milk. Maternal blood may also transmit hepatitis B and C, and milk can be a source of HTLV (human T cell lymphotropic virus types 1 and 2).

Here we describe infections that occur during pregnancy and around the time of birth, and discuss their effects on the mother, the fetus and the neonate.

INFECTIONS OCCURRING IN PREGNANCY

Immune and hormonal changes during pregnancy worsen or reactivate certain infections

The fetus may be considered as an immunologically incompatible transplant that must not be rejected by the mother. Reasons for the failure to reject the fetus include:

- the absence or low density of major histocompatibility complex (MHC) antigens on placental cells;
- a covering of antigens with blocking antibody;
- subtle defects in the maternal immune responses.

A severe or generalized immunosuppression in the mother would be undesirable because it would mean potentially disastrous susceptibility to infectious disease. Certain infections, however, are known to be more severe *(Fig. 23.1)*, and certain persistent infections reactivate *(Fig. 23.2)* during pregnancy. The hormonal changes that accompany pregnancy can also increase susceptibility. The picture is further complicated when there is malnutrition, which in itself impairs host defenses by weakening immune responses, decreasing metabolic reserves and interfering with the integrity of epithelial surfaces.

The fetus has poor immune defenses

Once the fetus is infected it is exquisitely susceptible because:

- IgM and IgA antibodies are not produced in significant amounts until the second half of pregnancy.
- There is no IgG antibody synthesis.
- Cell-mediated immune responses are poorly developed or absent, with inadequate production of the necessary cytokines.

Indeed if the fetus were able to generate a vigorous response to maternal antigens, a troublesome graft-versus-host reaction could be unleashed.

Most microorganisms have sufficient destructive activity to kill the fetus once it is infected, leading to spontaneous abortion, or stillbirth. Here, our interests focus on the few microorganisms that are capable of more subtle, non-lethal effects. They overcome the placental barrier by infecting it so that the infection then spreads to the fetus. They can then interfere with fetal development or cause lesions so that a live but damaged baby is born.

CONGENITAL INFECTIONS

Intrauterine infection may result in death of the fetus or congenital malformations

After primary infection during pregnancy, certain microorganisms enter the blood, establish infection in the placenta, and then invade the fetus. The fetus sometimes dies, leading to abortion, but when the infection is less severe, as in the case

INFECTIONS THAT ARE MORE SEVERE DURING PREGNANCY	
infection	**comments**
malaria	?depressed cell-mediated immunity
viral hepatitis	?additional metabolic burden of pregnancy
influenza	higher mortality during pandemics
poliomyelitis	paralysis more common
urinary tract infections	cystitis; pyelonephritis more common; atony of bladder and ureter leads to less effective flushing, emptying
candidiasis	vulvovaginitis
listeriosis	influenza-like illness
coccidioidomycosis	leading cause of maternal mortality in endemic areas in SW USA and Latin America

Fig. 23.1 The effect of pregnancy on the severity of infectious disease.

INFECTIONS THAT CAN REACTIVATE DURING PREGNANCY	
infection	**phenomenon**
polyomavirus (JC, BK)	viruses appear in urine
cytomegalovirus	increased shedding from cervix, virus in milk of nursing mother
herpes simplex virus	increased replication in cervical region
Epstein–Barr virus	increased antibody titers, increased shedding of virus in oropharynx

Fig. 23.2 Reactivation of persistent infections during pregnancy.

of a relatively non-cytopathic virus, or when it is partially controlled by the maternal IgG response, the fetus survives. It may then be born with a congenital infection, often showing malformations or other pathologic changes. The infant is generally small and fails to thrive. It produces specific antibodies, but often, for instance with cytomegalovirus (CMV), fails to generate an adequate virus-specific cell-mediated immune response, remaining infected for a long period. Hence, the lesions may progress after birth. It is a striking feature of these infections that they are generally mild or unnoticed by the mother.

Important causes of congenital infections are shown in *Figure 23.3*. Viruses that induce fetal malformations (i.e. act as teratogens) share certain characteristics with other teratogens such as drugs or radiation *(Fig. 23.4)*. The fetus tends to show similar responses (e.g. hepatosplenomegaly, encephalitis, eye lesions, low birth weight) to different infectious agents, and the diagnosis is difficult on purely clinical grounds. Most of these infections—herpes simplex virus (HSV)—rubella, CMV, syphilis—can also, at times, kill the fetus. They generally follow primary infection of the mother during pregnancy, so their incidence depends upon the proportion of non-immune females of childbearing age.

Routine antenatal screening for rubella antibody, treponemal antibody (which includes syphilis, yaws, pinta or bejel, which cannot be identified individually by serology), hepatitis B surface antigen and HIV antibody is being carried out to differing degrees worldwide. These tests help identify women who are infected with hepatitis B or HIV, infected or have been exposed in the past to treponemal infections, the most important of which is syphilis in this setting, or are susceptible to rubella.

Routine screening programs lead to clinical management issues for both the mother and child. For example, HIV diagnosis will lead to consideration of antiretroviral therapy for the mother and, immediately on birth, the child, offering a cesarean section delivery, and advising against breast feeding to reduce the risk of vertical transmission. In addition, the child will then be followed up for at least 12 months using sensitive tests to determine whether HIV has been transmitted vertically. Diagnosis of chronic hepatitis B infection will result in determination of the maternal level of infectivity, and a subsequent offer to the baby of an accelerated course of hepatitis B vaccine alone or, if the mother is highly infectious, vaccine and HBV-specific immunoglobulin. In addition, there are antiviral drugs for chronic hepatitis B that might be offered, together with long term follow-up, to the mother. Rubella susceptible women are offered rubella immunization postnatally. Women found to have been exposed to treponemal infection in pregnancy are offered antibiotic treatment and the baby is followed up for the first year using serology to identify active infection, as congenital syphilis can result from earlier untreated infection of the mother. In the case of CMV, which is not part of routine antenatal screening, an earlier infection can reactivate during pregnancy and lead to fetal infection. Partial control of the infection by maternal antibody under these circumstances means that the baby is generally unaffected, but a small percentage become symptomatic over the next couple of years.

The likelihood of fetal infection is increased when the mother develops a poor immune response, when the concentration of microbes in her blood is high (primary or secondary syphilis, e antigen positive hepatitis B carrier, HIV), or early after primary infection in the case of CMV.

There is no good evidence to suggest that maternal mumps, influenza or poliovirus infection during pregnancy leads to harmful effects in the fetus, but the human parvovirus

CONGENITAL (IN UTERO) INFECTIONS	
microorganism	**effects**
rubella virus	congenital rubella
cytomegalovirus (CMV)	congenital CMV – deafness, mental retardation
human immunodeficiency virus (HIV)	congenital infection – childhood AIDS; about 1 in 5 infants born to infected mothers are infected in utero*
varicella-zoster virus (VZV)	skin lesions; musculoskeletal, CNS abnormalities when fetus infected before 20 weeks. After later infection childhood zoster a common sequel**
herpes simplex virus (HSV)	neonatal HSV infection, often disseminated. Much higher risk when maternal infection primary rather than recurrent, infection in utero is rare
hepatitis B virus	congenital hepatitis B – persistent infection*†
parvovirus B19	after maternal infection 5–10% fetuses lost (abortion, hydrops fetalis)
Treponema pallidum	congenital syphilis – classical syndrome
Toxoplasma gondii	congenital toxoplasmosis
Listeria monocytogenes	congenital listeriosis – pneumonia, septicemia, meningitis**
Mycobacterium leprae	congenital infection common in mothers with lepromatous leprosy
*this figure is for resource poor countries wtih no intervention (no antiretroviral drugs, no cesarean section, or avoidance of breast feeding) **infection also occurs during and immediately after birth †protection of newborn by hepatitis B vaccine plus specific immunogloublin.	

Fig. 23.3 Maternal infections that are transmitted to the fetus. Congenitally infected babies may be symptomless, especially in cytomegalovirus infection. They are often small, fail to thrive or show detectable abnormalities later in childhood. In all cases the baby remains infected, often for long periods, and may infect others.

(see Chapter 26) occasionally causes fetal damage or death (in 5–10% of cases) following maternal infection in early pregnancy. The infected fetus develops severe anemia with pallor, ascites and hepatosplenomegaly (hydrops fetalis) as the virus infects progenitor erythroid stem cells. Intrauterine exchange blood transfusion is used to manage hydrops fetalis.

Congenital rubella

The fetus is particularly susceptible to rubella infection when maternal infection occurs during the first 3 months of pregnancy

At this time the heart, brain, eyes and ears are being formed and the infecting virus interferes with their development. If the fetus survives it may show certain abnormalities (*Fig. 23.5*). Not all fetuses are affected; in one study detectable congenital defects were seen in 15.3% of cases when maternal rubella occurred in the first month of pregnancy, 24.6% in the second month, 17.5% in the third month and 6.5% in the fourth month. The figure for the first month is relatively low because fetal death is a common sequel at this stage.

Congenital rubella can affect the eye, heart, brain and ear

Clinical manifestations of congenital rubella include low birth weight and eye (*Fig. 23.6*) and heart lesions. Effects on the brain and ears may not become detectable until later in childhood, in the form of mental retardation and deafness. Up to 80% of infected infants eventually suffer from deafness. About 25% of congenitally infected children develop insulin-dependent diabetes mellitus later in life (the virus replicates in the pancreas), but rubella is a very uncommon cause of this disease. There is a 15% mortality in infants showing signs of infection at birth, often associated with hypogammaglobulinemia.

Fetal rubella IgM is found in cord and infant blood

Infected fetuses produce their own IgM molecules to rubella virus, which can be detected in cord and infant blood. Maternal IgG antibodies are also present and together with interferons help control the spread of infection in the fetus. Virus can be isolated from the infant's throat or urine. The

COMPARISON BETWEEN TERATOGENIC VIRUSES AND OTHER TERATOGENS		
	viral teratogens (e.g. rubella)	other teratogens (e.g. drugs, radiation)
critical stages of susceptibility during pregnancy (organogenesis)	+	+
fetal death a possible outcome	+	+
maternal effects minimal or absent	+	+
cause retarded fetal growth	+	+
increase in frequency of naturally occurring abnormalities	−	+
influence of genetic factors in mother/fetus	−	+

Fig. 23.4 Teratogenic viruses show many similarities to other types of teratogen.

LESSONS IN MICROBIOLOGY

Rubella and the fetus

Dr Norman McAllister Gregg (1892–1966) was ophthalmic surgeon to the Royal Alexandra Hospital for Children in Sydney, and during the Second World War he noticed what he called an 'epidemic' of congenital cataract in infants. He went further and made the astute observation that all the mothers had suffered from rubella during early pregnancy. There were 78 infants with cataract, and 68 of the mothers had a history of rubella in early pregnancy. Many of the infants had heart defects, were small, and two thirds of them had microphthalmia. He published his findings in 1941, providing the first clear demonstration that an environmental factor could cause congenital malformations. It is a striking feature of the infection that, whereas the fetus suffers cruel malformations, the mother shows little or no signs of illness. We now know that several other viruses, notably CMV, can do this, as well as factors such as thalidomide and folate deficiency. Later studies on rubella revealed that congenitally infected infants also developed deafness and brain defects. Survivors were followed up until 1991 when they were 50, and other abnormalities have been observed, including the development of diabetes by the age of 25 years and certain vascular abnormalities.

It was not until 1962 that the causative virus was isolated and grown in cell culture. A rubella epidemic in the USA in 1964–5 left in its wake twenty thousand infants with the congenital rubella syndrome. By the late 1960s an effective live virus vaccine was available, and congenital rubella is now seen only when vaccination cover is poor. The fetus is exquisitely vulnerable to rubella during the first trimester of pregnancy. This is the critical stage in embryonic development when key organs (heart, ear, eye, brain) are being formed, and although the virus does no damage to the cells in which it grows, it interferes with mitosis. Interference with programmed mitosis in these major organs causes the malformations, vasculitis playing a part. The fetus is good at repairing damage but it cannot at a later stage compensate for the failure in basic organ development. The antimitotic action of the virus also means that the total number of cells in the body is reduced, and this is why the rubella-infected infants are smaller. Rubella virus remains in infected organs such as the lens and brain for more than a year, but eventually there is an adequate cell-mediated immune response and the virus is eliminated.

infant sheds virus into the throat and urine for several months and can infect susceptible individuals.

Congenital rubella is completely preventable by vaccination

Vaccination with live attenuated virus vaccine is given during childhood, usually with the combined MMR (mumps, measles and rubella) vaccine (see Chapter 34). Pregnancy is a contraindication to vaccination, and the only safe time during reproductive life is the immediate postpartum period. This is an interesting example of a vaccine that is given to protect an as-yet non-existent individual (the future fetus), the infection being only subclinical or mild in the mother. Until effective vaccines became available in the late 1960s, rubella was an important cause of congenital heart disease, deafness, blindness and mental retardation. The virus continues to circulate in the community and damage fetuses in countries with less extensive rubella vaccination programs.

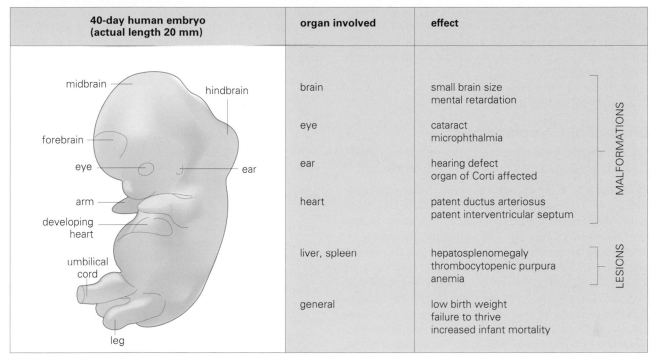

40-day human embryo (actual length 20 mm)	organ involved	effect	
	brain	small brain size mental retardation	MALFORMATIONS
	eye	cataract microphthalmia	
	ear	hearing defect organ of Corti affected	
	heart	patent ductus arteriosus patent interventricular septum	
	liver, spleen	hepatosplenomegaly thrombocytopenic purpura anemia	LESIONS
	general	low birth weight failure to thrive increased infant mortality	

Fig. 23.5 Organ involvement and effects in congenital rubella.

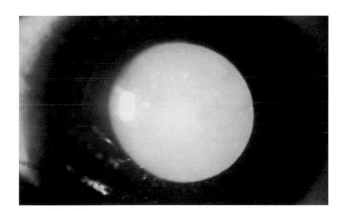

Fig. 23.6 Cataract in congenital rubella. (Courtesy of RJ Marsh and S Ford.)

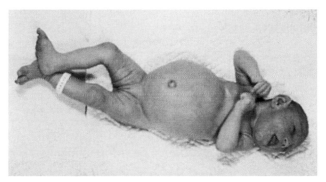

Fig. 23.7 Microcephaly with associated severe psychomotor retardation and hepatosplenomegaly in congenital cytomegalovirus infection. (Courtesy of WE Farrar.)

Congenital CMV infection

Mothers with a poor T cell proliferative response to CMV antigens are more likely to infect their fetus

After primary maternal infection during pregnancy, about 40% of fetuses are infected, and 5% of these show signs at birth. It is not known whether the fetus is especially vulnerable at certain stages of pregnancy. The fetus is also infected following CMV reactivation during pregnancy in women with previous CMV exposure, but fetal damage is then uncommon. As many as 1–2% of infants born in the USA are infected, and up to about 10% of these are symptomatic, with up to one million infectious doses of virus present per ml of urine. However, the incidence of congenital CMV infection is likely to be an underestimate worldwide.

Clinical features of congenital CMV include mental retardation, spasticity, eye abnormalities, hearing defects, hepatosplenomegaly, thrombocytopenic purpura and anemia

(Fig. 23.7). Deafness and mental retardation may not be detectable until later in childhood.

Diagnosis is by detecting CMV-specific IgM antibodies in infant blood within 3 weeks of delivery, and more reliably by virus isolation from the throat or urine. However, specialized cell lines are required. Molecular based methods of detecting viral genome may also be used. Live attenuated vaccines are being developed (AD169 and Towne strains), and in preliminary studies no-one who became pregnant after vaccination transmitted the virus to the infant.

Congenital syphilis

As a result of routine serologic screening for syphilis in antenatal clinics and treatment with penicillin (see Chapter 21), congenital syphilis is now rare, but is more common in developing countries.

Clinical features in the infant include rhinitis (snuffles), skin and mucosal lesions, hepatosplenomegaly, lymphadenopathy, and abnormalities of bones, teeth and cartilage (saddle-shaped nose). Pregnancy often masks the early signs of syphilis, but the mother will have serological evidence of treponemal infection, and treponemal IgM will be detected in the fetal blood.

Treatment of the mother before the fourth month of pregnancy prevents fetal infection.

Congenital toxoplasmosis

Acute asymptomatic infection by Toxoplasma gondii *during pregnancy can cause fetal malformation*

Approximately 35% of healthy adults have serological evidence of previous *Toxoplasma gondii* infection. Clinical features of congenital toxoplasmosis in the infant include convulsions, microcephaly, chorioretinitis, hepatospleno-megaly and jaundice, with later hydrocephaly, mental retardation and defective vision (see Chapter 25). There are often no detectable abnormalities at birth, but signs (e.g. chorioretinitis; see *Fig. 25.7*) generally appear within a few years. The incidence of fetal infection and damage (leading to abortion, stillbirth or disease in the newborn) increases from 14% when maternal infection is in the first trimester to 59% when in the third trimester.

Toxoplasma-specific IgM antibodies may be detected in cord blood. Treatment of a pregnant woman or an infected infant is with spiramycin or (with care to avoid toxicity) sulfonamide or pyrimethamine.

There is no vaccine. Prevention is by avoidance of primary infection which occurs via ingesting cysts from cat feces or lightly cooked meat during pregnancy.

Congenital HIV infection

In resource poor countries, approximately a quarter of infants born to mothers with HIV are infected: about a third of these in utero and the rest perinatally

Clinically congenital HIV infection manifests as poor weight gain, susceptibility to sepsis, developmental delays, lympho-cytic pneumonitis, oral thrush, enlarged lymph nodes, hepatosplenomegaly, diarrhea and pneumonia, and some infants develop encephalopathy and AIDS by 1 year of age. Since most infections take place during late pregnancy or during delivery, transmission rates are reduced by lowering the HIV load by offering antiretroviral drugs during pregnancy, especially during the last trimester or during labor, carrying out an elective cesarean section, and avoiding breastfeeding.

IgG antibodies present in the neonatal blood sample may be maternal in origin and can persist for at least 1 year. The mainstay of laboratory diagnosis therefore involves detection of HIV-1 proviral DNA or HIV-1 RNA by polymerase chain reaction (PCR), although these tests may not be positive until several months after birth, in conjunction with p24 antigen and HIV antibody detection.

Congenital and neonatal listeriosis

Maternal exposure to animals or foods infected with Listeria *can lead to fetal death or malformations*

Listeria monocytogenes is a small Gram-positive rod, which is motile and β-hemolytic. It is distributed worldwide in a great variety of animals including cattle, pigs, rodents and birds, and the bacteria occur in plants and in soil. Listeria can grow at regular refrigeration temperatures (e.g. 3–4°C). Transmission to man is by:

- contact with infected animals and their feces;
- consumption of unpasteurized milk or soft cheeses or contaminated vegetables.

In the USA there are about 1700 reported cases of listeriosis each year, about a third of them in newborn infants. Fecal carriage is uncommon, except in contacts of cases.

L. monocytogenes in the pregnant woman causes a mild influenza-like illness or is asymptomatic, but there is a bacteremia which leads to infection of the placenta and then the fetus. This may cause abortion, premature delivery, neo-natal septicemia or pneumonia with abscesses or granulomas. The infant can also be infected shortly after birth, for instance from other babies or from hospital staff, and this may lead to a meningitic illness.

L. monocytogenes is isolated from blood cultures, cerebro-spinal fluid (CSF) or newborn skin lesions.

Treatment is with ampicillin, which may need to be combined with gentamicin to achieve a bactericidal effect. There are no vaccines.

Pregnant women should avoid exposure to infected material, but the exact source of infection is generally unknown.

INFECTIONS OCCURRING AROUND THE TIME OF BIRTH

Effects on the fetus and neonate

The routes of infection in the fetus and neonate are shown in *Figure 23.8*.

Viral infections (e.g. rubella, CMV) are generally less damaging to the fetus when the maternal infection occurs late in pregnancy. Primary infection with varicella-zoster virus (VZV) in the first 20 weeks of pregnancy can lead to limb deformities and other severe lesions in the newborn. HSV infection in this setting is underdiagnosed and can lead to neonatal morbidity and mortality.

Bacterial infections originating from the vagina and perineum are more important than viral infections late in pregnancy, especially those occurring when the fetal mem-branes have been ruptured for more than 1–2 days, and result in chorioamnionitis, maternal fever, premature delivery and stillbirth. Infants of low birth weight (less than 1500 g) tend to be more severely affected. Bacteria involved include:

- group B hemolytic streptococci; 10–30% of pregnant women are colonized in rectum or vagina;
- *Escherichia coli;*
- *Klebsiella;*
- *Proteus;*
- *Bacteroides;*
- staphylococci;
- *Mycoplasma hominis.*

These infections may also be acquired after delivery to give later onset disease.

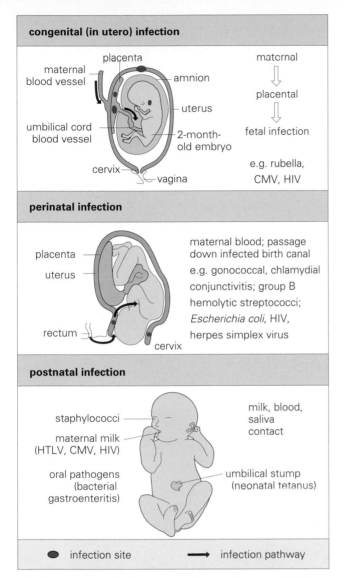

congenital (in utero) infection

maternal blood vessel — placenta — amnion — uterus — umbilical cord blood vessel — 2-month-old embryo — cervix — vagina

maternal ⇩ placental ⇩ fetal infection

e.g. rubella, CMV, HIV

perinatal infection

placenta — uterus — rectum — cervix

maternal blood; passage down infected birth canal e.g. gonococcal, chlamydial conjunctivitis; group B hemolytic streptococci; *Escherichia coli*, HIV, herpes simplex virus

postnatal infection

staphylococci — maternal milk (HTLV, CMV, HIV) — oral pathogens (bacterial gastroenteritis) — umbilical stump (neonatal tetanus)

milk, blood, saliva contact

● infection site → infection pathway

Fig. 23.8 Routes of infection in the fetus and neonate. (CMV, cytomegalovirus; HIV, human immunodeficiency virus; HTLV, human T cell lymphotropic virus.)

Neonatal septicemia often progresses to meningitis

Meningitis (see *Fig. 24.10*) is frequently fatal unless treated. Clinical diagnosis is difficult because the infant shows generalized signs such as respiratory distress, poor feeding, diarrhea and vomiting, but early diagnosis is essential and emergency treatment is required. 'Blind' antibiotic treatment should be started as soon as CSF (Gram stain and culture) and blood samples have been taken.

Fetal infection can occur during labor or breast feeding

Fetal infection during labor results from direct contact with the infecting microorganism as the fetus passes down an infected birth canal *(Fig. 23.9)*. For instance, cutaneous lesions of herpes simplex may develop 1 week after delivery with generalized infection and severe central nervous system (CNS) involvement. Approximately 80% of mothers with primary HSV infection (only about 10% with recurrent HSV)

have cervical lesions and about a third of their infants are infected. Gonococci *(Fig. 23.10)*, chlamydia or staphylococci (see Chapter 25) can infect the eye to cause ophthalmia neonatorum. Infection with group B streptococci generally occurs at this time.

In countries with high hepatitis B carrier rates, maternal blood is a major source of infection during or shortly after birth. More than 90% of infants from carrier mothers become infected and then carry the virus. This is preventable by giving the vaccine plus specific immunoglobulin to the newborn. Hepatitis C, in contrast, is not usually transmitted in this way, and less than 5% of children with carrier mothers are infected.

Human milk may contain rubella virus, CMV, human T cell lymphotropic virus (HTLV) and HIV. Virus titers are generally low and, except in the case of HTLV and HIV, milk is not thought to be an important source of infection. However, it makes sense to pasteurize milk in human milk banks, just as we pasteurize cows' milk.

Effects on the mother

Puerpural sepsis is prevented by aseptic techniques

After delivery (or abortion) a large area of damaged vulnerable uterine tissue is exposed to infection. Puerpural sepsis (childbed fever) was a major cause of maternal death in Europe in the 19th century. In 1843 Oliver Wendell Holmes made the unpopular suggestion that it was carried on the hands of doctors, and 4 years later Ignaz Semmelweiss in Vienna showed how it could be prevented if doctors and midwives washed their hands before attending a woman in labor and practiced aseptic techniques. This is because:

- Group A β-hemolytic streptococci were the major culprits and came from the nose, throat or skin of hospital attendants.
- Other possible organisms include anaerobes such as *Clostridium perfringens* or *Bacteroides*, *E. coli* and group B streptococci and originate from the mother's own fecal flora.

Puerpural sepsis carried a mortality rate of up to 10% until the 1930s, but now, like septic abortion, is uncommon in developed countries. Predisposing factors include premature rupture of the membranes, instrumentation and retained fragments of membrane or placenta. High vaginal swabs and blood cultures should be taken if there is postnatal pyrexia or an offensive discharge.

Other neonatal infections

Infection may be transmitted to the newborn infant during the first week or two after birth rather than during delivery as follows:

- Group B β-hemolytic streptococci and Gram-negative bacilli (see above) acquired by cross-infection in the nursery, can still cause serious infection at this time, often with meningitis (see Chapter 24).
- Herpes simplex virus may come from cold sores or herpetic whitlows of attending adults.
- Staphylococci from the noses and fingers of adult carriers may cause staphylococcal conjunctivitis or 'sticky eye' (see

NEONATAL INFECTIONS ACQUIRED DURING PASSAGE DOWN INFECTED BIRTH CANAL		
infectious agent	site of infection	phenomenon
Neisseria gonorrhoeae	conjunctiva	neonatal conjunctivitis (ophthalmia neonatorum)
Chlamydia trachomatis	conjunctiva, respiratory tract	neonatal conjunctivitis (ophthalmia neonatorum), neonatal pneumonia
herpes simplex virus	skin, eye, mouth	neonatal herpetic infection*
genital papillomavirus	respiratory tract	laryngeal warts in young children
group B streptococci** gram-negative bacilli (E. coli etc.)	respiratory tract	septicemia; death if not treated
Candida albicans	oral cavity	neonatal oral thrush
*although preventable by cesarean section, it is often difficult to detect maternal genital infection; infants can be treated prophylactically with aciclovir **up to 30% of women carry these bacteria in the vagina or rectum		

Fig. 23.9 Neonatal infections acquired during passage down an infected birth canal.

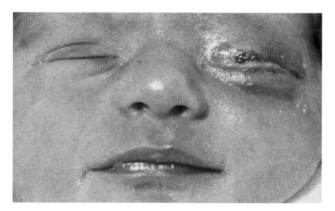

Fig. 23.10 Gonococcal ophthalmia neonatorum. Signs appear 2–5 days after birth. The inflammation and edema are more severe than with chlamydia infection. (Courtesy of JS Bingham.)

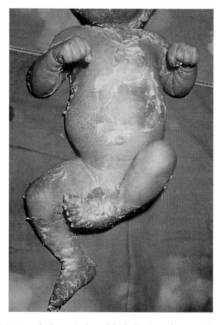

Fig. 23.11 Staphylococcal scalded skin syndrome. There are large areas of epidermal loss where bullae have burst. (Courtesy of L Brown.)

Chapter 25), skin sepsis in the neonate, and sometimes the staphylococcal 'scalded skin' syndrome *(Fig. 23.11)* due to a specific 'epidermolytic' staphylococcal toxin.

During the first week or two of life the nose of the neonate becomes colonized with *Staphylococcus aureus,* which can enter the nipple during feeding to cause a breast abscess. These infections are preventable if hospital staff pay vigorous attention to handwashing and aseptic techniques.

If hygienic practices are poor the umbilical stump, especially in developing countries, may be infected with *Clostridium tetani,* usually because instruments used to cut the cord are contaminated with bacterial spores, resulting in neonatal tetanus *(Fig. 23.12).* It can be prevented by immunizing mothers with tetanus toxoid.

In developing countries, gastroenteritis is an important problem during the neonatal period as well as during infancy

Diarrhea leading to water and electrolyte depletion is particularly serious in low birth weight infants. Causative agents include strains of *E. coli* and salmonellae rather than rotaviruses (Chapter 22). Breast feeding gives some protection by supplying specific antibodies and other less well characterized protective factors.

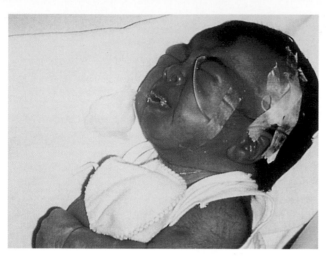

Fig. 23.12 Tetanus. Risus sardonicus in a newborn infant. (Courtesy of WE Farrar.)

KEY FACTS

- During pregnancy certain infections (coccidioidomycosis, influenza) can be more severe than usual, and there can be reactivation of certain persistent infections (polyomaviruses, CMV).

- A few infections are able to pass to the fetus via the placenta and cause damage. These infections are generally mild or subclinical in the mother (rubella, CMV, toxoplasmosis), but this is not always the case (syphilis).

- Once infected the fetus may die, but more importantly may survive and be born with the infection (HIV, toxoplasmosis), often showing characteristic malformations (rubella, syphilis).

- Infection of the infant during birth or shortly afterwards can cause local disease (conjunctivitis due to gonococci or chlamydia) or occasionally severe life-threatening illness (*E. coli* meningitis, herpes simplex virus or group B streptococcal infection).

- Life-threatening bacterial infection of the mother via the postpartum uterus (puerperal sepsis) used to be common but is now rare in developed countries.

QUESTIONS

1. A pediatrician is called to the postnatal ward by a midwife. She is anxious about a baby born 12 hours ago. The child is the mother's first baby. The labor was long and the delivery difficult and eventually forceps had to be used. The mother's membranes ruptured 12 hours before the baby was born. The mother had a fever of 38.5°C during the last stages of labor, which has persisted since her arrival on the postnatal ward. The baby had Apgar scores of 1 at 1 minute and 9 at 5 minutes. On examination, the baby is lethargic and pale. He has a faint systolic murmur, crepitations in both lung fields, and his liver is palpable below the costal margin. He is transferred to the Special Care Unit.

   a. What is the likely diagnosis?

   b. How would you investigate this baby?

   c. What are the risk factors in the mother's history?

2. Why are heart, brain, eyes and ears so commonly affected in congenital rubella?

3. In which of the following infections is human milk a common source?
   A. Herpes simplex
   B. HTLV1
   C. Syphilis
   D. Epstein–Barr virus
   E. *E. coli*

4. Which of the following congenital infections are prevented by vaccination?
   A. Syphilis
   B. HIV
   C. Rubella
   D. Listeriosis
   E. Toxoplasmosis

FURTHER READING

Demmler G. Congenital cytomegalovirus infection and disease. *Adv Pediatr Inf Dis* 1996; 11:134–62.

Kovar IZ. Neonatal and pediatric infections. *Curr Opin Infect Dis* 1990; 3:479–500.

Peckham C, Gibb D. Mother-to-child transmission of the human immunodeficiency virus. *N Engl J Med* 1995; 333:298–302.

Sever JL, Ellenberg JH, Ley ACX et al. Toxoplasmosis; maternal and pediatric findings in 23,000 pregnancies. *Pediatrics* 1988; 82:181–92.

Wilfert CM, Wilson W, Luzuriaga K. Pathogenesis of pediatric human immunodeficiency virus type 1 infection. *J Infect Dis* 1994; 170:286.

INTRODUCTION

Central nervous system infections are usually bloodborne or invade via peripheral nerves

The brain and spinal cord are protected from mechanical pressure or deformation by enclosure in rigid containers, the skull and vertebral column, which also act as barriers to the spread of infection. The blood vessels and nerves that traverse the walls of the skull and vertebral column are the main routes of invasion. Bloodborne invasion is the most common route of infection, for example by polioviruses or *Neisseria meningitidis*. Invasion via peripheral nerves is less common—for example by herpes simplex, varicella-zoster and rabies viruses. Local invasion from infected ears or sinuses, local injury or congenital defects such as spina bifida, also occurs, while invasion from the olfactory tract leading to amebic meningitis is rare.

Here we discuss the main routes of central nervous system invasion by microorganisms (see also Chapter 13) and the body's response, followed by a more detailed discussion of the diseases that result.

INVASION OF THE CENTRAL NERVOUS SYSTEM

Natural barriers act to prevent bloodborne invasion

Bloodborne invasion takes place across:

- the blood–brain barrier to cause encephalitis;
- the blood–cerebrospinal fluid (CSF) barrier to cause meningitis (*Fig. 24.1*).

The blood–brain barrier consists of tightly joined endothelial cells surrounded by glial processes, while the brain–CSF barrier at the choroid plexus consists of endothelium with fenestrations, and tightly joined choroid plexus epithelial cells. Microbes can traverse these barriers by:

- growing across, infecting the cells that comprise the barrier;
- being passively transported across in intracellular vacuoles;
- being carried across by infected white blood cells.

Examples of each route are seen in viral infections. Poliovirus, for instance, invades the central nervous system (CNS) across the blood–brain barrier. After oral ingestion of virus, a complex stepwise series of events leads to CNS invasion (*Fig. 24.2*). Poliovirus also invades the meninges after localizing in vascular endothelial cells, and can cross the blood–CSF barrier. Mumps virus behaves in the same way, as do circulating *Haemophilus influenzae*, meningococci or pneumococci. Once infection has reached the meninges and CSF, the brain substance can in turn be invaded if the infection crosses the pia. In poliomyelitis, for instance, a meningitic phase often precedes encephalitis and paralysis.

CNS invasion, however, is a rare event because most microorganisms fail to pass from blood to the CNS across the natural barriers. A large variety of viruses can grow and cause disease if introduced directly into the brain, but circulating viruses generally fail to invade, and CNS involvement by polio, mumps, rubella or measles viruses is seen in only a very small proportion of infected individuals. The factors that determine such CNS invasion are unknown.

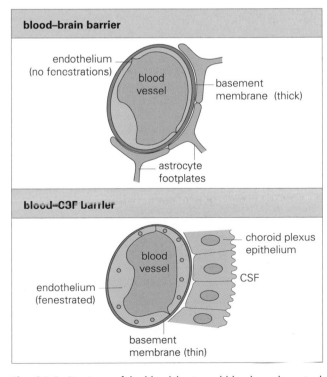

blood–brain barrier

endothelium (no fenestrations)

blood vessel

basement membrane (thick)

astrocyte footplates

blood–CSF barrier

endothelium (fenestrated)

blood vessel

choroid plexus epithelium

CSF

basement membrane (thin)

Fig. 24.1 Structures of the blood–brain and blood–cerebrospinal fluid (CSF) barriers.

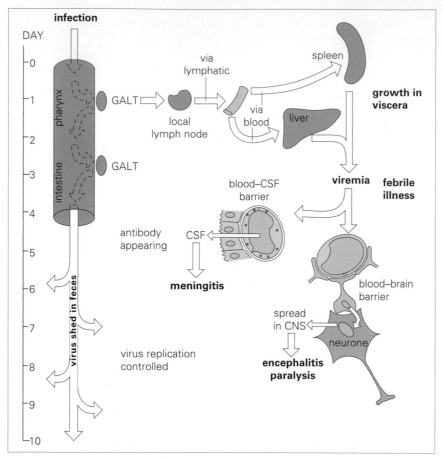

Fig. 24.2 The mechanism of central nervous system (CNS) invasion by poliovirus. (CSF, cerebrospinal fluid; GALT, gut-associated lymphoid tissue.)

Invasion of the CNS via peripheral nerves is a feature of herpes simplex, varicella-zoster and rabies virus infections

Herpes simplex virus (HSV) and varicella-zoster virus (VZV) present in skin or mucosal lesions (see Chapter 26), travel up axons using the normal retrograde transport mechanisms that can move virus particles (as well as foreign molecules such as tetanus toxin) at a rate of about 200 mm/day, to reach the dorsal root ganglia. Rabies virus, introduced into muscle or subcutaneous tissues by the bite of a rabid animal, infects muscle fibers and muscle spindles after the virus binds to the nicotinic acetylcholine receptor. It then enters peripheral nerves and travels to the CNS, to reach glial cells and neurones, where it multiplies.

THE BODY'S RESPONSE TO INVASION

CSF cell counts increase in response to infection

The response to invading viruses is reflected by an increase in lymphocytes, mostly T cells, and monocytes in the CSF (Fig. 24.3). A slight increase in protein also occurs, the CSF remaining clear. This condition is termed 'aseptic' meningitis. The response to pyogenic bacteria shows a more spectacular and more rapid increase in polymorphonuclear leukocytes

and proteins (Fig. 24.4), so that the CSF becomes visibly turbid. This condition is termed 'septic' meningitis. Certain slower growing or less pyogenic microorganisms induce less dramatic changes, such as in tuberculous or listerial meningitis.

The pathologic consequences of CNS infection depend upon the microorganism

In the CNS itself viruses can infect neural cells, sometimes showing a marked preference. Polio and rabies viruses, for instance, invade neurones whereas JC virus invades oligo-dendrocytes. Because there is very little extracellular space, spread is mostly direct from cell to cell along established nervous pathways. Invading bacteria and protozoa generally induce more dramatic inflammatory events, which limit local spread so that infection is soon localized to form abscesses.

Viruses induce perivascular infiltration of lymphocytes and monocytes, sometimes, as in the case of polio, with direct damage to infected cells. The pathogenesis of viral encephalo-myelitis is shown in *Figure 24.15*. Associated immune responses not only to viral, but also often to host CNS components, play a part in postvaccinial encephalitis. Infil-trating B cells produce antibody to the invading micro-organism, and T cells react with microbial antigens to release cytokines that attract and activate other T cells and macro-phages. The pathologic condition evolves over the course of

CSF CHANGES DURING CENTRAL NERVOUS SYSTEM INFECTION

	cells/ml	protein mg/dl	glucose mg/dl	causes
normal	0–5	15–45	45–85	—
septic (purulent) meningitis	200–20 000 (mainly neutrophils)	high (>100)	< 45	bacteria amebae brain abscess
aseptic* meningitis or meningoencephalitis	100–1000 (mainly mononuclear)	moderately high (50–100)	normal**	viruses, tuberculosis, leptospira, fungi, brain abscess, partly treated bacterial meningitis

*aseptic because the CSF is sterile on regular bacteriologic culture
**low (< 45) in the case of tuberculosis, fungi, leptospira

Fig. 24.3 Changes in cerebrospinal fluid (CSF) in response to invading microbes.

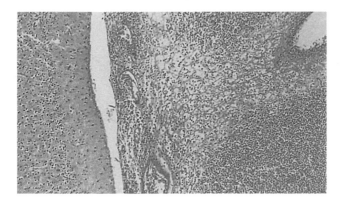

Fig. 24.4 Bacterial meningitis. Exudate of acute inflammatory cells in the subarachnoid space. Hematoxylin and eosin stain. (Courtesy of P Garen.)

several days and occasionally, when partly controlled by host defenses, over the course of years—for example subacute sclerosing panencephalitis (SSPE) caused by measles, which has both a virological and immunological pathogenesis. Bacteria cause more rapidly evolving pathologic changes, with local responses to bacterial antigens and toxins playing an important part.

In all cases, a degree of inflammation and edema that would be trivial in striated muscle, skin or liver may be life-threatening when it occurs in the vulnerable 'closed box' containing the leptomeninges, brain and spinal cord. It may be several weeks after clinical recovery before cellular infiltrations are removed and histologic appearances are restored to normal.

CNS invasion only rarely assists in the transmission of infection

From the point of view of a parasitic microorganism that needs to be transmitted to a fresh host, invasion of the CNS is generally foolish because it damages the host. The only occasions on which it makes sense are:

- When dorsal root ganglion neurones are invaded as an essential step in establishing latency (HSV and VZV). This

gives a mechanism for reactivation and further episodes of shedding from mucosal or skin lesions.
- In the case of rabies (see below), where CNS invasion in the animal host is necessary for two reasons. First, it enables the virus to spread from the CNS down peripheral nerves to the salivary glands, from which transmission takes place. Second, invasion of the limbic system of the brain causes a change in behavior of the infected animal so that it becomes less retiring, more aggressive and more likely to bite, thus transmitting the infection. Invasion of the limbic system can be regarded as a fiendish strategy on the part of rabies virus to promote its own transmission and survival.

MENINGITIS

Bacterial meningitis

Acute bacterial meningitis is a life-threatening infection, needing urgent specific treatment

Bacterial meningitis is more severe, but less common, than viral meningitis and may be caused by a variety of agents *(Figure 24.5)*. Prior to the 1990s, *Haemophilus influenzae* type b (Hib) was responsible for most cases of bacterial meningitis. However, the introduction of new vaccines into childhood immunization regimens has lowered overall Hib incidence in favor of *Neisseria meningitidis* and *Streptococcus pneumoniae*, which are now responsible for most bacterial meningitis. These three pathogens have several virulence factors in common *(Fig. 24.6)*, including possession of a polysaccharide capsule *(Fig. 24.7)*.

Meningococcal meningitis

Neisseria meningitidis is carried by about 20% of the population, but in epidemics higher rates are seen

Neisseria meningitidis is a Gram-negative diplococcus, which closely resembles *N. gonorrhoeae* in structure (see Chapter 21), but with an additional polysaccharide capsule that is antigenic and by which the serotype of *N. meningitidis* can be recognized. The bacteria are carried asymptomatically in the

NON-VIRAL MENINGITIS—CAUSES, TREATMENT AND PREVENTION		
pathogen	**treatment***	**prevention**
Neisseria meningitidis	penicillin (or chloramphenicol)	rifampin prophylaxis for close contacts polysaccharide vaccine (poor protection against group B)
Haemophilus influenzae	ampicillin,** ceftriaxone or cefotaxime (or chloramphenicol)	polysaccharide vaccine against type B (Hib)
Streptococcus pneumoniae	penicillin*** (or ceftriaxone or chloramphenicol)	prompt treatment of otitis media and respiratory infections polyvalent (23 serotypes), polysaccharide vaccine
Escherichia coli (and other coliforms), group B streptococci	gentamicin + cefotaxime or ceftriaxone (or chloramphenicol)**	no vaccines available
Listeria monocytogenes	penicillin or ampicillin + gentamicin	
Mycobacterium tuberculosis	isoniazid and rifampin and pyrazinamide ± streptomycin	BCG vaccination; isoniazid prophylaxis for contacts recommended in USA
Cryptococcus neoformans	amphotericin B and flucytosine	no vaccines available
*treatment should be initiated immediately and the susceptibility of the infecting isolate confirmed in the laboratory **if isolate is shown to be susceptible (10–20% of isolates are resistant because they produce a plasmid coded beta-lactamase) ***in areas of high prevalence of penicillin resistant pneumococci initial treatment with ceftriaxone may be advised until susceptibility of isolate is known		

Fig. 24.5 The important causative agents of non-viral meningitis, their treatment and prevention. (BCG, bacille Calmette–Guérin.)

BACTERIAL MENINGITIS – VIRULENCE FACTORS FOR MAJOR PATHOGENS			
virulence factor	**bacterial pathogen**		
	Neisseria meningitidis	*Haemophilus influenzae*	*Streptococcus pneumoniae*
capsule	+	+	+
IgA protease	+	+	+
pili	+	+	−
endotoxin	+	+	−
outer membrane proteins	+	+	−

Fig. 24.6 Virulence factors in bacterial meningitis.

population, up to 20% depending on geographic location, and are attached by their pili to the epithelial cells in the nasopharynx. Invasion of the blood and meninges is a rare and poorly understood event. The known virulence factors are summarized in *Figure 24.6*. People possessing specific complement-dependent bacterial antibodies to capsular antigens are protected against invasion. Those with C5–C9 complement deficiencies show increased susceptibility to bacteremia (as they do to *N. gonorrhoeae* bacteremia; see Chapter 21). Young children who have lost the antibodies acquired from their mother, and adolescents who have not previously encountered the infecting serotype, and therefore have no type-specific immunity, are those most often infected. Person to person spread takes place by droplet infection, and is facilitated by other respiratory infections, often viral, that cause increased respiratory secretions. Thus, conditions of overcrowding and confinement such as prisons, military barracks and college dormitories contribute to the frequency of infection in populations. During outbreaks of meningococcal meningitis, which most frequently occur in late winter and early spring, the carrier rate may reach 60–80%. Specific serotypes associated with infection exhibit some geographic variation. However, serotypes B, C and Y tend to predominate in more developed countries whereas serotypes A and

CAPSULES – IMPORTANT VIRULENCE FACTORS			
pathogen	capsule	important type	vaccine
Neisseria meningitidis	polysaccharide	A, B, C, Y, W-135	good for A and C; poor for B
Haemophilus influenzae	polysaccharide	b	Hib vaccine for <1 year olds
Streptococcus pneumoniae	polysaccharide	many	pneumovax:23-valent most common types
group B streptococcus	polysaccharide rich in sialic acid	(Ia, Ib, II) III in neonatal meningitis	– ? future
Escherichia coli		KI in meningitis	– ? future

Fig. 24.7 Polysaccharide capsules are important virulence factors in the pathogenesis of bacterial meningitis.

W-135 are more common in less developed regions. Available vaccines target serotypes A, C, Y and W-135 but not B *(Fig. 24.7)*. The UK was the first country to introduce the new meningitis C conjugate vaccine. It has been part of routine childhood immunization since November 1999. The UK Department of Health recommends that all first year university and college students and others between 20 and 24 years old should be immunized against meningitis C. However, the US Centers for Disease Control has taken steps to increase awareness and make the option for vaccination more available to college students living in student housing.

Clinical features of meningococcal meningitis include a hemorrhagic skin rash

After an incubation period of 1–3 days, the onset of meningo-coccal meningitis is sudden with a sore throat, headache, drowsiness and signs of meningitis which include fever, irritability, neck stiffness and photophobia. There is often a hemorrhagic skin rash with petechiae, reflecting the associated septicemia *(Fig. 24.8)*. In about 35% of patients this septicemia is fulminating, with complications due to disseminated intravascular coagulation, endotoxemia and shock, and renal failure. In the most severe cases there is an acute Addisonian crisis, with bleeding into the brain and adrenal glands referred to as Waterhouse–Friedrichsen syndrome. Mortality from meningococcal meningitis reaches 100% if untreated, but remains around 10% even if treated. In addition, serious sequelae such as permanent hearing loss may occur in some survivors *(Fig. 24.9)*.

A diagnosis of acute meningitis is usually suspected on clinical examination

Laboratory identification of the bacterial cause of acute meningitis is essential so that appropriate antibiotic therapy can be given and prophylaxis of contacts initiated. Preliminary microscopy results involving white cell counts and Gram staining for bacteria should be available within an hour of receipt of the CSF sample in the laboratory. Results of culture of CSF and blood should follow after 24 hours (see Chapter 32). Serology is not helpful in the diagnosis because the infection is too acute for an antibody response to be detectable.

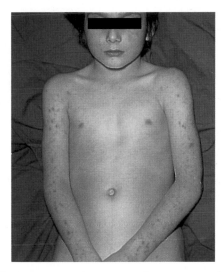

Fig. 24.8 Meningococcal septicemia showing a mixed petechial and maculopapular rash on the extremities and exterior surfaces. (Courtesy of WE Farrar.)

Bacterial meningitis is a medical emergency

Antibiotic therapy (penicillin or ampicillin) should be instigated if the diagnosis is suspected *(Fig. 24.5)*. Early treatment saves lives, although it may make recovery of viable organisms from specimens more difficult.

Close contacts in the family ('kissing contacts') should be given rifampin chemoprophylaxis for 2 days. Note that penicillin is not used for prophylaxis, because it does not eliminate nasopharyngeal carriage of meningococci. Patients should be given a course of rifampin to clear carriage after the acute phase of the infection has passed. Sulfonamides can no longer be relied upon for prophylaxis because resistance in meningococci is common.

Haemophilus meningitis

Type b H. influenzae *causes meningitis in infants and young children*

H. influenzae is a Gram-negative coccobacillus. 'Haemophilus' means 'blood-loving', and the name 'influenzae' was given because it was originally thought to be the cause of influenza, but is now known to be a common secondary invader in

BACTERIAL MENINGITIS – CLINICAL FEATURES				
pathogen	host (patient)	important clinical features	mortality (as % of treated cases)	sequelae (as % of treated cases)*
Neisseria meningitidis	children and adolescents	acute onset (6–24 hours) skin rash	7–10	< 1
Haemophilus influenzae	children < 5 years of age	onset often less acute (1–2 days)	5	9
Streptococcus pneumoniae	all ages, but especially children < 2 years of age and elderly	acute onset may follow pneumonia and/or septicemia in elderly	20–30	15–20
*major central nervous system deficit; in addition, up to 10% of patients develop deafness				

Fig. 24.9 Clinical features of bacterial meningitis.

the lower respiratory tract. There are six types (a–f) of *H. influenzae*, distinguishable serologically by their capsular polysaccharides:

- Unencapsulated strains are common and are present in the throat of most healthy people.
- The capsulated type b, a common inhabitant of the respiratory tract of infants and young children (where it may cause infection: see Chapter 18), very occasionally invades the blood and reaches the meninges.

Maternal antibody protects the infant up to 3–4 months of age, but as it wanes there is a 'window of susceptibility' until the child produces his/her own antibody. Anticapsular antibodies are good opsonins (see Chapter 14), which allow the bacteria to be phagocytosed and killed, but children do not generally produce them until 2–3 years of age, possibly because these antibodies are T independent. In addition to the capsule, *H. influenzae* has several other virulence factors, as shown in *Figure 24.6*.

Acute *H. influenzae* meningitis is commonly complicated by severe neurologic sequelae

The incubation period of *H. influenzae* meningitis is 5–6 days, and the onset is often more insidious than that of meningococcal or pneumococcal meningitis (*Fig. 24.9*). The condition is less frequently fatal, but, as with meningococcal infection, serious sequelae such as hearing loss, delayed language development, and mental retardation and seizures may occur (*Fig. 24.9*).

General diagnostic features are the same as for meningococcal meningitis, as explained above. For laboratory diagnosis, see Chapter 32. It is important to note that the organisms may be difficult to see in Gram-stained smears of CSF, particularly if they are present in small numbers.

Hib vaccine is effective for children from 2 months of age

General features of treatment are referred to above under meningococcal meningitis; details are summarized in

Figure 24.5. An effective *H. influenzae* vaccine (Hib), suitable for children 2 months of age and upwards, is available. Close contacts of patients are sometimes given rifampin prophylaxis.

Pneumococcal meningitis

Streptococcus pneumoniae is a common cause of bacterial meningitis, particularly in children and the elderly

Strep. pneumoniae was first isolated more than 100 years ago and has since received intensive study both as a pathogen and as the subject of early work on bacterial transformation. Despite this, relatively little is known about its virulence attributes apart from its polysaccharide capsule (*Figs 24.6 and 24.7*), and the pneumococcus remains a major cause of morbidity and mortality. (Pneumococcal respiratory tract infections are reviewed in Chapter 19.)

Strep. pneumoniae is a capsulate Gram-positive coccus carried in the throats of many healthy individuals. Invasion of the blood and meninges is a rare event, but is more common in the very young (less than 2 years of age), in the elderly, in those with sickle cell disease, in debilitated or splenectomized patients and following head trauma. Susceptibility to infection is associated with low levels of antibodies to capsular polysaccharide antigens: antibody opsonizes the organism and promotes phagocytosis, thereby protecting the host from invasion. However, this protection is type-specific and there are more than 85 different capsular types of *Strep. pneumoniae*.

The clinical features of pneumococcal meningitis are generally worse than with *N. meningitidis* and *H. influenzae* and are summarized in *Figure 24.9*. The general diagnostic features are the same as for meningococcal meningitis described above. Details are referred to in Chapter 32.

Treatment and prevention of pneumococcal meningitis are summarized in *Figure 24.5*. Since penicillin-resistant pneumococci have been observed worldwide, attention must be paid to the antibiotic susceptibility of the infecting strain, and empiric chemotherapy usually involves a combination of vancomycin and either cefotaxime or ceftriaxone.

An effective heptavalent protein-conjugate pneumococcal vaccine is available which the US Centers for Disease Control recommends for all children from 2 to 23 months of age (i.e. to be given with other recommended childhood vaccines) and for older children (24 to 59 months) who are at high risk (e.g. sickle cell disease, HIV infection, chronic illness or weakened immune systems) for serious pneumococcal infection. The older 23-valent polysaccharide vaccine remains available for children older than 5 years of age.

Listeria monocytogenes *meningitis*

Listeria monocytogenes *causes meningitis in immunocompromised adults*

Listeria monocytogenes is a Gram-positive coccobacillus and an important cause of meningitis in immunocompromised adults, especially in renal transplant and cancer patients. It also causes intrauterine infections and infections of the newborn, as summarized in Chapter 23. *L. monocytogenes* is less susceptible than *Strep. pneumoniae* to penicillin, and the recommended treatment is a combination of penicillin or ampicillin with gentamicin.

Neonatal meningitis

In general, neonates (especially those with low birth weight) are at increased risk for meningitis because of their immature immunological status, as illustrated by problems with, for example, humoral and cellular immunity, phagocytic capability, and inefficient alternative complement pathway. This is especially true as a result of medical advances in recent years which have greatly contributed to the increased survival of pre-term infants.

Though mortality rates due to neonatal meningitis in developed countries are declining the problem is still serious

Neonatal meningitis can be caused by a wide range of bacteria, but the most frequent are group B hemolytic streptococci (GBS) and *Escherichia coli* (Fig. 24.10; see also Chapter 23). This may occur by routes such as nosocomial infection. However, the infant may also be infected from the mother. For example, with women vaginally colonized by GBS, the infant may swallow maternal secretions such as infected amniotic fluid during delivery.

Neonatal meningitis often leads to permanent neurologic sequelae such as cerebral or cranial nerve palsy, epilepsy, mental retardation or hydrocephalus. This is partly because the clinical diagnosis of meningitis in the neonate is difficult, perhaps with no more specific signs than fever, poor feeding, vomiting, respiratory distress or diarrhea. In addition, due to the possible range of etiological agents, 'blind' antibiotic therapy in the absence of susceptibility tests may not be optimal, and adequate penetration of the antibiotic into the CSF is also an issue.

Tuberculous meningitis

Patients with tuberculous meningitis always have a focus of infection elsewhere, but approximately 25% may have no clinical or historic evidence of such an infection. In more than 50% of cases, meningitis is associated with acute miliary tuberculosis (Fig. 24.11). In areas with a high prevalence of tuberculosis, meningitis tends to be most commonly seen in children from 0 to 4 years of age. However, in areas where tuberculosis is less frequent, most meningitis cases are in adults.

Tuberculous meningitis usually presents with a gradual onset over a few weeks

There is a gradual onset of generalized illness beginning with malaise, apathy and anorexia and proceeding within a few weeks to photophobia, neck stiffness and impairment of consciousness. Occasionally the onset is much more rapid and may be mistaken for a subarachnoid hemorrhage. The variability of presentation means that the clinician needs to maintain an awareness of possible tuberculous meningitis to make the diagnosis. A delay in making the diagnosis and in starting appropriate antimicrobial therapy (Fig. 24.5) results in serious complications and sequelae.

Spinal tuberculosis is uncommon now except in developing countries; bacteria in the vertebrae destroy the intervertebral disks to form epidural abscesses. These compress the spinal cord and lead to paraplegia.

Fungal meningitis

Cryptococcus neoformans and *Coccidioides immitis* can invade the blood from a primary site of infection in the lungs and thence to the brain to cause meningitis. *Cryptococcus* has a marked tropism for the CNS and is the major cause of fungal meningitis. *C. neoformans* occurs as two varieties, each with two serotypes.

Cryptococcus neoformans *meningitis is seen in patients with depressed cell-mediated immunity*

It therefore occurs in AIDS patients and those undergoing clinical immune suppression. The onset is usually slow, over days or weeks. The capsulate yeasts can be seen in India-ink-stained preparations of cerebrospinal fluid (CSF) (Fig. 24.12) and can be cultured (see Chapter 32). Antigen detection is also a useful diagnostic tool and evidence of a decline in antigen and an increase in antibody levels in the CSF can be used as a measure of successful therapy. Treatment with the antifungal drugs amphotericin B and flucytosine in combination is recommended, the former penetrating poorly into CSF.

Coccidioides immitis *infection is common in particular geographic locations*

These locations are notably Southwest USA, Mexico and South America. CNS infection occurs in fewer than 1% of infected individuals, but is fatal unless treated. It may be part of the generalized disease or may represent the only extrapulmonary site. The organisms are rarely visible in the CSF, and cultures are positive in less than 50% of cases, but the diagnosis can be made by demonstrating complement-fixing antibodies in the serum. Treatment with amphotericin B, fluconazole or miconazole is recommended.

NEONATAL MENINGITIS		
group B streptococci and neonatal meningitis		
group B streptococci (*Streptococcus agalactiae*) are normal inhabitants of the female genital tract and may be acquired by the neonate		
	at or soon after birth	in the nursery
	early onset disease	**late onset disease**
age	< 7 days	1 week–3 months
risk factors	heavily colonized mother lacking specific antibody premature rupture of membranes pre-term delivery prolonged labor, obstetric complications	lack of maternal antibody exposure to cross-infection from heavily colonized babies poor hygiene in nursery
type of disease	generalized infection including bacteremia, pneumonia and meningitis	predominantly meningitis
type of group B streptococcus	all serotypes but meningitis mostly due to type III	90% type III
outcome	approximately 60% fatal; serious sequelae in many survivors	approximately 20% fatal
treatment	take blood and CSF for culture treat on suspicion gentamicin and ampicillin or cefotaxime/ceftriaxone	treat on suspicion take blood and CSF for culture gentamicin and ampicillin or cefotaxime/ceftriaxone
prevention	antibiotic treatment does not reliably abolish carriage in mother; not recommended 'blind' treatment of sick baby who has risk factors future: ?? immunize antibody-negative females of child-bearing age	good hygienic practices in nursery do not allow mothers to handle other babies

Fig. 24.10 Group B streptococci are a major cause of neonatal meningitis. (CSF, cerebrospinal fluid.)

Protozoal meningitis

Free-living amebae (*Naegleria* or *Acanthamoeba* spp.) can multiply in stagnant fresh water in warm countries, especially in the sludge at the bottom of lakes and swimming pools. If inhaled they can reach the meninges via the olfactory tract and cribriform plate. Primary amebic meningoencephalitis caused by *Naegleria* shows a rapid onset, and the mortality rate is high. *Acanthamoeba* causes a chronic condition (granulomatous amebic encephalitis). These slowly motile amebae can be seen on careful examination of a fresh wet sample of CSF. Treatment is not fully satisfactory. Amphotericin B, with miconazole and rifampin, has been used for *Naegleria*; a variety of drugs have been used for *Acanthamoeba*.

Viral meningitis

Viral meningitis is the most common type of meningitis

It is a milder disease than bacterial meningitis, with headache, fever and photophobia, but less neck stiffness. The CSF is clear in the absence of bacteria, and the cells are mainly lymphocytes, although polymorphonuclear leukocytes may be present in the early stages (*Fig. 24.3*). The causes of viral

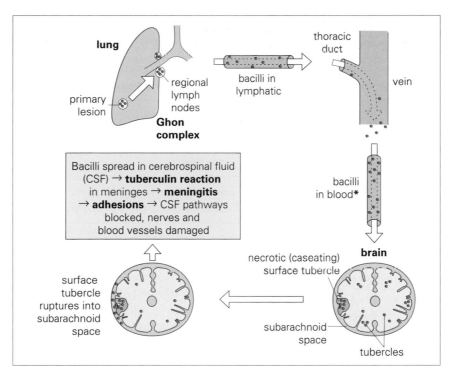

Fig. 24.11 The association between acute miliary tuberculosis and meningitis. (*Leads to miliary tuberculosis—Latin: *milium,* millet seed—each tubercle resembles a millet seed. Miliary tuberculosis also occurs in the lungs and elsewhere.)

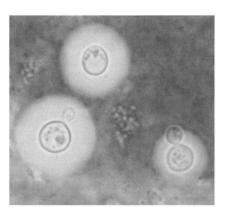

Fig. 24.12 *Cryptococcus neoformans* in India ink stained preparation of cerebrospinal fluid sediment. (Courtesy of AE Prevost.)

meningitis are listed in *Figure 24.13*, but viruses are isolated from the CSF in less than 50% of cases, which is why viral genome detection methods such as polymerase chain reaction (PCR) are used to make the diagnosis. As there are five groups of human enteroviruses which include the echoviruses, coxsackie Group A and B viruses, and the three polioviruses, and infection is commonly asymptomatic, a virus isolated from the throat or stool of a child with mild meningitis may be of no etiologic significance. However, the enteroviruses are common causes of seasonal aseptic meningitis. In contrast to bacterial meningitis, and despite there being only a few antiviral drugs for treatment, viral meningitis usually has a benign course, and complete recovery is the rule.

ENCEPHALITIS

Encephalitis is usually caused by viruses

The causes and pathogenesis of viral encephalitis are shown in *Figures 24.14* and *24.15*. Characteristically, there are signs of cerebral dysfunction, as the substance of the brain is affected, unlike meningitis where the lining of the brain is inflamed. Someone with an encephalitic illness will present with abnormal behavior, seizures and altered consciousness, often with nausea, vomiting and fever.

Toxoplasma gondii and *C. neoformans* can also cause life-threatening encephalitis or meningoencephalitis. This is particularly likely in those with defective cell-mediated immunity, and cerebral malaria as a complication of *Plasmodium falciparum* infection is frequently fatal. Encephalitis may occur in Lyme disease *(Borrelia burgdorferi)* and Legionnaires' disease *(Legionella pneumophila),* but the relative importance of bacterial invasion, bacterial toxins and immunopathology is unknown.

HSV encephalitis (HSE) is the most common form of severe sporadic acute focal encephalitis

It is thought that the incidence of HSE in the USA is about 1 per 250 000 to 500 000 population per year. A distinction is made between HSV infections of the CNS during the neonatal period and those in older children and adults. Neonates may acquire a primary and disseminated infection with a diffuse encephalitis after vaginal delivery from a mother shedding HSV-2 in the genital tract. Most HSE seen in older children and adults is due to HSV-1, of which most are due to virus

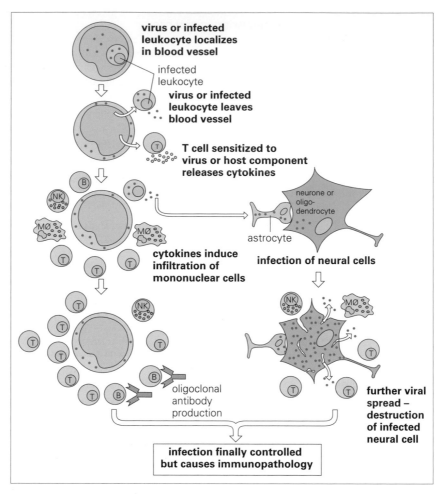

Fig. 24.15 The pathogenesis of viral encephalomyelitis. (Mφ, macrophage; NK, natural killer cell.)

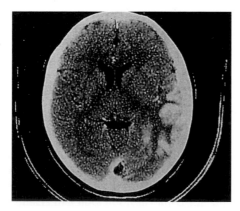

Fig. 24.16 Herpes simplex encephalitis. Computerized tomographic scan showing enhancement of gyral structures in the left temporal lobe and associated cerebral edema. (Courtesy of Dr J Curé.)

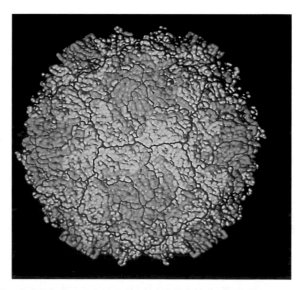

Fig. 24.17 Computer graphic model of the surface of a poliovirus based on X-ray diffraction studies. The capsid protein subunits visible on the surface of the virus particle are viral protein 1 (VP1) in blue, VP2 in green and VP3 in gray. (Courtesy of AJ Olson, Research Institute of Scripps Clinic, La Jolla, California.)

the clinical, epidemiologic, and virologic characteristics showed that the virus was a paramyxovirus which was transmitted to humans by close contact with infected pigs, probably by aerosol. The outbreak was ended by culling more than one million infected or exposed pigs in the local and surrounding regions in Malaysia. The Island flying fox, *Pteropus hypomelanus*, a fruit bat, was the likely reservoir as

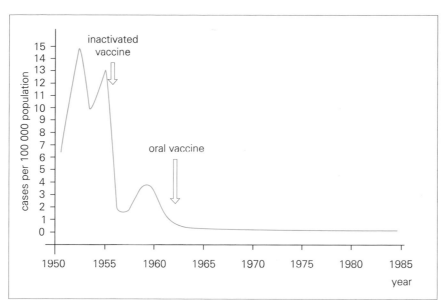

Fig. 24.18 The incidence of paralytic poliomyelitis in the USA from 1951 to 1985.

virus could be found in the urine and saliva of infected bats. The pigs were infected having eaten food contaminated by fruit bat secretions.

Rabies encephalitis

There are 35 000 cases of human rabies worldwide each year

The causative agent of rabies is a rhabdovirus, a bullet-shaped single-stranded RNA virus. The virus is excreted in the saliva of infected dogs, foxes, jackals, wolves, skunks, raccoons and vampire bats, and transmission to man follows a bite or salivary contamination of other types of skin abrasions or wounds. Some species of animal, such as foxes, are more infectious than others because larger amounts of virus, up to 10^6 infectious doses/ml, are present in their saliva. The infection is eventually fatal, although the course of the disease varies considerably between species. If an apparently healthy dog is still healthy 10 days after biting a human, rabies is extremely unlikely. However, the virus may be excreted in the dog's saliva before the animal shows any clinical signs of disease.

The virus can infect all warm-blooded animals. Rabies from vampire bats causes more than one million deaths per year in cattle in Central and South America. Dogs transmit most of the 35 000 cases of human rabies that occur in the world each year. In all the mainland masses, the infection maintains itself in non-human mammalian hosts; islands such as Australia, Great Britain, Japan, Hawaii, most of the Caribbean islands, and also Scandinavia, are free of rabies because of strict controls over the importation of animals such as dogs and cats, although this is changing. In the USA, the incidence of human rabies has been falling since the 1940s and 1950s, when most cases followed exposure to infected dogs. Since then the source has more often been non-domesticated animals such as skunks, raccoons and bats, or exposure to dogs in other countries.

Raccoon rabies spread slowly northwards from Florida in the 1950s, and in the 1980s caused an explosive epidemic in Virginia, Maryland and the District of Columbia. This outbreak was due to the importation of raccoons from infected areas for sporting purposes.

The incubation period in humans is generally 4–13 weeks, although it may occasionally be as long as 6 months, possibly due to a delay in virus entry into peripheral nerves. The virus travels up peripheral nerves and, in general, the further the bite is from the CNS, the longer the incubation period. For instance, a bite on the foot leads to a longer incubation period than a bite on the face.

While the virus is travelling up the axons of motor or sensory neurones, there is no detectable antibody or cell-mediated immune response, possibly because antigen remains sequestered in infected muscle cells. Hence, passively administered immunoglobulin may be given during the incubation period.

Once in the brain, the virus spreads from cell to cell until a large proportion of neurones is infected, but there is little cytopathic effect, even when viewed by electron microscopy, and almost no cellular infiltration. The striking symptoms of this disease are largely due to dysfunction rather than visible damage to infected cells. The change in behavior of infected animals results from virus invasion of the limbic system.

Clinical features of rabies include muscle spasms, convulsions and hydrophobia

After developing a sore throat, headache, fever and discomfort at the site of the bite, the patient becomes excited, with muscle spasms and convulsions. Involvement of the muscles of swallowing when attempting to drink water gave the old name for rabies—hydrophobia—as the symptoms are sometimes precipitated by the mere sight of water.

Once rabies has developed it is fatal, death occurring following cardiac or respiratory arrest. Paralysis is often a major feature of the disease. One or two patients treated in

INFECTIOUS DISEASES THAT MAY BE MANIFEST AS CHRONIC MENINGITIS OR BRAIN ABSCESS

bacterial	
tuberculosis	*Mycobacterium tuberculosis*
syphilis	*Treponema pallidum*
brucellosis	*Brucella abortus*
Lyme disease	*Borrelia burgdorferi*
nocardiosis*	*Nocardia asteroides*
actinomycosis*	*Actinomyces fumigatus*

fungal	
cryptococcosis	*Cryptococcus neoformans*
coccidioidomycosis	*Coccidioides immitis*
histoplasmosis	*Histoplasma capsulatum*
candidiasis	*Candida albicans*
blastomycosis*	*Blastomyces dermatitidis*

parasitic	
toxoplasmosis*	*Toxoplasma gondii*
cysticercosis*	*Taenia solium*

*disease manifest as brain abscess

Fig. 24.22 Infections causing chronic meningitis or brain abscess.

blocks the release of inhibitory mediators in spinal synapses, causing overactivity of motor neurones. It can also pass up sympathetic nerve axons and lead to overactivity of the sympathetic nervous system.

Clinical features of tetanus include muscle rigidity and spasms

After a period of 3–21 days, but sometimes longer, there are exaggerated reflexes, muscle rigidity and uncontrolled muscle spasms. Lockjaw (trismus) is due to contraction of jaw muscles. Dysphagia, 'risus sardonicus' (a sneering appearance), neck stiffness and opisthotonos (especially in neonatal tetanus; see Chapter 23) are also seen. Muscle spasms may lead to injury and eventually there is respiratory failure. Tachycardia and sweating can result from effects on the sympathetic nervous system. Mortality is up to 50%, depending on the severity and quality of treatment.

The diagnosis is clinical. Organisms are rarely isolated from the wound, and only a small number of bacteria are needed to form enough toxin to cause disease.

Human antitetanus immunoglobulin should be given as soon as tetanus is suspected clinically

The wound should be excised if necessary and penicillin given to inhibit bacterial replication. Muscle relaxants are used and, if necessary, respiratory support in an intensive care unit.

Immunization with toxoid prevents tetanus, the effects of the vaccine lasting for 10 years after the last dose. Thus, tetanus represents a vaccine-preventable disease that is unique in not being communicable but, instead, acquired from the environment as a result of exposure to *Cl. tetani* spores. Wounds should be cleansed, necrotic tissue and foreign bodies removed, and a tetanus toxoid booster given. Those with badly contaminated wounds should also be given tetanus immunoglobulin and penicillin.

In developing countries, routine immunization of women with tetanus toxoid and improved hygienic birth practices are having a significant impact in reducing the rates of neonatal tetanus.

Botulism

Spores of *Cl. botulinum* are widespread in soil and contaminate vegetables, meat and fish. When foods are canned or preserved without adequate sterilization (often at home), contaminating spores survive and can germinate in the anaerobic environment, leading to the formation of toxin.

Cl. botulinum *toxin blocks acetylcholine release from peripheral nerves*

Pre-formed botulinus toxin is ingested, then absorbed from the gut into the blood (see Chapter 22). It acts on peripheral nerve synapses by blocking the release of acetylcholine (see Chapter 17). It is therefore a type of food poisoning that affects the motor and autonomic nervous systems. Sometimes spores contaminate a wound and the toxin is then absorbed from this site. If the organism is ingested by infants, in the honey smeared on pacifiers for instance, it can multiply in the gut and produce the toxin, causing infant botulism.

Clinical features of botulism include weakness and paralysis

After an incubation period of 2–72 hours, there is descending weakness and paralysis, with dysphagia, diplopia, vomiting, vertigo and respiratory muscle failure. There is no abdominal pain, diarrhea or fever. Infants develop generalized weakness ('floppy babies'), but usually recover.

Botulism is treated with antibodies and respiratory support

A diagnosis of botulism is mainly clinical. The toxin can be demonstrated in contaminated food and occasionally in the patient's serum.

Since the specific *Cl. botulinum* strain(s) responsible are normally unknown, trivalent antitoxin (for type A, B and E toxins) must be given promptly together with respiratory support. The mortality is less than 20%, depending upon the success of the respiratory support.

Prevention is by avoiding imperfectly-sterilized canned or preserved food. Contaminated cans are often swollen due to the release of gas by clostridial enzymes. Home-preserved foods are often incriminated, but fruit, with its acidic pH, usually prevents the development of the spores. The toxin is heat labile and is destroyed by adequate cooking, for example boiling for 10 minutes. The spores can, however, survive boiling for 3–5 hours.

KEY FACTS

- Microbial invasion of the CNS is uncommon, due to the presence of the blood–brain and blood–CSF barriers, which limit the spread of infection.

- Once infectious agents have traversed these barriers they generally cause neurologic disease by involving the meninges (meningitis) or the brain substance (encephalitis).

- Viral meningitis is the commonest condition, bacterial meningitis the next commonest, with cerebral abscesses and viral encephalitis as rarities. The spinal cord (in myelitis) or peripheral nerves (in neuritis) are occasionally affected.

- Disease results from interference with the function of infected nerve cells (e.g. rabies), from direct damage to infected nerve cells (e.g. poliomyelitis), or from the inflammatory sequel to CNS invasion (e.g. bacterial meningitis, viral encephalitis).

- Because the anatomically defined compartments of the nervous system are adjacent or interconnected, more than one of them can be involved in a given infectious disease.

- CNS disease is sometimes seen in the helminth infections toxocariasis, hydatid disease and cysticercosis.

- CNS disease can also result when bacterial neurotoxins reach the CNS either from extraneural sites of growth (tetanus) or from contaminated food (botulism).

QUESTIONS

A 45-year-old bank manageress is brought to hospital by ambulance having collapsed in the street. She is unable to give a history, but a passerby had said that she suddenly collapsed having left a shop and then had a seizure. The police contact her husband who tells them that she has been complaining of a headache for the past few days and has been acting in a slightly strange way. She has no relevant past medical history, has not had a seizure before, and is on no medication. On examination she is drowsy, confused and has a temperature of 38°C. She has no focal neurologic signs, although her reflexes are brisk. The rest of her examination is normal. Fundoscopy reveals no papilledema, and examination of her oropharynx and ears is normal. Investigations include a full blood count, which is normal, and urea and electrolytes, including a blood glucose level, which are also normal.

1. What urgent investigations would you perform?

2. A CT scan shows an area of low density attenuation in the left temporal lobe and no evidence of cerebral edema or midline shift. Results of a lumbar puncture are: CSF appearance clear, white cell count $50/mm^3$ (all lymphocytes), zero red cells, protein 0.9 g/dl; CSF glucose 3.3 mmol/l; blood glucose 5 mmol/l; no organisms seen on Gram stain. What diagnoses would you consider in the light of these results and the clinical history?

3. How would you manage and treat her?

FURTHER READING

Chuka KB, Bellini WJ, Rota PA et al. Nipah virus: a recently emergent deadly paramyxovirus. *Science* 2000; 288:1432–5.

Cook TM, Protheroe RT, Handel JM. Tetanus: a review of the literature. *Br J Anaesth* 2001; 87:477–87.

Johnson RT. The pathogenesis of acute viral encephalitis and post infectious encephalomyelitis. *J Infect Dis* 1987; 155:359–64.

Lanciotti RW, Roehrig JT, Deubel V et al. Origin of West Nile virus responsible for an outbreak of encephalitis in the northeastern United States. *Science* 1999; 286:2333–7.

Mestel R. Putting prions to the test. *Science* 1996; 273:184–9.

Plotkin SA. Rabies. *Clin Infect Dis* 2000; 30:4–12.

Prusiner SB. Human prion diseases. In: *Principles and Practice of Clinical Virology*, 4th edition. Chichester: Wiley, 2000.

Shapiro RL, Hatheway C, Swerdlow DL. Botulism in the United States: a clinical and epidemiologic review. *Ann Intern Med* 1998; 129:221–8.

Tunkel AR. *Bacterial Meningitis*. Philadelphia: Lippincott Williams & Wilkins, 2001.

Whitley RJ, Gnann JW. Viral encephalitis: familiar infections and emerging pathogens. *Lancet* 2002; 359:507–14.

Infections of the eye

INTRODUCTION

Because the outer surface of the eye is exposed to the external world it is easily accessible to infective organisms. The conjunctiva is particularly susceptible. Not only is it a vulnerable epithelial surface, it is covered by the eyelids, which create a warm, moist, enclosed environment in which contaminating organisms can quickly establish and set up a focus of infection. The eyelids and tears protect the external surfaces of the eye, both mechanically and biologically; any interference with their function increases the chance of a pathogen becoming established.

Eyelid infections are generally due to *Staphylococcus aureus,* with involvement of the lid margins causing blepharitis, and eyelid glands or follicles causing styes or hordeolums.

The conjunctiva can be invaded by other routes, such as the blood or nervous system. The deeper tissues of the eye can also be invaded from within, particularly by protozoan and worm parasites.

CONJUNCTIVITIS

A wide variety of viruses and bacteria can cause conjunctivitis or pinkeye *(Fig. 25.1).* Some infections are common in children and resolve quickly, others are potentially more serious. Keratoconjunctivitis from adenovirus, herpes simplex virus or varicella-zoster virus can result in severe damage. An acute hemorrhagic conjunctivitis can follow infection with enterovirus 70 and coxsackie virus A24.

Chlamydial infections

Different serotypes of Chlamydia trachomatis *cause inclusion conjunctivitis and trachoma*

To establish infection on the conjunctiva, microorganisms must avoid being rinsed and wiped away in tears. The best way of achieving this is to have a specific mechanism of attachment to conjunctival cells. *Chlamydia,* for example, have surface molecules that bind specifically to receptors on host cells. This is one of the reasons that of all the organisms infecting the conjunctiva *(Fig. 25.1),* they are among the most successful. There are eight different serotypes of *Chlamydia trachomatis* responsible for inclusion conjunctivitis *(Fig. 25.2)* and another four serotypes responsible for trachoma, which is the most important eye infection in the world.

Six million people worldwide are blind because of trachoma

About 100–200 million people have trachoma, and six million are blinded by it, while many others suffer visual impairment. Trachoma was known in ancient Egypt four thousand years ago, and tweezers to remove inturned eyelashes *(Fig. 25.3)* have been found in royal tombs. Transmission of *C. trachomatis* is by contact, for example by contaminated flies, fingers and towels.

MICROBIAL INFECTIONS OF THE CONJUNCTIVA	
organism	**comments**
adenovirus	especially types 3,7, 8,19
measles virus	infection of conjunctiva via blood
herpes simplex virus	virus reactivating in ophthalmic division of trigeminal ganglia causes corneal lesion (dendritic ulcer)
varicella-zoster virus	may involve conjunctiva
enterovirus 70, coxsackie virus A24	acute hemorrhagic conjunctivitis
Chlamydia trachomatis (types A–C) (types D–K)	cause of trachoma and commonly blindness cause of inclusion conjunctivitis; infection via fingers etc. or in newborn via birth canal
Neisseria gonorrhoeae	infection of newborn via birth canal
Staphylococcus aureus	cause of eyelid infection (styes) and 'sticky eye' in neonates

Fig. 25.1 Microbial infections of the conjunctiva.

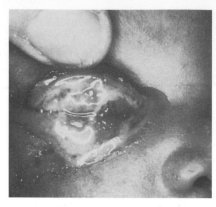

Fig. 25.2 Chlamydial conjunctivitis is the commonest form of neonatal conjunctivitis. (Courtesy of G Ridgway.)

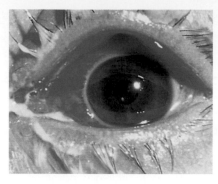

Fig. 25.4 Purulent discharge in bacterial conjunctivitis is often associated with infections by *Streptococcus pneumoniae*, *Haemophilus influenzae* or *Staphylococcus aureus*. (Courtesy of M Tapert.)

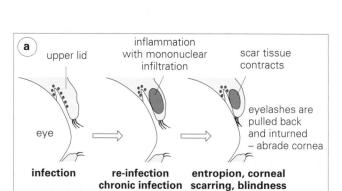

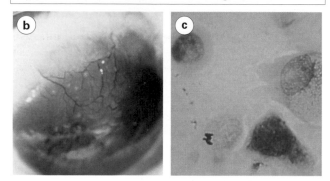

Fig. 25.3 *Chlamydia trachomatis* and blindness. The pathogenesis is outlined in (a). Scarring of the cornea (b) results from long-standing ocular trachoma. (Courtesy of RC Barnes.) Giemsa stain of an ocular scraping from trachoma (c) shows *C. trachomatis* as an intracellular inclusion. (Courtesy of G Ridgway.)

Trachoma itself is the result of chronic repeated infections (*Fig. 25.3*), which are especially prevalent when there is poor access to water, preventing regular washing of the hands and face. Under these circumstances, chlamydial infection is frequently spread from one conjunctiva to another and this can be referred to as 'ocular promiscuity', comparable with the spread of genital secretions in non-specific urethritis (see Chapter 21). Some chlamydial serotypes can infect the urinogenital tract (see Chapter 21) as well as the conjunctiva, and the conjunctiva or lungs of a newborn infant may become infected after passage down an infected birth canal (see Chapter 23). In this situation, systemic treatment with erythromycin is generally needed.

Chlamydial infections are treated with antibiotic and prevented by face washing

Laboratory diagnosis of chlamydial infections (see Appendix) can be carried out using conjunctival fluid or scrapings. Treatment is with topical or oral antibiotics (e.g. azithromycin, doxycycline, etc.). Because infection and re-infection are facilitated by overcrowding, shortage of water and abundant fly populations, the disease can be prevented by improvements in standards of hygiene. In many areas with high rates of endemic trachoma, disease leading to blindness has been sharply reduced or eliminated by socioeconomic development and specific intervention steps (e.g. face washing). This has led the World Health Organization to establish an international alliance for the global elimination of blinding trachoma by the year 2020.

In spite of many decades of research there are still no vaccines for chlamydial infections. This is partly because immunopathology itself makes a major contribution to the disease, and vaccine-induced immune responses could be harmful.

Other conjunctival infections

In developed countries, chlamydia account for only 20% of cases of conjunctivitis

Several bacteria (especially *Streptococcus pneumoniae*, *Haemophilus influenzae* and *Staphylococcus aureus*) can cause conjunctivitis (*Fig. 25.4*). A clone of *H. influenzae* biotype *aegyptius* causes Brazilian purpuric fever (BPF), which occurs up to several weeks after an acute attack of conjunctivitis with this strain. BPF is characterized by fever, purpura and massive vascular collapse, and is rapidly fatal. The pathogenesis is not clear. Originally described in Brazil, cases have now occurred in most parts of the world.

Infection by *Neisseria gonorrhoeae* is a hazard of birth through an infected birth canal, and can result in a severe purulent condition. It is seen on the first or second day of life (ophthalmia neonatorum) and requires urgent treatment with ceftriaxone (penicillin resistance is widespread). *Staph. aureus* also produces infections in newborns as well as in adults. The eyes of infants may be invaded by this organism if the organism is transferred from the child's own body or from an infected adult.

Direct infection of the eye may be associated with wearing contact lenses

Excessive wearing of contact lenses can lead to a reduction in the effectiveness of the eye's defense mechanisms, allowing pathogens to become established, but more likely hazards are the use of contaminated eye drops or cleaning solutions and the insertion of contaminated lenses. A number of bacteria can be transmitted directly in this way. The free-living ameba *Acanthamoeba* can multiply in unchanged lens cleaning fluids and be transferred when the lens is inserted, causing corneal damage.

Conjunctival infection may be transmitted by the blood or nervous system

Several organisms invade the superficial tissues of the eye after transport through the blood or, in the case of herpes simplex virus (HSV), by movement along the trigeminal nerve. Reactivation of this virus can result in the development of a keratitis with the formation of dendritic ulcers *(Fig. 25.5)*. Inadvertent use of topical steroids may aggravate this condition, and the resultant severe ulceration can lead to corneal destruction.

INFECTION OF THE DEEPER LAYERS OF THE EYE

The spectrum of organisms causing disease in the deeper layers of the eye is wider than that associated with the conjunctiva *(Fig. 25.6)*.

Entry into the deeper layers occurs by many routes

Trauma to the eye may result in the opportunistic establishment of a *Pseudomonas aeruginosa* infection, giving rise to

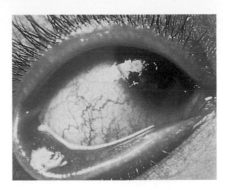

Fig. 25.5 Herpes simplex virus (HSV) keratitis. Dendritic ulcers, seen here on the cornea, are common in recurrent HSV infections. (Courtesy of MJ Wood.)

serious inner eye infection. This organism may also be introduced via contaminated eye drops. Rubella and cytomegalovirus (CMV) may invade the fetal eye in utero, the former causing cataracts and microphthalmia, the latter a severe chorioretinitis. CMV can also cause chorioretinitis in AIDS patients (see *Fig. 21.35e*). Congenital syphilis produces a retinopathy with quiescent lesions, and keratitis may appear in later life. Secondary syphilis is also associated with ocular inflammation.

Toxoplasmosis

Toxoplasma gondii infection can cause chorioretinitis leading to blindness

Chorioretinitis also occurs with toxoplasmosis. Infection occurs by swallowing oocysts released by infected cats (the primary host) or by eating meat containing tissue cysts. Although infection with this protozoan is widespread (see Chapter 5), it is not serious unless:

INFECTIONS OF THE DEEPER LAYERS OF THE EYE		
organism	**disease**	**route of infection**
rubella	cataracts, microphthalmia	infection in utero
cytomegalovirus	chorioretinitis	infection in utero; may occur in AIDS*
Pseudomonas aeruginosa	serious inner eye infection	after trauma foreign bodies in eye eye operations bacteria can contaminate eye drops
Toxoplasma gondii (toxoplasmosis)	chorioretinitis	infection in utero
Echinococcus granulosus (hydatid disease)	distortion of the eye by growth of larval tapeworm in hydatid cyst	transmission by eggs passed by dogs
Toxocara canis (ocular toxocariasis)	chorioretinitis, blindness	transmission by eggs passed by dogs
Onchocerca volvulus (river blindness)	sclerosing keratitis chorioretinitis	larvae transmitted by blood-feeding *Simulium* files

Fig. 25.6 Infections of the deeper layers of the eye. (*25% of patients with AIDS develop cytomegalovirus retinitis.)

- acquired in utero when the organism invades all tissues, especially the central nervous system (CNS);
- acquired (or reactivated) under immunosuppression.

Damage to the eye occurs primarily in congential toxoplasmosis. Women who become infected in pregnancy may transmit the infection to the fetus, as tachyzoites can cross the placenta. Tissue cysts can form in the retina of the fetus and undergo continuous proliferation, producing progressive lesions, particularly when levels of immunity are low. These lesions may also involve the choroid (*Fig. 25.7*) and lead ultimately to blindness. One or both eyes may be affected.

Parasitic worm infections

Toxocara canis *larvae cause an intense inflammatory response and can lead to retinal detachment*

Larval tapeworms (e.g. the hydatid cyst stage of *Echinococcus granulosus* transmitted by eggs passed from infected dogs) occasionally enter the eye, with growth of the cysts causing severe mechanical damage. Invasion by migratory larvae of the nematode *Toxocara canis* is more common. This parasite occurs naturally in the intestines of dogs, releasing thick-shelled resistant eggs into the environment. The eggs can

hatch if swallowed by humans, the larvae initiating, but failing to complete, their customary migration through the tissues. In the canine host, migration results in the worms re-entering the intestine where they mature. In humans, larvae can enter almost any organ, often the CNS or eye (*Fig. 25.8*), triggering an intense eosinophilic inflammatory response. In the eye, localized lesions in the retina may cause detachment. The misdiagnosis of such ocular lesions as retinoblastoma has led to enucleation. Anthelmintic treatment (albendazole, mebendazole) is beneficial.

Onchocerca volvulus *infection causes 'river blindness' and is transmitted by* Simulium *flies*

Onchocerca volvulus infection, the cause of 'river blindness' in Africa and Central America, is transmitted by biting *Simulium* flies, which take up microfilariae larvae from the skin of infected hosts and re-introduce the larvae after they have become infective, when next feeding. Adult worms live in subcutaneous nodules, and are comparatively harmless. The microfilariae, released by the females in enormous numbers, induce intense inflammatory reactions in the skin (see Chapter 26). The larvae migrate through the subcutaneous tissue, and invasion of the eye has been particularly common in certain regions of Africa as well as Central America.

The inflammatory responses in the eye cause a number of pathologic changes, which may affect both the anterior and posterior chambers (*Fig. 25.9*). These include:

- punctate and sclerosing keratitis;
- iridocyclitis;
- chorioretinitis;
- optic atrophy.

The disease is called river blindness because the *Simulium* flies develop in rivers, and people living near rivers are most affected. Blindness rates have reached 40% of the adult population in endemic areas, but vector control and ivermectin treatment have dramatically reduced the incidence of new infections in many African countries. Unfortunately the blindness is irreversible.

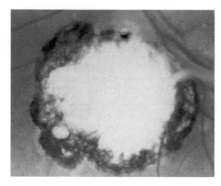

Fig. 25.7 Congenital toxoplasmosis. Fundal photograph showing the scar of healed chorioretinitis. (Courtesy of MJ Wood.)

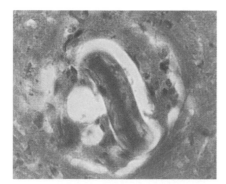

Fig. 25.8 *Toxocara canis.* Granuloma in the posterior pole of an infected eye. The larval nematode is clearly visible in the center of the granuloma. (Courtesy of D Spalton.)

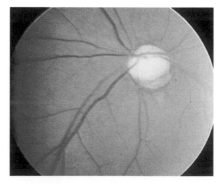

Fig. 25.9 Onchocerciasis. Sclerosis of the choroidal vessels caused by invading microfilaria of *Onchocerca volvulus*. (Courtesy of J Anderson.)

KEY FACTS

- The external surfaces of the eye are vulnerable to infection. They are protected by the eyelids and by factors such as lysozyme in tears.

- The consequences of eye infection are always potentially serious given that sight is dependent upon the presence of an intact transparent cornea.

- Microbes infecting the conjunctiva have specific attachment mechanisms.

- Inflammatory responses, though 'designed' to limit invasion and repair damage, can irreversibly damage conjunctival and corneal surfaces.

- Relatively few organisms invade the retina, and those that do are potentially sight-threatening.

- Some of the most serious infection-related diseases of the eye involve invasion by protozoan or helminth parasites. The diagnosis then often follows rather than precedes the development of visual impairment.

QUESTIONS

A 42-year-old homosexual man with AIDS complains of blurred vision. He has noticed that he has floaters and a visual field loss, which he describes as black patches in his vision. His last CD4 count was very low at 20 cells/mm³ and he has been admitted to hospital for treatment of *Pneumocystis jiroveci* (formerly *P. carinii*) pneumonia and Kaposi's sarcoma. Fundoscopy reveals areas of white infiltrates and hemorrhages consistent with a diagnosis of retinitis. Examination of his visual fields reveals a single scotoma (a blind spot) in the inferotemporal part of his retina.

1. What infections are associated with a choroidoretinitis?

2. How would you make the diagnosis?

3. How would you treat a patient with CMV retinitis?

FURTHER READING

Cox FEG et al., eds. *Parasitology.* vol. 5 of Collier LH et al., eds, *Topley & Wilson's Microbiology and Microbial Infections,* 9th edition. London: Arnold, 1998.

Harding SP. Viral infections of the eye. *Rev Med Virol* 1993; 3:161–71.

Holmes KK. The chlamydia epidemic. *J Am Med Assoc* 1981; 245:1718–23.

Weiss A, Brinser JH, Nazar-Stewart V. Acute conjunctivitis in childhood. *J Pediatr* 1993; 122:10–14.

Wilcox ADP, Stapleton F. Ocular bacteriology. *Rev Med Microbiol* 1996; 7:123–31.

Infections of the skin, soft tissue, muscle and associated systems

INTRODUCTION

Healthy intact skin protects underlying tissues and provides excellent defense against invading microbes

The microbial load of normal skin is kept in check by various factors, as shown in *Figure 26.1*. Alterations in these factors (e.g. prolonged exposure to moisture) upsets the ecologic balance of the commensal flora, and predisposes to infection.

A small number of microbes cause diseases of muscle, joints or the hemopoietic system. Invasion of these sites is generally from the blood, but the reason for localization to particular tissues is often obscure. Circulating microbes tend to localize in growing or damaged bones (acute osteomyelitis) and in damaged joints, but we do not know why coxsackieviruses or *Trichinella spiralis* invade muscle. On the other hand some viruses infect a given target cell, and plasmodia invade erythrocytes because they have specific attachment sites for these cells.

Infections of the skin

In addition to being a structural barrier, the skin is colonized by an array of organisms which forms its normal flora. The relatively arid areas of the forearm and back are colonized with fewer organisms, predominantly Gram-positive bacteria and yeasts. In the moister areas, such as the groin and the armpit, the organisms are more numerous and more varied and include Gram-negative bacteria. The normal flora of the skin plays an important role, as does the normal flora in other body sites, in defending the surface from 'foreign invaders'.

FACTORS CONTROLLING THE SKIN'S MICROBIAL LOAD
the limited amount of moisture present
acid pH of normal skin
surface temperature < optimum for many pathogens
salty sweat
excreted chemicals such as sebum, fatty acids and urea
competition between different species of the normal flora

Fig. 26.1 The number of bacteria on the skin vary from a few hundred per cm² on the arid surfaces of the forearm and back, to tens of thousands per cm² on the moist areas such as the axilla and groin. This normal flora plays an important role in preventing 'foreign' organisms from colonizing the skin, but it too needs to be kept in check.

An appreciation of the structure of the skin helps in understanding the different sorts of infection to which the skin and its underlying tissues are prone *(Fig. 26.2)*. If organisms breach the stratum corneum the host defenses are mobilized, the epidermal Langerhans' cells elaborate cytokines, neutrophils are attracted to the site of invasion, and complement is activated via the alternative pathway.

Microbial disease of the skin may result from any of three lines of attack

These lines of attack are:

- breach of intact skin, allowing infection from the outside;
- skin manifestations of systemic infections, which may arise as a result of bloodborne spread from the infected focus to the skin or by direct extension (e.g. draining sinuses from actinomycotic lesions, or necrotizing anaerobic infection from intra-abdominal sepsis);
- toxin-mediated skin damage due to production of a microbial toxin at another site in the body (e.g. scarlet fever, toxic shock syndrome).

The sequence of events in the pathogenesis of mucocutaneous lesions caused by bacterial, fungal and viral infections is outlined in *Figure 26.3*. Breaches in the skin range from microscopic to major trauma, which may be accidental (e.g. lacerations or burns) or intentional (e.g. surgery). Hospitalized patients are liable to other skin breaches (e.g. pressure sores and intravenous catheter insertions), which may become infected (see Chapter 36). Infections in compromised individuals such as patients with burns are discussed in Chapter 30. Here we will consider primary infections of the skin and underlying soft tissues, together with mucocutaneous lesions resulting from certain systemic viral infections. Systemic bacterial and fungal infections that cause mucocutaneous lesions are summarized in *Figure 26.4*.

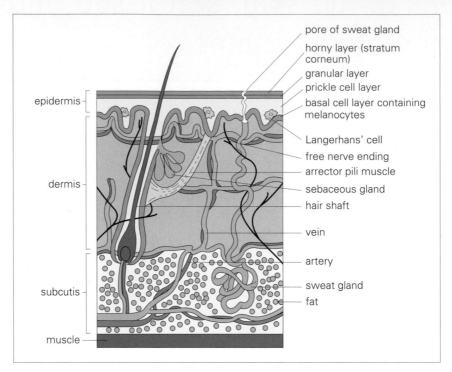

Fig. 26.2 Infection of the skin and soft tissue can be related to the anatomy of the skin. Pathogens usually enter the lower layers of the epidermis and dermis only after the skin surface has been damaged.

BACTERIAL INFECTIONS OF SKIN, SOFT TISSUE AND MUSCLE

These can be classified on an anatomic basis

The classification depends upon the layers of skin and soft tissue involved, although some infections may involve several components of the soft tissues:

- Abscess formation. Boils and carbuncles are the result of infection and inflammation of the hair follicles in the skin (folliculitis).
- Spreading infections. Impetigo is limited to the epidermis and presents as a bullous, crusted or pustular eruption of the skin. Erysipelas involves the blocking of dermal lymphatics and presents as a well-defined, spreading erythematous inflammation, generally on the face, legs or feet, and often accompanied by pain and fever. If the focus of infection is in the subcutaneous fat, cellulitis, a diffuse form of acute inflammation, is the usual presentation.
- Necrotizing infections. Fasciitis describes the inflammatory response to infection of the soft tissue below the dermis. Infection spreads, often with alarming rapidity, along the fascial planes causing disruption of the blood supply. Gangrene or myonecrosis may follow infection associated with ischemia of the muscle layer. Gas resulting from the fermentative metabolism of anaerobic organisms may be palpable in the tissues (gas gangrene).

The common causative organisms are shown in *Figure 26.5*. Note that the same pathogen (e.g. *Streptococcus pyogenes*) can cause different infections in different layers of the skin and soft tissue.

Staphylococcal skin infections

Staphylococcus aureus *is the most common cause of skin infections and provokes an intense inflammatory response*

Staphylococcus aureus causes minor skin infections such as boils or abscesses as well as more serious postoperative wound infection. Infection may be acquired by 'self-inoculation' from a carrier site (e.g. the nose) or acquired by contact with an exogenous source, usually another person. People who are nasal carriers of virulent *Staph. aureus* may suffer from recurrent boils, but an inoculum of about 100 000 organisms is thought to be required in the absence of a wound or foreign body. *Staph. aureus* can also cause serious skin disease due to toxin production (scalded skin syndrome, toxic shock syndrome; see below).

A boil begins, within 2–4 days of inoculation, as a superficial infection in and around a hair follicle (folliculitis; *Fig. 26.6*). In this site the organisms are relatively protected from the host defenses, multiply rapidly and spread locally. This provokes an intense inflammatory response with an influx of neutrophils. Fibrin is deposited, and the site is walled off. Abscesses typically contain abundant yellow creamy pus formed by the massive number of organisms and necrotic white cells. They continue to expand slowly, eventually erode the overlying skin, 'come to a head' and drain. Drainage inwards can result in seeding of the staphylococci to

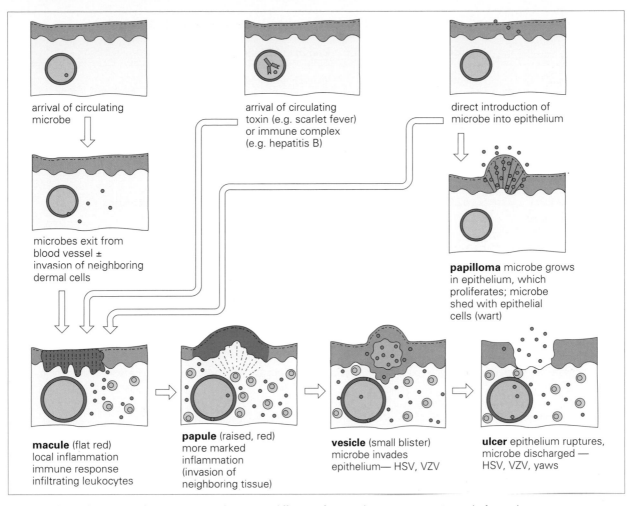

arrival of circulating microbe

↓

microbes exit from blood vessel ± invasion of neighboring dermal cells

arrival of circulating toxin (e.g. scarlet fever) or immune complex (e.g. hepatitis B)

direct introduction of microbe into epithelium

↓

papilloma microbe grows in epithelium, which proliferates; microbe shed with epithelial cells (wart)

macule (flat red) local inflammation immune response infiltrating leukocytes

papule (raised, red) more marked inflammation (invasion of neighboring tissue)

vesicle (small blister) microbe invades epithelium— HSV, VZV

ulcer epithelium ruptures, microbe discharged — HSV, VZV, yaws

Fig. 26.3 The pathogenesis of mucocutaneous lesions. In different infections the starting point (arrival of microbe or toxin or immune complex) and the final picture (e.g. maculopapular rash, vesicle) will be different. (HSV, herpes simplex virus; VZV, varicella-zoster virus.)

underlying body sites to cause serious infections such as peritonitis, empyema or meningitis.

Staph. aureus *infections are often diagnosed clinically and treatment includes drainage and antibiotics*

Staph. aureus is the most common cause of boils, and diagnosis is made on clinical grounds. Isolation and further identification of the infecting staphylococcus in hospital patients and staff is important in the investigation of hospital infections (see Chapter 36).

Treatment involves drainage and this is usually sufficient for minor lesions, but antibiotics may be given in addition when the infection is severe and the patient has a fever. Most *Staph. aureus* are beta-lactamase producers, but methicillin-susceptible *Staph. aureus* (MSSA) can be treated with enzyme-stable penicillins such as nafcillin. Isolates resistant to these compounds (i.e. methicillin-resistant *Staph.* aureus (MRSA); see Chapter 33) may be treated with vancomycin, linezolid or quinopristin–dalfoprisin. Treatment with these agents does not necessarily eradicate carriage of the staphylococci.

Recurrent infections may be treated in nasal carriers of *Staph. aureus* with nasal creams containing antibiotics. For example, mupirocin has been used successfully for carriers of methicillin-resistant staphylococci (see Chapter 36). Good skin care and personal hygiene should be encouraged.

Staphylococcal scalded skin syndrome is caused by toxin-producing Staph. aureus

This condition, also known as 'Ritter's disease' in infants and 'Lyell's disease' or 'toxic epidermal necrolysis' in older children, occurs sporadically and in outbreaks. It is caused by strains of *Staph. aureus* producing a toxin known as 'exfoliatin' or 'scalded skin syndrome toxin'. The initial skin lesion may be minor, but the toxin causes destruction of the intercellular connections and separation of the top layer of the epidermis. Large blisters are formed, containing clear fluid, and within one or two days the overlying areas of skin are lost (Fig. 26.7) leaving normal skin underneath. The baby is irritable and uncomfortable, but rarely severely ill. However, treatment should take into account the risk of increased loss of fluid from the damaged surface, and fluid replacement may be needed. As mentioned above, antimicrobial chemotherapy would employ beta-lactamase stable penicillins (e.g. nafcillin) against MSSA whereas vancomycin, linezolid or quinopristin–dalfoprisin would be used for MRSA.

SKIN MANIFESTATIONS OF SYSTEMIC INFECTIONS CAUSED BY BACTERIA AND FUNGI		
organism	**disease**	**skin manifestation**
Salmonella typhi *Salmonella schottmuelleri*	enteric fever	'rose spots' containing bacteria
Neisseria meningitidis	septicemia, meningitis	petechial or maculopapular lesions containing bacteria
Pseudomonas aeruginosa	septicemia	ecthyma gangrenosum, skin lesion pathognomonic if infected by this organism
Treponema pallidum *Treponema pertenue*	syphilis yaws	disseminated infectious rash seen in secondary stage of disease, 2–3 months after infection
Rickettsia prowazeki *Rickettsia rickettsii* *Rickettsia conori*	typhus spotted fevers	macular or hemorrhagic rash
Streptococcus pyogenes	scarlet fever	erythematous rash caused by erythrogenic toxin
Staphylococcus aureus	toxic shock syndrome	rash and desquamation due to toxin
Blastomyces dermatitidis	blastomycosis	papule or pustule develops into granuloma lesions containing organisms
Cryptococcus neoformans	cryptococcosis	papule or pustule, usually on face or neck

Fig. 26.4 Skin lesions are often associated with systemic infection with particular bacteria and fungi. The lesions may provide useful diagnostic aids. Sometimes they are a site from which organisms are shed.

Toxic shock syndrome is caused by toxic shock syndrome toxin-producing Staph. aureus

This systemic infection came to prominence through its association with tampon use by healthy women, but it is not confined to women and can occur as a result of *Staph. aureus* infection at non-genital sites (e.g. a wound). Toxic shock syndrome (TSS) involves multiple organ systems and is characterized by fever, hypotension and a diffuse macular erythematous rash followed by desquamation of the skin, particularly on the soles and palms *(Fig. 26.8)*. TSS is caused by exotoxins of *Staph. aureus,* most commonly TSST1, which behaves as a superantigen (stimulating T cell proliferation and cytokine release; see Chapter 16). While the prevalence of TSS in the USA is currently estimated at 6000 cases per year, greater than 90% of adults carry antibodies to TSST1. Treatment of TSS includes steps to open the infected site (e.g. drainage), fluid replacement and antistaphylococcal chemotherapy.

Streptococcal skin infections

Streptococcal skin infections are caused by Strep. pyogenes *(group A streptococci)*

Streptococcal impetigo develops independently of streptococcal upper respiratory tract infection, and although up to 35% of patients carry the same strain in their nose or throat, colonization may well occur after the skin has become infected. The organisms are acquired through contact with other people with infected skin lesions and may first colonize and multiply on normal skin before invasion through minor breaks in the epithelium and the development of lesions. The various risk factors involved in the development of streptococcal impetigo are shown in *Figure 26.9*. *Strep. pyogenes* may also cause erysipelas, an acute deeper infection in the dermis. About 5% of patients with erysipelas go on to develop bacteremia which carries a high mortality if untreated. As discussed previously, impetigo may also be caused by *Staph. aureus* and occasionally presents in more extreme bullous form (i.e. bullous impetigo) as blisters resembling localized scalded skin syndrome (see above).

Strep. pyogenes possesses certain surface proteins (M and T) which are antigenic. The species can be subdivided (typed) on the basis of these antigens, and it has been recognized that certain M and T types are associated with skin infection (and these differ from the types associated with sore throats). T proteins play no known role in virulence, and their function is unknown. M proteins are important virulence factors because they inhibit opsonization and confer on the bacterium resistance to phagocytosis. A variety of additional factors contribute to the virulence of the organism, such as lipoteichoic acid and F protein which facilitate binding to epithelial cells.

DIRECT ENTRY INTO SKIN OF BACTERIA AND FUNGI		
structure involved	**infection**	**common cause**
keratinized epithelium	ringworm	dermatophyte fungi (*Trichophyton*, *Epidermophyton* and *Microsporum*)
epidermis	impetigo	*Streptococcus pygenes* and/or *Staphylococcus aureus*
dermis	erysipelas	*Strep. pyogenes*
hair follicles	folliculitis boils (furuncles) carbuncles	*Staph. aureus*
subcutaneous fat	cellulitis	*Strep. pyogenes*
fascia	necrotizing fasciitis	anaerobes and microaerophiles, usually mixed infections
muscle	myonecrosis gangrene	*Clostridium perfringens* (and other clostridia)

Fig. 26.5 Direct introduction of bacteria or fungi into the skin is the most common route of skin infection. Infections range from mild, often chronic, conditions such as ringworm to acute and life-threatening fasciitis and gangrene. Relatively few species are involved in the common infections.

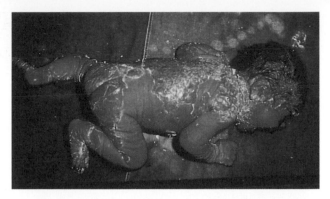

Fig. 26.7 Scalded skin syndrome results from infection of the skin with strains of *Staphylococcus aureus* producing a specific toxin, which destroys the intercellular connections in the skin, resulting in large areas of desquamation. The appearance may be confused with a burn. (Courtesy of A du Vivier.)

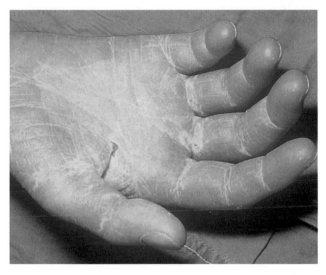

Fig. 26.8 Toxic shock syndrome results from systemic infection with *Staphylococcus aureus*, but has skin manifestations in the form of desquamation, particularly of the palm and soles. (Courtesy of MJ Wood.)

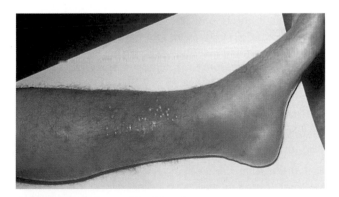

Fig. 26.6 Folliculitis. A superficial infection shown here localized in the hair follicles on the leg. The boils contain creamy-yellow pus and masses of bacteria. *Staphylococcus aureus* is the most common cause. (Courtesy of A du Vivier.)

Clinical features of streptococcal skin infections are typically acute

They develop within 24–48 hours of skin invasion and trigger a marked inflammatory response as the host attempts to localize the infection (*Figs 26.10* and *26.11*). *Strep. pyogenes* elaborates a number of toxic products and enzymes, such as hyaluronidase, which help the organism to spread in tissue. Lymphatic involvement is common, resulting in lymphadenitis and lymphangitis.

Lysogenic strains of *Strep. pyogenes* produce pyrogenic exotoxins (formally called erythrogenic toxins). As with TSST1 in *Staph. aureus* (discussed previously) these toxins are superantigens with a potent influence on the immune system. The toxins also act on skin blood vessels to cause the diffuse erythematous rash of scarlet fever, which may occur with streptococcal pharyngitis. *Strep. pyogenes* may also cause a form of toxic shock syndrome which has been especially

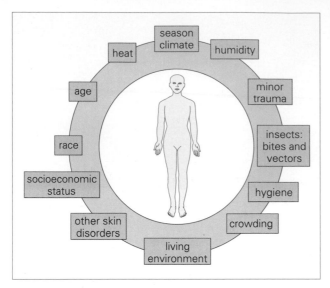

Fig. 26.9 Various factors are involved in the development of streptococcal skin infections. Particular M types of *Streptococcus pyogenes* have a predilection for skin, but various factors predispose the host (usually a child) to infection. Mixed infections with *Staphylococcus aureus* are also common.

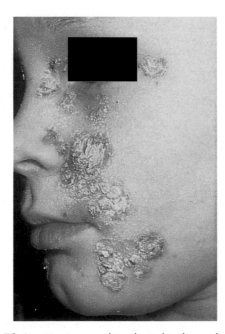

Fig. 26.10 Impetigo is a condition limited to the epidermis, with typically yellow, crusted lesions. It is commonly caused by *Streptococcus pyogenes* either alone or together with *Staphylococcus aureus*. (Courtesy of MJ Wood.)

associated with the production of the pyrogenic exotoxin SpeA.

Certain M types (e.g. M49) of Strep. pyogenes are associated with acute glomerulonephritis

Acute glomerulonephritis (AGN) occurs more often after skin infections than after infections of the throat (see Chapter 18). It is characterized by the deposition of immune complexes on the basement membrane of the glomerulus, but the precise role of the streptococcus in the causation is still unclear

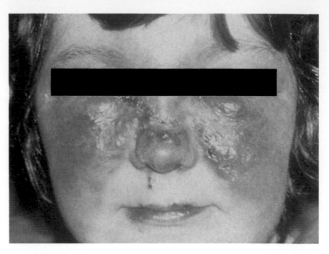

Fig. 26.11 Erysipelas. Infection with *Streptococcus pyogenes* involving the dermal lymphatics and giving rise to a clearly demarcated area of erythema and induration. When the face is involved there is often a typical 'butterfly-wing' rash, as shown here. (Courtesy of MJ Wood.)

(see Chapter 17); 10–15% of individuals infected with a nephritogenic strain will develop AGN about 2–3 weeks after the primary infection. Most people recover completely, and recurrence after a subsequent streptococcal infection is rare. Rheumatic fever (see Chapter 18) very rarely follows skin infections with *Strep. pyogenes*.

Streptococcal skin infections are usually diagnosed clinically and treated with penicillin

Gram stains of pus from vesicles in impetigo show Gram-positive cocci, and culture reveals *Strep. pyogenes* sometimes mixed with *Staph. aureus* (*Fig. 26.12*). In erysipelas, skin cultures are often negative, although culture of fluid from the advancing edge of the lesion may be successful.

Penicillin is the drug of choice, although eythromycin or an oral cephalosporin may be used for penicillin-allergic patients. However, the prevalence of resistance in streptococci is increasing, and these drugs are not effective in mixed infections with *Staph. aureus*. Severe infections may require hospitalization.

Impetigo is prevented by improving the host factors associated with acquisition of the disease, as illustrated in *Figure 26.9*. Since AGN rarely recurs on subsequent streptococcal infection, long-term prophylaxis with penicillin is not indicated (in contrast to the long-term prophylaxis following rheumatic fever; see Chapter 18).

Cellulitis and gangrene

Cellulitis is an acute spreading infection of the skin that involves subcutaneous tissues

Cellulitis extends deeper than erysipelas and usually originates either from superficial skin lesions such as boils or ulcers or following trauma. It is rarely bloodborne, but conversely it may lead to bacterial invasion of the bloodstream. Infection develops within a few hours or days of trauma and quickly produces a hot red swollen lesion (*Fig. 26.13*). Regional

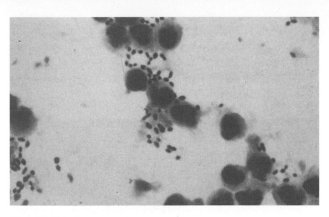

Fig. 26.12 Gram-positive cocci in pus.

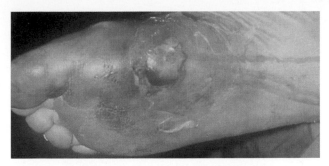

Fig. 26.14 Severe progressive cellulitis of the foot. Such cellulitis is usually caused by anaerobic bacteria or a mixture of aerobes and anaerobes and is a particular problem in diabetic patients with peripheral vascular and neuropathic damage. (Courtesy of JD Ward.)

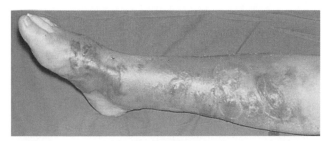

Fig. 26.13 When the focus of infection is in the subdermal fat, cellulitis—a severe and rapidly progressive infection—is the typical presentation. Large blisters and scabs may also be present on the skin surface. (Courtesy of MJ Wood.)

lymph nodes are enlarged and the patient suffers malaise, chills and fever.

The great majority of cases of cellulitis are caused by *Strep. pyogenes* and *Staph. aureus*. Occasionally, in patients who have had particular environmental exposure, other organisms may be implicated. For example, *Erysipelothrix rhusiopathiae* is associated with cellulitis in butchers and fishmongers, while *Vibrio vulnificus* and *Vibrio alginolyticus* may complicate traumatic wounds acquired in salt water environments.

The pathogen causing cellulitis is isolated in only 25–35% of cases, and initial therapy should cover streptococci and staphylococci. Attempts can be made to confirm the clinical diagnosis by culture of:

- aspirates from the advancing edge of the cellulitis;
- the site of trauma (if present);
- skin biopsies;
- blood.

Treatment should be initiated on the basis of the clinical diagnosis because of the rapid progression of the disease, particularly when caused by *Strep. pyogenes*. Initial therapy should cover both streptococci and staphylococci.

Anaerobic cellulitis may develop in areas of traumatized or devitalized tissue

Such damaged tissue is associated with surgical or traumatic wounds or is found in ischemic extremities. Diabetic patients are particularly prone to anaerobic cellulitis of their feet (*Fig. 26.14*). The causative organisms depend upon the circumstances of the trauma: infections in the lower parts of the body are most often caused by organisms from the fecal flora whereas wounds from human bites are infected with oral organisms. Foul-smelling discharge, marked swelling and gas in the tissues are characteristic of anaerobic cellulitis, and a mixture of organisms is usually cultured from the wound. Treatment needs to be aggressive to halt the spread of infection, and both antibiotics and surgical debridement are required. Osteomyelitis (see below) is a common sequela.

Synergistic bacterial gangrene is a relentlessly destructive infection

This rare infection is caused by a mixture of organisms, typically microaerophilic streptococci and *Staph. aureus*. The gangrene most commonly follows surgery in the groin or genital area, starting at the site of a drain or suture. Cellulitis develops in the surrounding skin and extends rapidly (within hours), leaving a black necrotic center. The condition is often fatal, and treatment requires radical excision of the necrotic area and systemic antibiotic therapy.

Necrotizing fasciitis, myonecrosis and gangrene

Necrotizing fasciitis is a frequently fatal mixed infection caused by anaerobes and facultative anaerobes

Although apparently resembling synergistic bacterial gangrene, necrotizing fasciitis is a much more acute and highly toxic infection, causing widespread necrosis and undermining of the surrounding tissues, such that the underlying destruction is more widespread than the skin lesion (*Fig. 26.15*). While caused by a variety of organisms, necrotizing fasciitis has been most prominently linked by the popular media with *Strep. pyogenes*, where it has been frequently termed 'flesh-eating bacteria'. Patients with necrotizing fasciitis deteriorate rapidly and frequently die. Radical excision of all necrotic fascia is an essential part of therapy, along with antibiotics given both locally to the wound and systemically.

Traumatic or surgical wounds can become infected with Clostridium species

Clostridium tetani gains access to the tissues through trauma to the skin, but the disease it produces is entirely due to the production of a powerful exotoxin (see Chapter 17).

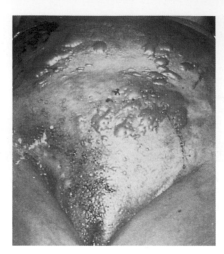

Fig. 26.15 Necrotizing fasciitis of the abdominal wall. In patients such as this, infection can be seen rapidly spreading from its origin and causing deep and widespread necrosis. Complete debridement and intensive antimicrobial therapy is required, but the condition is often fatal. (Courtesy of WM Rambo.)

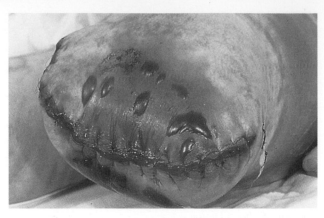

Fig. 26.16 Gas gangrene caused by *Clostridium perfringens*. Organisms from the fecal flora may contaminate a wound and grow and multiply in poorly perfused (anaerobic) tissue. Infection spreads rapidly, and gas can be felt in the tissue and seen on radiographs. (Courtesy of J Newman.)

Gas gangrene or clostridial myonecrosis can be caused by several species of clostridia, but *Clostridium perfringens* is the most common. The organism and its spores are found in the soil and in human and animal feces, and can therefore gain access to traumatized tissues by contamination from these sources. Infection develops in areas of the body with poor blood supply (anaerobic), and the buttocks and perineum are common sites, particularly in patients with ischemic vascular disease or peripheral arteriosclerosis. The organisms multiply in the subcutaneous tissues, producing gas and an anaerobic cellulitis, but a characteristic feature of clostridial infection is that the organisms invade deeper into the muscle, where they cause necrosis and produce bubbles of gas, which can be felt in the tissue and sometimes seen in the wound *(Fig. 26.16)*. The infection proceeds very rapidly and causes acute pain. Much of the damage is due to the production by *Cl. perfringens* of a lecithinase (also known as alpha toxin), which hydrolyzes the lipids in cell membranes resulting in cell lysis and death *(Fig. 26.17)*. The presence of dead and dying tissue further compromises the blood supply, and the organisms multiply and produce more toxin and more damage. Other extracellular enzymes may also play a role in helping the clostridia to spread. If the toxin escapes from the affected area and enters the bloodstream, there is massive hemolysis, renal failure and death.

Amputation may be necessary to prevent further spread of clostridial infection

Because of the rapid progression and fatal outcome of this type of clostridial infection, gangrenous areas require immediate surgery to excise all the affected tissue, and amputation may be necessary. Anti-alpha toxin may help if given early enough, and treatment in a hyperbaric oxygen chamber has also been recommended to improve the oxygenation of the tissue.

Antibiotics (e.g. penicillin) are adjuncts to, not replacements for, surgical debridement.

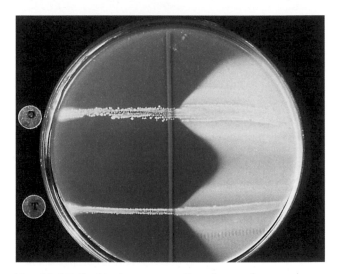

Fig. 26.17 The Nagler reaction. *Clostridium perfringens* produces alpha toxin, which is a lecithinase. If the organism is grown on a medium containing egg yolk (lecithin), enzyme activity can be detected as opacity around the line of growth (right). If anti-alpha toxin is applied to the surface of the plate before inoculation of the organism, the action of the toxin is inhibited (left). This test can be used to confirm the identity of a clostridial isolate.

Prevention of infection is of foremost importance. Wounds should be cleansed and debrided early to remove dead and poorly perfused tissue, which the anaerobes favor. Prophylactic antibiotics should be given preoperatively to patients having elective surgery of body sites liable to contamination with fecal flora (see Chapters 33 and 36).

Propionibacterium acnes and acne

P. acnes *goes hand in hand with the hormonal changes of puberty which result in acne*

An increased responsiveness to androgenic hormones leads to increased sebum production plus increased keratinization and desquamation in pilosebaceous ducts. Blockage of ducts

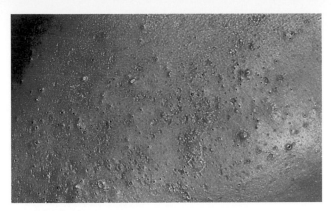

Fig. 26.18 Typical lesions of acne. 'Blackheads' are seen when plugs of keratin block the pilosebaceous duct. (Courtesy of A du Vivier.)

turns them into sacs in which *P. acnes* and other members of the normal flora (e.g. micrococci, yeasts, staphylococci) multiply. *P. acnes* acts on sebum to form fatty acids and peptides, which together with enzymes and other substances released from bacteria and polymorphs, cause the inflammation *(Fig. 26.18).* Comedones are greasy plugs composed of a mixture of keratin, sebum and bacteria and capped by a layer of melanin (blackheads in popular terminology) *(Fig. 26.19).*

Treatment of acne includes long-term administration of oral antibiotics

The antibiotics used to treat acne are usually one of the tetracyclines, or erythromycin. Other treatments include skin care, keratolytics and, in severe cases, synthetic vitamin A derivatives such as isotretinoin. Orally administered antibiotics reduce the surface numbers of *P. acnes* with a concomitant lowering of the free fatty acids, which act as skin irritants, which result from the activity of bacterial enzymes on sebum. Acne can be a problem for teenagers, but often disappears in older age groups as the sebaceous follicles become less active.

Other Gram-positive rods related to *P. acnes,* such as corynebacteria and brevibacteria, can also cause skin infections.

MYCOBACTERIAL DISEASES OF THE SKIN

Leprosy

Leprosy affects millions of people worldwide

Leprosy has been recognized since biblical times, but in the past the word was a generic term applied to several different diseases and also implying 'moral uncleanliness'. Leprosy is thought to have spread to Europe in the 6th century, and by the 13th century there were some two hundred leper hospitals in England. Over the centuries that followed leprosy declined in incidence, and by the 15th century was no longer endemic in England; in contrast tuberculosis was on the increase. Now leprosy is rare in the UK and USA. However, in the late 1990s the worldwide estimate of cases was 1–2 million, especially concentrated in southeast Asia, Africa and the Americas. The total number of new cases reported each year is approximately 500 000 to 800 000.

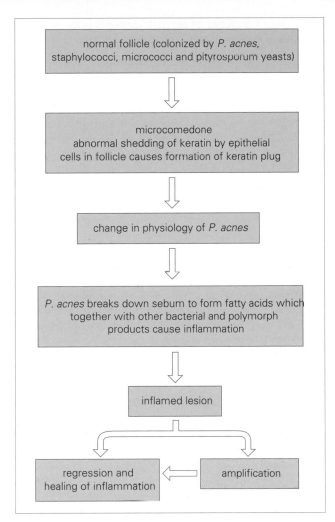

Fig. 26.19 The proposed mechanism of the pathogenesis of acne. Hormonal changes in the host initiate the formation of comedones from normal follicles and thereby change the environment of *Propionibacterium acnes* and its physiologic properties. *P. acnes* is also known to be an immunostimulator.

Leprosy is caused by Mycobacterium leprae

Mycobacterium leprae was discovered by GA Hansen in 1873, who identified it as the first bacterial agent capable of causing human disease. Leprosy (Hansen's disease) appears to be confined to humans. *M. leprae* is found in nine-banded armadillos, chimpanzees and mangabey monkeys; however, epidemiologic studies have not demonstrated a significant link between this carriage and human disease. Transmission of infection is directly related to overcrowding and poor hygiene and occurs by direct contact and aerosol inhalation. Relatively few organisms are shed from skin lesions, but nasal secretions of patients with lepromatous leprosy are laden with *M. leprae*. Arthropod vectors may play a role in transmission. Leprosy is not highly contagious, and prolonged exposure to an infected source is necessary; it seems that children living under the same roof as an open case of leprosy are most at risk. Ironically, because the lesions of leprosy are more obvious, patients were in the past excluded from the community and gathered in leper colonies, whereas tuberculosis is much more contagious, but people with tuberculosis were not shunned.

The clinical features of leprosy depend upon the cell-mediated immune response to M. leprae

M. leprae cannot be grown in artificial culture media, and little is known about its mechanism of pathogenicity. Two animal models have been used: infection in the armadillo and in the footpads of mice. The organism grows better at temperatures below 37°C, hence its concentration in the skin and superficial nerves, and it grows extremely slowly; in the mouse footpad the generation time is 11–13 days. Likewise in man the incubation period may be many years.

M. leprae grows intracellularly, typically within skin histiocytes and endothelial cells and the Schwann cells of peripheral nerves. The immune response is all important in deciding the type of disease.

M. leprae shares many pathobiologic features with *M. tuberculosis*, but the clinical manifestations of the diseases are quite different. After an incubation period of several years, the onset of leprosy is gradual and the spectrum of disease activity is very broad depending upon the presence or absence of a cell-mediated immune (CMI) response to *M. leprae* *(Fig. 26.20)*. At one end of the spectrum is tuberculoid leprosy (TT), characterized by blotchy red lesions with anesthetic areas on the face, trunk and extremities *(Fig. 26.21)*. There is palpable thickening of the peripheral nerves because the organisms multiply in the nerve sheaths. The local anesthesia

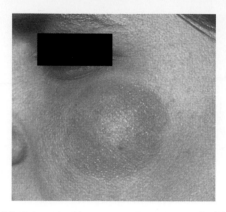

Fig. 26.21 Tuberculoid leprosy—a characteristic dry blotchy lesion on the face, but the diagnosis needs to be confirmed by microscopic examination of skin biopsy *(Fig. 26.24)*. (Courtesy of the Institute of Dermatology.)

renders the patient prone to repeated trauma and secondary bacterial infection. This disease state is equivalent to secondary tuberculosis (see Chapter 19), with a vigorous CMI response leading to phagocytic destruction of bacteria, and exaggerated allergic responses. TT carries a better prognosis than lepromatous leprosy (LL) and in some patients is self-limiting, but in others may progress across the spectrum towards LL.

In LL there is extensive skin involvement with large numbers of bacteria in affected areas. As the disease progresses there is loss of eyebrows, thickening and enlargement of the nostrils, ears and cheeks, resulting in the typical leonine (lion-like) facial appearance *(Fig. 26.22)*. There is progressive destruction of the nasal septum, and the nasal mucosa is loaded with organisms *(Fig. 26.23)*. This form of the disease is equivalent to miliary tuberculosis (see Chapter 19) with a weak CMI response and many extracellular organisms visible in the lesions. The gross deformities characteristic of late disease result primarily from infectious destruction of the nasomaxillary facial structures, and secondarily from pathologic changes in the peripheral nerves predisposing to repeated trauma of the hands and feet and subsequent superinfection with other organisms.

Whether a patient develops TT or LL may in part be genetically determined. Patients with intermediate forms of the disease may progress to either extreme.

M. leprae *are seen as acid-fast rods in nasal scrapings and lesion biopsies*

An alertness to the possibility of leprosy when confronted with a patient with dermatologic, neurologic or multisystem complaints is of fundamental importance. Although the majority of cases are in people who are not native to Europe or the USA, the diagnosis should also be considered in those who have worked in endemic areas.

Nasal scrapings and biopsies of skin lesions should be stained by Ziehl–Neelsen or auramine stain (see Appendix) to demonstrate acid-fast rods. In LL these are numerous, but in TT few if any organisms are seen, but the appearance of granulomas is sufficiently typical to allow the diagnosis to be made *(Fig. 26.24)*. Remember that, in contrast to *M. tuberculosis*, the organism cannot be grown in vitro.

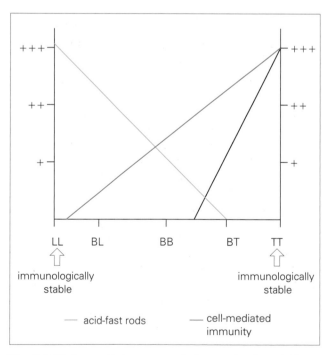

Fig. 26.20 Immunologic responses in leprosy. In tuberculoid leprosy (TT) the patient is capable of mounting an effective cell-mediated immune (CMI) response, which makes it possible for macrophages to destroy the organisms and contain the infection. At the other extreme, in lepromatous leprosy (LL) the patient is incapable of producing a CMI response and the organisms multiply unhindered. These patients have many acid-fast rods in their skin and nasal secretions, and are much more infectious than TT patients. Borderline lepromatous (BL), borderline borderline (BB), and borderline tuberculoid (BT) responses are found between these extremes.

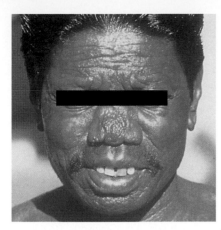

Fig. 26.22 Extensive skin involvement in lepromatous leprosy results in a characteristic leonine appearance. (Courtesy of DA Lewis.)

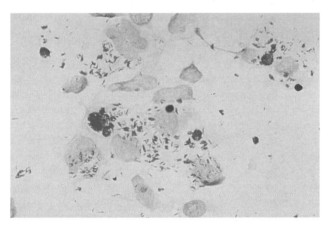

Fig. 26.23 In lepromatous leprosy the nasal mucosa is packed with *Mycobacterium leprae*, seen here in an acid-fast stain (Ziehl–Neelsen) of nasal scrapings. (Courtesy of I Farrell.)

Treatment

Leprosy is treated with dapsone given as part of a multidrug regimen to avoid resistance

If the disease is diagnosed early and treatment initiated promptly the patient has a much better prognosis. Dapsone (see Chapter 33) had long been the mainstay of therapy, but multidrug therapy is now used because of dapsone resistance:

- For LL, triple therapy with dapsone, rifampin and clofazimine is given for a minimum of 2 years and may be lifelong or until all skin scrapings and biopsies are negative for acid-fast rods.
- For TT, a combination of dapsone and rifampin for 6 months is recommended, the rationale being that in this form of disease there are many fewer organisms and therefore less chance of emergence of resistant mutants.

As a result of multidrug therapy, which is reasonably cheap, well tolerated and effects a complete cure, steady progress is being made towards the elimination of leprosy as a public health problem.

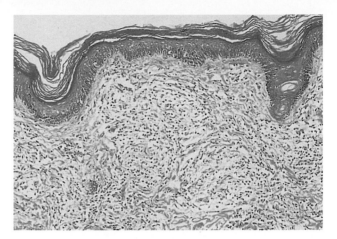

Fig. 26.24 In tuberculoid leprosy the organisms are much more sparse but characteristic granulomas form in the dermis, as shown in this histologic preparation. (Courtesy of CJ Edwards.)

Destruction of the organisms by effective antimicrobial therapy may result in an inflammatory response, erythema nodosum leprosum, which may be severe and, occasionally, fatal. Treatment with corticosteroids or thalidomide may be indicated.

Vaccine trials with bacille Calmette-Guérin (BCG) and heat-killed *M. leprae* for the prevention of leprosy have shown conflicting results.

Other mycobacterial skin infections

Mycobacterium marinum, M. ulcerans *and* M. tuberculosis *also cause skin lesions*

Mycobacterium marinum and *M. ulcerans* are two slow-growing mycobacterial species that prefer cooler temperatures and cause skin lesions. As its name suggests, *M. marinum* is associated with water and marine organisms. Human infections follow trauma, often minor such as a graze acquired while climbing out of a swimming pool or while cleaning out an aquarium, which becomes contaminated with mycobacteria from the wet environment. After an incubation period of 2–8 weeks, initial lesions appear as small papules, which enlarge and suppurate and may ulcerate. Histologically, the lesions are granulomas and hence the name 'swimming pool granuloma' or 'fish-tank granuloma' *(Fig. 26.25)*. Sometimes the nodules follow the course of the draining lymphatic and produce an appearance that may be mistaken for sporotrichosis (see below).

M. ulcerans causes chronic, relatively painless cutaneous ulcers known as 'Buruli ulcers'. This disease is prevalent in Africa and Australia, but is rarely seen elsewhere.

Tuberculosis of the skin is exceedingly uncommon. Infection can occur by direct implantation of *M. tuberculosis* during trauma to the skin (lupus vulgaris) or may extend to the skin from an infected lymph node (scrofuloderma).

FUNGAL INFECTIONS OF THE SKIN

Fungal infections may be confined to the very outermost layers of the skin and hairshafts or penetrate into the keratinized layers of the epidermis, nails and hair (the superficial and

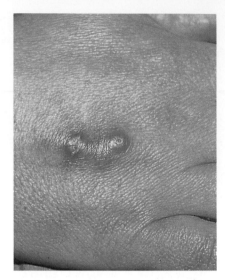

Fig. 26.25 Fish-tank granuloma caused by *Mycobacterium marinum* infection of a lesion acquired while cleaning out a fish tank. (Courtesy of MJ Wood.)

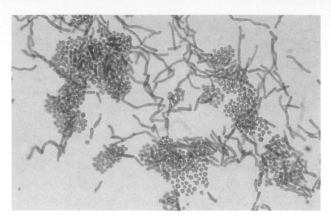

Fig. 26.26 Infected skin scales stained to show the thick-walled yeast forms of *Malassezia furfur* and the short angular hyphae. (Courtesy of Y Clayton and G Midgley.)

cutaneous mycoses); others develop in the dermal layers (subcutaneous mycoses). In addition, some systemic fungal infections acquired by the airborne route have skin manifestations *(Fig. 26.4)*.

Superficial and cutaneous mycoses

These are some of the most common infections in humans. Superficial infections of the skin and hair (pityriasis versicolor, tinea nigra, black and white piedras) mainly cause cosmetic problems; cutaneous infections (ringworm, tineas) caused by the dermatophyte fungi are more significant. The important causative agents are the superficial yeast *Malassezia furfur* and the cutaneous dermatophytes *Epidermophyton*, *Trichophyton* and *Microsporum*.

Pityriasis versicolor

M. furfur *is the cause of pityriasis or tinea versicolor*

The yeast *M. (Pityrosporum) furfur* is a common skin inhabitant. The change from commensalism to pathogenicity appears to be associated with the phase change from yeast to hyphal forms of the fungus, but the stimulus for this is unknown. Infections are usually confined to the trunk or proximal parts of the limbs and are associated with hypo- or hyperpigmented macules that coalesce to form scaling plaques. The lesions are not usually itchy and in some patients they resolve spontaneously.

Pityrosporum yeasts are also thought to be involved in the pathogenesis of seborrheic dermatitis.

Diagnosis of pityriasis versicolor can be confirmed by direct microscopy of scrapings

Direct microscopy of scrapings shows characteristic round yeast forms *(Fig. 26.26)*, and treatment with a topical azole antifungal (see below) or with selenium sulfide (2%) lotion is appropriate.

Cutaneous dermatophytes

Dermatophyte infections are acquired from many sources and are spread by arthrospores

Species of dermatophytes are described as anthropophilic, zoophilic or geophilic depending upon their primary source (human, animal or soil). The species concerned differ in their geographic distribution, in their predilection for different body sites and in the degree of host response elicited in humans. The source of an infection determines its route of transmission to humans and, to some extent, its distribution in human populations *(Fig. 26.27)*, although population movements are changing established patterns. For example immigration from Latin America replaced *Microsporum audouinii* by *Trichophyton tonsurans* as the common cause of tinea capitis in the USA, but the latter (which responds poorly to treatment) is again increasing.

The anthropophilic species are the most common causes of dermatophyte infections. In temperate countries, *Trichophyton verrucosum* from cattle, *T. mentagrophytes* from rodents, and *Microsporum canis* from cats and dogs, are the most common zoophilic causes of human infection. Geophilic species such as *Microsporum gypseum* are uncommon causes of human disease, but are seen in people who have appropriate exposure, such as gardeners and agricultural workers. Zoophilic and geophilic species tend to cause a greater inflammatory response than anthropophilic species.

Infections are spread by contact with arthrospores, the thick-walled vegetative cells formed by dermatophyte hyphae *(Fig. 26.28)*, which can survive for months. In anthropophilic and zoophilic species these are shed from the primary host in skin scales and hair.

Dermatophytes invade skin, hair and nails

The dermatophytes are keratin-loving organisms and invade the keratinized structures of the body (i.e. skin, hair and nails). The arthrospores adhere to keratinocytes, germinate and invade. The latin word 'tinea' (meaning a maggot or grub) or 'ringworm' is used for these infections because they were originally thought to be caused by a worm-like parasite. Thus tinea capitis affects the hair and skin of the scalp, tinea

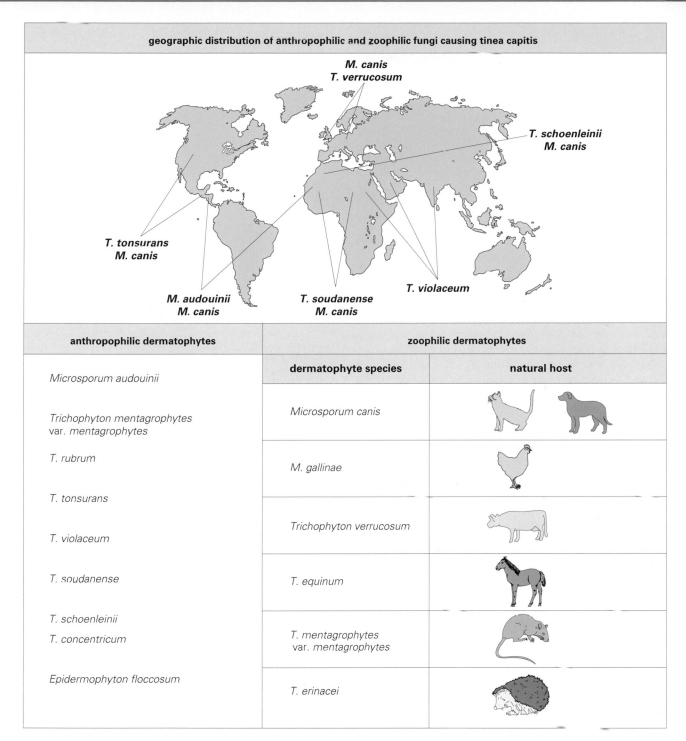

Fig. 26.27 Three genera of dermatophytes are important causes of disease: *Microsporum*, *Trichophyton* and *Epidermophyton*. Within each genus there are anthropophilic, zoophilic and geophilic species. The natural host and therefore distribution of anthropophilic species varies. *Microsporum gypseum* is the geophilic species of importance.

corporis the body, tinea cruris the crotch, tinea manuum the hands, tinea unguium the nails and tinea pedis the feet (*Fig. 26.29*).

The typical lesion is an annular or serpentine scaling patch with a raised margin. The main symptom is itching, but this is variable in degree. The skin is often dry and scaly and sometimes cracks (e.g. between the toes in tinea pedis), while infections of hair cause hair loss (*Fig. 26.30*). The degree of associated inflammation varies with the infecting species,

usually being greater with zoophilic than with anthropophilic species. Individuals also differ in their susceptibility to infection, but the factors determining these differences are not clearly understood. Similarly, dermatophyte species differ in their ability to elicit an immune response; some, such as *Trichophyton rubrum*, cause chronic or relapsing conditions, whereas other species induce long-term resistance to reinfection. In some patients, circulating fungal antigens give rise to immunologically mediated hypersensitivity phenomena in

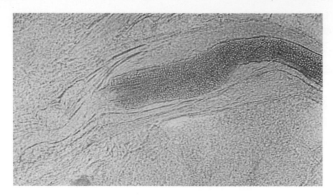

Fig. 26.28 Arthrospores of *Trichophyton tonsurans* in an infected hair shaft. These thick-walled spores are the form in which infection is spread. They can survive in the environment for weeks or months before infecting a new host. (Courtesy of AE Prevost.)

the skin (e.g. erythema or vesicles) known as dermatophytid reactions. When the skin becomes cracked and macerated as a result of infection, it is liable to superinfection with other organisms such as Gram-negative bacteria in moist sites.

Very rarely, dermatophytes invade the subcutaneous tissues via the lymphatics, causing granulomas, lymphedema and draining sinuses. Further extension to sites such as the liver and brain may be fatal.

Most dermatophyte species fluoresce under ultraviolet light

This feature can be used as a diagnostic aid, particularly for tinea capitis, in the clinic. Laboratory diagnosis depends upon microscopic examination for fungal hyphae and culture on Sabouraud agar of scrapings or clippings from lesions *(Fig. 26.31;* see Appendix). Dermatophytes infecting hair show a characteristic distribution, which may be helpful for identification:

- Some, such as most *Microsporum* species, form arthrospores on the outside of the hair shaft (ectothrix infections).

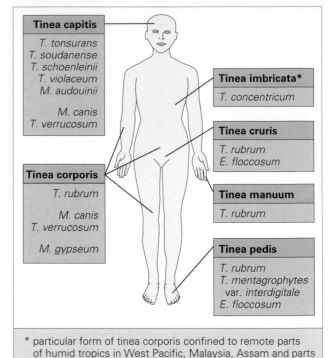

Tinea capitis	
T. tonsurans	
T. soudanense	
T. schoenleinii	
T. violaceum	
M. audouinii	
M. canis	
T. verrucosum	

Tinea imbricata*
T. concentricum

Tinea cruris
T. rubrum
E. floccosum

Tinea corporis	
T. rubrum	
M. canis	
T. verrucosum	
M. gypseum	

Tinea manuum
T. rubrum

Tinea pedis
T. rubrum
T. mentagrophytes
var. *interdigitale*
E. floccosum

* particular form of tinea corporis confined to remote parts of humid tropics in West Pacific, Malaysia, Assam and parts of the Amazon basin in Brazil

Fig. 26.29 Tinea (or ringworm) is the disease of skin, hair and nails caused by dermatophyte fungi. Different species have predilections for different body sites. (E., *Epidermophyton*; M., *Microsporum*; T., *Trichophyton*.)

- The majority of *Trichophyton* infections form arthrospores within the hair shaft (endothrix infection, *Fig. 26.32*).

Confirmation of identity depends upon the colonial and microscopic characteristics of the fungi cultured on Sabouraud agar *(Fig. 26.33)*. Growth may take up to 2 weeks, but identification is not difficult and is useful for determining the source of infection.

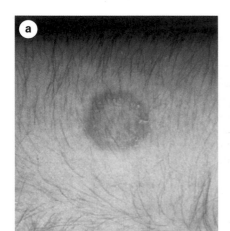
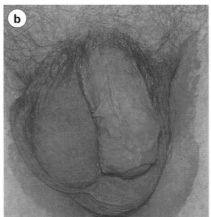
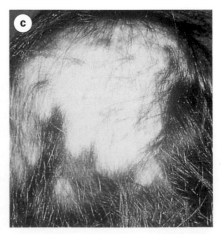

Fig. 26.30 (a) Classic annular lesion of tinea corporis, caused here by infection with a *Microsporum* species. (Courtesy of AE Prevost.) (b) Tinea cruris or 'jock itch' is a scaly rash on the thighs; the scrotum is usually spared. (Courtesy of MJ Wood.) (c) Tinea capitis is characterized by scaling on the scalp and hair loss. Some dermatophytes fluoresce under ultraviolet light, and this can be an aid to diagnosis. (Courtesy of MH Winterborn.)

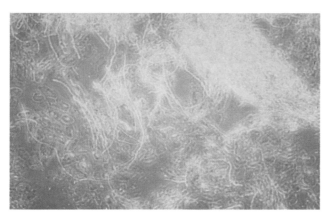

Fig. 26.31 Dermatophyte infection. Samples of skin, hair and nails need to be be 'cleared' by treatment with potassium hydroxide before examining under the microscope for the presence of fungal hyphae. (Courtesy of RY Cartwright.)

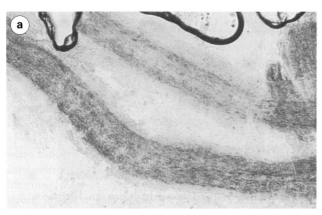

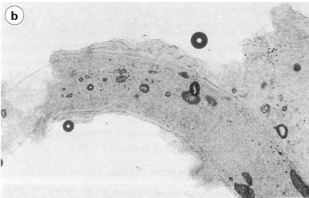

Fig. 26.32 Dermatophytes may form arthrospores within the hair shafts (endothrix infection) as shown in (a) and less commonly outside the shaft (ectothrix infection) as shown in (b). (Courtesy of Y Clayton and G Midgley.)

Dermatophyte infections are treated topically if possible

However, infections of nails and hair are better treated by oral antifungal drugs. A range of agents is available for topical treatment (see Chapter 33), both antifungals (e.g. miconazole) and keratolytic agents such as Whitfield's ointment (a mixture of salicylic and benzoic acids). The orally administered agent most commonly used is griseofulvin. Scalp infections take

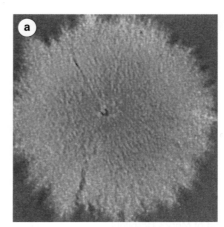

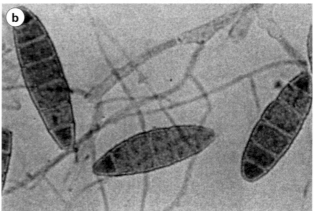

Fig. 26.33 (a) Macroscopic growth (colony) and (b) microscopic preparation showing the macroconidia of *Microsporum gypseum*.

6–12 weeks to respond, fingernail infections up to 6 months and toenail infections 1 year or longer. The relapse rate of treated nail infections is high, and many physicians advise against treatment unless there is pain or more widespread skin involvement.

Candida and the skin

Candida *requires moisture for growth*

The relative dryness of most areas of skin limits the growth of fungi such as *Candida* that require moisture. *Candida* is found in low numbers on healthy intact skin, but rapidly colonizes damaged skin and intertriginous sites (apposed skin sites which are often moist and become chafed, Fig. 26.34). *Candida* also colonizes the oral and vaginal mucosa and overgrowth may result in disease in these sites (thrush, see Chapter 21). However, a substantial lowering of host resistance (e.g. neutropenia) is necessary for *Candida* to invade deeper subcutaneous tissue, and disseminated candidiasis does not often originate from skin infection unless there is instrumentation through infected areas (see Chapter 30).

Subcutaneous mycoses

Subcutaneous fungal infections can be caused by a number of different species

Lesions usually develop at sites of trauma (a thorn, a bite) where the fungus becomes implanted. With the exception of

Fig. 26.38 A characteristic cutaneous burrow in scabies. (Courtesy of MJ Wood.)

inflammatory masses in which fungal infections may establish. Good personal hygiene prevents infestation; use of insecticidal creams, lotions, shampoos and powders containing malathion or carbaryl helps to clear the insects directly.

The scabies mite has a more intimate contact with the human host than lice, living its whole life in burrows within the skin. The female lays eggs into these burrows, and so the area of infection can spread to cover large areas of the body from the original site, which is usually on the hands or wrists (*Fig. 26.38*; see Chapter 21). Infection causes a characteristic rash with itching, and secondary infections may follow scratching. Very heavy infections may develop in immuno-compromised individuals or in people who are unable to care adequately for themselves. Under these conditions there is extensive thickening and crusting of the skin (Norwegian

scabies). Treatment with malathion or gamma benzene hexa-chloride is recommended; benzyl benzoate can also be used on unbroken skin.

MUCOCUTANEOUS LESIONS CAUSED BY VIRUSES

Mucocutaneous lesions caused by viruses can be divided into:

- those in which the virus remains restricted to the body surface at the site of initial infection;
- those in which the virus causes mucocutaneous lesions after spreading systemically through the body (*Fig. 26.39*).

The infections that spread systemically can in turn be divided into:

- those in which the skin lesions (vesicular) are sites of virus replication and are infectious;
- those in which the skin lesions (maculopapular) are non-infectious and immunologically mediated, although the virus can be shed from other sites.

The skin rash has a characteristic distribution in many infectious diseases, but with the exception of zoster the reason for this is unknown.

Rashes are particular features of human infection and are rare in animals. This is because human skin is naked and is a turbulent, highly reactive tissue in which immune and inflammatory events are clearly visible. Rashes are not often in themselves a source of suffering but they may be very helpful for the clinician who needs to make a diagnosis. The veterinarian is less privileged because the skin of most other mammals is largely covered with fur, and skin lesions

MUCOCUTANEOUS LESIONS CAUSED BY VIRUSES			
	virus	**lesion**	**virus shedding from lesion**
no systemic spread	papilloma (wart)	common wart	+
		plantar wart	
		genital wart	
	molluscum contagiosum (poxvirus)	fleshy papule	+
	orf (poxvirus from sheep, goats)	papulovesicular	+
systemic spread	herpes simplex, varicella-zoster	vesicular (neural spread and latency)	+
	coxsackievirus A (9, 16, 23)	vesicular, in mouth (herpangina)	+
	coxsackievirus A16	vesicular (hand, foot and mouth disease)	+
	erythrovirus (formerly human parvovirus) B19	facial maculopapular (erythema infectiosum)	–
	human herpesvirus 6	exanthem subitum (roseola infantum)	–
	measles	maculopapular skin rash	–
	rubella, echoviruses (4, 6, 9, 16)	maculopapular not distinguishable clinically	–
	dengue and other arthropod transmitted viruses	maculopapular	–

Fig. 26.39 Mucocutaneous lesions caused by viruses. The pathogenesis of these diseases is illustrated in *Figure 26.3*. Papillomas and vesicular lesions are generally sites of virus shedding. The distribution as well as the nature of the lesion can be important in diagnosis (e.g. varicella), but many maculopapular rashes are clinically indistinguishable.

generally involve hairless areas such as udders, scrotums, ears, prepuces, teats, noses or paws, which have the human properties of thickness, sensitivity and vascular reactivity.

Papillomavirus infection

About 70 different types of papillomavirus can infect humans

Papillomaviruses are 55 nm diameter, icosahedral, double-stranded DNA viruses and cause skin papillomas (warts). The 70 different types that can infect humans show less than 50% cross-hybridization of DNA, although not all types are common. Human papillomaviruses (HPV) are species-specific and distinct from animal papillomaviruses. They are highly adapted to human skin and mucosa and are ancient associates of our species; therefore for most of the time they cause little or no disease. They show some adaptation to definite sites on the body:

- At least 25 types, including HPV 6, 11, 16, and 18, can infect the genital areas and are sexually transmitted.
- HPV 1 and 4 tend to cause plantar warts.
- HPV 2, 3 and 10 cause warts on the knees and fingers.

Papillomaviruses are generally transmitted by direct contact, but they are stable and can also be spread indirectly. For instance, plantar warts can be acquired from contaminated floors or from the non-slip surfaces at the edges of swimming pools, and in a given individual warts can be spread from one site to another by shaving.

Papillomavirus infects cells in the basal layers of skin or mucosa

After entering the body via surface abrasions the virus infects cells in the basal layers of the skin or mucosa *(Fig. 26.3)*. There is no spread to deeper tissues. Virus replication is slow and is critically dependent upon the differentiation of host cells. Viral DNA is present in basal cells, but viral antigen and infectious virus are produced only when the cells begin to become squamified and keratinized as they approach the surface. The infected cells are stimulated to divide and finally, 1–6 months after initial infection, the mass of infected cells protrudes from the body surface to form a visible papilloma or wart *(Fig. 26.40)*. There is marked proliferation of prickle cells, and vacuolated cells are present in the more superficial layers. Warts can be:

- filiform with finger-like projections;
- flat topped;
- flat because they grow inwards due to external pressure (plantar warts);
- a cauliflower-like protuberance (e.g. genital warts);
- a flat area of dysplasia on the cervix.

Immune responses eventually bring virus replication under control and, several months after infection, the wart regresses. Antibodies are demonstrable, but CMI responses are more important in recovery. It seems likely that viral DNA remains in a latent state in the basal cell layer, infecting an occasional stem cell, and is therefore retained within the layer as epidermal cells differentiate and are shed from the surface. Hence, when patients are subsequently immunocompromised (e.g. post-transplant) crops of warts may result from reactivation of latent virus in the skin.

Papillomavirus infections are associated with cancer of the cervix, vulva, penis and rectum

The association between genital warts and cancer of the cervix, vulva, penis and rectum is referred to in Chapter 17. It is not clear whether this association is causal or merely casual. There is no evidence that regular skin warts are involved in the development of skin cancer. There is, however, a rare autosomal recessive disease, epidermodysplasia verruciformis, characterized by multiple warts containing many different HPV types which are not normally seen, and causing skin warts and poorly understood immunologic defects. Warts may undergo malignant change (squamous cell carcinomas) in nearly 30% of these patients, usually in sun-exposed sites.

Diagnosis of papillomavirus infection is clinical and there are many treatments

Wart viruses cannot be cultivated in the laboratory, and at present serologic tests are neither useful nor available. HPV DNA detection methods can be used to examine samples not only for the HPV type but also to quantify the viral load.

An astounding variety of treatments have been used for warts, some of them doubtless seeming effective because skin warts eventually disappear without treatment. Post-hypnotic suggestion has at times been successful. Current treatments of skin warts include the application of karyolytic agents such as salicylic acid and destruction of wart tissue by cryotherapy, freezing with dry ice (solid carbon dioxide) or with liquid nitrogen. The latter is the most commonly used and most effective treatment. Genital intraepithelial lesions, especially cervical, can lead to malignant disease, and treatment to eliminate the infection may involve laser therapy, loop excision, and surgery.

Molluscum contagiosum is an umbilicated lesion caused by a poxvirus

The poxvirus infects epidermal cells to form a fleshy lesion, often with an umbilicated center *(Fig. 26.41)*. It only infects humans and is spread by contact, or in the case of genital

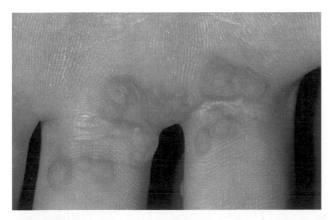

Fig. 26.40 Common warts (papillomas) on the hand. (Courtesy of MJ Wood.)

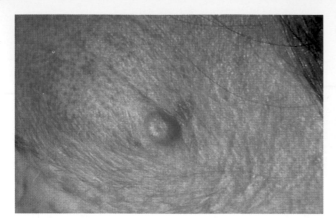

Fig. 26.41 Single umbilicated lesion in molluscum contagiosum. (Courtesy of MJ Wood.)

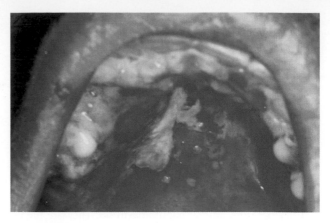

Fig. 26.42 Primary herpes simplex virus infection. There are shallow ulcers with white exudate on the palate and gums. (Courtesy of JA Innes.)

lesions, by sexual intercourse. There are two antigenically distinct types. Poxvirus particles can be seen by electron microscopy (see Chapter 3).

Orf is a papulovesicular lesion caused by a poxvirus

Orf (contagious pustular dermatitis) is an uncommon infection of the epidermis and is acquired by direct contact with infected sheep or goats. There is a papulovesicular lesion, generally on the hands, which may ulcerate. It is a clinical diagnosis and can be confirmed by electron microscopy.

Herpes simplex virus infection

Herpes simplex virus infection is universal and occurs in early childhood

Herpes simplex virus (HSV) is a medium-sized (120 nm) double-stranded DNA virus of the herpesvirus group. Two types, HSV-1 and HSV-2, are distinguishable antigenically. They cause a wide variety of clinical syndromes, the basic lesion being an intraepithelial vesicle, from which the virus is shed. Infection is usually transmitted from the saliva or cold sores of other individuals and frequently by kissing.

Clinical features of HSV infection are vesicles and latency

After infection the virus replicates in cells in the oral mucosa and forms virus-rich vesicles. The patient suffers at most a mild febrile illness. The vesicles ulcerate and become coated with a whitish-grey slough (Fig. 26.42).

During the primary infection, virus particles enter sensory nerve endings in the lesion and are transported to the dorsal root (trigeminal) ganglion, where they initiate latent infection in sensory neurones (see Chapter 16). The lesion resolves as antibody and CMI responses develop. The latent virus remains in the sensory ganglion for life, and under certain circumstances can reactivate and spread down sensory nerves to cause cold sores at the site of the original infection (Fig. 26.43).

Primary infection can also occur in:

- the eye, to cause conjunctivitis and keratitis, often with vesicles on the eyelids (see Chapter 25);
- the finger, to cause herpetic whitlow;
- other skin sites following direct contact with infected

individuals where there is rubbing or trauma, for instance in rugby football ('scrum pox') or in wrestlers ('herpes gladiatorum');
- the genital tract (see Chapter 21). Although HSV-2 arose as a sexually transmitted variant of HSV-1, the sites infected by the two types are now less clearly distinct.

Serious complications associated with HSV infection include:

- herpetic infection of eczematous skin areas leading to severe disease in young children (Fig. 26.44);
- acute necrotizing encephalitis following either primary infection or reactivation (see Chapter 24);
- neonatal infection acquired from the genital tract of the mother (see Chapter 23);
- primary or reactivating HSV infection in immuno-compromised individuals, causing very severe disease (see Chapter 30).

HSV reactivation is provoked by a variety of factors

In healthy individuals HSV reactivation is provoked by:

- certain febrile illnesses (e.g. common cold, pneumonia);
- direct sunlight;
- stress;
- trauma;
- menstruation;
- immunocompromise.

Reactivation is more severe in immunocompromised patients (see Chapter 30).

A sensory prodrome in the affected area which may include feeling pins and needles, pain, burning, and itching precedes the appearance of the lesion and is due to virus activity in sensory neurones. The lesion, a so-called 'cold sore', generally occurs around the mucocutaneous junctions in the nose or mouth (Fig. 26.45). Less commonly, when the ophthalmic branch of the trigeminal ganglion is involved, the lesion is a dendritic ulcer of the cornea. Large amounts of virus are shed in the cold sore, which scabs over and heals over the course of about 1 week. Occasionally the sensory prodrome occurs without proceeding to a cold sore (see also varicella-zoster virus recurrence below).

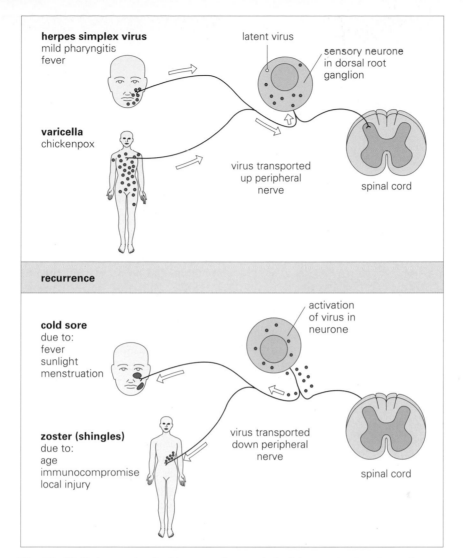

Fig. 26.43 Pathogenesis of cold sores and zoster. In both herpes simplex virus and varicella-zoster virus infections the virus in mucocutaneous nerve endings travels up the axon to reach the sensory neurones, where it becomes latent. Recurrences are due to reactivation of the virus within the neurone to become infectious followed by passage of virus down the axon to mucocutaneous site(s) and local spread and replication to form clinical lesion(s).

HSV is readily isolated from vesicle fluid, and infection is treated with aciclovir

HSV is also readily isolated from saliva, conjunctival fluid and lesions at affected sites. The majority of samples sent to hospital laboratories are from genital lesions, and the virus causes a distinct cytopathic effect when isolated in the laboratory using cell culture lines such as human embryo lung. Typing by immunofluorescence can be carried out, and HSV types 1 and 2 DNA detection can also be used to make the diagnosis in different clinical settings, which has been shown to be more sensitive than virus culture.

Aciclovir has revolutionized the treatment of HSV infection (see Chapter 33) and can be used either topically or systemically. It is relatively non-toxic and acts specifically in virus-infected cells. Recurrent herpetic eruptions have been successfully treated with low doses of aciclovir given twice daily for 6 to 12 months, at which time treatment can be stopped and the frequency of recurrent infection reassessed.

Other antiviral treatment options include valaciclovir and famciclovir. Aciclovir must be given intravenously when treating severe HSV infections such as herpes simplex encephalitis or disseminated HSV infection in immunocompromised individuals. Alternative antivirals such as ganciclovir, foscarnet or cidofovir may be used when antiviral resistance is being considered.

Varicella-zoster virus (VZV) infection

VZV causes chickenpox (varicella) and zoster (shingles) and is highly contagious

VZV is a medium-sized (100–200 nm diameter) double-stranded DNA virus of the herpesvirus group and is morphologically indistinguishable from HSV. There is only

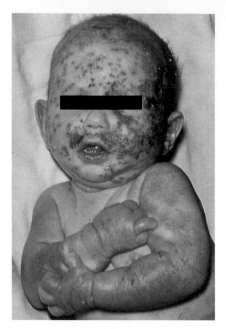

Fig. 26.44 Eczema herpeticum due to herpes simplex virus infection in an infant. (Courtesy of MJ Wood.)

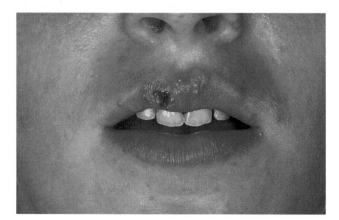

Fig. 26.45 Recurrent herpes simplex virus vesicles on the mucocutaneous margin of the lip. (Courtesy of A du Vivier.)

one serologic type. The virus grows more slowly than HSV and is not released from the infected cell. Infection is by inhalation of droplets from respiratory secretions and saliva, or by direct contact from skin lesions. Primary infection with VZV causes varicella (chickenpox). Immunity develops and prevents re-infection (a second attack of varicella), but the virus persists in the body, and later in life, after reactivation, causes zoster (shingles). Nearly all humans in resource rich countries are infected during childhood, but there are many areas of the world where the incidence of chickenpox in children is low, e.g. Africa and the Caribbean islands. The vesicles of zoster are an important source of varicella in the community (see Chapter 16).

Varicella is characterized by crops of vesicles that develop into pustules and then scab

After primary infection, the virus passes across surface epithelium in the respiratory tract to infect mononuclear cells, and is then carried to lymphoid tissues. There are no

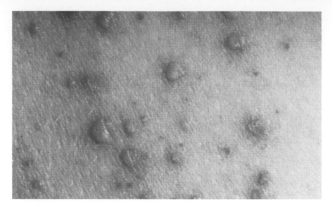

Fig. 26.46 Early rash in varicella (chickenpox), with macules, papules and vesicles. (Courtesy of MJ Wood.)

symptoms and no detectable lesions at the site of entry into the body. The virus slowly replicates in lymphoreticular tissues for about a week, and then enters the blood in association with mononuclear cells and is seeded out to epithelial sites. These are mainly the respiratory tract and the skin, but also include the mouth, often the conjunctiva, and probably also the alimentary and urinogenital tracts. In the skin, for unknown reasons, the trunk, face and scalp are especially involved. At these epithelial sites the virus exits from small blood vessels, infecting subepithelial and finally epithelial cells. Multinucleated giant cells with intranuclear inclusions are present in the lesions. In the oropharynx and respiratory tract the virus reaches the surface and is shed to the exterior to infect other individuals about 2 weeks after initial infection. In the skin it takes a day or two longer, and it is at this stage, when the characteristic varicella vesicles appear, that a clinical diagnosis can be made *(Fig. 26.46)* The mean incubation period is 14 days (range 10–23 days).

The patient remains well until a day or two before the rash, when there may be slight fever and malaise, but the illness is usually mild and often unnoticed. The vesicles appear first on the trunk, then on the face and scalp, and less commonly on the arms and legs. They often come in 'crops' over the course of several days and all stages of lesions occur simultaneously, then develop into pustules, break down, and scab over. The lesions are deeper than with HSV, and scarring is more common. Lesions in the mouth may be painful.

Varicella is usually more severe and more likely to cause complications in adults

The skin lesions of varicella can become infected with staphylococci or streptococci to produce secondary impetigo, but varicella in a child is characteristically a very mild illness. The main complications are:

- interstitial pneumonia, which can be detected radiologically, although it is often subclinical, in up to 20% of adults with varicella; secondary bacterial pneumonia can also occur;
- CNS involvement, which may consist of a lymphocytic meningitis or an encephalomyelitis (see Chapter 24).

Thrombocytopenia can occur, but it is usually symptomless. In immunocompromised patients, particularly children with leukemia, varicella can be a life-threatening disease.

After primary infection during pregnancy the virus may infect the fetus (see Chapter 23), but maternal antibody is present by then and the infection is generally without serious consequences. Congenital varicella syndrome is seen in up to 1–2% if maternal infection occurs in the first or second trimester. Clinical features include skin scarring, hypoplastic limbs, and other stigmata involve the eyes and brain. When the mother is infected a few days before or after delivery the infant is exposed without the protection of maternal antibody and can suffer a serious disease. Passive immunization with varicella-zoster immune globulin (VZIG) may prevent or attenuate the infection in the infant.

Zoster results from reactivation of latent VZV

During primary infection, VZV in mucocutaneous lesions enters sensory nerve endings and establishes latent infection in sensory neurones in dorsal root ganglia (Fig. 26.43). Later in life, reactivation can occur to cause zoster in the dermatome at the site of the reactivation. Thoracic dermatomes are most commonly affected because these are the most common sites for the original varicella lesions. Zoster is unilateral because the reactivation is a localized event in a single dorsal root ganglion. Zoster therefore originates from inside the body and is not directly acquired from either varicella or zoster in other individuals. During reactivation in sensory neurones (Fig. 26.43), there is paresthesia and pain. Pain may be severe and precedes the development of the erythematous rash in which virus-rich vesicles appear (Fig. 26.47) by several days. It takes a few days for the virus to travel down peripheral nerves and multiply in the skin. Fever and malaise may accompany the rash. Sometimes the immune response controls the reactivating virus before skin lesions have had time to form, and in this case the sensory phenomena occur without the skin eruption.

Conditions that predispose to zoster include:

- Increasing age. Although zoster is very occasionally seen in childhood, its incidence increases with increasing age, rising from 3/1000/year in 50–59-year-olds to 10/1000/year in 80–89-year-olds.
- Immunocompromise due to leukemia, lymphoma, AIDS, solid organ transplant or other drug-induced immunosuppression. For instance, zoster occurs in about 20% of patients with Hodgkin's disease.
- Trauma or tumors affecting the brain or spinal cord.

The skin areas affected by zoster reflect the distribution of the original varicella rash, as might be expected from its pathogenesis (Fig. 26.43). Hence the trunk is most commonly involved. Ophthalmic zoster involving the upper eyelid, forehead and scalp is a particularly unpleasant manifestation which can be sight-threatening.

Postherpetic neuralgia is a common complication of zoster

In the healthy host, postherpetic neuralgia (also known as zoster-associated pain, ZAP) is common, especially in the elderly. The pain, which can be severe early in the illness, continues for up to several months after the lesions have resolved. It is difficult to treat, although antiviral agents reduce the incidence, duration and severity of ZAP if started as soon as possible after zoster occurs.

Zoster may be severe in immunocompromised patients. A few days after the localized eruption, the virus, with inadequate control by cell-mediated immunity, spreads via the blood to produce skin and visceral lesions throughout the body. Hemorrhagic complications and pneumonia may occur.

Laboratory diagnosis of VZV

It is a clinical diagnosis that can be assisted by carrying out immunofluorescence tests on skin lesion scrapings using VZV-specific monoclonal antibodies, using molecular tests to detect VZV DNA, or by isolating VZV in cell culture, although the cytopathic effect may take a couple of weeks. Herpesvirus particles can be seen by electron microscopy in vesicle fluid, but are indistinguishable from other herpesviruses and in particular HSV, which also causes vesicular lesions. Past infection is determined by detecting VZV IgG by enzyme-linked immunosorbent assay (ELISA) or other methods. A VZV IgM result may be helpful if the skin lesions have healed and the diagnosis needs to be made for clinical reasons.

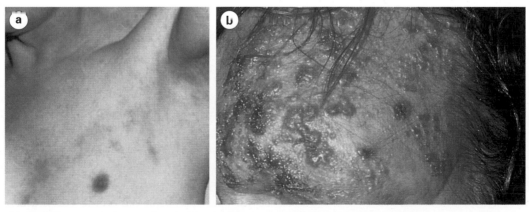

Fig. 26.47 Zoster rash. (a) A band of faint erythema, an early sign of shingles, along an intercostal nerve. (b) Rash affecting the ophthalmic division of the trigeminal nerve. (Courtesy of MJ Wood.)

Treatment of varicella and zoster infection

Varicella skin lesions are treated with baths and soothing applications to relieve itching and to prevent scratching and secondary infection. VZV is much less sensitive than HSV to aciclovir, but this drug, or the more readily bioavailable valaciclovir or famciclovir, can be used orally to treat varicella and zoster. Treatment is often not considered, as chickenpox is thought of as a mild infection that causes little discomfort. However, varicella can cause complications in adolescents and adults, and antiviral treatment should be offered, especially as new lesion formation, viral shedding and symptoms will be reduced. Severe infections must be treated with intravenous aciclovir, especially in high risk groups. VZIG contains a high titer of human antibody to the virus, and is used to prevent varicella in susceptible individuals at risk of complications (e.g. immunocompromised patients) after exposure.

A live attenuated vaccine is licensed in a number of countries, and universal childhood immunization was started in the USA in 1995.

Rashes caused by coxsackieviruses and echoviruses

Coxsackieviruses and echoviruses cause a variety of exanthems (skin rashes)

Sometimes such infections are accompanied by an enanthem (lesions on internal epithelial surfaces such as the oral cavity). These infections are generally seen in young children, are not usually distinguishable on clinical examination, and are not severe. These viruses are also responsible for illnesses affecting the CNS (see Chapter 24), the upper respiratory tract (see Chapter 18), and striated and heart muscle (see below).

Coxsackievirus A lesions are usually vesicular and occur mostly on the buccal mucosa and the tongue. Most children complain of a sore mouth or tongue and there is slight fever. When vesicular lesions are also seen on the skin, principally on the hands and feet, the condition is called 'hand, foot and mouth disease' (Fig. 26.48). The virus is present in the lesions, and coxsackievirus A16 is the most common cause.

Maculopapular rashes resembling rubella and often occurring in the summer are common manifestations of some coxsackie A and echovirus infections.

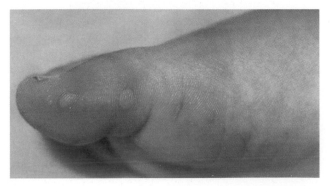

Fig. 26.48 Vesicular lesions on the foot in hand, foot and mouth disease. (Courtesy of MJ Wood.)

Rashes caused by human erythrovirus (formerly parvovirus) B19

Erythrovirus B19 causes slapped cheek syndrome

Parvoviruses are very small (22 nm diameter) single-stranded DNA viruses. The defective parvoviruses (see Appendix) require a helper (adeno-) virus to replicate, and are called 'adeno-associated viruses'; there are four serotypes and infection is common, but they have not been implicated in any human disease. However, erythrovirus B19 grows in mitotically active cells and causes a febrile illness in children with a characteristic maculopapular rash on the face ('slapped cheek syndrome'). The condition is referred to as 'erythema infectiosum' and sometimes 'fifth disease', it being the fifth of the six common exanthematous infections recognized by 19th century physicians.

Symptomless erythrovirus B19 infection is common and spreads by respiratory droplets

Nearly 50% of the population has B19 antibodies. The virus grows in hemopoietic cells in the bone marrow, and although this normally causes no more than a temporary and barely detectable fall in hemoglobin levels, it can lead to serious consequences in those with chronic anemia. In children with sickle cell anemia for instance, the effect on erythropoiesis may cause an aplastic crisis. The virus can also cause arthralgia when it infects adults. Laboratory diagnosis is made by testing sera for erythrovirus B19-specific IgM. Molecular tests may be used to detect B19 DNA in fetal blood when hydrops fetalis is suspected. Erythrovirus B19 cannot be isolated in cell culture.

Rashes caused by human herpesviruses 6 and 7 (HHV-6 and -7)

HHV6 is present in the saliva of over 85% of adults and causes roseola infantum

HHV6 was first isolated in 1986—the preceding five HHV being HSV1, HSV2, VZV, CMV and EBV—and its behavior and natural history are still being studied. Infection occurs in most of the population in the first 3 years of life. The virus replicates in T and B cells and also in the oropharynx, from where it is shed into saliva. The virus persists in the body after initial infection.

HHV6 is the cause of exanthem subitum (also called roseola infantum), a very common acute febrile illness in infants and young children. After an incubation period of about 2 weeks, children develop a high fever which lasts for several days. The disease is mild, and within 2 days of the fever subsiding a maculopapular rash is seen (Fig. 26.49).

HHV7 is present in the saliva of over 75% of adults

HHV7 has been isolated from CD4-positive T cells. Infection occurs later than HHV6 during infancy and early childhood. The virus persists in the saliva, but it is not yet known whether it is a significant cause of disease, although exanthema subitum has been reported with HHV7.

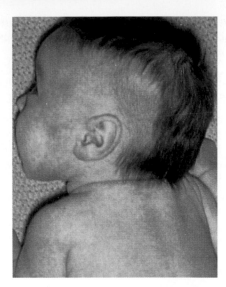

Fig. 26.49 Maculopapular rash in roseola infantum. (Courtesy of MJ Wood.)

HHV8 is associated with all forms of Kaposi's sarcoma skin lesions

After a number of epidemiologic reports, it had been thought that a transmissible agent was involved in the development of Kaposi's sarcoma (KS), a skin malignancy more common in some Mediterranean areas and parts of Africa in addition to AIDS-associated KS. A number of molecular technology developments allowed the identification of HHV8 in 1994 in the endothelial cells of KS lesions. It has also been associated with two other rare malignancies.

It is a clinical diagnosis. The incidence of AIDS-associated KS has dropped since the advent of highly active antiretroviral therapy. In addition, retrospective studies have shown that ganciclovir and foscarnet treatment has resulted in a reduction of KS lesions.

SMALLPOX

Smallpox (variola) was a major scourge of humankind for at least three thousand years. It was caused by a poxvirus and spread from person to person by contact with skin lesions and via the respiratory tract. The disease was severe, with a generalized rash *(Fig. 26.50)*, and was fatal in up to 40% of cases, depending upon the strain of virus.

Global smallpox eradication was officially certified in December 1979

During the first part of the 20th century, smallpox was largely eradicated from Oceania, North America and Europe by widespread vaccination, as originally developed by Edward Jenner (see Chapter 34), using a live attenuated strain of virus (vaccinia virus), together with strict controls at frontiers. In 1967, the WHO started a campaign to eradicate smallpox from the world, focusing on South America, Africa, India and Indonesia, making use of vaccination, surveillance and containment of cases. Despite such daunting difficulties as cultural barriers, warfare and transport to remote areas, the campaign was successful. Occasional cases had continued to

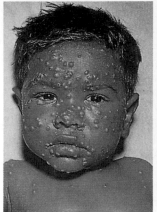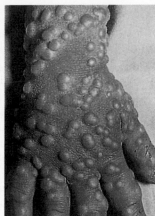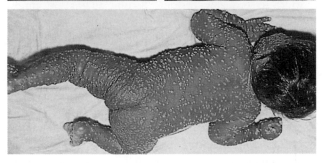

Fig. 26.50 Smallpox. These pictures were used as smallpox recognition cards by the World Health Organization during its smallpox eradication campaign. After upper respiratory tract infection, the virus reached the skin, where it replicated to cause a widespread vesiculopustular rash, with later scarring, especially on the face. The fatality rate was up to 40%, depending on the age of the host and the strain of the virus. (Courtesy of the World Health Organization.)

occur in the USA until the 1940s, and in 1974 there were 218 000 cases worldwide, mostly in Asia, but the last case was recorded in Somalia in October 1977. The total cost to the WHO was about $US 150 million.

Global eradication of smallpox was possible for a variety of reasons

These reasons are as follows:

- There were no subclinical infections, so cases could be readily identified.
- The virus was eliminated from the body on recovery, with no carriers.
- Humans were the only host (no animal reservoir).
- An effective vaccine was available.

For a few years there were concerns about monkeypox, a simian disease caused by a similar virus and acquired by contact with infected monkeys in Africa. It is, however, poorly transmitted from human to human. However, over 80 people were believed to have contracted monkeypox in the USA in 2003. This was thought to be due to contact with infected prairie dogs. Concerns about the use of smallpox by bioterrorists have resulted in countries making contingency plans for the potential threat, which include the stockpiling of smallpox vaccine.

MEASLES

Measles has several special features as follows:

- Nearly all infected individuals become unwell and develop disease. This is in contrast to most other viral infections, in which a significant proportion of individuals undergo an asymptomatic or subclinical infection.
- The disease is so characteristic that a clinical diagnosis can nearly always be made without the need for laboratory help. We can recognize measles as described one thousand years ago by the Arabian physician Rhazes.
- There is only one antigenic type of measles virus.
- After infection there is complete resistance to re-infection, which is probably lifelong. Second attacks are almost unknown.
- Measles is highly infectious, and nearly all susceptible children contract the disease on exposure. Until recently measles was regarded as a routine inescapable part of childhood, and more than 99% of individuals were infected.
- There is a striking contrast between measles in well-nourished children with good access to medical care (i.e. in developed countries) and measles under conditions of malnutrition or starvation or with poor medical services (i.e. developing countries, *Fig. 26.51*).

Etiology and transmission

Measles outbreaks occur every few years in unvaccinated populations

The basic virology of this paramyxovirus is described in Chapter 3 and in the Appendix. Transmission takes place readily via respiratory droplets. Although the virus is soon inactivated as it dries on surfaces, it is more stable in droplets suspended in the air. In unvaccinated populations, outbreaks tend to occur every few years when the number of susceptible children reaches a high enough level.

Clinical features of measles include respiratory symptoms, Koplik's spots and a rash

The inhaled virus enters the body at unknown sites in the upper or lower respiratory tract and spreads to subepithelial and local lymphatic tissues, without causing detectable lesions or symptoms. During the next few days the virus slowly spreads and multiplies in lymphoid tissues elsewhere in the body, including the spleen. The virus then enters the blood in larger amounts and about one week after infection disseminates to a variety of epithelial sites. Clinical signs soon appear in the respiratory tract where there are only one or two layers of epithelial cells to traverse. The patient is well until 9–10 days after infection and then develops an acute respiratory illness with a runny nose, fever and cough. Conjunctivitis is also a feature, and as a result of the large amounts of virus being shed in respiratory secretions, the patient is highly infectious. The diagnosis may be suspected during this prodromal illness, especially after known exposure to measles, It takes a day or two longer for the foci of infection at mucosal and skin surfaces to cause lesions. Koplik's spots appear inside the cheek (*Fig. 26.52*), and shortly afterwards the unmistakable maculopapular rash (*Fig. 26.53*) is seen, first on the face, then spreading down the body to the extremities. The diagnosis is now clear.

Measles rash results from a cell-mediated immune response

Antibodies are formed, but a cell-mediated immune (CMI) response is needed to control the growth of virus in the lungs and elsewhere. Without it the virus continues to grow and

CLINICAL IMPACT OF MEASLES		
site of virus growth	**well-nourished child; good medical care**	**malnourished child; poor medical care**
lung	temporary respiratory illness	life-threatening pneumonia
ear	otitis media quite common	otitis media more common, more severe
oral mucosa	Koplik's spots	severe ulcerating lesions
conjunctiva	conjunctivitis	severe corneal lesions, secondary bacterial infection, blindness may result
skin	maculopapular rash	hemorrhagic rashes may occur ('black measles')
intestinal tract	no lesions	diarrhea – exacerbates malnutrition, halts growth, impairs recovery
urinary tract	virus detectable in urine	no known complications
overall impact	**serious disease in a small proportion of those infected**	**major cause of death in childhood (estimated one million deaths/year worldwide)**

Fig. 26.51 The clinical impact of measles depends upon the host. Measles is a much more serious disease in malnourished children with poor access to medical care. The same epithelial surfaces are infected, but more extensively and with more serious sequelae.

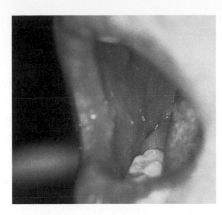

Fig. 26.52 Koplik's spots seen as minute white dots on the inflamed buccal mucosa of a patient with measles. (Courtesy of MJ Wood.)

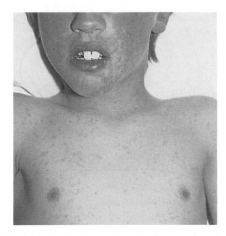

Fig. 26.53 Maculopapular rash on the face and trunk of a patient with measles. (Courtesy of MJ Wood.)

gives rise to giant cell pneumonia (see Chapter 19). The CMI response is also responsible for the skin lesions, which are not seen in patients with serious defects in this type of immunity. Children with agammaglobulinemia, on the other hand, have a normal course of disease, develop normal immunity, and can be protected by vaccination. In uncomplicated cases recovery is rapid.

During measles, as in a variety of other acute infections, there are temporary defects in immune responses to unrelated antigens. For instance, at about the time the rash appears, individuals who are known to be tuberculin-positive give negative skin test responses to tuberculin. This returns to normal in about a month. During the 'virgin-soil' epidemic, when measles reappeared after a long absence in Southern Greenland, in 1953, and adults as well as children were infected, there was increased mortality in those previously infected with tuberculosis.

Complications of measles are particularly likely among children in developing countries

Complications of measles include:

- opportunistic bacterial superinfections, which are quite common, especially otitis media and pneumonia, as a result of virus damage to respiratory surfaces;
- a primary measles virus pneumonia (giant cell pneumo-

nia), which is seen in patients with serious CMI response defects;
- encephalitis, which occurs in about 1 in 1000 cases (see Chapter 24);
- very rarely, subacute sclerosing panencephalitis (SSPE). This develops 1–10 years after apparent recovery from acute infection.

Children in countries where there is poor medical care and malnutrition develop a more serious disease *(Fig. 26.51)*, especially during famine. This is attributable to:

- poor local mucosal defenses, which can be improved by vitamin A administration;
- impaired immune defenses due to protein–calorie malnutrition, with the added impact of measles virus-induced immunosuppression;
- poor medical services, with less ready availability of antibiotics to control secondary infection;
- high levels of bacterial contamination of the environment;
- exposure to a larger virus dose—a possible factor if others with severe measles shed larger amounts of virus from the respiratory tract.

Diagnosis, treatment and prevention

Measles is usually diagnosed clinically; there is no antiviral treatment, but there is a vaccine

Although the clinical diagnosis should be clear, the rash is similar to a number of other viral exanthems which affect the same age group. In addition, with the success of the vaccine, the incidence of measles infection has fallen and it is less likely that healthcare workers will see children with measles in resource rich countries. Therefore, the measles IgM assay is helpful in confirming the diagnosis either on blood or saliva samples. Virus isolation in cell culture is rarely necessary.

A live attenuated vaccine has been available since 1963. It is effective, safe and long-lasting, and is combined with mumps and rubella vaccines (MMR vaccine; see Chapter 34). Before a vaccine became available, measles killed 7–8 million children each year worldwide. By 1996 this was reduced to 1 million, and if the mass immunization programs used in the Americas and Europe are applied to developing countries, the WHO suggests that measles could be eliminated from the world by the year 2010.

RUBELLA

Rubella virus infection causes a multisystem infection, but its main impact is on the fetus

There is only one serotype of this single-stranded RNA togavirus, and its principal impact is on the fetus (see Chapter 23). It is transmitted by droplet infection, and is less contagious than measles, but more so than mumps.

After entering the body silently at unknown sites in the respiratory tract, the virus grows for a period in local lymphoid tissues, followed by spread to the spleen and to lymph nodes elsewhere in the body. One week after infection further multiplication in these tissues leads to viremia and localization of virus in the respiratory tract and skin, and sometimes the placenta, joints and kidney. The pathogenesis

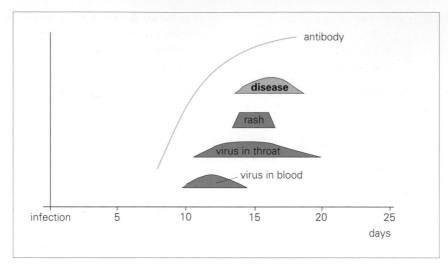

Fig. 26.54 The pathogenesis of rubella. Rubella is generally a very mild, often subclinical infection, but it can cause arthritis and has a major impact when it infects the fetus.

of rubella is outlined in *Figure 26.54*, and the clinical consequences of infection in various tissues of the body are shown in *Figure 26.55*.

After an incubation period of 14–21 days there is a mild disease, with fever, malaise and an irregular maculopapular rash lasting 3 days. Enlarged lymph nodes are often evident behind the ear, but the infection is commonly subclinical.

Rubella is diagnosed serologically; there is no treatment, but there is a vaccine

Clinical diagnosis of rubella is sometimes possible but should be confirmed in the laboratory. Laboratory diagnosis is made by demonstrating rubella-specific IgM antibodies (see Chapter 32). Virus isolation from the throat is rarely indicated —virus isolation requires specialized cell lines, and indirect methods are needed to demonstrate its growth. Viral RNA can be detected in samples from different sites.

There is no antiviral treatment. A live attenuated rubella vaccine that is safe and effective is given by injection, generally in combination with measles and mumps vaccines (MMR vaccine). Prevention of congenital rubella is referred to in Chapter 23.

The maculopapular rashes seen in certain arthropod-borne virus infections (e.g. dengue) and in zoonotic virus infections (e.g. Marburg disease) are referred to in Chapters 27 and 28. A maculopapular rash may be seen in the prodromal stage of hepatitis B virus infection (see Chapter 22), and is immune complex-mediated.

OTHER INFECTIONS PRODUCING SKIN LESIONS

Other bacterial, fungal and rickettsial infections produce a variety of rashes or other skin lesions

Most of these are referred to elsewhere in this book, and they are listed in *Figure 26.4*. Rashes in rickettsial infections are often striking, as in the case of Rocky Mountain spotted fever or typhus (see Chapter 27). Most rickettsia invade vascular endothelial cells, from whence they are shed into the blood to infect blood-sucking arthropod vectors. Invasion of vascular endothelial cells in the skin provides the basis for the skin rash but is not a source of direct shedding to the exterior.

PATHOGENESIS OF RUBELLA		
site of virus growth	result	comment
respiratory tract	virus shedding but symptoms minimal (mild sore throat, coryza, cough)	patient infectious five days before to three days after symptoms
skin	rash	often fleeting, atypical; immunopathology involved (Ag–Ab complexes)
lymph nodes	lymphadenopathy	more common in posterior triangle of neck or behind ear
joints	mild arthralgia, arthritis	immunopathology involved (circulating immune complexes)
placenta/fetus	placentitis, fetal damage	congenital rubella

Fig. 26.55 Clinical consequences of rubella virus invasion of different body tissues.

KAWASAKI SYNDROME

Kawasaki syndrome is an acute vasculitis and is probably caused by superantigen toxins

The Kawasaki syndrome is a childhood illness of uncertain etiology. Patients, who are generally less than 4 years of age, develop fever, conjunctivitis and a rash. There is dryness and redness of the lips and red palms and soles with some edema, desquamation of fingertips, often arthralgia and myocarditis, which gives a case mortality of about 2%. The basic pathology is an acute vasculitis, and 20% of untreated patients develop coronary artery aneurysms. The disease is commoner in those of Asian ancestry, but occurs worldwide. There is no clear evidence for person to person transmission, but it is thought to be of infectious origin, and is probably due to the superantigen toxins (see Chapter 16) of *Staph. aureus* or *Strep. pyogenes*.

Treatment, which prevents the aneurysms if given early enough, is high dose intravenous immunoglobulin.

VIRAL INFECTIONS OF MUSCLE

Viral myositis, myocarditis and pericarditis

Some viruses, particularly coxsackievirus B, cause myocarditis and myalgia

Group B, and to a lesser extent group A, coxsackieviruses and certain enteroviruses are the main viral causes of acute myocarditis and pericarditis. Both conditions are seen principally in adult males and are important because they can be mistaken for myocardial infarction, yet the prognosis is good and complete recovery is the rule. There is also evidence for persistent infection linked with chronic myocarditis and chronic dilated cardiomyopathy. The most common cause of viral myocarditis in infants is the coxsackievirus B group and may be rapid in onset and fatal. These infections are transmitted by the fecal–oral route and occasionally from pharyngeal secretions. Ingested coxsackieviruses spread from the pharynx or gut wall to the lymphatics and then to the blood. Invasion of striated muscles, heart or pericardium takes place across small blood vessels and results in acute inflammation. In the heart and pericardium this gives rise to dyspnea, pain in the chest, and sometimes mimics a myocardial infarction. Coxsackievirus may be isolated from throat swabs, fecal specimens or occasionally pericardial fluid. Alternatively, viral RNA detection methods may be used, for example in-situ hybridization on endomyocardial biopsy tissue. Mumps and influenza are less common causes of myocarditis or pericarditis. Rubella (see Chapter 23) can cause myocarditis and associated congenital lesions in the fetus.

Group B coxsackieviruses also cause pleurodynia or epidemic myalgia. This condition is sometimes called 'Bornholm disease', after the Danish island where there was an extensive outbreak in 1930. There is pain and inflammation involving intercostal or abdominal muscles.

Influenza (especially influenza B in children) can cause pain and tenderness in muscles, but it is not known whether this is associated with viral invasion of muscle. Myalgias are also seen in dengue and in rickettsial and other febrile infections and are probably caused by circulating cytokines.

Laboratory diagnosis in these settings can be difficult, as serology and virus isolation can only give circumstantial evidence for association between that virus infection and a specific organ. Direct detection methods in affected tissue may be more helpful.

The use of antiviral drugs such as pleconaril is being investigated for treating enterovirus infections. There are no specific vaccines for coxsackievirus infections.

Postviral fatigue syndrome

It has been difficult to establish postviral fatigue syndrome as a clinical entity

The postviral fatigue syndrome or chronic fatigue syndrome is sometimes referred to as myalgic encephalomyelitis, but this is inappropriate because there is no evidence for CNS pathology. It consists of:

- chronic and severe muscle weakness, lasting at least 6 months, often as a sequel to an acute febrile illness;
- severe tiredness;
- less regularly associated symptoms such as depression, headache and anxiety.

It is more reliably identified when the first two symptoms appear in a previously healthy individual with no history of psychosomatic illness. Several viruses have been suggested as causes. There have been repeated claims for the role of coxsackie B viruses, based on antibody tests and on the detection of a virus-specific protein in the serum of patients, but these results have not been widely confirmed, and the picture remains unclear. A small proportion of cases appear to be due to chronic infection with Epstein–Barr virus (EBV). Occasional reports have associated the condition with HHV6 and with other viruses. It has also been suggested that it is due to 'allergic reactions' triggered by virus infections.

PARASITIC INFECTIONS OF MUSCLE

Relatively few protozoan or helminth parasites invade muscle tissues or cause serious disease. Three of the more common are described here to illustrate the variety of organisms and the range of pathology.

Trypanosoma cruzi infection

Trypanosoma cruzi is a protozoan and causes Chagas' disease

Chagas' disease is also known as American trypanosomiasis (see Chapter 27). The disease is restricted to Central and South America, where it affects an estimated 10–12 million people. It is a zoonosis, and *Trypanosoma cruzi* has been isolated from more than 150 species of mammal. The parasite is carried by blood-sucking bugs, which deposit infective trypomastigote stages on to the skin as they defecate while feeding. If these are rubbed into mucous membranes or wounds, the parasites penetrate cells, transform into amastigotes and proliferate. The infected cells then burst, liberating trypomastigotes, and a local lesion is formed. The parasite is dispersed around the body to re-invade other cells. Major sites of infection include the CNS, intestinal myenteric plexus, reticuloendothelial system and cardiac muscle.

Chagas' disease is complicated by heart failure many years later

Disease occurs as an acute febrile phase, with intense inflammatory changes, and as a chronic phase that becomes apparent years later. In the chronic phase there is gradual tissue destruction with autoimmune damage playing an important role. The parasite invades the myofibrils of the heart (see *Fig. 27.19*) causing myocarditis, and muscle fibrils and Purkinje fibers may be replaced by fibrous tissue. As a result of the conduction defects this causes, the heart enlarges, there are cardiac arrhythmias, and heart failure can occur.

Nifurtimox and benznidazole are used to treat the acute phase, but the chronic disease is irreversible. At present no vaccine is available, and prevention of infection is the most important measure.

Taenia solium infection

The larval stages of Taenia solium *invade body tissues*

Tapeworms are intestinal parasites, but the larval stages of several species may invade deeper tissues. The most important of these are:

- *Echinococcus granulosus* (which causes hydatid disease, see Chapters 24 and 28);
- the pork tapeworm *Taenia solium*.

Humans acquire *T. solium* infection by eating undercooked infected pig meat in which the cysticercus larvae are found as small, bladder-like structures in the muscle tissue. These larvae are digested out in the intestine and mature into the adult tapeworm, which may reach a length of several meters. *T. solium* is unusual in that its eggs can hatch directly in the human intestine. This may result from accidental swallowing of water contaminated with eggs, but can occur directly from the eggs released by adult worms. If hatching occurs, the larvae cross the intestinal wall and are carried via the blood to internal organs. Sites of development include the CNS and body muscles. In the latter, the cysts eventually become calcified and can be seen on radiography *(Fig. 26.56)*. Muscle infection is not serious, being largely asymptomatic. Infections are common in many parts of the world, particularly South and Central America and Asia. Avoidance of undercooked pork products is the safest precaution, and infections can be treated with praziquantel.

Trichinella spiralis infection

The larvae of Trichinella *spiralis invade striated muscle*

This nematode has many unique features. It is able to infect almost any warm-blooded animal, and has a lifecycle in which a complete generation (infective stage to infective stage) develops within the body of a single host. Transmission depends upon the ingestion of muscle tissue containing viable infective larvae. As far as humans are concerned, the

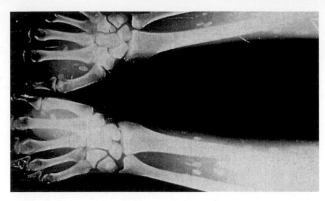

Fig. 26.56 Radiograph showing numerous calcified cysts of *Taenia solium* in the forearms. (Courtesy of R Muller and JR Baker.)

commonest route of transmission is through infected pig meat, but many other meat sources have been known to transmit infection (e.g. bear, boar, horse). Infections occur worldwide. When infected undercooked meat is eaten, the larvae are digested out in the small intestine and develop rapidly into the adult worms. These live in the mucosa, each female releasing about one thousand newborn larvae directly into the intestinal tissues, from where they are carried in blood or lymph around the body. Eventually the larvae penetrate striated muscles and mature into the infective stage, transforming muscle cells into a parasite-sustaining nurse cell (see *Fig. 28.12*).

Light infections are asymptomatic, but the migration and penetration of the larvae is associated with inflammatory reactions, which can be severe and life-threatening when a person is heavily infected. A variety of symptoms are associated with this phase, of which fever, muscle pains, weakness and eosinophilia are characteristic. Myocarditis may also occur, although the parasite does not develop in the heart.

Diagnosis by symptoms usually occurs after the parasites have invaded the muscles and treatment then is difficult. Mebendazole can be used, but corticosteroids may also be required.

Sarcocystis

Sarcocystis *is a rare muscle parasite*

The cyst stages of *Sarcocystis*, a protozoan related to *Toxoplasma*, are occasionally reported in human muscles. Infection is acquired from the meat of infected food animals and may cause myositis.

JOINT AND BONE INFECTIONS

Joints and bones will be considered separately for convenience, but joint lesions often spread to involve neighboring bone, and vice versa (e.g. in tuberculosis).

Reactive arthritis, arthralgia and septic arthritis

Arthralgia and arthritis occur in a variety of infections and are often immunologically mediated

Examples of such infections are outlined in *Figure 26.57*. Joints can become infected by the hematogenous route or

ARTHRALGIA AND ARTHRITIS IN INFECTIOUS DISEASES		
	infectious agent	comments
viral arthritis	hepatitis B rubella mumps Ross River and other togaviruses parvovirus	occurs in prodromal period; due to circulating immune complexes especially in young women, often follows live virus vaccine unusual, mostly in men mosquito-transmitted infections in Australia (Ross River) and Africa may follow adult infection

reactive arthritis	*Campylobacter, Yersinia,* salmonellae,
	   shigellae, *Chlamydia trachomatis*
	   (Reiter's syndrome*)
		'post-infectious' arthritis, HLA B27-associated, no bacterial invasion
		   of joint, immune mediated

septic arthritis	*Staphylococcus aureus* salmonellae *Haemophilus influenzae* *Neisseria gonorrhoeae* *Mycobacterium tuberculosis* *Borrelia burgdorferi* streptococci, *Pseudomonas aeruginosa* *Mycoplasma hominis* *Sporothrix schenckii*	commonest cause of suppurative arthritis occurs in children occurs in children may affect multiple joints often with bone lesions, especially weight bearing joints and bones arthritis a late feature of Lyme disease uncommon bacteria can enter maternal blood during delivery and invade joints; uncommon fungal infection of joints
*urethritis, arthritis,uveitis, mucocutaneous lesions; complicates 1–2% of cases of chlamydial urethritis		

Fig. 26.57 Arthralgia and arthritis in infectious diseases.

directly following trauma or surgery, but in many cases the condition is immunologically mediated rather than due to microbial invasion of the joint. The microbe responsible is at a distant site in the body and causes a 'reactive arthritis'. Reactive arthritis and arthralgia occur after certain enteric bacterial infections, and the arthralgia in rubella and hepatitis B infections is of similar origin. In this type of arthritis more than one joint is usually affected.

Ankylosing spondylitis is associated with *Klebsiella* infection, and it has been suggested that the antigenic similarity between *Klebsiella* and HLA B27 antigens provokes a cross-reactive immune response that causes the disease. So far there is no evidence that rheumatoid arthritis is caused by either viruses or other microbes.

Circulating bacteria sometimes localize in joints, especially following trauma

Such bacterial localization can then cause a suppurative (septic) arthritis. Generally a single joint is involved. Joints are very susceptible, particularly if they are already damaged, for instance by rheumatoid arthritis, or if a prosthesis has been inserted. Knees are most commonly affected, followed by hips, ankles (see *Fig. 21.11b*) and elbows. Signs include a fever, joint pain, limitation of movement and swelling, and usually a joint effusion. Bacteria can be isolated from the joint fluid or seen in the centrifuged deposit, and the commonest organism is *Staph. aureus*. Sometimes the source of the circulating bacteria is obvious (e.g. a septic skin lesion), but often no source is apparent.

Osteomyelitis

Bone can become infected by adjacent infection or hematogenously

As with joints, infection can be by the direct route (e.g. from a nearby focus of infection, after fractures, after orthopedic surgery) or from circulating microbes. The commonest cause of hematogenous osteomyelitis is *Staph. aureus*, but when infection is from a neighboring site it is generally mixed, with Gram-negative rods and occasionally anaerobes also present. There seems to be no equivalent to reactive arthritis, in which inflammation is due to infection at a distant site.

Acute osteomyelitis typically involves the growing end of a long bone, where sprouting capillary loops adjacent to epiphyseal growth plates promote the localization of circulating bacteria. It therefore tends to be a disease of children and adolescents, and may follow non-penetrating injury to the bone.

Osteomyelitis results in a painful tender bone lesion and a general febrile illness.

Osteomyelitis is treated with antibiotics and sometimes surgery

The infection is diagnosed from blood cultures taken before the start of antimicrobial therapy or, if there is an open lesion, from a bone biopsy. Periosteal reaction and bone loss may be visible radiologically (*Fig. 26.58*). Treatment is begun on a 'most likely' basis (e.g. nafcillin for MSSA, see above) as soon as microbiologic samples have been taken.

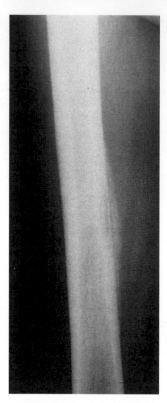

Fig. 26.58 Acute staphylococcal osteomyelitis in the femur of a 24-year-old woman. There is a well-defined periosteal reaction in relation to the midshaft of the femur and an underlying lucency. (Courtesy of AM Davies.)

Osteomyelitis can become chronic, especially when there are necrotic bone fragments to act as a continued source of infection. Surgical intervention for debridement and drainage, as well as prolonged courses of antibiotics, may be necessary.

Tuberculosis may affect the spine, the hip, the knee and the bones of the hands and feet, and in developed countries is particularly seen in immigrants from the Indian subcontinent. Constitutional disturbances are often absent, but the site is generally painful and pressure from a tuberculous abscess in the spine can cause paraplegia.

INFECTIONS OF THE HEMOPOIETIC SYSTEM

Many infectious agents cause changes in circulating blood cells

Examples of such agents include:

- *Bordetella pertussis*, which causes lymphocytosis;
- EBV and cytomegalovirus infections, which cause mononucleosis;
- *Plasmodium* spp. which cause anemia and thrombocytopenia.

A smaller number of infectious agents act directly on cells in the bone marrow (human parvovirus) or cause malignant transformation of lymphocytes—for example human T cell lymphotropic virus (HTLV) type 1. The range of possibilities is summarized in *Figure 26.59*. HTLV1 and HTLV2 are mentioned in Chapters 21 and 24, but are described more fully below.

HTLV1 infection

HTLV1 is mainly transmitted by maternal milk

HTLV1 was first isolated in 1980 from a patient with adult T cell leukemia (ATLL). Infection is widespread, especially in certain islands in the West Indies and Japan, where 5–15% of the population are infected, and also in South America and parts of Africa. Transmission is primarily via maternal milk, less effectively via sexual intercourse, and by blood-contaminated equipment in intravenous drug misusers.

HTLV1 infects T cells, and up to 5% of those infected develop T cell leukemia

HTLV1 infects T cells and persists. The *tax* gene product, a transcriptional activator protein, stimulates transcription of host genes controlling production of interleukin 2 (IL-2), IL-2 receptor and other molecules, thus affecting cell replication. Infected T cells proliferate, and if in addition there are certain chromosomal abnormalities, malignant transformation takes place.

Clinically, the patient develops a mild febrile disease with lymphadenopathy. The skin is often involved, with nodule and plaque formation, and pleural effusion or aseptic meningitis can occur. There is also increased susceptibility to opportunist infections such as *Pneumocystis jiroveci* and *Strongyloides stercoralis*. Depressed delayed hypersensitivity responses to tuberculin is associated. Polymyositis has been described. Up to 5% of infected individuals eventually develop T cell leukemia, which has a high and rapid mortality rate, and a similar proportion progress to 'tropical' spastic paraparesis (TSP), also known as HTLV-associated myelopathy (HAM), in which there is primary demyelination (see Chapter 24). Neural cells do not appear to be infected, and it is not known how the virus causes a neurologic disease.

Detection of HTLV1 and HTLV2 specific antibody is based on serological methods with type differentiation by immunoblot. Antiretroviral agents other than protease inhibitors have been shown to inhibit viral replication and are under investigation as part of the management of individuals with ATLL or TSP. Other treatments have been examined with limited success. HTLV antibody positive individuals are assumed to be infectious and should not donate blood or organs. HTLV antibody screening of blood donors is now included in many countries.

HTLV2 infection

HTLV2 was first isolated in 1982 from a patient with T cell hairy leukemia, although it is not the usual cause of this condition. HTLV2 is closely related to HTLV1, is transmitted by similar routes and has been reported in intravenous drug misusers and native Amerindian tribes in North, Central and South America. It has been associated with a number of neurological conditions including occasional reports of myelopathy.

MICROBES AFFECTING BLOOD CELLS OR HEMOPOIESIS			
microbe	**disease**	**effect**	**mechanism**
Plasmodium spp.	malaria	anemia	replication in erythrocytes
Babesia spp.	babesiosis (uncommon, tick-borne)	anemia	replication in erythrocytes
Bartonella brucelliformis	oroya fever* (rare, sandfly-transmitted, occurs in Peru)	anemia	replication in erythrocytes
Ehrlichia sp. (Rickettsiae)	human ehrlichiosis (tick transmitted in Southern USA and Japan)	leucopenia, thrombocytopenia	replication in leukocytes
human parvovirus	erythema infectiosum	temporary fall in hemoglobin levels aplastic crisis (individual with chronic anemia)	replication in erythropoietic cells
Colorado tick fever virus	Colorado tick fever	no effect on survival of infected erythrocytes	replication in erythropoietic cells
human T cell lymphotropic virus (HTLV)1, HTLV2	T cell leukemia, lymphoma	malignant transformation of infected T cells	replication in T cells
HIV**	AIDS	immunosuppression	infection of CD4-positive T cells
Epstein–Barr virus (EBV)	infectious mononucleosis	thrombocytopenia, anemia	autoantibody to platelets, erythrocytes
cytomegalovirus (CMV)	congenital CMV complication of adult infection	anemia, thrombocytopenia	infection of, or autoantibody to, erythrocytes, platelets

*a cutaneous form (Verrugas) also occurs; in 1885 a Peruvian medical student, Daniel Carrion, demonstrated the common bacterial origin by inoculating himself with infected blood from the cutaneous form of the disease and developing oroya fever

**many other viruses infect immune cells and depress immune responses less dramatically (e.g. CMV, measles)

Fig. 26.59 Microbes affecting blood cells or hemopoiesis.

KEY FACTS

- The intact skin is an invaluable barrier that defends the body against invasion.
- A wide range of organisms is associated with skin infection and disease.
- Bacteria, fungi and viruses usually gain access through breaches of the barrier caused by trauma.
- Some parasites initiate their own penetration into the skin (leptospirosis, schistosomiasis).
- Other microbes are introduced into the skin by arthropod vectors.
- Once in the skin, microbes cause local infections or disseminate through the body to distant sites.
- Pathogens may be acquired by other routes, disseminate in the body and then localize in the skin or cause toxic or immunopathologic manifestations in the skin.
- Superficial infections of the skin are among the commonest human infections (boils, impetigo, warts, acne, ringworm).
- Invasion of pathogens deeper into dermal and subdermal tissues may produce severe infections that can be rapidly fatal, as in gangrene, or slow but progressive deformation and destruction, as in leprosy.
- Infections of muscle usually arise from invasion from the outside, whereas infections of joints are more often bloodborne.
- Bone infections may arise either by local spread from an infected joint or as a result of hematogenous seeding.
- Bone marrow cells or leukocytes may be invaded by viruses that interfere with hemopoiesis (parvovirus), cause malignant transformation (HTLV1 and 2), or interfere with the immune system (EBV, HIV).

QUESTIONS

A 19-year-old philosophy student sees the college doctor because she has been feeling tired since starting her third term 3 weeks previously. She has been feverish and sweaty, and has had a sore throat and some abdominal discomfort. On examination she has a temperature of 38.5°C, cervical lymphadenopathy, a few palatal petechiae, an inflamed pharynx, and tender smooth splenomegaly. The results of investigations are: hemoglobin 14 g/dl; white cell count 4×10^9/l with atypical lymphocytes; alanine transaminase 300 IU/l; aspartate transaminase 350 IU/l.

1. What is the differential diagnosis?

2. How would you investigate this woman for EBV infection?

3. The results of the monospot test are as follows: agglutination with unadsorbed serum to which the indicator horse red blood cells are added; agglutination with guinea pig (antigen) cells to which horse red blood cells are added; no agglutination with ox cell stroma cells to which horse red blood cells are added; VCA IgM positive; VCA IgG. How would you interpret these results?

4. What are the more common complications of EBV infection?

5. What would be your advice to this patient?

A 4-year-old boy has been referred to the clinic with a history of a painful arm. He fell while on a climbing frame 5 days ago and lacerated his right forearm. He has become more unwell in the last 24 hours with a fever, vomiting and abdominal pain. On examination he is miserable, dehydrated and feverish. His right forearm is exquisitely tender over the area of the wound. His abdomen is tender, but there is no rebound tenderness or guarding. His chest is clear.

1. What is the likely diagnosis?

2. What investigations would you perform?

3. The results of investigations are hemoglobin 15 g/dl and white cell count 24×10^9/l with 90% neutrophils, and blood cultures grow *Staph. aureus* sensitive to nafcillin. A radiograph of the forearm shows soft tissue swelling over the affected area of the forearm. How would you treat this condition?

A 2-year-old girl develops a fine erythematous rash together with the sudden onset of a high fever. She is up to date with her immunization schedule, and her doctor sees her at home. On examination she is unwell with a fever and rash. There are no other findings of note.

1. What is the differential diagnosis?

2. The diagnosis is invariably a clinical diagnosis, but if this child is admitted to hospital she may be further investigated. What investigations would you perform if she is admitted?

FURTHER READING

Harahap M. *Diagnosis and Treatment of Skin Infections.* Oxford: Blackwell, 1997.

Lesher JL. *An Atlas of Microbiology of the Skin.* Boca Raton: CRC Press, 2000.

Mandal S, Berendt AR, Peacock SJ. Staphylococcus aureus bone and joint infection. *J Infect* 2002; 44:143–51.

Noble WC. Skin bacteriology and the role of Staphylococcus aureus in infection. *Br J Dermatol* 1998; 139(Suppl 53):9–12.

Park KC, Han WS. Viral skin infections: diagnosis and treatment considerations. *Drugs* 2002; 62:479–90.

Saliba EK, Oumeish OY, Oumeish I. Epidemiology of common parasitic infections of the skin in infants and children. *Clin Dermatol* 2002; 20:36–43.

Seal DV, Hay RJ, Middleton K. *Skin and Wound Infections.* London: Taylor and Francis, 2000.

Tan HH, Goh CL. Parasitic skin infections in the elderly: recognition and drug treatment. *Drugs Aging* 2001; 18:165–76.

Thestrup-Pedersen K. Bacteria and the skin: clinical practice and therapy update. *Br J Dermatol* 1998; 139(Suppl 53):1–3.

Trent JT, Federman D, Kirsner RS. Common viral and fungal skin infections. *Ostomy Wound Manage* 2001; 47:28–34.

Vector-borne infections

INTRODUCTION

A number of important human diseases, caused by organisms ranging from viruses to worms, are transmitted by blood-feeding arthropods. These vectors inject the organisms into humans as they take a blood meal. Two classes of arthropods make the major contribution to disease transmission, the six-legged insects and the eight-legged ticks and mites. Arthropod-transmitted infections are commonest in warmer countries, but occur worldwide. Schistosomiasis, a major topical disease, is also vector-transmitted, but in this case the vectors are aquatic snails

Transmission of disease by vectors

In sparsely populated areas transmission by insects is an effective means of spread

Disease transmission by insects has major implications for the host, the vector and the parasite. To consider the parasite first, it requires the organism to be present in the right place (in the blood) and at the right time (some insects, for example, bite only at night). Blood is an inhospitable environment, and this may require quite subtle evasion mechanisms for parasite survival. In addition, the conditions found in the vector are likely to be extremely different from those in the human host, and the parasite may have to make a remarkably complex transition in a short time. With the larger protozoal and helminth parasites this transition often involves clearly-visible changes in appearance and is responsible for much of the complicated nomenclature of parasite lifecycles. Since some insect vectors have lifespans hardly longer than those of their parasites, there is considerable wastage due to death of the vector before the parasite has matured to the infective stage for man. A difference of a few days in a mosquito's lifespan can make an enormous difference in the effectiveness of malaria transmission, and indeed this simple factor is believed to underly much of the difference between the African pattern of endemic infection and the Indian pattern of sporadic epidemics. However, what may be lost from wastage is more than compensated for by the enormously increased distance over which dissemination of the parasite can occur.

Vector transmission of disease means that the disease may be controlled by controlling the vector

This is, however, much easier said than done, as was discovered during the attempts to eradicate malaria by dichlorodiphenyltrichloroethane (DDT) spraying of the mosquito breeding areas. In the event the mosquitoes developed resistance and more damage was done to the environment than to the insects. Nevertheless, vector control remains a highly desirable goal in relation to the diseases discussed in this chapter and is, for instance, a major reason why malaria is not endemic in many European countries.

A potential advantage of this type of transmission for the host is that it is sometimes possible to immunize specifically against the transmission stages of the parasite. Again malaria can serve as an example—vaccines against the sporozoites, gametocytes and gametes having been clearly shown to block transmission in animal models. Once transmission is blocked, there is a mathematically calculable possibility that the disease will die out.

ARBOVIRUS INFECTIONS

Arboviruses are arthropod-borne viruses

A wide range of about five hundred different viruses is transmitted by arthropods such as ticks, mosquitoes and sandflies. These arboviruses multiply in the arthropod vector, and for each virus there is a natural cycle involving vertebrates (various birds or mammals) and arthropods. The virus enters the arthropod when the latter takes a blood meal from the infected vertebrate, and passes through the gut wall to reach the salivary gland where replication takes place. Once this has occurred, 1–2 weeks after ingesting the virus, the arthropod becomes infectious, and can transmit virus to another vertebrate during a blood meal. Certain arboviruses that infect ticks are also transmitted directly from adult tick to egg (vertical transmission), so that future generations of ticks are infected without the need for a vertebrate host.

Only a small number of arboviruses are important causes of human disease

Arboviruses tend to replicate in vascular endothelium, the central nervous system (CNS), skin and muscle, and are therefore multisystem infections. They are generally named after the clinical disease (e.g. yellow fever) or the place where they were first discovered (e.g. Rift Valley fever, Japanese encephalitis). A few (e.g. Ross River virus in Australia and the Pacific) cause arthritis.

The human stage of the virus cycle may be essential (urban yellow fever, dengue), there being no other vertebrate host, or it may be 'accidental' from the virus's point of view, with

PRINCIPAL RICKETTSIAL DISEASES OF HUMANS

	organism	disease	arthropod vector	vertebrate reservoir	clinical severity	geographic distribution
spotted fevers***	R. rickettsii	Rocky Mountain spotted fever	tick*	dogs, rodents	+	Rocky Mountain states, eastern USA
	R. akari	rickettsial pox	mite*	mice	–	Asia, Far East, Africa, USA
	R. conorii	Mediterranean spotted fever	tick	dogs	+	Mediterranean
typhus	R. prowazekii	epidemic typhus	louse	human**	++	Africa, South America
	R. typhi	endemic typhus	flea	rodents	–	worldwide
	Orientia tsutsugamushi	scrub typhus	mite*	rodents	++	Far East
others	Coxiella burnetii	Q fever	none	sheep, goats, cattle	+	worldwide
	Bartonella quintana	trench fever	louse	human	+	Asia, Africa, Central and South America†
	Ehrlichia chaffeensis††	fever (ehrlichiosis)	tick	?	+	USA, Japan (E. sennetsu)

*vertically transmitted in arthropod
**non-human vertebrates are possibly also involved
***other rickettsiae cause similar tick-borne fevers in Africa, India, Australia
†multiply extracellularly; 1 million soldiers infected in the First World War
††isolated at Fort Chaffe, Arkansas; parasitizes lymphocytes, monocytes, neutrophils

Fig. 27.5 The principal rickettsial diseases in humans.

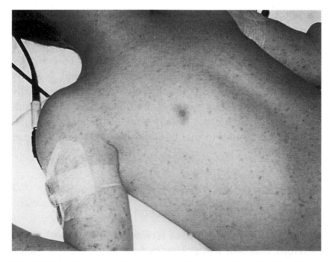

Fig. 27.6 Generalized maculopapular rash with petechiae in Rocky Mountain spotted fever. (Courtesy of TF Sellers, Jr.)

Epidemic typhus

Epidemic typhus is transmitted by the human body louse

Epidemic typhus is transmitted from person to person by *Pediculus corporis*. The rickettsiae (*R. prowazekii*) multiply in the gut epithelium of the louse and are excreted in feces during the act of biting. The rickettsiae enter the skin when the bite is scratched. The disease cannot maintain itself unless enough people are infested with lice. Epidemic typhus is therefore classically associated with poverty and war, when clothes and bodies are washed less frequently. There were 30 million cases in Eastern Europe and the Soviet Union from 1918 to 1922. The disease is seen in Africa, Central and South America, and to a lesser extent in the USA. As there is no direct person-to-person spread, outbreaks can be terminated by delousing campaigns.

Untreated epidemic typhus has a mortality as high as 60%

Rickettsiae proliferate at the site of the bite and then spread in the blood to infect vascular endothelium in skin, heart, CNS, muscle and kidney. About 1 week after the louse bite (there is no eschar) the infected person develops fever, headache and flu-like symptoms. The generalized maculopapular rash appears 5–9 days later and sometimes there is severe meningo-encephalitis with delirium and coma. In untreated cases mortality can range from 20% in healthy individuals to as high as 60% in elderly or compromised patients, due to peripheral vascular collapse or secondary bacterial pneumonia.

Convalescence may take months. In some individuals the rickettsiae are not eliminated from the body on clinical recovery and remain in the lymph nodes. As much as 50 years later, the infection can reactivate to cause Brill–Zinsser disease, and the patient once again acts as a source of infection for any lice that may be present.

Endemic typhus

Endemic typhus is caused by *Rickettsia typhi* and is transmitted to humans by the rat flea. The disease is similar to epidemic typhus, but is less severe.

Scrub typhus

Scrub typhus is caused by *Orientia tsutsugamushi* and is transmitted to humans by trombiculid mites (chiggers). It occurs only in the Far East; cases were seen in American soldiers in Vietnam. The rickettsiae are maintained in the mites by transovarial transfer and are transmitted to humans or rodents during feeding. There is an eschar, and a macular rash appears after about 5 days of illness.

BORRELIA INFECTIONS

Relapsing fever

The epidemic form of relapsing fever is caused by Borrelia recurrentis, *which is transmitted by human body lice*

Borrelia recurrentis is a Gram-negative spirochete consisting of an irregular spiral, 10–30 µm long, and is highly flexible, moving by rotation and twisting.

Epidemics of relapsing fever *(Fig. 27.7)* are due to transmission of infection by the human body louse. Bacteria multiply in the louse, and when louse bites are rubbed the lice are crushed and the bacteria are introduced into the bite wound. Lice are essential for person-to-person transmission of louse-borne relapsing fever. As with other louse-borne infections (e.g. typhus), spread of the disease in humans is favored when people rarely wash and when clothes are not changed (e.g. in wars, natural disasters). The last great epidemic in North Africa and Europe during the Second World War caused fifty thousand deaths.

The endemic form of relapsing fever in humans is transmitted by tick bites

Infection with other species of *Borrelia* is endemic in rodents in many parts of the world, including western USA, and

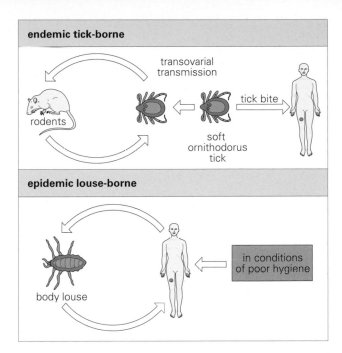

Fig. 27.7 Transmission in relapsing fever.

Borrelia is transmitted by soft ticks of the genus *Ornithodoros*. In the tick, the bacteria are transmitted transovarially from generation to generation. Also, ticks survive for up to 15 years between feeds, which helps maintain the endemic cycle of tick-borne relapsing fever.

Relapsing fever is characterized by repeated febrile episodes due to antigenic variation in the spirochetes

The bacteria multiply locally and enter the blood. After an incubation period of 3–10 days there is a sudden onset of illness with chills and fever, lasting for 3–5 days *(Fig. 27.8)*. The afebrile period lasts about a week before there is a second attack of fever, which is followed by another afebrile period. Generally there are 3–10 such episodes, of diminishing severity. More serious illness can occur if there is extensive growth of bacteria in the spleen, liver and kidneys.

Agglutinating and lytic antibodies are formed against the infecting bacteria, which are cleared from the blood. Under the 'pressure' of this immune response a new antigenic type emerges and is free to multiply and cause a fresh febrile episode.

Antigenic variation involves switching of variable proteins on the bacterial surface. The *Borrelia* have arrays of genes (Variable Large Proteins [Vlp] and Variable Small Proteins [Vsp]) that are altered and activated by gene conversion involving plasmids carrying collections of these genes. The result is that a single cloned bacterium can give rise spontaneously to approximately 30 serotypes and switching occurs at a rate of 1:1000–1:10 000 per cell generation. Similar phenomena are seen in trypanosomes. Direct person-to-person transmission does not occur. Mortality with endemic (tick-borne) relapsing fever is less than 5%, but may be up to 40% in epidemic (louse-borne) relapsing fever.

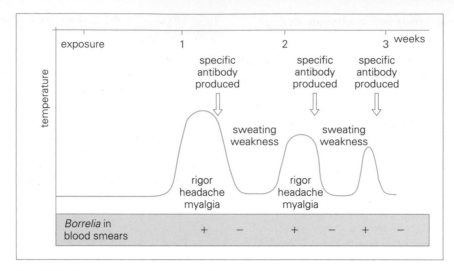

Fig. 27.8 Course of events in relapsing fever.

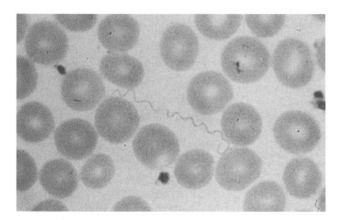

Fig. 27.9 Tightly coiled helical spirochetes of *Borrelia recurrentis* in the blood of a patient with relapsing fever. (Courtesy of TF Sellers.)

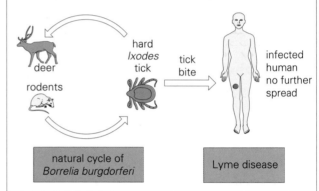

Fig. 27.10 Transmission of Lyme disease.

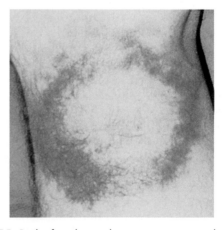

Fig. 27.11 Rash of erythema chronicum migrans on the leg in Lyme disease. (Courtesy of E Sahn.)

Relapsing fever is diagnosed in the laboratory and treated with tetracycline

The bacteria can be cultivated in the laboratory and can be seen in Giemsa-stained smears of blood taken during the febrile period *(Fig. 27.9)*. Complement fixation antibody tests are available, but are rarely useful because of the problem of antigenic variation.

Tetracycline is used in treatment and to prevent relapses. The best preventative measure is avoidance of arthropod vectors.

Lyme disease

Lyme disease is caused by Borrelia *spp. and is transmitted by* Ixodes *ticks*

Lyme disease occurs in Europe, the USA and most continents of the world, and is named after the town in Connecticut, USA where the first cases were recognized in 1975. It is caused by *Borrelia burgdorferi* (USA) or other species of *Borrelia*. The natural cycle of infection takes place in mice and deer in whom it is transmitted by hard ticks of the genus *Ixodes*

(Fig. 27.10). Human infection follows the bite of an infected tick (larval, nymph or adult form). In Europe and the USA, infection is more common in summer months when recreational exposure to infected ticks is more likely. Person-to-person transmission does not occur.

Erythema chronicum migrans is a characteristic feature of Lyme disease

The bacteria multiply locally, and after an incubation period of about 1 week fever, headache, myalgia, lymphadenopathy and a characteristic lesion at the site of the tick bite develop. The skin lesion is called 'erythema chronicum migrans' (Fig. 27.11), its name describing its main features. It begins as a macule and enlarges over the next few weeks, remaining red and flat, but with the center clearing, until it is several inches in diameter. In 50% of patients fresh transient lesions appear on the skin elsewhere in the body. Immunologic findings include circulating immune complexes and sometimes elevated serum IgM levels and cryoglobulins that contain IgM.

Lyme disease commonly causes additional disease 1 week to 2 years after the initial illness

In 75% of untreated patients, in spite of antibody and T cell responses to the *Borrelia*, there are additional later manifestations of disease. These are seen from 1 week to more than 2 years after the onset of illness. The first of these manifestations to appear are neurologic (meningitis, encephalitis, peripheral neuropathy) and cardiologic (heart block, myopericarditis). The second of these manifestations to appear are arthralgia and arthritis, which may persist for months or years. Immune complexes are found in affected joints. These late manifestations are immunologic in origin and are probably due to antigenic cross-reactivity between *Borrelia* and host tissues. The *Borrelia* themselves are rarely detectable at this stage.

Lyme disease is diagnosed serologically and treated with antibiotic

The *Borrelia* are rarely seen in skin biopsies but can sometimes be isolated from biopsies obtained at an early stage, although this may take weeks. Thus, Lyme disease is primarily diagnosed on clinical presentation and known exposure. When indicated, serologic tests such as enzyme-linked immunosorbent assay (ELISA) and indirect fluorescent antibody (IFA) are useful. Specific IgM antibodies are detected 3–6 weeks after infection, and IgG antibodies at a later stage. Antigenic cross-reactivity may result in false positive results.

Doxycycline or amoxicillin are effective in treatment of early disease. Late disease, especially with neurologic complications, may require more aggressive therapy with intravenous penicillin or ceftriaxone for several weeks.

Prevention of Lyme disease is by avoidance of tick bites.

PROTOZOAL INFECTIONS

Malaria

Malaria is initiated by the bite of an infected female anopheline mosquito

Malaria is restricted to areas where these mosquitoes can breed, i.e. the tropics between 60°N and 40°S (except areas higher than about 2000 m). It is of major importance in Africa, India, the Far East and South America. Because of drug and insecticide resistance, malaria is now on the increase globally. About 35% of the world's population is estimated to

HUMAN MALARIA PARASITES				
species	**Plasmodium falciparum**	**P. vivax**	**P. malariae**	**P. ovale**
major distribution	West, East and Central Africa, Middle East, Far East, South America	India, North and East Africa, South America, Far East	tropical Africa, India, Far East	tropical Africa
common name	malignant tertian	benign tertian	quartan	ovale tertian
duration of liver stage (incubation period)	6–14 days	12–17 days (with relapses up to 3 years)	13–40 days (with relapses up to 20 years)	9–18 days (with rare relapses)
duration of asexual blood cycle (fever cycle)	48 hours	48 hours	72 hours	50 hours
major complication	cerebral malaria anemia hypoglycemia jaundice pulmonary edema shock	–	nephrotic syndrome	–

Fig. 27.12 Human malaria parasites. The most important and life-threatening complications occur with *Plasmodium falciparum*, hence its old name 'malignant tertian malaria'.

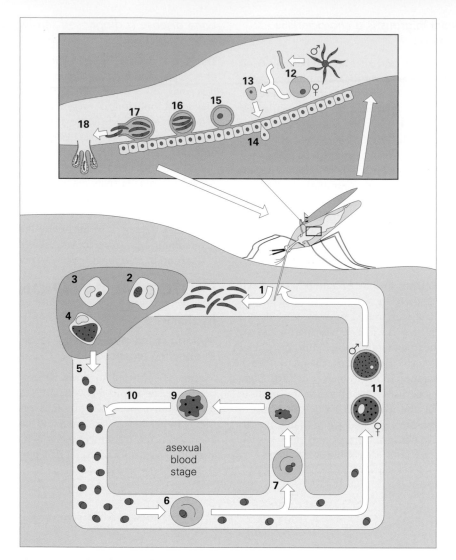

Fig. 27.13 The lifecycle of malaria in man and mosquito. In the symptomless pre-erythrocytic stage, sporozoites from the saliva of an infected *Anopheles* mosquito are injected into the human bloodstream when the mosquito bites (1). They then enter the parenchymal cells of the liver (2), where they mature in approximately 2 weeks into tissue schizonts (4), finally rupturing to produce 10 000 to 40 000 merozoites (5). These circulate in the blood for a few minutes before entering the red blood cells (6) to initiate the asexual blood stage. Some parasites, however, remain within the liver to lie dormant as hypnozoites (3), which are the cause of relapses. Once in the red blood cells, the merozoites mature into the ring form (7), trophozoite (8) and schizont (9), which complete the cycle by maturing to release merozoites back into the circulation (10). This cycle may last for months or even years. Some merozoites, however, go on to initiate the sexual stage, maturing within the red blood cells to form male and female gametocytes (11), which can be taken up by the *Anopheles* mosquito on feeding. On entering the gut of the insect, the male gametocyte exflagellates (12) to form male microgametes, which fertilize the female gamete to form the zygote (13). This then invades the gut mucosa (14), where it develops into an oocyst (15). This develops to produce thousands of sporozoites (16), which are released into the gut (17), finally migrating to the salivary glands of the insect (18), whence the cycle begins again.

be infected, with some 10 million new cases annually and perhaps two million deaths. Increased air travel means new cases are regularly seen in the developed world, and unless the diagnosis is constantly borne in mind, vital treatment may be withheld, with fatal results. Malaria can also be transmitted by blood transfusion, needle accidents or, very rarely, from mother to fetus.

The lifecycle of the malaria parasite comprises three stages

Four species of *Plasmodium* cause malaria in man, of which *P. falciparum* is the most virulent *(Fig. 27.12)*. All have similar lifecycles, which are the most complex of any human infection, comprising three quite distinct stages and

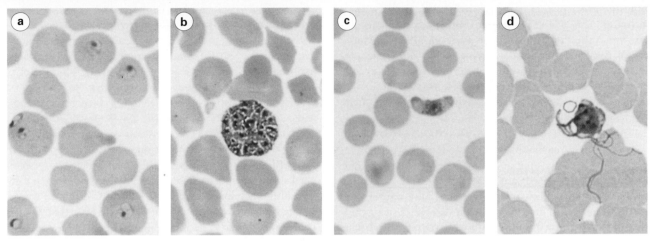

Fig. 27.14 Different stages of the malaria parasites. (a) *Plasmodium falciparum* ring forms in red blood cells. (b) *Plasmodium vivax* erythrocytic schizont. (c) *P. falciparum* female gametocyte. (d) *P. vivax* male gametocytes exflagellating to form microgametes 20–25 μm long.

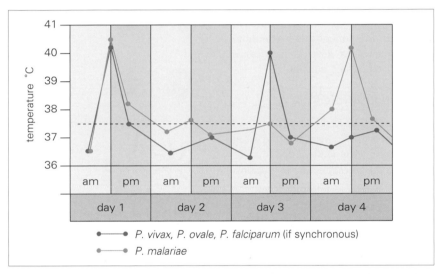

Fig. 27.15 Malaria fever charts showing cyclical fluctuations in temperature. The peaks coincide with the maturation and rupture of the intraerythrocytic schizonts, occurring every 48 hours (*Plasmodium falciparum, Plasmodium vivax* and *Plasmodium ovale*) or every 72 hours (*Plasmodium malariae*), when the cycles are synchronized.

characterized by alternating extracellular and intracellular forms (*Figures 27.13* and *27.14*).

Invasion of red cells requires at least two separate receptor –ligand interactions; the lack of one red cell surface receptor, the 'Duffy' antigen, explains the resistance to *P. vivax* of most West Africans. Other genetic traits that contribute to resistance to malaria include hemoglobin S (sickle cell), β-thalassemia, and glucose-6-phosphate dehydrogenase deficiency.

Clinical features of malaria include a fluctuating fever and drenching sweats

Symptoms range from fever to fatal cerebral or renal disease and are associated exclusively with the asexual blood stage (*Fig. 27.13*). The clinical picture depends upon the age and immune status of the patient, as well as the species of parasite. The most characteristic feature is fever, which follows rupture of erythrocytic schizonts and is mainly due to the induction of cytokines such as interleukin 1 (IL-1) and tumor necrosis factor (TNF). The synchronous cycle in red cells means that the different species of malaria give characteristic patterns of fever, with either a 48-hour (tertian: days 1 and 3) or 72-hour (quartan: days 1 and 4) periodicity (*Fig. 27.15*). A typical paroxysm starts with a feeling of intense cold with shivering, followed by a hot dry stage and finally a period of drenching sweats. Headache, muscle pains and vomiting are common. *P. falciparum* infections may cause a daily evening fever due to superimposed non-synchronous parasite cycles. In such cases diagnosis may be missed and the symptoms attributed to influenza or some other pyrexial disease. Enlargement of the spleen and liver is common and anemia almost invariable.

Complications of malaria include cerebral malaria, severe anemia, hypoglycemia, lactic acidosis and glomerulonephritis

In the absence of re-infection, *P. vivax, P. ovale* and *P. malariae* malarias are normally self-limiting infections, but relapses may occur. *P. falciparum* malaria, however, is frequently fatal during the first 2–3 weeks due to a variety of complications *(Fig. 27.12)*. Relapses may occur after months or even years, especially in *P. vivax* because of parasites that lie dormant in the liver ('hypnozoites').

Complicated *P. falciparum* malaria is most common in children aged between 6 months and 5 years, and in pregnant, particularly primigravid, women. However, it can occur at any age in the non-immune (e.g. tourists). The most dangerous complication is 'cerebral malaria', with progressive headache, neck stiffness, convulsions and coma. Possible causes include binding of parasitized red cells in cerebral capillaries, increased permeability of the blood–brain barrier, and excessive induction of cytokines such as TNF. If successfully treated, there is usually little or no impairment of cerebral function, although neurologic and psychiatric sequelae may occur in 5–10% of childhood cases.

Severe anemia is also common, due partly to red cell destruction and partly to dyserythropoiesis in the bone marrow. Of the other complications, hypoglycemia and lactic acidosis are thought to be important contributors to mortality. Immune complex glomerulonephritis is common, and there is a particular tendency to develop progressive nephrotic disease in *P. malariae* (quartan) malaria.

Malaria has an immunosuppressive effect

The strong epidemiologic correlation between malaria and endemic Burkitt's lymphoma probably reflects reduced T cell cytotoxicity against Epstein–Barr virus (EBV)-infected cells. Malaria may also interfere with the efficacy of vaccines against common viral or bacterial infections.

Immunity to malaria develops gradually and seems to need repeated boosting

Immunity to malaria develops in stages, and in endemic areas children who survive early attacks become resistant to severe disease by about 5 years. Parasite levels fall progressively until adulthood when they are low or absent most of the time. However, 1 year spent away from exposure is sufficient for most of this immunity to wane, i.e. repeated boosting is needed to maintain it. The actual mechanisms are still controversial and seem to involve both antibody and cell-mediated immunity *(Fig. 27.16)*.

Malaria is diagnosed by finding parasitized red cells in a blood film

The blood film may need to be thick; alternatively bone marrow may be used. Later (schizont) stages may be sequestered in deep tissues, so parasites may be deceptively scarce in, or even absent from, the blood. Any case of fever, especially with anemia, splenomegaly or cerebral signs, in a patient who conceivably could have malaria is therefore best treated as malaria. However, the presence of parasites in the blood of an ill patient from an endemic area does not mean malaria is the cause of the illness, since parasitemia may be asymptomatic. The demonstration of antibody by immuno-fluorescence or ELISA confirms previous exposure, and a predominance of IgM would suggest a recent attack.

stage	mechanism
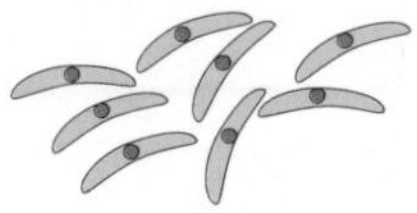 sporozoites	antibody
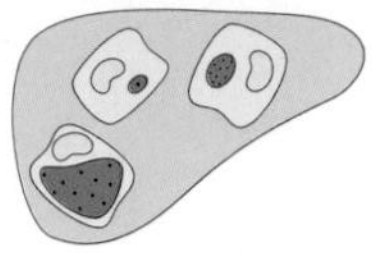 liver stage	cytotoxic T cells TNF IFN-α IL-1
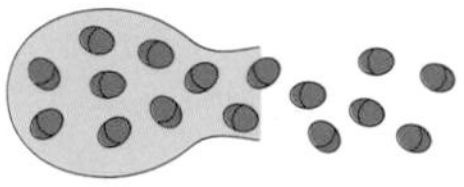 merozoites	antibody
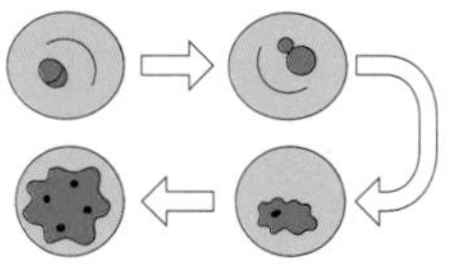 asexual erythrocyte stage	antibody ROI RNI ECP TNF
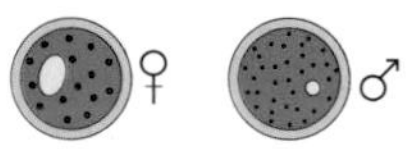 gametocytes	antibody ?cytokines
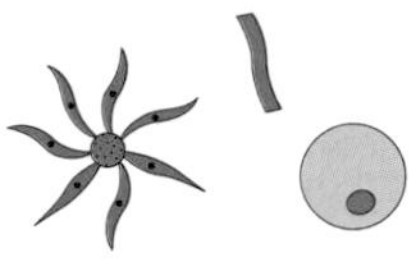 gametes	antibody

Fig. 27.16 Immunity to malaria. The principal mechanisms thought to be responsible for immunity at each stage of the cycle. (IFN, interferon; IL, interleukin; TNF, tumor necrosis factor; ROI, reactive oxygen intermediates; RNI, reactive nitrogen intermediates; ECP, eosinophil cationic proteins.)

Quinine is the drug of choice for life-threatening malaria

Quinine remains the drug of choice for life-threatening malaria. Complications of quinine treatment include massive intravascular hemolysis ('blackwater fever'). Other major drugs are chloroquine (to which *P. falciparum* is increasingly resistant) and the Chinese drug quinghaosu (artemisin), with primaquine for preventing relapses.

The most promising forms of prevention are bednets impregnated with mosquito repellents. The prospects for a malaria vaccine are discussed in Chapter 34.

Trypanosomiasis

Three species of the protozoan Trypanosoma cause human disease

Trypanosoma brucei gambiense and *T. b. rhodesiense* cause African trypanosomiasis or sleeping sickness, and *T. cruzi* causes South American trypanosomiasis or Chagas' disease. The diseases differ quite markedly in:

- the insect vector;
- the localization of the parasite;
- the effects on the immune system.

African trypanosomiasis

African trypanosomiasis is transmitted by the tsetse fly and restricted to equatorial Africa

The vector of African trypanosomiasis is the tsetse fly *Glossina*, and there is a reservoir of infection in several domestic and wild animals (cattle, pigs, deer). In humans, *T. brucei* remains extracellular, first in the tissues near the insect bite and then in the blood, where it divides rapidly and continuously.

Clinical features of African trypanosomiasis include lymphadenopathy and 'sleeping sickness'

Following an infected bite a swollen chancre develops at the site, with widespread lymph node enlargement, especially in the back of the neck (Winterbottom's sign; *Fig. 27.17a*). The parasite establishes in the blood and multiplies rapidly, with fever, splenomegaly and, often, signs of myocardial involvement. The CNS may become involved (more acutely in the East African *T. b. rhodesiense* than the West African *T. b. gambiense*), with the gradual development of headache, psychologic changes ('silent grief'), voracious appetite and weight loss, and finally coma ('sleeping sickness'; *Fig. 27.17b*) and death. Unlike malaria, cured trypanosomiasis can leave the patient with severe residual neurologic and mental disability.

T. brucei evades host defenses by varying the antigens in its glycoprotein coat

T. brucei survives freely in the blood because of its remarkable degree of antigenic variation, based on switching between some one thousand different genes for the glycoprotein coat. A high concentration of IgM is found in the blood, and later in the cerebrospinal fluid (CSF), and this is manufactured by the plasma cells (Mott cells), which are a feature of the lymphocytic infiltrate seen as 'perivascular cuffing' around blood vessels in the brain (*Fig. 27.18*).

African trypanosomiasis is diagnosed by demonstrating parasites microscopically and can be treated with a variety of drugs

T. brucei can be demonstrated in lymph nodes (by puncture) or in late cases in CSF. A raised serum IgM (up to 16-times normal concentration) supports diagnosis.

Arsenical drugs such as tryparsamide and melarsoprol have been the mainstay of treatment, especially in chronic disease, and several non-arsenicals are used in the acute stages (e.g. suramin, nitrofurazone, pentamidine). Pentamidine is the drug of choice for prophylaxis.

Control of the tsetse fly vector is difficult, though insecticides are widely used. Bed nets are ineffective as the flies feed during daylight hours.

Chagas' disease

T. cruzi is transmitted by the reduviid ('kissing') bug

T. cruzi is transmitted by non-flying reduviid ('kissing') bugs, which restricts the disease to areas of poor housing. Almost all

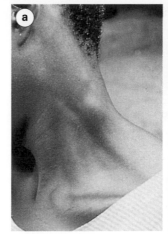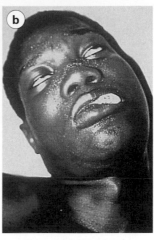

Fig. 27.17 African trypanosomiasis. (a) Enlargement of the lymph nodes in the neck (Winterbottom's sign). (Courtesy of PG Janssens.) (b) Coma (sleeping sickness) due to generalized encephalitis. (Courtesy of ME Krampitz and P de Raadt.)

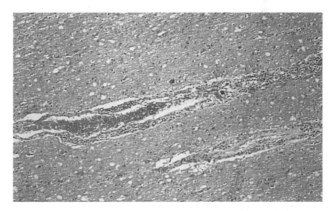

Fig. 27.18 Lymphocytic infiltration around a blood vessel in the brain in *Trypanosoma brucei* infection. (Hematoxylin and eosin stain.) (Courtesy of R Muller and JR Baker.)

species of mammal can act as reservoirs of infection. The parasite invades host cells, notably macrophages and cardiac muscle cells.

Chagas' disease has serious long-term effects, which include fatal heart disease

Chancres ('chagomas') may develop at the site of infection, with a transient febrile illness, that may rarely lead to death by heart failure. Following invasion of host cells, the disease pursues an extremely slow and chronic course. The two major symptoms, which can take years to appear, involve the heart and the intestinal tract. The major cause of death is myocarditis, with progressive weakening and dilation of the ventricles due to destruction of cardiac muscle by the parasite (*Fig. 27.19*) and probably also to autoimmune mechanisms induced by cross-reacting antigens. Dilation of the intestinal tract is due to similar processes in nerve cells, and the organs become incapable of proper peristalsis; mega-esophagus and megacolon are the two commonest manifestations.

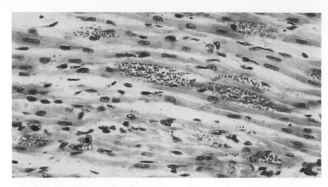

Fig. 27.19 Amastigote forms of *Trypanosoma cruzi* in cardiac muscle in Chagas' disease. (Hematoxylin and eosin stain.) (Courtesy of H Tubbs.)

Chronic Chagas' disease is usually diagnosed serologically

In the acute phase, parasites may be seen in a blood film, but the chronic disease is usually diagnosed serologically or by 'xenodiagnosis'. Clean reduviid bugs are fed on the patient and their rectal contents examined 1–2 months later, or homogenized and injected into mice, in which even a single trypanosome will produce a patent infection. In the late stages, muscle biopsy may also be diagnostic. Polymerase chain reaction (PCR) techniques are being developed.

Chagas' disease is very difficult to cure. Several drugs, including arsenicals, are effective against the blood stage (trypomastigote), but usually fail to eliminate the intracellular stage (amastigote). Prevention is ideally achieved by improved housing and living standards. Vector control by insecticides is difficult, and a vaccine, though under investigation, is in practical terms many years away.

Leishmaniasis

Leishmania *parasites are transmitted by sandflies and cause New World and Old World leishmaniasis*

Several species of *Leishmania* parasites cause disease in both the New World and the Old World; *(Fig. 27.20)*. In the latter areas especially, dogs can act as an important reservoir of infection. All are transmitted by sandflies.

Leishmania *is an intracellular parasite and inhabits macrophages*

Leishmania evades the killing mechanisms of macrophages *(Fig. 27.21)* unless they are strongly activated—for example by interferon-gamma (IFNγ). The two principal sites of parasite growth are:

- the liver and spleen (visceral leishmaniasis);
- the skin (cutaneous leishmaniasis).

Untreated visceral leishmaniasis (kala-azar) causes liver failure

Visceral leishmaniasis or 'kala-azar' usually develops slowly, with fever and weight loss, followed months or years later by hepatomegaly and, especially, splenomegaly; untreated patients will die of liver failure. Skin lesions may appear following treatment; these contain massive numbers of

LEISHMANIA SPECIES AND CLINICAL SYNDROMES		
species	distribution	disease
L. donovani L. infantum	Africa, India, Mediterranean	visceral leishmaniasis
L. chagasi	South America	
L. major L. tropica L. aethiopica	Africa, India, Mediterranean	cutaneous leishmaniasis
L. mexicana L. braziliensis L. peruviana	South and Central America	

Fig. 27.20 *Leishmania* species—their distribution and clinical syndromes.

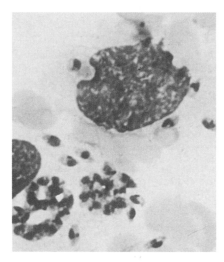

Fig. 27.21 *Leishmania* within macrophages in aspirate from a lesion of New World leishmaniasis. (Courtesy of MJ Wood.)

parasites, and the syndrome is known as 'post-kala-azar dermal leishmaniasis' (PKDL).

Cutaneous leishmaniasis is characterized by a large ulcer and immunity to reinfection

Classical cutaneous leishmaniasis also progresses insidiously, from a small papule at the site of infection to a large ulcer. This may eventually heal with considerable scarring *(Fig. 27.22)* leaving the patient relatively immune to reinfection. Old World leishmaniasil lesions are known as 'Oriental sores' (also 'Baghdad boil' and 'Delhi sore') and in the New World leishmaniasis as 'espundia' (mucocutaneous) and 'chiclero ulcer' (the ear).

Immunodeficient patients may suffer more severe leishmaniasis

In immunodeficient patients widespread chronic skin lesions can occur—diffuse cutaneous leishmaniasis—analogous to lepromatous leprosy. Visceral leishmaniasis is now a major

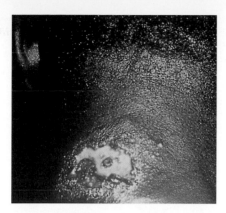

Fig. 27.22 Cutaneous lesion on the neck in *Leishmania braziliensis* infection. (Courtesy of PJ Cooper.)

complication of HIV infection not only in the tropics, but also around the Mediterranean.

Leishmaniasis is diagnosed by demonstrating the organism microscopically and is treated with antimonials

Demonstration of the organism in biopsies of marrow, spleen or skin lesions (depending upon the clinical picture) is definitive proof of leishmaniasis. A positive delayed hypersensitivity reaction to leishmanial antigens (Montenegro test) can be useful if parasites are not found.

Apart from the simple self-healing cutaneous lesion, leishmaniasis requires prolonged treatment with antimonial compounds (sodium stibogluconate, meglumine antimonate); if these fail, pentamidine or amphotericin B may be successful. Impregnated bed nets are effective against the sandfly vector, and the animal reservoir can be eliminated by dog control.

The prospects for vaccination against the cutaneous disease are quite promising.

HELMINTH INFECTIONS

Schistosomiasis

Schistosomiasis is transmitted through a snail vector

All digenetic trematodes (the flukes) must pass through a mollusc intermediate host in order to complete their larval development. However, schistosomes are the only group in which larvae penetrate directly into the final host after release from the snail.

The lifecycle of schistosomes is illustrated in *Figure 27.23*. Infected snails, which are always aquatic, release fork-tailed larvae into the surrounding water. These penetrate the host's skin, enter the dermis and pass via the blood, through the lungs to the liver, where they mature and form permanent male and female pairs before relocating to their final site:

- the veins surrounding the bladder for *Schistosoma haematobium*;
- the mesenteric veins around the small intestine for *Schistosoma japonicum* and *Schistosoma mansoni*.

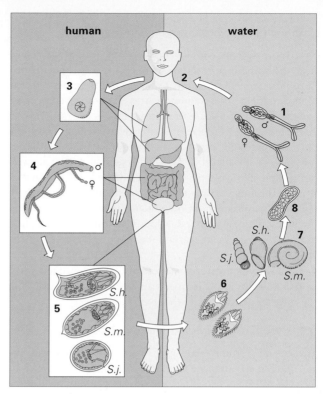

Fig. 27.23 Lifecycle of schistosomes. Free-swimming cercariae in water (1) penetrate unprotected skin. (2) During penetration they lose their tails to become schistosomulae. (3) These migrate through the bloodstream via the lungs and liver to the veins of the bladder (*Schistosoma haematobium*) or bowel (*Schistosoma mansoni, Schistosoma japonicum*), where they mature (4) to produce characteristic eggs (5) within 6–12 weeks. The eggs then penetrate the bladder or colon, to be passed in the urine or the feces (6). Eggs released into fresh water are taken up by snail intermediate hosts (7) where they mature into sporocysts (8). These release cercariae (1) into the water to complete the cycle.

The cycle is completed when eggs laid by the female worms move across the walls of the bladder or bowel and leave the body.

Clinical features of schistosomiasis result from allergic responses to the different lifecycle stages

The stages of skin penetration, migration and egg production are each associated with pathologic changes, collectively affecting many body systems. Penetration can cause a dermatitis, which becomes more severe on repeated re-infection. The developmental stages are associated with the onset of allergic symptoms (fever, eosinophilia, lymphadenopathy, spleno- and hepatomegaly, diarrhea), but the most severe pathology arises following the onset of egg laying. The body becomes hypersensitive to antigens released by the eggs as they pass through tissues to the outside world, or become trapped in other organs after being swept away in the bloodstream:

- In urinary schistosomiasis caused by *S. haematobium*, movement of eggs through the bladder wall causes hemorrhage. With time the bladder wall becomes inflamed and infiltrated, polyps develop, and malignant changes may follow; nephrosis may also occur (see Chapter 20).

- Release of the eggs of *S. japonicum* and *S. mansoni* similarly causes intestinal hemorrhage and inflammation.

A more serious consequence of these infections results from the inflammatory responses to eggs that become trapped in other organs of the body, primarily the liver, but also the lung and CNS. These consequences do not develop in all patients, but if they do, severe disease may ensue (see Chapter 22). Formation of granulomas by delayed hypersensitivity reactions around eggs in the presinusoidal capillaries interferes with blood flow and, together with extensive portal fibrosis (Symmer's pipestem fibrosis), leads to portal hypertension. As a consequence there is hepatosplenomegaly, collateral connections form between the hepatic vessels, and fragile esophageal varices develop. The collateral circulation can lead to eggs being washed into the capillary bed of the lungs.

Intense inflammatory reactions are also provoked when worms killed by anthelmintic treatment are carried back from the mesenteric vessels into the liver.

Schistosomiasis is treated with praziquantel

Treatment of individuals with praziquantel removes the worms, but in advanced cases the pathology is irreversible. Vaccine research is making progress, but a vaccine may be more useful in reducing pathology than preventing infection

Control of infection at a population level is achieved by breaking the transmission cycle, through avoidance of infected water and improvement in sanitation.

Filariasis

Filarial nematodes depend upon blood-feeding arthropod vectors for transmission

The filarial nematodes parasitize the deeper tissues of the body (see Chapter 6). The most important species can be divided into those located in the lymphatics (*Brugia, Wuchereria*) and those in subcutaneous tissues (*Onchocerca*). A number of less harmful species also occur. In all species, the female worms release live microfilaria larvae, which are picked up by the vector from the blood (lymphatic species) or skin (*Onchocerca*). Both groups can cause severe inflammatory responses, reflected in a variety of pathologic responses in the skin and lymph nodes, but each is associated with additional and characteristic pathology. Descriptions of the diseases caused by *Onchocerca* are given in Chapters 25 and 28).

Lymphatic filariasis caused by Brugia and Wuchereria is transmitted by mosquitoes

The mosquitoes introduce the infective larvae into the skin as they feed. These larvae develop slowly into long thin adult worms (females 80–100 mm × 0.25 mm), found in the lymph nodes and lymphatics of the limbs (usually lower) and groin. Infections become patent after about a year, when sheathed microfilariae appear in the blood. Infected individuals may show few clinical signs or have acute manifestations such as fever, rashes, eosinophilia, lymphangitis, lymphadenitis (Fig. 27.24) and orchitis. Later chronic obstructive changes, caused by repeated episodes of lymphangitis, may block lymphatics, leading to hydrocele and to the gross enlargement

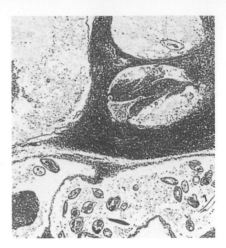

Fig. 27.24 Lymph node containing adult *Wuchereria*, showing dilated lymphatics and tissue reaction in the vessel walls. (Courtesy of R Muller and JR Baker.)

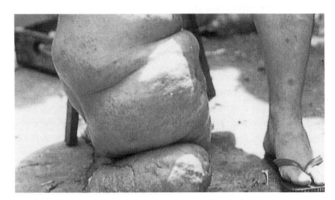

Fig. 27.25 Elephantiasis of the leg, caused by *Brugia malayi*. (Courtesy of AE Bianco.)

of breasts, scrotum and limbs, the latter condition being known as 'elephantiasis' (Fig. 27.25). Recent evidence suggest that some of the inflammatory responses to infection are triggered by symbiotic *Wohlbachia* bacteria that live within the nematodes.

A feature of filarial infections in endemic regions is that not everyone exposed develops symptomatic infections. Many, although microfilaremic, remain asymptomatic, and relatively few show gross pathology (Fig. 27.26). Some individuals develop pulmonary symptoms known as 'tropical pulmonary eosinophilia' (see Chapter 19).

Few drugs are really satisfactory for treating filariasis

Diethylcarbamazine, which primarily kills microfilariae, has long been used, but can result in a violent allergic response (Mazzotti reaction). Suramin kills adult worms, but is toxic. Ivermectin is effective against onchocerciasis and may be useful for lymphatic filariasis as well. Albendazole is currently used as part of a WHO campaign to eliminate the disease. Antibiotics, which kill the *Wohlbachia* symbionts, also are effective against the worms

It is difficult to prevent transmission of filariasis, although this can be minimized by vector control and prevention of biting.

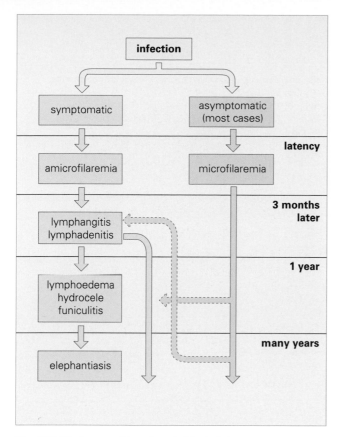

Fig. 27.26 Course of lymphocytic filariasis in symptomatic cases. (Redrawn from Muller and Baker, 1990.)

KEY FACTS

- Many important infections (arboviruses, rickettsiae, *Borrelia*, protozoa, helminths) are transmitted by vectors—insects, ticks or snails.

- Some are chronic (Lyme disease, leishmaniasis, schistosomiasis) or can be lethal (malaria, viral encephalitis).

- Often they are restricted to tropical countries because of the distribution of the vector. Global warming may alter this distribution and therefore the diseases transmitted.

- Strong immune responses are mounted, often leading to immunopathologic complications. Treatment is usually by chemotherapy.

- Vector control is difficult, but can lead to disease eradication.

- With very few exceptions (yellow fever), vaccines are not available for this group of diseases.

QUESTIONS

A 42-year-old businessman is admitted to hospital with a fever, sore throat, chills, headache, muscle aches, abdominal pain, nausea and vomiting. He returned from a 3-month trip to West Africa 2 weeks ago and has taken antimalarial prophylaxis. On examination he has a fever of 38°C, a mildly inflamed pharynx, a regular pulse rate of 100 beats/minute and a blood pressure of 110/70 mmHg. The only other features of note are splenomegaly and a tender, mildly enlarged liver.

1A. What differential diagnosis must you consider immediately?

1B. What immediate investigations would you perform?

1C. How would you manage this patient?

2. A person bitten by ticks while on vacation in the USA is at risk from:
A. West Nile encephalitis
B. Eastern equine encephalitis
C. Relapsing fever
D. Lyme disease
E. St Louis encephalitis

3. Which disease is transmitted by mosquitoes?
A. Lymphatic filariasis
B. Leishmaniasis
C. Chagas' disease
D. Epidemic typhus
E. Western equine encephalitis

4. Which of the following statements about malaria is correct?
A. Infection is transmitted by *Culex* mosquitoes
B. Once infected, immunity is lifelong
C. Infection only occurs in Africa
D. The most dangerous species is *Plasmodium vivax*
E. The parasites develop first in the liver

FURTHER READING

Cook GC, ed. *Manson's Tropical Diseases,* 20th edition. London: WB Saunders, 1996.

Fisher-Hoch S. Viral hemorrhagic fever. *Med Int* 1988; 54:2240–7.

Hoffman SL, ed. *Malaria Vaccine Development.* Washington DC: ASM Press, 1996.

Muller R, Baker JR. *Medical Parasitology.* London: Gower Medical Publishing, 1990.

Nimmanitya S. Dengue fever and dengue hemorrhagic fever. *Med Int* 1988; 54:2247–51.

Rahn DW, Evans J, eds. *Lyme Disease.* Philadelphia: American College of Physicians, 1998.

Service MW, ed. *Encyclopedia of Arthropod-Transmitted Infections of Man and Domesticated Animals.* Wallingford, Oxon: CABI Publishing, 2001.

Tsai TF. Arboviral infections in the United States. *Infect Dis Clin N Am* 1991; 5:73–102.

INTRODUCTION

Some multisystem infections in man are animal diseases (i.e. zoonoses)

In these infections, a non-human vertebrate host is the reservoir of infection and humans are involved only incidentally. The human infection follows contact with the reservoir host, but is not essential for the microbe's lifecycle or for its maintenance in nature. One striking feature of zoonotic infections, and of the arthropod-borne infections described in Chapter 27, is that few are transmitted effectively from human to human.

Sometimes, however, the zoonotic origin of these infections is less clear. For example, tularemia can be acquired either by direct contact with the reservoir host or from an arthropod vector, and is included in this chapter. Plague is included because it is transmitted from infected rats via the rat flea, although it is also transmissible directly from human to human.

Other zoonoses are dealt with in their relevant chapters (e.g. toxoplasmosis in Chapter 23, rabies in Chapter 24, salmonellosis in Chapter 22, psittacosis in Chapter 19).

ARENAVIRUS INFECTIONS

Arenaviruses are transmitted to humans in rodent excreta

Many zoonoses are caused by enveloped single-stranded RNA viruses called arenaviruses. On electron microscopy (Fig. 28.1) these pleomorphic virus particles can be seen to contain sand-like granules, giving rise to the name 'arena' (Latin: *arena*, sand). Arenaviruses are parasites of various species of rodent in which they cause a harmless lifelong infection with continuous excretion of virus in urine and feces of apparently healthy infected animals. Humans infected from this source may develop severe and often lethal disease. The arenaviruses and the diseases they cause are included in *Figure 28.2*. As with most zoonoses, infection is not transmitted, or is transmitted with low efficiency, from human to human. However, doctors and nurses have been infected by direct contact with blood or secretions from patients infected

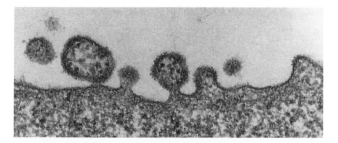

Fig. 28.1 Electron micrograph of lymphocytic choriomeningitis virus budding from the surface of an infected cell. The sand-like granules in the virus particles are characteristic of arenaviruses. (Courtesy of K Mannweiler and F Lehmann–Grübe.)

with Lassa fever virus. The usual incubation period is 5–10 days.

Arenavirus infection is diagnosed by serology, virus isolation or viral genome detection

Diagnosis by testing for specific antibodies or viral genome, or by isolating viruses, can be carried out in special centers.

Prevention of infection by reducing exposure to the virus concerned was dramatically illustrated when rodent trapping terminated outbreaks of Bolivian hemorrhagic fever (see panel). Treatment with the antiviral agent ribavirin has been successful if used early in Lassa fever.

Lymphocytic choriomeningitis virus occurs worldwide

Lymphocytic choriomeningitis (LCM) has caused sporadic infection in people living in mouse-infested dwellings, and once or twice in children possessing apparently normal, but infected hamsters. There is generally a non-specific febrile illness, but occasionally an aseptic lymphocytic meningitis occurs, with recovery.

Lassa fever virus is an arenavirus that infects a bush rat in parts of west Africa

Human exposure to infected rats, *Mastomys natalensis*, or their urine results in a febrile disease, which is generally not very severe. There are about 300 000 cases with 5000 deaths/year, and Lassa fever is the commonest febrile illness in hospitals in parts of Sierra Leone. Transfer of virus from hospital patient to healthcare worker via blood or tissue fluids often gives rise to a more severe illness with high mortality. This involves hemorrhage, capillary damage, hemoconcentration and collapse, and was seen when the disease was first recognized in Americans in the village of Lassa in 1969. However, person-

VIRAL FEVERS AND HEMORRHAGIC DISEASES ACQUIRED FROM VERTEBRATES OR FROM UNKNOWN SOURCES					
virus	virus group	disease	animal of origin	lethality	geographic distribution
lymphocytic choriomeningitis (LCM)	arenavirus	LCM	mouse, hamster	–	worldwide
Lassa fever	arenavirus	Lassa fever	African bush rat (*Mastomys natalensis*)	+	West Africa
Machupo	arenavirus	Bolivian hemorrhagic fever	bush mouse (*Calomys callosus*)	+	NE Bolivia
Junin	arenavirus	Argentinian hemorrhagic fever	*Calomys* spp., mice	+	Argentina
Hantaan	bunyavirus	hemorrhagic fever fever with renal syndrome (Korean hemorrhagic fever) severe pulmonary syndrome	mice, rats	+	Far East, Scandinavia, E Europe SW USA
Marburg	filovirus	Marburg disease	unknown	++	Africa (lab. infections in Marburg, Germany)
Ebola	filovirus	Ebola disease	unknown	++	Africa (Sudan, Zaire)

Fig. 28.2 Viral fevers and hemorrhagic diseases acquired from vertebrates or from unknown sources.

to-person transmission via droplet spread is thought to be rare.

Outbreaks have been reported in Central Africa, Liberia, Nigeria and Sierra Leone. A recent outbreak in Sierra Leone, from January 1996 to April 1997, involved 823 cases with a mortality rate of 19%. The incubation period of 6–21 days would allow an infected individual to carry the disease anywhere in the world. Therefore, Lassa fever must be considered in travelers from these endemic areas with fevers of unknown origin.

KOREAN HEMORRHAGIC FEVER

The Hantaan virus causes Korean hemorrhagic fever and infects rodents

The Hantaan virus is a bunyavirus that causes a harmless persistent infection in various species of mice and rats. After exposure to the urine of infected animals there is a febrile illness, often with hypotension, hemorrhage and a renal syndrome. Many American soldiers suffered severe infections in Korea, and a milder disease is seen in eastern Europe and Scandinavia. Related viruses are present in mice and rats in the USA, and outbreaks in southwestern USA caused 26 deaths with severe pulmonary disease. Laboratory diagnosis is by the detection of specific IgM or IgG antibody.

MARBURG AND EBOLA HEMORRHAGIC FEVERS

The source of Marburg and Ebola hemorrhagic fevers is unknown

Marburg and Ebola hemorrhagic fevers occur in central and east Africa and are caused by filoviruses, long filamentous single-stranded RNA viruses. Patients develop fever, hemorrhage, rash, and disseminated intravascular coagulation (see Chapter 17). There is no specific treatment and no vaccine, and the reservoir of origin and natural cycle of maintenance for both viruses is unknown.

Infection with Marburg virus was first recognized in 1967 in Marburg, Germany, after exposure of laboratory workers to infected African green monkeys from Uganda. However, these monkeys are not the natural hosts, and the ultimate source of the infection is still unknown. Mortality was about 20% and, as with Ebola virus infection, it was noted that the virus could be detected in semen for months after clinical recovery; one patient transmitted the infection to his wife by this route. Altogether, 31 infections have been recorded, 8 of which were fatal.

Outbreaks of a similar disease occurred in 1976 in southern Sudan and in the region of the Ebola river in Zaire (now Democratic Republic of the Congo). Overall, there were

LESSONS IN MICROBIOLOGY

Bolivian hemorrhagic fever: a lesson in ecology

In 1962 there was an outbreak of a severe and often lethal infectious disease in the small town of San Joachim, Bolivia. Patients developed fever, myalgia and an enanthem, followed by capillary leakage, hemorrhage, shock and a neurologic illness. This disease was termed 'Bolivian hemorrhagic fever' and had a mortality rate of 15%. Extensive investigations failed to incriminate an arthropod vector, but the evidence pointed to a role for mice in the epidemic. Acting on this possibility, hundreds of mouse traps were airlifted to the beleagured town, and it was soon shown that trapping mice had a dramatic effect on the incidence of the disease. The epidemic was completely halted. Quite separately, a virus was isolated from the tissues of a trapped local bush mouse *(Calomys callosus)*. The virus was shown to cause a harmless lifelong infection in this animal, with continued excretion of virus in urine and feces. The virus (given the name 'Machupo') was an arenavirus, a group that includes lymphocytic choriomeningitis (LCM) virus (infecting mice and hamsters) and Lassa fever virus (infecting an African bush rat). These viruses cause a harmless persistent infection in the natural rodent host, but an often severe disease in humans exposed to infected animals.

This outbreak of Bolivian hemorrhagic fever provided an important lesson in ecology. Because of the high incidence of malaria in the San Joachim area, extensive dichlorodiphenyltrichloroethane (DDT) spraying had been carried out to control mosquitoes. As a result, geckos (small lizards that eat insects) accumulated DDT in their tissues and the local cats that preyed on geckos began to die with lethal concentrations of DDT in their livers. The shortage of cats, in turn, allowed the bush mice to invade human

dwellings. The close vicinity of infected mice to humans and human food led to the epidemic *(Fig. 28.3)*.

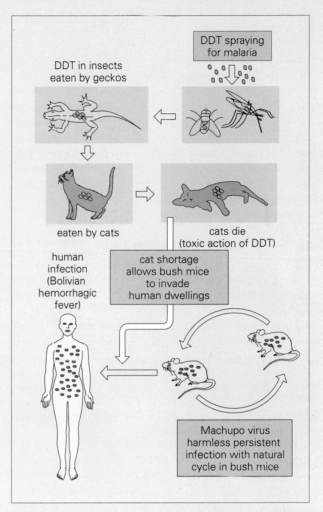

Fig. 28.3 Bolivian hemorrhagic fever—a lesson in ecology. (DDT, dichlorodiphenyltrichloroethane.)

602 cases and 397 deaths. Person-to-person transmission took place in local hospitals via contaminated syringes and needles. In 1989 monkeys infected with a similar virus were inadvertently imported into the USA from the Philippines. A number of the monkeys died but, although at least four people were infected, none developed disease.

A large epidemic was seen in Kikwit, Zaire in 1995 with 315 cases and 244 deaths. Outbreaks occurred in Gabon in February and July 1996 and northern Uganda in 2000. Excluding the most recent outbreak, approximately 1500 cases with over 1000 deaths have been reported.

Q FEVER

Coxiella burnetii *is the rickettsial cause of Q fever*

The disease Q fever was first recognized in Australia in 1935, but the cause was unknown for several years—hence Q (query) fever. The causative rickettsia, *Coxiella burnetii*, differs from other rickettsiae (see Chapter 27) in the following ways:

- It is not transmitted to humans by arthropods.
- It is relatively resistant to desiccation, heat and sunlight, and is therefore stable enough to be acquired from infected material by inhalation.

- Its main site of action is the lung rather than vascular endothelium elsewhere in the body, so that there is usually no rash.

C. burnetii *is transmitted to man by inhalation*

C. burnetii can infect many species of wild and domestic animals. In many countries (e.g. USA) infection of livestock is quite common, but there are few human cases (less than 50/year reported in the USA). People who come into contact with infected animals, especially their placentas (e.g. veterinarians, farmers, abattoir workers) are at risk from aerosolized organisms. Unpasteurized milk and tissue fluids from infected stock can also transmit the disease.

After inhalation, the microbe multiplies in the terminal airways of the lung, and about 3 weeks later the patient develops fever, severe headache, and often respiratory symptoms and an atypical pneumonia. The rickettsia can also spread to the liver, commonly causing hepatitis. Recovery is usually complete in 2 weeks, but the disease can become chronic. The heart is then sometimes involved (endocarditis), with thrombocytopenia and purpura in some patients, and this condition is fatal if untreated.

Q fever is diagnosed serologically and treated with antibiotics

A four-fold or greater rise in complement-fixing antibody titer is significant. There are two antigenic forms of the rickettsial lipopolysaccharide (LPS): phase 1 and phase 2. Antibody to phase 2 is seen in acute Q fever, and to both phase 1 and phase 2 in chronic disease. The Weil–Felix test (see Chapter 27) is not used.

Acute infection is treated with oral tetracyclines, chronic infections may require drug combinations such as rifampin and doxycycline or trimethoprim–sulfamethoxazole. A killed vaccine is available for those at risk. The rickettsiae are destroyed when milk is pasteurized.

ANTHRAX

Anthrax is caused by Bacillus anthracis *and is primarily a disease of herbivores*

Bacillus anthracis is a large Gram-positive rod and is aerobic and non-motile. Most members of the genus *Bacillus* are harmless saprophytes, present in soil, water, air and vegetation. *Bacillus cereus* is a cause of food poisoning, but *B. anthracis* is the principal pathogen and is unique in having an antiphagocytic capsule made of D-glutamic acid. It forms spores, which survive for years in soil.

Anthrax is a disease of herbivores such as sheep, goats, cattle and horses, and bacilli are excreted in feces, urine and saliva. Humans are relatively resistant. The disease is largely confined to developing countries (parts of Asia, Africa, Middle East), human infection occurring following direct contact with infected animals, or by contact with spores present in animal products. The spores can enter the body via the skin and mucous membranes or, less commonly, via the respiratory tract. In developed countries, where animal infection is now uncommon, human infection is rare and has been due to exposure to contaminated imported goods such as hides,

skin, wool, goat hair and bristles, bones and bone-meal in fertilizers. Spores have also been used in bioterrorism.

Anthrax is characterized by a black eschar, and the disease can be fatal if untreated

B. anthracis spores germinate in tissues at the site of entry. The bacteria then multiply and produce the anthrax toxin, which consists of a protective antigen, an edema factor (an adenylate cyclase) and a lethal factor; all are plasmid-coded. Toxic activity requires the protective antigen and at least one of the other two. Host defenses are inhibited by the antiphagocytic capsule surrounding the bacillus (see Chapter 14).

The skin is the usual site of entry. As the toxic material accumulates, there is edema and congestion, and a papule develops within 12–36 hours. The papule ulcerates, the center becoming black and necrotic to form an eschar or 'malignant pustule' (although there is no pus) which is painless and is often surrounded by a ring of vesicles *(Fig. 28.4)*. The bacilli spread to the lymphatics and in about 10% of cases reach the blood to cause septicemia. Continued multiplication and production of the toxin causes generalized toxic effects, edema and death.

When the spores are inhaled and enter alveolar macrophages, bacterial growth in the lung leads to pulmonary edema and mediastinal hemorrhage, with spread to the blood and death. Pulmonary anthrax is now very rare in most developed countries, where it was referred to as 'woolsorter's disease'.

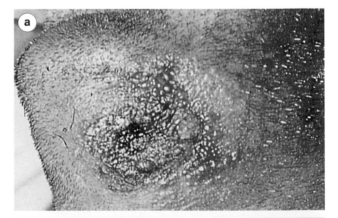

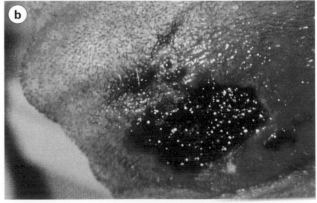

Fig. 28.4 Anthrax. (a) Characteristic black eschar surrounded by a ring of vesiculation. (b) Eight days later, the eschar has enlarged to cover the previously vesicular area, and the surrounding edema has diminished. (Courtesy of FJ Nye.)

Anthrax is diagnosed by culture and treated with penicillin

Films from skin lesions show Gram-positive bacilli, but the diagnosis is confirmed and the organism distinguished from non-pathogenic bacilli by culture on blood agar. Antibodies to toxin antigens indicate presence of the bacillus.

Anthrax is successfully treated by penicillin, given early and in large doses. Erythromycin or chloramphenicol can be given where there is penicillin allergy. Cutaneous anthrax is fatal in 10–20% of cases when untreated.

Anthrax can be prevented and is now mainly a disease of developing countries

Animals can be protected by vaccination with live avirulent bacteria. Infected animals are isolated, killed and buried or cremated without autopsy. A vaccine consisting of purified protective antigen is available for humans at high risk. Human infection is reduced by rigidly controlled disinfection of imported animal products such as hides, hair and wool.

PLAGUE

The plague is caused by Yersinia pestis, which infects rodents and is spread to man by fleas

Yersina pestis is a small Gram-negative rod with a surrounding antiphagocytic capsule that is associated with virulence. The sylvatic reservoirs are rodents such as rats, squirrels, gerbils and field mice, in which the infection is generally mild, the bacteria being spread between animals and to humans by fleas *(Fig. 28.5)*. Infections in urban rats have been the most important sources of plague in humans, and the disease has at times decimated populations and influenced the course of history. In the 14th century about 25% of the population of Europe died in plague epidemics (see panel). Early in the 20th century the disease arrived in North America and is at present endemic in wild rodents in western USA. Plague is now extremely rare in Europe and uncommon in the USA.

The rat flea (*Xeopsylla cheopsis*) carries infection from rat to rat and from rat to human. *Y. pestis* causes blood to clot in the gut of the flea, multiplies profusely in the clot and eventually blocks the lumen, so that the flea regurgitates infected material as it attempts to feed. As infected rats sicken, their fleas leave and may bite humans thus transmitting 'bubonic' plague. This disease is not generally transmitted from person to person. However, when there is extensive replication of bacteria in the lung, with bronchopneumonia and large numbers of bacteria in the sputum, the infection can spread from person to person by droplets, causing 'pneumonic' plague, with extremely rapid onset.

Rodent infection is endemic in India, southeast Asia, South Africa, South America, Mexico and the western states of the USA. Sporadic plague continues to occur in these parts of the

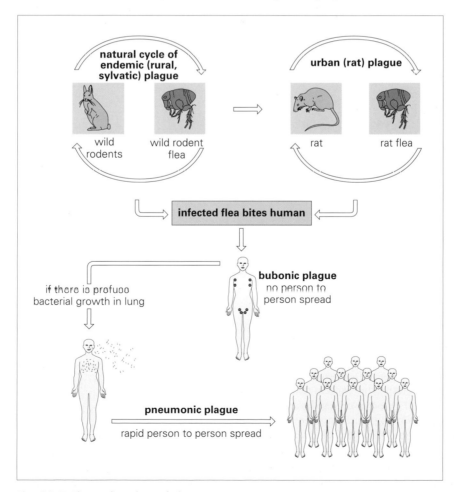

Fig. 28.5 The epidemiology of plague.

The Black Death in 14th century England

For thousands of years, *Yersinia pestis* has been endemic in rodents in the Far East, with occasional epidemic spread into Europe and elsewhere. In January 1348, three galleys laden with spices from the East brought the plague to the port of Genoa, Italy. The disease, for reasons that are not clear, became known as 'The Black Death' and soon spread to the rest of Europe, arriving in London in December 1348. To the medieval mind, the speed and violence with which the illness passed from person to person (in the pneumonic form in the winter) was its most terrifying feature. The bubonic form was also important, especially in the warmer summer months, there being at least one family of black rats per household and three fleas to a rat.

The disease was attributed to earthquakes, to the movement of the planets, to a Jewish or Arab plot (350 massacres of Jews took place during the Black Death in Europe), and most commonly to God's punishment for human wickedness. You could become infected without touching a plague victim, and to many it seemed that there was something—a miasma or a poison—in the air. Physicians wore strange masks, and infected houses were labeled and boarded up, together with the inhabitants. But it was impossible to isolate all those who were sick. Rich and poor perished.

The population of England was about four million, and over a period of 2.5 years, approximately 35% (more than a million) died. The clergy, for unknown reasons, suffered an even greater mortality of nearly 50%. Altogether in Europe at least 25 million people

died. The Black Death was a major human disaster, with lasting effects on economic and social structure. There were a further five, less severe, outbreaks in England in the 14th century. The epidemic in 1665, the year before the Great Fire of London, was graphically described by Daniel Defoe (who was only 5 at the time) in his *Journal of a Plague Year in London*. The last pandemic arose in China and reached Hong Kong in 1894, where Yersin and (independently) Kitasato described the causative bacillus.

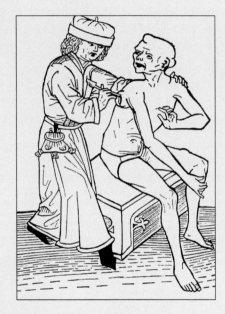

Fig. 28.6 Fifteenth century German woodcut showing incision of a bubo. (Courtesy of the World Health Organization.)

world, for instance in hunters exposed to infected prairie dogs in the USA and in rural populations elsewhere.

Clinical features of plague include buboes, pneumonia and a high death rate

The infecting bacteria multiply at the site of entry in the skin, and spread via the lymphatics to local and regional lymph nodes. They produce a number of virulence factors, including an antiphagocytic capsular antigen (fraction 1, coded by a plasmid), endotoxin and various other protein toxins. Lymph nodes in the armpit or groin become very tender and enlarge to form 'buboes' with hemorrhagic inflammation 2–6 days after the flea bite. The patient develops fever. In mild forms the infection is arrested at this stage, but spread to the blood often occurs, with septicemia, hemorrhagic illness and multisystem involvement (spleen, liver, lungs, CNS).

Common complications are disseminated intravascular coagulation, pneumonia and meningitis. The death rate is about 50% in untreated bubonic plague, and nearly 100% in pneumonic plague. On recovery there is solid immunity, and bacteria are eliminated from the body.

Plague is diagnosed microscopically and treated with antibiotic

Organisms can be recovered in fluid aspirated from lymph nodes, or from sputum in pneumonic plague and stained with Giemsa, Gram or fluorescent antibody (the staining is bipolar); they can also be cultivated.

Streptomycin and/or tetracycline are used to treat plague.

Plague has been prevented by the following measures:

- classically, by quarantine measures in ports and on ships;
- by rodent control, especially of rats at the site of entry of ships and aircraft into plague-free countries;

- by strict isolation of patients with plague;
- by chemoprophylaxis (tetracycline) during an epidemic or visit to an affected area;
- by vaccination of military personnel and of certain workers in endemic areas.

The vaccine consists of formalin-killed bacteria and gives partial protection.

YERSINIA ENTEROCOLITICA INFECTION

Yersinia enterocolitica is a cause of diarrheal disease (see Chapter 22) and is mentioned here because it has a reservoir in rodents, rabbits, pigs and other livestock.

TULAREMIA

Tularemia is caused by Francisella tularensis *and is spread by arthropods from infected animals*

Tularemia is caused by the small Gram-negative rod *Francisella tularensis*, first isolated from rodents in Tulare County, California in 1912 and later shown by Edward Francis to cause human disease. It is present in rodents and in a wide variety of other wild animals in many countries in the northern hemisphere, including the USA (especially Arkansas and Missouri), Russia, Scandinavia and Spain, and can occur in contaminated water. The variety found in North America causes a more severe disease than that found in Europe and Asia. In the infected animal it causes a plague-like disease and is spread via ticks, mites, lice and biting flies. In *Dermacentor* ticks, the bacteria are transmitted vertically by infected female ticks to her offspring via the ovum. Human infection is sporadic, the normal means of infection being contact with the carcass of an infected animal (e.g. skinning of hares, rabbits, muskrats) or the bite of an arthropod vector. There is no spread from person to person.

Clinical features of tularemia include painful swollen lymph nodes

F. tularensis parasitizes the reticuloendothelial system and lives intracellularly in macrophages, inhibiting phagosome–lysosome fusion. It spreads at the site of entry, aided by an antiphagocytic capsule, and after 3–5 days forms a skin ulcer. There is a febrile illness, and lymphatic spread results in swollen painful regional lymph nodes. Blood invasion and involvement of lungs, gastrointestinal tract and liver is not uncommon, with the formation of granulomatous nodules around infected reticuloendothelial cells. There may be a rash. Mortality in untreated patients is 5–15%. The conjunctiva or oral mucosa can be infected via contaminated fingers, resulting in ocular or oral manifestations. Infection by inhalation is less common and gives a febrile illness with respiratory symptoms.

Tularemia is diagnosed serologically and treated with streptomycin

Infected tissues can be examined by fluorescent antibody staining, but isolation of bacteria is not often attempted, because of the high risk of laboratory infection. Antibody tests are more commonly used in diagnosis.

Streptomycin is an effective treatment, and a live attenuated bacterial vaccine is available for people with an occupational risk (e.g. fur trappers). Handling animals with gloves, particularly when skinning or eviscerating, gives protection, and contact with ticks should be avoided.

PASTEURELLA MULTOCIDA INFECTION

Pasteurella multocida *is part of the normal flora of cats and dogs and is transmitted to man by an animal bite*

Pasteurella multocida is an encapsulated Gram-negative rod and is distributed worldwide. A number of capsular types exist. It is part of the normal oral flora in cats, dogs and other domestic and wild animals, in which it can also cause pneumonia and septicemia. It is transmitted to humans by animal bites (especially cat bites) or scratches.

P. multocida *infection causes cellulitis, is diagnosed by microscopy and treated with penicillin*

Local multiplication of bacteria leads within a day or two to cellulitis and lymphadenitis; other types of bacteria including anaerobes are often present in the lesion. Infection can become systemic in patients with compromised immune systems. Virulence factors include endotoxin and the capsule.

P. multocida can be cultivated and identified in material from the wound.

Penicillin is an effective treatment, and ampicillin has been used in prophylaxis after cat or dog bites. Bite wounds should be cleansed and debrided.

LEPTOSPIROSIS

Leptospirosis is caused by the spirochete Leptospira interrogans, *which infects mammals such as rats*

Leptospira are tightly coiled spirochetes 5–15 μm long. They show active rotational movement and have two flagella, originating at each end but located within the cell as in *Borrelia*. Their delicate outline is best seen by dark field microscopy because they are not very well stained by dyes. There are two well-defined species, each with several serotypes, but others may exist. *Leptospira biflexa* is free-living, *L. interrogans* is pathogenic. The ends of *L. interrogans* are bent into a question-mark shape, hence the specific name. This species infects many domestic and wild mammals in various parts of the world *(Fig. 28.7)*, dogs and rats being important sources of infection. Infected animals develop a chronic kidney infection with excretion of large numbers of bacteria in urine. The spirochetes are soon killed on drying, heating and exposure to detergents or disinfectants, but they remain viable for several weeks in stagnant alkaline water or wet soil. Humans are infected by ingestion of, or exposure to, contaminated water or food. The bacteria, aided by their motility, enter through breaks in skin or mucosae, so infection can be acquired by swimming, working or playing in contaminated water.

LEPTOSPIRA INTERROGANS DISEASES			
leptospiral serogroup	animal host	distribution	clinical features
canicola	dog	worldwide	influenza-like illness ('canicola fever', '7-days fever') is the commonest; can progress to aseptic meningitis, liver and kidney damage (Weil's disease)
icterohaemorrhagiae	rat	worldwide	
hebdomadis	mice voles rats cattle	Japan, Europe	

Fig. 28.7 Diseases caused by the three main serogroups of *Leptospira interrogans*. There are 19 different serogroups of this organism, other serogroups including seroja (pigs) and pomona (swine and cattle in USA and Europe). Among the serogroups there are 172 different serotypes.

Therefore, miners, farmers, sewage workers, and watersports enthusiasts are especially at risk. There are about 60 cases/year in England and Wales, and about 100/year are reported in the USA. Bacteria are excreted in human urine, but person-to-person transmission is rare. Immunity is serotype specific.

Clinical features of leptospirosis include kidney and liver failure

The bacteria reach the blood and, after an incubation period of 1–2 weeks, cause a febrile, influenza-like illness. In about 90% of cases this resolves uneventfully, but multiplication can cause:

- hepatitis, jaundice and hemorrhage in the liver;
- uremia and bacteriuria in the kidney;
- aseptic meningitis and conjunctival or scleral hemorrhage in the cerebrospinal fluid (CSF) and the aqueous humor (*Fig. 28.8*).

The main clinical signs result from damage to the endothelia of blood vessels, the clinical picture depending to some extent upon the particular type of leptospire involved. Weil's disease, the severe form with hemorrhagic complications and kidney and liver failure, occurs in only 5–10% of patients with leptospirosis.

Leptospirosis is diagnosed by microscopy and serologic tests and treated with antibiotics

There is often a history of exposure. Bacteria can be isolated from blood, CSF and urine, and a rise in agglutinating serotype-specific antibody can be demonstrated.

Penicillin and tetracyclines have been valuable in treatment when given within a day or two of the onset of illness, and doxycycline will prevent disease in those exposed to infection.

Measures for prevention include:

- rodent control;
- protective clothing;
- prophylactic penicillin after cuts and abrasions in those at risk.

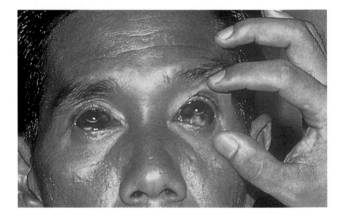

Fig. 28.8 Conjunctival hemorrhages in a jaundiced patient with leptospirosis. (Courtesy of D Lewis.)

RAT BITE FEVER

Rat bite fever is caused by bacteria transmitted to humans by a rodent bite

This uncommon but worldwide condition is caused by one of two species: *Spirillum minor* (or *minus*), a Gram-negative spiral-shaped organism (spirillar fever), or *Streptobacillus moniliformis*, a Gram-negative filamentous bacillus (streptobacillary fever). These bacteria are found in the oropharyngeal flora of 50% of healthy wild and laboratory rats and also in other rodents. Transmission to humans is by biting.

Clinical features of rat bite fever can include endocarditis and pneumonia

After an incubation period of 7–10 days there is an onset of fever, headache and myalgia. Bacteria multiply at the site of the bite, and in the case of *S. moniliformis*, cause an inflamed local lesion. Spread of infection to lymph nodes and the blood leads to lymphadenopathy, rash and arthralgia. Fever may be recurrent if untreated.

Complications include endocarditis and pneumonia, and there is a mortality of up to 10% in untreated patients.

Rat bite fever is diagnosed by microscopy or culture and is treated with antibiotics

S. moniliformis can be cultured from the wound site, lymph nodes and blood, but *Spirillum minor* cannot be cultivated and must be demonstrated in tissues by dark field microscopy.

Penicillin and streptomycin are effective treatments.

Measures for prevention include:

- rodent control;
- prevention of rat bites in laboratory workers.

BRUCELLOSIS

Brucellosis occurs worldwide and is caused by Brucella species

Brucellae are small Gram-negative non-motile coccobacilli, adapted to intracellular replication. Four 'species' cause disease in humans—*Brucella abortus*, *B. melitensis*, *B. suis*, *B. canis*—but these are probably all variants of *B. melitensis*. The first three share common A and M antigens (*B. abortus* primarily A and *B. melitensis* primarily M); *B. canis* is distinct.

Brucellae are primarily animal pathogens, infecting humans after contact with infected animals or their products (*Fig. 28.9*).

- *B. abortus* infects cows worldwide, but has been eliminated from several developed countries. It causes mild disease in humans.
- *B. melitensis* infects goats and sheep and is common in Malta and other Mediterranean countries, Mexico and South America. It causes more severe disease in humans.
- *B. suis* infects pigs in the USA (the most important cause of brucellosis), in South America and southeast Asia. It causes severe disease with destructive lesions in humans.
- *B. canis* infects dogs and is an uncommon cause of mild disease.

In cows and goats, brucellae localize in the placenta, causing contagious abortion, and also in mammary glands, from where they are shed for long periods in milk. They are present in uterine discharges, feces and urine.

Human brucellosis (undulant fever, Malta fever) occurs when the bacteria enter the body via abrasions in the skin, via the alimentary tract or, most commonly, via the respiratory tract. Infection is therefore more common in farmers, veterinarians and abbatoir workers. Unpasteurized cows' milk (UK, USA), goats' milk or cheese (Mediterranean countries) are less frequent sources of infection. There is no spread from person to person. Infection is common worldwide, but incidence is low in the developed world.

Clinical features of brucellosis are immune-mediated and include an undulant fever and chronicity

The infecting bacteria pass from the site of entry into local and regional lymph nodes, the thoracic duct and thus the blood (septicemic phase). Reticuloendothelial cells are infected (liver, spleen, bone marrow, lymphoid tissues) and here the bacteria can survive for prolonged periods. The result is an inflammatory (granulomatous) reaction with epithelioid and giant cells, central necrosis and peripheral fibrosis.

Quite commonly the infection is subclinical. The symptoms of acute brucellosis begin after an incubation period of 1–3 weeks with a gradual onset of malaise, fever, drenching sweats, aching and weakness. A rising and falling (undulant) fever is seen in a minority of patients. Enlarged lymph nodes and spleen may be detected and hepatitis can occur (*Fig. 28.10*). The bone marrow lesions may progress to osteomyelitis, and cholecystitis, endocarditis and meningitis are occasionally seen. Abortion occurs in infected cows, sows and goats, but not in humans, who lack the sugar compound erythritol, that stimulates bacterial growth in the placenta.

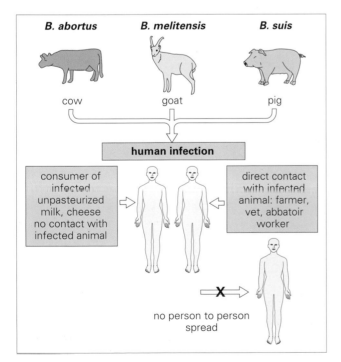

Fig. 28.9 Transmission of brucellosis. Human infection follows contact with infected animals or consumption of infected animal products.

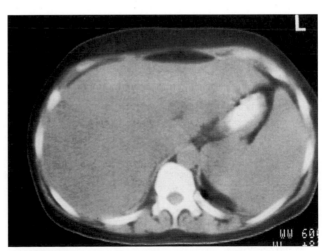

Fig. 28.10 Computerized tomographic scan showing hepatosplenomegaly in *Brucella melitensis* infection. (Courtesy of H Tubbs.)

The patient generally recovers after a few weeks or months, but a chronic stage (more than one year's illness) can develop with tiredness, aches and pains, anxiety, depression and occasional fever. Relapses and remissions may occur. Brucellae cannot be isolated at this stage, and chronic brucellosis is often a difficult diagnosis. Agglutinin titers are generally high, but antibodies are less relevant than cell-mediated immunity for this intracellular parasite.

Brucellosis is diagnosed by serologic tests and treated with antibiotics

Brucellae can be isolated in some cases from blood cultures (or from bone marrow or lymph nodes), and urine culture may be successful. This takes up to 4 weeks. IgM antibodies are present in acute brucellosis, IgG and IgA in chronic brucellosis. A rising titer suggests a current infection.

Brucellae are susceptible to tetracycline and streptomycin; co-trimoxazole is also used. Because of the intracellular location of the bacteria, prolonged courses of treatment (3 months) are needed.

Brucellae in milk are destroyed by pasteurization. In the USA and UK, brucellosis has gradually declined (about 100 cases/year now reported in the USA) following eradication and control programs. Protective clothing and goggles may be used by those in close contact with infected animals (farmers, veterinarians, abattoir workers). There is no satisfactory vaccine available for humans. Indeed, veterinarians may develop a mild illness when accidentally infected with the live S19 animal vaccine.

HELMINTH INFECTIONS

Few helminth infections are true multisystem diseases

It is a somewhat arbitrary decision to include a particular helminth infection in a chapter on multisystem zoonotic infections. Many of the worm parasites that can be acquired from animals have stages that invade a number of the body systems. Others are primarily located in a particular organ, but cause pathologic changes that can be widespread in their effects. Conversely, although stages of certain worms may be widely distributed in the body, their pathologic effects are most commonly associated with a particular organ.

For example:

- The larvae of the pork tapeworm *Taenia solium*, which cause the disease cysticercosis, develop in a variety of tissues, including muscle. However, the most serious pathology is caused by larvae found in the CNS. Accordingly, this infection is discussed in Chapter 24.
- After infection with eggs of the dog nematode *Toxocara canis*, larvae migrate throughout the body, causing the condition known as 'visceral larval migrans'. Again, the most serious effects are associated with larvae that localize in the CNS (see Chapter 24) and the eye (see Chapter 25).

However, three helminths can be considered as genuinely multisystem in their effects. These are:

- the tapeworm *Echinococcus granulosus*;
- the nematode *Trichinella spiralis*;
- the nematode *Strongyloides stercoralis*.

Echinococcus

Echinococcus adults are tiny tapeworms in dogs, and their larvae cause hydatid cysts in humans

The adults of this species live as tiny (3–5 mm long) tapeworms in the intestine of the dog. Eggs laid by the worm are passed in feces, surviving for long periods. If swallowed (by sheep or accidentally by humans), the eggs hatch, releasing larvae which then penetrate the small intestine mucosa to enter a blood vessel. Larvae then lodge in a capillary bed, usually in the liver, but also in the body cavity, lung, brain, eye, spinal cord or long bones. They then grow slowly into large, thick-walled, fluid-filled (hydatid) cysts, the pathologic signs being largely due to the mechanical pressure exerted by the cysts (*Fig. 28.11*).

Echinococcosis (hydatid disease) is diagnosed by scans, by microscopy or serologically and treated with praziquantel and surgery

Cysts can be detected by radiography, ultrasound or CT scans. Serologic tests can assist diagnosis, but sensitivity and specificity are variable. Finding hooklets and scolices in aspirated cyst fluid provides confirmation. Although drug treatment (praziquantel) is available, surgical removal, where possible, is the most satisfactory way of dealing with the infection. Great care must be taken during removal to prevent leakage of fluid from the cysts. Not only may this trigger anaphylactic responses in sensitized individuals, but the numerous larvae

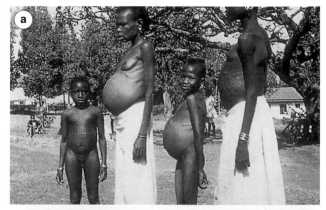

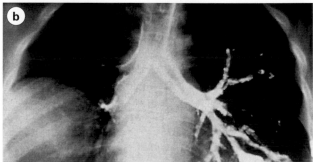

Fig. 28.11 Hydatid cysts. (a) Patients showing marked abdominal swelling caused by hydatid cysts in the liver. (Courtesy of GS Nelson.) (b) Bronchogram showing blockage of a bronchus by a cyst of *Echinococcus granulosus* in the lower left medial region. (Courtesy of RB Holliman.)

in the fluid (produced by asexual division) can cause metastatic infections in other sites.

Echinococcus multilocularis closely resembles *E. granulosus*, but results in the formation of a multilocular cyst consisting of hundreds of small vesicles, without a fibrous outer capsule. The parasite generally occurs as a fox–rodent cycle in North Europe, Siberia and parts of North America, and infections occur via contamination by fox feces. Liver involvement leads to jaundice and weight loss, and the condition is usually inoperable.

Trichinella

Trichinella spiralis *is transmitted in undercooked pork and causes the disease trichinosis*

T. spiralis is perhaps the most widely distributed of all nematode parasites, being capable of infecting almost any warm-blooded animal. Its natural cycle involves predators (e.g. bears, seals) and their prey, or scavengers and the carrion they feed on, but a domestic cycle has become established in pigs and rats.

Humans are infected by eating undercooked meat (pork or wild animal) containing the encysted infected larval stages. These larvae mature rapidly into adults in the small intestine, their invasion of the mucosa causing an acute enteritis.

The clinical features of trichinosis are mainly immunopathologic in origin

Female worms release live larvae into the mucosa, which invade the blood vessels and become distributed around the body. Bacteremia may occur at this stage. The larvae attempt to invade the cells of many organs (including the heart and CNS), although they can mature only in striated muscles, where they form the characteristic cysts *(Fig. 28.12)*. There is a wide spectrum of pathologic signs, such as fever, joint and muscle pains, eosinophilia, periorbital edema, myositis, petechial hemorrhage; encephalitis and cardiac abnormalities may also occur. These signs are mainly caused by hypersensitivity and inflammatory responses.

Trichinosis is diagnosed by microscopy and serologically and treated with anthelmintics and anti-inflammatories

Diagnosis of trichinosis is by muscle biopsy and demonstration of specific antibody by ELISA. Treatment is possible with benzimidazoles, but symptomatic treatment with anti-inflammatories may also be necessary.

Strongyloides

Strongyloides *infections are most often passed between humans, but can develop in animal hosts including dogs*

Strongyloides infection is acquired by the penetration of infective larvae through the skin. The larvae migrate to the lung, enter the alveoli, pass up the bronchi and trachea, and are then swallowed. Only females develop parthenogenetically in the host, and they lay strings of eggs into the intestinal mucosa *(Fig. 28.13)*. The eggs hatch within the intestine to release larvae that pass out with the feces and require warm

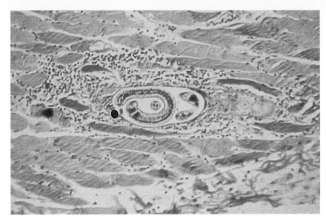

Fig. 28.12 Inflammatory reaction around a cyst containing a coiled larva of *Trichinella spiralis*. Trichrome stain. (Courtesy of IG Kagan.)

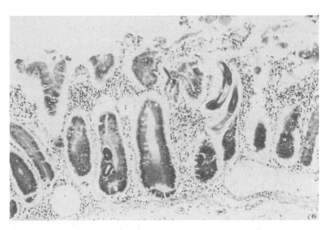

Fig. 28.13 *Strongyloides stercoralis*. Adults and larvae in the mucosa of small intestine, showing disruption of the villous surface.

moist soil to become infective. The geographic distribution of strongyloidiasis is similar to that of hookworm (tropical areas and in rural southern states of the USA).

Infections are most often passed between humans, but the two species can also develop in animal hosts including dogs (*S. stercoralis*) and African primates (*S. fulleborni*). Fecal larval stages may develop directly into the infective stage and penetrate the mucosa or perianal skin to reinfect the host—the process of autoinfection.

Strongyloides *infections are usually asymptomatic, but can cause disseminated disease in association with T cell deficiencies or malnutrition*

Autoinfection is unimportant in immunocompetent hosts, and most infected individuals are asymptomatic, though vomiting or diarrhea may occur. However, in T cell deficiencies or malnutrition, autoinfection can lead to 'hyperinfection' or 'disseminated strongyloidiasis', the larvae invading almost all organs and causing severe, and sometimes fatal, pathology. Infected patients may show vomiting, abdominal pain, diarrhea with malabsorption and dehydration, eosinophilia, pneumonitis and other 'allergic' signs. Disseminated strongyloidiasis can arise long after initial infection. It has been firmly established that infections can persist for many years (more than 30), being maintained by low-level autoinfection until the patient's immune defenses are reduced. HTLV1 antibody testing should be considered in this setting as the two infections are associated.

Strongyloides infection is diagnosed by microscopy and treated with anthelmintics

Laboratory diagnosis depends upon finding the larvae in the feces; anthelmintics such as thiabendazole or levamisole are used for treatment.

KEY FACTS

- The multisystem infections described in this chapter are zoonoses, being maintained naturally in a reservoir of non-human vertebrates.

- Humans are infected incidentally, generally from rodents (arenaviruses, hantaviruses, plague, tularemia, leptospirosis) or from domestic animals (brucellosis, hydatid disease, leptospirosis, echinococcosis, trichinosis).

- There is generally no transmission from person to person.

- The nature and the extent of human–animal contact are determining factors.

- Some of these infections are highly virulent.

- When the reservoir host is common in crowded human communities (e.g. plague), disease epidemics have been major events in history.

- When humans have less extensive contact with the reservoir host, the infection, even when virulent, has less impact (e.g. Lassa fever, Ebola fever).

- Most of these infections are now less frequent in developed countries (e.g. anthrax, brucellosis, hydatid disease), but remain as frequent causes of disease in other parts of the world.

- There are satisfactory antimicrobial agents for most of the non-viral infections, but effective vaccines are generally not available.

QUESTIONS

A 39-year-old sailor who has visited the Far East and then Africa, has felt unwell for a previous month with a fever, headaches, tiredness and sweats. While at sea he had a temperature of 38°C. He has no other symptoms of note. On examination he had a temperature of 39°C, tenderness in the left upper quadrant of the abdomen and one fingerbreadth splenomegaly. Hospital investigations showed: hemoglobin 14 g/dl, white cell count 1.8×10^9/l; platelets 250×10^9/l; blood films, no malarial parasites seen; erythrocyte sedimentation rate 40 mm/hour; urea and electrolytes normal; liver function tests normal; chest radiograph normal; blood cultures, no growth after 48 hours; early morning urine, no growth of *Mycobacterium tuberculosis*. Questions revealed a history of eating unpasteurized dairy products while in Africa. What is the most probable diagnosis?
A. Q fever
B. Anthrax
C. Trichinosis
D. Brucellosis
E. Leptospirosis

FURTHER READING

Hugh-Jones ME. *Outline of Zoonotic Diseases*. Ames: Iowa State University Press, 2002.

Palmer SR, Soulsby EJL, Simpson DIH, eds. *Zoonoses*. Oxford: Oxford University Press, 1998.

Fever of unknown origin

INTRODUCTION

Fever is an abnormal increase in body temperature and may be continuous or intermittent

The homeostatic mechanisms of the body maintain a constant body temperature with daily fluctuations (circadian temperature rhythm) not exceeding ± 1–1.5°C. Although 37°C (98.6°F) is taken as 'normal', individuals vary in their body temperature; in some it may be as low as 36°C, in others as high as 38°C. Fever is defined as an abnormal increase in body temperature—an oral temperature higher than 37.6°C (100.4°F) or a rectal temperature higher than 38°C (101°F)—and may be continuous or intermittent:

- In continuous fever the body temperature is elevated over the whole 24-hour period and swings less than 1°C; this is characteristic of, for example, typhoid and typhus fever.
- In an intermittent fever the temperature is above normal throughout the 24-hour period, but swings more than 1°C during that time. A swinging fever is typical of pyogenic infections, abscesses and tuberculosis.

Fever may be produced in response to:

- exogenous pyrogen such as endotoxin in Gram-negative cell walls;
- endogenous pyrogen such as interleukin 1 (IL-1) released from phagocytic cells.

It is thought that fever may be a protective response by the host *(Fig. 29.1)*.

DEFINITIONS OF FEVER OF UNKNOWN ORIGIN

Fever is a common complaint of patients presenting to a doctor. The cause is usually immediately apparent or is discovered within a few days, or the temperature settles spontaneously. However, if the patient's fever is greater than 38.3°C (101°F) on several occasions and continues for more than 3 weeks despite 1 week of intensive evaluation, a provisional diagnosis of 'fever of unknown origin' (FUO) is made. This is the classical definition of FUO, but as an increasing number of patients with serious underlying diseases are successfully kept alive by modern medicine, FUO in patients in particular risk groups has also been defined *(Fig. 29.2)*.

CAUSES OF FUO

Infection is the most common cause of FUO

For centuries, fever has been recognized as a characteristic sign of infection, and infection is the single most common cause of FUO, accounting for 30–40% of FUO in adults and up to 50% in children. However, there are important non-infectious causes of fever, most notably:

- malignancies;
- collagen-vascular diseases *(Fig. 29.3)*.

These non-infectious causes need to be differentiated from infections during the investigation of a patient with a FUO. Despite intense and prolonged investigations, the cause of fever remains undiagnosed in 5–15% of patients. However, in the absence of significant weight loss or indication of severe underlying disease the outcome, though potentially long term, is generally positive. A further 10% of patients may have a factitious fever (produced artificially by the patient; e.g. in Munchausen syndrome).

Infective causes of classical FUO

The most common infective causes of classical FUO are shown in *Figure 29.4*. These can be divided into two main groups:

- infections such as tuberculosis and typhoid fever caused by specific pathogens;
- infections such as urinary tract infections, biliary tract infections and abscesses, which can be caused by a variety of different pathogens.

Most of these infections are described in detail elsewhere in this book. Bacterial endocarditis is discussed below.

Significant infection may be present in the absence of fever in some groups of patients, notably:

- seriously ill neonates;
- the elderly;
- patients with uremia;

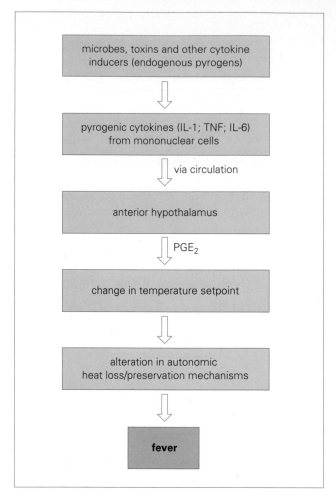

Fig. 29.1 Mechanisms of fever. Fever may be induced either by exogenous pyrogens such as microbes or their toxins or by endogenous pyrogens released in the host, and may have a protective effect. (IL-, interleukin; PG, prostaglandin; TNF, tumor necrosis factor.)

- patients receiving corticosteroids;
- those taking antipyretic drugs continuously.

In these people other signs and symptoms of infection have to be sought. This chapter deals only with patients whose presenting complaint is fever.

INVESTIGATION OF CLASSICAL FUO

Steps in the investigative procedure

Because of the many possible causes of FUO, both infectious and non-infectious, it is clearly not practicable to attempt specific investigations for each at the outset. The diagnostic pathway can be divided into a series of stages, each stage attempting to focus the investigation on the likely causes (*Fig. 29.5*).

Stage 1 comprises careful history-taking, physical examination and screening tests

Careful history-taking is essential and should include questions about travel, occupation, hobbies, exposure to animals and known infectious hazards, antibiotic therapy

within the previous 2 months, substance misuse and other habits. Some of the infections listed in *Figure 29.4* are zoonoses (e.g. leptospirosis, spotted fevers), whereas others are vector-borne (e.g. malaria, trypanosomiasis) and/or of limited geographic distribution (e.g. histoplasmosis). Hence the importance of a travel history.

In the light of the history and the differential diagnosis, a complete physical examination of the patient with FUO is essential. In particular:

- The skin, eyes, lymph nodes and abdomen should be examined.
- The heart should be auscultated.

It is also important to confirm that the patient does have a fever. In some series, as many as 25% of patients whose presenting complaint was a FUO did not have a fever, but had a naturally exaggerated circadian temperature rhythm. Up to 10% may have a factitious fever.

Routine investigations such as chest radiography and blood tests should be performed at this stage.

Stage 2 involves reviewing the history, repeating the physical examination, specific diagnostic tests and non-invasive investigations

A review of the patient's history, particularly after discussion with colleagues and perhaps carried out by a second physician, is valuable to check for omissions such as exposure to particular risk factors in the recent or more distant past. The physical examination should also be repeated because rashes and other signs of infection can be transient.

Clues to the diagnosis elicited by careful history-taking should direct specific investigations. As the most common cause of unexplained fever is infection, collection and careful examination of appropriate specimens are essential. Skin tests may also be appropriate at this stage. The most important specimens include:

- Blood for culture.
- Blood for examination of antibodies. A sample of serum collected when the patient presents should also be stored for comparison with later samples to detect rising antibody titers even if the patient is some weeks into the infection. Serologic tests are helpful, particularly in the diagnosis of cytomegalovirus (CMV) and Epstein–Barr virus (EBV) infection, toxoplasmosis, psittacosis and rickettsial infections. Positive results in syphilis serology should be viewed with caution as other infections can cause biologic false-positives (see Chapter 21).
- Direct examination of blood to diagnose malaria, trypanosomiasis and relapsing fever.

Repeated sampling of blood, urine and other body fluids is often required, and the laboratory should be alerted to search for unusual and fastidious organisms (e.g. nutritionally variant streptococci as a cause of endocarditis; see below). If possible, serial cultures should be collected before antimicrobial therapy is commenced.

Technical advances in diagnostic imaging techniques have provided the physician with a wide range of non-invasive investigative methods (e.g. ultrasound, CT scan, MRI, etc.). Some radiologic procedures such as chest radiographs are

DEFINITIONS OF FEVER OF UNKNOWN ORIGIN		
definition	**symptoms**	**diagnosis**
classical FUO	fever (> 38.3°C) on several occasions and more than 3 weeks' duration	uncertain despite appropriate investigations after at least three outpatient visits, 3 days in hospital, or 1 week of intensive ambulatory investigation
nosocomial (hospital-acquired) FUO	fever (> 38.3°C) on several occasions in a hospitalized patient receiving acute care; infection not present or incubating on admission	uncertain after 3 days despite appropriate investigations, including at least 2 days incubation of microbiologic cultures
neutropenic FUO	fever (> 38.3°C) on several occasions; neutrophil count < 500/mm³ in peripheral blood, or expected to fall below that number within 1–2 days	uncertain after 3 days despite appropriate investigations, including at least 2 days' incubation of microbiologic cultures
HIV-associated FUO	fever (> 38.3°C) on several occasions; fever of more than 4 weeks' duration as an outpatient or more than 3 days' duration in hospital; confirmed positive HIV serology	uncertain after 3 days despite appropriate investigations, including at least 2 days' incubation of microbiologic cultures

Fig. 29.2 Definitions of fever of unknown origin (FUO). The classical definition of FUO requires that the fever is of 3 or more weeks' duration, but in compromised patients infections frequently progress rapidly because of inadequate host defenses. Consequently the pace of the investigations needs to be rapid if appropriate therapy is to be initiated.

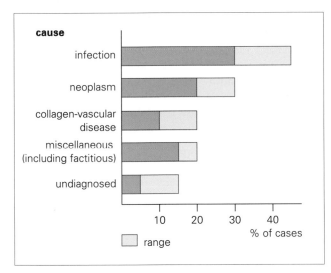

Fig. 29.3 Causes of fever of unknown origin. The results of several retrospective studies show that infection is the single most common cause. A significant number of fevers remained undiagnosed.

routine in the work-up of patients with FUO *(Fig. 29.6)*, while others such as gallium or technetium scans are applied in the light of the likely diagnosis *(Fig. 29.7)*.

Stage 3 comprises invasive tests

Biopsy of liver and bone marrow should always be considered in the investigation of classical cases of FUO, but other tissues such as skin, lymph nodes and kidney may also be sampled. It is undesirable or impossible to repeat biopsies, and there-

fore it is important to organize the laboratory examination of material carefully to maximize the information obtained.

Stage 4 involves therapeutic trials

Trials of corticosteroids (e.g. prednisone, dexamethasone) or prostaglandin inhibitors (e.g. aspirin, indometacin) may be indicated if a non-infectious cause is suspected. There are few indications for empiric antimicrobial or cytotoxic chemotherapy in the management of classical FUO. However, a trial of antituberculous drugs may be advocated in patients with a history of tuberculosis in the absence of supporting microbiologic evidence. Infections can progress very rapidly in people who are neutropenic or have AIDS, and 'blind' therapy is warranted (see below).

TREATMENT OF FUO

The investigation and management of a patient with FUO requires persistence and an informed and open mind in order to reach the correct diagnosis. As the range of infective causes of FUO is enormous the correct diagnosis is an essential prelude to the choice of appropriate treatment. As soon as the cause has been identified, specific therapy, if available, should be given.

FUO IN SPECIFIC PATIENT GROUPS

The main difference between FUO in these groups and classical FUO is the time course

As mentioned above, an increasing number of people are surviving with severe underlying disease that predisposes

INFECTIVE CAUSES OF FEVER OF UNKNOWN ORIGIN	
infection	usual cause
Bacterial	
tuberculosis	*Mycobacterium tuberculosis*
enteric fevers	*Salmonella typhi*
osteomyelitis	*Staphylococcus aureus* (also *Haemophilus influenzae* in young children, *Salmonella* in patients with sickle-cell disease)
endocarditis	oral streptococci, *Staph. aureus*, coagulase-negative staphylococci
brucellosis	*Brucella abortus, B. melitensis* and *B. suis*
abscesses (esp. intra-abdominal)	mixed anaerobes and facultative anaerobes from gut flora
biliary system infections	Gram-negative facultative anaerobes, e.g. *E. coli*
urinary tract infections	Gram-negative facultative anaerobes, e.g. *E. coli*
Lyme disease	*Borrelia burgdorferi*
relapsing fever	*Borrelia recurrentis*
leptospirosis	*Leptospira icterohaemorrhagiae*
rat bite fever	*Spirillum minus (Spirillum minor)*
typhus	*Rickettsia prowazekii*
spotted fevers	*Rickettsia rickettsii, Rickettsia conori*
psittacosis	*Chlamydophila psittaci*
Q fever	*Coxiella burnetii*
Parasitic	
malaria	*Plasmodium* species
trypanosomiasis	*Trypanosoma brucei*
amebic abscesses	*Entamoeba histolytica*
toxoplasmosis	*Toxoplasma gondii*
Fungal	
candidiasis	*Candida albicans*
cryptococcosis	*Cryptococcus neoformans*
histoplasmosis	*Histoplasma capsulatum*
Viral	
AIDS	HIV
infectious mononucleosis	Epstein–Barr virus, cytomegalovirus
hepatitis	hepatitis viruses

Fig. 29.4 Representative infective causes of fever of unknown origin (FUO). A wide range of infections can present as FUO. Some, such as brucellosis, are zoonoses, and many are vector-borne. Therefore the patient must have had appropriate exposure to contract these infections. For example, there are about 2000 cases of malaria annually in the UK (ca. 700 in the USA), but all are contracted outside the country. A travel history is therefore very important. (*E. coli, Escherichia coli.*)

INVESTIGATION OF CLASSICAL FUO	
Stage 1	history physical examination screening tests
Stage 2	review history repeat physical examination specific diagnostic tests non-invasive investigations
Stage 3	invasive tests
Stage 4	therapeutic trials

Fig. 29.5 The diagnostic pathway for the investigation of a patient with fever of unknown origin (FUO) can be divided into several stages.

them to infection or are receiving treatment such as cytotoxic drugs that compromises their defenses against infection. These groups of patients are discussed in more detail in Chapter 30, but are included here because, in addition to classical FUO, newer classifications of FUO (*Fig. 29.2*) define:

- nosocomial FUO;
- neutropenic FUO;
- HIV-associated FUO.

Classically a FUO may exist for weeks or months before a diagnosis is made, whereas for hospital-acquired (noso-comial) FUO and in neutropenic patients the time course is hours to days. The more common infective causes of FUO in these groups are shown in *Figure 29.8*.

Investigation should proceed in the stages listed above, but with the particular emphasis depending upon the patient. In hospital patients the emphasis will depend upon:

- the type of operative procedures performed; fever is a common complaint in patients who have received transplants and may indicate graft-versus-host disease rather than infection;
- the presence of foreign bodies, especially intravascular devices;
- drug therapy, as drug fevers are a common non-infective cause of FUO;
- the underlying disease and stage of chemotherapy in neutropenic patients;
- the presence of known risk factors such as intravenous drug misuse, travel and contact with infected individuals in patients with HIV. Although the major opportunist infections in people with AIDS are well described (see Chapter 30), common infections can present atypically and new infections continue to emerge.

INFECTIVE ENDOCARDITIS

Infective endocarditis is an uncommon disease that often presents as a FUO and is fatal if untreated. The infection involves the endothelial lining of the heart, usually including

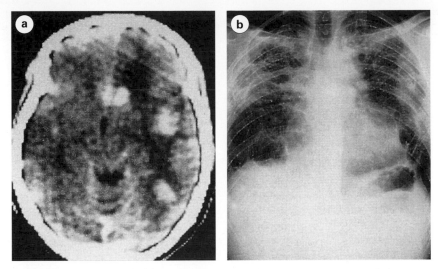

Fig. 29.6 Computerized tomography (CT) scans help in the demonstration of abscesses. The patient in (a) has a tuberculoma of the brain, but the CT appearance is not sufficiently characteristic to distinguish this from a pyogenic abscess or a meningioma. (Courtesy of J Ambrose.) The chest radiograph in (b) shows a patient with sarcoidosis. The differential diagnosis between infective and non-infective causes of granulomas is important, and can be difficult in the early stages of the investigation. (Courtesy of M Turner-Warwick.)

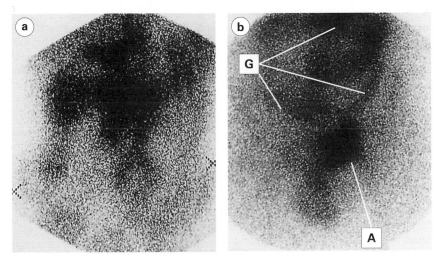

Fig. 29.7 Gallium concentrates in many inflammatory and neoplastic tissues and is a useful non-invasive technique in the investigation of a patient with fever of unknown origin. (a) Retroperitoneal lymphadenopathy of Hodgkin's disease highlighted by a gallium scan. (Courtesy of H Tubbs.) (b) Intra-abdominal abscess shown by a gallium scan. (A, abscess; G, gallium in colon.) (Courtesy of WE Farrar.)

the heart valves. It may occur as an acute, rapidly progressive disease or in a subacute form. The majority of these patients have a pre-existing heart defect, either congenital or acquired (e.g. as a result of rheumatic fever), or a prosthetic heart valve in situ. However, the patient may be unaware of any defect before the infection.

Almost any organism can cause endocarditis, but native valves are usually infected by oral streptococci and staphylococci

Infection of native valves is most commonly caused by species of oral streptococci (viridans group) such as *Streptococcus sanguis*, *Strep. oralis* and *Strep. mitis* and by *Staph. aureus*. Intra-

venous drug misusers have the added complication of infection due to organisms they inject into themselves. Coagulase-negative staphylococci are common causes of early prosthetic valve endocarditis and are probably acquired at the time of surgery. The species causing late infections—more than 3 months after cardiac surgery—are somewhat more like those causing native valve endocarditis (*Fig. 29.9*).

Endocarditis is an endogenous infection acquired when organisms entering the bloodstream establish themselves on the heart valves. Therefore, any bacteremia can potentially result in endocarditis. Most commonly streptococci from the oral flora enter the bloodstream, for example during dental procedures or vigorous teeth cleaning or flossing, and adhere

INFECTIVE CAUSES OF FUO IN SPECIFIC PATIENT GROUPS		
category of FUO	**infection**	**usual cause**
nosocomial	vascular-line related other device related transfusion-related cholecystitis and pancreatitis pneumonia (related to assisted ventilation) postoperative abscesses, e.g. intra-abdominal postgastric surgery	staphylococci staphylococci, *Candida* cytomegalovirus Gram-negative rods Gram-negative rods, including *Pseudomonas* Gram-negative rods and anaerobes systemic candidiasis
neutropenic	vascular-line related oral infection pneumonia soft tissue, e.g. perianal abscess	staphylococci *Candida*, herpes simplex virus Gram-negative rods, *Candida*, *Aspergillus*, CMV mixed aerobes and anaerobes
HIV-associated	respiratory tract central nervous system gastrointestinal tract genital tract or disseminated	cytomegalovirus, *Pneumocystis*, *Mycobacterium tuberculosis*, *M. avium-intracellulare* *Toxoplasma* *Salmonella*, *Campylobacter*, *Shigella* *Treponema pallidum*, *Neisseria gonorrhoeae*

Fig. 29.8 Representative infective causes of fever of unknown origin (FUO) in specific patient groups. Patients who contract their FUO in hospital are most likely to be infected with 'hospital pathogens', either from their own normal flora or from the hospital environment. This also applies to neutropenic patients if they are hospitalized, but some are treated as outpatients and may therefore be exposed to a wider range of pathogens. People with AIDS commonly become infected with opportunist pathogens, though an increasing range of organisms is now implicated. It is important to take a detailed history, as latent infections can become florid as the patient's immune status deteriorates. (CMV, cytomegalovirus.)

to damaged heart valves. It is thought that fibrin–platelet vegetations are present on damaged valves before the organisms implant, and that adherence is probably associated with the ability of the organisms to produce dextran as well as adhesins and fibronectin-binding proteins. Having attached themselves to the heart valve, the organisms multiply and attract further fibrin and platelet deposition. In this position they are protected from the host defenses, and vegetations can grow to several centimeters in size. This is probably quite a slow process and correspondingly the time period between the initial bacteremia and the onset of symptoms averages around 5 weeks (*Fig. 29.10*).

A patient with infective endocarditis almost always has a fever and a heart murmur

The signs and symptoms of infective endocarditis are very varied, but relate essentially to four ongoing processes:

- the infectious process on the valve and local intracardiac complications;
- septic embolization to virtually any organ;
- bacteremia, often with metastatic foci of infection;
- circulating immune complexes and other factors.

The patient almost always has a fever and a heart murmur and may also complain of non-specific symptoms such as anorexia, weight loss, malaise, chills, nausea, vomiting and night sweats, symptoms that are common to many of the causes of FUO listed in *Figure 29.4*. Peripheral manifestations may also be evident in the form of splinter hemorrhages and

Osler's nodes (*Fig. 29.11*). Microscopic hematuria resulting from immune complex deposition in the kidney is characteristic (see Chapter 17).

Blood culture is the most important test for diagnosing infective endocarditis

Microbiologic and cardiologic investigations are of critical importance. The blood culture is the single most important laboratory test. Ideally three separate samples of blood should be collected within a 24-hour period and before antimicrobial therapy is administered. Methods for processing blood cultures are described in the Appendix. Isolation of the causative organism is essential so that antibiotic susceptibility tests can be performed and optimum therapy prescribed. Nutritionally variant strains of oral streptococci are known to cause infective endocarditis. These may fail to grow in blood culture media unless pyridoxal is added to the broth. Alternatively they grow as satellite colonies around *Staph. aureus* colonies on blood agar.

The mortality of infective endocarditis is 20–50% despite treatment with antibiotics

Although the majority of species causing infective endocarditis are highly susceptible to a range of antibiotics, complete eradication takes several weeks to achieve, and relapse is not uncommon. This is probably due to factors such as:

- relative inaccessibility of the organisms within the vegetations both to antibiotics and to host defenses;

MAJOR ETIOLOGIC AGENTS OF INFECTIVE ENDOCARDITIS	
native valve	1. oral streptococci and enterococci 2. *Staph. aureus* 3. coagulase-negative staphylococci 4. Gram-negative (enteric) rods 5. fungi (mainly *Candida*)
intravenous drug misuser	1. *Staph. aureus* 2. oral streptococci and enterococci 3. Gram-negative (enteric) rods 4. fungi (mainly *Candida*) 5. coagulase-negative staphylococci
prosthetic valve (early)	1. coagulase-negative staphylococci 2. *Staph. aureus* 3. Gram-negative (enteric) rods 4. oral streptococci and enterococci 5. fungi (mainly *Candida*)
prosthetic valve (late)	1. oral streptococci and enterococci 2. coagulase-negative staphylococci 3. *Staph. aureus* 4. Gram-negative (enteric) rods 5. fungi (mainly *Candida*)

Fig. 29.9 Causative agents of endocarditis in different groups of patients (in rank order of decreasing importance). Although almost any organism can cause endocarditis, the majority of cases are caused by a relatively small range of species. The relative importance of these species varies depending upon whether the patient has his/her own heart valves or a prosthetic valve.

- the organism's high population density and relatively slow rate of multiplication.

Before the advent of antibiotics infective endocarditis had a mortality of 100%, and even today despite treatment with appropriate antibiotics, the mortality remains at 20–50%.

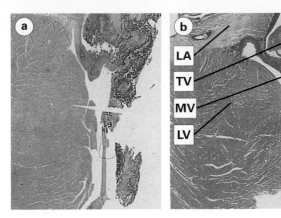

Fig. 29.10 Bacteria circulating in the bloodstream adhere to, and establish themselves on, the heart valves. Multiplication of the microbes is associated with destruction of valve tissue and the formation of vegetations, which interfere with, and may severely compromise, the normal function of the valve. These histologic sections show the virtual destruction of the leaflet at the mitral valve by staphylococci. (a) Gram stain. (b) Eosin–Van Geisen stain. (LA, left atrium; LV, left ventricle; MV, remnant of mitral valve; TV, thrombotic vegetation.) (Courtesy of RH Anderson.)

The antibiotic treatment regimen for infective endocarditis depends upon the infecting organism

For penicillin-susceptible streptococci, high dose penicillin is the treatment of choice. Patients with a good history of penicillin allergy can be treated with ceftriaxone or vancomycin. MIC (minimum inhibitory concentration) and MBC (minimum bactericidal concentration) tests (see Chapter 33) should be performed to detect organisms that are less susceptible or tolerant to penicillin (inhibited, but not killed; e.g. MBC $\geq 32 \times$ MIC). These organisms and enterococci, which are always more resistant to penicillin, should be treated with a combination of penicillin (or ampicillin) and an aminoglycoside. Combinations such as these act synergistically against streptococci and enterococci (see Chapter 33).

Staphylococcal endocarditis, particularly in prosthetic valve endocarditis when the organisms may be hospital-acquired and consequently often resistant to many antibiotics, often presents a more difficult therapeutic challenge. A β-lactamase

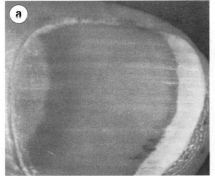
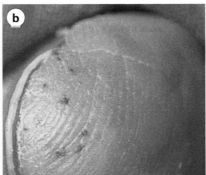
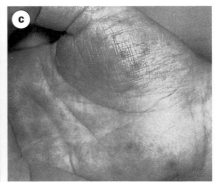

Fig. 29.11 Outward signs of endocarditis may be helpful in suggesting the diagnosis. These result from the host's response to infection in the form of immune complex-mediated vasculitis, focal platelet aggregation and vascular permeability. (a and b, different views) Splinter hemorrhages in the nailbed and petechial lesions in the skin. (c) Osler's nodes. These are tender nodular lesions that tend to affect the palms and fingertips. (Courtesy of H Tubbs.)

stable penicillin such as nafcillin is often suitable and may be given in combination with an aminoglycoside or rifampicin. Glycopeptide antibiotics (e.g. vancomycin) should be used for penicillin-allergic patients and for treating methicillin-resistant staphylococci. Detailed treatment regimens are published by the American Heart Foundation and the British Society for Antimicrobial Chemotherapy.

People with heart defects need prophylactic antibiotics during invasive procedures

People with known heart defects should be given prophylactic antibiotics to protect them during dental surgery and any other invasive procedure that is likely to cause a transient bacteremia.

Most people with a FUO have a treatable disease presenting in an unusual manner

The clinical investigation needs to be individualized, but this chapter outlines the essential stages in the investigation of every patient and draws attention to the important infective causes of FUO.

Although classically a patient with FUO presents with a long history (weeks or months of fever), patients also present with fevers that are not immediately diagnosed by routine laboratory investigations. For these groups (nosocomial, neutropenic and HIV-associated), new definitions of FUO have been proposed. The list of pathogens causing fever in these patients is growing.

The clinician's aim in the investigation of every patient with FUO should be to discover the cause, i.e. to change a FUO to a fever of known origin, and to initiate appropriate treatment.

KEY FACTS

- Fever is the body's response to exogenous and endogenous pyrogens. It is a common symptom and may have a protective effect.

- The term fever of unknown origin (FUO) is used when the cause of fever is not obvious, has classically exceeded 3 weeks' duration, and is not revealed by routine clinical and laboratory investigations.

- The increase in numbers of immunocompromised patients has prompted definition of FUO groups other than classical (i.e. nosocomial, neutropenic and HIV-associated FUO).

- Among the causes of FUO, infection is the most common, but neoplasms and autoimmune diseases are also significant. As many as 15% of cases may remain undiagnosed.

- The list of infective causes is long, therefore the first stage of investigation (i.e. the patient's history and results of physical examination and screening tests) are critical pointers to subsequent specific diagnostic tests.

- Therapeutic trials may be indicated if a diagnosis has not been achieved, but may confuse the results of further tests.

- The correct diagnosis is paramount to direct appropriate specific therapy.

- Infective endocarditis is an uncommon, but classic, example of a FUO. It is usually caused by Gram-positive cocci, the species depending upon the patient's underlying predisposition, and is fatal unless treated.

QUESTIONS

A 60-year-old woman presents to the clinic with a 7-day history of malaise, nausea and loss of appetite. Ten years previously she had been admitted with an aortic root dissection. This was corrected successfully at operation and her aortic root and valve were replaced. She has been quite well until now, although she is a poor complier and it has been difficult to stabilize her anticoagulant therapy. On examination her temperature is 38°C and she is flushed and unwell. Her pulse rate is 110 beats/min, and her blood pressure is 80/60 mmHg. A prosthetic valvular click and a systolic murmur are heard on auscultation. Her chest is otherwise clear, and abdominal examination is unremarkable. The results of initial investigations are: hemoglobin, 8.3 g/dl normochromic, normocytic film; white cell count, 14.6×10^9/l with 60% neutrophils; platelets, 192×10^9/l.

1. What is the probable diagnosis and what further investigations are critical?

2. What is the most common pathogen responsible for this condition?

3. What are the crucial components of management of this condition?

4. What are the possible complications of this condition?

5. What guidelines are available to reduce the risk of this disease occurring?

FURTHER READING

Akpede GO, Akenzua GI. Aetiology and management of children with acute fever of unknown origin. *Paediatr Drugs* 2001; 3:169–93.

Akpede GO, Akenzua GI. Management of children with prolonged fever of unknown origin and difficulties in the management of fever of unknown origin in children in developing countries. *Paediatr Drugs* 2001; 3:247–62.

Armstrong WS, Katz JT, Kazanjian PH. Human immunodeficiency virus-associated fever of unknown origin: a study of 70 patients in the United States and review. *Clin Infect Dis* 1999; 28:341–5.

Arnow PM, Flaherty JP. Fever of unknown origin. *Lancet* 1997; 350:575–80.

Bayer AS, Bolger AF, Taubert KA et al. Diagnosis and management of infective endocarditis and its complications. *Circulation* 1998; 98:2936–48.

Collazos J, Guerra E, Mayo J, Martinez E. Tuberculosis as a cause of recurrent fever of unknown origin. *J Infect* 2000; 41:269–72.

Davies GR, Finch RG. Fever of unknown origin. *Clin Med* 2001; 1:177–9.

Hirschmann JV. Fever of unknown origin in adults. *Clin Infect Dis* 1997; 24:291–300.

Majeed HA. Differential diagnosis of fever of unknown origin in children. *Curr Opin Rheumatol* 2000; 12:439–44.

Mayo J, Collazos J, Martinez E. Fever of unknown origin in the setting of HIV infection: guidelines for a rational approach. *AIDS Patient Care STDs* 1998; 12:373–8.

Tal S, Guller V, Gurevich A, Levi S. Fever of unknown origin in the elderly. *J Intern Med* 2002; 252:295–304.

INTRODUCTION

The human body has a complex system of protective mechanisms to prevent infection, involving both the adaptive (cellular and humoral) immune system and the innate defense system (e.g. skin, mucous membranes). These have been described in detail in earlier chapters (see Chapters 9 and 10). So far we have concentrated on the common and serious infections occurring in people whose protective mechanisms are largely intact. In these circumstances the interactions between host and parasite are such that the parasite has to use all its guile to survive and invade the host, and the healthy host is able to put up a fight against such an invasion. In this chapter we will consider the infections that arise when the host–parasite equation is weighted heavily in favor of the parasite, in other words when the host is compromised.

THE COMPROMISED HOST

Compromised hosts are people who have one or more defects in their body's natural defenses against microbial invaders. Consequently they are much more liable to suffer from severe and life-threatening infections. Modern medicine has effective methods for treating at least half of all serious cancers, has perfected organ transplantation and has developed technology that enables people with otherwise fatal diseases to lead prolonged and productive lives. A consequence of these achievements, however, is an increasing number of compromised people prone to infection. In addition there is a growing population of people with HIV infection and AIDS.

The host can be compromised in many different ways

Compromise can take a variety of forms, falling into two main groups:

- defects, accidental or intentional, in the body's innate defense mechanisms;
- deficiencies in the adaptive immune response.

These disorders of the immune system can be further subclassified as 'primary' or 'secondary' (Fig. 30.1):

- Primary immunodeficiency is inherited or occurs by exposure in utero to environmental factors or by other unknown mechanisms. It is rare, and varies in severity depending upon the type of defect.
- Secondary or acquired immunodeficiency is due to an underlying disease state (Fig. 30.2) or occurs as a result of treatment for a disease.

Primary defects of innate immunity include congenital defects in phagocytic cells or complement synthesis

Congenital defects in phagocytic cells confer susceptibility to infection, and of these perhaps the best known is chronic granulomatous disease (Fig. 30.3), in which an inherited failure to synthesize cytochrome b_{245} leads to a failure to produce reactive oxygen intermediates during phagocytosis.

The central role of complement in the innate defense mechanisms is undisputed, and inability to generate classical C3 convertase (see Chapter 10) through congenital defects in the synthesis of the early components, particularly C4 and C2, is associated with a high frequency of extracellular infections.

Secondary defects of innate defenses include disruption of the body's mechanical barriers

A variety of factors can disrupt the mechanical non-specific barriers to infection. For example, burns, traumatic injury and major surgery destroy the continuity of the skin and may leave poorly vascularized tissue near the body surface, providing a

WHAT MAKES A HOST COMPROMISED	
factors affecting innate systems	
primary	complement deficiencies phagocyte cell deficiencies
secondary	burns, trauma, major surgery, catheterization, foreign bodies (e.g. shunts, prostheses), obstruction
factors affecting adaptive systems	
primary	T cell defects, B cell deficiencies, severe combined immunodeficiency
secondary	malnutrition, infectious diseases, neoplasia, irradiation, chemotherapy, splenectomy

Fig. 30.1 Factors that make a host compromised.

INFECTIONS THAT CAUSE IMMUNOSUPPRESSION	
viral	**bacterial**
measles	*Mycobacterium tuberculosis*
mumps	*Mycobacterium leprae*
congenital rubella Epstein–Barr virus cytomegalovirus HIV1, HIV2	*Brucella* spp.

Fig. 30.2 Infections that cause immunosuppression.

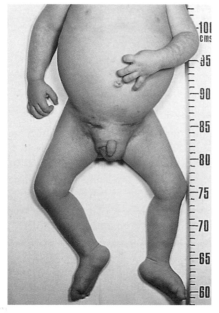

Fig. 30.3 Bilateral draining lymph nodes in an 18-month-old boy with chronic granulomatous disease. Abscesses caused by *Staphylococcus aureus* had developed in both groins and had to be surgically drained. (Courtesy of AR Hayward.)

relatively defenseless site for microbes to colonize and invade. In health, the mucosal barriers of the respiratory and alimentary tract are vital to prevent infection. Damage sustained, for example through endoscopy, surgery or irradiation therapy, provides easy access for infecting organisms. Devices such as intravascular and urinary catheters, or procedures such as lumbar puncture or bone marrow aspiration, allow organisms to bypass the normal defenses and enter normally-sterile parts of the body. Foreign bodies such as prostheses, e.g. hip joints or heart valves, and cerebrospinal fluid (CSF) shunts alter the local non-specific host responses and provide surfaces that microbes can colonize more readily than the natural equivalents.

The adage 'obstruction leads to infection' is a valuable reminder that the defenses of many body systems work partly through the clearance of undesirable materials, e.g. by urine flow, ciliary action in the respiratory tract, and peristalsis in the gut. Interference with these mechanisms as a result of pathologic obstruction, central nervous system dysfunction or surgical intervention tends to result in infection.

Primary adaptive immunodeficiency results from defects in the primary differentiation environment or in cell differentiation

The major congenital abnormalities arising in the adaptive immune system are depicted in *Figure 30.4*. A defect in the stromal microenvironment in which lymphocytes differentiate may lead to failure to produce B cells (Bruton-type agammaglobulinemia) or T cells (DiGeorge syndrome).

Differentiation pathways themselves may also be affected. For example, a non-functional recombinase enzyme will prevent the recombination of gene fragments that form the B cell antibody or the T cell receptor variable regions for antigen recognition, with a resulting severe combined immunodeficiency (SCID).

The most common form of congenital antibody deficiency—common variable immunodeficiency—is characterized by recurrent pyogenic infections and is probably heterogenous. Although the number of immature B cells in the marrow tends to be normal, the peripheral B cells are either low in number or in some cases absent. Where present they are unable to differentiate into plasma cells in some cases or to secrete antibody in others.

Transient hypogammaglobulinemia of infancy, characterized by recurrent respiratory infections, is associated with a low serum IgG concentration, which often normalizes abruptly by 3–4 years of age (*Fig. 30.5*).

Immunoglobulin deficiency occurs naturally in human infants as the maternal serum IgG concentration decays and can become a serious problem in very premature babies.

Causes of secondary adaptive immunodeficiency include malnutrition, infections, neoplasia, splenectomy and certain medical treatments

Worldwide, malnutrition is a common and the most important cause of acquired immunodeficiency. The major form, protein–energy malnutrition (PEM) presents as a wide range of disorders, with kwashiorkor and marasmus at the two poles. It results in:

- drastic effects on the structure of the lymphoid organs (*Fig. 30.6*);
- gross reductions in the synthesis of complement components;
- sluggish chemotactic responses of phagocytes;
- lowered concentrations of secretory and mucosal IgA;
- reduced affinity of IgG;
- in particular, a serious deficit in circulating T cell numbers (*Fig. 30.7*), leading to inadequate cell-mediated responses.

Infections themselves are often immunosuppressive (*Fig. 30.2*), and none more so than HIV infection, which gives rise to AIDS (see Chapter 21). Neoplasia of the lymphoid system frequently induces a state of reduced immunoreactivity, and splenectomy, for whatever reason, results in impaired humoral responses.

Treatment of disease can also cause immunosuppression. For example:

- Cytotoxic agents such as cyclophosphamide and azathioprine cause leukopenia or deranged T and B cell function.
- Corticosteroids reduce the number of circulating leuko-

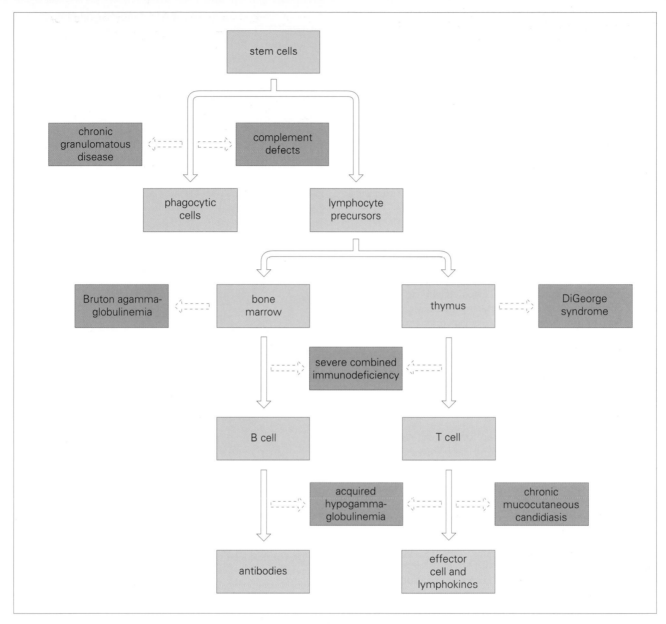

Fig. 30.4 The major primary cellular immunodeficiencies. The deficiency states (shown in purple boxes) derive either from defects in the primary differentiation environment (bone marrow or thymus) or during cell differentiation (shown as dashed arrows derived from the differentiation state indicated).

cytes, monocytes and eosinophils and suppress leukocyte accumulation at sites of inflammation.

- Irradiation therapy adversely affects the proliferation of lymphoid cells.

Therefore a patient receiving treatment for neoplastic disease will be immunocompromised as a result of both the disease and the treatment.

It is important to recognize immunodeficiencies and to understand which procedures are likely to compromise the natural defenses of a patient. Due to improvements in medical technology, many immune defects, particularly immuno-suppression resulting from irradiation or cytotoxic drugs, are transient, and patients who survive the period of immuno-suppression have a good chance of a complete recovery.

Microbes that infect the compromised host

Compromised people can become infected not only with any pathogen able to infect non-compromised individuals, but also with opportunist pathogens—microbes that are incapable of causing disease in a healthy person, but able to infect when the host defenses are lowered, often with fatal consequences. Different types of defect predispose to infection with different pathogens depending upon the critical mechanisms operating in the defense against each microorganism *(Fig. 30.8)*. Here we will concentrate mainly on the opportunist infections and refer to other chapters for information about other pathogens.

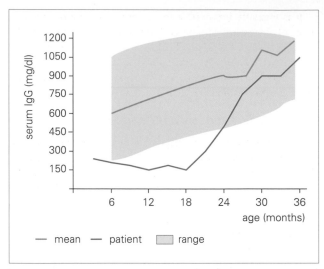

Fig. 30.5 Serum immunoglobulin concentrations in a boy with transient hypogammaglobulinemia compared with the range of normal controls. The patient developed mild paralytic polio when immunized at 4 months of age with attenuated (Sabin) vaccine.

INFECTIONS OF THE HOST WITH DEFICIENT INNATE IMMUNITY DUE TO PHYSICAL FACTORS

Burn wound infections

Burns damage the body's mechanical barriers, neutrophil function and immune responses

Burn wounds are sterile immediately after the burn is inflicted, but inevitably become colonized within hours with a mixed bacterial flora. Burn injuries cause direct damage to the mechanical barriers of the body and abnormalities in neutrophil function and immune responses. In addition there is a major physiologic derangement with loss of fluids and electrolytes. The burn provides a highly nutritious surface for organisms to colonize, and the incidence of serious infection varies with the size and depth of the burn and the age of the patient. Modern topical antimicrobial therapy should prevent infection of burns of less than 30% of the total body area, but larger burns are always colonized. Non-invasive infection is confined to the eschar, which is the non-viable skin debris on the surface of deep burns. It is characterized by rapid separation of the eschar from the underlying tissue and a heavy exudate of purulent material from the burn wound. The systemic symptoms are usually relatively mild. However, organisms can invade from heavily colonized burn eschars into viable tissue beneath and rapidly destroy the tissue, converting partial thickness burns into full skin thickness destruction. From here it is a small step to invasion of the lymphatics and thence to the bloodstream or direct invasion of blood vessels, and to septicemia. Septicemia in patients with burns is often polymicrobial.

The major pathogens in burns are aerobic and facultatively anaerobic bacteria and fungi

The most important pathogens in burn wounds are:

- *Pseudomonas aeruginosa* and other Gram-negative rods;
- *Staphylococcus aureus*;

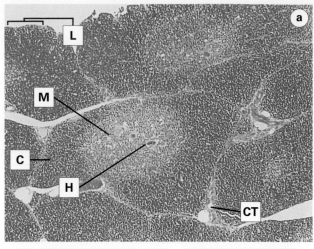

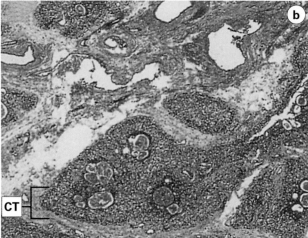

Fig. 30.6 Thymic histology in normal children and children with protein–energy malnutrition (PEM). (a) Normal thymus showing well-demarcated cortex and medullary zones. (b) Acute involution in PEM characterized by lobular atrophy, loss of distinction between cortex and medulla, depletion of lymphocytes and enlarged Hassall's corpuscles. (C, cortex; CT, connective tissue; H, Hassall's corpuscle; L, lobule; M, medulla.) (Courtesy of RK Chandra.)

- *Streptococcus pyogenes*;
- other streptococci;
- enterococci.

Candida spp. and *Aspergillus* together account for about 5% of infections. Anaerobes are rare in burn wound infections. Viral infections, mostly herpesvirus and cytomegalovirus (CMV), have been reported, but their clinical significance is uncertain.

P. aeruginosa *is a devastating Gram-negative pathogen of burned patients*

Ps. aeruginosa is an opportunist Gram-negative rod that has a long and infamous association with burn infections. It grows well in the moist environment of a burn wound, producing a foul, green-pigmented discharge and necrosis. Invasion is not uncommon, and the characteristic skin lesions (ecthyma gangrenosum) that are pathognomonic of *P. aeruginosa* septicemia may appear on non-burned areas (see *Fig. 30.8*). Host factors predisposing to infection include:

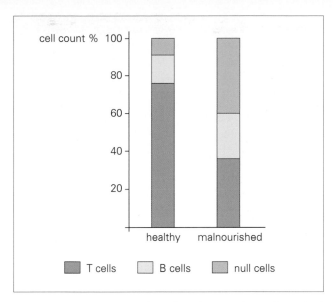

Fig. 30.7 The proportion of T cells is decreased in malnourished patients compared with healthy controls. B cell counts are usually unaltered, and lymphocytes lacking T and B cell markers are increased.

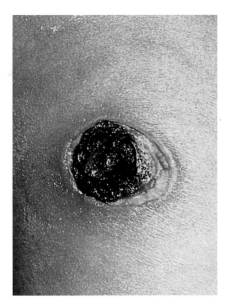

Fig. 30.8 Ecthyma gangrenosum in a child with *Pseudomonas* septicemia associated with immunodeficiency. (Courtesy of H Tubbs.)

- abnormalities in the antibacterial activities of neutrophils;
- deficiencies in serum opsonins.

Added to these are the virulence factors of the organism, which include the production of elastase, protease and exotoxin. This combination makes *P. aeruginosa* the most devastating Gram-negative pathogen of burned patients. Treatment is difficult because of the organism's innate resistance to many antibacterial agents. A combination of aminoglycoside, usually gentamicin or tobramycin, with one of the beta-lactams such as azlocillin, ceftazidime or imipenem is usually favored, but several units have reported strains resistant to these agents.

It is virtually impossible to prevent colonization. Prevention of infection depends largely upon inhibiting the multiplication of organisms colonizing the burn by applying topical agents such as silver nitrate. Both active and passive immunization have been tried, the latter appearing to hold more promise at present.

Staph. aureus *is the foremost pathogen of burn wounds*

The most important predisposing factor to *Staph. aureus* infection in burns patients appears to be an abnormality of the antibacterial function of neutrophils. Infections follow a more insidious course than streptococcal infections (see below), and it may be several days before the full-blown infection is apparent. The organism is capable of destroying granulation tissue, invading and causing septicemia. *Staph. aureus* infections of skin are discussed in detail in Chapter 26. Treatment with antistaphylococcal agents such as cloxacillin or nafcillin (or a glycopeptide if methicillin-resistant *Staph. aureus* is isolated) should be administered if there is evidence of invasive infection. Every effort should be made to prevent the spread of staphylococci from patient to patient. Although transmissible by both airborne and contact routes, the contact route is by far the more important.

The high transmissibility of Strep. pyogenes *makes it the scourge of burns wards*

Strep. pyogenes (group A strep) infections of skin and soft tissue are discussed in some detail in Chapter 23. *Strep. pyogenes* was the most common cause of burn wound infection in the pre-antibiotic era and is still to be feared in burns wards. The infection usually occurs within the first few days of injury and is characterized by a rapid deterioration in the state of the burn wound and invasion of neighboring healthy tissue. The patient may become severely toxic and will die within hours unless treated appropriately. *Strep. pyogenes* rarely infects healthy granulation tissue, but freshly grafted wounds may become infected, resulting in destruction of the graft. Every effort should be made to prevent spread. Penicillin is the drug of choice for treatment, and erythromycin or vancomycin can be used for penicillin-allergic patients.

Beta-hemolytic streptococci of other Lancefield groups (notably groups C and G; see Appendix) and enterococci are also important pathogens of burn wounds.

Traumatic injury and surgical wound infections

Both accidental and intentional trauma destroy the integrity of the body surface and leave it liable to infection. Accidental injury may result in microbes being introduced deep into the wound. The species involved will depend upon the nature of the wound, as discussed in Chapter 26.

Staph. aureus *is the most important cause of surgical wound infection*

Staph. aureus surgical wound infection (see Chapter 36) may be acquired during surgery or postoperatively and may originate from the patient or from another patient or staff member. The wound is less well defended than normal tissue; it may have a damaged blood supply and there may be foreign bodies such as sutures. Classic studies of wound infections have shown that far fewer staphylococci are needed to initiate infection around a suture than in normal healthy skin. Wound infections can be severe and the organisms can invade the bloodstream, with consequent seeding of other sites such as the heart valves, causing endocarditis (see Chapter 29) or bones, causing osteomyelitis (see Chapter 26), thereby further compromising the patient.

Catheter-associated infection of the urinary tract is common

Urinary catheters disrupt the normal host defenses of the urinary tract and allow organisms easy access to the bladder. Such catheter-associated infection of the urinary tract is especially common if catheters are left in place for more than 48 hours (see Chapter 20). The organisms involved are usually Gram-negative rods from the patient's own fecal or periurethral flora, but cross-infection also occurs (see Chapter 36).

Staphylococci are the most common cause of intravenous and peritoneal dialysis catheter infections

Intravenous and peritoneal dialysis catheters breach the integrity of the skin barrier and allow organisms from the skin flora of the patient or hands of the carer easy access to deeper sites. Staphylococci are the most common cause of infection, but coryneforms, Gram-negative rods and *Candida* are also implicated.

Coagulase-negative staphylococci, particularly *Staph. epidermidis*, account for more than 50% of the infections (Fig. 30.9). These opportunists are members of the normal skin flora and for many years were considered to be harmless. However, they have a particular propensity for colonizing plastic and can therefore seed sites adjacent to plastic devices and thence cause invasive infections. Their virulence factors are not well understood, but their ability to produce an adhesive slime material and grow as biofilms on plastic surfaces is likely to be important. Infections are characteristically more insidious in onset than those caused by the more virulent *Staph. aureus*, and recognition is hampered by the difficulty in distinguishing the infecting strain from the normal flora. Treatment is also difficult because many *Staph. epidermidis* carry multiple antibiotic resistances, and agents such as a glycopeptide (vancomycin or teicoplanin) and rifampicin may be required (see Chapter 33). Whenever possible the plastic device should be removed.

Infections of plastic devices in situ

The technical developments in plastics and other synthetic materials have enabled many advances in medicine and surgery, but in the process have produced further ways of introducing infectious agents. *Staph. epidermidis* is an important cause of infection of cardiac pacemakers, vascular grafts and CSF shunts.

Staph. epidermidis is the most common cause of prosthetic valve and joint infections

Patients with prosthetic heart valves or prosthetic joints are compromised by:

INFECTIONS INVOLVING *STAPHYLOCOCCUS EPIDERMIDIS*	
infection of:	% of infections caused by *Staph. epidermidis*
prosthetic heart valve early (< 2 months postoperatively)	30–70
late (> 2 months postoperatively)	20–30
prosthetic hip	10–40
cerebrospinal fluid shunt	30–65
vascular grafts	5–20
peritoneal dialysis related	30
intravascular catheters	10–50

Fig. 30.9 Percentage of infections caused by *Staph. epidermidis* in patients with plastic devices in situ. (Data from Gemmell and McCartney, 1990.)

- the surgery to implant the prosthesis;
- the continued presence of a foreign body.

Staph. epidermidis is again the most common pathogen, either gaining access during surgery or from a subsequent bacteremia originating from, for example, an intravascular line infection. Endocarditis associated with prosthetic heart valves is discussed in Chapter 29.

The most common complication of joint replacement is loosening of the prosthesis, while infection is the second most common complication and is much more likely to lead to permanent failure of the procedure. The difficulties of treatment have been outlined above, but there is understandably great reluctance to remove a prosthetic device, even though it is sometimes the only way to eradicate an infection.

Infections due to compromised clearance mechanisms

Stasis predisposes to infection, and in health the body functions to prevent stasis. In the respiratory tract, damage to the ciliary escalator predisposes the lungs to invasion, particularly in patients with cystic fibrosis, who are infected with *Staph. aureus* and *Haemophilus influenzae* and later with *P. aeruginosa* (see Chapter 19).

Obstruction and interruption of normal urine flow allows Gram-negative organisms from the periurethral flora to ascend the urethra and to establish themselves in the bladder. Septicemia is an important complication of urinary tract infection superimposed on obstruction.

INFECTIONS ASSOCIATED WITH SECONDARY ADAPTIVE IMMUNODEFICIENCY

The underlying immunodeficiency state determines the nature and severity of any associated infection, and in some cases infection is the presenting clinical feature in a patient with an immunologic deficit. However, septicemia and related infectious complications of immunodeficiency are most commonly encountered in patients hospitalized for chemotherapy for malignant diseases or organ transplantation. In these patients, infection continues to be a major cause of morbidity and mortality (Fig. 30.10). Increasingly these infections are iatrogenic and caused by opportunist pathogens acquired in hospital.

Hematologic malignancy and bone marrow transplant infections

A lack of circulating neutrophils following bone marrow failure predisposes to infection

Susceptibility to infection of patients with leukemia is primarily due to the lack of circulating neutrophils that inevitably follows bone marrow failure. Septicemia may be the presenting feature, but is much more common when the patient has been exposed to chemotherapy to induce a remission of the disease (remission-induction chemotherapy). Neutropenia (defined as a count of less than 0.5×10^9 neutrophils/l may persist for a few days to several weeks. Similarly, prolonged periods of neutropenia occur after bone marrow transplantation.

The length of time for which the patient is neutropenic influences the nature of any associated infection and the frequency with which it occurs—for example, fungal infections are much more common in patients who are neutropenic for more than 21 days. Although Gram-negative rods such as *Escherichia coli* and *P. aeruginosa* from the bowel flora have in the past been the most common cause of septicemia in neutropenic patients, Gram-positive organisms—staphylococci, streptococci and enterococci—are gaining in importance. *Staph. epidermidis* septicemia associated with intravascular catheters (see above) is common. Infections caused by fungi are also increasing, partly because more patients are surviving the early neutropenic period with the aid of modern antibacterial agents and granulocyte transfusions. Severe CMV infections are an important feature of bone marrow transplantation and are associated with graft-versus-host reactions as well as immunosuppressive therapy.

Solid organ transplant infections

Most infections occur within 3–4 months of transplantation

Suppression of a patient's cell-mediated immunity is necessary to prevent rejection of a grafted organ, and the cytotoxic regimens used usually suppress humoral immunity to some extent as well. In addition, high doses of corticosteroids to suppress inflammatory responses are required. The combination of these factors results in a severely compromised host, and those that have an effect on infection in recipients of solid organ transplants (e.g. kidney, heart, lung, liver) include:

OPPORTUNISTIC PATHOGENS IN NEUTROPENIC PATIENTS AND ORGAN TRANSPLANT RECIPIENTS
bacteria

Gram-positive
    Staphylococcus aureus
    coagulase-negative staphylococci
    streptococci
    Listeria spp.
    Nocardia asteroides
    Mycobacterium tuberculosis
    Mycobacterium avium-intracellulare

Gram-negative
    Enterobacteriaceae
    Pseudomonas aeruginosa
    Legionella spp.
    Bacteroides spp.

fungi
Candida spp. *Aspergillus* spp. *Cryptococcus neoformans* *Histoplasma capsulatum* *Pneumocystis jiroveci***
parasites
Toxoplasma gondii *Strongyloides stercoralis*
viruses
herpesviruses, e.g. HSV, CMV, VZV, EBV, HHV6, HHV7 hepatitis B hepatitis C polyomaviruses, e.g. BKV, JCV adenoviruses HIV*
*HIV has been transmitted via organ transplantation and   unscreened blood **formerly *P. carinii*

Fig. 30.10 Opportunistic pathogens in neutropenic patients and organ transplant recipients. (CMV, cytomegalovirus; EBV, Epstein–Barr virus; HHV, human herpes virus; HSV, herpes simplex virus; VZV, varicella-zoster virus.)

- the underlying medical condition of the patient;
- the patient's previous immune status;
- the type of organ transplant;
- the immunosuppressive regimen;
- the exposure of the patient to pathogens.

The organisms that cause the most common and most severe infections are shown in *Figure 30.10*. Some of the viral

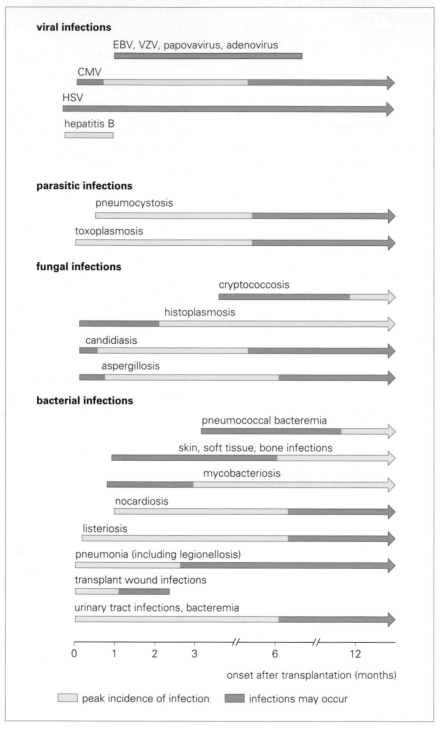

Fig. 30.11 This timetable shows the time of onset and peak incidence of infections in patients after renal transplantation. The patient is at risk of some infections, particularly hepatitis B and wound infections, for a limited period only, immediately post-transplant. Other infections may develop after several weeks of immunosuppression, but the majority constitute a risk throughout the period of immunosuppression. Note that *Pneumocystis jiroveci,* previously known as *Pneumocystis carinii* (pneumocystosis), is now thought to be a fungus. (CMV, cytomegalovirus; EBV, Epstein–Barr virus; HSV, herpes simplex virus; VZV, varicella-zoster virus.) (Adapted from Reese and Douglas, 1986.)

infections lie latent and reactivate when cell-mediated surveillance is suppressed.

From 3–4 months after transplantation the risk of infection is reduced, but remains for as long as the patient is immunosuppressed *(Fig. 30.11)*.

AIDS infections

The clinical definition of AIDS includes the presence of one or more opportunistic infections

People with AIDS are often infected concomitantly with multiple pathogens, which they fail to eradicate despite prolonged, appropriate and aggressive antimicrobial chemotherapy. Most of the pathogens involved are intracellular microbes that require an intact cell-mediated immune response for effective defense. As the HIV-infected individual progresses to AIDS (see Chapter 21), the immunodeficiency deepens and organisms that are usually controlled by cell-mediated immunity are able to reactivate to cause disseminated infections not seen in the immunologically normal individual.

Many of the pathogens that cause infections in the immunocompromised host (see *Fig. 30.10*) are described elsewhere in this book. Other opportunist pathogens are described in more detail below.

OTHER IMPORTANT OPPORTUNIST PATHOGENS

Fungi

Candida is the most common fungal pathogen in compromised patients

This yeast is an opportunist pathogen in a variety of patients and in various body sites. It is the cause of:

* vaginal and oral thrush (see Chapter 21);
* skin infections (see Chapter 26);
* endocarditis, particularly in drug addicts (see Chapter 29).

Candida manifests itself in different ways depending upon the nature of the underlying compromise:

* *Chronic mucocutaneous candidiasis.* This is rare and is a persistent but non-invasive infection of mucous membranes, hair, skin and nails in patients, often children, with a specific T cell defect rendering them anergic to *Candida (Fig. 30.12)*. It may be controlled by intermittent courses of ketoconazole.
* *Oropharyngeal and esophageal candidiasis.* This is seen in a variety of compromised patients, including people with ill-fitting dentures, diabetes mellitus or on antibiotics or corticosteroids, and now characteristically in people with HIV *(Fig. 30.13)*. Treatment with antifungal mouthwashes (nystatin or an azole compound) is recommended, particularly in the immunocompromised in whom the gastrointestinal tract probably serves as one of the routes for disseminated disease (see below).
* *Gastrointestinal candidiasis.* This is seen in patients who have undergone major gastric or abdominal surgery and in those with neoplastic disease. The organism can pass through the intestinal wall and spread from a gastrointestinal focus. Antemortem diagnosis is difficult, and as many as 25% of patients do not have any symptoms in the early stages of disease. If there is dissemination from the gut, blood cultures may become positive and *Candida* antigens may be detectable in the serum. A high index of suspicion is required to initiate antifungal therapy early in these patients, but disseminated disease is often fatal.
* *Disseminated candidiasis.* This is probably acquired via the gastrointestinal tract, but also arises from intravascular catheter-related infections. Patients with lymphoma and leukemia are most at risk. Bloodborne spread to almost any

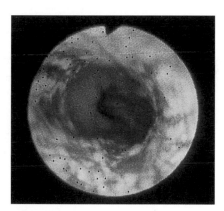

Fig. 30.13 *Candida* esophagitis. Endoscopic view showing extensive areas of whitish exudate. (Courtesy of I Chesner.)

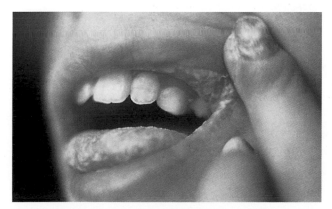

Fig. 30.12 Chronic mucocutaneous candidiasis in a child with impaired T cell response to antigens. (Courtesy of MJ Wood.)

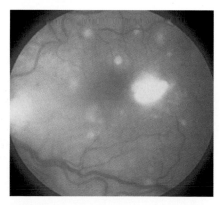

Fig. 30.14 *Candida* endophthalmitis. Fundal photograph showing areas of white exudate. (Courtesy of AM Geddes.)

organ can occur. Infections of the eye (endophthalmitis; *Fig. 30.14*) and the skin (nodular skin lesions; see Chapter 26) are important because they provide diagnostic clues, and without these the non-specific symptoms of fever and septic shock make early diagnosis difficult. Immuno-compromised patients are often given antifungal therapy 'blindly' if they have a fever and fail to respond to broad spectrum antibacterial agents *(Fig. 30.15)*.

Cryptococcus neoformans *infection is most common in people with impaired cell-mediated immunity*

C. neoformans is an opportunistic yeast with a worldwide distribution. It can cause infection in the immunocompetent host, but infection is seen more frequently in people with impaired cell-mediated immunity. The onset of disease may be slow and usually results in lung infection or meningo-encephalitis; occasionally other sites such as skin, bone and joints are involved (see Chapter 26).

C. neoformans can be demonstrated in the CSF and is characterized by its large polysaccharide capsule (see *Fig. 24.12*). Rapid identification can be made by antigen detection in a latex agglutination test using specific antibody-coated latex particles. Treatment involves a combination of amphotericin and flucytosine (see Chapter 33) and can be monitored by detecting a fall in CSF antigen concentration. The prognosis depends largely upon the patient's underlying disease; in the severely immunocompromised, mortality is approximately

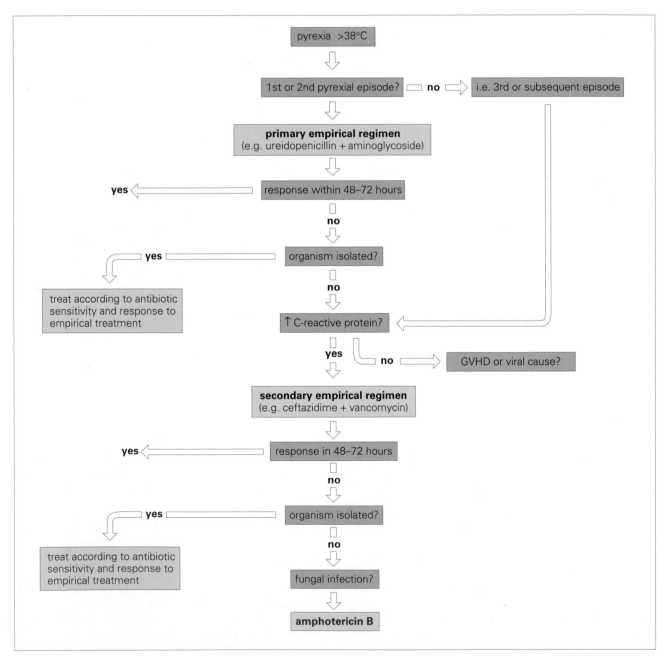

Fig. 30.15 Neutropenic patients succumb very rapidly to infections, and decisions to treat have to be made on an empiric basis. This figure shows one example of such a decision-making tree. (GVHD, graft-versus-host disease.) (Adapted from Rogers, 1989.)

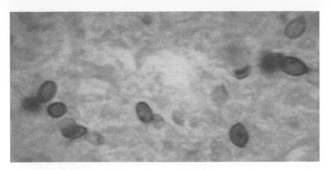

Fig. 30.16 Histologic section of the lung showing yeast forms of *H. capsulatum*. Methenamine silver stain. (Courtesy of TF Sellers, Jr.)

50%. In patients with AIDS it is almost impossible to eradicate the organism even with intensive treatment.

Disseminated Histoplasma capsulatum *infection may occur years after exposure in immunocompromised patients*

This is a highly infectious fungus that causes an acute but benign pulmonary infection in healthy people, but can produce a chronic progressive disseminated disease in the compromised host. The organism is endemic only in tropical parts of the world and notably in the so-called 'histo belt' of the central USA, particularly in the Ohio and Mississippi river valleys. The natural habitat of the organism is the soil. It is transmitted by the airborne route and the fungal spores are deposited in the alveoli, from whence the fungus spreads via the lymphatics to the regional lymph nodes. As disseminated disease may occur many years after the initial exposure in immunocompromised patients it may present in patients who have long since left endemic areas. The infection is also seen in people with HIV who have visited endemic areas.

Cultures of blood, bone marrow, sputum and CSF may yield *Histoplasma*, but biopsy and histologic examination of bone marrow, liver or lymph nodes is often required to make the diagnosis *(Fig. 30.16)*. Approximately 50% of cases of progressive disease in the immunocompromised are successfully treated with amphotericin.

Invasive aspergillosis is usually a fatal disease in the compromised patient

The role of *Aspergillus* spp. in diseases of the lung has been outlined in Chapter 19, but this fungus is now increasingly reported as a cause of invasive disease in compromised patients, usually in profoundly neutropenic patients or those receiving high dose corticosteroids *(Fig. 30.17)*. Like *Histoplasma*, aspergilli are found in soil, but have a worldwide distribution. Infection is spread by the airborne route, and the lung is the site of invasion in almost every case. Dissemination to other sites, particularly the central nervous system *(Fig. 30.18)* and heart, occurs in about 25% of compromised individuals with lung infection. Because of the ubiquitous nature of the fungus, diagnosis depends upon demonstrating tissue invasion, and this usually entails a lung biopsy.

Although invasive aspergillosis is usually fatal in the compromised patient, early diagnosis and institution of treatment—amphotericin is the drug of choice (see Chapter

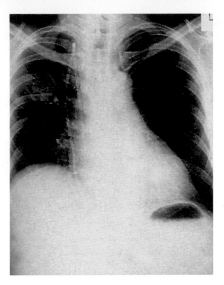

Fig. 30.17 Chest radiograph showing invasive aspergillosis in the right lung of a patient with acute myeloblastic leukemia. (Courtesy of C Kibbler.)

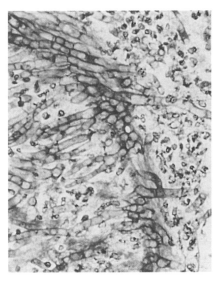

Fig. 30.18 Numerous septate hyphae invading a blood vessel wall in cerebral aspergillosis. Periodic acid–Schiff stain. (Courtesy of WE Farrar.)

33)—together with a reduction in corticosteroid and cytotoxic therapy wherever possible, appear to improve the prognosis. Outbreaks of hospital-acquired infection have been reported (see Chapter 36), especially in relation to recent building work.

Pneumocystis jiroveci *(formerly* P. carinii) *only causes symptomatic disease in people with deficient cellular immunity*

P. jiroveci is an atypical fungus which appears to be widespread, a large proportion of the population have antibodies to the organism, but it only causes symptomatic disease in people whose cellular immune mechanisms are deficient. There is therefore a high incidence of *P. jiroveci* pneumonia in patients receiving immunosuppressive therapy to prevent transplant rejection and in people with HIV. It is very rare to

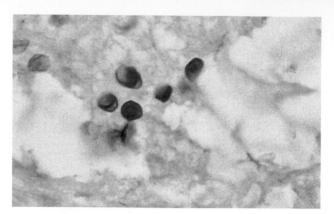

Fig. 30.19 Darkly staining cysts of *Pneumocystis jiroveci* in an open lung biopsy from an AIDS patient with pneumonia. Grocott silver stain. (Courtesy of M Turner-Warwick.)

find *Pneumocystis* infection in any other site in the body, but the reason for this is unknown.

Diagnosis is not easy and requires a high index of suspicion. The symptoms are non-specific and can mimic a variety of other infectious and non-infectious respiratory diseases. In addition, unlike the other fungi described above, the organism cannot be isolated in expectorated sputum using conventional culture methods, and invasive techniques such as bronchoalveolar lavage or open lung biopsy are required. In samples obtained by these techniques the organism can be demonstrated by silver or immunofluorescent stains *(Fig. 30.19)*. DNA amplification by the polymerase chain reaction improves the sensitivity of the diagnostic tests.

Treatment is with high dose co-trimoxazole (trimethoprim–sulfamethoxazole) or pentamidine (see Chapter 33), and co-trimoxazole has been used prophylactically with some success.

Bacteria

Nocardia asteroides *is an uncommon opportunist pathogen with a worldwide distribution*

The family Actinomycetes, relatives of the mycobacteria, but resembling fungi in that they form branching filaments, contain two pathogenic genera, *Actinomyces* and *Nocardia*. Actinomycosis is discussed in Chapter 22. *N. asteroides*

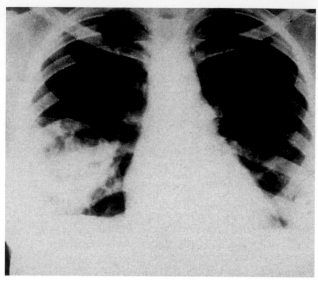

Fig. 30.20 Pulmonary nocardiosis. Chest radiograph showing a large rounded lesion in the right lower zone with multiple cavities. (Courtesy of TF Sellers, Jr.)

infections have been reported in the immunocompromised, especially in renal transplant patients. The lung is usually the primary site, but infection can spread to the skin, kidney or central nervous system *(Fig. 30.20)*. As with *Aspergillus*, hospital outbreaks of nocardiosis have been described.

Nocardia can be isolated on routine laboratory media, but is often slow to grow and is consequently easily overgrown by commensal flora. Therefore the laboratory staff should be informed if nocardiosis is suspected clinically, so that appropriate media are inoculated. The organism is a Gram-negative branching rod and weakly acid fast *(Fig. 30.21)*.

Sulfonamides or co-trimoxazole are the drugs of choice, but treatment can be difficult and various other regimens involving tetracycline, aminoglycosides or imipenem have been described.

Mycobacterium avium-intracellulare *disease is often a terminal event in AIDS*

Although mycobacterial infections are well documented in immunosuppressed patients, it is the association between

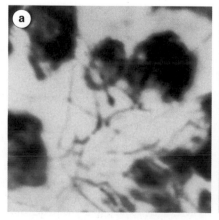
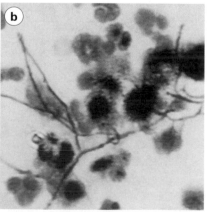

Fig. 30.21 *Nocardia asteroides* in sputum. (a) Acid-fast stain. (Courtesy of TF Sellers, Jr.) (b) Gram's stain. (Courtesy of HP Holley.)

AIDS and mycobacteria that is now most prominent. This includes disseminated infection with *Mycobacterium tuberculosis* and *Mycobacterium avium-intracellulare* (*Mycobacterium avium* complex or MAC), and these organisms can be isolated from blood cultures from patients with AIDS. *M. tuberculosis* has been described in detail in Chapter 19. *M. avium-intracellulare* belongs to the so-called 'atypical' mycobacteria or mycobacteria other than tuberculosis (MOTT). It resembles *M. tuberculosis* in that it is slow-growing, but it is resistant to the conventional antituberculous drugs. Multidrug therapy with combinations such as clofazimine or rifamycin derivatives together with macrolides such as azithromycin or clarithromycin, quinolones, isoniazid, ethambutol, cycloserine or pyrazinamide have been recommended.

Protozoa and helminths

Cryptosporidium and Isospora belli *infections cause severe diarrhea in AIDS*

Cryptosporidium (Fig. 30.22) is a protozoan parasite that causes human disease, and is well known to veterinarians as an animal pathogen. It causes significant but self-limiting diarrhea in healthy normal people (see Chapter 22), but severe and chronic diarrhea in people with AIDS. Effective treatment is difficult, but spiramycin is currently the first choice (see Chapter 33).

Isospora belli (Fig. 30.23) is a parasite very similar to *Cryptosporidium* and also produces severe diarrhea in people with AIDS. Unlike *Cryptosporidium*, however, it is susceptible to co-trimoxazole.

Immunosuppression may lead to reactivation of dormant Strongyloides stercoralis

Strongyloides stercoralis is a parasitic roundworm that remains dormant for years following initial infection, but may be reactivated to produce massive autoinfection in the immunosuppressed patient. Although rare in the UK and most of the USA, it should be borne in mind in patients who have lived in endemic areas such as the tropics and southern USA, even if this was many years before their immunosuppression.

Viruses

Certain virus infections are both more common and more severe in compromised patients, and regular surveillance is critical

The virus infections that are more common or more severe in the compromised patient (see *Fig. 30.10*) have been described in detail elsewhere in this book. Many of these represent reactivation of latent infections. Pre-transplantation baseline serology is carried out to determine both the donor and recipient status for a number of virus infections, including HIV, hepatitis B and C, CMV, EBV and HSV. Suppression of specific virus infections using antiviral agents is part of the management of the recipient in conjunction with regular virological surveillance post-transplantation using viral genome or antigen detection methods. As part of a pre-emptive treatment stategy, blood samples are collected for early detection of viremia or antigenemia which precedes disease. For example, transplant donors and recipients are

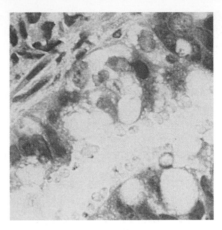

Fig. 30.22 Numerous organisms in the brush border of the intestine in cryptosporidiosis. (Courtesy of J Newman.)

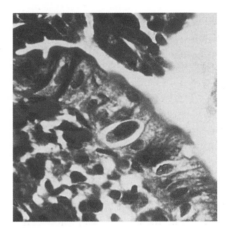

Fig. 30.23 Human coccidiosis, with a single *Isospora belli* organism within an epithelial cell and a chronic inflammatory reaction in the lamina propria. (Courtesy of GN Griffin.)

screened for CMV IgG. CMV causes a broad spectrum of clinical disease in this setting, including pneumonitis, esophagitis, colitis, hepatitis and encephalitis. If there is a transplant mismatch, i.e. the donor is CMV IgG positive and the recipient CMV IgG negative, the infection may be acquired from the donor organ or bone marrow. If possible, transplant centers try to avoid this situation, as the risk of a primary CMV infection in the first month post-transplantation is extremely high, as is the morbidity and mortality. In this case, CMV DNA or CMV antigen monitoring is carried out on blood samples on a regular basis post-transplantation to detect early infection and start antiviral therapy as soon as possible. Some centers offer antiviral therapy in the immediate post-transplant period in this clinical setting to delay the onset of infection to a time when the recipient is less immunosuppressed. CMV IgG positive recipients are at risk of reactivation or re-infection and will also be monitored regularly post-transplantation. Reactivation usually occurs at 8 to 12 weeks post-transplantation.

Antiviral prophylaxis for HSV reactivation is often given to bone marrow transplant recipients for prolonged periods post-transplantation. Episodes may be recurrent and generally occur in the immmediate post-transplantation period. Virus surveillance is therefore not carried out, but if a breakthrough infection occurs it is important to collect material from the lesions for virus isolation or genome sequence analysis to determine the antiviral susceptibility. Herpetic lesions can be persistent and involve the lips, esophagus and other parts of the gastrointestinal tract, and may cause a pneumonitis, hepatitis or encephalitis.

Herpes zoster, a reactivation of VZV infection, may occur within a few months post-transplantation, affecting the skin dermatome supplied by the involved nerve. Sometimes the distribution may be multidermatomal and dissemination can occur to other sites.

HHV6 and HHV7 infection, re-infection or reactivation have been reported in transplant recipients, in particular with neurologic conditions including encephalitis. HHV8 has been associated with the development of Kaposi's sarcoma (KS) in individuals with AIDS as well as classic and endemic KS in HIV-uninfected individuals.

EBV infection can lead to tumor development

EBV infection has been associated with the development of Hodgkin's disease, non-Hodgkin's lymphomas in individuals with HIV infection, post-transplantation lymphoproliferative disease and smooth-muscle tumors in immunosuppressed children. EBV-associated post-transplant lymphoproliferative disorder (PTLD) has a broad spectrum of clinical syndromes ranging from infectious mononucleosis to malignancies containing clonal chromosomal abnormalities with a high mortality rate, especially with the monoclonal tumors. The risk factors recognized for PTLD development in solid organ transplant recipients include post-transplantation primary EBV infection, mismatched donor and recipient CMV status, CMV disease, and intensity and type of immunosuppressive therapy. With respect to EBV infection, EBV-susceptible recipients have a 10–76-fold higher risk of PTLD compared with recipients with previous EBV exposure.

As the two peaks of primary EBV infection are in children and adolescents, the incidence of PTLD is higher in pediatric transplant recipients. The prevalence of PTLD in pediatric liver transplant recipients ranges from 4% to 14% depending on the immunosuppressive regimen. Retrospective studies have shown that up to 50% of pediatric transplant recipients with primary EBV infections are at risk of developing PTLD. The infection may be acquired in the community or, in the transplant setting, from the donor organ or blood products. The natural history of EBV infection and pathophysiology of post-transplant EBV-driven lymphoproliferation is not well understood. Diagnostic criteria for EBV-associated PTLD have been developed. However, in the absence of randomized, placebo-controlled trials, there is little information on the efficacy of specific treatment protocols. A number of investigations of the treatment of post-transplant lymphomas by adoptive transfer of EBV-specific cytotoxic T lymphocytes have been reported.

Adenovirus infection has a high mortality rate

Primary and reactivated adenovirus infections can result in disseminated disease in immunocompromised hosts, in particular pediatric and adult bone marrow transplant recipients. Hepatitis and pneumonia are most frequently reported. Again, adenovirus surveillance is often carried out in centers by collecting blood samples post-transplantation which are tested for adenovirus DNA in order to detect early viremia. Where adenovirus viremia is detected, management options include reducing immunosuppression and treating with an antiviral agent such as ribavirin or cidofovir. However, there are few reports of successful outcomes.

Hepatitis B infection may be detected after engraftment

Hepatitis B virus infection has an immunopathological basis, with jaundice occurring after cytotoxic T cells have lysed the hepatitis B surface-antigen-bearing hepatocytes. Therefore, bone marrow transplant recipients with an acute HBV infection (or reactivation in those with evidence of previous HBV exposure) pre-transplantation become symptomatic after engraftment. Hepatitis C virus infection is associated with veno-occlusive disease in bone marrow transplant recipients.

Polyoma viruses can cause hemorrhagic cystitis and progressive multifocal leukoencephalopathy

Polyomavirus infections, by BK or JC viruses, acquired via the respiratory tract and latent in the kidney, are often detected in the urine of bone marrow transplant recipients (see Chapter 20). They are often asymptomatic, although BK viruria is associated with hemorrhagic cystitis. JC virus, which can reactivate and disseminate to cause progressive multifocal leukoencephalopathy in people with AIDS, is less commonly seen since the advent of highly active antiretroviral therapy.

KEY FACTS

- A compromised person is one whose normal defenses against infection are defective. Immunodeficiences may involve the innate or adaptive immune systems and may be primary or secondary.

- Compromised patients can be infected with any of the pathogens capable of infecting immunocompetent individuals. In addition they suffer many infections caused by opportunist pathogens. The type of infection is related to the nature of the compromise.

- Effective antimicrobial therapy is often difficult to achieve in the absence of a functional immune response, even when the pathogen is susceptible to the drug in vitro.

- Important bacterial opportunists include *P. aeruginosa*, especially in neutropenic patients and those with major burns, and *Staph. epidermidis* in patients with plastic devices in situ. In AIDS the predominant bacterial opportunists are intracellular pathogens benefiting from the lack of cell-mediated immunity.

- AIDS, and neutropenia (particularly following cytotoxic therapy), predispose to fungal infections (e.g. *Candida*, *Aspergillus* and *Cryptococcus*) especially when the patient has received previous antibacterial therapy.

- Viral infections are more common and severe in immunodeficient patients than in normal patients, particularly reactivation of latent infections (e.g. herpes simplex virus, CMV, JC virus).

QUESTIONS

A 24-year-old man with HIV visits his doctor with a 6-week history of recurrent and worsening headaches. His CD4 count is 80/mm^3 and he has been well since being diagnosed as HIV1 seropositive in 1987. On examination he has no focal neurologic signs and fundoscopy is normal. He has oral candidiasis. A computerized tomographic head scan is normal, and a lumbar puncture is performed. The results are: CSF appearance, clear; white cells, 150/mm^3, predominantly lymphocytic;

CSF glucose, 2.2 mmol/l; blood glucose, 3.8 mmol/l; protein, 0.4 g/dl.

1. What is the most likely diagnosis, and what diagnostic tests would you perform?

2. What other confirmatory investigations might you ask for?

3. How would you manage him?

FURTHER READING

Brostoff J, Scadding GK, Male D, Roitt IM. *Clinical Immunology.* London: Mosby International, 1991.

Gemmell CG, McCartney AC. Coagulase-negative staphylococci within the hospital environment. *Rev Med Microbiol* 1990; 1:213–18.

Orr KE, Gould FK. Infection problems in patients receiving solid organ transplants. *Rev Med Microbiol* 1992; 3:96–103.

Reese RE, Douglas RG, eds. A *Practical Approach to Infectious Diseases.* Baltimore/Toronto: Little, Brown & Co, 1986.

Rogers TR. Management of septicaemia in the immunocompromised with particular reference to neutropenic patients. In: Shanson DC, ed. *Septicaemia and Endocarditis.* Oxford: Oxford Medical Publications, 1989.

Diagnosis and control

5

31. Strategies for control—an introduction   *441*

32. Diagnosis of infection and assessment of host defense mechanisms   *453*

33. Attacking the enemy: antimicrobial agents and chemotherapy   *473*

34. Vaccination   *513*

35. Passive and non-specific immunotherapy   *539*

36. Hospital infection, sterilization and disinfection   *545*

INTRODUCTION

Infectious diseases can be controlled by drugs, immunization and a 'healthy' environment

One of the great achievements of applied medical research has been its success in controlling so many infectious diseases; smallpox has been eradicated and other infections are now controlled effectively in many parts of the world. This control has been accomplished in three main ways:

- by the use of drugs (chemotherapy);
- by vaccines (immunization);
- by improving the environment (e.g. better sanitation, nutrition) *(Fig. 31.1)*.

In general, chemotherapy is used to control infectious diseases in individuals, whereas immunization and environmental improvements are used for control in populations. Understanding the ways in which these diseases arise, spread and can be controlled requires detailed epidemiologic studies to provide an accurate basis for assessment of risks and for planning intervention. These studies are based on knowledge of the infectious agents and their patterns of association with their hosts, but require the collection and analysis of data, in conjunction with the use of mathematical models, to produce useful pictures of disease transmission and control. Where the causal links between a clinical condition and an infectious agent or its mode of transmission are unknown, epidemiologic investigations can establish this link and thus determine appropriate control strategies.

EPIDEMIOLOGIC CONSIDERATIONS

Understanding the biology of the infectious agent—microparasites and macroparasites

Microparasites reproduce directly within the host and are typically transient

Microparasites (viruses, bacteria, fungi and protozoans) reproduce directly within the host, often at very high rates. They are usually small and have a short generation time. Recovery from infection usually gives immunity against re-infection, in the case of viral infections this may be lifelong. With some important exceptions (e.g. herpes, HIV), the duration of infection is short relative to the lifespan of the host. Microparasitic infections are, therefore, typically transient.

In defining the epidemiology of these diseases, and to describe how infections flow through a host population, it is useful to divide hosts into four classes of individuals: (1) susceptible; (2) infected but latent (i.e. non-infectious); (3) infected and infectious; (4) recovered and immune *(Fig. 31.2)*. The *incubation period* (time between infection and disease), the *latent period* (time between infection and infectiousness) and the generation time (the sum of the latent and infectious periods) are also useful *(Fig. 31.3)*. In some infections, infectiousness may be intermittent (e.g. herpes viruses), or vary widely throughout the incubation period

(e.g. HIV). Average latent and infectious periods of some common microparasitic infections are listed in *Figure 31.4*.

Macroparasites do not reproduce directly within the host and are typically not transient

Macroparasites (helminths and arthropods) do not reproduce directly within the host, but produce transmission stages that pass to the exterior to complete the lifecycle. They are typically large, and their generation times can often be a significant fraction of the host's lifespan. Immunity tends to be of a relatively short duration once the parasites are removed, and hosts may be continually re-infected.

The spread of infection is related to the reproductive rate of the infectious agent

The reproductive rate of an organism provides a useful measure of its biological success. Because microparasites in the body cannot be counted accurately the basic reproductive rate of a microparasite, R_0, is defined as the average number of secondary cases of infection produced by one primary case in a completely susceptible population, and is also referred to as the *case reproductive rate* or the *transmission potential*. For macroparasites, where numbers can be counted, R_0 is the average number of female offspring produced throughout the lifetime of a mature female.

These definitions apply to infections in idealized situations where the host population is completely susceptible, but this

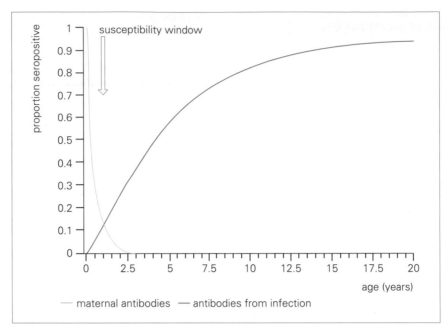

Fig. 31.6 An age-stratified serologic profile recording the presence or absence of antibodies specific to the antigens of a directly transmitted childhood viral infection (average age at infection is 5 years). There is a susceptibility window between the decay in maternally derived antibody and the rise in seroprevalence due to infection.

Influence of behavior on the spread of infection

For an infection—except a sexually transmitted disease—to take hold, the density of susceptible people must exceed a critical value

Transmission of directly transmitted infections requires contact between susceptible and infectious persons. The degree of contact is determined by the density of susceptible people in the community, which must exceed a critical value that can be calculated. This concept clarifies the target vaccination cover for mass campaigns, which should aim to reduce the density of susceptibles below this value.

R0 of sexually transmitted diseases (STDs) depends upon the average rate of acquisition of new sexual partners

Behavioral factors are of particular importance for STDs such as gonorrhea or HIV infection since the rate at which individuals acquire different sexual partners varies *(Fig. 31.8).* R_0 can be greatly influenced by the variance in sexual activity. Those who have many sexual partners are both more likely to acquire and to transmit infection and play a key role in the persistence of such infections in the community of sexually active individuals. People with many sexual partners are therefore an obvious target for treatment and education about safer sex practices.

Transmission between groups

Patterns of population mixing are important in designing policies to control infection. Intensity of transmission will

AVERAGE AGE AT INFECTION FOR DIFFERENT INFECTIONS IN DIFFERENT LOCALITIES		
infectious disease	**average age at infection A (years)**	**source of data**
measles	5–6	USA, 1955–58
	4–5	England and Wales, 1948–68
	1–2	Thailand, 1967
	2–3	India, 1978
rubella	9–10	Sweden, 1965
	9–10	Manchester, UK, 1970–82
	2–3	Gambia, 1976
	6–7	Poland, 1970–88
varicella	6–8	USA, 1921–28
poliomyelitis	12–17	USA, 1955
pertussis	4–5	England and Wales, 1948–68
	4–5	USA, 1920–60
mumps	6–7	England and Wales, 1975–77
	6–7	Netherlands, 1977–79

Fig. 31.7 Average age at infection *(A)* for different infections at different localities before widescale immunization.

LESSONS IN MICROBIOLOGY

The science of epidemiology

Epidemiology is the study of the occurrence, spread and control of diseases. It is based upon the collection of detailed statistical information and can be undertaken at several levels, from the purely descriptive to the analytical and experimental, in which mathematical modeling plays an increasingly important part. Epidemiologic data can be used to record the diseases affecting a population and, where infectious, to identify their causes and modes of transmission. They can also be used to predict the future likelihood of infection, to identify risk factors, and to plan control programs.

Like all sciences, epidemiology has its own jargon and specialized use of terms

Infection is the term used to indicate the presence of an infectious organism in an individual or population. The term *disease* is used only when infection has detectable clinical consequences, whether mild or severe. The time interval between exposure to infection and appearance of disease is the *incubation period.* Individuals who are infected and can transmit infection to others are *infectious.* Infectiousness may persist after disease has disappeared, the individuals concerned being known as *carriers.* The carrier state may also occur without disease ever having been apparent. Spread of infection—*transmission*—occurs in many ways, but depends upon direct or indirect contact between infectious individuals and individuals who are susceptible (see Chapter 13).

Infection may lead to an acquired immunity, and immune individuals are then often *resistant* to further infection.

In populations, infection or disease is described as *endemic* if it occurs regularly at low or moderate frequency, or *hyperendemic* if frequency is high. *Epidemics* occur when there are sudden increases in frequency above endemic levels; *pandemics* are global epidemics. *Prevalence* describes the number of cases of infection or disease in members of a population, either at a given point in time (*point* prevalence) or over a given period (*period* prevalence). *Seroprevalence* refers to the number of individuals who are antibody positive for a particular infection. The appearance of such antibodies in individuals is called *seroconversion. Incidence* refers to the number of new cases arising in a population over a defined period of time. *Age-specific* prevalence or incidence refers to infection or disease within particular age groups. Prevalence and incidence may show periodic fluctuations or trends over time (often referred to as longitudinal trends).

Secular trends are long-term changes over periods of years, whereas *periodic* trends are shorter term (months to a few years). *Seasonal* trends are annual or monthly changes, reflecting climatic or behavioral factors, and acute trends are those that result in epidemic outbreaks.

Descriptive epidemiologic data can be collected during outbreaks or collected subsequently

The more complete the data, the more fruitful analysis is likely to be. Accordingly, it is necessary to record not only data relating to the infection itself, but also demographic, geographic, climatic, socioeconomic, behavioral and personal data. Division or *stratification* of a population by such parameters is a useful way of seeing whether infection is associated with particular characteristics.

Analytical epidemiology uses two basic approaches: case control and cohort studies

Case control studies are *retrospective*, taking a group in which infection or disease is present and comparing with a matching control group in which it is absent in order to identify cause and effect. Cohort studies are normally *prospective.* They monitor the appearance of infection or disease in carefully defined groups over a prolonged period. Again, comparison with a control group is used to identify cause and effect. A third form of analysis is *epidemiologic investigation*, the study of epidemics as they occur. This involves collection of all relevant data in an attempt to identify the infectious agent and its transmission and to define control measures.

Experimental epidemiology applies epidemiologic methods to experimental systems

Such experimental systems include drug or vaccine trials, in which individuals with or without disease, or exposed or non-exposed to infectious agents, are given specific therapy, and the results compared with those of individuals given placebos or alternative therapy. Experimental epidemiology requires detailed statistical planning and analysis.

Mathematical modeling is a powerful tool in epidemiology

Mathematical modeling of infection and disease in populations is applied in descriptive, analytical and experimental epidemiology and is a powerful interpretive as well as a predictive tool with very wide applicability to disease control.

LESSONS IN MICROBIOLOGY

Surveillance

In many countries, public health authorities carry out continuing epidemiologic surveys of particular diseases in the national population (e.g. the Centers for Disease Control (CDC) of the US Public Health Service, and the Communicable Diseases Surveillance Centres (CDSC) of the Health Protection Agency in the UK). The World Health Organization performs a similar role internationally. At a national level, surveillance is often based on notifiable diseases, practitioners being obliged to report these diseases when they occur in their patients (*morbidity* data). Surveillance records can also be taken from notified causes of death (*mortality* data), from reports sent in by diagnostic laboratories, from population surveys and from detailed case investigations. Such data are then published regularly, for example in the *American Morbidity and Mortality Weekly Report* (MMWR) and the weekly *UK Communicable Diseases Report* (CDR), so that the medical community is alerted to trends in patterns of disease, and recommendations for control are made quickly and efficiently.

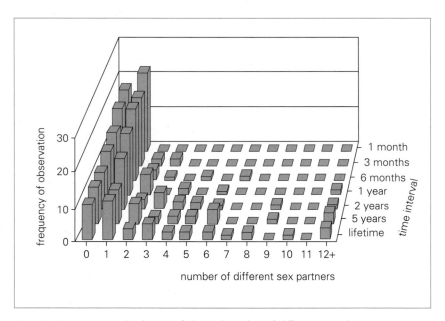

Fig. 31.8 Frequency distribution of claimed number of different sexual partners over various time periods (1 month to lifetime) recorded in a survey of male and female students in 1987 in the UK.

differ within different groupings but, equally importantly, contact between groups can also play a key role in determining patterns of infection and disease. In these circumstances, R_0 will be influenced by the likelihood of an individual in one group making contact with someone in the same group or in another group. Different patterns of mixing are of great importance in the design of policies for the control of infection.

Patterns of mixing are influenced by the timing of school terms and vacations

For directly transmitted infections such as measles, rubella, mumps and pertussis, high rates of transmission can occur among young children attending primary or secondary schools (5–15-year-olds), and this age group serves to seed infection via family contacts to younger and older persons. In countries with a generally high level of vaccination coverage in children, pockets of infection persist in poor communities or ethnic minorities in major urban centers with low rates of vaccine uptake. Targeting vaccination at children before they enter primary school, and at young children in poor urban centers, is an effective way of minimizing between-group transmission.

Changes in incidence of infection

Many common directly transmitted viral and bacterial infections show regular peaks in incidence

Epidemiologic data accumulated over many years make it possible to measure the mean *inter-epidemic period* (the time interval between major peaks in incidence). A striking feature of many common directly transmitted viral and bacterial infections is the regularity of such peaks in incidence. They are usually of two kinds:

- seasonal (e.g. the effects of school terms and vacations on childhood infections);
- longer term. Before mass vaccination, the longer term inter-epidemic period for measles in the UK was 2 years whereas for pertussis it was 3–4 years (Fig. 31.9 and see Chapter 34).

These intervals are determined by interactions between the infectious agent and its host, generating fluctuations in the value of R, below and above unity. At the start of an epidemic cycle the infectious agent spreads rapidly. As the susceptible pool is depleted the value of R falls below unity and incidence begins to decline. This continues until the pool of susceptibles is replenished by new births, the density of susceptibles eventually rising to a level sufficient to trigger the next epidemic.

Transmission success

The transmission success of an infection will vary between communities because of differences in demography (net birth rate) and behavior (patterns of mixing). For example, the inter-epidemic period for measles in large urban centers in Africa or India before the introduction of mass vaccination was often 1 year. In contrast, in the UK and the USA the period was typically 2 years. The difference is a direct reflection of difference in the average age at infection (Fig. 31.7). Mass vaccination acts to increase the average age at infection. The implications of this are discussed in Chapter 34, but one consequence is an increase in the inter-epidemic period (Fig. 31.9). Therefore mass vaccination not only alters the incidence of infection, but affects the age distribution of cases and the pattern of fluctuations.

DETECTION AND DIAGNOSIS

Understanding the epidemiology of an infection can help to define the correct strategies for control at the population level. However this understanding, and decisions about control, both depend heavily upon the the ability to recognize outbreaks of disease, to follow their progress and to identify the causative organism concerned. Detection and diagnosis are therefore key activities here as they are for treatment of infection at the level of the individual.

Descriptive epidemiology involves asking questions about an outbreak of disease that will help to identify the pathogen and the source of infection. It is important to have a *case definition*, which includes the symptoms of the disease as well as details of the individuals involved and the timing of events. Analysis of these data should make it possible to say where and how the outbreak has arisen, who is at risk and what treatment is necessary to control further infection (see panel on legionnaires' disease for an example). Measures used may involve antibiotic treatment of those immediately affected, or vaccination if a large number are at risk (e.g. the meningitis outbreaks in UK university students). For sexually transmitted disease (see above) an important element of detection is to establish contact patterns, or mixing matrices, so that individuals who may acquire an infection can be treated and further transmission prevented.

This approach to outbreaks of known or new disease follows their chance discovery as a result of clinical observations, exemplified by the discovery of AIDS in 1981 through the increased occurrence of *Pneumocystis carinii* (now known as *Pneumocystis jiroveci*) infection and of Kaposi's sarcoma in homosexual males. A more systematic approach to detection relies on a regular notification system—a surveillance system that routinely records episodes of a number of legally notifiable diseases. Such systems operate nationally through government or federal health organizations as well as internationally through the World Health Organization for diseases such as cholera, yellow fever and plague. Regular monitoring of this kind makes it easier to identify outbreaks, because it provides the baseline against which 'the occurrence of cases in excess of expectancy' (the definition of an epidemic) can be measured.

Once outbreaks of infectious disease have been detected, the pathogen concerned can be identified by conventional diagnostic procedures (see Chapter 32) to ensure that the appropriate antibiotic or vaccination is given.

CHEMOTHERAPY VERSUS VACCINATION

The concept of selectivity—or specificity—is central to both chemotherapy and vaccination

Although they appear so different (Fig. 31.10), both chemotherapy and vaccination developed together from the intensive study that followed the demonstration in the late

infectious disease	inter-epidemic period *T* (years)	source of data
measles	2 1 1	England and Wales, 1948–68 Yaounde, Cameroun, 1968–75 Ilesha, Nigeria, 1958–61
rubella	3–5	Manchester, UK, 1961–83
mumps	3	England and Wales, 1960–80
poliomyelitis	3–5	England and Wales, 1948–82
pertussis	3–4	England and Wales, 1948–85

INTER-EPIDEMIC PERIOD OF SOME COMMON INFECTIONS

Fig. 31.9 Inter-epidemic period (T) of some common infections, at different localities.

LESSONS IN MICROBIOLOGY

LEGIONNAIRES' DISEASE—A CASE STUDY

Background

War veterans of the Pennsylvania American Legion held their convention at a hotel in Philadelphia on July 21–24 1976. By early August an outbreak of severe pneumonia (cause unknown) among participants was reported. Deaths occurred despite antibiotic treatment.

Case definition

- Attendance at the convention or presence at the hotel between July 1st and August 18th.
- Onset between those dates of cough, fever, verified pneumonia.

182 patients met this definition, of whom 149 had attended the convention and 9 had been at the hotel for other conventions in the time period. An additional 39 patients had the clinical condition, but had not been in the hotel. They had, however, been within one block of the hotel in the relevant time period.

The epidemic

Cases appeared in late July, peaking between the 25th and 27th. 78% of the cases were male, most were older than 50. The incubation period was between 2 and 10 days. A significant proportion of cases had spent time in the lobby or stood outside the hotel to watch the parade. There was no significant person-to-person spread.

Conclusion

The evidence pointed to an airborne infectious agent, most likely acquired in the hotel lobby or immediately outside, entering the body via respiration. Initially, although the clinical evidence suggested a bacterial infection (large numbers of neutrophils in the sputum) no organisms could be demonstrated. *Legionella,* a previously unknown bacterium (see p. 223) was isolated and identified shortly afterwards. Erythromycin was found to be effective. The biology of *Legionella* pointed to control through disinfection and high temperature treatment of water supplies and air-conditioning plant.

1800s that diseases could be caused by microbes. Pasteur (see *Fig. 31.11*) showed that killed or weakened microbes (e.g. anthrax, rabies) could be used to induce immunity that was active against that disease, while Ehrlich's work with histologic dyes led him to the idea that particular chemicals ('drugs') might bind specifically to particular microbial structures and damage them, thus being active against several diseases (see Chapter 33). Both therefore established the concept of selectively or specifically targeting infectious organisms within the body as a means of controlling disease.

The specificity of an antimicrobial drug resides in its ability to damage the microbe and not the host

Antimicrobial drugs should ideally bind to a molecule present only in the microbe to ensure specificity for the microbe and not the host (see also Chapter 33). The extent to which this can be achieved varies from microbe to microbe. Bacteria, with their prokaryotic cell structure, are much more remote from humans than fungi, protozoa or worms (which are all eukaryotic). It is not surprising, therefore, that the most effective antibiotics are generally those used against bacteria. There are four major sites in the bacterial cell that are sufficiently different from human cells that they can be targeted by antimicrobial agents. These are:

- the cell wall;
- the bacterial ribosome;

CHEMOTHERAPY AND VACCINES COMPARED		
	chemotherapy	**vaccination**
specificity	usually high	very high
toxicity	potentially high	usually low
duration of effect	usually short	usually long
duration of treatment	may be prolonged	usually short, but may need boosting
effectiveness	bacteria: high viruses ⎤ fungi ⎬ moderate parasites ⎦	viruses: high bacteria ⎤ fungi ⎬ low/ parasites ⎦ moderate

Fig. 31.10 Comparison of chemotherapy and vaccination.

- the nucleic acid synthetic pathway;
- the cell membrane (*Fig. 31.12*).

Many antimicrobial agents are products of microbes themselves or derivatives of these products. It is presumed that they form part of the self-preservation mechanism by

LESSONS IN MICROBIOLOGY

Louis Pasteur (1822–1895)

The science of microbiology was established in the 19th century by the work of many distinguished scientists. However one such scientist, Louis Pasteur, may legitimately be regarded as a founding father of this discipline *(Fig. 31.11)*. He, along with Robert Koch, a German doctor (see Chapter 12), was able to show that living organisms or 'microbes' were the cause of disease, and provided a firm scientific basis for their study and control.

Pasteur began work at a time when spontaneous generation was still an accepted explanation for the appearance of microorganisms in decaying material. His elegant experiments showed that sterile organic infusions would not putrify or ferment if there was no subsequent contact with airborne contaminants,

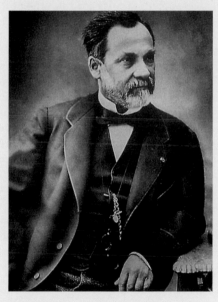

Fig. 31.11 Louis Pasteur (1822–1895).

proving that spontaneous generation did not occur, and that all microbes must come from pre-existing microbes. This discovery contributed to many fields of science, both basic and applied. Perhaps most important was the contribution Pasteur made to the work of Lister on antiseptics, which revolutionized approaches to surgery.

Pasteur worked in an amazing variety of microbiologic fields, from fermentation in the brewing of beers and production of wines, to identification of silkworm diseases, bringing to each a penetrating scientific insight and making discoveries that brought him national and international reknown. His understanding of the roles of organisms in causing diseases, and his acute scientific perception, enabled him to grasp from a series of 'mishaps' with experiments on chicken cholera that attenuated microbes could induce not disease, but immunity from disease. His ideas generated powerful opposition, but his belief then was strong enough to encourage him in 1881 to take part in a public trial of his vaccine against anthrax in domestic animals. Later, he used his insight into rabies, caused by organisms he could not see or culture, to develop an attenuated vaccine made from the dried spinal cords of infected rabbits. This was proven effective in humans in 1885 when Pasteur inoculated Joseph Meister, a 9-year-old boy who had been badly bitten by a rabid dog. Meister survived, and Pasteur's views on vaccination became universally accepted.

Pasteur ended his life as a national hero in his native France, and with a worldwide reputation for his work. His name is immortalized not only in the process of sterilization—'pasteurization'—that he developed, but in the Institut Pasteur in Paris, which remains one of the most important international centers of microbiologic work.

---

which the microbes prevent overcrowding with their own or other species.

Although it is possible to administer antimicrobial agents in ways that prolong their presence in the body, they are no longer active once concentrations fall below a critical threshold. Continuing antimicrobial activity therefore requires repeated administration.

The specificity of a vaccine depends upon the body's exquisite recognition of foreignness

The body has a battery of T and B lymphocyte receptors that can recognize almost any foreign antigen. Vaccine specificity therefore depends upon the introduction into the body of

molecules from the pathogen that can trigger responses against that organism but not against host tissues (see also Chapter 34). Once triggered, responses not only persist for some time, but the immune system will now remember its experience of the antigens concerned and the body will respond more actively if these are re-introduced as a consequence of infection. In contrast to chemotherapy, therefore, vaccination can give long term protection without readministration.

Both drugs and vaccines can have drawbacks

Although the specificity of antimicrobial compounds and vaccines should minimize problems with their use, neither

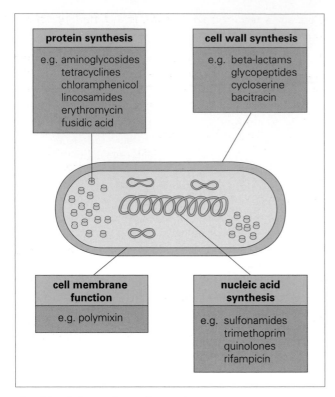

Fig. 31.12 Targets for antibacterial action.

is completely risk free. Incorrect use of antibiotics (e.g. overdosing) can give rise to acute toxicity, and prolonged treatment may produce a chronic toxicity. The ratio between the minimum dose level that has antimicrobial activity and the minimum dose to produce toxic effects in the host is termed the *therapeutic index*. The preferred drugs have a high index, i.e. are much more toxic to the pathogen than to the host. Antibiotics are relatively complex molecules and as such can become the target of immune responses. Hypersensitivity to drugs such as penicillin is relatively common (5–10% of the population) and can result in very severe consequences. Vaccines, likewise, can cause unexpected effects in certain individuals, generating immunologically-mediated side effects that can produce lasting damage, which is most severe if it affects the brain. For both vaccines and antibiotics, the element of risk is generally very small and has to be set against the much more serious and more probable consequences of the infections they are designed to treat.

Viruses have been particularly difficult targets for chemotherapy since so much of the viral lifecycle uses host components

However a few susceptible points do exist, notably the enzymes necessary for viral replication, and the development of aciclovir for herpesviruses (targeting DNA polymerase) and zidovudine (AZT, targeting reverse transcriptase) for HIV are excellent examples of tailor-made chemotherapy. Many virus infections, however, are successfully controlled by vaccination. Of those that are not, HIV remains the most pressing target.

Microbe resistance can develop to both drugs and vaccines

The development of resistance is, in effect, a change in balance in favor of the microbe, and affects both drugs and vaccines. It can occur in a variety of different ways, for example:

- Penicillin resistance is often due to the production of an enzyme, beta-lactamase, by the microbe. This enzyme breaks the penicillin beta-lactam ring.
- Chloroquine resistance in malaria is due to the development of a mechanism that pumps the drug out of the parasite at an increased rate.
- Resistance to the protective effects of vaccination by variants of influenza virus is due to small changes in the surface hemagglutinin and neuraminidase molecules.

Usually drugs have to be given regularly, while vaccines often have to be given only once

A major difference between drugs and vaccines is that drugs are designed to treat disease, and have to be given on a regular basis, whereas vaccines are designed to prevent it, and need to be given only a few times, often only once. There are, of course, exceptions to this: passive antibody can be used to treat acute infection just as a drug can, while drugs like pyrimethamine and chloroquine are used for prophylaxis against malaria almost as if they were short-term vaccines. However, in most cases there is a clear-cut distinction between the one- or two-shot vaccine, conferring protection for years, and the daily or twice-daily drug dose. Naturally, patients and doctors favor the former, whereas the pharmaceutical industry prefers the latter. Therefore, while drug development is carried out by industry without the need for external encouragement, vaccine development needs an outside stimulus in the form of earmarked funding—a field in which the World Health Organization, in particular, has performed with great distinction.

CONTROL VERSUS ERADICATION

Control and eradication are different objectives, although eradication is always an ideal endpoint

Many infections are controlled (at least in some parts of the world) by antimicrobial treatment or prevented by vaccination, but are certainly not eradicated, even in those countries where control is most effective. Epidemiologic theory predicts that once transmission rates fall below a threshold value the infection should die out, and this may certainly be true at a local levels. However, reservoirs of infection persist where treatment is non-existent or ineffective, or infection is re-introduced by the movement of peoples, and new epidemics may therefore develop. To date only one disease—smallpox—has been taken to the point at which the organism has been eliminated. What are the chances that other infectious diseases will follow smallpox into oblivion? Various factors are important in determining the effectiveness of any eradication program (*Fig. 31.13*).

FACTORS FAVORING GLOBAL ERADICATION OF AN INFECTIOUS DISEASE	
factor	**rationale**
disease limited to humans	no re-invasion by microbe from animal or arthropod host
no long term carrier state	no re-invasion by microbe from human carriers
cases easily recognized clinically	surveillance possible
one or few serotypes	a single vaccine is adequate
stable, cheap, effective vaccine available	worldwide program possible
eradication program is cost-effective	program likely to be undertaken

Fig. 31.13 Factors favoring global eradication of infectious disease. Smallpox fitted all categories, whereas some diseases pose problems with numbers of unrecognized cases (e.g. polio and rubella) and others with cost-effectiveness (e.g. measles and shigellosis).

Realism is required when considering the long term aims of control strategies

Hopes raised by the early success of antibiotics were soon dashed by the emergence of resistance, and far from the microbial load borne by the human race being diminished in recent years, it has if anything increased. Many infections covered in this book—HIV, legionnaires' disease, Lyme disease, cryptosporidiosis, to name but a few—do not feature in older textbooks of microbiology. Effective vaccines for some important infections remain elusive. Approaches to the control of infectious diseases is therefore a matter of identifying priorities such as:

- Which diseases could, with suitable effort, be eradicated?
- Would the cost of eradication be justified?
- Which diseases need urgent measures to stop them getting worse?
- Which diseases are responsible for the most human suffering and economic loss?

Inevitably, some diseases will not feature strongly on any such list, and it must be accepted that they may always be with us.

KEY FACTS

- Epidemiology contributes to the understanding of infection and disease in populations and assists approaches to treatment and control.

- Each parasite has a characteristic basic reproductive rate (R_0) that determines its ability to spread in fully susceptible populations. Many factors constrain R_0 and these determine the actual (effective) reproductive rate (R).

- Knowledge of the values for R_0 and R allow predictions about the spread of epidemics, the effectiveness of control measures and the implementation of vaccination programs.

- Different epidemiologic approaches are needed when dealing with infections caused by microparasites (e.g. viruses) and macroparasites (e.g. worms) and for diseases that are sexually transmitted.

- Detection and diagnosis are crucial activities for the identification and control of infectious diseases.

- Chemotherapy, vaccination and environmental measures all have their place in the control of infectious disease. The most appropriate measure for controlling an infectious disease will depend upon many factors, as described in Chapters 33–36.

QUESTIONS

1. What are the advantages and disadvantages of chemotherapy compared with vaccination?

2. An infection that appears suddenly and then spreads globally is termed:
   A. Epidemic
   B. Endemic
   C. Hyperendemic
   D. Pandemic
   E. Hypoendemic

3. The term basic reproductive rate (R_0) describes:
   A. The maximum reproductive rate of an infectious organism
   B. The reproductive rate achievable in real hosts in real situations
   C. The number of progeny of a pathogen produced before the disease is apparent clinically
   D. The reproductive rate required to produce clinical symptoms
   E. The reproductive rate of an infectious organism seen after vaccination

4. An important factor responsible for the differences in epidemiology between measles and HIV is:
   A. There is no vaccine against HIV
   B. Measles never affects adults
   C. Measles is transmitted by respired droplets
   D. The two infections are caused by different groups of viruses
   E. HIV infects lymphocytes

5. Which childhood disease has the shortest inter-epidemic interval?
   A. Rubella
   B. Measles
   C. Mumps
   D. Pertussis
   E. Poliomyelitis

6. Louis Pasteur was associated with:
   A. Vaccination against anthrax
   B. Fermentation in brewing
   C. Silkworm disease
   D. Vaccination against rabies
   E. All of these

FURTHER READING

Anderson RM, May RM. *Infectious Diseases of Humans: Dynamics and Control.* Oxford: Blackwell Scientific, 1992.

Giesecke J. *Modern Infectious Disease Epidemiology.* London: Edward Arnold, 1994.

Gordis L. *Epidemiology.* Philadelphia: WB Saunders, 1996.

Scott ME, Smith G. *Parasitic and Infectious Diseases: Epidemiology and Ecology.* New York: Academic Press, 1994.

Diagnosis of infection and assessment of host defense mechanisms

INTRODUCTION

Good quality specimens are needed for reliable microbiologic diagnoses

The precise identification of the causative organism in infection has become increasingly important now that therapeutic intervention is possible. The ability to achieve this depends upon a positive interaction between the clinician and the microbiologist; the clinician must be aware of the complexity of the tests and the time required to achieve a result. In turn, the microbiologist must appreciate the nature of the patient's condition and be able to assist the clinician in interpreting the laboratory report. A fundamental step in any diagnosis is the choice of an appropriate specimen, which ultimately depends upon an understanding of the pathogenesis of infections.

Microbiology differs from other clinical laboratory disciplines in the amount of interpretative input required. When a specimen is received, the microbiologist must decide on the appropriate processing pathway, and when the result is received it must be interpreted in relation to the specimen and the patient.

AIMS OF THE CLINICAL MICROBIOLOGY LABORATORY

The aims of the microbiology laboratory are:

- to provide accurate information about the presence or absence of microorganisms in a specimen that may be involved in a patient's disease process;
- where relevant, to provide information on the antimicrobial susceptibility of the microorganisms isolated.

Identification is achieved by detecting the microorganism or its products or the patient's immune response

Laboratory tests are carried out:

- to detect microorganisms or their products in specimens collected from the patient;
- to detect evidence of the patient's immune response (production of antibodies) to infection.

The tests fall into three main categories:

- *Identification of microorganisms by isolation and culture.* Microorganisms may grow in artificial media or, in the case of viruses, in cell cultures. In some instances, quantification is important (e.g. more than 10^5 bacteria/ml of urine is indicative of infection whereas lower numbers are not; see Chapter 20). Once an organism has been isolated in culture, its susceptibility to antimicrobial agents can be determined.
- *Identification of a specific microbial product.* Non-cultural techniques that do not depend upon the growth and multiplication of microorganisms to detect microorganisms have the potential to yield more rapid results. These techniques include the detection of structural components of the cell (e.g. cell wall antigens) and extracellular products (e.g. toxins). Alternatively, specific gene sequences can be detected by the application of DNA probes to clinical specimens. These techniques are becoming more widely used, especially with the possibilities for amplification of DNA by the polymerase chain reaction (PCR; see below). They are potentially applicable to all microorganisms, but antimicrobial susceptibilities cannot be determined without culture (although the presence of resistance genes may be detectable by specific probes).
- *Detection of specific antibodies to a pathogen.* This is especially important when the pathogen cannot be cultivated in laboratory media (e.g. *Treponema pallidum*, many viruses) or when culture would be particularly hazardous to laboratory staff (e.g. culture of *Francisella tularensis*, the cause of tularemia, or the fungus *Coccidioides immitis*). Detection of IgM and/or IgG antibodies in a single serum collected during the acute phase of illness can be helpful in diagnosis of, for example, rubella-specific IgM, hepatitis A IgM and hepatitis B surface antigen, or in rare diseases such as Lassa fever. The classic diagnostic method is by detection of a rise (four-fold or greater) in antibody titer between 'paired' sera, collected in the acute phase of an infection (5–7 days after onset of symptoms) and in convalescence (after 3–4 weeks). Such tests therefore tend to result in a delayed or retrospective diagnosis and are therefore of limited help.

SPECIMEN PROCESSING

Specimen handling and interpretation of results is based upon a knowledge of normal flora and contaminants

Specimens intended for cultivation of microorganisms can be divided into two types:

- those from sites that are normally sterile;
- those from sites that usually have a commensal flora (*Fig. 32.1*; see also Chapter 8).

A thorough knowledge of the microorganisms normally isolated from specimens from non-sterile sites, and the common contaminants of specimens collected from sterile sites, is important to ensure that specimens are properly handled and the results are correctly interpreted. Some specimens from sites that should be sterile (e.g. bladder urine, sputum from the lower respiratory tract) are usually collected after passage through orifices that have a normal flora, which may contaminate the specimens. This needs to be considered when interpreting the culture results of these specimens.

In an ideal world each specimen arriving in the laboratory would be considered in turn together with the information provided about the patient on the request form so that the microbiologist could assess the pathogens likely to be present and devise an 'individualized' processing plan. However, in reality this approach is not practicable because of constraints on time and money. Thus, specimens tend to be processed by type (e.g. urine, blood, feces) and the microbiologist looks for easily cultivated pathogens known to be associated with each sample type. However, if the laboratory is provided with suitable information, such as a statement of possible etiology, more fastidious or unusual pathogens can be sought and relevant antibiotic susceptibilities assessed. Additional information regarding the schemes used for the basic processing of specimens are outlined below and described in detail in the Appendix.

To obtain a test result that correctly identifies the infection, it is important to collect an appropriate specimen, to use the appropriate transport conditions and to deliver specimens rapidly to the laboratory. These conditions all affect the accuracy of the laboratory report, and therefore its value to the clinician and ultimately to the patient. Key points to remember about specimen collection are summarized in *Figure 32.2*.

Culture takes at least 18 hours to produce a result

Time is a key factor because the conventional methods of microbiologic diagnosis depend upon growth and identification of the pathogen. Results of culture cannot be achieved in less than 18 hours and may take much longer (e.g. several weeks) for a minority of pathogens such as the mycobacteria which grow very slowly. Thus specimen processing can be categorized according to the time required to achieve a result and the method—cultural or non-cultural. An alternative route to the diagnosis of an infection is an immunologic one, relying on the detection of an antibody response to the putative pathogen in the patient's blood. These diagnostic routes are summarized in *Figure 32.3*, but rapid technologies (e.g. PCR, nucleic-acid probes, microarrays, etc.) are having a major influence on this process.

SAMPLING SITES AND THE NORMAL FLORA
body sites that are normally sterile
blood and bone marrow
cerebrospinal fluid
serous fluids
tissues
lower respiratory tract
bladder
body sites that have a normal commensal flora
mouth, nose and upper respiratory tract
skin
gastrointestinal tract
female genital tract
urethra

Fig. 32.1 Sampling sites and interpretation of results. Some sites in the body are sterile in health so that growth of any organism is indicative of infection provided that the specimen has been properly collected and transported, and examined in the laboratory without delay. The significance of isolates from sites that have a commensal flora depends upon the identity of the isolate and the quantity, as well as the immune status of the patient.

AIDE-MEMOIRE FOR SPECIMEN COLLECTION
take the appropriate specimen; e.g. blood and cerebrospinal fluid in suspected meningitis
collect the specimen at the appropriate time, during the acute phase of the disease; e.g. malarial films, virus isolation, viral genome detection, IgM detection
if possible collect specimen before patient receives antimicrobials
collect enough material and an adequate number of samples, e.g. enough blood/serum for more than one set of blood cultures
avoid contamination (a) from normal flora; e.g. midstream urine (b) from non-sterile equipment
use the correct containers and appropriate transport media
label specimens properly
complete request form with enough clinical information and a statement of possible etiology
talk to the microbiologist and inform the laboratory if special tests are required
transport specimens rapidly to the laboratory

Fig. 32.2 Important steps in specimen collection and delivery to the laboratory. The responsibility of the clinician does not end with collection of the specimen and requesting tests. Good communication with the microbiologist is essential.

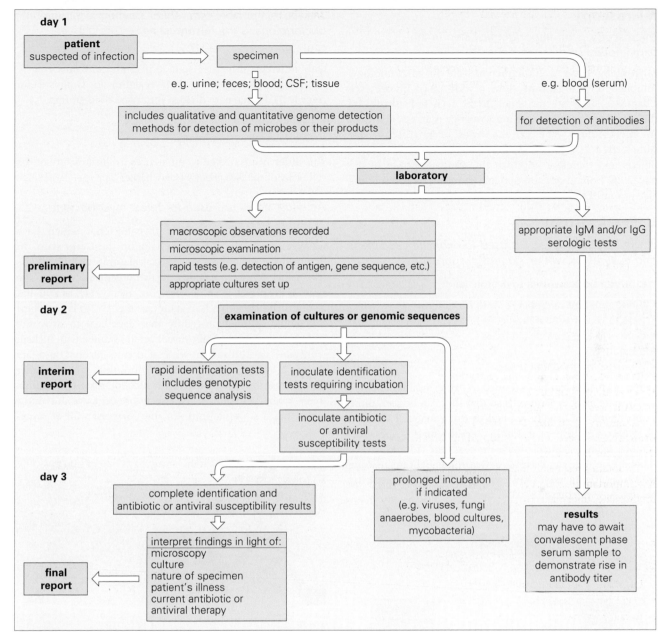

Fig. 32.3 Route from patient to microbiologic diagnosis. This scheme shows an overview of the key steps in specimen processing. Some tests can be performed on the specimen immediately and yield 'same day' results. Culture of specimens involves a minimum of 18 hours' incubation before colonies are visible and can be identified. Antibiotic susceptibility tests involve a further incubation period. Alternatively the diagnosis may be based on the detection of specific antibodies in serum samples. (CSF, cerebrospinal fluid.)

NON-CULTURAL TECHNIQUES FOR THE LABORATORY DIAGNOSIS OF INFECTION

Non-cultural techniques do not require microorganism multiplication before detection

Although medical microbiology has long been synonymous with the cultivation of microorganisms from patients' specimens, these techniques are labor-intensive and slow to produce results (days rather than hours) because replication of organisms is a necessary, but rate-limiting, step. In addi-

tion, some microorganisms cannot be cultured in artificial media, and viable organisms may be difficult to recover from specimens of patients who have received antimicrobial therapy. Non-cultural techniques do not require multiplication of the microorganism before its detection. Some techniques, such as microscopy and detection of microbial antigens in specimens, can provide very rapid results (i.e. within 2 hours). Other non-cultural methods such as the use of DNA probes and amplification of DNA by the polymerase chain reaction (PCR) may also provide a rapid answer in a matter of hours.

Microscopy

Microscopy is an important first step in the examination of all specimens

Microscopy plays a fundamental role in microbiology. Although microorganisms show a wide range in size (see Chapter 1) they are too small to be seen individually by the naked eye, and therefore a microscope is an essential tool in microbiology. The various types of microscopy are summarized in *Figure 32.4*. The light microscope magnifies objects and therefore improves the resolving power of the naked eye from about 100 000 nm (0.1 mm) to 200 nm; the electron microscope can improve this to 0.1 to 1.0 nm.

Light microscopy

Bright field microscopy is used to examine specimens and cultures as wet or stained preparations

Wet preparations are used to demonstrate:

- blood cells and microbes in fluid specimens such as urine, feces or cerebrospinal fluid (CSF);
- cysts, eggs and parasites in feces;
- fungi in skin;
- protozoa in blood and tissues.

Living organisms can be examined to detect motility.

Dyes are used to stain cells so that they can be seen more easily. Stains are usually applied to dried material that has been fixed (by heat or alcohol) onto the microscope slide. Samples from specimens themselves, or pure cultures can be stained. The slide can then be viewed in the light microscope with an oil immersion lens, which improves the resolving power of the microscope.

The most important differential staining technique in bacteriology is the 'Gram' stain

Differential staining procedures exploit the fact that cells with different properties stain differently and thus can be distinguished. Based on their reaction to Gram's stain (*Fig. 32.5*), bacteria are divided into two broad groups:

- Gram positive (stain purple);
- Gram negative (stain pink).

This difference is related to differences in the structure of the cell walls of the two groups (see Chapter 2).

Acid-fast stains are used to detect mycobacteria

Some organisms, particularly mycobacteria, which have waxy cell walls, do not readily take up the Gram stain. To demonstrate their presence, special staining techniques are used which rely on the ability of such organisms to retain the stain in the presence of 'decolorizing' agents such as acid and alcohol. The Ziehl–Neelsen stain (see *Fig. 19.24*) is a classical differential staining procedure that uses heat to drive the fuchsin stain into the cells; mycobacteria stained with fuchsin withstand decolorization with acid and alcohol and are therefore known as 'acid-' and 'alcohol-fast', whereas other bacteria lose the stain after acid and alcohol treatment. Alternatively, many laboratories use the fluorescent dye auramine, which has a strong affinity for the waxy cell wall of myco-

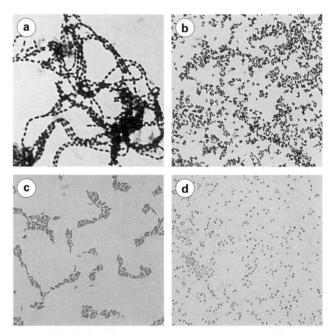

Fig. 32.5 The Gram stain is the most important stain for studying bacteria. The combination of the violet dye (crystal violet) and iodine (acting as a mordant) binds to the cell wall. Gram-positive cells retain the stain when challenged with acetone and remain purple. Gram-negative cells lose the purple stain and appear colorless until stained with a pink counterstain (neutral red or safranin). Examination of Gram-stained films also allows the shape of the cells to be noted. Some examples are shown: (a) Gram-positive cocci in chains (streptococci); (b) Gram-positive rods (*Listeria*); (c) Gram-negative rods (*Escherichia coli*); (d) Gram-negative cocci (*Neisseria*).

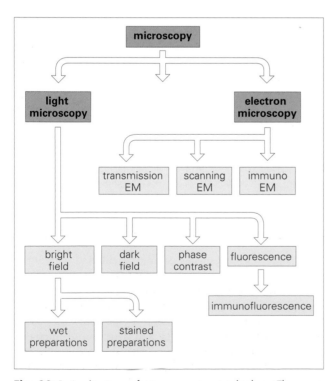

Fig. 32.4 Applications of microscopy to microbiology. The scheme shows the different uses of light and electron microscopy (EM) for looking at microbes.

bacteria, to demonstrate these organisms by fluorescence microscopy *(Fig. 32.6)*.

Other staining techniques can be used to demonstrate particular features of cells

Examples of such features to aid identification include the volutin (polyphosphate) storage granules in *Corynebacterium* spp. and lipid in *Bacillus* spp. *(Fig. 32.7)*. Protocols for these staining methods are given in the Appendix.

Dark field (dark ground) microscopy is useful for observing motility and thin cells such as spirochetes

The light microscope may be adapted by modifying the condenser so that the object appears brightly lit against a dark background. Living organisms can be examined by dark field microscopy and thus motility can be observed. The method is also used for visualizing very thin cells such as spirochetes because the light reflected from the surface of the cells makes

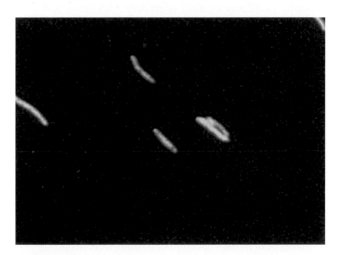

Fig. 32.6 Fluorochrome stain of *Mycobacterium tuberculosis* with a mixture of auramine O and rhodamine B. Mycobacteria appear fluorescent under ultraviolet light. (Courtesy of DK Banerjee.)

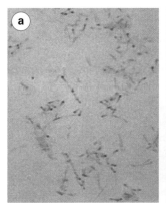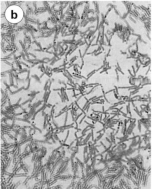

Fig. 32.7 Special staining techniques can be used to demonstrate particular features of bacterial cells. (a) Corynebacteria stained to demonstrate polymetaphosphate storage granules (volutin granules), which appear as dark spots in blue-green cells (Albert's stain). (b) Lipid storage granules in *Bacillus cereus* stained with Sudan black (black lipid against red cells).

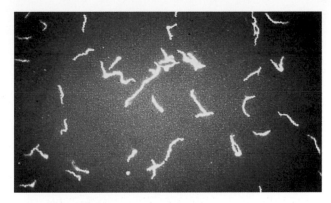

Fig. 32.8 Spirochetes visualized by dark ground microscopy. Spirochetes and leptospires are much thinner than most bacterial cells (approximately 0.1 μm diameter compared with 1 μm for *Escherichia coli*), but they appear larger when viewed by dark ground illumination.

them appear larger and therefore more easily visible than when examined by bright field microscopy *(Fig. 32.8)*.

Phase contrast microscopy increases the contrast of an image

This technique enhances the very small differences in refractive index and density between living cells and the fluid in which they are suspended and therefore produces an image with a higher degree of contrast than that achieved by bright field microscopy.

Fluorescence microscopy is used for substances that are either naturally fluorescent or have been stained with fluorescent dyes

If light of one wavelength shines on a fluorescent object, it emits light of a different wavelength. Some biological substances are naturally fluorescent; others can be stained with fluorescent dyes and viewed in a microscope with an ultraviolet light source instead of white light *(Fig. 32.6)*.

Fluorescence microscopy is widely used in microbiology and immunology and has been developed to detect microbial antigens in specimens and tissues by 'staining' with specific antibodies tagged with fluorescent dyes (immunofluorescence). The method can be made more sensitive or can be adapted to the detection of antibody by labeling a second antibody in an indirect test *(Fig. 32.9)*.

Electron microscopy

The specimen needs to be cut into thin sections for electron microscopy

The electron microscope uses a beam of electrons instead of light, and magnets are used to focus the beam instead of the lenses used in a light microscope. The whole system is operated under a high vacuum. Electron beams penetrate poorly, and a single microbial cell is too thick to be viewed directly. To overcome this the specimen is fixed and mounted in plastic and cut into thin sections, which are examined individually. Electron-dense stains such as osmium tetroxide, uranyl acetate or glutaraldehyde, are applied to the specimen to improve contrast. The electrons pass through the section

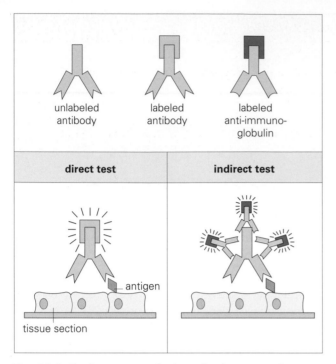

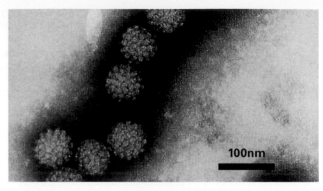

Fig. 32.10 Electron micrograph of papillomavirus, the human wart virus. (Courtesy of the Regional Virus Laboratory, Birmingham, UK.)

Fig. 32.9 The fluorescent antibody test for detection and identification of microbial (or tissue) antigens or antibodies directed against them. In the *direct* test, antibody labeled with a fluorescent dye is applied to a tissue section bearing the antigen, unbound antibody is washed away, and the bound antibody showing the presence and location of the antigen is visualized by fluorescence microscopy. In the *indirect* test, antigen is revealed by successive treatments with unlabeled antibody and then fluorescent-labeled anti-immunoglobulin which amplifies the signal (thus if the first antibody is human, the labeled antibody will be an anti-human Ig).

and produce an image on a fluorescent screen. Images are photographed and enlarged so that the original specimen is magnified many thousandfold *(Fig. 32.10)*.

Electron microscopy can be used to identify virus particles

Direct examination of specimens allows rapid identification of virus particles and detection of viruses that are difficult or impossible to cultivate (e.g. rotaviruses). Fluid for examination is dried onto a copper grid and examined. About one million virus particles per ml are needed if they are to be detectable. The sensitivity can be increased by reacting the fluid with antiviral antibody so that clumps of virus particles are visible. This is known as immunoelectron microscopy, a technique analogous to immunofluorescence in light microscopy.

Detection of microbial antigens in specimens

Detection of specific microbial antigens can be a more rapid method for detecting the presence of an organism than attempting to grow and identify the microbe. The methods include:

- those that detect antigens by their interaction with specific antibodies;
- those that detect microbial toxins.

They are summarized in *Figure 32.11*. Detection of microbial genes using DNA probes is discussed later in this chapter.

Specific antibody coated onto latex particles will react with the organism or its product, resulting in visible clumping

For example, the common causative agents of bacterial meningitis (*Streptococcus pneumoniae*, *Haemophilus influenzae* and *Neisseria meningitidis* types A and C) can be detected in CSF by mixing the specimen with specific antibody coated onto latex particles. If the antigen (i.e. the organism or its product) is present the particles will clump together *(Fig. 32.12)*. These tests give results within minutes of receipt of the specimen, but their sensitivity is not significantly greater than that of the Gram stain, and false positive results may occur because of cross-reacting antigens. However, they can be a useful diagnostic aid when the patient has received antibiotics and organisms may appear morphologically unidentifiable in the CSF and fail to grow in culture.

Immunoassay can be used to measure antigen concentration

Antigens can be measured by their binding to a standard amount of antibody, the fractional occupancy of the available antibody binding sites being a measure of the antigen concentration *(Fig. 32.13)*. Usually, the antibody is adsorbed for convenience to a solid phase and the amount of antigen bound assessed using a second antibody labeled with an enzyme *(Fig. 32.14)* or a fluorescent probe.

- The test employing an enzyme label is referred to as an enzyme-linked immunosorbent assay (ELISA).
- The use of chemiluminescent or time-resolved fluorescent labels gives assays of very high sensitivity.

Earlier forms of immunoassay used labeling with a radio-isotope rather than an enzyme or a fluorescent probe.

Monoclonal antibodies can distinguish between species and between strains of the same species on the basis of antigenic differences

Monoclonal antibodies *(Fig. 32.15)* are used as diagnostic tools. In direct ELISA (see above), enzyme-conjugated monoclonal

NON-CULTURAL TECHNIQUES
non-specific techniques for detection of microbial products fatty acid end-products of metabolism of anaerobes can be detected in fluid specimens (e.g. pus, blood) by gas liquid chromatography
antigen detection detection of soluble carbohydrate antigens by agglutination of antibody-coated latex particles or red blood cells (*Fig. 32.12*) e.g. *Streptococcus pneumoniae* capsule *Haemophilus influenzae* type b capsule ⎤ in CSF *Neisseria meningitidis* capsule ⎟ and urine *Cryptococcus neoformans* capsule ⎦ *Strep. pyogenes* group antigen in throat swabs
detection of particular antigens by binding to antibodies labelled with: enzyme (*Fig. 32.14*) e.g. ELISA for hepatitis B, rotavirus fluorescent molecule (*Fig. 32.9*) detection of genes encoding microbial products with DNA probes (*Fig. 32.17*)
toxin detection detection of exotoxins *Clostridium botulinum* toxin by injection of patient's serum into mice (unprotected and protected with specific antiserum) *Clostridium difficile* cytotoxin in feces by addition of suspension to cell culture *Clostridium perfringens* and *Staphylococcus aureus* enterotoxins in feces by agglutination of antitoxin-coated latex particles *Escherichia coli* enterotoxin detected by tissue culture or animal model
detection of endotoxin endotoxin from cell walls of Gram-negative bacteria detected by *Limulus* lysate assay (clotting of extracts of amebocytes of the horseshoe (*Limulus*) crab)

Fig. 32.11 Non-cultural techniques for detection of microbial products. Identification of specific microbial products can be a more rapid method for detecting microorganisms than isolation and culture. The available techniques vary in their specificity. Toxins may be detected either by virtue of their antigenic properties or by demonstrating their action. (CSF, cerebrospinal fuid; ELISA, enzyme-linked immunosorbent assay.)

bacteria in CSF or urine
sample with surface
antigen on bacterial cells

specific antibody
bound to inert carrier
particles (e.g. latex beads)

agglutination
of carrier
particles

Fig. 32.12 When a specimen of cerebrospinal fluid (CSF) containing bacteria (e.g. *Haemophilus influenzae*) is mixed with a suspension of latex particles coated with specific antibody (e.g. *H. influenzae* anticapsular antibodies), the interaction between antigen and antibody causes an immediate agglutination of particles, which is visible to the naked eye.

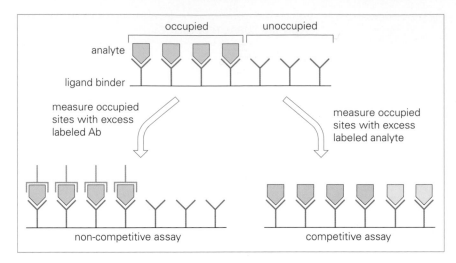

Fig. 32.13 The principle of ligand-binding assays. The ligand-binding agent may be in the soluble phase or bound to a solid support as shown, the advantage of the latter being the ease of separation of bound from free analyte. After exposure to analyte, the fractional occupancy of the ligand-binding sites can be determined by competitive or non-competitive assays using labeled reagents (in orange) as shown.

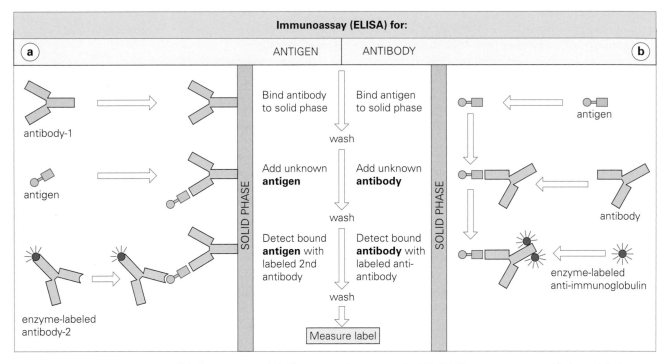

Fig. 32.14 Immunoassay on a solid phase (enzyme-linked immunosorbent assay, ELISA). (a) The test antigen is added to solid phase antibody-1 and the occupancy (see *Figure 32.13*) measured by adding an enzyme-labeled second antibody and reading bound enzyme (e.g. peroxidase or alkaline phosphatase) through a colorimetric or luminometric reaction. In some cases, particularly with small antigens, unoccupied sites can be detected by adding a standard amount of labeled antigen. (b) Antibody to be tested is added to solid phase antigen and is detected by addition of an enzyme-labeled anti-immunoglobulin (see the indirect test in *Figure 32.13*, which uses a fluorescent anti-immunoglobulin to detect bound antibody. Similarly the label in the above assays can be a fluorescent probe rather than an enzyme).

antibodies are frequently employed to detect antigens in specimens from patients. Rotaviruses, HIV, hepatitis B virus, herpes virus and respiratory syncytial virus (RSV) can all be detected directly with monoclonal antibodies in ELISAs. *Chlamydia trachomatis* infection can be diagnosed within a few hours by a direct fluorescent antibody test employing a mono-clonal antibody labeled with fluorescein (see Chapter 21).

Detection of microbes by probing for their genes

Organisms carrying genes for virulence factors can be detected by nucleic acid probes for the virulence factors

A gene probe is a nucleic acid molecule that when in the single-stranded state and labeled, can be used to detect a complemen-

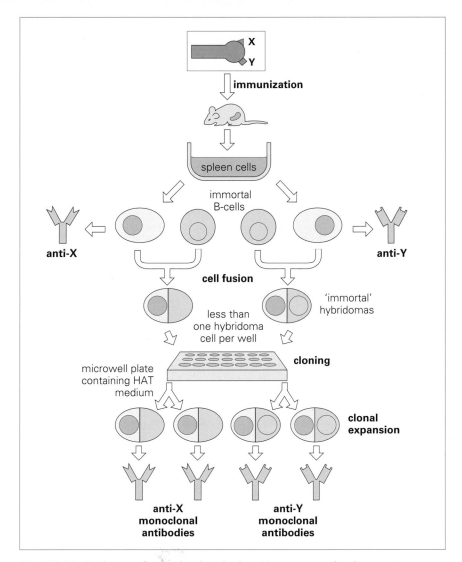

Fig. 32.15 Production of monoclonal antibodies. Mice immunized with an antigen bearing, for example, two epitopes, X and Y, develop spleen cells making anti-X and anti-Y, which appear as antibodies in the serum. The spleen is removed and the individual B cells fused in polyethylene glycol with constantly dividing (i.e. 'immortal') B tumor cells selected for a purine deficiency and often for their inability to secrete immunoglobulin to form hybridoma cells. The resulting cells are distributed into microwell plates in HAT (hypoxanthine, aminopterin, thymidine) medium which kills off the perfusion partners (but not the fused hybridoma cells) at such a high dilution that, on average, each well will contain less than one hybridoma cell. A hybridoma is the fusion product of a single antibody-forming cell and a tumor cell; each hybridoma has the ability of the former to secrete a single species of antibody and the immortality of the latter, enabling it to proliferate continuously. The clonal progeny thus provide an unending supply of antibody with a single specificity—the monoclonal antibody. These monoclonal antibodies can be 'labeled' with enzymes or fluorescent molecules and can then be visualized when they bind to specific antigens (e.g. on virus particles).

tary sequence of DNA by hybridizing to it. Polynucleotide probes may be obtained from naturally occurring DNA by cloning DNA fragments into appropriate plasmid vectors and then isolating the cloned DNA. However, if the sequence of the gene of interest is known, oligonucleotide probes can be synthesized or generated by PCR (see below). Probes are labeled either with a radioactive isotope or with compounds that give color reactions in suitable conditions (e.g. biotin streptavidin).

Depending on whether the material to be queried is DNA or RNA, several approaches have been used to probe for the detection of specific nucleic acid target sequences (Fig. 32.16).

At present, probes are commercially available for the rapid detection (e.g. 2 to 4 hours) of a variety of pathogenic microorganisms, either in clinical samples or for culture confirmation, including chlamydia, group A streptococci, *N. gonorrhoeae*, mycobacteria, fungi and human papillomavirus.

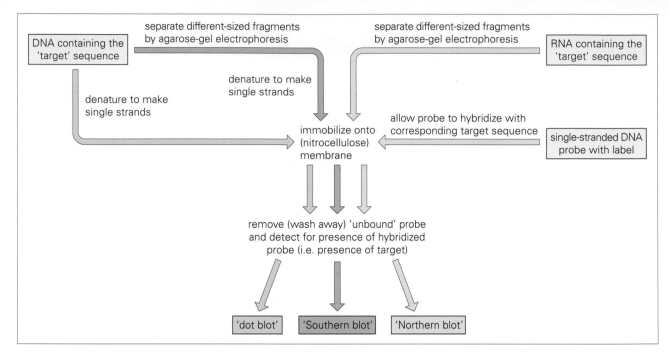

Fig. 32.16 Principal approaches to nucleic acid hybridization. Denatured (i.e. single stranded) target DNA may be directly immobilized onto a solid support (e.g. nitrocellulose membrane) where it is allowed to hybridize with a specific single-stranded DNA probe sequence which is labeled to enable subsequent detection (dot blot). Alternatively, different-sized DNA fragments may first be separated by agarose-gel electrophoresis, denatured, and then transferred to the membrane for probe hybridization and detection (Southern blot). When performed with electrophoretically separated RNA molecules the process is referred to as a Northern blot.

Nucleic acid probes alone are of limited use for small numbers of organisms

While gene probes are an important addition to the diagnostic armamentarium, they may be insufficiently sensitive in circumstances where only a small number of organisms are available for detection (i.e. where there are few copies of the gene). In such circumstances the combination of gene amplification by the polymerase chain reaction (PCR; see below) followed by hybridization with oligonucleotide probes is a potential solution. In addition, PCR may be used to detect directly the presence of microbial pathogens, which is especially useful for organisms that are slow or difficult to grow in the laboratory.

PCR can be used to amplify a specific DNA sequence to produce millions of copies within a few hours

Although PCR theoretically can detect a single gene sequence (*Fig. 32.17*), such sensitivity is seldom achieved in clinical specimens, but very small numbers of bacteria (e.g. 10 or fewer depending on the sample size) can be detected by standard PCR techniques, and more sophisticated methods can detect one viral sequence. A further advantage is the speed with which this can be achieved (i.e. only a few hours). Post-PCR analysis (e.g. confirmation of the PCR product by agarose-gel electrophoresis) adds additional time to the process. However, the use of specifically constructed PCR primers that fluoresce when incorporated into PCR-generated amplicons has allowed the development of 'real-time' PCR protocols that detect the product as it is being generated without the the need for post-PCR analysis. RNA (e.g. retrovirus) may be amplified after it has been converted to DNA by the enzyme reverse transcriptase (termed RT-PCR).

The specificity of PCR is determined by careful choice of primers

These primers (oligonucleotides) are complementary to the target DNA—therefore in order to synthesize suitable primers, the sequence of the target must be known. PCR is currently available for the detection of a variety of pathogens including *C. trachomatis*, *N. gonorrhoeae*, *M. tuberculosis* and viruses such as cytomegalovirus, hepatitis C virus, herpes simplex virus and HIV (*Fig. 32.18*). Both qualitative and quantitative detection can be carried out (e.g. HIV-1 RNA load).

CULTIVATION (CULTURE) OF MICROORGANISMS

Bacteria and fungi can be cultured on solid nutrient or liquid media

While cultures can be made in liquid media (broth), it is not possible to tell whether there is more than one species present. Therefore, solid media are more useful in diagnostic microbiology. Bacteria and fungi grow on the surface of solid nutrient media (agar-based) to produce colonies composed of thousands of cells derived from a single cell implanted on the surface. Colonies of different species often have characteristic appearances, which can give a clue to their likely identity (*Fig. 32.19*).

Different species of bacteria and fungi have different growth requirements

It is possible to grow the majority of species of bacteria and fungi of medical importance in artificial media in the laboratory, but there is no one universal culture medium that

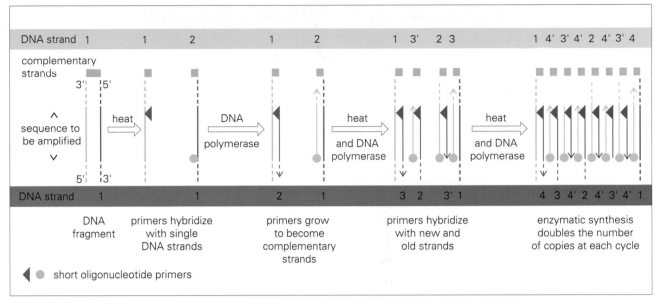

Fig. 32.17 The polymerase chain reaction. The short oligonucleotide primers hybridize with the nucleotide sequences on complementary strands at each end of the DNA fragment to be expanded. These, together with a heat-stable polymerase, produce rapidly increasing numbers of fragments consisting of the sequence to be amplified, and after several cycles millions of copies can be obtained. (The individual strands are numbered in the figure so that their fate can be followed with each succeeding cycle). After the initial cycles, copies (superscripted) identical to the sequence to be amplified are formed.

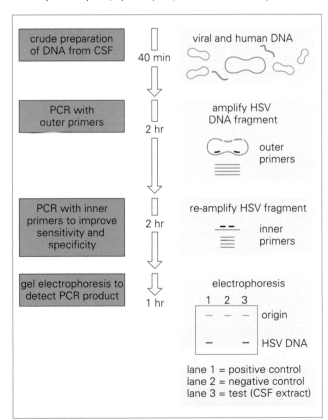

Fig. 32.18 Detection of herpes simplex virus (HSV) DNA in cerebrospinal fluid (CSF) from a patient with encephalitis by nested polymerase chain reaction (PCR). Nested PCR is a modification of the original PCR technique in which the DNA of interest is amplified first with two primers which recognize sequences some distance apart and then, in a second reaction, with a further pair of primers which recognize sequences within the length of the DNA amplified by the first pair. This technique improves the sensitivity and specificity of PCR.

will support the growth of them all, and there are still some species that can only be grown in experimental animals (e.g. *Mycobacterium leprae* and *Treponema pallidum*). Some bacteria that cannot be cultivated on artificial media (e.g. chlamydia and rickettsia) can be grown in cell cultures (see below).

Many culture media are designed not only to support the growth of the desired organisms, but also to inhibit the growth of others (i.e. they are 'selective media'). The important media used in the diagnostic laboratory and schemes using these media for processing different clinical specimens are outlined in the Appendix.

Specimens collected from body sites that have a normal commensal flora will contain a mixture of organisms from which the pathogen has to be recognized. Specimens are 'plated out' on a carefully chosen range of nutrient and selective media to produce single colonies to insure a pure culture. These are subcultured to fresh media for identification and antibiotic susceptibility tests (see below), a procedure which can take 48 hours or longer by conventional (non-molecular) approaches (*Fig. 32.3*).

Parasites such as *Leishmania*, *Trypanosoma* and *Trichomonas* can be cultivated in liquid media to allow small numbers present in the original specimen (e.g. blood or vaginal secretions) to multiply and thus become easier to detect by microscopic examination. Parasites do not form colonies on solid media in the same way as bacteria and fungi.

Viruses, chlamydia and rickettsia must be grown in cell or tissue cultures

This is because these organisms are incapable of a free-living existence. Most cell cultures used in the diagnostic laboratory are continuous cell lines—human or animal cells adapted to growth in vitro that can be stored at –80°C until required. The

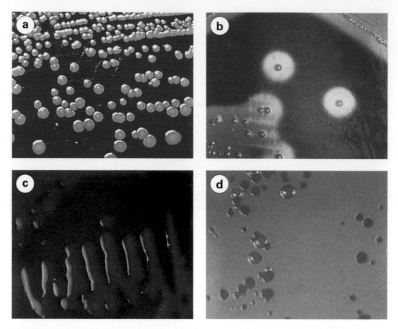

Fig. 32.19 Bacterial colonies. A bacterial cell implanted on a solid nutrient medium will multiply to produce a colony containing millions of cells. Different species produce characteristically different colonies, and this feature can be used as a preliminary clue to the identity of the organism. (a) Golden colonies of *Staphylococcus aureus*. (b) Additional features such as the ability to lyse red blood cells can be demonstrated by culturing bacteria on blood-containing media. Here, β-hemolysis (complete hemolysis) is produced by *Streptococcus pyogenes* on horse blood agar. (c) Culture media can be made selective by including agents that are inhibitory to some species. For example, MacConkey agar contains bile salts so only those organisms tolerant to bile will grow. In addition it contains lactose and a pH indicator. Species that ferment lactose change the indicator to bright pink. (d) Non-lactose-fermenting species, such as *Salmonella* and *Shigella*, form yellowish colonies.

specimen is introduced into the cell culture medium and the presence of viruses detected by observing the cells for a 'cytopathic effect' (CPE).

Cell culture techniques are specialized and labor intensive, and some viruses either cause no CPE or cause a CPE that takes a week or more to evolve (e.g. cytomegalovirus, although CMV antigens can be detected after 1–2 days in cells). Therefore, alternative methods such as antigen detection (see above), antibody detection (see below) and PCR-based approaches are important for diagnosis.

IDENTIFICATION OF MICROORGANISMS GROWN IN CULTURE

Bacteria are identified by simple characteristics and biochemical properties

A preliminary identification of many of the bacteria of medical importance has traditionally been made on the basis of the following few simple characteristics of the cells *(Fig. 32.20)*:

- Gram reaction;
- cell morphology (e.g. rod or coccus) and arrangement (e.g. pairs or chains);
- ability to grow under aerobic or anaerobic conditions;
- growth requirements (simple or fastidious).

Further identification is made on the basis of biochemical properties such as:

- ability to produce enzymes that can be detected by simple tests;
- ability to metabolize sugars oxidatively or fermentatively (aerobically or anaerobically);
- ability to use a range of substrates for growth (e.g. glucose, lactose, sucrose).

While these tests can be done individually (e.g. in broth media containing the specifically required reagents) they are more commonly performed using commercial kits or automated systems which have the potential to give a rapid (e.g. 2–4 hours) indication of pathogen identity based on biochemical profiles.

Some species are identified on the basis of their antigens by reacting cell suspensions with specific antisera. The key tests for species of medical importance are given in the Appendix.

Antibiotic susceptibility can only be determined after the bacteria have been isolated in a pure culture

A variety of methods are available for antimicrobial susceptibility testing, including broth microdilution and automated instrument approaches. However, the most widely employed method assesses antibiotic susceptibility by applying filter paper disks, which contain different antibiotics, onto a lawn

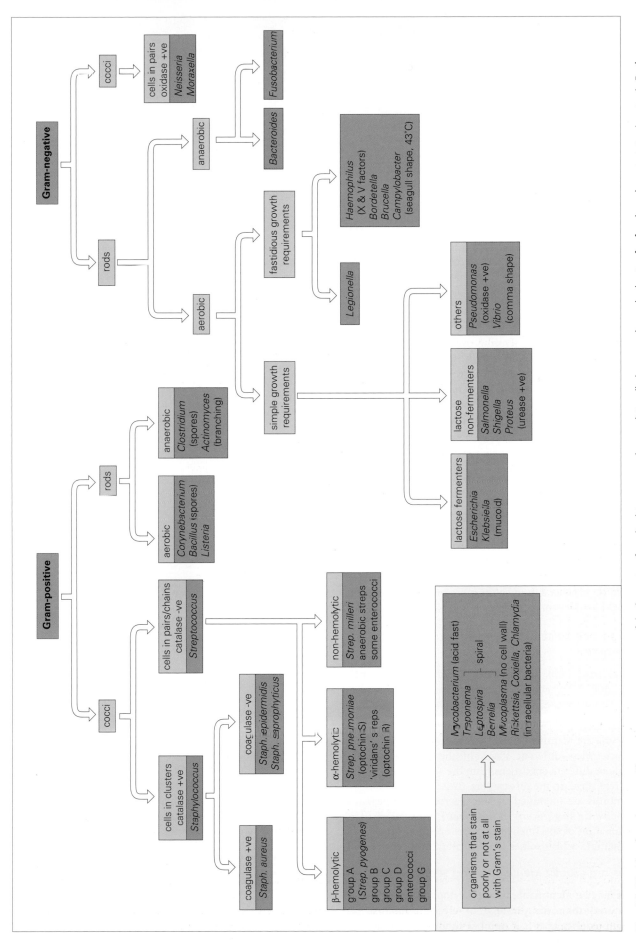

Fig. 32.20 Identifying bacteria. The preliminary investigation of the bacteria of medical importance has traditionally been made on the basis of a few key characteristics (see text). Further identification may then be made on the basis of biochemical and serologic tests.

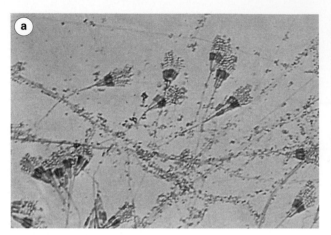
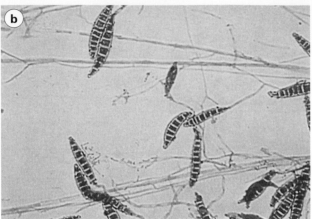

Fig. 32.21 Fungi under the microscope. Fungi can be grown on agar culture media in the same way as bacteria, but most species grow much more slowly than bacteria and it may take up to 2 weeks for a colony to form. Colonial characteristics (such as color) are helpful in the identification of fungi, but confirmation depends upon microscopic examination of the hyphae and sporing structures. (a) *Penicillium* in a wet preparation showing the conidiophores and free conidia. (b) Macroconidia of *Microsporum canis* stained with lactophenol cotton blue.

of the test organism which has been seeded onto an agar plate (i.e. disk diffusion). During overnight incubation the organisms grow and multiply and the antibiotics diffuse out from the disks and inhibit growth around the disk. Therefore, after isolation of bacteria from a specimen, a further incubation period (overnight for disk diffusion testing) is required before antibiotic susceptibility results are available. Methods for antibiotic susceptibility tests are described in more detail in Chapter 33.

Fungi are identified by their colonial characteristics and cell morphology

Fungi are identified from colonies or pure cultures largely on the basis of colonial characteristics (e.g. color) and the morphology of the individual cells viewed under the microscope *(Fig. 32.21)*. Biochemical tests (substrate assimilation) can be used for detailed identification of yeasts of medical importance. In general, fungi grow more slowly than bacteria, and final identification may take up to 2 weeks.

Protozoa and helminths are identified by direct examination

Many protozoa and parasites can be identified by direct examination of specimens without resort to culture, and therefore the results can be obtained on the day of receipt of the specimen in the laboratory:

- Protozoa are identified on the basis of their morphologic characteristics—different stages of the lifecycle may be visible in different specimens from the same patient and at different stages in the disease *(Fig. 32.22)*.
- Helminths are identified by the macroscopic appearance of the worm (e.g. *Ascaris* or *Enterobius*) or by microscopic examination of specimens (e.g. feces or urine) for eggs of, for example, schistosomes (see Chapter 22).

Viruses are usually identified using serologic tests

Viruses may be identifiable by their cytopathic effect in cell culture and their morphology in electron microscopic preparations *(Fig. 32.10)*. A number of viruses may now be

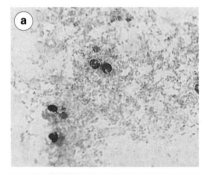
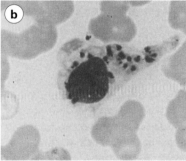

Fig. 32.22 Although some parasites can be cultivated in the laboratory, identification is usually based on microscopic appearances in the specimen. (a) Acid-fast stain of *Cryptosporidium* in feces. Like mycobacteria, this organism is able to retain the pink carbol fuchsin stain when challenged with acid alcohol. (b) *Leishmania donovani* (Donovan bodies) in a stained preparation from a specimen of bone marrow.

identified by nucleic-acid-based tests (e.g. probes and PCR; see above), but diagnosis is also often made by detecting viral antigens or by testing for the presence of specific antibodies in the patient's serum (see below).

ANTIBODY DETECTION METHODS FOR THE DIAGNOSIS OF INFECTION

Serologic tests (the study of antigen–antibody interactions) are used:

- to diagnose infections;
- to identify microorganisms (see above);
- to type blood for blood banks and tissues for transplantation.

Diagnoses based on detecting antibodies in patients' sera are retrospective

The major disadvantage of a diagnosis based on the detection of antibodies in a patient's serum is that it is retrospective, as 2–4 weeks must elapse before IgG antibodies produced in response to the infection are detectable. What is more, a positive result indicates only that the patient has come into contact with the infection at some time in the past. However, IgM antibodies are detected earlier in the infection (7–10 days) and are usually indicative of active, as opposed to past, infection. It may also help to show that the patient has 'seroconverted' by demonstrating a four-fold or greater rise in antibody titer between sera collected in the acute and convalescent phases of the disease.

Antibody detection can be invaluable for identifying organisms that grow either slowly or with difficulty

Despite the drawbacks mentioned above, antibody detection is the main method for the laboratory diagnosis of viral infections. The techniques employed often allow several different infections to be screened for simultaneously (e.g. causes of atypical pneumonia, see Chapter 19). Sera should be collected during the acute phase of the disease and stored at –20°C until a convalescent phase serum is available; the two sera are then tested in parallel. Few diagnoses can be made with any confidence on the results of single serum samples, but sometimes early testing is justified if there is a clinical suspicion of a rare infection that the patient is unlikely to have encountered before (e.g. legionellosis). Previous immunization makes it difficult if not impossible to interpret some serologic tests, because antibodies detected may be the result of immunization or infection (e.g. the Widal test for the serologic diagnosis of enteric fever, see Chapter 22).

Common serologic tests used in the laboratory to diagnose infection

Precipitation reactions are based on the precipitation of antigen–antibody aggregates

When antigen and antibody meet in solution at sufficiently high concentrations, their multivalency results in the formation of aggregates which usually precipitate. These precipitation reactions can be visualized more sensitively by allowing the antigen and antibody to diffuse towards each other through agar gels (Fig. 32.23). Provided there is no immunochemical relationship (i.e. cross-reaction between the antigens), each antigen reacts with a corresponding set of antibodies present within the serum to form separate lines of precipitation in the gel. A practical example is the Elek test for the detection of diphtheria toxin from isolates of *Corynebacterium diphtheriae* (note that a PCR-based method is now available which directly detects the toxin gene in clinical samples).

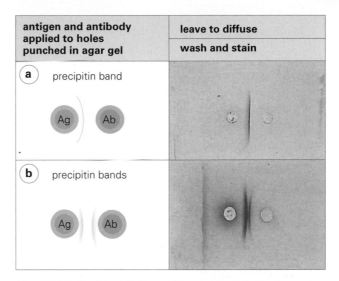

antigen and antibody applied to holes punched in agar gel	leave to diffuse
	wash and stain
a precipitin band	
b precipitin bands	

Fig. 32.23 Double diffusion and immunoprecipitation in agar gels. The opaque lines can be better visualized by staining. (a) Precipitin band formed with a single antigen. The two independent antigens in (b) give separate precipitation bands with their corresponding antibody sets (Abs) coexisting within the complex.

Hemagglutination can be used to detect antibodies against any antigen that can be linked to the surface of red cells

Antibodies directed against antigens on the surface of red cells cause cross-linking in such a way that when the cells are allowed to sediment in a microtiter agglutination tray, they form a mat on the bottom of the well rather than a tight button (Fig. 32.24). This system can be used to detect antibodies against any antigen that can be linked, whether covalently or non-covalently, to the surface of the red cell or even to other particles such as latex. It can also be used to detect antigens (e.g. hepatitis B surface antigens) if specific antibody has been linked to the particle surface. This assay is a classic technique only in use in reference laboratories.

Antibodies can also mask viral molecules such as the influenza hemagglutinins, which are involved in specific adherence to cells, allowing the development of a hemagglutination inhibition test (Fig. 32.25). This assay is a classic technique only in use in reference laboratories.

Complement consumption can form the basis of a test for either antigen or antibody

Complement consumption can be used provided the immune complex is capable of activating the complement system. The complement fixation test (CFT) is carried out as shown in Figure 32.26. This is another classic assay that is mostly helpful in making a retrospective diagnosis. Serum to be tested for antibody is mixed with the known antigen. If antibodies are present, complexes will be formed, which will consume some or all of the complement subsequently added. The consumption of complement is measured by adding indicator red cells coated with a subagglutinating amount of erythrocyte antibody; any residual complement will lyse these indicator cells. Alternatively, with a standard antiserum the system can be used to look for antigen in a given sample.

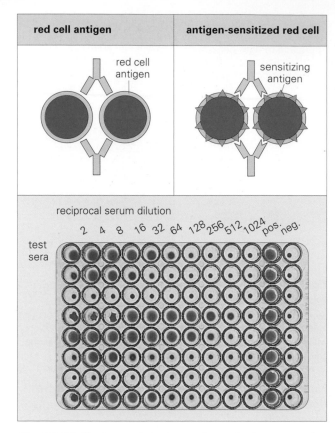

Fig. 32.24 The hemagglutination test for antibodies using red cells sensitized by antigen. Doubling dilutions of sera are made (horizontal row), with positive and negative controls in vertical rows 11 and 12, respectively. A tight button of cells indicates a negative reaction. Agglutinated cells form a carpet over the bottom of the well. A rapid microagglutination method is used for the detection of antibodies to *Legionella* in the patient's serum.

ELISAs can be used to assay antibody in a given sample

These assays have been described previously (*Fig. 32.14*). The amount of antibody binding to the solid phase antigen is a measure of the antibody content of the original sample, and can be detected by adding a second antibody conjugated with an enzyme (e.g. phosphatase or peroxidase) that produces a color reaction with a given substrate.

A variety of tests assess the ability of antibodies to inhibit microbial activity

A number of tests focus on the ability of antibodies in a patient's serum to inhibit some biologic faculty of the micro-organism in question. An example is the anti-streptolysin O test, in which the streptolysin O toxin is neutralized by antibody. The extent to which the test serum can be diluted before it fails to prevent the toxin from lysing red cells provides a convenient titer (*Fig. 32.27*). The ability of a patient's serum containing specific antibody to immobilize motile bacteria—for example the *Treponema pallidum* inhibition (TPI) test—is another example.

Antibodies to cytopathic viruses can be detected by the ability of the patient's serum to prevent virus infectivity

In the case of cytopathic viruses, antibodies can be detected by the ability of the patient's serum to prevent the development of a cytopathic effect. These antibodies are called neutralizing antibodies. The important applications of these methods are referred to in the appropriate systems chapters (see Chapters 18–30).

ASSESSMENT OF HOST DEFENSE SYSTEMS

The opsonic activity and activities of individual components of complement can also be assessed

Although assessment of overall serum complement activity is a relatively uncommon procedure at the present time, it is often of value to assess the opsonic activity of complement in the serum sample by measuring its ability to facilitate the uptake of a microbial particle by a phagocytic cell (*Fig. 32.28*).

The activities of individual components of the complement system can be evaluated either by:

- their ability to be titrated into a complement-dependent lytic system in which the component to be tested is lacking;
- direct immunochemical measurement, often using gel precipitation reactions.

The nitroblue tetrazolium (NBT) test is used to assess phagocytic activity

The ability of neutrophils to become phagocytic and to concurrently reduce molecular oxygen can be assayed by the nitroblue tetrazolium (NBT) test. When yellow NBT dye is added to blood, it forms complexes with heparin or fibrinogen in the sample. These complexes are then phagocytosed by neutrophils that have been activated by the addition of exogenous endotoxin. The dye complex is taken into the stimulated neutrophils and substitutes for oxygen by acting as a substrate for the reduction process, forming as a result a blue insoluble formazan (*Fig. 32.29*).

Lymphocytes

Lymphocytes are counted and classified by detecting their cell surface molecules

Lymphocyte differentiation is accompanied by the expression of related molecules on the cell surface. Detection of these molecules by immunofluorescent techniques allows their enumeration and, in addition, their classification into different subpopulations (*Fig. 32.30*). Monoclonal antibodies are widely used to define these differentiation molecules, and increasing use is being made of the technique of flow cytofluorimetry (*Fig. 32.31*), which is a more rapid and less laborious means of analyzing lymphocyte subpopulations than conventional fluorescent microscopy.

The development of T effector cells to an antigen can often be revealed by intradermal challenge with that antigen

Such an intradermal challenge usually gives rise to erythema and induration, peaking at around 48 hours (*Fig. 32.32*).

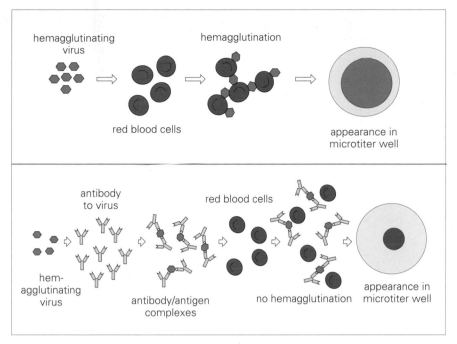

Fig. 32.25 Hemagglutination inhibition. Some viruses (e.g. influenza) have hemagglutinin molecules on their outer surface, and when virus particles are mixed with red blood cells they cause hemagglutination. In the presence of specific antibody, however, hemagglutination is inhibited. This test can therefore be used to detect the presence of antibodies to influenza virus in a patient's serum.

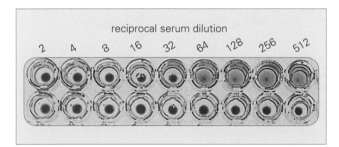

Fig. 32.26 Complement fixation tests (CFTs) are available for the serologic diagnosis of a range of infections. If antigen plus a source of complement (usually guinea pig serum) is added to a test serum, any antibodies present will bind the antigen and in most cases the complexes formed will 'fix' the complement, which is now unavailable to cause lysis of the antibody-coated red cells used as indicators. (Remember that, as described in Chapter 10, the 'classical pathway' activation of complement by antigen–antibody complexes leads to generation of membrane attack complexes which in the present case would lyse the red cells.) Therefore lysis of red cells is a negative reaction; no lysis is a positive test for antibodies. This figure shows a CFT for antibodies to *Coxiella burnetii* (a cause of atypical pneumonia). In the top row using dilutions of acute serum, complement has been fixed only in the first five wells (i.e. the antibody titer is 1/32), whereas with convalescent serum in the second row there is no lysis of the red blood cells at any dilution of serum and so the antibody titer is equal to or greater than 1/512. This demonstrates a four-fold rise in titer between acute and convalescent phase sera, indicating infection with *Coxiella burnetii*. CFTs are rather cumbersome, and there is a tendency to replace them with other more modern tests such as enzyme-linked immunosorbent assays (ELISAs).

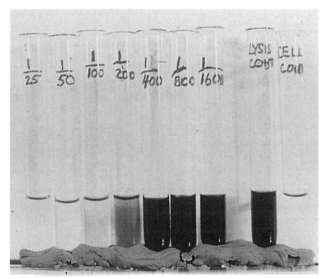

Fig. 32.27 Anti-streptolysin O (ASO) test. The O-toxin lyses red cells. Test serum is diluted until the antibodies it contains it no longer inhibit lysis by a standard concentration of toxin. Positive and negative controls are included in the test (right).

This time course has led to the reaction being described as 'delayed-type hypersensitivity'.

Overall responsiveness of the T cell population can be probed by using materials such as phytohemagglutinin or concanavalin A, which are polyclonal stimulators in the sense that they activate T cell populations independently of their precise antigen specificity. However, when peripheral blood

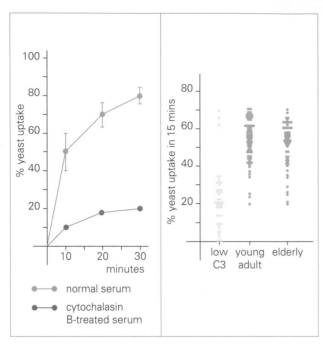

Fig. 32.28 Opsonic activity of serum. (a) Time course for the uptake of yeast opsonized with a normal serum by polymorphonuclear neutrophil leukocytes (PMNs) from 12 healthy donors, and uptake of yeast by PMNs from one donor after treatment with cytochalasin B (40 mg/ml), which inhibits phagocytosis. (b) The distribution of opsonic activity for 150 sera from young healthy, elderly and pathologic sera. (Redrawn from Kerr et al. 1983.)

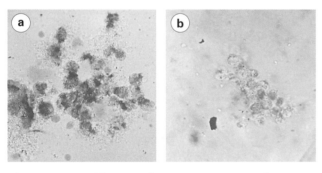

Fig. 32.29 Nitroblue tetrazolium (NBT) test. In normal polymorphs and monocytes, reactive oxygen intermediates (ROIs) are activated by phagocytosis, and yellow NBT is converted to purple-blue formazan (a). Patients with chronic granulomatous disease (CGD) cannot form ROIs and so the dye stays yellow (b). (Courtesy of AR Hayward.)

cells are incubated with antigen in vitro, the specifically sensitized T cells, which represent only a very small fraction of the total, become activated and divide. Examination of the cultures will reveal blast cells and mitotic divisions, but the most convenient way of assessing the response is by the incorporation of radiolabeled thymidine, which provides a measure of cell proliferation *(Fig. 32.33).*

Cytokines can now be studied in great detail

Stimulated T cells also release cytokines. Originally, cytokines were recognized by their activity within a biologic assay, with specificity being confirmed by abrogation of activity with a

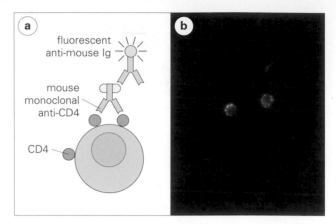

Fig. 32.30 Visualization of lymphocyte surface differentiation molecules by immunofluorescence. (a) The double antibody test using mouse monclonal antibodies to the required surface molecule. (b) Direct demonstration of antibody receptors on the surface of two B lymphocytes by fluorescent anti-immunoglobulin. Aggregation and capping of the surface receptors by the anti-immunoglobulin reagent is evident.

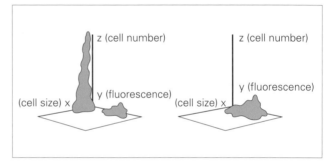

Fig. 32.31 Flow cytofluorimetry. Cells in the sample are stained with specific fluorescent reagents to detect surface molecules and then stream one at a time past a laser. Each cell is measured for size (forward light scatter) and granularity (90° light scatter), as well as for red and green fluorescence, to detect two different surface markers. The three-dimensional plots show a whole lymphocyte population (left) and a CD8+ population obtained by cell sorting (right), stained with anti-CD8.

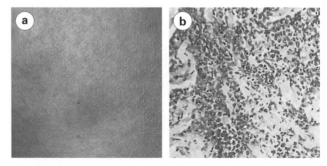

Fig. 32.32 Tuberculin-type delayed sensitivity. The dermal response to antigens of leprosy bacillus in a sensitive subject (the Fernandez reaction) is characterized by (a) red induration maximal at 48–72 hours and (b) dense infiltration of the injection site with lymphocytes and macrophages. (Hematoxylin and eosin, × 80.)

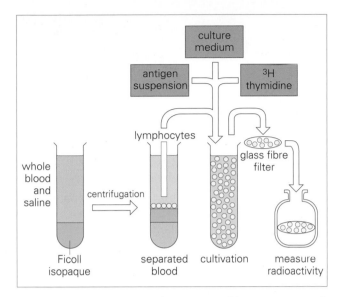

Fig. 32.33 Lymphocyte stimulation assessed by incorporation of radioactive thymidine. A high count indicates that lymphocytes have proliferated and confirms their sensitivity to the antigen.

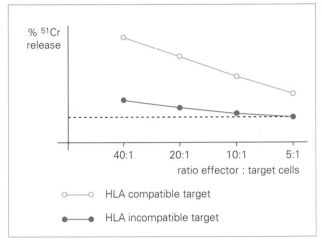

Fig. 32.34 Measurement of cytotoxic activity of human lymphocytes against influenza-infected target cells. Only those targets that share human leukocyte antigens (HLA) haplotype with the cytotoxic cell donor are attacked (haplotype restriction) with consequent release of ^{51}Cr. The dotted line indicates background release of isotype from target cells incubated in the absence of effector cells.

specific antibody. However, with the advent of cloned cytokines and monoclonal antibodies directed against them, there is a strong move towards immunoassay of the individual cytokines and cytokine receptors.

The ability of cytotoxic T cells to attack targets is conventionally assayed using a radioisotope

Cytotoxic T cells attack targets such as virally infected cells, and this ability is conventionally assayed by prelabeling the target with a radioisotope such as ^{51}Cr, and then looking for release of the isotope into the supernatant from damaged cells (*Fig. 32.34*).

PROTOCOLS FOR SPECIMEN PROCESSING

There are basic protocols used in the diagnostic laboratory for processing specimens of:

- urine;
- feces;
- genital tract specimens;
- skin and soft tissue specimens;
- eye swabs;
- respiratory tract specimens, including nose, throat and ear swabs, and sputum;
- CSF;
- pus;
- other fluids such as pleural and pericardial fluids and joint aspirates;
- blood;
- bone marrow and other biopsy specimens;
- autopsy and forensic specimens.

These are detailed in the Appendix.

KEY FACTS

- Microbiologic confirmation of a clinical diagnosis of infection depends upon the collection of high quality specimens and their rapid despatch to the laboratory with all the necessary supporting information.

- Laboratory tests detect microorganisms or their products or evidence of a patient's immune response to infection.

- While coming from different perspectives, culture and serologic methods are important, cooperative, approaches to the identification of clinically important pathogens.

- Newer molecular techniques (e.g. involving PCR and probes) are increasingly used to detect pathogens rapidly; however, antimicrobial susceptibility can only be determined and appropriate treatment information provided by isolating organisms in pure culture.

- Growth of bacteria requires at least 18 hours (isolation of viruses and of fungi may take much longer); culture results cannot therefore be expected in less than 24 hours.

- Interpretation of culture results depends upon the source of the specimen. From sites that are normally sterile, any isolated organism is significant. From sites colonized by commensal flora, isolating and identifying the pathogen can be more difficult.

- Good communication between the clinician and the microbiologist is extremely important.

QUESTIONS

1. List three body sites that are sterile in health and three that have normal commensal flora.

2. Which specimens would you collect to assist in the diagnosis of (a) urinary tract infection, (b) meningitis, (c) osteomyelitis and (d) malaria?

3. What specimens would you collect to detect antibodies? What is important about the timing of these specimens?

4. What is the shortest time you would expect it to take to get a result from the laboratory for (a) significant bacteriuria in a midstream urine specimen from a patient with dysuria, (b) microscopic evidence of infection in the CSF of a young patient with a stiff neck, and (c) antibiotic susceptibility of *Staphylococcus aureus* isolated from a blood culture of a febrile patient?

FURTHER READING

Forbes BA, Sahm DF, Weissfeld A. *Bailey & Scott's Diagnostic Microbiology*, 11th edition. St Louis: Mosby, 2002.

Henry JB, ed. *Clinical Diagnosis and Management by Laboratory Methods.* Philadelphia: WB Saunders, 2001.

Kerr MA, Falconer JS, Bashey A et al. The effect of C3 levels on yeast opsonization by normal and pathological sera; identification of a complement-dependent opsonin. *Clin Exp Immunol* 1983; 54:793–800.

Larone D. *Medically Important Fungi: a Guide to Identification*, 4th edition. Washington: American Society for Microbiology, 2002.

Murray PR, Barron EJ, Pfaller MA et al., eds. *Manual of Clinical Microbiology*, 8th edition. Washington: American Society for Microbiology, 2003.

Rose NR. *Manual of Clinical Laboratory Immunology*, 6th edition. Washington: American Society for Microbiology, 2002.

Singleton P. *DNA Methods in Clinical Microbiology.* Dordrecht: Kluwer, 2000.

INTRODUCTION

The interactions between host, microbial pathogen and antimicrobial agent can be considered as a triangle, and any alteration in one side will inevitably affect the other two sides *(Fig. 33.1)*. In this chapter two sides of the triangle will be examined in greater detail:

- the interactions between antimicrobial agents and microorganisms;
- the interactions between antimicrobial agents and the human host.

Laboratory aspects of antibiotic susceptibility tests and assays will also be outlined. The third side of the triangle, the interactions between microorganisms and the human host, has been considered in detail in the preceding chapters. The concluding part of the present chapter will draw together the three sides of the triangle.

SELECTIVE TOXICITY

The term 'selective toxicity' was proposed by the immuno-chemist Paul Ehrlich (see panel, *Fig. 33.2*). Selective toxicity is achieved by exploiting differences in the structure and metabolism of microorganisms and host cells; ideally the antimicrobial agent should act at a target site present in the infecting organism, but absent from host cells. This is more likely to be achievable in microorganisms that are prokaryotes than in those that are eukaryotes, as the former are structurally more distinct from the host cells. (A comparison of the cellular organization of prokaryotic and eukaryotic cells is given in Chapter 1.) At the other end of the spectrum, viruses are difficult to attack because of their obligate intra-cellular lifestyle—a successful antiviral agent must be able to enter the host cell, but inhibit and damage only a virus-specific target. The desirable features of ideal antimicrobial agents are summarized in *Figure 33.3*.

DISCOVERY AND DESIGN OF ANTIMICROBIAL AGENTS

The term 'antibiotic' has traditionally referred to natural metabolic products of fungi, actinomycetes and bacteria that kill or inhibit the growth of microorganisms. Antibiotic production has been particularly associated with soil micro-organisms and in the natural environment is thought to provide a selective advantage for organisms in their compe-tition for space and nutrients. Although the majority of antibacterial agents in clinical use today are derived from natural products of fermentation, most are then chemically modified (i.e. semi-synthetic) to improve their antibacterial or pharmacologic properties. However, some agents are totally synthetic (e.g. sulfonamides, quinolones). Therefore the term 'antibacterial' or 'antimicrobial' agent is often used in preference to 'antibiotic'. Agents used against fungi and parasites can also be included under antimicrobials, but the terms antifungals, antiprotozoans and anthelmintics are more often used.

The discovery of new antimicrobial agents used to be entirely a matter of chance. Pharmaceutical companies under-took massive screening programs searching for new soil microorganisms that produced antibiotic activity. In the light of our greater understanding of the mechanisms of action of existing antimicrobials the processes have become rational-ized, searching either for new natural products by target-site-directed screening or synthesizing molecules predicted to interact with a microbial target. More recently, genomic approaches to the identification of new (unexploited) targets have been applied. The steps in a rational design program are summarized in *Figure 33.4*.

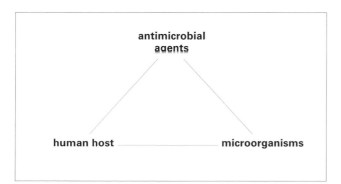

Fig. 33.1 The interactions between antimicrobial agents, microorganisms and the human host can be viewed as a triangle. Any effect on one side of the triangle will have effects on the other two sides.

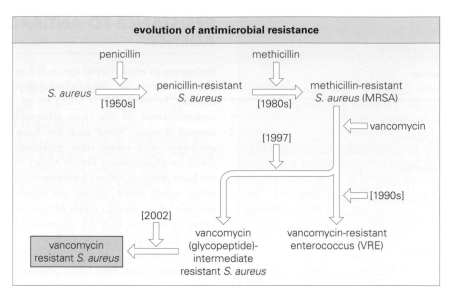

Fig. 33.5 'Time line' illustrating the chronological emergence of antibiotic resistance in Gram-positive cocci.

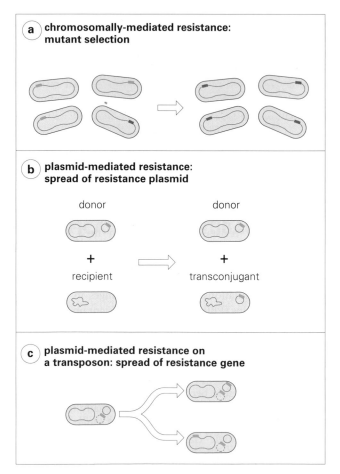

Fig. 33.6 A chromosomal mutation (a) can produce a drug-resistant target, which confers resistance on the bacterial cell and allows it to multiply in the presence of antibiotic. Resistance genes carried on plasmids (b) can spread from one cell to another more rapidly than cells themselves divide and spread. Resistance genes on transposable elements (c) move between plasmids and the chromosome and from one plasmid to another, thereby allowing greater stability or greater dissemination of the resistance gene.

(*Fig. 33.6b*; see also Chapter 2). Such plasmids often code for resistance determinants to several unrelated families of antibacterial agents. Therefore a cell may acquire 'multiple' resistance to many different drugs (i.e. in different classes) at once, a process much more efficient than chromosomal mutation. This so-called 'infectious resistance' was first described by Japanese workers studying enteric bacteria, but is now recognized to be widespread throughout the bacterial world. Some plasmids are promiscuous, crossing species barriers, and the same resistance gene is therefore found in widely different species. For example, TEM-1, the most common plasmid-mediated beta-lactamase in Gram-negative bacteria, is widespread in *E. coli* and other enterobacteria and also accounts for penicillin resistance in *Neisseria gonorrhoeae* and ampicillin resistance in *H. influenzae*.

Resistance may be acquired from transposons and other mobile elements

Resistance genes may also occur on transposons; the so-called 'jumping genes', which by a replicative process are capable of generating copies which may integrate into the chromosome or into plasmids (see Chapter 2). The chromosome provides a more stable location for the genes, but they will be disseminated only as rapidly as the bacteria divide. Transposon copies moving from the chromosome to plasmids are disseminated more rapidly. Transposition can also occur between plasmids, for example from a non-transmissible to a transmissible plasmid, again accelerating dissemination (*Fig. 33.6c*).

'Cassettes' of resistance genes may be organized into genetic elements called integrons

As discussed previously, antibiotic-resistance genes may individually reside on plasmids, the chromosome, or on transposons found in both locations. However, in some instances multiple resistance genes may come together in a structure known as an integron. As shown in *Figure 33.7a*, the integron encodes a site-specific recombination enzyme (*int* gene; integrase) which allows insertion (and also excision)

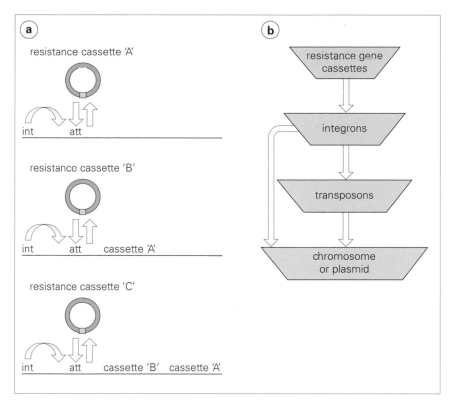

Fig. 33.7 (a) Basic integron structure and (b) overall interrelationship between integrons and other DNA elements. (att, integron attachment site; int, integrase.)

of antibiotic-resistance gene 'cassettes' (resistance gene plus additional sequences including an 'attachment' region) into the integron attachment site *(att)*. In classic operon fashion, a strong integron promoter controls transcription of the inserted genes. Based on their integration mechanism (integrase, etc.), integrons have been organized into different classes found in both Gram-negative and Gram-positive organisms. Whether acting as independent mobile genetic elements or inserted into transposons, integrons are capable of moving into a variety of DNA molecules, the overall hierarchy of which is depicted in *Figure 33.7b*. With their ability to capture, organize and rearrange different antibiotic-resistance genes, integrons represent an important mechanism for the spread of multiple antibiotic resistance in clinically important microorganisms.

Mechanisms of resistance

Resistance mechanisms can be broadly classified into three main types. These are summarized below and in *Figure 33.8* and described in more detail where relevant for each antibiotic in later parts of this chapter. Where bacterial mechanisms of antimicrobial resistance have been elucidated they appear to involve the synthesis of new or altered proteins. As mentioned above, the genes encoding these proteins may be found on plasmids or the chromosome.

The target site may be altered

The target may be altered so that it has a lowered affinity for the antibacterial, but still functions adequately for normal metabolism to proceed. Alternatively an additional target (e.g. enzyme) may be synthesized.

Access to the target site may be altered (altered uptake or increased exit)

This mechanism involves decreasing the amount of drug that reaches the target by either:

- altering entry, for example by decreasing the permeability of the cell wall;
- pumping the drug out of the cell (known as an efflux mechanism).

Enzymes that modify or destroy the antibacterial agent may be produced (drug inactivation)

There are many examples of such enzymes, the most important being:

- beta-lactamases;
- aminoglycoside-modifying enzymes;
- chloramphenicol acetyl transferases.

These will be described in the relevant parts on these antibiotics.

CLASSES OF ANTIBACTERIAL AGENTS

The following parts of this chapter deal with groups of antibacterial agents based on their target site and chemical structure. In each case, the discussion attempts to summarize the answers to the questions set out in *Figure 33.9*, reviewing the interactions between antibacterial agent and bacteria and between the antibacterial and the host (i.e. two sides of the triangle in *Figure 33.1*).

RESISTANCE TO ANTIMICROBIAL AGENTS			
antibacterial	**mechanism of resistance**		
	altered target	altered uptake	drug inactivation
beta-lactams	+	+	+
glycopeptides	+		
aminoglycosides	+	+	+
tetracyclines	+	+	
chloramphenicol		+	+
macrolides	+	+	+
lincosamides	+		
streptogramins	+		
oxazolidinones	+		
fusidic acid	+		
sulfonamides/ trimethoprim	+	+	
quinolones	+	+	
rifampicin	+		

Fig. 33.8 Mechanisms of resistance can be classified into three main types. For antibiotics where more than one mode of resistance exists, drugs vary as to which is more frequently encountered.

INHIBITORS OF CELL WALL SYNTHESIS

Peptidoglycan, a vital component of the bacterial cell wall (see Chapter 2), is a compound unique to bacteria and therefore provides an optimum target for selective toxicity. Synthesis of peptidoglycan precursors starts in the cytoplasm; wall subunits are then transported across the cytoplasmic membrane and finally inserted into the growing peptidoglycan molecule. Several different stages are therefore potential targets for inhibition *(Fig. 33.10)* The antibacterials that inhibit cell wall synthesis are varied in chemical structure. The most important of these agents are the beta-lactams, the largest group, and the glycopeptides which are active only against Gram-positive organisms. Bacitracin (primarily used topically) and cycloserine (mainly used as a 'second-line' medication for treatment of tuberculosis, discussed later in this chapter) have many fewer clinical applications.

Beta-lactams

Beta-lactams contain a beta-lactam ring and inhibit cell wall synthesis by binding to penicillin-binding proteins (PBPs)

Beta-lactams comprise a very large family of different groups of bacteriocidal compounds all containing the beta-lactam ring. The different groups within the family are distinguished by the structure of the ring attached to the beta-lactam ring—in penicillins this is a five-membered ring, in cephalosporins a six-membered ring—and by the side chains attached to these rings *(Fig. 33.11)*.

PBPs are membrane proteins (e.g. carboxypeptidases, transglycosylases and transpeptidases) capable of binding to penicillin (hence the name PBP) and are responsible for the final stages of cross-linking of the bacterial cell wall structure. Inhibition of one or more of these essential enzymes results in an accumulation of precursor cell wall units, leading to activation of the cell's autolytic system and cell lysis *(Fig. 33.12)*.

Most beta-lactams have to be administered parenterally

Although the majority of beta-lactams have to be administered intramuscularly or intravenously, there are some orally active agents. Most achieve clinically useful concentrations in the cerebrospinal fluid (CSF) when the meninges are inflamed (as in meningitis) and the blood–brain barrier becomes more permeable. In general, they are not effective against intracellular organisms.

A few of the cephalosporins, notably cefotaxime, are metabolized to compounds with less microbiologic activity. All beta-lactams are excreted in the urine, and for some, such

WHAT DO WE NEED TO KNOW ABOUT AN ANTIBACTERIAL AGENT?	
What is it?	chemical structure natural or synthetic product
What does it do?	target site mechanism of action
Where does it go? (and therefore preferred route of administration)	absorption, distribution, metabolism and excretion of the drug in the body of the host
When is it used?	spectrum of activity and important clinical uses
What are the limitations to its use?	toxicity to the human host lack lack of toxicity, i.e. resistance of the bacteria
How much does it cost?	great variation between agents but cost is a serious limitation on availability of some agents in developing countries

Fig. 33.9 In order to understand the nature and optimum use of an antibacterial agent, the questions listed here must be answered.

as benzylpenicillin, this is very rapid—hence the need for frequent doses. Probenecid can be administered concurrently to slow down excretion and maintain higher blood and tissue concentrations for a longer period of time.

Different beta-lactams have different clinical uses, but are not active against species that lack a cell wall

A vast array of beta-lactam antibiotics are currently registered for clinical use. Some, such as penicillin, are active mainly against Gram-positive organisms, whereas others (e.g. semi-synthetic penicillins, carboxypenems, monobactams, second, third and fourth generation cephalosporins) have been developed for their activity against Gram-negative rods. Only the more recent beta-lactams are active against innately more resistant organisms such as *Pseudomonas aeruginosa* (Fig. 33.13)

It is important to remember that beta-lactams are not active against species that lack a cell wall (e.g. *Mycoplasma*) or those with very impenetrable walls such as mycobacteria, or intracellular pathogens such as *Brucella*, *Legionella* and *Chlamydia*.

Resistance to beta-lactams may involve one or more of the three possible mechanisms

Resistance by alteration in target site

Methicillin-resistant staphylococci (e.g. *Staph. aureus*, *Staph. epidermidis*—MRSA, MRSE, respectively) synthesize an additional PBP, which has a much lower affinity for

beta-lactams than the normal PBPs and is therefore able to continue cell wall synthesis when the other PBPs are inhibited. Although the *mecA* gene which codes for the additional PBP is present on the chromosome in all cells of a resistant population, in many instances it may only be transcribed in a proportion of the cells, resulting in a phenomenon known as 'heterogeneous resistance'. In the laboratory, special cultural conditions are used to enhance expression and demonstrate resistance. Methicillin-resistant staphylococci are resistant to all other beta-lactams. The majority of strains also produce beta-lactamase (see below).

Other organisms such as *Streptococcus pneumoniae*, *Neisseria gonorrhoeae* and *Haemophilus influenzae* may also utilize PBP changes to achieve beta-lactam resistance which may vary depending on the compound employed.

Resistance by alteration in access to the target site

This mechanism is found in Gram-negative cells where beta-lactams gain access to their target PBPs by diffusion through protein channels (porins) in the outer membrane. Mutations in porin genes result in a decrease in permeability of the outer membrane and hence resistance. Strains resistant by this mechanism may exhibit cross-resistance to unrelated antibiotics that use the same porins.

Resistance by production of beta-lactamases

Beta-lactamases are enzymes that catalyze the hydrolysis of the beta-lactam ring to yield microbiologically inactive products. Genes encoding these enzymes are widespread in the bacterial kingdom and are found on the chromosome and on plasmids.

The beta-lactamases of Gram-positive bacteria are released into the extracellular environment (Fig. 33.12a) and resistance will only be manifest when a large population of cells is present. The beta-lactamases of Gram-negative cells, however, remain within the periplasm (Fig. 33.12b).

To date, hundreds of different beta-lactamase enzymes have been described. All have the same function but with differing amino acid sequences that influence their affinity for different beta-lactam substrates. Some enzymes specifically target penicillins or cephalosporins while others are especially troublesome in broadly attacking most beta-lactam compounds (i.e. extended-spectrum beta-lactamases, ESBLs). Some beta-lactam antibiotics (e.g. cloxacillin, ceftazidime, imipenem) are hydrolyzed by very few enzymes (beta-lactamase stable), whereas others (e.g. ampicillin) are much more labile. Beta-lactamase inhibitors such as clavulanic acid (Fig. 33.14) are molecules that contain a beta-lactam ring and act as 'suicide inhibitors', binding to beta-lactamases and preventing them from destroying beta-lactams. They have little bactericidal activity of their own.

Side effects

Toxic effects of beta-lactam drugs include mild rashes and immediate hypersensitivity reactions

Statistics regarding allergy to beta-lactam drugs are complicated by the fact that the problem historically involves self reporting by patients who are often mistaken in their

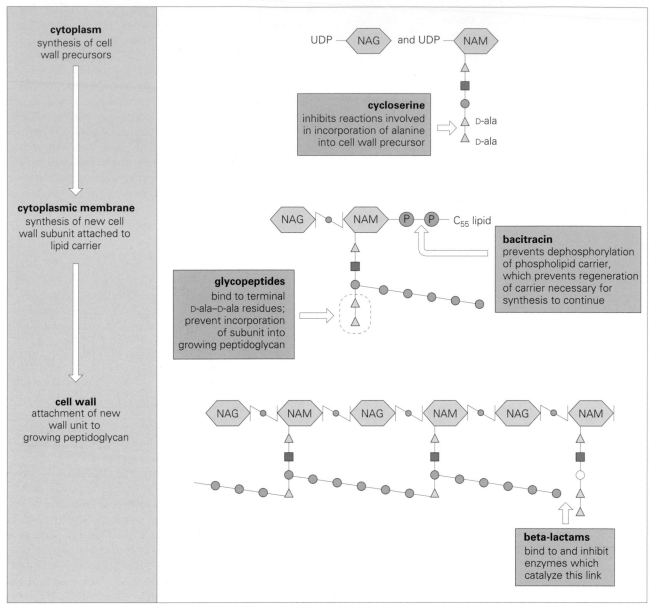

Fig. 33.10 The synthesis of peptidoglycan is a complex process that begins in the cytoplasm, proceeds across the cytoplasmic membrane and leads to the attachment of new wall units to the growing peptidoglycan chain. This synthetic pathway can be inhibited at a variety of points by antibacterial agents. The precise mechanism of inhibition caused by glycopeptides such as vancomycin is unknown, but the mechanism of action of beta-lactams has now been fully elucidated (see text). (NAG, N-acetyl glucosamine; NAM, N-acetyl muramic acid; UDP, uridine diphosphate.)

'diagnosis.' Nevertheless, serious allergy to beta-lactam drugs in the form of an immediate (type 1) hypersensitivity reaction may occur in 0.5–2% of patients, although anaphylaxis occurs much less frequently (ca. 0.002% of treatment courses). Mild idiopathic reactions, usually in the form of a rash, are more common (ca. 25% of treatment courses), especially with ampicillin. Patients who are allergic to penicillin are often allergic to cephalosporins (less with third generation compounds) and vice versa, but aztreonam, a monobactam, shows negligible cross-reactivity.

Benzylpenicillin can produce neurotoxicity if given in high doses, particularly in patients with renal impairment. This toxicity is manifest as fits, unconsciousness, myoclonic spasms and hallucinations. Carbenicillin can cause platelet dysfunction and sodium overload (because it is given as a sodium salt), especially in patients with liver failure, renal failure and congestive heart failure.

Glycopeptides

Glycopeptides are large molecules and act at an earlier stage than beta-lactams

Glycopeptides include vancomycin and teicoplanin. Both are very large molecules and therefore have difficulty penetrating into Gram-negative cells. Teicoplanin is a natural complex of five different but closely related molecules.

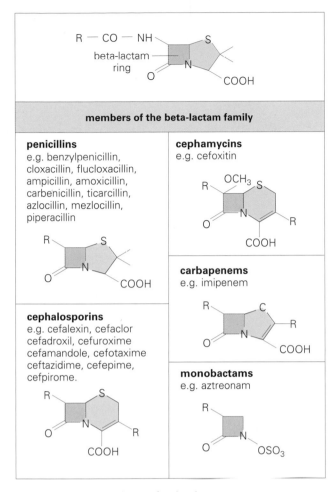

Fig. 33.11 The beta-lactam family. The ring structure is common to all beta-lactams and must be intact for antibacterial action. Enzymes (beta-lactamases) that catalyze the hydrolysis of the beta-lactam bond render the agents inactive. The penicillins and cephalosporins are the major classes of beta-lactam antibiotics, but other members of the family, particularly the carbapenems and monobactams, are the focus of new developments.

Glycopeptides are bacteriocidal and interfere with cell wall synthesis by binding to terminal D-alanine–D-alanine at the end of pentapeptide chains that are part of the growing bacterial cell wall structure *(Fig. 33.10)*. This binding inhibits the transglycosylation reaction and prevents incorporation of new subunits into the growing cell wall. As glycopeptides act at an earlier stage than beta-lactams, it is not useful to combine glycopeptides and beta-lactams in the treatment of infections.

Vancomycin and teicoplanin must be given by injection for systemic infections

Vancomycin and teicoplanin are not absorbed from the gastrointestinal tract and do not penetrate the CSF in patients without meningitis. However, bactericidal concentrations are achieved in most patients with meningitis because of the increased permeability of the blood–brain barrier. Excretion is via the kidney.

Both vancomycin and teicoplanin are active only against Gram-positive organisms

Vancomycin and teicoplanin are used mainly for:

- the treatment of infections caused by Gram-positive cocci and Gram-positive rods that are resistant to beta-lactam drugs, particularly multiresistant *Staphylococcus aureus* and *Staphylococcus epidermidis*;
- for patients allergic to beta-lactams;
- the treatment of *Clostridium difficile* in antibiotic-associated colitis, although concerns that this may promote emergence of glycopeptide-resistant enterococci in the gut flora have led to the increasing use of alternative compounds.

Resistance

Some organisms are intrinsically resistant to glycopeptides

As mentioned previously, Gram-negative bacteria are 'naturally' resistant to the glycopeptides since these compounds are too large to efficiently move through the outer membrane to the peptidoglycan. Other organisms have an altered glycopeptide target, such as pentapeptides terminating in D-alanine–D-lactate (e.g. *Erysiplothrix*, *Leuconostoc*, *Lactobacillus* and *Pediococcus*) or D-alanine–D-serine (e.g. *Enterococcus gallinarum*, *Enterococcus casseliflavus*).

Organisms may acquire resistance to glycopeptides

Historically, the most clinically relevant acquired glyco-peptide resistance has been observed in *Enterococcus faecium* and *Enterococcus faecalis* (vancomycin-resistant enterococci; VRE), first reported by investigators in the United Kingdom in 1986. Since that time, a variety of resistance phenotypes have been described which can be differentiated by transferability (e.g. plasmid association), inducibility and extent of resistance *(Fig. 33.15)*. The genes associated with the highest levels of glycopeptide resistance are *vanA*, *vanB*, and *vanD* which encode a ligase producing pentapeptides terminating in D-alanine–D-lactate.

VanA is the best understood mechanism of acquired glycopeptide resistance

VanA-type glycopeptide resistance has been the most extensively studied and is characterized by inducible high level resistance to both vancomycin and teicoplanin. VanA is associated with transposable elements related to Tn*1546* (ca. 11 kb in size) which may be chromosomal or plasmid (transferable) in nature.

VanB is associated with inducible high-level resistance to vancomycin but not teicoplanin (although teicoplanin resistance can be induced by prior exposure to vancomycin). VanB resistance may be chromosomal or plasmid linked and is associated with a very large (34 kb) transposable element, Tn*1549*.

VanD is chromosomal in nature and thus non-transferable, resulting in constitutive resistance to high levels of vanco-mycin but low levels of teicoplanin.

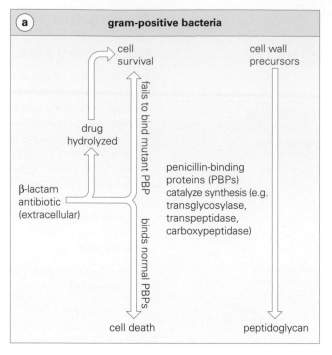

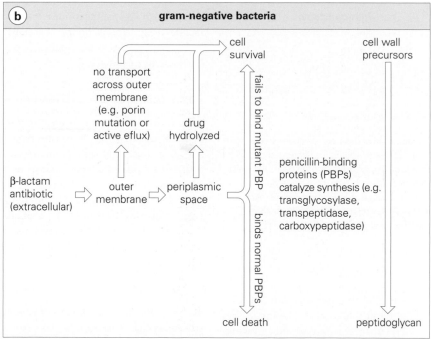

Fig. 33.12 Penicillin-binding proteins (PBPs) play a key role in the final stages of peptidoglycan synthesis. They catalyze the cross-linkage of wall subunits, which are then incorporated into the cell wall. Beta-lactams are able to enter the cell (e.g. through pores in the outer membrane of Gram-negatives) and bind to the PBP. This prevents it from catalyzing the cross-linkage of subunits, leading to their accumulation in the cell and the release of autolytic enzymes, which causes cell lysis. Within the periplasmic space of Gram-negatives (b1) beta-lactamases can inactivate beta-lactams before they reach their target PBPs, thereby protecting the cell from antibiotic action. Alternatively, mutant PBPs fail to bind beta-lactase thus allowing peptidoglycan synthesis to occur. In Gram-positive bacteria (b2) beta-lactams may be extracellularly destroyed by beta-lactamases or rendered ineffective, as in Gram-negatives, by mutant PBPs.

CHARACTERISTICS OF REPRESENTATIVE BETA-LACTAMS		
drug class	**category**	**general spectrum of activity**
penicillins		
penicillin G, V*	natural penicillin	Gram-positive bacteria

cloxacillin*
dicloxacillin*
nafcillin*
oxacillin*
	semisynthetic
	  (beta-lactamase
	  resistant) penicillin
		Gram-positive bacteria (incl. beta-lactamase
		  producers)

amoxicillin*,**
ampicillin*,**
	semisynthetic
	  (amino) penicillin
		Gram-positive bacteria
		Gram-negative bacteria, including spirochetes, *Listeria
		  monocytogenes, Proteus mirabilis* and some *Escherichia coli*

carbenicillin*
ticarcillin**
	semisynthetic
	  (carboxy) penicillin
		Gram-positive bacteria
		enhanced coverage of Gram-negatives, including *Pseudomonas*
		  and *Klebsiella*

mezlocillin piperacillin**	semisynthetic (ureido) penicillin	
cephalosporins		
cefadroxil* cefazolin cefalexin* cephalothin cephradine*	first generation	Gram-positive bacteria
cefaclor* cefamandole cefmetazole cefonicid cefotetan cefprozil* cefuroxime*	second generation	
cefdinir* cefditoren* cefoperazone cefpodoxime* cefotaxime ceftazidime ceftibuten* ceftizoxime ceftriaxone	third generation	
cefepime cefpirome	fourth generation	improved activity against Gram-negative bacteria

Fig. 33.13 Although there are many beta-lactam agents available, the most commonly used ones are listed, together with their main indications.

CHARACTERISTICS OF REPRESENTATIVE BETA-LACTAMS		
drug class	**category**	**general spectrum of activity**
cephamycin[†]		
cefmetazole cefotetan cefoxitin		Gram-positive bacteria improved activity against *Bacillus fragilis*
carbapenems		
ertapenem imipenem meropenem		Gram-positive and Gram-negative bacteria
monobactams		

*oral formulation available
**can be formulated in combination with beta-lactamase inhibitors (see *Fig. 33.14*)
[†]often classified with second generation cephalosporins

Fig. 33.13, cont'd.

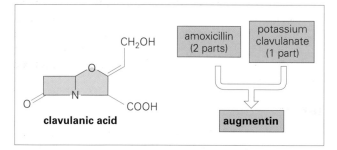

Fig. 33.14 Clavulanic acid, a product of *Streptomyces clavuligerus*, inhibits the most common beta-lactamases (e.g. TEM enzymes) and allows amoxicillin to inhibit cells producing these enzymes. Augmentin is the most widely used of these combination drugs. Other combinations include ticarcillin and clavulanic acid, and piperacillin and tazobactam.

Glycopeptide resistance in the staphylococci occurs by mutation or by acquisition from the enterococci

Within the coagulase-negative staphylococci (CNS), *Staphylococcus epidermidis* and *Staphylococcus haemolyticus* are especially prone to development of glycopeptide resistance by mechanisms which remain incompletely understood. Nevertheless, resistant clinical and laboratory-generated isolates have been shown to differ from their susceptible counterparts in a variety of ways including changes in glycopeptide binding capacity, membrane proteins and cell wall synthesis and composition.

Coagulase-positive staphylococci (i.e. *Staphylococcus aureus*) showing decreased susceptibility to glycopeptides (but not fully resistant) were first described by Japanese investigators in 1996. The reduced susceptibility of these vancomycin-intermediate or glycopeptide-intermediate isolates (VISA or GISA, respectively) may be either homogeneously or

CHARACTERISTICS OF GLYCOPEPTIDE RESISTANCE IN THE ENTEROCOCCI			
type	**resistance**	**expression**	**transmissible**
VanA	vancomycin teicoplanin	inducible	+
VanB	vancomycin	inducible	+
VanD	vancomycin (variable) teicoplanin (variable)	constitutive	–

Fig. 33.15 Characteristics of glycopeptide resistance in enterococci.

heterogeneously expressed. In either case, 'resistance' is not associated with VanA, B, or D but, instead, appears to involve other mechanisms affecting cell wall composition (e.g. leading to increased thickness, etc.).

Unfortunately, high level glycopeptide resistance has also been observed in *Staph. aureus*. This is due to the *vanA* gene (apparently acquired from VRE) residing on a staphylococcal plasmid.

Side effects

The glycopeptides are potentially ototoxic and nephrotoxic

Vancomycin is usually given by intravenous infusion, administered slowly to avoid 'red-man' syndrome due to histamine release. Particular care must be taken to prevent toxic concentrations accumulating in patients with renal impairment. Oral vancomycin is used for treatment of antibiotic-associated pseudomembranous colitis due to *Clostridium difficile*. Teicoplanin is less toxic than vancomycin and can be given by intravenous bolus and by intramuscular injection.

INHIBITORS OF PROTEIN SYNTHESIS

Although protein synthesis proceeds in an essentially similar manner in prokaryotic and eukaryotic cells, it is possible to exploit the differences (e.g. 70S vs 80S ribosome) to achieve selective toxicity. The process of translation of the messenger RNA (mRNA) chain into its corresponding peptide chain is complex, and a range of antibacterial agents act as inhibitors, although the full details of their mechanisms of action are not yet known *(Fig. 33.16)*.

Aminoglycosides

The aminoglycosides are a family of related molecules with bacteriocidal activity

The aminoglycosides contain either streptidine (streptomycin) or 2-deoxystreptamine (e.g. gentamicin; *Fig. 33.17*). The original structures have been modified chemically by changing the side chains to produce molecules such as amikacin and netilmicin that are active against organisms that have developed resistance to earlier aminoglycosides.

Aminoglycosides act by binding to specific proteins in the 30S ribosomal subunit, where they interfere with the binding of formylmethionyl-transfer RNA (fmet-tRNA) to the ribosome *(Fig. 33.16)* thereby preventing the formation of initiation complexes from which protein synthesis proceeds. In addition, aminoglycosides cause misreading of mRNA codons and tend to break apart functional polysomes (protein synthesis by multiple ribosomes tandemly attached to a single mRNA molecule) into non-functional monosomes.

Aminoglycosides must be given intravenously or intramuscularly for systemic treatment

Aminoglycosides are not absorbed from the gut, do not penetrate well into tissues and bone, and do not cross the blood–brain barrier. Thus, they are usually administered as an intravenous infusion. Intrathecal administration of streptomycin is used in the treatment of tuberculous meningitis, and gentamicin may be administered by this route in the treatment of Gram-negative meningitis in neonates. Aminoglycosides are excreted via the kidney.

Gentamicin and the newer aminoglycosides are used to treat serious Gram-negative infections

Gentamicin, tobramycin, amikacin and netilmicin are important for the treatment of serious Gram-negative infections, including those caused by *P. aeruginosa* (*Fig. 33.18*). They are not active against streptococci or anaerobes, but are active against staphylococci. Tobramycin is slightly more active than gentamicin against *P. aeruginosa*. Amikacin and netilmicin are both less active, but may be active against strains resistant to gentamicin and tobramycin (see below).

Streptomycin is now reserved almost entirely for the treatment of mycobacterial infections. Neomycin is not used for systemic treatment, but can be used orally in gut decontamination regimens in neutropenic patients.

Production of aminoglycoside-modifying enzymes is the principal cause of resistance to aminoglycosides

Although relatively uncommon, resistance to aminoglycoside antibiotics may occur by alteration of the 30S ribosomal target protein (e.g. a single amino acid change in the P12 protein prevents streptomycin binding). Resistance may also arise through alterations in cell wall permeability or in the energy-dependent transport across the cytoplasmic membrane.

Production of aminoglycoside-modifying enzymes is the most important mechanism of acquired resistance (*Fig. 33.19*). The genes for these enzymes are often plasmid-mediated, located on transposons, and transferable from one bacterial species to another. The enzymes alter the structure of the aminoglycoside molecule, thus inactivating the drug. The type of enzyme determines the spectrum of resistance of the organism containing it.

The aminoglycosides are potentially nephrotoxic and ototoxic

The therapeutic 'window' between the serum concentration of aminoglycoside required for successful treatment and that which is toxic is small. Blood concentrations should be monitored regularly, particularly in patients with renal impairment. Netilmicin is reported to be one of the less toxic aminoglycoside antibiotics.

Tetracyclines

Tetracyclines are bacteriostatic compounds that differ mainly in their pharmacological properties rather than in their antibacterial spectra

Tetracyclines are a family of large cyclic structures that have several sites for possible chemical substitutions (*Fig. 33.20*).

Tetracyclines inhibit protein synthesis by binding to the small ribosomal subunit in a manner that prevents aminoacyl transfer RNA from entering the acceptor sites on the ribosome (*Fig. 33.16*). While this process may occur with both prokaryotic and eukaryotic ribosomes, the selective action of tetracyclines is due to their much greater uptake by prokaryotic cells.

Tetracyclines are usually administered orally. Doxycycline and minocycline are more completely absorbed than tetracycline, oxytetracycline and chlortetracycline and so result in higher serum concentrations and less gastrointestinal upset because there is less inhibition of normal gut flora. Tetracyclines are well distributed and penetrate host cells to inhibit intracellular bacteria. They are excreted primarily in bile and urine.

Tetracyclines are active against a wide variety of bacteria, but their use is restricted due to widespread resistance

Tetracyclines are used in the treatment of infections caused by mycoplasmas, chlamydiae and rickettsiae. Resistance in other

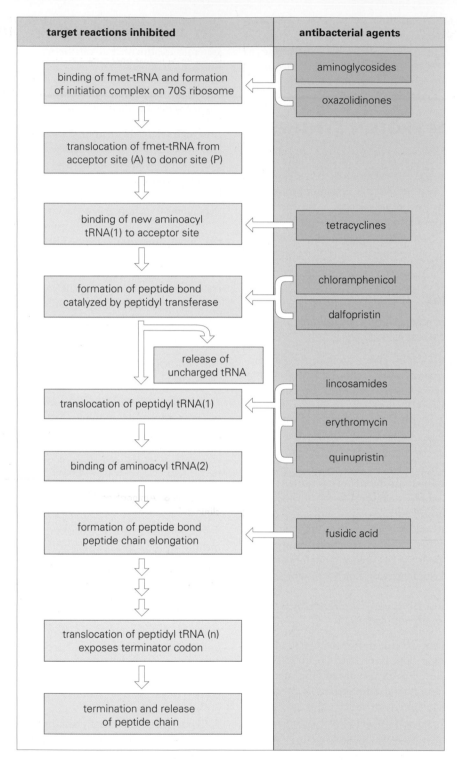

Fig. 33.16 The synthetic pathway leading to the production of new protein in bacterial cells is extremely complex and still not fully elucidated. A number of different groups of antibacterial agents act by inhibiting proteins with specific reactions in this synthetic pathway. They can be grouped into those that act on the 30S subunit of the ribosome (e.g. aminoglycosides and tetracyclines) and those that act on the 50S subunit (e.g. chloramphenicol, lincosamides, erythromycin and fusidic acid). (fmet-tRNA, formylmethionyl-transfer RNA.)

CHEMICAL GROUPS OF AMINOGLYCOSIDES	
4, 6-disubstituted 2-deoxystreptamines	
gentamicin*	complex of 3 closely related structures; first aminoglycoside with broad spectrum
tobramycin**	activity very similar to gentamicin but slightly better against *Pseudomonas aeruginosa*
kanamycin**	no longer in clinical use
amikacin	semi-synthetic derivative of kanamycin; active against many gentamicin-resistant Gram-negative rods
netilmicin*	activitiy spectrum similar to amikacin; probably least toxic of aminoglycosides
4, 5-disubstituted 2-deoxystreptamines	
neomycin**	too toxic for parenteral use but has topical uses in decontaminating mucosal surfaces
streptidine-containing	
streptomycin**	oldest aminoglycoside; now use restricted to treatment of tuberculosis
*micins from *Micromonospora* species **mycins from *Streptomyces* species	

Fig. 33.17 Aminoglycoside-aminocyclitol antibiotics can be classified according to their chemical structure. They are also differentiated by the genus of microorganisms that produces them, and this is reflected in the spelling of the names.

INDICATIONS FOR AMINOGLYCOSIDE THERAPY
Basic rule: use only in severe, life-threatening infections
Gram-negative septicemia (including *Pseudomonas*) usually in combination with beta-lactam
Septicemia of unknown* etiology arising from: hospital-acquired infection malignancy immunosuppressive therapy major trauma, major surgery or major burns intravenous catheter urinary catheter extremes of age
Bacterial endocarditis for synergy with penicillin
Staphylococcus aureus septicemia in combination with beta-lactam
Pyelonephritis for difficult cases
Post-surgical abdominal sepsis in combination with anti-anaerobe therapy
*every effort should be made to establish etiology

Fig. 33.18 Aminoglycosides are valuable additions to the clinician's armamentarium despite their potential toxicity. They are important agents active against Gram-negative facultative bacteria and are often used in combination with beta-lactams to broaden the spectrum to include streptococci and some anaerobes, which are not susceptible to aminoglycosides alone. Resistance to aminoglycosides, particularly among enterobacteria and staphylococci, is mediated by the production of aminoglycoside-modifying enzymes, which react with groups on the aminoglycoside molecule to yield an altered aminoglycoside product. This competes with the unmodified aminoglycoside for uptake into the cell and binding to the ribosome.

genera is common, due partly to the widespread use of these drugs in humans and also to their use as growth promoters in animal feed. The resistance genes are carried on a transposon and new cytoplasmic membrane proteins are synthesized in the presence of tetracycline. As a result tetracycline is positively pumped out of resistant cells (efflux mechanism).

Tetracyclines should be avoided in pregnancy and in children under 8 years of age

Tetracyclines suppress normal gut flora, resulting in gastro-intestinal upset and diarrhea and encouraging overgrowth by resistant and undesirable bacteria (e.g. *Staph. aureus*) and fungi (e.g. *Candida*).

Interference with bone development and brown staining of teeth occurs in the fetus and in children. Systemic administration may cause liver damage.

Chloramphenicol

Chloramphenicol contains a nitrobenzene nucleus and prevents peptide bond synthesis, with a bacteriostatic result

Chloramphenicol is a relatively simple molecule containing a nitrobenzene nucleus, which is responsible for some of the toxic problems associated with the drug (see below). Other derivatives have been produced, but none is in widespread clinical use.

Chloramphenicol has affinity for the large (50S) ribosomal subunit where it blocks the action of peptidyl transferase, thereby preventing peptide bond synthesis *(Fig. 33.16)*. The drug has some inhibitory activity on human mitochondrial ribosomes (which are also 70S) which may account for some of the dose-dependent toxicity to bone marrow (see below).

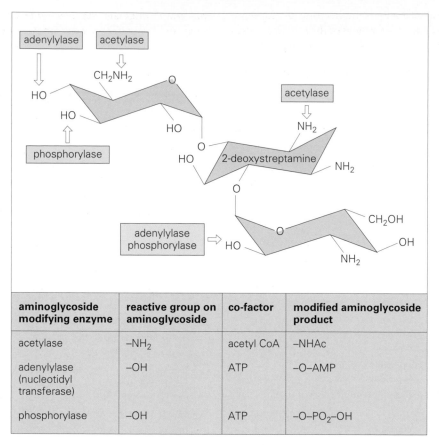

aminoglycoside modifying enzyme	reactive group on aminoglycoside	co-factor	modified aminoglycoside product
acetylase	–NH$_2$	acetyl CoA	–NHAc
adenylylase (nucleotidyl transferase)	–OH	ATP	–O–AMP
phosphorylase	–OH	ATP	–O–PO$_2$–OH

Fig. 33.19 Prototype structure of aminoglycoside consisting of aminohexoses linked via glycosidic linkage to a central 2-deoxystreptamine nucleus. Hydroxyl and amino groups are sites at which these compounds can be inactivated by phosphorylation, adenylation or acetylation catalyzed by enzymes produced by resistant strains.

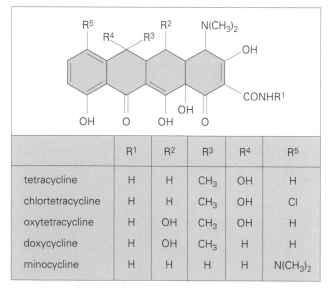

	R^1	R^2	R^3	R^4	R^5
tetracycline	H	H	CH$_3$	OH	H
chlortetracycline	H	H	CH$_3$	OH	Cl
oxytetracycline	H	OH	CH$_3$	OH	H
doxycycline	H	OH	CH$_3$	H	H
minocycline	H	H	H	H	N(CH$_3$)$_2$

Fig. 33.20 Tetracyclines are four-ring molecules with five different sites for substitution, thereby giving rise to a family of molecules with different substituents at different sites. Members of the family differ more in their pharmacologic properties than in their spectrum of activity.

Chloramphenicol is well absorbed when given orally, but can be given intravenously if the patient cannot take drugs by mouth. Topical preparations are also available. It is well distributed in the body and penetrates host cells. Chloramphenicol is metabolized in the liver by conjugation with glucuronic acid to yield a microbiologically inactive form that is excreted by the kidneys.

The main indication for chloramphenicol has been for Salmonella typhi, though resistance is limiting its effectiveness

Chloramphenicol has been used in the treatment of bacterial meningitis (particularly *H. influenzae*) since the drug achieves satisfactory concentrations in the CSF. Topical preparations are used for eye infections. Chloramphenicol is active against a wide variety of bacterial species, both Gram-positive and Gram-negative, aerobes and anaerobes, including intracellular organisms. However, its potential serious toxic effects (see below) and issues of resistance have all but eliminated the systemic use of chloramphenicol in countries where alternative agents are readily available.

The most common mechanism of chloramphenicol resistance involves the inactivation of the drug by a plasmid-mediated enzymatic mechanism which is easily transferred within Gram-negative bacterial populations. Chloramphenicol acetyl transferases produced by resistant bacteria (*Fig. 33.21*) are intracellular, but are capable of inactivating all chloramphenicol in the immediate environment of the cell. Acetylated chloramphenicol fails to bind to the ribosomal target.

The most important toxic effects of chloramphenicol are in the bone marrow

Nitrobenzene is a bone marrow suppressant, and the structurally similar chloramphenicol molecule has similar effects. This toxicity takes two forms:

- dose-dependent bone marrow suppression, which occurs if the drug is given for long periods and is reversible when treatment is stopped;
- an idiosyncratic reaction causing aplastic anemia, which is not dose dependent and is irreversible. It can occur after treatment has stopped, but is fortunately very rare, occurring in about 1 in 30 000 patients treated.

Chloramphenicol is also toxic to neonates, particularly premature babies whose liver enzyme systems are incompletely developed. This can result in 'gray baby syndrome'. Thus, chloramphenicol serum concentrations should be monitored in neonates.

Macrolides, lincosamides and streptogramins

These three groups of antibacterial agents share overlapping binding sites on ribosomes, and resistance to macrolides confers resistance to the other two groups. The clinically important drugs are the macrolide erythromycin, and the lincosamide clindamycin; some streptogramins (e.g. pristinamycin) are currently under development.

Macrolides

Erythromycin is the most widely used macrolide and prevents the release of transfer RNA after peptide bond formation

The macrolides are a family of large cyclic molecules all containing a macrocyclic lactone ring *(Fig. 33.22)* and bacteriostatic in activity. Erythromycin is the best known and most widely used, but some of the newer agents, such as azithromycin and clarithromycin, with improved activity and pharmacology may substitute erythromycin for specific indications. Spiramycin is another macrolide used almost exclusively for the treatment of cryptosporidiosis and in the prevention of congenital toxoplasmosis.

Erythromycin binds to the 23S ribosomal RNA (rRNA) in the 50S subunit of the ribosome and blocks the translocation step in protein synthesis, thereby preventing the release of transfer RNA after peptide bond formation *(Fig. 33.16)*.

Erythromycin is usually administered by the oral route, but can also be given intravenously. It is well distributed in the body and penetrates mammalian cells to reach intracellular organisms. The drug is concentrated in the liver and excreted in the bile. A small proportion of the dose is recoverable in the urine.

Erythromycin is an alternative to penicillin for streptococcal infections, but resistant strains of streptococci are common

Erythromycin is active against Gram-positive cocci and is an important alternative treatment of infections caused by streptococci in patients allergic to penicillin. It is active against *Legionella pneumophila* and *Campylobacter jejuni*. It is also active against mycoplasmas, chlamydiae and rickettsiae and is therefore an important drug in the treatment of atypical pneumonia and chlamydial infections of the urinogenital tract.

Resistance is primarily due to either plasmid-encoded *mef* or *erm* genes, for efflux or alteration in the 23S rRNA target by methylation of two adenine nucleotides in the RNA, respectively. The methylase enzyme may be either inducible or constitutively expressed. Erythromycin is a better inducer of resistance than the lincosamides, but strains resistant to erythromycin will also be resistant to lincomycin and clindamycin, so-called 'MLS (macrolide–lincosamide–streptogramin) resistance'. Induction also varies between bacterial species, and resistant strains of Gram-positive cocci such as staphylococci and streptococci are common. In contrast to methylation, efflux is only active against macrolide drugs and does not confer lincosamide and streptogramin resistance.

Erythromycin is relatively free of serious toxic side effects

Erythromycin causes nausea and vomiting after oral administration in a significant number of patients. Jaundice is associated with some formulations of the drug.

Fig. 33.21 Resistance to chloramphenicol is mediated in some organisms by the production of a chloramphenicol acetyl transferase enzyme, which catalyzes the addition of acetyl groups to the chloramphenicol molecule. This is a two-stage reaction producing acetylated chloramphenicol, which is inactive.

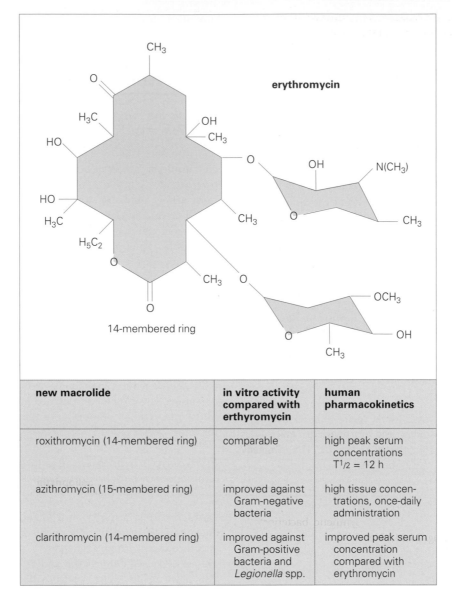

new macrolide	in vitro activity compared with erthyromycin	human pharmacokinetics
roxithromycin (14-membered ring)	comparable	high peak serum concentrations T$\frac{1}{2}$ = 12 h
azithromycin (15-membered ring)	improved against Gram-negative bacteria	high tissue concentrations, once-daily administration
clarithromycin (14-membered ring)	improved against Gram-positive bacteria and Legionella spp.	improved peak serum concentration compared with erythromycin

Fig. 33.22 The macrolides are antibacterial agents composed of large structures, which may be 14-, 15- or 16-membered rings. Erythromycin is the oldest and most widely used of these, but new agents with improved activity and fewer side effects are being developed.

Lincosamides

Clindamycin inhibits peptide bond formation

Clindamycin is a chlorinated more active derivative of lincomycin and represents the most important drug in this class.

Lincosamides bind to the 50S ribosomal subunit and inhibit protein synthesis in a manner similar to erythromycin (Fig. 33.16), hence the MLS resistance combination noted above. The selectively toxic action results from a failure to bind to the equivalent mammalian ribosomal subunit.

Clindamycin is usually given orally, but can be administered intramuscularly or intravenously. It penetrates well into bone, but not into CSF, even when the meninges are inflamed. Clindamycin is actively transported into polymorphonuclear leukocytes and macrophages. It is metabolized in the liver to several products with variable antibacterial activity,

and clindamycin activity persists in feces for up to 5 days after a dose.

Clindamycin has a spectrum of activity similar to that of erythromycin

Clindamycin is much more active than erythromycin against anaerobes, both Gram-positive (e.g. Clostridium spp.) and Gram-negative (e.g. Bacteroides). However, Cl. difficile is resistant and may be selected in the gut, causing pseudomembranous colitis (see below). The activity of clindamycin against Staph. aureus and its penetration into bone makes it a valuable drug in the treatment of osteomyelitis. Clindamycin is not active against aerobic Gram-negative bacteria, because of poor penetration of the outer membrane.

As clindamycin is a less potent inducer of 23S rRNA methylase (see MLS resistance above), erythromycin-resistant strains may appear susceptible to clindamycin in vitro. However, resistance will be manifest in vivo.

Pseudomembranous colitis caused by Cl. difficile *was first noted following clindamycin treatment*

Pseudomembranous colitis caused by *Cl. difficile* follows treatment with many antibiotics. The pathogenesis of this complication is described in Chapter 22, and it should be treated with metronidazole or oral vancomycin.

Streptogramins

The streptogramins formulation currently available is a mixture of streptogramin B and A compounds—quinupristin–dalfopristin, respectively *(Fig. 33.23)*—that are bacteriostatic individually but synergistically bacteriocidal in combination. Both compounds bind to 23S RNA in the large (50S) ribosomal subunit (dalfopristin facilitates binding of quinupristin). Dalfopristin inhibits protein synthesis at an earlier stage than quinupristin *(Fig. 33.16)*, and they together interfere with elongation and extension of peptide chains.

Resistance is relatively uncommon but may develop by altering the quinupristin binding site (MLS resistance described above), enzymatic inactivation, or efflux.

The quinupristin–dalfopristin combination is active against Gram-positive cocci, including multidrug-resistant isolates. Activity is good against *Enterococcus faecium* but not *E. faecalis* (most probably due to an intrinsic efflux mechanism).

Quinupristin–dalfopristin is administered intravenously and primarily metabolized in the liver.

Oxazolidinones

Oxazolidinones are a new class of synthetic bacteriostatic antimicrobial agents *(Fig. 33.24)*. Linezolid, the oxazolidinone currently available, is active against a wide range of Gram-positive bacteria, including multiresistant strains. Linezolid inhibits initiation of protein synthesis *(Fig. 33.16)* by targeting 23S ribosomal RNA in the 50S subunit in a manner which prevents formation of a functional 70S complex.

Due to the drug's unique mechanism of action, resistance mutations (i.e. altered target) are rare and seen primarily in *Enterococcus faecium*.

Linezolid is administered orally or intravenously and is metabolized in the liver.

Fusidic acid

Fusidic acid is a steroid-like compound that inhibits protein synthesis

Fusidic acid is a bacteriostatic agent that inhibits protein synthesis by forming a stable complex with elongation factor EF-G (the bacterial equivalent of the human EF-2), guanosine diphosphate and the ribosome.

Fusidic acid can be administered orally or intravenously. It is well absorbed and penetrates well into tissues and bone, but not into the CSF. Topical preparations are also available, but their use should not be encouraged, because of the rapid emergence of resistance (see below). Fusidic acid is metabolized in the liver and excreted in the bile.

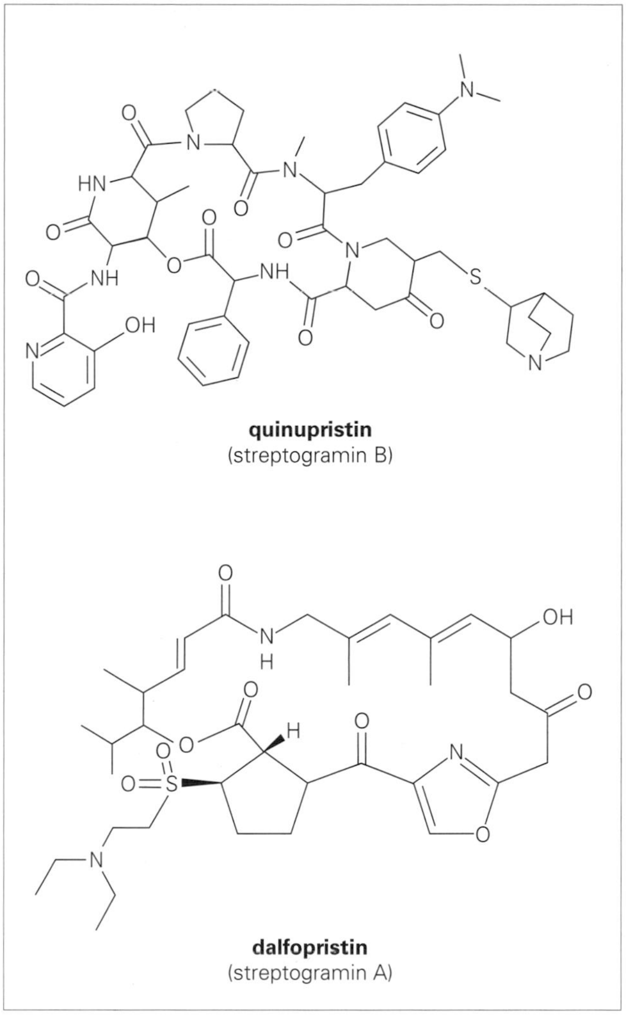

quinupristin
(streptogramin B)

dalfopristin
(streptogramin A)

Fig. 33.23 Chemical structure of the streptogramins.

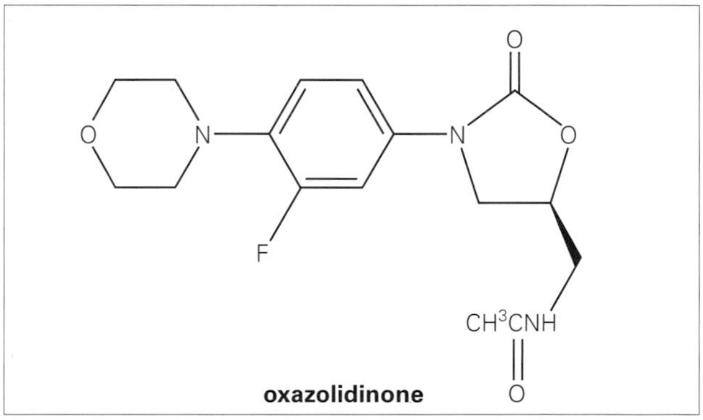

oxazolidinone

Fig. 33.24 Chemical structure of oxazolidinones.

Fusidic acid is a treatment for staphylococcal infections, but should be used with other antistaphylococcal drugs to prevent emergence of resistance

Fusidic acid is active against Gram-positive cocci, and its most important use is in the treatment of staphylococcal infections resistant to beta-lactams or in patients who are allergic to alternative staphylococcal agents. Fusidic acid should be given

INHIBITORS OF NUCLEIC ACID SYNTHESIS
inhibitors of DNA repliction
quinolones
inhibitors of RNA polymerase
rifampicin
antimetabolites inhibiting precursor synthesis
sulfonamides
trimethoprim

Fig. 33.25 Inhibition of nucleic acid takes place at different stages in its synthesis and function, and different groups of antimicrobial agents are involved.

in combination with another antistaphylococcal agent to prevent the emergence of resistant mutants with altered EF-G, which emerge rapidly in staphylococcal populations exposed to the drug.

Fusidic acid has few side effects

Occasionally, fusidic acid causes jaundice and gastrointestinal upset.

INHIBITORS OF NUCLEIC ACID SYNTHESIS

Antibacterial agents that act as inhibitors of nucleic acid synthesis do so in one of three main ways as listed in *Figure 33.25*.

Quinolones

Quinolones are synthetic agents that interfere with replication of the bacterial chromosome

Quinolones represent a large family of bacteriocidal synthetic agents which, in a manner similar to the cephalosporins, can be generally grouped in categories or 'generations' based on their spectrum of activity (*Fig. 33.26*). Nalidixic acid is the first generation prototype, but the addition of fluorine at position 6 of the main quinolone ring (i.e. fluoroquinolones) (*Fig. 33.27*) has improved antibacterial activity, leading to the synthesis of many additional compounds.

The antibacterial activity of quinolones is due to their ability to inhibit the activity of bacterial DNA gyrase and topoisomerases. During replication of the bacterial chromosome, DNA gyrase produces and removes supercoils in DNA ahead of the replication fork to maintain the proper 'tension' required for efficient DNA duplication. Topoisomerase IV similarly acts to remove supercoils and to separate newly formed DNA 'daughter' strands after replication (*Fig. 33.28*). These enzymes thus act in concert to insure that the DNA molecule has the proper conformation for efficient replication and packaging within the cell. Quinolones are able to interfere with these essential enzymes in bacteria while not affecting their counterparts in mamalian cells.

Resistance to quinolones is chromosomally mediated

An important feature is that so far there have been no substantiated reports of plasmid-mediated resistance. However,

CHARACTERISTICS OF REPRESENTATIVE QUINOLONES		
drug	category*	general spectrum of activity
nalidixic acid	first generation	Gram-negative bacteria (excluding *Pseudomonas*)
ciprofloxacin enoxacin lomefloxacin norfloxacin ofloxacin	second generation	first generation coverage but including *Pseudomonas* spp., and some Gram-positives (*Staphylococcus aureus* but not *Streptococcus pneumoniae*)
levofloxacin gatifloxacin moxifloxacin sparfloxacin	third generation	second generation coverage but improved Gram-positive coverage (penicillin-sensitive and -resistant *Strep. pneumoniae*) and some activity against anaerobes
trovafloxacin	fourth generation**	third generation coverage expanded activity against anaerobes

*all but first generation compounds are fluoroquinolones
**associated with cases of acute liver failure; use reserved for life-threatening situations

Fig. 33.26 Characteristics of representative quinolones. The most commonly used agents are listed, together with their main indications.

chromosomally mediated resistance occurs and is exhibited in two forms:

- mutations which change the target enzymes in a manner that affects quinolone binding;
- changes in cell wall permeability, resulting in decreased uptake, or by efflux. These mechanisms may also lead to cross-resistance to other unrelated agents affected by the same process.

Because of their safety and tolerability, quinolones are commonly used as alternatives to beta-lactam antibiotics for treating a variety of infections

Quinolones are primarily administered orally since they are readily absorbed from the gastrointestinal tract, achieving significant serum concentrations and good distribution throughout the body compartments. Excretion is mostly in the urine, though a small proportion is excreted in the feces.

Nalidixic acid does not achieve antibacterial systemic concentrations. It is only active against enterobacteria, and, although occasionally employed in treatment of urinary tract

nalidixic acid

ciprofloxacin

moxifloxacin

trovafloxacin

Fig. 33.27 The quinolones form a large group of synthetic antibacterial agents.

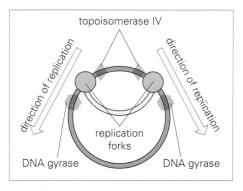

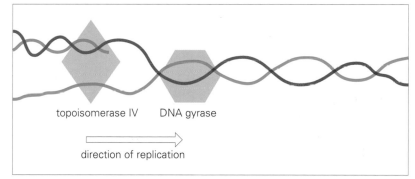

Fig. 33.28 An overview (a) and enlarged view (b) of the role played by bacterial gyrase and topoisomerase enzymes in replication of the bacterial chromosome.

infections (see Chapter 20), its use has largely been replaced by the newer fluorinated compounds.

The newer quinolones have improved activity against Gram-negative rods, including *P. aeruginosa*. In addition to the treatment of urinary tract infections the newer quinolones are useful for systemic Gram-negative infections and in the treatment of chlamydial and rickettsial infections. They are also useful in infections caused by other intracellular organisms such as *L. pneumophila* and *S. typhi*, and in combination with other agents for 'atypical' mycobacteria. They have activity against staphylococci, but overall have only limited use against streptococci and enterococci (*Fig. 33.26*).

Fluoroquinolones are not recommended for children or pregnant or lactating women because of possible toxic effects on cartilage development

Gastrointestinal disturbances are the most common side effect of quinolones. Neurotoxicity and photosensitivity

reactions are less common. However, a notable exception is the potential for liver toxicity associated with trovafloxacin (*Fig. 33.26*) which has prompted severe restrictions on its use.

Rifamycins

Rifampicin is clinically the most important rifamycin and blocks the synthesis of mRNA

Rifampicin is the most important member of the rifamycin family in clinical use. It is a large molecule with a complex structure. Other family members such as rifabutin and rifapentine are also available. All are bacteriocidal in activity.

Rifampicin binds to DNA-dependent RNA polymerase and blocks the synthesis of mRNA. Selective toxicity is based on the far greater affinity for bacterial polymerases than for the equivalent human enzymes.

Rifampicin is administered orally, is well absorbed and is very well distributed in the body. It crosses the blood–brain barrier and reaches high concentrations in saliva. It also appears to have an affinity for plastics, which can be valuable in the treatment of infections involving prostheses.

Rifampicin is metabolized in the liver and excreted in bile. The compound is red, and urine, sweat and saliva of treated patients turns orange. This is harmless, although disturbing for the patient, but is good evidence of patient compliance.

The newer rifamycins, rifabutin and rifapentine, are excreted more slowly than rifampicin, thereby allowing less frequent administration—a feature particularly attractive in the treatment of tuberculosis.

The primary use for rifampicin is in the treatment of mycobacterial infections, but resistance is increasing

While used primarily against mycobacteria, rifampicin may also be used for the prophylaxis of close contacts of meningococcal and *Haemophilus* meningitis. However highly resistant meningococcal strains may emerge, thus short courses only (maximum 48 hours) should be given (see Chapter 24).

While staphylococci rapidly develop resistance to rifampicin, the drug can be efficacious if used in combination with another agent, particularly in the treatment of prosthetic valve endocarditis (see Chapter 29).

Resistance is provided by chromosomal mutations that alter the RNA polymerase target, which then has lowered affinity for rifampicin and escapes inhibition. The prevalence of rifampicin-resistant *M. tuberculosis* is increasing, threatening the future of its use in antituberculous therapy.

Rashes and jaundice are side effects of rifampicin treatment

Intermittent rifampicin can lead to hypersensitivity reactions.

ANTIMETABOLITES AFFECTING NUCLEIC ACID SYNTHESIS

Several commonly used antimicrobial agents inhibit bacterial metabolic pathways including those which produce precursors for nucleic acid synthesis.

Sulfonamides

Sulfonamides are structural analogues of and act in competition with para-aminobenzoic acid

This group of molecules are produced entirely by chemical synthesis (i.e. they are not natural products). In 1935, the parent compound sulfanilamide became the first clinically effective antibacterial agent. The *p*-amino group is essential for activity, but modifications to the sulfonic acid side chain have produced many related agents (*Fig. 33.29*).

Sulfonamides are bacteriostatic compounds that act in competition with *para*-aminobenzoic acid, PABA, for the active site of dihydropteroate synthetase, an enzyme that catalyzes an essential reaction in the synthetic pathway of tetrahydrofolic acid (THFA), which is required for the synthesis of purines and pyrimidines and therefore for nucleic acid synthesis (*Fig. 33.30*). Selective toxicity depends on the fact that many bacteria synthesize THFA whereas human cells lack this capacity and depend on an exogenous supply of folic

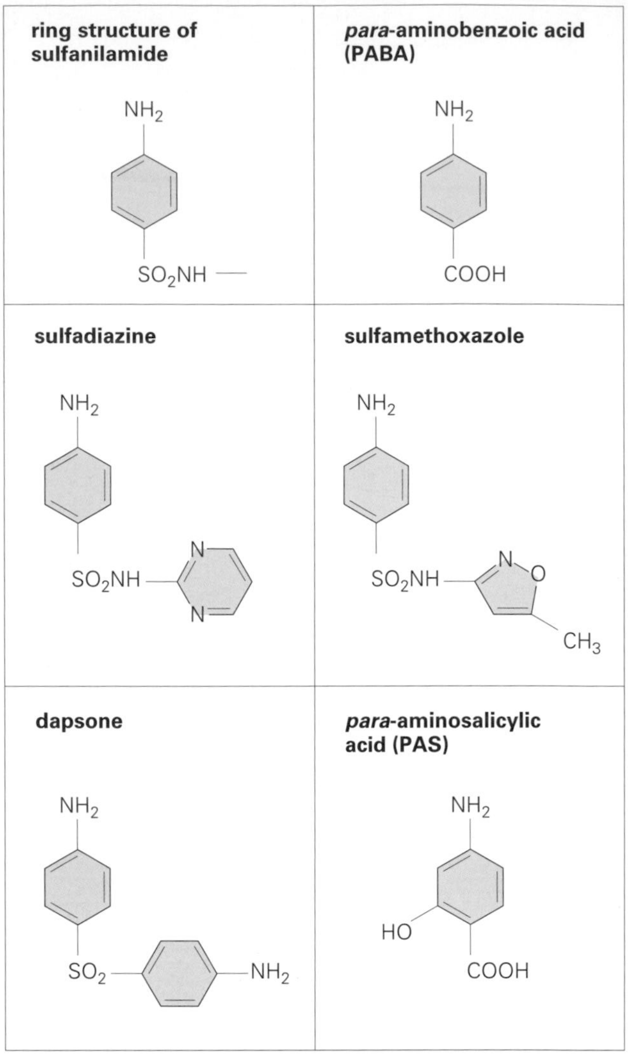

Fig. 33.29 The ring structure of the sulfonamides is very similar to the structure of the normal substrate (PABA) of the dihydropteroate synthetase enzyme, which the sulfonamides inhibit. There are many different sulfonamides available and they differ in their pharmacologic properties more than in their spectrum of activity. Relatively few are now in common clinical use. Dapsone is important in the treatment of *Mycobacterium leprae*, and para-aminosalicylic acid is used for the treatment of *M. tuberculosis*.

acid. Bacteria that can use preformed folic acid are similarly unaffected by sulfonamides.

Sulfonamides are usually administered orally, often in combination with trimethoprim as co-trimoxazole (see below). Different molecules within the family differ in their solubility and penetrability. Metabolism occurs in the liver, and free and metabolized drug are excreted by the kidneys.

Sulfonamides are useful in the treatment of urinary tract infection, but resistance is widespread

The sulfonamides have a spectrum of activity primarily against Gram-negative organisms (except *Pseudomonas*). They are therefore useful in the treatment of urinary tract infections (see Chapter 20). However, susceptibility cannot be assumed, as resistance is widespread with plasmid-mediated genes coding for an altered dihydropteroate synthetase. This is

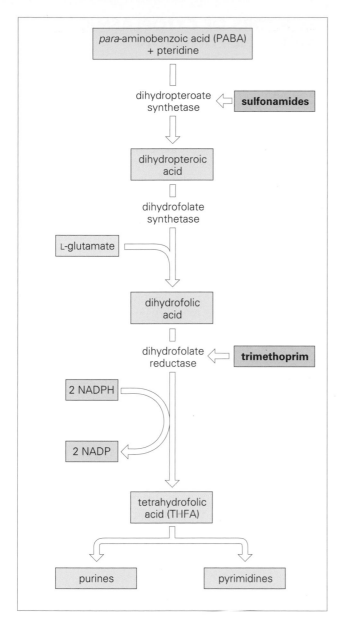

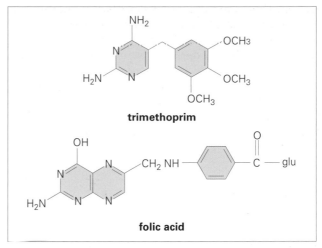

Fig. 33.31 Trimethoprim resembles the aminohydroxypyrimidine moiety of folic acid and in this way antagonizes the enzyme dihydrofolate reductase.

Fig. 33.30 Sulfonamides and trimethoprim inhibit in series the steps in the synthesis of tetrahydrofolic acid by interacting with key enzymes in the pathway.

moiety of the folic acid molecule *(Fig. 33.31)*. Other agents with a similar structure and mechanism of action include the antimalarial pyrimethamine and the anticancer drug methotrexate.

Trimethoprim, like sulfonamides, prevents THFA synthesis, but at a later stage by inhibiting dihydrofolate reductase *(Fig. 33.30)*. This enzyme is present in mammalian cells as well as bacterial and protozoan cells, and selective toxicity depends upon the far greater affinity of trimethoprim for the bacterial enzyme.

Trimethoprim is often given in combination with sulfamethoxazole as co-trimoxazole. The advantages of this combination over either drug alone are:

- Mutant bacteria resistant to one agent are unlikely to be resistant to the other (i.e. double mutation).
- The two agents act synergistically against some bacteria (i.e. the action of the combination is greater than the action of either agent alone).

Trimethoprim can be given orally (either alone or as co-trimoxazole) or by intravenous infusion (alone or accompanied by sulfonamide). Trimethoprim is excreted in urine, and in patients with severe renal failure it is excreted more rapidly than sulfonamide so that the synergistic ratio of the combination may be lost.

Trimethoprim is often given with sulfamethoxazole as co-trimoxazole, and both are used for urinary tract infections

Trimethoprim alone is active against Gram-negative rods with the exception of *Pseudomonas* spp. and its main use is in the treatment (and long term prophylaxis) of urinary tract infection (see Chapter 20).

Co-trimoxazole is active against a wide range of urinary tract pathogens and against *S. typhi*. This combination is also valuable for the treatment of pneumonia caused by the fungus *Pneumocystis jiroveci* (formerly *P. carinii*), although pentamidine, another pyrimidine derivative, is probably the preferred alternative (see Chapter 30). Co-trimoxazole is also

essentially unchanged in its affinity for PABA, but has a greatly decreased affinity for the sulfonamide. A resistant cell therefore possesses two distinct enzymes: a sensitive chromosome-encoded enzyme and a resistant plasmid-encoded enzyme.

Rarely, sulfonamides cause Stevens–Johnson syndrome

Sulfonamides are relatively free of toxic side effects, but rashes and bone marrow suppression can occur.

Trimethoprim (and co-trimoxazole)

Trimethoprim is a structural analogue of the aminohydroxypyrimidine moiety of folic acid and prevents the synthesis of THFA

Trimethoprim is one of a group of pyrimidine-like molecules analogous in structure to the aminohydroxypyrimidine useful for the treatment of nocardiosis (see Chapter 30) and chancroid (see Chapter 21).

Resistance to trimethoprim is provided by plasmid-encoded dihydrofolate reductases

Plasmid-encoded dihydrofolate reductases with altered affinity for trimethoprim allow the synthesis of THFA to proceed unhindered by the presence of trimethoprim. The 'replacement enzymes' are approximately 20 000-fold less susceptible to trimethoprim while retaining their affinity for the normal substrate. Bacteria that are resistant to sulfonamide and trimethoprim are also resistant to co-trimoxazole.

People with AIDS seem to be more prone to the side effects of trimethoprim and co-trimoxazole

Trimethoprim alone and in combination with sulfamethoxazole can cause neutropenia. Nausea and vomiting may occur.

OTHER AGENTS THAT AFFECT DNA

Nitroimidazoles

Metronidazole is a nitroimidazole with antiparasitic and antibacterial properties

After entry into the microbial cell the molecule is activated by reduction, and the reduced intermediate products are responsible for antimicrobial activity, probably through interaction with, and breakage of, the cell's DNA. The reactive intermediates are short-lived and decompose to non-toxic inactive end-products. Metronidazole is active only against anaerobic organisms because only these can produce the low redox potential necessary to reduce the parent drug.

Metronidazole has also been used as a hypoxic cell sensitizer in radiotherapy.

Metronidazole is usually given orally or rectally. It is well absorbed and well distributed in tissues and CSF. The drug is metabolized and most of the parent compound and metabolites are excreted in the urine

Metronidazole was originally introduced for the treatment of the flagellate parasite Trichomonas vaginalis

Metronidazole is also effective against other protozoan parasites such as *Giardia lamblia* and *Entamoeba coli*. It is an important agent for the treatment of infections caused by anaerobic bacteria.

Metronidazole resistance is relatively rare and appears to involve either an alteration in uptake or a decrease in cellular reductase activity, thereby slowing the activation of the intracellular drug.

Rarely, metronidazole causes central nervous system side effects

The most serious side effects of metronidazole involve the central nervous system and include peripheral neuropathy. However, these are relatively uncommon and usually seen only in patients on large doses or prolonged treatment.

INHIBITORS OF CYTOPLASMIC MEMBRANE FUNCTION

The cytoplasmic membranes that encompass all kinds of living cells perform a variety of vital functions. The structure of these membranes in bacterial cells differs from that in mammalian cells and allows the application of some selectively toxic molecules, but these are few in number compared with those acting at other target sites. The most important are the polymyxins, which act on the membranes of Gram-negative bacteria. The polyene antifungal agents (amphotericin B, nystatin) also act by inhibiting membrane function (see below).

Polymyxins

Polymyxins are bacteriocidal cyclic polypeptides that disrupt the structure of cell membranes

The free amino groups of polymyxins act as cationic detergents, disrupting the phospholipid structure of the cell membrane. Polymyxin B and E are the most common members of the family still in clinical use.

In the past they have been used systemically, but due to poor distribution in tissues, neurotoxicity and nephrotoxicity, they have been superseded by less toxic agents.

Polymyxins are primarily used topically but have also been used for gut decontamination, wound irrigation and as a bladder washout

Polymyxins are active against Gram-negative organisms except *Proteus* spp. They are mostly used topically in ointments, and for wound irrigation or as a bladder washout. After oral administration, polymyxins are not absorbed from the gut, and polymyxin E (colistin) has been used in some gut decontamination regimens for neutropenic patients.

Resistance due to chromosomally mediated alterations in membrane structure or antibiotic uptake has been reported.

URINARY TRACT ANTISEPTICS

Nitrofurantoin and methenamine inhibit urinary pathogens

Nitrofurantoin and methenamine are both synthetic compounds that, when taken orally, are absorbed and excreted in the urine in concentrations high enough to inhibit urinary pathogens. Nitrofurantoin has activity only in acid urine. Methenamine is hydrolyzed at acid pH to produce ammonia and formaldehyde; it is the formaldehyde that has the antibacterial activity. Nitrofurantoin is used to treat uncomplicated urinary tract infection, and both agents are used to prevent recurrent urinary tract infections. They have the advantage that in susceptible bacterial populations resistance rarely develops.

ANTITUBERCULOUS AGENTS

M. tuberculosis and other mycobacterial infections need prolonged treatment

The treatment of infections caused by *M. tuberculosis* and other mycobacteria presents an enormous challenge to medicine and the pharmaceutical industry because these organisms:

- Have a waxy outer layer that makes them naturally very impermeable and difficult to penetrate with antibiotics.
- Have an intracellular location, often in cells surrounded by a mass of caseous material, that also makes it difficult for antibiotics to get to them.
- Grow and multiply extremely slowly, and effective inhibition (and therefore cure) takes weeks or months to achieve. Long term therapy is therefore a challenge for drug delivery, and orally administrable drugs are consequently highly desirable. It also follows that the emergence of resistance among the mycobacteria and toxicity in the patient are more likely than with the 'short sharp shock' treatment more often administered for bacterial infections.
- Are common and increasing in the wake of the AIDS epidemic in developing countries, where the cost of drug treatment can be prohibitive.

A number of antituberculous agents are now available. Most are restricted to treating mycobacteria to prevent resistance emerging in other species or because their toxicity makes them unattractive for general use.

The drugs for first line therapy of tuberculosis are isoniazid, ethambutol, rifampicin, pyrazinamide and streptomycin

Treatment regimens vary between countries but, with susceptible strains, a 9-month course of isoniazid and rifampicin is an approach that has been used with good success. Pending results of susceptibility tests, a three- or four-drug combination is the common initial treatment, and this is continued for resistant isolates. The structure and mechanism of action of rifampicin and streptomycin have been described in preceding parts of this chapter.

Isoniazid

Isoniazid inhibits mycobacteria and is given with pyridoxine to prevent neurologic side effects

Isoniazid is isonicotinic acid hydrazide, a compound that inhibits mycobacteria, but does not affect other species of bacteria or humans to any great extent. Its bacteriocidal activity results from inhibition of mycolic acid synthesis, which also accounts for its specificity. It is well absorbed after oral administration, and a single daily dose is usually prescribed except in more difficult cases such as meningitis or miliary tuberculosis. The main toxic effects in humans are neurologic complications, which can be prevented by the concurrent administration of pyridoxine, and hepatitis.

Ethambutol

Ethambutol inhibits mycobacteria, but can cause optic neuritis

Ethambutol is a synthetic molecule that inhibits, but does not kill, mycobacteria. It acts by inhibiting the polymerization of arabinoglycan, a critical constituent of the mycobacteria cell wall. It is well absorbed after oral administration and well distributed in the body, including the CSF. Resistance appears fairly rapidly if the drug is used alone. Thus, it is combined with other drugs in antituberculous therapy. An important

toxic side effect is optic neuritis, and visual acuity should be monitored during therapy.

Pyrazinamide

Pyrazinamide is a synthetic analogue of nicotinamide. The mechanism of its bactericidal activity is not understood. After oral administration, the drug is readily absorbed from the gastrointestinal tract and well distributed in body tissues and fluids. It is primarily metabolized in the liver and excreted by the kidney. As with ethambutol, resistance during monotherapy requires that the drug be used in combination with other first line agents. The most important toxic side effect of pyrazinamide is hepatotoxicity.

Mycobacterial resistance

Drug resistance and immunocompromised patients complicate tuberculosis therapy

Despite the use of antibiotics in combination, the incidence of resistance among mycobacteria is a persistent and increasing problem. Infections with mycobacteria other than *M. tuberculosis* are on the increase as opportunist infections in people with AIDS, and these organisms tend to be innately more resistant than *M. tuberculosis*.

Treatment of leprosy

Widespread use of dapsone monotherapy for leprosy has led to resistance, so it is now often combined with rifampicin

Infection caused by *M. leprae* is characterized by persistence of the organism in the tissues for years and necessitates very prolonged treatment to prevent relapse. For many years dapsone, related to the sulfonamides *(Fig. 33.29)*, has been used. This drug has the advantages that it is given orally and it is cheap and effective. However, widespread monotherapy has resulted in the emergence of resistance, and a combination of dapsone, rifampicin and clofazime, a phenazine compound, is now commonly used as multidrug therapy.

ANTIBACTERIAL AGENTS IN PRACTICE

It is clear from the preceding sections of this chapter that although there are certain 'rules of thumb' about the resistance of bacteria to an antibiotic, it is often impossible to do more than guess in the absence of laboratory tests. Susceptibility tests performed in the laboratory examine the interaction between antibiotics and bacteria in an isolated and rather artificial fashion. At best the results are a helpful guide to the likely outcome of therapy, at worst they are misleading. Patient factors such as age, underlying disease, and renal and liver impairment, must be taken into account in the antibiotic management of an infection.

Susceptibility tests

Laboratory tests for antibiotic susceptibility fall into two main categories:

- diffusion tests;
- dilution tests.

Diffusion tests involve seeding the organism on an agar plate and applying filter paper disks containing antibiotics

The isolate to be tested is seeded over the entire surface of an agar plate, and filter paper disks containing the antibiotics are applied. After overnight incubation the plate is observed for zones of inhibition around each antibiotic disk *(Fig. 33.32)*. The amount of antibiotic in the disk is related to, among other things, the achievable serum concentration and therefore differs for different antibiotics. In addition, antibiotics differ in their ability to diffuse in agar, so the size of the inhibition zone (and not simply its presence) is an indicator of susceptibility of the isolate. The zone sizes are compared with those for reference organisms (either tested in parallel or established previously and published in reference tables) and the result recorded as 'S' (susceptible), 'I' (intermediate) or 'R' (resistant). An 'I' result indicates that the isolate is less susceptible than the norm, but may respond to higher doses of antibiotic or in sites where the antibiotic is concentrated (e.g. in urine in the bladder for antibiotics excreted by the kidneys).

A dilution test provides a quantitative estimate of susceptibility to an antibiotic

A more quantitative estimate of the susceptibility of an organism to an antibiotic can be achieved by performing a MIC (minimum inhibitory concentration) test (i.e. a test to find the lowest concentration that will inhibit visible growth of the bacterial isolate in vitro). Serial dilutions of the test antibiotic are prepared in broth or agar medium and inoculated with a suspension of the test organism. After overnight incubation, the MIC is recorded as the highest dilution in which there is no macroscopic growth *(Fig. 33.33)*. These tests can be performed in a microtiter plate format and form the basis of some automated susceptibility test systems. An alternative approach is the E-test in which a filter paper strip impregnated with a gradient of antibiotic is laid on an agar plate seeded with the test isolate. The concentration on the strip at which growth is inhibited indicates the MIC.

MIC tests are clearly more costly than diffusion tests in terms of time and materials and are not required for every isolate from every patient, but they yield useful information for the management of difficult infections or for patients who are failing to respond to apparently appropriate therapy.

An advantage of an MIC test is that it can be extended to determine the MBC (minimum bacterial concentration), which is the lowest concentration of an antibiotic required to kill the organism. In order to discover whether the agent has actually killed the bacteria rather than simply inhibited their growth, the test dilutions are subcultured onto a fresh drug-free medium and incubated for a further 18–24 hours *(Fig. 33.33)*. The antibacterial agent is considered to be bactericidal if the MBC is equal to or not greater than fourfold higher than the MIC.

Killing curves provide a dynamic estimate of bacterial susceptibility

One of the disadvantages of MIC and MBC tests is that the result is read at only one point in time. A more dynamic estimate of bacterial susceptibility can be gained by measuring the decrease in viability of the population with time *(Fig. 33.34)*. As with MIC tests, it is not feasible to perform killing curves manually for every test isolate, but they can provide useful information for difficult treatment problems. A number of the automated susceptibility test systems use a measure of bacterial viability (e.g. turbidity, electrical impedance) in the presence of an antibacterial as their indicator system. These machines can produce results more rapidly (within about 4 hours) than conventional susceptibility tests. However, automated systems do not work well with fastidious organisms (e.g. pneumococcus, *N. meningitidis*, etc.) or with resistance that is characteristically difficult to detect (e.g. borderline oxacillin MICs in *Staphylococcus aureus*, ESBLs in Gram-negative isolates, etc.)

Combining antibacterial agents can lead to synergism or antagonism

Hospital patients frequently receive more than one antibacterial agent, and these agents may interact with each other (and also with other drugs such as diuretics).

Antibacterial combinations are described as:

- 'synergistic' if their activity is greater than the sum of the individual activities;
- 'antagonistic' if the activity of one drug is compromised in the presence of the other.

Both diffusion and dilution tests allow the action of combinations of antibiotics to be studied. Although synergy can often be demonstrated in vitro *(Fig. 33.35)*, it is difficult to confirm in vivo. Co-trimoxazole is an example of a combination that is frequently used (see above). Another example is the combination of penicillin (or ampicillin) with gentamicin in the treatment of endocarditis caused by *Enterococcus* spp., as this combination has been shown to be clearly superior to the effect of the beta-lactam alone *(Fig. 33.36)*.

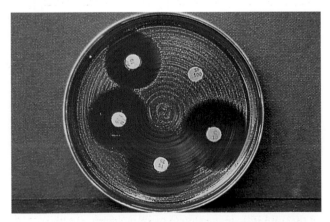

Fig. 33.32 The antibiotic susceptibility of an organism can be tested by the application of filter paper impregnated with antibiotic onto a lawn of the organisms seeded on an agar plate. After overnight incubation the organism grows and the antibiotics diffuse to produce a zone of inhibition that indicates the degree of susceptibility: disk susceptibility test indicating sulfonamide resistance (SF100 is the sulfonamide disk) (Courtesy of DK Banerjee.)

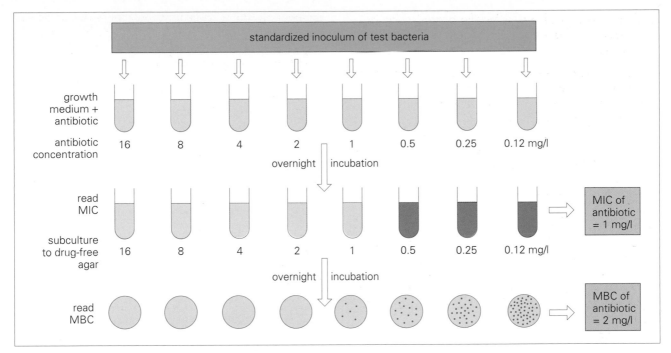

Fig. 33.33 More precise measures of the amount of antibiotic required to inhibit and kill a bacterial population can be estimated by establishing the minimum inhibitory concentration (MIC) and minimum bactericidal concentration (MBC) of the antibiotic. Using the standard method as outlined in this illustration, the MIC result is available after 24 hours and the MBC result after 48 hours. A number of variables such as the inoculum size, the growth medium and the interpretation of the results affect the outcome of MIC tests.

Antagonism can be demonstrated between some pairs of antibiotics in vitro but is rarely evident in vivo.

ANTIBIOTIC ASSAYS

In the preceding parts of this chapter the pharmacokinetic properties (absorption, distribution, excretion) of antibacterial agents have been summarized. Some antibacterials have a narrow 'therapeutic index'—that is, the concentration required for successful treatment and the concentration toxic to the patient are not very different. The concentrations of such antibiotics should be monitored both to prevent toxicity and to ensure that therapeutic concentrations are achieved. Other less toxic agents should be monitored in some circumstances in some patients (*Fig. 33.37*). Serum concentrations are usually measured, but urine, CSF and other body fluids can be assayed if applicable.

Antibiotic assays may be performed by a variety of methods such as high performance liquid chromatography and direct assays for biological activity (bioassay). However, the most common approach uses immunologic methods which can be automated. In this method, the antibiotic in the patient specimen is an 'antigen' that competes with a specific level of labeled 'tracking' antibiotic for binding sites on an 'anti-drug' antibody. Thus, increased antibiotic levels in a patient sample result in decreased binding of tracking antibiotic, etc. Such assays are rapid, require only small volumes of serum, and are highly specific. However, they are obviously only applicable to instances where specific antidrug antibody is available.

ANTIVIRAL THERAPY

The last 15 years has seen a range of new antiviral agents licensed for use against a number of virus infections, including HIV, hepatitis B (HBV), hepatitis C (HCV) and influenza A and B (*Fig. 33.38*). The current antivirals for treating individuals with virus infections are all virustatic rather than virucidal. The problem in developing new antivirals has been mostly due to the difficulty of interfering with viral activity in the cell without adversely affecting the host. This is because viruses are dependent on the host cell's protein synthetic machinery. In addition, early diagnosis of short incubation period viral infections, such as the respiratory viruses, is critical for antiviral chemotherapy to be successful. Virus-specific replication steps can be identified (*Fig. 33.39*), and more of these will doubtless be exploited, such as identifying virus-induced enzymes.

Antiviral resistance occurs with varying prevalence in different patient populations: for example, aciclovir-resistant HSV and ganciclovir-resistant CMV are mostly seen in immunocompromised individuals at a low level. Antiretroviral resistance is seen across all the main classes of agents—nucleoside reverse transcriptase inhibitors, non-nucleoside reverse transcriptase inhibitors, and protease inhibitors—with increasing frequency in resource rich countries. Lamivudine-resistant HBV is well recognized and is usually detected after a couple of years of treatment. One issue with antiviral resistance is that the replication fitness of the drug-resistant variants is often less than the wild type strain. In addition, in the case of a number of viruses, including HBV and HCV, the response varies depending on the viral genotype.

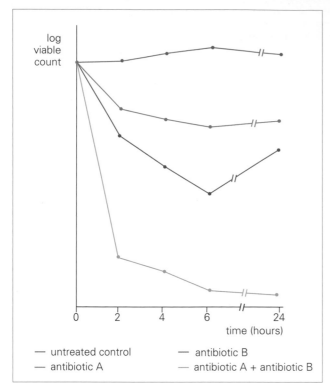

Fig. 33.34 A more dynamic picture of the interaction between an antibiotic and a bacterial population can be gained from producing killing curves. In these experiments a culture of 2×10^6 colony forming units/ml was treated with antibiotics A and B alone and in combination. Compared with the untreated control both A and B inhibit the growth of the bacterial culture, but B is more active than A. However, in combination, the activity of A plus B is synergistic (i.e. it is more active than the sum of the activities of the two antibiotics alone). The combination also prevents the regrowth seen after 6–24 hours when the antibiotics are used singly.

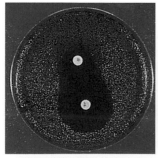
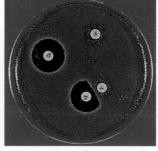

Fig. 33.35 (a) Synergy of two antibacterials. Disks containing sulfonamide and trimethoprim have been placed to demonstrate the synergistic activity of these two agents against *Escherichia coli*. Synergy can be recognized by the fact that the zones of inhibition become continuous between the two disks. (b) Antagonism. Nitrofurantoin is capable of antagonizing the activity of nalidixic acid. When the disks are placed far apart, nalidixic acid inhibits the test organism, but when placed close together this inhibition is antagonized by the presence of nitrofurantoin, as demonstrated by the foreshortening of the zone of inhibition.

USE OF ANTIBIOTIC COMBINATIONS
to obtain a synergistic effect, e.g. co-trimoxazole
to prevent or delay emergence of persistent organisms, e.g. isoniazid, rifampicin and ethambutol for tuberculosis
to treat polymicrobial infections, e.g. intra-abdominal abcesses where the different microbes have different susceptibilities
to treat serious infections in the stage before the infectious agent is identified

Fig. 33.36 Reasons for using antibiotic combinations. Ideally, single drugs are used, but antibiotic combinations are justifiable under certain circumstances.

ANTIBIOTIC ASSAYS ARE IMPORTANT
when an antibiotic has a narrow therapeutic index, e.g. aminoglycosides
when the normal route of excretion of antibiotic is impaired, e.g. in patients with renal failure for agents excreted via the kidney
when the absorption of the antibiotic is uncertain, e.g. after oral administration
to ascertain concentrations in sites of infection into which penetration of antibiotic is irregular or unknown, e.g. in CSF
in patients receiving prolonged therapy for serious infections, e.g. endocarditis
in neonates with serious infections
in patients who fail to respond to apparently appropriate therapy
to check on patient compliance

Fig. 33.37 Assays of antibiotics in clinical practice are particularly important when the antibiotic is potentially toxic, but there is a variety of other situations in which assays are important. (CSF, cerebrospinal fluid.)

Some viral infections have an immunopathologic basis, such as CMV pneumonitis, in which case an antiviral is given in combination with an immunoglobulin preparation. This may be human normal imunoglobulin or virus-specific immunoglobulin, i.e. CMV hyperimmune globulin. Moreover, an immunomodulator may be given in conjunction with an antiviral such as pegylated interferon and ribavirin to treat hepatitis C infection.

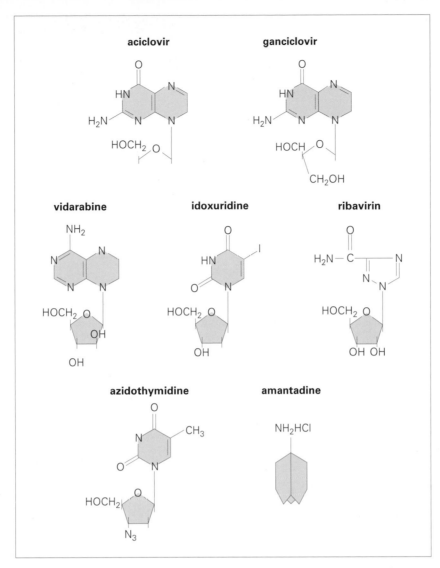

Fig. 33.38 Antiviral agents are few in number and narrow in their spectrum of activity—for example, amantadine is effective against influenza A, but not influenza B, while aciclovir is effective against herpes simplex virus (HSV) and varicella-zoster virus (VZV), but not cytomegalovirus (CMV) or Epstein–Barr virus (EBV).

Palivizumab is an example of a humanized monoclonal antibody produced to prevent infection. It is directed against the respiratory syncytial virus (RSV) fusion protein and has potent neutralizing and fusion inhibitory activity. It is used in specific clinical settings to prevent severe lower respiratory tract infections caused by RSV requiring hospitalization in children born at 35 weeks' gestation or less who are less than 6 months old at the onset of the RSV season. In addition, it may be used in children less than 2 years of age with specific respiratory and cardiac conditions such as bronchopulmonary dysplasia.

Finally, in the case of some viral respiratory tract infections, antibiotics are often given to control or act as prophylaxis against a secondary bacterial infection. Influenza infection is an example where staphylococcal and streptococcal pneumonia may occur after the initial virological insult.

Aciclovir (acycloguanosine)

Aciclovir inhibits HSV and varicella-zoster virus (VZV) DNA polymerase

Aciclovir is used in the treatment of HSV and VZV infections. A number of other agents are now licensed, including valaciclovir, the L-valyl ester of aciclovir, and famciclovir. Aciclovir is inactive until phosphorylated and is an example of a prodrug. Aciclovir (Fig. 33.40) is phosphorylated by the herpesvirus thymidine kinase and the monophosphate is then converted by cellular kinases to the triphosphate, which inhibits the herpesvirus DNA polymerase. As it is taken up and efficiently phosphorylated by HSV infected cells, the action on cellular DNA polymerase is minimal and toxic side effects such as neutropenia and thrombocytopenia are usually not severe. The drug is also incorporated into viral DNA,

replication stage	drugs available
1 Adsorption	fusion inhibitors, e.g. T-20*
2 Penetration and uncoating	amantadine
3 Viral DNA/RNA synthesis	examples include: aciclovir zidovudine lamivudine nevirapine ribavirin
4 Viral protein synthesis	interferons
5 Assembly	protease inhibitors
6 Release	none available

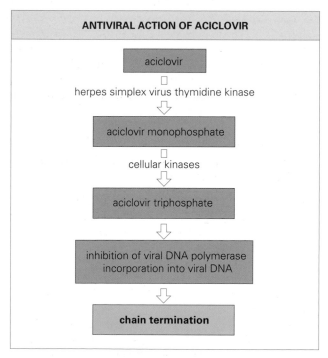

Fig. 33.39 The site of action of antiviral agents. Resistance to agents is uncommon, but does occur (e.g. cytomegalovirus strains resistant to ganciclovir, herpes simplex virus strains resistant to aciclovir). Adsorption of virus to cell can be blocked by virus-specific antibody. *T-20 binds to the HIV gp41 site, preventing attachment to the T cell.

ANTIVIRAL ACTION OF ACICLOVIR

aciclovir

herpes simplex virus thymidine kinase

aciclovir monophosphate

cellular kinases

aciclovir triphosphate

inhibition of viral DNA polymerase incorporation into viral DNA

chain termination

Fig. 30.40 The activity of an antiviral agent against different herpes viruses is correlated with the ability of the viruses to induce a thymidine kinase, hence aciclovir is most active against herpes simplex virus and least active against cytomegalovirus.

resulting in chain termination. As it is excreted by the kidney, the drug can crystallize in the renal tract in individuals with renal failure, causing acute tubular necrosis. Otherwise, aciclovir has an excellent safety profile.

Systemic aciclovir has revolutionized the treatment of HSV encephalitis, and HSV and VZV infections in immuno-compromised patients. It is effective in treating primary and recurrent genital herpes. In shingles (herpes zoster), recovery is accelerated and post-zoster pain reduced. As with HSV, the virus remains latent in ganglia and can reactivate.

As the oral bioavailablilty is only 15–20%, aciclovir is given intravenously in a number of clinical settings initially. Valaciclovir and famciclovir have improved bioavailability profiles in comparison with aciclovir, resulting in less frequent daily dosages.

Ganciclovir (dihydroxypropoxy-methylguanine, DHPG)

Ganciclovir is structurally similar to aciclovir but has an extra hydroxyl group. The range of activity is broader than that of aciclovir, and the drug is active against CMV infections. CMV does not encode a thymidine kinase, but the drug is monophosphorylated by a virus UL97 gene-specified kinase and then further phosphorylated by cellular kinases. However, selective toxicity is not seen, and it is myelosuppressive, its main adverse effect being bone marrow toxicity. Ganciclovir triphosphate inhibits CMV DNA polymerase. It is given intravenously because of limited oral bioavailability. However, an improved oral agent, valganciclovir, has been produced.

Ganciclovir is given to treat CMV infections such as retinitis, encephalitis and gastrointestinal disease seen in immunocompromised individuals. It is also used as pre-emptive therapy in bone marrow transplant as well as solid organ transplant recipients, who are monitored regularly for the presence of CMV in their blood as this leads to CMV dissemination.

Foscarnet (phosphonoformate)

This compound attaches to the pyrophosphate-binding site of the herpesvirus DNA polymerase, preventing nucleotide binding and therefore inhibiting viral replication. It is used in treating CMV infections and is active against HSV and VZV. It is nephrotoxic and is often used as a second line agent.

Nucleoside and nucleotide reverse transcriptase inhibitors

The following have similar modes of action and are mostly used in conjunction with the other main classes of antiretroviral drugs—the non-nucleoside reverse transcriptase inhibitors and protease inhibitors—to treat HIV-infected individuals.

Zidovudine (azidothymidine, AZT)

Zidovudine is an analogue of the nucleoside thymidine in which the hydroxyl group on the ribose is replaced by an azido group. After conversion to the triphosphate by cellular enzymes (Fig. 33.41) it acts as an inhibitor of, and substrate for, the viral reverse transcriptase. The azido group prevents the formation of phosphodiester linkages. Proviral DNA formation is blocked because AZT triphosphate is incorporated into the DNA with resulting chain termination.

Zidovudine is given orally. Toxicity is a problem, with bone marrow suppression (anemia, neutropenia, leukopenia) and less commonly nausea, vomiting, myalgia and malaise. This was more often seen in the early days of HIV treatment when the drug was given at a high dose. Regular blood tests are necessary to detect anemia and myelosuppression.

Drug resistance is well recognized and can lead to cross-resistance to other nucleoside analogues.

Zalcitabine (ddC, deoxycytidine), didanosine (ddI, deoxyinosine), lamivudine (3TC, thiacytidine), stavudine (d4T, didehydrodideoxyuridine), abacavir, tenofovir

Like zidovudine, these nucleoside analogues are converted to triphosphates and inhibit the HIV reverse transcriptase. Some of these agents have been combined: Combivir (AZT and 3TC) and Trizivir (AZT, 3TC and abacavir). Tenofovir is a nucleotide reverse transcriptase inhibitor.

There are a number of adverse effects shared by this class of drugs but the more specific side effects include pancreatitis (ddI), peripheral neuropathy (ddC, d4T, ddI), lipodystrophy, i.e. fatty tissue redistribution from subcutaneous areas such as the face and limbs, to the neck and abdominal viscera (d4T), and hypersensitivity (abacavir). Mitochondrial toxicity due to inhibition of the mitochondrial DNA polymerase and lactic acidosis is also reported.

Drug resistance is well recognized and can lead to cross-resistance to other nucleoside analogues.

Non-nucleoside reverse transcriptase inhibitors

Nevirapine and efavirenz (DMP)

These are used in combination with the nucleoside analogues and may be used as first line drugs before moving to the protease inhibitor class. This is because they lead to a rapid fall in the plasma HIV RNA load, especially in those individuals with very high HIV loads for whom protease inhibitor treatment is being considered, and have fewer side effects. They act as non-competitive inhibitors of HIV1 reverse transcriptase by binding to a hydrophobic pocket proximal to the enzyme catalytic site. They are inactive against HIV2. The most common adverse effect with nevirapine is a skin rash. Efavirenz may cause vivid dreams and sleep disturbance initially.

A single mutation in the reverse transcriptase leads to resistance to both drugs, effectively removing this class of drug from the treatment regimen.

Protease inhibitors

Nelfinavir, saquinavir, indinavir, ritonavir, Kaletra, amprenavir

The protease enzyme acts in the post-translational cleavage of the *gag* and *gag–pol* polyproteins into the structural proteins and enzymes critical for viral replication. The result of protease inhibition is the production of immature, defective viral particles. Protease inhibitors are very potent drugs which lead to a rapid fall in the plasma HIV RNA load, especially in those individuals with very high HIV loads, and are usually given in combination with nucleoside analogues. They are metabolized and excreted rapidly and have to be taken several times daily. Side effects include gastrointestinal disturbances, the lipodystrophy syndrome (body fat redistribution), increased triglycerides, and insulin resistance leading to diabetes.

Drug resistance is well recognized and a number of protease mutations result in cross-resistance. A protease inhibitor that has been licensed is a combination of lopinavir and ritonavir (Kaletra), which looks very promising in terms of a lesser degree of drug resistance developing. Fusion inhibitor T-20 blocks HIV before it enters the host cell by binding to gp41, the transmembrane glycoprotein.

Ribavirin (tribavirin)

This guanosine analogue is triphosphorylated by cellular enzymes. It has various actions including inhibition of

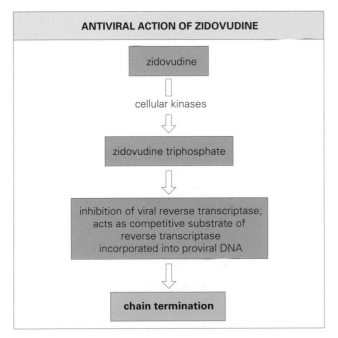

Fig. 33.41 HIV reverse transcriptase is 100 times more sensitive than host cell DNA polymerase to zidovudine triphosphate, but toxic effects are not uncommon.

production of guanosine triphosphate pools needed for viral nucleic acid synthesis. It is used clinically as an aerosol for severe respiratory syncytial virus (RSV) infection in infants and for arenavirus infections such as Lassa fever (see Chapter 26). It is active against measles.

Influenza virus inhibitors

Amanatidine and rimantadine have been joined by a new class of agents, the neuraminidase inhibitors, which have increased the range of activity by inhibiting both influenza A and B.

Amantidine

It has been known since the 1960s that amantidine specifically inhibits the replication of influenza A viruses, but has no effect on influenza B and other respiratory viruses. It acts by inhibiting the penetration of virus into the cell, or its uncoating. Fusion of the viral envelope with a cell membrane, which normally occurs at a low pH, is prevented. Amantadine raises the pH in intracellular vacuoles and therefore blocks infection. The standard dose can cause minor neurologic side effects such as insomnia, dizziness and headache, especially in elderly patients, and this has discouraged its widespread use. Amantadine can be given prophylactically during community outbreaks of influenza A. It can also be used for treatment, and if taken within 48 hours of symptoms there is a reduction in disease severity.

Neuraminidase inhibitors: zanamivir and oseltamivir

Neuraminidase is one of the two surface glycoproteins studded on the influenza virus surface and cleaves sialic acid residues from the host cell, thus releasing the virus and allowing further spread in the respiratory tract.

The neuraminidase inhibitors act as competitive reversible inhibitors of the active enzyme site. Zanamivir is an inhaled agent which is a sialic acid analogue. Oseltamivir is an oral drug cleaved by esterases to the active carboxylate form. Both interact in different ways at the enzyme active site and act on influenza A and B.

These drugs reduce viral shedding, disease severity, duration and symptoms if given early in infection and can be used as prophylaxis.

Agents against hepatitis B and C viruses

Although interferons have been used to treat individuals with these chronic infections, success has been limited for reasons outlined below. In addition, relapse often occurs on discontinuing treatment.

Studies have shown greater success in treating HCV infections by combining pegylated interferon with ribavirin, and with HBV using antivirals such as lamivudine and adefovir.

Development of antivirals

Directions being taken in the development of new antivirals include:

- Blocking adsorption of virus to the cell by coating the virus with analogues or peptides of the cell receptor molecule (e.g. the CD4 molecule on T cells in the case of HIV) or coating cells with viral attachment proteins (e.g. gp120 in the case of HIV).
- Blocking viral mRNA with short nucleotide sequences that are complementary to viral sequences. These antisense oligonucleotides bind to newly transcribed viral RNA and block its action.
- Using compounds that inactivate virus when used topically.

Uses of interferons in human infection

Interferons (IFNs; see Chapter 9) show a dramatic effect on virus replication in vitro (at pg/ml of IFN) and are active against certain experimental virus infections. However, their clinical use has been disappointing. One problem has been that their very short half-life in the circulation makes it difficult to deliver adequate amounts to the sites of infection. Very large doses have an established role in the treatment of chronic hepatitis B and C infection. IFNs have an effect on papillomavirus infections, given by intralesional injection, but are not used routinely.

Interferons, especially IFNγ, also have important actions on the immune system and a potential for use as immunomodulators.

Many patients experience flu-like symptoms with IFNs

Flu-like symptoms of fever, myalgia and headache are side effects of IFNs, even with genetically engineered IFNs. Indeed such symptoms in virus infections have been attributed to the action of endogenously produced IFNs. Leukopenia, thrombocytopenia, and central nervous system effects have also been noted with IFN treatment, especially with high dose treatment.

ANTIFUNGAL AGENTS

Compared with antibacterials, the number of suitable antifungal drugs is very limited. Selective toxicity is much more difficult to achieve in the eukaryotic fungal cells than in the prokaryotic bacteria, and although the available antifungals have greater activity against fungal cells than they do against human cells the difference is not as marked as it is for most antibacterial agents. Treatment of fungal infections is further hampered by problems of solubility, stability and absorption of the existing drugs, and the search for new agents is a high priority. Drug resistance is also increasing.

Antifungals can be classified on the basis of target site and chemical structure

Like antibacterials, antifungals can be classified on the basis of target site and chemical structure. This immediately reveals a major difference between antibacterial and antifungal agents, with the major antifungals acting on the synthesis or function of the intracellular membranes. The exceptions are flucytosine (5-fluorocytosine) and griseofulvin, which interfere with DNA synthesis. There are currently no inhibitors of fungal protein synthesis that do not also inhibit the equivalent mammalian pathway.

Azole compounds and echinocandins inhibit cell membrane synthesis

Azole antifungals act by inhibiting lanosterol C14-demethylase, an important enzyme in sterol biosynthesis. Clotrimazole and miconazole are useful as topical preparations. Ketoconazole has become the agent of choice for many serious fungal infections (Fig. 33.42), and fluconazole is increasingly used in the treatment of *Candida* infections. Resistance to the azoles is becoming more widespread and threatens to compromise this group of compounds Further azole compounds (e.g. posaconazole, voriconazole) are currently being tested. The more recent echinocandin antifungals offer new therapeutic options against infections such as *Aspergillus*, *Candida* and *Pneumocystis*.

Polyenes inhibit cell membrane function

Amphotericin B and nystatin act by binding to sterols in cell membranes, resulting in leakage of cellular contents and cell death. Their preferential binding to ergosterol over cholesterol is the basis for selective toxicity. Amphotericin remains the drug of choice for the treatment of serious systemic fungal infections despite its serious toxic side effects; lipid formulations have lower toxicity. Nystatin is used only in topical formulations.

Flucytosine and griseofulvin inhibit nucleic acid synthesis

Flucytosine (5-fluorocytosine) is deaminated to 5-fluorouracil, which inhibits DNA synthesis. Selective toxicity is based on the preferential uptake by fungal cells compared with host cells. Flucytosine is active only on yeasts (e.g. *Candida* spp. and *Cryptococcus*). Resistance emerges rapidly to flucytosine, which should therefore be used in combination with amphotericin B (whereby it is sometimes possible to reduce the dose of amphotericin B and therefore the toxic side effects).

Griseofulvin appears to inhibit nucleic acid synthesis and to have antimitotic activity, possibly by inhibiting microtubule assembly. It may also have effects on cell wall synthesis by inhibiting chitin synthesis. In the host, griseofulvin binds specifically to newly formed keratin and is active in vivo only against dermatophyte fungi (see Chapters 4 and 20).

Other topical antifungal agents include Whitfield's ointment, tolnaftate, ciclopirox, haloprogin and naftifine

A variety of agents such as Whitfield's ointment (a mixture of benzoic and salicylic acids), tolnaftate, ciclopirox, haloprogin and naftifine, are available as creams for the topical treatment of superficial mycoses. These are usually available over the counter, and there is little to choose between them.

No single antifungal agent is ideal

The main uses and adverse effects of antifungals are summarized in *Figure 33.42*. Although there are several effective preparations available, some conditions such as ringworm infection of the nails or recurrent vaginal candidiasis are frequently intractable to treatment. The number of antifungal agents for systemic fungal infections is limited, and their adverse effects are considerable.

Fungi develop resistance to antifungal agents

Although much less studied than resistance to antimicrobials used against bacteria, there is evidence that many similar mechanisms operate in resistance to antifungals. These include:

- enzyme modification;
- target modification;
- reduced permeability;
- active efflux pumps;
- failure to activate antifugal agents.

Resistance involving some or all of these mechanisms has been described in *Aspergillus*, *Candida* and *Cryptococcus*, particularly in the case of the azole compounds.

There is an urgent need for safer more efficacious antifungal agents

Invasive fungal infections are a significant cause of morbidity and mortality in patients undergoing chemotherapy, immune suppression and transplantation. The incidence of these infections is increasing in parallel with the increasing numbers of such patients and their improved survival due to effective antibacterial therapy. New agents to control these infections (particularly *Aspergillus*) are needed.

ANTIPARASITIC AGENTS

Parasites pose particular problems

Any consideration of antiparasitic agents must take into account the very large number of different parasites capable of infecting man, the complexities of their lifecycles and the differences between them in their metabolic pathways. Thus, drugs acting against protozoa are usually inactive against helminths and vice versa. Additionally, protozoans and helminths are eukaryotes and therefore metabolically more similar to humans than are bacteria. Although some antibacterials do have antiprotozoan activity (e.g. metronidazole, tetracycline), in general antibacterials are ineffective against parasites. A major challenge has been to identify targets where there are sufficient differences between host and parasite to facilitate safe drug activity. Some of these targets include:

- unique drug uptake—choloroquine, mefloquine, primaquine in malaria;
- differences in folic acid metabolism—pyrimethamine in malaria, sulfonamides in toxoplasmosis, trimethoprim in cyclosporidiosis;
- polyamine uptake—pentamidine in leishmaniasis and toxoplasmosis;
- unique trypanothione-dependent reduction mechanisms—fluoromethylornithine against trypanosomes;
- unique neurotransmitters—piperazine, ivermectin, pyrantel against nematodes;

THERAPEUTIC APPLICATIONS OF ANTIFUNGAL AGENTS			
infection	antifungal of choice	route of administration	adverse effects
superficial mycoses			
ringworm (dermatophytes)	griseofulvin	oral	nil
	ketoconazole	oral	anorexia, nausea, vomiting; dose-dependent depression of serum testosterone leading to gynecomastia
candidiasis	fluconazole	oral	inhibits metabolism of ciclosporin when given at high doses
	nystatin	topical	nil
systemic mycoses			
histoplasmosis	ketoconazole	oral	see above
blastomycosis	ketoconazole	oral	see above
coccidioidomycosis	ketoconazole (amphotericin B for CNS involvement) fluconazole	oral	do not use ketoconazole and amphotericin B together (some evidence of antagonism)
paracoccidioido-mycosis	ketoconazole	oral	see above
aspergillosis	amphotericin B fluconazole caspofungin acetate	IV (now available in liposomes)	nephrotoxicity and potassium loss; acute reactions within $\frac{1}{2}$–$1\frac{1}{2}$ h of injection include rigors and hypotension
candidiasis	fluconazole amphotericin B 1 flucytosine	oral IV oral	flucytosine may cause neutropenia and jaundice; emergence of resistant mutants is common if drug is used alone; combination with amphotericin B can be synergistic
cryptococcosis	amphotericin B 1 flucytosine	IV oral	
zygomycosis	amphotericin B	IV	
pneumocystis pneumonia	trimethoprim–sulfamethox-azole pentamidine isetionate	oral	low toxicity

Fig. 33.42 The major therapeutic applications of antifungal drugs. Orally active agents are important for the treatment of superficial mycoses, which are often minor but troublesome infections and may require prolonged treatment. Amphotericin is the most important agent for the treatment of severe systemic mycoses, but is toxic. The azoles, particularly fluconazole and ketoconazole and some of the newer agents, provide suitable alternative therapy in some instances.

- cytoskeletal proteins (tubulin)—benzimidazoles against nematodes;
- intracellular calcium levels—praziquantel against flukes and tapeworms;
- oxidative phosphorylation—niclosamide against tapeworms.

Despite differences between host and parasite in these targets, it remains true that a number of the more effective anti-

parasite drugs carry the risk of significant toxicity, and their use has to balance benefit against cost.

The wide array of different drugs that have been developed is summarized in *Figures 33.43* and *33.44*.

Drug resistance is an increasing problem

As with the antibacterials, drug resistance is a significant problem in the treatment of parasitic infections, particularly with malaria. Malaria treatment is based on four different regimes:

- prophylactic—to prevent infection;
- therapeutic—to treat infection;
- radical cure—to treat infection and prevent relapse;
- control of gametocytes—to prevent transmission.

Chloroquine is one of the drugs of choice for prophylactic and therapeutic treatment, but there is now worldwide resistance of *Plasmodium falciparum* to this drug, and *P. vivax* also shows resistance. The usual alternative to chloroquine has been mefloquine or combined pyrimethamine/sulfadoxine, but there is now significant resistance to the antifolate compounds. Quinine, the original antimalarial is now the resort for severe malaria, although this can have serious side effects. Development of antimalarials from natural products provides the prospect of new compounds, the most important being derivatives of artemisinin (the Chinese drug quinghaosu). Drug resistance is less of a problem with other protozoans and, although widespread in animal parasitic nematodes, has yet to become a serious issue with human infections.

Protozoans make use of enzyme and target modification to develop resistance (e.g. against antifolates and sulfonamides), but in addition active efflux pumps have been described in resistance of *P. falciparum* to chloroquine, mefloquine and artemisinin. Resistance to benzimidazole anthelmintics involves target modification, arising from mutations in cuticular tubulins.

USE AND MISUSE OF ANTIMICROBIAL AGENTS

Much has been said in this chapter about the interactions between antimicrobial agents and microbes—the mechanisms of selective toxicity and the defenses put up by resistant organisms. The distribution, metabolism and excretion of agents by the host have been considered briefly, together with the important toxic side effects of the agents.

The choice of antimicrobial for treating specific infections is dealt with in the appropriate systems chapter (see Chapters 18–30). Dosage regimens have not been included because they vary with the agent, the infection, the age and the underlying condition of the patient, and sometimes from one country to another. Practitioners should consult appropriate local pharmacy guidelines.

Antimicrobial agents should only be used appropriately for prophylaxis or treatment

In conclusion we should stand back and ask 'Is antimicrobial therapy necessary for this patient, and if so which agent is appropriate?'. Antimicrobial agents can be used:

- to help prevent infection (prophylaxis);
- to treat infection.

Prophylactic use of antibiotics is appropriate only in a few clearly defined circumstances and is usually of limited duration (e.g. 1–2 days). Specific examples include (i) patients of normal susceptibility who have been exposed to specific pathogens (e.g. bacterial meningitis or tuberculosis), (ii) individuals with increased susceptibility to infection (e.g. neutropenic patients) and (iii) perioperative antibiotic 'cover' for patients undergoing surgery.

Antimicrobial use results in the selection of resistant strains

If antibiotic treatment is necessary, several factors must be considered, and these are summarized in *Figure 33.45*. It is important to recognize that during treatment not only the infecting microbe, but also the patient and all his or her normal microbial flora are being exposed to the effects of the antimicrobial agent. Use of antimicrobials has been clearly shown to select for resistant strains, both in the individual and in the community, and overuse or inappropriate use only increases this risk. History suggests that microbes will never run out of ways of developing resistance, but we may run out of effective antimicrobials.

THERAPEUTIC APPLICATIONS OF MAJOR ANTI-PROTOZOAL DRUGS			
disease/site	agent	route of administration	safety
amebiasis			
lumen	diloxanide furoate	oral	safe
tissue	metronidazole	oral	treatment of chronic mild infection and of extra-
	tinidazole	oral	intestinal infections, all safe
	dehydroemetine	IM	treatment of acute and hepatic infections
	chloroquine	oral	dehydroemetine has some toxicity
amebic meningoencephalitis	amphotericin B	IV	nephrotoxic, fever
cryptosporidiosis	spiramycin	oral	fully effective agent awaited
	paramomycin		
cyclosporosis	trimethoprim– sulfamethoxazole	oral	low toxicity
giardiasis	metronidazole	oral	safe
	tinidazole	oral	safe
	furazolidone	oral	toxic; hypersensitivity reactions
leishmaniasis	antimonials	IV/IM	
	pentamidine	IM	toxic
	amphotericin B	IV	
malaria			
pre-erthyrocytic stages	primaquine	oral	radical cure, some toxicity (risk of favism in G6PDH-deficient patients)
blood stages	chloroquine	oral	generally safe
	quinine	oral, IM	some toxicity, used against drug resistant *P. falciparum*
	proguanil	oral	used with chloroquine
	pyrimethamine		used in combination with sulfadoxine
	tetracycline	oral	used against drug resistant *Plasmodium falciparum*
	mefloquine	oral	mild side effects
toxoplasmosis	pentamidine	IM and aerosolized	toxic IM, shock
microsporidiosis	metronidazole	oral	safe—temporary improvement
trichomoniasis	pyrimethamine	oral	safe, but long-term treatment may produce anemia
	sulfadiazine		
	metronidazole	oral	safe
	tinidazole	oral	safe
trypanosomiasis			
African	suramin	IV	toxic
	pentamidine	IM	toxic
	melarsoprol	IV	toxic, passes blood–brain barrier
	tryparsamide	IV	toxic, passes blood–brain barrier
American	nifurtimox	oral	side effects common
	benznidazole	oral	side effects common

Fig. 33.43 Therapeutic applications of the major antiprotozoan drugs. Several are potentially toxic and must be given under supervision. Some also have antibacterial activity and have been described in detail earlier in the chapter. Drug resistance is a problem, particularly in the treatment of malaria. (G6PDH, glucose-6-phosphate dehydrogenase.)

THERAPEUTIC APPLICATIONS OF MAJOR ANTHELMINTIC DRUGS		
disease	agent	safety
cestodes (tapeworms)		
adult stage infection	niclosamide	safe
	praziquantel	safe, can prevent cysticercosis following infection with *Taenia solium*
larval stage (e.g. hydatid disease, cysticercosis)	benzimidazole carbonates	safe, but limited use
trematodes (flukes)		
schistosomiasis and intestinal flukes	praziquantel oxamniquine	⎱ safe, mild side effects
liver and lung fluke infection	praziquantel	⎰
nematodes (roundworms)		
ascariasis and pinworm infection	mebendazole	⎱ all are safe drugs[†],
	albendazole	⎰ mebendazole drug of choice
	flubendazole	
	pyrantel pamoate	safe[†], mild side effects, not used in children <1 year
	piperazine	safe[†], except in epilepsy
hookworm infection	mebendazole	⎱ all are safe drugs[†]
	albendazole	⎰ mebendazole drug of choice
	flubendazole	
	pyrantel pamoate	safe[†], mild side effects, not used for children <1 year
strongyloidiasis	thiabendazole	mild side effects[†]
trichinosis	mebendazole	⎱ all are safe drugs[†]
	albendazole	⎰ mebendazole drug of choice
	flubendazole	
	thiabendazole	mild side effects[†]
trichuriasis	mebendazole	safe[†]
cutaneous larva migrans (infection with animal hookworm)	albendazole	safe[†]
	thiabendazole*	mild side effects[†]
toxocariasis (visceral larva migrans)	thiabendazole	mild side effects[†]
	mebendazole	safe[†]
lymphatic filariasis	diethyl carbamizine	allergic side effects
	ivermectin	mild side effects
aberrant or unusual species	mebendazole	⎱ drugs of choice for
	thiabendazole	⎰ majority of infections
*topical administration [†]not used in pregnancy		

Fig. 33.44 Therapeutic applications of the major anthelmintic drugs. All are administered orally except thiabendazole for larva migrans, which is administered topically. Note that many of these drugs are not safe in pregnancy.

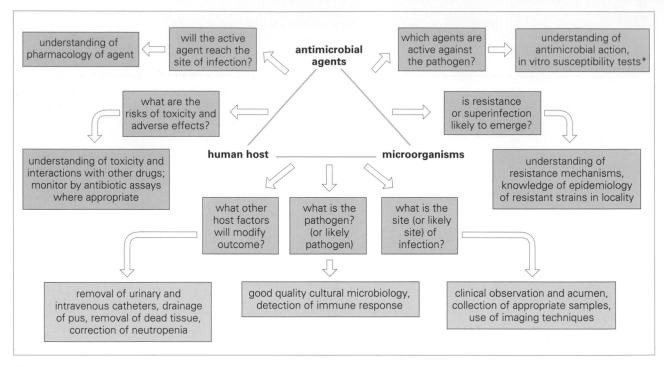

Fig. 33.45 The interactions between antimicrobial agents, microorganisms and the human host can be summarized by examining the answers to several questions affecting each side of the triangle of interaction. *Other tests include phenotypic and genotypic antiviral susceptibility tests and viral load tests.

 KEY FACTS

- Infection is unique among the diseases which afflict mankind because it involves two distinct biological systems. Antimicrobial agents are designed to inhibit one system (the microbe) while doing minimal damage to the other (the patient). Antimicrobial agents require selective toxicity.

- Antimicrobial agents are often themselves products of microorganisms (natural products) although most are chemically modified to improve their properties. Other agents are entirely synthetic. Antibacterials are the most numerous; designing antiviral, antifungal and antiparasitic drugs which are selectively toxic provides much greater challenges.

- Antibacterials are classified by their target site and their chemical family; this helps us to understand better their mode of action and the mechanisms of resistance.

- Antibacterials have four possible sites of action in the bacterial cell: cell wall, protein, nucleic acids and cell membrane. The majority act at the cell wall or inhibit protein or nucleic acid synthesis. At each site there are many different molecular targets (enzymes or substrates) which can be specifically inhibited.

- Development of resistance is the major limiting factor of antibacterials. It arises through random mutation of bacterial chromosomal genes but, more importantly through acquisition, from other bacteria, of resistance genes on integrons, transposons and plasmids.

- Mutated or acquired genes confer resistance by altering the target site of the antibacterial, altering the uptake of the drug, or producing drug-destroying enzymes.

- The emergence of AIDS has provided an enormous stimulus to research in antivirals (especially anti-HIV drugs). Selective toxicity is again a major challenge. Drug combinations show promise in the treatment of HIV, but there is no specific therapy for the majority of viral diseases. Effective therapy is available for other viral infections, including hepatitis B and C, influenza A and B, HSV and CMV.

- The number of classes of antifungal molecules is very limited. Toxicity (all), difficulty of formulation (polyenes), and emerging resistance (azoles) make effective treatment of serious fungal infections a real challenge.

KEY FACTS

- Although there are many antiparasitic drugs available, a number show toxicity and others are becoming increasingly ineffective because of the development of resistance. This is particularly acute in malaria infections, where parasites show resistance to almost all drugs presently available.

- Bacteria can be tested in the laboratory for their susceptibility to antibacterials. The results of well-controlled tests provide a valuable guide to appropriate treatment. In vitro tests with antifungals are less reliable and are rarely performed with antivirals in the clinical laboratory setting.

QUESTIONS

1. List the main classes of antibacterial agents in clinical use and give an example in each class.

2. List the main mechanisms by which resistance to antibacterials is exhibited and give an example of each.

3. Why is selective toxicity an issue in the development of effective antiviral, antifungal and antiparasitic compounds?

FURTHER READING

Gilbert DN, Moellering RC, Sande MA. *The Sanford Guide to Antimicrobial Therapy.* Hyde Park, Vermont: Antimicrobial Therapy Inc., 2002.

Greenwood D. *Antimicrobial Chemotherapy.* Oxford: Oxford University Press, 2000.

Murray P et al. *Manual of Clinical Microbiology,* 7th edition. Washington, DC: American Society for Microbiology, 1999.

Sande MA, Gilbert DN, Mollering RC. *The Sanford Guide to HIV/AIDS Therapy.* Hyde Park, Vermont: Antimicrobial Therapy Inc., 2002.

Vaccination

INTRODUCTION

Vaccination aims to prime the adaptive immune system to the antigens of a particular microbe so that a first infection induces a secondary response

'Never in the history of human progress,' wrote the pathologist Geoffrey Edsall, 'has a better and cheaper method of preventing illness been developed than immunization at its best'. It is a sobering thought that the greatest success story in medicine, the elimination of smallpox, began before either immunology or microbiology were recognized as disciplines—indeed before the existence of microbes or the immune system was even suspected. As a result of the pioneering work of Jenner with vaccinia (see *Fig. 34.3*) all forms of specific, actively induced immunity are now referred to as 'vaccination'.

The principle of vaccination is simple: to induce a 'primed' state so that on first contact with the relevant infection a rapid and effective secondary immune response will be mounted, leading to prevention of disease. Vaccination depends upon the ability of lymphocytes, both B and T cells, to respond to specific antigens and develop into memory cells, and therefore represents a form of actively enhanced adaptive immunity. The passive administration of preformed elements such as antibody is considered in Chapter 35.

An important aspect of vaccination programs is the generation of *herd immunity*—that is, raising the overall level of immunity in a population to a point at which there are insufficient susceptible individuals to maintain effective transmission. Successful vaccination programs therefore rest not only on the development and use of vaccines themselves, but also on an understanding of the epidemiologic aspects of disease transmission.

Despite the increasing number of licenced vaccines, and the many successes, there are still considerable challenges, such as to develop effective vaccines to prevent the estimated 5.2 million annual deaths from three major infectious killers *(Fig. 34.1)*.

AIMS OF VACCINATION

The aims of vaccination vary from blocking transmission and preventing symptoms to eradication of disease

The most ambitious aim of vaccination is eradication of the disease. This has been achieved for smallpox, the eradication of polio is in sight, and there has clearly been a dramatic downward trend in the incidence of most of the diseases against which vaccines are currently in use *(Fig. 34.2)*. However, as long as any focus of infection remains in the community, the main effect of vaccination will be protection of the individual against infection.

In certain cases the aim of vaccination may be more limited: namely, to protect the individual against symptoms or pathology. For example, diphtheria and tetanus vaccines only induce immunity against the toxins produced by the bacteria, as it is the effect of these toxins rather than the simple presence of the microbe itself that is harmful.

Finally, in the case of vector-borne diseases with a well-defined infective stage (e.g. malaria), one can visualize a vaccine that will block transmission without directly benefiting the vaccinated individual at all—an 'altruistic' vaccine.

INFECTIOUS AGENTS THAT ARE MAJOR KILLERS		
organism	**disease**	**estimated annual deaths (millions)**
HIV	AIDS	2.6
Mycobacterium tuberculosis	tuberculosis	1.5
Plasmodium spp.	malaria	1.1
		Total 5.2

Fig. 34.1 Infectious agents that are major killers. We currently lack effective vaccines against these organisms, although bacillus Calmette–Guérin (BCG) vaccination can provide protection against tuberculosis in some parts of the world. Source: Global Alliance for Vaccines and Immunization (GAVI), 2002 (from WHO, 1999).

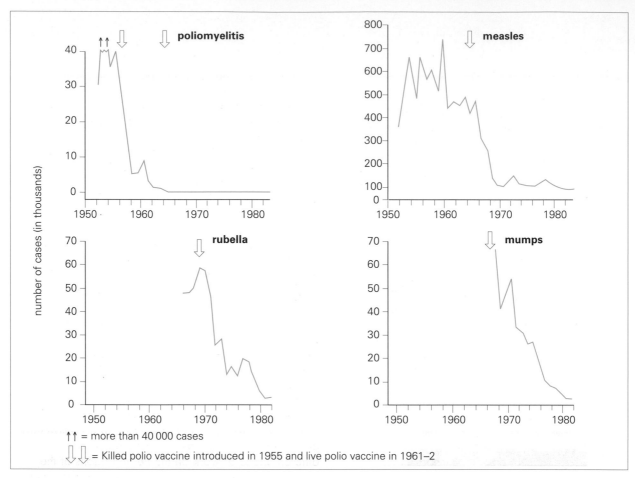

Fig. 34.2 The effect of vaccination on the incidence of various viral diseases in the USA. Most infections have shown a dramatic downward trend after the introduction of a vaccine (arrows). (Redrawn from Mims and White, 1984.)

REQUIREMENTS OF A GOOD VACCINE

The ideal vaccine should be effective, safe, stable and of low cost

To be effective a vaccine must not only induce an adequate immune response, but the response must also be of the right type. Therefore:

- A purely antibody response is unlikely to be of benefit against an intracellular infection such as tuberculosis. T-cell-mediated immunity is required.
- A purely cell-mediated response is unlikely to be of benefit against streptococcal pneumonia. Opsonizing antibodies are essential for immunity.
- High levels of serum antibody may be irrelevant to mucosal protection against polio. Secretory IgA concentrations will be more important.
- Activation of cytotoxic T cells may be harmful in hepatitis. They could induce liver damage.

The duration of response is of prime importance

For short-term protection (e.g. a tourist about to visit a disease area), the primary antibody response arising from the vaccine itself may be perfectly adequate and memory cells may not be strictly necessary. On the other hand, for protection against exposure at some time in the future, the induction of immunologic memory is essential. Diseases with a longer incubation period will be easier to protect against, because the immune system has more time to mount a secondary response. Immunologic memory is often naturally boosted by periodic outbreaks of disease in the community (e.g. the annual measles and mumps epidemics), but as diseases gradually die out this can no longer be relied upon. Paradoxically, therefore, the less disease there is in the population, the more important it is to be vaccinated—a point that parents often do not appreciate.

In general, living vaccines induce stronger and more lasting immunity than non-living vaccines (see below).

The safety of vaccines is a major consideration

The very high cost of the awards that can follow successful litigation for vaccine-induced damage has been an element in the retreat of several commercial organizations from vaccine production and development, coupled with the fact that vaccination is inherently less profitable than chemotherapy (see below). In addition, vaccines are the only compounds routinely given to healthy people. In fact, considering the enormous number of vaccine administrations the safety record is extremely good. Nevertheless there have been a few

LESSONS IN MICROBIOLOGY

Edward Jenner (1749–1823)

The English physician Edward Jenner *(Fig. 34.3)* is regarded as the founder of modern vaccination, but he was by no means the first to try the technique. The ancient practice of 'variolation' dates back to 10th century China, and arrived in Europe in the early 18th century by way of Turkey. The technique involved the inoculation of children with dried material from healed scabs of mild smallpox cases, and was a striking foretaste of the principles of

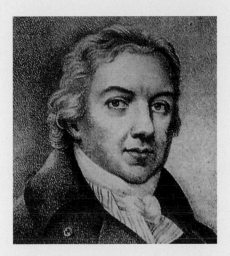

Fig. 34.3 Edward Jenner (1749–1823).

modern attenuated viral vaccines. This practice was, however, both inconsistent and dangerous, and Jenner's innovation was to show that a much safer and more reliable protection could be obtained by deliberate inoculation with cowpox (vaccinia) virus. Milkmaids exposed to this infection were traditionally known to be resistant to smallpox and so retained their smooth complexions. In 1796, Jenner tested his theory by inoculating 8-year-old James Phipps with liquid from a cowpox pustule on the hand of Sarah Nelmes. Subsequent inoculation of the boy with smallpox produced no disease. (Note that such an experiment could not even be considered today!) Jenner's book 'An Inquiry into the Causes and Effects of the Variolae Vaccinae, a Disease Discovered in some of the Western Counties of England, particularly Gloucestershire, and Known by the Name of the Cow Pox', published in 1798, is a classic of its kind—lively, stylish and well argued. Although greeted with skepticism at first, Jenner's ideas soon became accepted, and he went on to inoculate thousands of patients in a shed in the garden of his house at Berkeley, Gloucestershire. He ultimately achieved world fame, though his fellowship of the Royal Society was conferred for a quite different piece of work on the nesting habits of the cuckoo! His house at Berkeley is now preserved as a museum and is used for small symposia by the British Society of Immunology.

---

serious vaccine accidents, such as the Lubeck disaster of 1926 (see Chapter 15), and safety testing is now rigorous, requiring extensive quality control and animal trials, prior to trials in man. Some of the problems encountered in assuring the safety of vaccines are summarized in *Figure 34.4*.

Stability is particularly critical with living attenuated vaccines

Stability is a requirement of all compounds destined to remain on the shelf for long periods. Maintenance of the 'cold chain' between the factory and the clinic—which may be a small field hospital thousands of miles away—is not easy, and in one study with measles vaccine in Cameroon, only one dose in six actually reached the patient in an active form. The attenuated live polio vaccine has been shown to be stable for 1 year at 4°C, but for only a few days at 37°C.

The cost of a vaccine is relative, but cannot be high for use in developing countries

One might think that US$80 spent on a vaccine that prevented hepatitis B, a potentially fatal infection and one of the major causes of liver carcinoma, is money well spent.

PROBLEMS WITH VACCINE SAFETY
live attenuated vaccines
• insufficient attenuation
• reversion to wild type
• administration to immunodeficient patient
• persistent infection
• contamination by other viruses
• fetal damage
non-living vaccines
• contamination by toxins
• allergic reactions
• autoimmunity
genetically engineered vaccines
• possible inclusion of oncogenes

Fig. 34.4 Both living and non-living vaccines require rigorous quality and safety control. Some of the more common problems are listed.

However, in terms of the health budget of a typical developing country, such vaccines—and indeed many much cheaper vaccines—are clearly out of reach of the ordinary population or the health systems in such countries. Whether vaccines made by new technology will be cheaper to produce than those currently in use or be more expensive is discussed below.

TYPES OF VACCINE

A vaccine should contain some (or at least one) of the protective antigens of the microbe

The vaccines in use today are of different types, each of which has its mertis and drawbacks:

- microbes with artificially reduced virulence ('attenuated');
- microbes with naturally reduced virulence for man;
- killed organisms;
- subcellular fragments.

The smallpox vaccine, vaccinia, was in many ways the ideal vaccine

Smallpox vaccination worked well because the vaccinia virus, a natural animal ('heterologous') virus, shares antigens with the smallpox virus. In animal experiments, non-virulent strains of some microbial parasites will induce protection against virulent strains, and several veterinary vaccines are based on the same idea. For example, herpesvirus from turkeys has been used to protect chickens, and monkey and calf-derived rotavirus has been tried with some success in human infants.

Live attenuated vaccines make up the bulk of successful viral vaccines

Some of the attenuated virus vaccines in current use have been produced by the selection of mutants induced at random—'genetic roulette' as it has been termed. Two principal methods are used:

- serial passage in cells cultured in vitro;
- adaptation to low temperatures.

For oral polio vaccine (OPV), attenuation was by passage through monkey kidney cells or human embryo fibroblasts, virulence being checked for by signs of neurotoxicity in monkeys *(Fig. 34.5)*. Analogous methods have been used for measles, rubella, mumps and yellow fever *(Fig. 34.6)*.

The unpredictable character of random mutants is illustrated by the three serotypes of attenuated poliovirus (the 'Sabin' oral vaccine):

- Type 1 contains 57 separate base substitutions.
- Types 2 and 3 contain only a few base substitutions, of which all but two are probably unrelated to the loss of virulence.

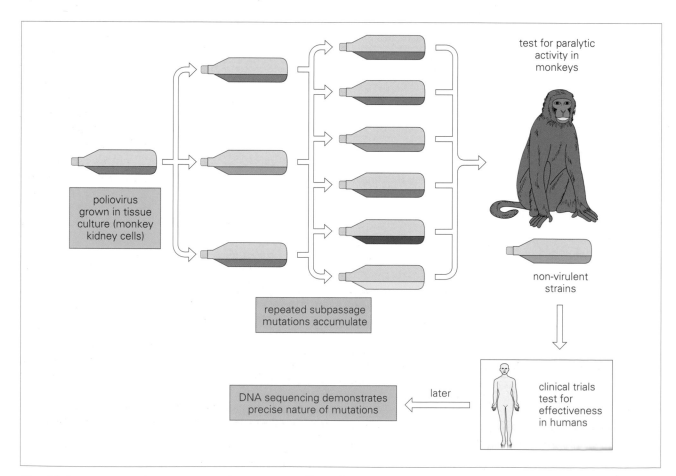

Fig. 34.5 Live attenuated vaccines (e.g. polio) were originally produced by allowing viruses to grow in unusual conditions, and selecting the randomly occurring mutants that had lost virulence.

LIVE ATTENUATED VACCINES	
organism	**method of attenuation**
viruses	
standard	
poliovirus	passage in monkey kidney, human embryo cell lines
measles	passage in human kidney, amnion, chick embryo
rubella	passage in rabbit kidney, human diploid cells
mumps	passage in chick fibroblasts
yellow fever	passage in monkey, mouse, egg
varicella	passage in human diploid cells
experimental	
influenza	
respiratory	
syncytial virus	cold adaptation
rotavirus	
cytomegalovirus	
herpesvirus	passage in human embryo fibroblasts
bacteria	
standard	
Mycobacterium bovis BCG	passage for 10 years in glycerol–bile–potato medium
Salmonella typhi	chemical mutagenesis
experimental	
Shigella	chemical mutagenesis
Vibrio cholerae	toxin deleted

Fig. 34.6 Several different approaches are used to produce today's live attenuated vaccines. Passage through cell lines produces random mutants that can be selected for loss of virulence.

GENETIC DELETIONS IN DIFFERENT STRAINS OF BCG VACCINE				
strain	**region**			
	RD1	**RD2**	**RD8**	**RD14**
M. bovis	+	+	+	+
M. bovis BCG (pre-1931)	–	–	+	+
M. bovis BCG Glaxo	–	–	+	+
M. bovis BCG Danish	–	–	+	+
M. bovis BCG Pasteur	–	–	+	–
M. bovis BCG Connaught	–	–	–	+

Fig. 34.7 A number of genetic regions have been deleted from different BCG strains since the original attenuation. Regions RD1, 2, 8 and 14 contain 9, 11, 4 and 8 open reading frames, respectively. (Data from Behr MA et al. *Science* 1999; 284: 1502.)

chemical mutagen was found to revert rather easily to the wild type, and the same problem occurred with a respiratory syncytial virus vaccine.

Randomly induced attenuation of bacteria has not been achieved to the same extent, but the development by Calmette and Guérin of an attenuated strain of bovine tuberculosis after more than 10 years (1908–1918) of culture on glycerol–bile–potato medium shows that it is possible. The bacille Calmette–Guérin (BCG) is the one well-established attenuated bacterial vaccine and has not reverted to virulence in over 70 years; recent studies have shown that BCG had suffered deletions of a number of regions of its chromosome by 1931, and that different strains of the vaccine such as the Pasteur and Danish strains have independently undergone further gene loss (see *Fig. 34.7*). BCG vaccination is now given to approximately 90% of the world's babies at birth, and protects against the most severe disseminated forms of tuberculosis such as TB meningitis, even if its effectiveness against pulmonary TB in adults is more variable (see below). A more recent development is the production of an attenuated strain of *Salmonella typhi*, produced by exposure to chemical mutagens, which has proved to be at least as good as the older killed typhoid vaccine.

Genetically engineered or 'site-directed' mutation shows great promise in both viruses and bacteria. The majority are deletion mutants in which a gene related to virulence has been inactivated. Examples range from an experimental poliovirus type 2 strain with a single base change, through *Salmonella* strains with mutations in the *aroA* or *galE* enzyme gene, to pseudo-rabies virus lacking the entire thymidine kinase gene, and cholera organisms lacking the gene for the A toxin subunit.

Killed or 'inactivated' organisms are used where living vaccines are not available

In some cases living vaccines may not be available because attenuation has not been achieved or reversion to the wild

This explains why reversion to the wild-type virulent virus is more common with types 2 and 3 (though still rare at less than one per million vaccinations). This can be a problem when there are many unvaccinated people in a population—an outbreak of polio in Haiti and the Dominican Republic in 2000–2001 seems to have come from OPV given to one child several years earlier. Some countries, such as the USA, still prefer to use the less effective inactivated polio vaccine to avoid the possibility of such reversion.

Interestingly, the polio and measles vaccines produced in this way turned out to be temperature-sensitive mutant strains. In other cases, temperature sensitivity has been deliberately selected for by the process of cold adaptation, during which the virus is encouraged to grow at low temperatures, for example 25°C, which usually means that it grows less well, if at all, at body temperature. Such a virus might then colonize the upper respiratory tract, but not warmer tissues such as the lungs. An influenza vaccine made in this way has given promising results. However, another temperature-sensitive influenza mutant induced by a

INACTIVATED VACCINES	
organism	**method of inactivation**
viruses	
rabies	β-propiolactone
influenza	β-propiolactone
polio (Salk)	formaldehyde
hepatitis A	formaldehyde
bacteria	
Salmonella typhi	heat plus phenol or acetone
Vibrio cholerae	heat
Bordetella pertussis	heat or formaldehyde
E. coli (experimental)	colicin
Yersinia pestis	formaldehyde

Fig. 34.8 Several methods are in use to produce inactivated vaccines. One of the most famous, the rabies vaccine, dates back to the time of Pasteur. Colicin is a potent endonuclease that destroys chromosomal and plasmid DNA, leaving intact cells with a normal complement of antigens.

type occurs too easily. Killed vaccines have the advantage of non-infectivity and therefore relative safety, but the disadvantage of generally lower immunogenicity and the consequent need for several doses.

A variety of methods are available for inactivation *(Fig. 34.8)*. With the older viral vaccines such as influenza and polio (Salk), formaldehyde was used but, more recently, β-propiolactone and various ethylenimines and psoralens are being used (e.g. for the current rabies vaccine). Ultraviolet light is not regarded as fully reliable, because it only selectively damages the viral nucleic acid, which can be repaired. Formaldehyde, phenol, acetone or simple heating are all used for bacteria and are equally successful.

Subcellular fractions can be used as vaccines if protective immunity is directed against a particular part of an organism

Established examples of vaccines that are subcellular fractions include: the polysaccharide capsules of pneumococci, haemophilus and meningococci; the surface coat of the hepatitis B virus, which is produced by recombinant DNA technology; and the fragmented virus or purified surface antigens of influenza virus vaccines. Vaccines based on the protein filaments (pili) used by *Escherichia coli* and *Neisseria gonorrhoeae* to attach to urinary tract epithelium are still experimental. Removal of all live infectious material is obviously a vital element in ensuring the safety of such vaccines.

Toxoids are inactivated bacterial toxins that can induce protective antibody

Bacterial toxins that have been inactivated (usually by formaldehyde) so that they are no longer toxic, but still induce protective antibody, are called toxoids. Two such toxoids—diphtheria and tetanus—are among the most successful and

widely used of all vaccines. In combination with killed *Bordetella pertussis*, they constitute the well-known triple vaccine, DTP (diphtheria, tetanus, pertussis). There is some evidence that omission of the pertussis component reduces the antibody response to the two toxoids; thus pertussis acts as an 'adjuvant' as well as a specific vaccine.

With the use of small peptides as potential vaccine antigens (see below), tetanus toxoid has been widely suggested as a useful 'carrier' protein. The idea is that most patients have been previously immunized to the toxoid and therefore possess tetanus-specific T memory cells, which will help the peptide-specific B cells to make antibody. This approach is useful for inducing a good primary response, but less useful for memory responses, in which T cells need to be recalled by the proteins of the infection rather than by those of tetanus.

The same approach led to the development of conjugate *H. influenzae* type b (Hib) vaccine. Tetanus or diphtheria toxoids are conjugated with capsular polysacchandes of *H. influenzae* to improve the immunogenicity of this vaccine in infants and young children.

The other common toxin-inducing bacterium is *Vibrio cholerae*, and vaccines containing the B subunit of cholera toxin plus killed organisms have had some success, particularly in the induction of mucosal immunity following immunization.

A variety of viruses and bacteria can be used as vectors for cloned genes

The idea of using expression vectors (e.g. *E. coli*, yeast) to express genes coding for potentially immunogenic proteins is as old as recombinant DNA technology itself. More recently, however, an ingenious modification has been introduced in which the expression vector, complete with inserted gene(s), is itself the vaccine. Following injection into the patient, it will proliferate sufficiently to release an immunizing amount of the foreign protein, but without inducing disease itself.

The first vector to be proposed in 1982 was the vaccinia virus. This had the advantage of being already established as a highly effective vaccine and of possessing a large enough (DNA) genome for insertion of several foreign genes without disrupting virus structure or function. However, it also had the disadvantage that a large proportion of the world's population was immune to vaccinia and would probably eliminate the virus before it had produced the desired amount of foreign gene product. There was also the problem that vaccinia itself could induce complications (principally encephalitis) in about one case in 100 000. Nevertheless, in a pioneer experiment in chimpanzees, vaccinia containing the gene for hepatitis B surface antigen (HBsAg) gave excellent protection against a challenge infection, and similarly for influenza and herpes simplex virus (HSV). A modified form of the virus, called modified vaccinia virus Ankara (MVA) is now being used to develop new vaccines for malaria and tuberculosis *(Fig. 34.9)*.

Several other viruses have subsequently been considered as vectors, including attenuated yellow fever virus, adenovirus, herpes simplex virus (HSV) and varicella-zoster virus (VZV); successful insertion has been achieved for genes from a variety

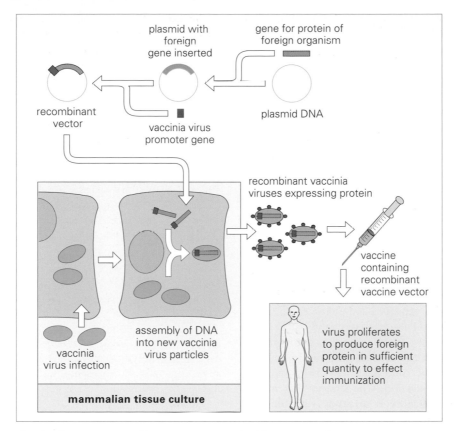

Fig. 34.9 It is now possible to insert genes coding for antigens of one or more microorganisms into a large virus such as modified vaccinia virus Ankara so that they replicate and are released into the host.

of viruses including respiratory syncytial virus, Epstein–Barr virus, rabies virus, dengue virus and Lassa fever virus.

Bacteria are also good candidates as vectors, the two leading ones being the attenuated salmonellae mentioned earlier and BCG. *S. typhi* has the advantage of being an intestinal infection so when given orally (with a dose of bicarbonate to prevent inactivation by gastric acid) it will induce mucosal immunity in the gut. Avirulent mutants of *S. typhi* might therefore act as general vectors for vaccines against all enteric diseases—a field in which current vaccines are far from adequate.

BCG is the latest vector to be proposed, and the advantages are:

- The very large genome.
- The fact that BCG is now the most widely used of all vaccines, being given, usually just after birth, to about 90% of all children in the world.
- Another special merit is that it induces predominantly cell-mediated immunity, both to itself and to other antigens given with it, so it could be the ideal vector for antigens from all persistent intracellular organisms—a large and important category that includes in addition to *Mycobacterium tuberculosis* and *Mycobacterium leprae*, *Brucella*, *Leishmania*, *Toxoplasma*, *Histoplasma*, *Listeria*, rickettsiae and chlamydiae, many viruses and, possibly (in its liver stage), malaria. Perhaps in the future a single vector containing all required antigens may become available—although giving too many antigens at once may lead to antigenic competition.

Gene cloning and peptide synthesis aim to produce immunogenic peptides for use as vaccines

The technologies involved are now reasonably standard, though there is considerable debate about which expression vector to use for cloning genes. The first successful vaccine made in this way was against foot and mouth disease (although the emergency vaccine currently available in the UK consists of inactivated virus with adjuvant). First by gene cloning in *E. coli* and soon afterwards by chemical synthesis, it was shown that a 20-amino-acid peptide from one of the capsid proteins could protect guinea pigs against infection.

Synthetic peptides are now available from a wide range of microbes, and there is extensive research into how to select the right peptide and how to make it as immunogenic as possible. One approach is to attach peptides to larger carrier molecules such as tetanus toxin (see above), but whenever possible the attempt is made to include sequences in the peptide that can themselves trigger T cells. These 'T cell epitopes' can to some extent be predicted from the known sequence of the molecule. Where they are not available, the strategy is to construct new sequences including one or more T cell epitopes as well as the epitope against which antibody is required (the 'B cell epitope'). A further refinement has been to couple together several copies of separate T and B epitopes into 'multiple antigen peptides', using a branching core of lysines and up to eight attached peptides—the so-called 'octopus' molecule. In one study, four each of the T cell and B cell epitopes gave the best results. Even then, it has usually been found that an adjuvant is needed to enhance immunogenicity.

Problems with these approaches are:

- The variation in peptide response from patient to patient and the existence of genetic non-responders. The role of major histocompatibility complex (MHC) antigens in this is discussed below.
- It is more difficult to replicate a discontinuous B cell epitope than a linear epitope.

DNA vaccines

Much interest has been generated by the surprising discovery that intramuscular injection of microbial DNA itself, with a suitable promoter, can immunize laboratory animals against infections such as influenza and malaria. It is thought that the corresponding antigen is expressed and presented on muscle cells, but much work is still needed to verify this and to ensure that there is not a risk of side effects such as autoimmunity or microbial tolerance. DNA vaccines tend to promote cell-mediated immunity, but conditions have been found to encourage antibody production. One strategy that induces good immunological memory is to prime with the DNA vaccine and then boost with the protein itself, perhaps presented by a viral vector such as modified virus Ankara or fowlpox. At present, no DNA vaccine has been approved for routine human or veterinary use, but DNA vaccines are currently being developed against a number of viruses such as influenza, cytomegalovirus and herpes simplex virus. DNA vaccination against influenza has given impressive protection against virus challenge in animal models.

Other strategies for making vaccines against non-protein antigens

Expressing a foreign protein or epitope within a viral or bacterial vector is much easier than getting a vector to make a complex carbohydrate or lipid antigen, which often requires a complex series of enzymic modifications that may be species specific. There are, however, other ways in which the immune system can be primed to make an immune response to such antigens. These include selecting for peptide epitopes that mimic the same shape as that recognized by a monoclonal antibody, in a technique called phage display. Another approach is to use anti-idiotype molecules. This is possible because antibodies can recognize structures related to each other's combining sites (idiotypes; see Chapter 11), just as they can recognize antigens; thus a first antibody against an antigen can be used to raise second antibodies, some of which will have idiotypes resembling the original antigen. One advantage of such 'surrogate antigens' is that, being large proteins, they behave as T-dependent antigens, even when the original antigen was T-independent—a polysaccharide, for example. This strategy has been successfully applied to the vaccination of mice against streptococcal, hepatitis B and trypanosomal antigens, and to raise secondary antibody responses to endotoxin.

LIVING VERSUS NON-LIVING VACCINES		
	living	non-living
preparation	attenuation (not always feasible)	inactivation
administration	may be natural route (e.g. oral) may be single dose	injection usually multiple doses
adjuvant	not required	usually required
safety	may revert to virulence	requires safe method of inactivation
heat lability (for tropical use)	requires cold chain	satisfactory
cost	low	high
duration of immunity	usually years	may be long or short
immune response	IgG, IgA cell-mediated	mainly IgG, little or no cell-mediated unless given will appropriate adjuvant

Fig. 34.10 Living and non-living vaccines each have advantages and disadvantages.

SPECIAL CONSIDERATIONS

Both living and non-living vaccines have advantages and disadvantages

Living versus non-living vaccines is one of the most keenly debated topics in vaccinology, and some general points can be made, as well as some that apply specifically to particular vaccines. These are summarized in *Figure 34.10*.

The issue can be appreciated most clearly with those diseases that normally induce good long-term immunity following recovery from infection (e.g. the common childhood viruses). Here, live attenuated vaccines are much more likely to be effective, since they reproduce many of the features of the infection itself, including:

- replication of the virus;
- localization to the appropriate part of the body (e.g. gut, lung);
- efficient induction of cytotoxic T cells, which may be related to the fact that for microbial peptides to become associated with MHC class I molecules it is usually necessary for the peptides to have been synthesized in the

cell rather than taken in by endocytosis, as a non-living vaccine antigen would be.

A further theoretic advantage is the possibility that attenuated strains will spread through the population by normal transmission routes, protecting those who have not been vaccinated.

The principal disadvantages of living attenuated vaccines are:

- the possibility of reversion to virulence;
- the danger that they may cause severe disease in immunocompromised patients.

Many natural infections do not leave the patient with solid immunity (e.g. influenza). This can be for a variety of reasons, prominent among them being antigenic diversity, antigenic variation, immunosuppression, and the induction of responses that protect the microbe. In such cases the rationale for using a living attenuated vaccine is weaker, and a sub-cellular component that induces strong immunity, which attacks the microbe at a weak spot (e.g. a polysaccharide capsule or a vital attachment molecule), possibly in the form of a mixture of antigenic types, is more likely to work. The problem of correct localization will then need to be addressed by other means, such as aerosols for the lung and enteric capsules for the gut.

Polio is the only disease at present for which live and killed vaccines compete on approximately equal terms (see poliomyelitis, Chapter 22).

Many polysaccharide antigens fail to stimulate T cells and therefore induce only primary responses

Most complex antigens contain both T and B cell epitopes, so T cells are induced that cooperate with B cells, leading to T and B cell memory, immunoglobulin switching (e.g. IgM→IgG), and affinity maturation—all features of the secondary response, and essential for a vaccine to be effective. Polysaccharide antigens that fail to stimulate T cells (T-independent antigens) induce only primary responses no matter how often they are administered. Such antigens are particularly ineffective in children under 2 years of age. The current strategy is to conjugate the polysaccharide to a suitable protein, preferably from the same microorganism. The results of this are discussed below in relation to pneumo-coccal and meningococcal vaccines. Another approach to this problem, although still largely experimental, is the use of anti-idiotypic antibody as a 'surrogate' antigen (see above).

MHC class II molecules are needed for T cell responses

Antigens that do stimulate T cells may be less effective in some individuals than in others. This is especially a feature of small peptides and is due to the very precise binding required between the peptide, the MHC class II—human leukocyte antigen (HLA)-D—molecule on the antigen-presenting cell, and the T cell receptor. HLA antigens are extremely poly-morphic, and it is quite common to find that a particular HLA molecule fails to bind a particular peptide. If none of an individual's available MHC class II molecules (two each of DP, DQ and DR) binds a particular peptide, the individual will be a 'non-responder' and will not mount T cell responses. Similar MHC restriction could apply to peptide epitopes designed to induce cytotoxic T cell immunity, where peptides are presented by MHC class I molecules.

It is not known to what extent MHC restriction contributes to the failure of a certain percentage of individuals to respond well to almost all standard vaccines, and it may be that the problem has been overemphasized even where small peptides are concerned. For example, a 21-amino-acid malaria peptide has been found from which peptides of 11–14 amino acids stimulate only T cells from a few DR types, whereas a 15-amino-acid sequence stimulates all the DR types tested. Such peptides that bind to a variety of DR types are called 'promiscuous'. This suggests that it may often be possible to confer a broader range of MHC responsiveness by adding to or modifying a few amino acids in a peptide.

Pathologic consequences of vaccination may be due to the vaccine or the immune response

Vaccine causes of pathology include:

- Contamination of attenuated viruses with other viruses growing in the same cell lines, particularly since monkey cells are often used, and several monkey viruses are lethal for humans.
- Hypersensitivity to egg proteins with living viral vaccines grown in chick embryo cells. Children with a history of egg sensitivity should be skin-tested with diluted vaccine and may have to be immunized in stages with lower than usual doses or, if anaphylaxis is expected, not at all.

A more complicated situation arises where the vaccine antigen itself induces a pathologic response such as hypersensitivity or autoimmunity. Hypersensitivity reactions to the older killed measles vaccines were a stimulus to the development of a living attenuated replacement. It appeared that although the killed vaccine induced good non-neutral-izing antibodies to the hemagglutinin, it failed to induce antibody to the fusion (F) protein, which was destroyed by the inactivation process. The F protein is responsible for viral cell-to-cell spread. As a result, during infection large amounts of virus were produced together with high titers of non-neutralizing antibody. The resulting immune complexes caused severe type III hypersensitivity during the attack of measles, so the patient's illness was actually made worse. A similar response occurred to the killed respiratory syncytial virus vaccine. The fever and malaise that follow vaccination with killed typhoid organisms is due to the endotoxin, and mediated by cytokines such as interleukin 1 (IL-1) and tumor necrosis factor-alpha (TNFα).

Autoimmunity during infections can sometimes be traced to antigenic similarity ('mimicry') between host and microbe, and the same is theoretically possible with vaccine antigens. However, this does not seem to have been observed with the present vaccines, but could occur if strong T cell epitopes are conjugated to weak antigens, such as polysaccharides, which might cross-react with host molecules. Where the cross-reacting component can be identified, it should be removed before a vaccine is considered for use; Chagas' disease is a case in point.

PATHOLOGIC COMPLICATIONS OF VACCINATION	
complication	vaccine
hypersensitivity to egg antigens to viral antigens	live measles, mumps killed measles, RSV
convulsions, encephalitis	pertussis, measles (1 per million)
meningitis	mumps (1 per million)
arthritis	rubella

Fig. 34.11 Complications are rare with modern vaccines, but the physician must always be aware of the possibility. (RSV, respiratory syncytial virus.)

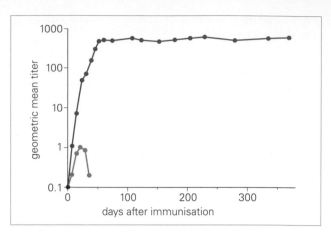

Fig. 34.12 Effects of adjuvants on antibody responses of mice to egg albumin. Mice were injected subcutaneously with egg albumin in saline or in Freund's incomplete adjuvant. Antibody titers at intervals over time are shown. The blue symbols represent antigen in saline, and the red symbols antigen in adjuvant. (From Hunter, *Vaccine* 2002; 20:S7–S12).

Perhaps the most widely publicized complication of vaccination is the occurrence of fits and brain damage, notably after vaccination for pertussis (see Chapter 19). Whether or not this is truly due to the vaccine is discussed below. *Figure 34.11* lists the major reported complications of other vaccines.

Living vaccines should not usually be given to immunocompromised people

The most absolute contraindications to using living vaccine in immunocompromised people are the use of vaccinia or BCG in patients with severe T cell deficiency. Indeed it was the spreading and eventually fatal vaccinia infections that alerted the New York pediatrician DiGeorge to the occurrence of the athymic syndrome that bears his name. Measles, mumps and rubella (MMR) vaccine is generally not advised for other T cell deficiencies of childhood, including those following treatment with glucocorticosteroids or immunosuppressive drugs. People with impaired immunity resulting from cancer, diabetes mellitus or treatment with immunosuppressive drugs should not be given live vaccines (measles, oral polio, yellow fever, BCG). For example, hypogammaglobulinemic patients unable to make antibody responses can become persistently infected following vaccination with live polio vaccine.

The spread of the HIV epidemic worldwide has made vaccination more problematic, particularly as it may not be possible to identify HIV-infected children without appropriate screening. The current recommendations (in 2002) are that asymptomatic HIV-infected children can be given childhood vaccines as normal. Some vaccines can also be given to symptomatic HIV-infected individuals (measles, oral polio, the risk of complications being on balance less than the risk of death from the natural infection), but the live yellow fever and BCG vaccines are not recommended.

Non-living vaccines are less of a problem in the immunocompromised host since, although they may be ineffective, they are unlikely to be dangerous. Vaccines aimed specifically at the induction of antibody (e.g. capsular polysaccharides, hepatitis B) are recommended in all but the most severe B cell deficiencies, but the alternative of passive immunization (see Chapter 35) should also be considered. Extra vaccines are recommended for individuals who do not have a functional spleen—such as Hib, meningitis, pneumococcal vaccine and influenza vaccines—as such people may be more susceptible to these infections.

Adjuvants

Many adjuvants will enhance the immune response when administered with antigen

It has been known since the 1920s that certain substances will enhance the consequent immune response when administered simultaneously with antigen. For example, it was found that giving antigen in Freund's incomplete adjuvant, a water-in-oil emulsion, dramatically enhanced antibody responses (*Fig. 34.12*). The first such substances that were shown to be safe, convenient and effective were aluminum salts, which form a repository of antigen within the tissue. Aluminum adjuvants are currently used in the DPT vaccine, hepatitis B vaccine, some but not all of the Hib vaccines, and vaccines against Lyme disease, anthrax and rabies. However although aluminum adjuvants seem to be safe, numerous other materials are being considered or tried experimentally for clinical use. The word 'adjuvant' is also sometimes used in a slightly different sense to denote a substance that, when given alone, enhances some immune function such as inhibition of tumor growth or recovery from infection. This type of non-specific immunostimulant is discussed in Chapter 35.

Many years of work in animals have established that a wide range of materials are effective as vaccine adjuvants, and these are briefly described here since the clinical adjuvants of the future are likely to be drawn from among them (*Fig. 34.13*).

Alum-precipitated antigens are especially effective at inducing antibody responses, but much less active in inducing cell-mediated immunity

The powerful adjuvanticity of aluminum salts has not been fully explained. Some of it is no doubt due to the formation of small inflammatory lesions, which may progress to granulomas,

VACCINE ADJUVANTS
inorganic salts
aluminum hydroxide (alhydrogel)*
aluminum phosphate*
calcium phosphate*
beryllium hydroxide
delivery systems
liposomes**
ISCOMs**
non-ionic block co-polymers
slow release formulations**
bacterial products
BCG
killed mycobacteria (complete Freund's adjuvant)†
MDP†
RIBI
*Bordetella pertussis** (with diphtheria, tetanus toxoids)
natural mediators **
IL-1
IL-2
IFNγ
IL-12
*routinely used in man   **experimental
†too toxic for human use

Fig. 34.13 A variety of foreign and endogenous substances can act as adjuvants, but only aluminum and calcium salts and pertussis are routinely used in clinical practice. (BCG, bacille Calmette-Guérin; IFN, interferon; IL, interleukin; ISCOMs, immune-stimulating complexes; MDP, muramyl dipeptide; RIBI, lipid A derivative emulsified in mycobacterial trehalose dimycolate and cell wall.)

with consequent trapping of antigen and slow release with exposure to large numbers of macrophages and other antigen-presenting cells. Antigens (e.g. toxoids) were originally entrapped in 'floccules' of the salt by adding them during its chemical preparation. Such antigens are described as 'alum precipitated'. Now, however, it is more usual to add the antigen to a preformed gel of aluminum hydroxide or phosphate.

A variety of novel formulations in which antigen is presented on the surface of small spherical structures are also used as adjuvants

A similar 'depot' effect is thought to account for the adjuvanticity of these novel formulations, which include:

- liposomes, which are single- or multiple-walled phospholipid vesicles;
- ISCOMs (immune-stimulating complexes), which are micelles composed of a saponin derivative, QUIL A, which traps amphipathic proteins;
- block non-ionic co-polymers of polyoxyethylene and polyoxypropylene.

Depending upon the precise formulation and the nature of the antigen used, these have all been shown to be highly effective, and many are in veterinary use. It is too early to say which, if any, will become standard clinical adjuvants, and this may depend upon safety testing as much as immunologic efficacy.

Mycobacteria and other bacteria can be effective adjuvants

The adjuvanticity of mycobacteria is remarkable, and was used by Freund in his famous preparation 'complete Freund's adjuvant' (CFA), in which mycobacteria are emulsified with water in an oil vehicle. CFA is particularly effective in boosting cell-mediated immune responses such as delayed type hypersensitivity (DTH) to antigens that are normally weak inducers. Unfortunately, as several accidental injections have shown, CFA is too toxic for use in man, causing chronic non-healing granulomas. The water-in-oil emulsion without mycobacteria is known as 'incomplete Freund's adjuvant' (IFA), and this has been used in man with no apparent undesired side effects, but without the great potency of CFA for cell-mediated immune responses. An extensive study of the role played by the mycobacteria in CFA has yielded the small water-soluble molecule muramyl dipeptide (MDP), which is claimed to retain most of the benefit of mycobacteria without being so toxic.

Numerous other bacterial derivatives are being investigated as adjuvants and, as already mentioned, the killed pertussis organisms in the 'triple' DPT vaccine appear to act as adjuvants for the diphtheria and tetanus toxoids.

The most recent development in the adjuvant field has been the use of cytokines

It had always been suspected that adjuvants such as CFA and MDP acted partly by inducing cytokines important for inducing inflammation, and when purified recombinant cytokines became available it was found that many cytokines were indeed effective adjuvants when added to vaccines. IL-2, IL-12, IFNγ and granulocyte–macrophage colony stimulating factor (GM-CSF) have been shown to be effective in a number of experimental studies. There are also recent data that IL-15 and IL-18 can enhance the response to DNA vaccines. In man, IL-1 and IFNγ have been shown to be particularly useful in cases where the response to a vaccine is impaired (e.g. in hemodialysis patients immunized against hepatitis B).

Dendritic cells have been proposed as natural adjuvants

If a peptide antigen is targeted so that it is taken up by the antigen-presenting dendritic cells, it induces a far better immune response than one delivered in a non-specific adjuvant such as Freund's incomplete adjuvant. Another benefit of dendritic cell presentation of vaccine adjuvants is that they can induce MHC class-I-restricted CD8-mediated T cell immunity through a process called cross-priming. This type of approach works well in animal models but is not very practical for general use in man, although it may be useful in cancer.

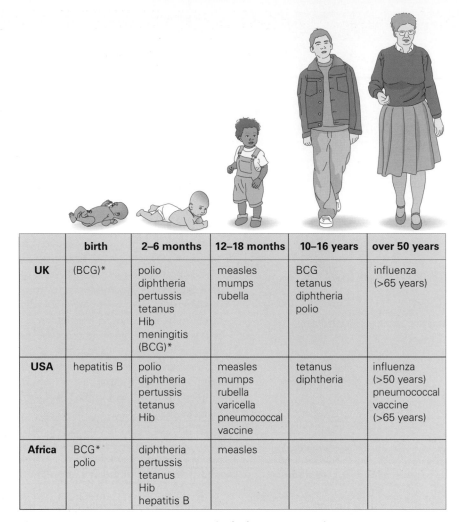

	birth	2–6 months	12–18 months	10–16 years	over 50 years
UK	(BCG)*	polio diphtheria pertussis tetanus Hib meningitis (BCG)*	measles mumps rubella	BCG tetanus diphtheria polio	influenza (>65 years)
USA	hepatitis B	polio diphtheria pertussis tetanus Hib	measles mumps rubella varicella pneumococcal vaccine	tetanus diphtheria	influenza (>50 years) pneumococcal vaccine (>65 years)
Africa	BCG* polio	diphtheria pertussis tetanus Hib hepatitis B	measles		

Fig. 34.14 Current vaccine practice. Risk of infection varies with age.

When to vaccinate

The age of those vaccinated depends upon the age of the vulnerable population

Since most of the diseases that vaccines are designed to prevent affect young children *(Fig. 34.14)*, vaccination is carried out as early as possible, bearing in mind that:

- The presence of maternally derived antibody reduces the effectiveness of some vaccines, which are therefore usually delayed until the third month of life or later.
- Live attenuated vaccines (including vaccinia when it was used) can cause severe disease in immunodeficiency states, which may not be diagnosed immediately after birth.
- If the disease is mainly a risk to the elderly (e.g. pneumococcal pneumonia), vaccination is usually given at a late age.

Further details of when various vaccines are given will be found in the discussions of individual vaccines below.

Can the vaccination of newborn babies affect the development of their immune system?

Some vaccines can safely be given to babies within a few days of birth. These include BCG, oral polio vaccine, and hepatitis

A and B vaccines. However there are some concerns that the introduction of antigens from these vaccines into the developing immune system may have profound effects beyond the induction of specific immunity. For example, BCG vaccination, which induces TH1 T cell immunity, might affect the TH1/TH2 cytokine balance to other diseases. Some recent work from west Africa suggests that measles vaccination may reduce morbidity from all causes in young children—although further work is needed to confirm how generally applicable this is in other settings, and to elucidate the mechanism responsible. It is also worth noting that although today's children can receive 11 or more different vaccines, the total number of antigens these contain is still probably less than the large number of antigens that were contained in the smallpox vaccine.

COMMUNITY-BASED CONTROL BY VACCINATION

We will now consider the epidemiologic effects of vaccination, before moving on to discuss individual vaccines in more detail.

CRITICAL VACCINATION COVERAGE TO BLOCK TRANSMISSION OF CERTAIN CHILDHOOD INFECTIONS

infectious disease	average age at infection before immunization* (years)	case reproductive rate (R_0)	critical vaccination coverage (p_c)
measles	4–5	15–17	92–95%
pertussis	4–5	15–17	92–95%
mumps	6–7	10–12	90–92%
rubella	9–10	7–8	85–87%
diphtheria	11–14	5–6	80–85%
poliomyelitis	12–15	5–6	80–85%
*in developed countries			

Fig. 34.15 Estimates of vaccination coverage necessary to block transmission of certain vaccine-preventable childhood viral and bacterial infections.

Different vaccination coverage is needed to eradicate different infections

Other things being equal, the higher the reproductive rate of an infection (the larger the value of R_0—i.e. the larger the number of people subsequently infected by one infected individual—see Chapter 31), the harder it will be to eradicate an infection by mass vaccination. Where transmission occurs by random contacts between infectious and susceptible individuals (e.g. childhood viral infections), eradication will be achieved if the percentage successfully immunized (p), exceeds a critical value (p_c), at which too few susceptibles remain to perpetuate transmission. This value is related to R_0 ($p_c = 100-[100/R_0]$), so that the higher the value of R_0 the higher the vaccine coverage (p_c) needed to eliminate infection. p_c values for various vaccine-preventable childhood viral and bacterial infections are listed in *Figure 34.15*.

Global eradication of measles, with its R_0 of 15–17 and p_c of 92–95%, will almost certainly be more difficult than the eradication of smallpox (R_0 of 2–4). In the USA, where measles/mumps/rubella (MMR) vaccination is essentially compulsory before entry to primary school, the average age at infection for rubella before immunization was about 9 years, compared with around 5 years for measles. The R_0 value for rubella is roughly half that for measles, and rubella has been effectively eradicated by the vaccination program. The incidence of measles on the other hand has declined more slowly and continues to show local flare-ups in urban centers with low vaccine uptake.

Average age at vaccination must be less than average age at infection for eradication

For most live vaccines (e.g. MMR) efficacy is reduced if high titers of maternal antibodies are present. These typically decay to undetectable levels at around 6 months to 1 year (Fig. 34.16). The subsequent rise in seropositivity in an un-vaccinated community reflects immunity acquired via natural infection. The trough in seropositivity at about 1 year is obviously the optimum age to vaccinate, but high efficacy or high potency vaccines, such as those recently developed against measles and mumps, allow effective vaccination at younger ages when maternal antibodies are still present. This is particularly important in high transmission areas in developing countries, where the susceptibility age window for vaccination may be very narrow.

When vaccination does not take place soon after birth or when a broad age range of children is immunized, the estimation of the critical fraction to be immunized to eliminate infection must take account of the average age at vaccination. For eradication to be possible the average age at vaccination must be less than the average age at infection, and cohort vaccination should therefore focus on young infants, taking account of vaccine performance in those with maternal antibodies.

A two-stage vaccination program can eradicate certain infections

There are difficulties in eradicating infections such as measles in major urban centers in some developing countries where the average age at infection is often 1–2 years (see *Fig. 34.16*). To block transmission, more than 97% of infants would have to be effectively immunized before their first birthday. In practice this is impossible. An alternative approach is a two-stage vaccination program—for example, targeted at infants around 1 year of age and then young children at around 2–3 years of age:

- The first stage acts to reduce transmission efficiency (but not to block transmission) and hence widens the age window of susceptibility in which vaccine can be administered.
- The second stage attempts to block transmission via the creation of very high levels of herd immunity.

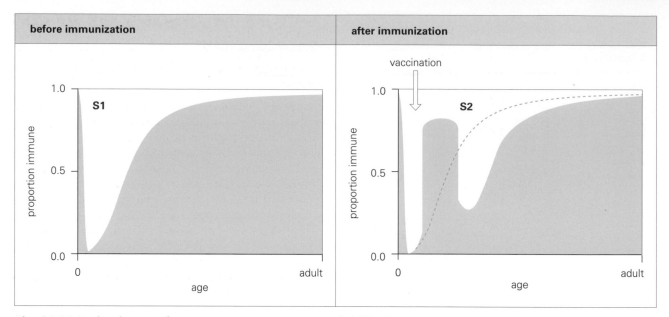

Fig. 34.16 Predicted impact of mass immunization against a typical childhood viral or bacterial infection on the age distribution of susceptibility in a population. Before immunization there is a 'valley' of susceptibility (S1) in the young age classes when infection can occur. Vaccination reduces the rate of transmission, creating an upward shift in the age (S2) at which susceptibles may acquire natural infection.

100% vaccination coverage is not needed to eradicate infection

Immunization has both a direct and an indirect effect. The direct effect protects those successfully immunized and, by reducing the incidence of infection, results in fewer infected individuals to transmit infection to those still susceptible. The latter therefore benefit indirectly from those who have been immunized. As long as the proportion of the population immunized is sufficiently large, even though it is less than 100%, the number of susceptibles will eventually fall below the level required to maintain $R > 1$.

Mass immunization at levels below those needed to block transmission obviously reduces the incidence of infection, but, surprisingly, it will have little impact on the total number of individuals remaining susceptible *(Fig. 34.16)*. With immunization at sub-threshold levels, and as long as the infection remains endemic, the fraction remaining susceptible depends only on the organism's reproductive R_0 and not on whether those gaining immunity did so as a result of immunization or natural infection.

Mass vaccination can have indirect effects

Mass vaccination at below eradication levels reduces the probability of an unimmunized individual acquiring infection. In consequence, infection tends to be acquired at an older average age than before vaccination *(Fig. 34.16)*. If the risk of disease associated with infection increases with age, a program of immunization at levels below that required to block transmission (i.e. below p_c) can have perverse complications. The outcome depends upon precisely how the risk of serious disease per case of infection changes with age *(Fig. 34.17)*. For example, all levels of vaccination coverage

reduce the incidence of encephalitis from measles, but low vaccination rates increase the overall incidence of serious disease from rubella and mumps acquired at a later age.

Mass vaccination can increase the risk of serious disease associated with rubella

Rubella can damage babies whose mothers are infected in the first trimester of pregnancy. The risk of this damage is therefore proportional to the age-specific fertility profile for a given country *(Fig. 34.17a)*. Vaccinating, say, 50% of all 2 year olds would reduce the total number of cases of rubella but push the average age of those who do become infected towards the childbearing years. If very high levels of coverage can be attained (under a compulsory program, as in the USA, or a highly coordinated system of recall, incentives and surveillance, as in the UK), eradication can be achieved by vaccinating successive cohorts of 1–2 year olds. If levels of vaccine uptake under a voluntary scheme only reach 60–70% (as in the UK earlier in the rubella vaccination campaign), vaccination against rubella should be confined to early teenage girls before they join the 'pregnancy' age classes, so that infection can spread and confer immunity at younger ages. How can we tell at what level of coverage to switch from one strategy to the other? Epidemiologic calculations suggest that a switch to the mass cohort strategy (where MMR is offered to 1–2 year olds) is advisable provided that more than 70% of boys and girls can be immunized by 2 years of age. Adding MMR vaccination of 1–2-year-old boys and girls to an existing strategy focused only on teenage girls would have little effect on disease, provided uptake in 12–13-year-old girls was already high (80–90%). Some benefit will accrue over 10 years or more once the uptake of MMR in 1–2 year olds reaches very high levels (90% or more).

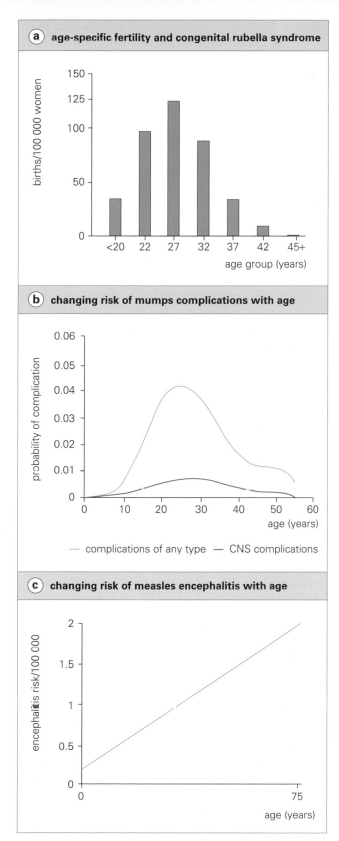

Fig. 34.17 Age-dependent risk of complications from infection. (a) Age-specific fertility of women, as shown, directly influences the risk of congenital rubella syndrome in infants. (Data for the UK.) (b) Changes in the absolute risk of complications from mumps infection in the UK relative to age. (c) Changes with age in the risk of measles encephalitis in the USA.

FACTORS INFLUENCING THE SUCCESS OF VACCINATION

Vaccination success is influenced by population density

The design of immunization programs, particularly in developing countries, is influenced by variations in population density. In small villages in rural areas, population density and the associated net birth rates may be too low for the endemic maintenance of infections such as measles or pertussis (see Chapter 13). However, people living in these regions are at risk from contact with large urban centers. One solution is to target vaccination coverage in relation to group size, with dense groups receiving the highest levels of coverage. In some circumstances transmission can be blocked by high levels of mass immunization in the urban centers alone, since they provide the reservoir of infection for the low density rural regions.

High vaccine coverage in infants and children, particularly in poor communities, must be a central aim in national immunization programs

Programs in developed countries may be influenced by regional variation in vaccine uptake. In the USA, disadvantaged minorities in large urban centers create pockets of susceptibility (due to low vaccine uptake) that prevent the elimination of infections such as measles and pertussis. Serologic surveillance, in both urban and rural areas, is a key component in the identification of weaknesses in current programs.

The rate at which susceptibles acquire many common vaccine-preventable childhood infections varies with age

For many common vaccine-preventable childhood infections, such as measles, mumps and rubella, the per capita rate at which susceptibles acquire infection varies with age. For rubella *(Fig. 34.18)* the rate changes from an infection rate of 80/1000 susceptibles/year in the 0–4 year olds via a higher level in the 5–14 year olds back to the lower level in adults. This reflects social patterns of behavior, the high rates in the 5–14 year olds reflecting frequent and intimate contact within school environments. These age-dependent variations can reduce the predicted level of cohort vaccination required to block or eliminate transmission. This is because immunization increases the average age at infection (see above). Susceptibles who avoid vaccination and infection may move from an age class with a high rate of infection to an older one with a lower rate.

The risks of infection must outweigh any risk associated with vaccination

Most vaccines have some small risk of inducing serious complications. Any assessment of the benefit from an immunization program must therefore include a comparison of the number of cases of serious disease prevented by mass vaccination with the number of cases due to vaccination itself. Such calculations are not straightforward because they depend upon the interrelation between various factors such as:

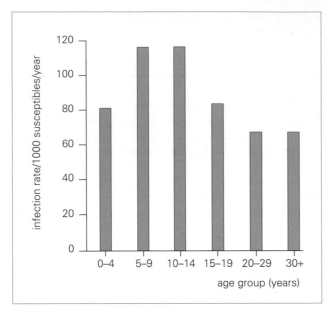

Fig. 34.18 Age-related changes in the rate of infection with the rubella virus.

- vaccine efficacy and safety;
- proportion of each cohort of children immunized;
- average age of immunization;
- indirect effects of mass vaccination on the rate of transmission of the infectious agent.

Typically, the risks from infection and from vaccination change as vaccination coverage increases. When infection is common and vaccination rare, the risks due to the former are invariably greater, often by many orders of magnitude. When infection is very rare as a result of vaccination, the reverse may be true. Ultimately, the risk of vaccination will always be greater once vaccination has eliminated infection.

The new, more immunogenic vaccines provide better protection, but may be less safe

A factor relevant to concerns about vaccine-associated complications is the development of high potency live virus vaccines, which provide protection for the vast majority of those immunized and allow vaccination at an age (around 6 months) when maternally derived antibodies are still present. Although the new, more immunogenic vaccines provide better protection, their use may be associated with increased reactogenicity or lower safety, exacerbating the conflict between individual and community interests. Are there circumstances in which a higher efficacy vaccine should be used, even though it may lead to more cases of vaccine-associated disease? In the case of mumps, for example, the high potency 'Urabe Am 9' vaccine is estimated to have an efficacy of approximately 98%, while the lower potency 'Jeryl Lynn' vaccine has an efficacy of around 94%, and evidence suggests higher complication rates with the former. At levels of vaccine coverage high enough to block transmission, the sensible option is to use the lower potency vaccine. However, if high uptake cannot be achieved, then the total incidence of serious disease (both vaccine- and infection-produced) is reduced to a greater extent by the high potency vaccine.

Epidemiologic understanding assists the design of vaccination programs

The development of a safe, effective and cheap vaccine or drug is only the first step, albeit a vital one, towards the control of an infectious disease within a community. The interaction between a population of hosts and an infectious agent is inherently non-linear. For example, when population density doubles, the prevalence of many directly transmitted viral and bacterial infections may increase by more than two-fold. Complex patterns of change in the incidence of infection can arise when immunization programs with partial coverage are initiated. The many variables that influence rates of transmission often hinder the assessment of the likely impact of a given control program. Epidemiologic analysis at the level of the population biology of the interaction between host and infectious agent is critical for the development of community-based programs. Appreciation of the components that determine the transmission potential of an infectious agent, as measured by the basic reproductive rate R_0, is vital.

Means of infection control other than vaccines

In the search for new vaccines, we must not lose sight of the fact that some diseases can be controlled equally well by other means. In the developed world, public health measures rather than vaccines (or antibiotics) eliminated malaria and cholera and reduced the incidence of tuberculosis, and it could be argued that tropical diseases such as schistosomiasis or Chagas' disease could also be controlled by reducing contact with the snail or insect vector. However, vector control is not easy in practice and, like chemotherapy but unlike vaccination, needs to be maintained more or less indefinitely.

With certain diseases the chance of infection is so slight that a successful vaccine can never justify the cost and effort of producing it, and passive immunization after exposure may be a better approach (e.g. as for snakebite).

CURRENT VACCINE PRACTICE

Vaccines in general use

Diphtheria toxoid is almost universally given with tetanus toxoid and alum, and usually with pertussis vaccine

Although diphtheria toxin loses some antigenicity when converted (by formaldehyde) to the toxoid, it remains a highly effective vaccine. Surprisingly, for a vaccine aimed at the disease rather than the bacterium, it has also reduced the number of carriers of diphtheria, which may imply that the toxin plays a role in the survival or spread of the organism. Diphtheria toxoid is almost universally given with tetanus toxoid and alum, usually with pertussis, in three injections starting at 1.5–3 months of age plus a later boost. A booster may be given at 3–4 years of age, and in some countries, such as the USA, a booster with just tetanus and diphtheria is then given every 10 years. Protection is usually 90% or better.

Tetanus toxoid is also highly effective, and is in universal use

However, there are some differences in policy regarding booster injections and the treatment of patients after exposure. In most countries, following the three injections of young children, a booster is given at entry to school, and another is recommended every 5–10 years. Where exposure is suspected and a booster has not been given within 5 years, a booster can be given combined with antitoxin if the wound is dirty (see passive immunization, Chapter 35). Reactions to the vaccine are limited to mild hypersensitivity in repeatedly boosted patients, so tetanus toxoid can be considered one of the safest and most effective vaccines.

It is not clear whether pertussis vaccine can cause brain damage, but it does prevent deaths from whooping cough

Mass vaccination against whooping cough was introduced in Britain in 1957, using the whole heat- or formalin-killed vaccine developed during the 1940s. This is given with diphtheria and tetanus toxoid as part of the DTP or 'triple' vaccine, though the later boosts are not given since whooping cough is only a serious disease in young children.

Controversy has surrounded the use of this vaccine. There is no doubt that the incidence of whooping cough has diminished dramatically where the vaccine has been used, but several trials were required to establish statistical evidence for a protective effect. This was partly due to the omission of one of the three serotypes from some batches. In addition, there is no standard vaccine in general use. A more serious controversy concerns undesirable reactions to the vaccine. Mild reactions such as pain, inflammation and fever are quite common, probably due to the endotoxin and other toxins, but in the 1970s studies were published in the UK that claimed that severe screaming attacks, fits and permanent brain damage could follow pertussis vaccination in approximately 1/100 000 injections. The debate still continues about whether this is genuinely cause and effect, but meanwhile the understandable alarm of parents led to a fall of vaccine acceptance to as low as 30% in some areas. Predictably, a severe epidemic of whooping cough soon followed in the winter of 1978–1979, with over 100 000 cases and many deaths (Fig. 34.19). This perhaps constitutes the best evidence that the vaccine is in fact effective, but the controversy undoubtedly damaged the reputation of this vaccine, and of vaccines generally, in the mind of the public. There have also been suggestions that giving the component DPT vaccines separately may reduce the risk of complications, but this has not been proved.

A new two-component acellular pertussis vaccine has now been licensed in some countries such as the USA, consisting of the pertussis toxoid and filamentous haemagglutinin. The acellular vaccine causes significantly fewer reactions and gives greater vaccine efficacy.

Measles is now being considered to be a candidate for worldwide eradication

Live attenuated measles vaccine was introduced in the USA in 1963, and since that time the incidence of the disease, which used to kill over 500 children a year, has shrunk to almost nil. Worldwide eradication could therefore be possible (Fig 31.13), but the vaccine would require a considerably better uptake in most other countries than at present. An inactivated measles vaccine, also introduced in 1963, was withdrawn as it did not provide protection. The original live attenuated Edmonston B vaccine has since been replaced by a series of other more attenutated strains, which cause fewer reactions (fever and rashes).

The principal debate surrounding measles vaccine concerns the best age at which to give the vaccine. Maternal antibody can prevent proper immunization with measles, so it is necessary to wait until at least 6 months of age. However, even by the age of 9 months the vaccine gives only about 80% protection, so in countries where measles is uncommon it is usual to wait until about 1 year. However, in developing countries, where measles is still widespread, children are likely to be exposed before this age, so the vaccine is generally

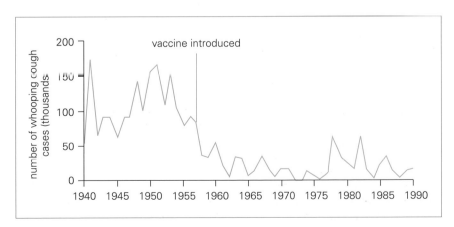

Fig. 34.19 The number of cases of whooping cough notified fell steadily after the introduction of mass immunization in 1958, although epidemics continued to occur at approximately 4-year intervals. Following the scare about the possible adverse effects of pertussis vaccine, the number of cases rose, and there was a large epidemic in the winter of 1978–1979.

given at around 9 months, followed by another dose at 1 year to protect those who do not respond well to the first. The duration of protection against measles appears to be at least 21 years, though this may be partly due to boosting during natural epidemics, so that as measles disappears from the population, adults may become susceptible again. If so, a logical strategy would be to give a boost as a routine, perhaps at primary or secondary school entry.

Mumps vaccine is most conveniently given with measles and rubella vaccines

What has been said about measles also applies to the live attenuated mumps vaccine. Some countries have questioned the need for a mumps vaccine, but in its absence about 1000 cases per year of mumps meningitis can be expected in the UK, while another calculation predicted 40 deaths and 95 cases of deafness per year in the USA. Mumps vaccine is most conveniently given as part of the MMR vaccine. The importance of receiving both doses of MMR is illustrated by a recent outbreak of mumps in Northern Ireland, where 55.4% of the confirmed cases had received one dose, but only 0.9% had received two doses of MMR.

Rubella vaccine is given to both boys and girls even though boys do not themselves need such vaccination

Rubella is a relatively mild disease that illustrates vividly the issues that can arise when setting the benefit to the individual against that of the population. In the UK it has until recently been considered that boys do not need vaccinating against rubella and so should not be exposed to the slight risk of vaccine complications; in addition, circulation of wild rubella in the population as a whole is useful in boosting immunity in girls. Therefore the live attenuated vaccine was given only to girls at adolescence to protect them against developing the disease while pregnant and transmitting it to the fetus, resulting in the congenital rubella syndrome.

However, because of its high reproduction rate (see Chapter 26), rubella will maintain its presence in the population indefinitely unless well over 50% of the population are protected. In the USA, therefore, rubella vaccine has been given to boys as well, and this approach (i.e. immunization with MMR vaccine at about 1 year) has recently been adopted in the UK. There is, however, the danger that as the level of infection in the community falls, cases will occur at a later age, therefore actually increasing the chance of fetal damage. Therefore until the disease is eradicated vaccine strategy needs to be carefully tailored to the prevailing situation in each country.

Both oral polio vaccine and inactivated polio vaccine have advantages and disadvantages

The remarkable decline in poliomyelitis is due to the use of one or other of two vaccines:

- the killed virus (Salk 1954),
- the live attenuated virus (Sabin 1957).

Both these vaccines are effective, and their advantages and disadvantages are listed in *Figure 34.20*.

ORAL AND INACTIVATED POLIO VACCINES COMPARED		
	inactivated (IPV)	**attenuated (OPV)**
introduced	Salk 1954	Sabin 1957
in use	Sweden, Finland, Holland, Iceland, USA	most other countries
dosage schedule	injection plus alum	oral at 2, 4, 6 months also at birth in endemic countries
risks	if inadequately killed (very rare) otherwise safe	in immunodeficiency reversion to virulence ?interference by other viruses cold chain failure
advantages	can be added to other childhood vaccines	IgA boosted herd immunity cheaper than Salk vaccine

Fig. 34.20 Poliomyelitis is unusual in that both live attenuated and killed vaccines are available and widely used. Three doses of the attenuated virus vaccine are given, as the three types of virus present in the vaccine interfere with each others' replication in the intestine. The repeated doses ensure an adequate response to each type. (IPV, inactivated polio vaccine; OPV, oral polio vaccine.)

The live attenuated oral polio vaccine (OPV) has become the first choice in most countries. Its main advantages are:

- its lower cost;
- the fact that (as with all live vaccines) immunity is induced in the right place: namely, the mucosal surfaces;
- the prediction that by spreading within the population it will induce 'herd' immunity—this is borne out by the fact that vaccine strains are now more common (e.g. in sewage) in the USA than wild strains.

Against these advantages is the risk of reversion to virulence, particularly by types 2 and 3, which as described earlier, do not differ as much from the wild strains as might be desired. Wild virus has been isolated from the stools within days of vaccination, and there have been several cases of paralytic poliomyelitis, especially in contacts of the vaccine; one estimate put these at 1–2 cases per million. OPV is, of course, not used in immunocompromised patients.

The above-mentioned considerations have led to the rejection of OPV in favor of an inactivated polio vaccine (IPV) in certain countries, notably Sweden, Finland, Holland and Iceland. Here it is argued that in practice:

- IPV induces equally good immunity—the pathology of polio does not occur in the gut.
- IPV might even be more effective in developing countries, where OPV has been somewhat disappointing, presumably

because, as was shown for measles, the 'cold chain' between factory and clinic was not adequately maintained.

Surprisingly, the duration of immunity following OPV is not demonstrably longer than with IPV, perhaps reflecting the relatively shorter duration of mucosal than systemic immunity. However, in the absence of substantial herd immunity, a high rate of IPV uptake would be essential for eradication.

Clearly, then, although polio vaccination has been highly successful, there is room for further improvements. Two current lines of development are the production of better and cheaper vaccines, both attenuated and inactivated, and the use of combined regimens (e.g. IPV followed by OPV in various sequential combinations).

Polio is the next disease that may be eradicated—Europe was declared polio free in 2002, and the Global Polio Eradication Initiative aims to certify the world as polio-free by the end of 2005. In 2000, polio infections occurred in only 20 countries, with fewer than 3000 cases diagnosed worldwide. To certify the world as free of polio, there must be no wild polio virus transmission for 3 years. Even when eradication is achieved, vaccination may not be stopped immediately, as some immunosuppressed individuals can shed live virus for a number of years.

Calmette and Guérin's attenuated tubercle bacillus (BCG) has been in use for over 70 years

However, despite this longstanding use, BCG still inspires fierce debate about its usefulness. This matter is important considering that tuberculosis kills some approximately 1.5 million people a year worldwide and is increasing in countries where AIDS is pandemic.

In its favor is the fact that BCG has given clear protection in controlled trials such as that carried out in the UK (1950) and in the USA on American Indians and Puerto Ricans in the 1970s. Efficacies of 70% or better have also been reported from several South American and African countries. In addition, the same vaccine appeared to be equally effective against leprosy in Uganda and, to a lesser extent, in other countries.

Immunization strategy varies according to the likelihood of infection:

- at birth in high-risk countries;
- at entry to secondary school, such as in the UK (but only to those with a negative or weakly positive Mantoux test; see Chapter 19).

One disadvantage of using BCG in countries where tuberculosis is rare is that by causing Mantoux (tuberculin) conversion, it destroys the diagnostic value of this test.

One problem with trials of BCG is the shifting background level of infection, which is dependent upon factors other than vaccination, notably general public health and anti-tuberculous chemotherapy. In countries with a low incidence of disease it would now be impossible to carry out a satisfactory trial based on clinical protection, and there is no rapid test that accurately predicts protection. The tuberculin skin test, widely used as a predictor of protection, has been shown to vary independently of actual protection, and is probably better regarded as a measure of mycobacterial exposure rather than immunity (see Chapter 14).

Another problem is that in other equally well controlled trials, BCG had little or no protective effect. Indeed in two trials, in southern India (1980) and southern parts of the USA, BCG has actually seemed to increase the incidence of tuberculosis. Numerous explanations have been put forward for these extraordinary discrepancies, which are unmatched by any other vaccine. These include differences between vaccine strains (there is no agreed world standard), genetic differences between the human populations, differences in the prevalent clinical pattern of disease, and differences in the type and number of environmental mycobacteria which might modulate the level of immunity in the population. At present, most experts think that exposure to environmental mycobacteria is most likely to affect the protection seen with BCG vaccination—a recent study carried out in young adults in parallel in the UK, where BCG vaccination gives protection, and in Malawi, where it does not, showed that the Malawians had strong T cell immunity to environmental mycobacterial antigens before they were vaccinated and that vaccination caused little enhancement. In contrast most of the UK children were immunologically naïve before vaccination, and vaccination induced strong T cell immunity.

Quite apart from these debatable effects on tuberculosis, BCG has three other potential uses:

- as an adjuvant for other vaccines;
- as a vector for cloned genes from other organisms;
- as a general non-specific immunostimulant (see Chapter 35).

To overcome the shortcomings of BCG, over 200 new vaccines have now been tested in animals, although few seem to give better protection than BCG. These include recombinant BCG vaccines, attenuated strains of M. tuberculosis, prime-boost vaccines using a DNA vaccine and a recombinant virus or two different recombinant viruses, and subunit vaccines consisting of secreted proteins.

Hepatitis B virus vaccine was the first vaccine in human use to be made by recombinant DNA technology

The first vaccine to be used for hepatitis B virus (HBV) vaccine was unusual in several ways. This plasma-derived vaccine consisted of a non-living antigenic preparation derived from the blood of virus carriers; the surface coat antigen (HBsAg) is overproduced by the virus, and circulates as free, non-infectious, 22 nm diameter spherical particles (up to 10^{13}/ml of blood; *Fig. 34.21*). When purified and inactivated, so as to

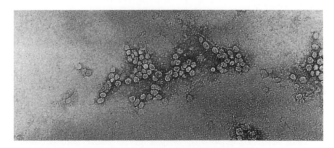

Fig. 34.21 Electron micrograph of purified 22 nm hepatitis B surface antigens expressed in yeast cells. (Courtesy of JR Pattison.)

be scrupulously free of DNA, the vaccine was shown to be at least 95% protective in a controlled trial in American male homosexuals in 1980, and licensed in the following year. This vaccine had three disadvantages:

- Being derived from human blood, it had to be purified with exceptional care because of the risk of transmitting live HBV or other viruses.
- Even after three doses, antibody levels started to fall 1–2 years later, so boosting was necessary. An antibody level of 100 units/l is considered to be protective.
- Finally, it was extremely expensive to make, and limited supplies mainly restricted its use to healthcare professionals.

Meanwhile, a second vaccine was produced via recombinant DNA technology—the first such vaccine to go into human use. The same antigen (HBsAg) is involved, the gene being cloned into a yeast vector which produces large amounts of the antigenic protein. As well as being safer and cheaper—about 50% of the cost of the plasma-derived vaccine when introduced—this recombinant vaccine appears to be equally effective. Recent refinements include the insertion of other ('pre-S') genes into the vector, to code for proteins involved in the infectious process. The idea of incorporating HBV genes into a living attenuated vector is also under consideration.

Initially, hepatitis B vaccination was only given to high risk groups such as medical personnel, those handling blood products, intravenous drug users and gay men, but it is now given to all babies at birth in the USA. Babies born to mothers known to be hepatitis surface antigen positive are also given a dose of hepatitis B immunoglobulin. Over 95% of vaccine recipients make an antibody response to hepatitis B surface antigen, but the remaining 5% can fail to respond to a second course of vaccination. Some of these non-responders may be chronically infected with hepatitis B.

HBV is now clearly a candidate for eventual eradication

In Africa, HBV is typically acquired during early childhood, so the vaccine is given at the same time as the usual childhood ones, the major problem being to keep the cost within affordable limits. At present, US$1/dose is about the minimum. In the Far East, on the other hand, HBV is commonly transmitted to newborns by mothers who are chronic carriers. Here a course of vaccine injections (at 1 week, 5 weeks, 9 weeks and 1 year) is combined with passive immunization with immune globulin. Early results show good protection, and it is hoped that the number of carriers will progressively fall, and with it the incidence of liver carcinoma.

Hepatitis A vaccine is now available, but there is no vaccine yet for hepatitis C

Travelers to countries where hepatitis A is endemic can be immunized with a vaccine derived from human diploid cells that has been formaldehyde inactivated. Until this vaccine became available, passive immunization with pooled normal human immunoglobulin, which gives good but transient protection, was the standard method. As the new inactivated whole virus vaccine has been shown to be very effective,

inducing 94% protection against clinical hepatitis A in Thai children, it is now recommended that it should be given to children of 2 years or older in areas where the annual incidence of hepatitis A is 20/100 000 population or higher. It is hoped that a vaccine will ultimately be available for the more recently discovered hepatitis C virus.

Rabies is the only disease where post-exposure vaccination is successful, because of its long incubation period

The rabies vaccine is famous for Pasteur's courageous demonstration in 1885 that a desiccated (air-killed) preparation of spinal cord from rabid rabbits would protect humans against rabies, even after infection with the virus (see Chapter 31).

Over one century later, neuro-tissue vaccine (NTV) is still used in some countries, but elsewhere has been replaced by virus grown in human diploid cells or duck embryos, and then inactivated with propiolactone. Three doses of vaccine give adequate antibody titers for protection. No safe attenuated virus is yet available, though an attenuated or a genetically engineered vaccine is still a possibility.

For post-exposure cases, a course of 5–6 intramuscular injections, starting as soon as possible, the first combined with an injection of human hyperimmune globulin (20 IU/kg), gives virtually complete protection. Pre-exposure (i.e. for travelers to high-risk areas), 2–3 doses are usually sufficient, with a boost every few years where the risk is maintained (e.g. veterinarians and other animal handlers). Eradication might seem an unattainable goal, but schemes to introduce an attenuated virus to wildlife via infected food bait have been tried out in Switzerland and neighboring countries, as well as Canada, and have had some remarkable success.

Vaccines are available for some arbovirus infections, but notably not for dengue fever

Arbovirus infections are vector-borne fevers and include yellow fever, dengue, south east Asian hemorrhagic fever and Japanese encephalitis. They are among the most virulent virus infections (see Chapter 28), and good vaccines are highly desirable. An attenuated yellow fever virus was developed in 1937, and this '17D' strain remains the standard highly effective vaccine for yellow fever. A single subcutaneous dose, with a boost every 10 years for residents in the tropics, or frequent visitors, gives excellent protection and is a requirement for all travelers to countries where the disease does not occur but where it might become established if virus brought in by a traveler infected the mosquito or non-human primate hosts. This requirement for vaccination can even apply to travelers in transit at an airport!

Vaccines are also available against Japanese encephalitis (inactivated virus is used in all countries except China, which uses a live attenuated virus as vaccine) and Rift Valley fever. However, no vaccine is currently available for dengue fever, and this is now recognized as a high priority. One problem is the existence of four serotypes, but a more serious complication is the possibility that one manifestation of the disease may be immunopathologic. This is the 'hemorrhagic shock syndrome' seen in patients infected with a second serotype

CHANGING FORMULATIONS OF INFLUENZA VIRUS VACCINES			
	H3N2	**H1N1**	**B**
1999–2000	A/Sydney/5/1997	A/Beijing/262/1995	B/Beijing/184/1993
2000–2001	A/Moscow/10/1999	A/New Caledonia/20/1999	B/Beijing/184/1993
2001–2002	A/Moscow/10/1999	A/New Caledonia/20/1999	B/Sichuan/379/1999
2002–2003	A/Moscow/10/1999	A/New Caledonia/20/1999	B/Hong Kong/330/2001

Fig. 34.22 Changing formulations of influenza virus vaccines. The A strains are described in terms of the type of hemagglutinin (H) and neuriminidase (N) antigens they express. The strain designation denotes: influenza virus type/location of isolation/isolate number/year of isolation. (Reproduced with permission from Palese and Garcia-Sastre, *J Clin Invest* 2002; 110:10.)

following earlier exposure to a first. Whatever the mechanism of this condition, there is an obvious possibility that a vaccine that did not protect fully against all serotypes might precipitate the condition.

Vaccines currently used for influenza are only partially effective

Unlike most of the diseases considered so far, influenza does not induce good long-lasting immunity even after recovery from infection in healthy people. This is mainly due to its ability to undergo antigenic 'shift' and 'drift' (see Chapters 16 and 19), but also to the curious tendency for responses to different strains to be dominated by antibody against the strain first encountered by the individual ('original antigenic sin'). However, influenza is such an important cause of morbidity and mortality (estimated at 150/million in the USA), that a range of only partially effective vaccines is in use, pending the development of something better.

The most widely used influenza vaccines are formalin- or β-propiolactone-killed viral vaccines, usually including two subtypes of influenza A and one of B, and containing the hemagglutinin (H) and neuraminidase (N) prevalent or anticipated in the population (*Figure 34.22*). This vaccine is offered to high-risk groups such as nursing and ancillary staff, the elderly, and patients with chronic respiratory, cardiac or renal disease, anemia, diabetes mellitus or immunodeficiency. In such patients, efficacy is estimated at about 70% in terms of reducing severity, but only about 30% if total prevention is the criterion. Revaccination in subsequent years is required to maintain antibody levels, but whether with the same or a different strain does not give a further boost of titer.

Trials with live cold-adapted strains are in use in Russia and have shown some protection, but up to 30% of normal patients may fail to produce antibody and would presumably not be protected. Temperature-sensitive mutants designed to grow in the upper but not the lower respiratory tract have been disappointing, due to reversion to wild type.

An alternative is a recombinant virus containing portions of RNA coding for appropriate H and N antigens. A theoretic advantage of recombinant and other live vaccines would be the induction of cytotoxic T cell memory, which is generally poor or absent with killed viruses. However, viral antigens entrapped in ISCOMs have recently been shown to induce good cytotoxic T cell responses.

A live attenuated VZV vaccine has been shown to be highly protective

Chickenpox, caused by VZV, can occasionally lead to severe complications and is a life-threatening disease in children with leukemia; a successful vaccine might also prevent zoster (shingles) in older people. A live attenuated VZV vaccine, derived from the Oka strain, was obtained by passage in human and guinea pig cell lines. This vaccine induces detectable antibody titers in 97% of children, and antibody is maintained for at least 6 years in over 90% of healthy children, although vaccination gives considerably less protection in leukemic children on chemotherapy. Trials of a heat-inactivated preparation of the childhood VZV vaccine have shown that it can help prevent the reactivation of the virus in cancer patients receiving hemopoietic cell transplants.

Pneumococcal vaccines need to protect against many different serotypes

Antigenic diversity is a problem with pneumococcal infection. However, since the 84 serotypes of *Streptococcus pneumoniae* are stable in the population and do not show the rapid changes of influenza, it is theoretically possible to produce a complete vaccine containing them all. In practice it has been found that less than half this number is sufficient to protect against the majority of infections.

The antigen used is the capsular polysaccharide prepared from large scale bacterial culture. Currently available vaccines contain polysaccharide antigens from 23 different serotypes, and induce antibodies in 80% of healthy adults. The indications for vaccination are similar to those for influenza, and in the USA the vaccine is strongly recommended for the elderly, being appreciably cheaper than the treatment for pneumonia. In children under 2 years, the other main high risk group, the response to the vaccine is generally poor, since the IgG2 class of antibody, which predominates in responses to carbohydrate antigens, develops late and the polysaccharides behave as T-independent antigens.

Conjugation to a protein carrier has been shown to improve the response, presumably by allowing T cells to participate, and a vaccine with purified capsular polysaccharide from seven serotypes of *Strep. pneumoniae* is now available, which induces antibodies in virtually all immunized infects. Conjugate vaccines under development would increase coverage to 9 or 11 serotypes. A large field trial of three doses of the nine-valent vaccine is underway in The Gambia, west Africa, to see if the incidence of X-ray-confirmed pneumonia can be reduced.

Meningococcal vaccines are only partially effective and not available for all serotypes

Here the principle, using a capsular polysaccharide as antigen, is the same as with the pneumococcus athough again the response is less than optimal, particularly in younger children. Vaccines are currently available for *N. meningitidis* strains A, C, Y and W-135. Vaccination against meningitis is now mandatory for pilgrims visiting Mecca in Saudi Arabia for the Umrah and Haj pilgrimages, and some countries also require returning pilgrims to be vaccinated. This is to prevent outbreaks such as that of *N. meningitis* W-135 which occurred in pilgrims in 2000. So far it has not been possible to develop an effective vaccine against group B strains, as the type B polysaccharide, which is largely composed of sialic acid, is poorly immunogenic. This is a problem as group B strains cause most of the meningitis cases in the USA and Europe. An alternative to using the capsular polysaccharide as the vaccine antigen may be to use membrane proteins that have now been identified during genomic sequencing.

A problem that has been noted with both pneumococcal and meningococcal vaccines is that other infections, notably even quite mild malaria, interfere with the normal response to the vaccine. Thus it was found in a Nigerian trial that treatment of malaria with chloroquine 1 week before vaccination improved the anti-polysaccharide responses. This emphasizes the desirability of a malaria vaccine (see below).

Like pneumococcal and meningococcal vaccine, Haemophilus influenzae *vaccine is a capsular polysaccharide vaccine*

The b serotype of *Haemophilus influenzae* (Hib) is responsible for the most serious disease. Its capsule, a phosphodiester-linked polymer of ribose and ribitol, suffers from the same problems as the other polysaccharides, and the first polysaccharide vaccine gave low immunogenicity in children under 2 years. Various polysaccharide–protein conjugates are now available, using either tetanus or diphtheria toxoid, given either alone (2–3 doses subcutaneously at 2–6 months) or with the triple DTP vaccine. These appear to induce good antibody and memory responses (the conjugation changes the polysaccharide from a T-independent to a T-dependent antigen) and, encouragingly, poor initial responders may respond well to later boosting. A large-scale trial in Finland showed 94% efficacy, and it is very rare to have invasive Hib disease in an infant that has been completely vaccinated.

The TY21a strain of typhoid gives 60–90% protection against typhoid for at least 5 years

For nearly a century travelers to the tropics, and particularly military personnel, have been subjected to the 'TAB' vaccine,

consisting of heat-, phenol-, alcohol- or acetone-killed whole *S. typhi* and *S. paratyphi* organisms, injected intramuscularly once or twice. Not only was the vaccine fairly unpleasant, with local pain and general malaise due to the endotoxin content, but its efficacy has repeatedly been questioned. In various controlled trials, protection has been estimated at 10–70%, depending partly upon the size of the infecting dose. There is therefore a considerable demand for new and better typhoid vaccines.

Two candidates have emerged:

- a live attenuated organism;
- a capsular polysaccharide.

The first attenuated typhoid bacillus (TY21a) was produced by random chemical mutagenesis, but current attention focuses on enzyme-deficient strains with mutations in either the galactose epimerase (GalE) or the aromatic amino acid synthesis pathway (AroA). These mutations allow the bacilli to survive and proliferate for a few days only, so that when given orally they induce local immunity in the intestine, but not systemic disease. All these mutant strains appear to be safe and effective (7 years after the final dose, the protective efficacy was still 67% in vaccinees living in endemic areas), and the latter two have the added advantage of being suitable vectors for inserted genes derived from other organisms. The TY21a strain is given either with a tablet of sodium bicarbonate or in enteric-coated capsules.

The polysaccharide vaccine is composed of purified 'Vi' (virulence) antigen. A single dose of 25 µg has given protection in the 72% range after 1.5 years, which declined to 50% 3 years after vaccination.

New V. cholerae *vaccines may give better protection than the original heat-killed vaccine*

The original heat-killed whole *V. cholerae* vaccines suffered from the same disadvantages as the older typhoid vaccines—unpleasant reactions and only approximately 50% protection for 6 months. Vaccination was therefore not recommended, nor legally required for foreign travel. Two new cholera vaccines (live and killed) are now licensed and available in a limited number of countries. The killed vaccine, which can be given orally, seems to give good (> 85%) protection for 6 months after the second dose, and protection is still > 60% 3 years later in vaccine recipients over 5 years of age. Interestingly the killed vaccine gives some degree of cross-protection against *E. coli*, therefore giving additional protection against traveler's diarrhea.

New and experimental vaccines

A live heterologous rotavirus vaccine is a possibility

As mentioned earlier, rotavirus infection might be amenable to a live heterologous vaccine, as was the case with smallpox. Bovine and monkey strains of the virus have been tried as oral vaccines in infants, with 70–80% reported protection. The first licensed rhesus-based rotavirus tetravalent vaccine was withdrawn in 1999 following reports of intussusception (a blockage of the intestine), but a bovine rotavirus vaccine is undergoing further trials for both safety and efficacy. The possibility of using the 'naturally' attenuated human strains that can appear in nurseries is also being explored. Prospects are therefore quite favorable for the eventual availability of a rotavirus vaccine.

A shigella vaccine might be possible using mutated Shigella strains or by inserting shigella antigens into other vectors

Live, randomly attenuated shigella organisms, though fairly effective as oral vaccines, never came into general use because of the short duration of protection and occasional side effects. Current research is concentrated on deliberately mutated strains and on the insertion of shigella antigens into S. typhi or other vectors.

A variety of types of E. coli vaccines are being investigated

A fully successful vaccine against E. coli infection has not yet emerged, because of the serotypic diversity of both surface antigens and toxins. However, trials have been conducted with toxoids based on the enterotoxins, purified fimbriae,

whole killed organisms and live attenuated strains, all of which give some protection. The combined killed cholera/B toxin subunit vaccine mentioned above also gave significant protection against E. coli because of cross-reaction between the two toxins.

Despite trials, there is still no effective malaria vaccine

At the time of writing, several clinical trials of a malaria vaccine have been published, and more will certainly follow. Peptides, recombinant protein and DNA-modified virus (prime boost) vaccines, mainly targeting the sporozoite and liver stages, have all been tested in humans. Although some trials have shown statistically significant protection, vaccine eficacy was low (below 30%) and was not reproducible. Other potential targets for attack within the unusually complex malaria lifecycle (see Chapter 27) include the liver stage itself, the merozoite (infective for the red cell), the sexual stages (gametocytes and gametes) and the soluble molecules thought to be responsible for inducing pathology (Fig. 34.23). This wide range of choices clearly increases the

stage	vaccine strategy
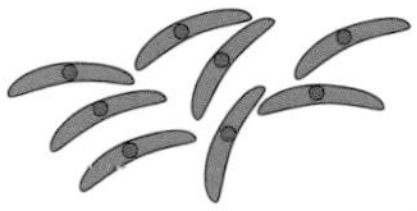 sporozoites	sporozoite vaccine to induce blocking antibody, already field-tested in humans
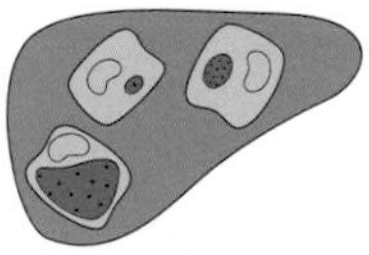 liver stage	sporozoite vaccine to induce cell-mediated immunity to liver stage, already tested in humans
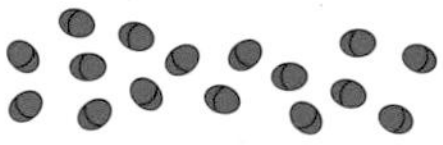 merozoites	merozoite (antigen) vaccine to induce invasion inhibitory antibody
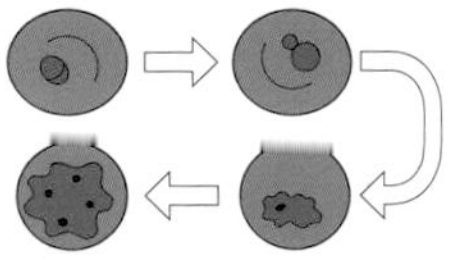 asexual erythrocyte stage	asexual stage (antigen) vaccine to induce other responses to red cell stage, and against toxic products ('anti-disease vaccine')
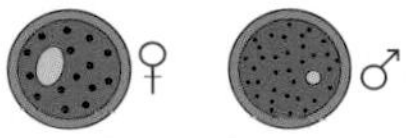 gametocytes	vaccines to interrupt sexual stages – 'transmission blocking' vaccine
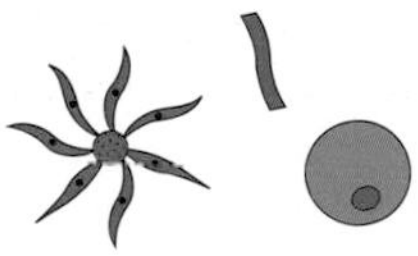 gametes	

Fig. 34.23 Malaria vaccine strategies. A number of different approaches are being investigated, reflecting the complexity of the lifecycle and of immunity to this parasite (see Chapter 27).

chance of success, but each approach has its problems: for example, extensive antigenic variation in the blood stage, and the need for 100% efficacy with the hepatic and prehepatic stages; also the sexual stage vaccines would only block transmission, protecting the community, but not the vaccinee. Each approach has its vigorous proponents, but it seems likely that a successful vaccine will contain antigens from several or all stages.

Three different approaches have given some protection against cutaneous leishmaniasis

These three approaches are:

- 'Leishmanization', an ancient Middle Eastern practice in which children are deliberately infected in an inconspicuous skin site with *Leishmania tropica* from a mild case, resulting in a self-healing lesion ('Oriental sore') and subsequent immunity to more widespread disease. This had some popularity in the former Soviet Union and Israel, but protection is variable, and non-virulent disease can never be guaranteed.
- Use of killed promastigotes (the invasive stage), 2–3 times intramuscularly. Up to 80% protection was claimed in a Brazilian trial, but this was of uncertain duration.
- Injection of killed promastigotes plus BCG, which produced the most dramatic results. In a Venezuelan trial over 90% protection was induced, but it is too soon to say for how long this protection lasts, and another trial in Sudan failed to show that the combined vaccine was any better than BCG alone in protecting against visceral leishmaniasis.

Meanwhile a much more novel type of vaccine is being tested. This uses a saliva protein from the sandfly vector that when used as a vaccine induces strong DTH responses and protection in mice. This approach would have the advantage that people would be repeatedly boosted when bitten by sandflies, whether infected or uninfected, but whether it could ever completely prevent infection is less clear.

Vaccines still awaited

There remains a long list of important infectious diseases for which vaccines, although desirable, are not yet available (*Fig. 34.24*). In some cases it is probably only a matter of time, but in others there are fundamental problems. With the adenoviruses and rhinoviruses, for example, the serotypic diversity (about 40 and 110, respectively) makes it difficult to imagine a fully effective vaccine. With the live herpes virus vaccines there is the danger of latency with reactivation, and with the killed vaccines the difficulty of obtaining large amounts of virus (except with herpes simplex). With respiratory syncytial virus, the problem has been reversion of attenuated strains and enhancement of disease by killed vaccines. With the bacterial diseases listed in *Figure 34.24*, it is the lack of convincing immunity following natural infection that is discouraging, syphilis perhaps being the outstanding example. The same applies to the protozoa and helminths, though research is proceeding in a variety of directions, and some quite effective vaccines have been produced for veterinary use (e.g. hookworm in dogs, lungworm in cattle).

IMPORTANT INFECTIOUS DISEASES FOR WHICH THERE IS NO SATISFACTORY VACCINE	
organism	**disease**
HIV	AIDS
hepatitis C	hepatitis
herpes simplex virus	genital infection
cytomegalovirus	effect on fetus
Epstein–Barr virus	glandular fever
rhinoviruses	common cold
dengue virus	dengue fever
Neisseria gonorrhoeae	gonorrhea
*Mycobacterium tuberculosis**	tuberculosis
*Mycobacterium leprae**	leprosy
Treponema pallidum	syphilis
Chlamydia trachomatis	trachoma, urethritis
Plasmodium spp.	malaria
Trypanosoma spp.	trypanosomiasis
Filaria spp.	filariasis, onchocerciasis
Leishmania spp.	leishmaniasis
Schistosoma spp.	schistosomiasis
*BCG vaccination provides variable protection against tuberculosis but does provide some protection against leprosy	

Fig. 34.24 Important infectious diseases for which a satisfactory vaccine is not yet available.

The most concentrated effort is probably being directed against HIV, where the production of a vaccine to limit the spread or progression of AIDS is literally a race against time. By 2002, there had been over 30 candidate vaccines tested in phase I/II clinical trials, and phase III efficacy trials are ongoing in several developing countries. Most workers have focused on the gp160 molecule by which the virus attaches and fuses itself to cells, and a recombinant gp120 vaccine is being tested in Thailand—although the extraordinarily extensive antigenic variation of this molecule makes success quite problematic. Another vaccine being tested in Kenya consists of a DNA prime followed by a modified vaccinia virus Ankara boost containing the gag p24/p17 antigens from the A clade of the HIV virus as well as a string of cytotoxic T cell epitopes.

Will we need new vaccines against bioterrorism?

New vaccines, and some old ones, may be needed to protect us against the threat of bioterrorism. Vaccines against *Bacillus anthracis* (anthrax) and *Yersinia pestis* (plague) are available, but only for those at high risk of occupational exposure. Smallpox vaccine is also being produced again, leading to debates as to whether mass vaccination or vaccination of only those exposed to the virus and their contacts would be better.

However, we also need to better exploit the vaccines we do have available—it is disturbing that many deaths worldwide still occur from vaccine-preventable diseases *(Fig. 34.25)*. Thus the better implementation of existing vaccines remains an important goal.

New methods of delivery

The vaccines of the future may use totally new means of delivering the antigen.

Transcutaneous vaccination using skin patches

A novel approach to vaccination is the development of skin patches impregnated with antigen. The antigen is taken up by the many Langerhans' cells in the epidermis, which will carry it to the local draining lymph node. Even recombinant viral vectors expressing vaccine antigens can be adsorbed onto the skin in this way. One clever idea is to use a vaccine antigen togther with cholera toxin as an adjuvant on the patch, thus protecting against two diseases at once.

Edible plant vaccines

A novel approach to vaccination is to express the genes for bacterial or viral antigens in edible plant tissues. This could be a much cheaper way of making vaccines than the existing fermentation or cell cuture methods, as the transgenic plant will make the vaccine antigen as it grows. The plant will also deliver the vaccine, as the vaccinee only has to eat some of the transgenic plant to get immunized. Potatoes, tomatoes and tobacco plants have been used in experiments to make edible vaccines, with promising results. A number of problems still need to be overcome but maybe one day eating a transgenic banana will protect us against a battery of human pathogens, since the plant could be engineered to express multiple genes!

GLOBAL DEATHS FROM EIGHT VACCINE-PREVENTABLE DISEASES	
	annual deaths (estimate)
polio	720
diphtheria	5 000
pertussis	346 000
measles	888 000
tetanus*	410 000
Haemophilus influenzae b	400 000
hepatitis B	900 000
yellow fever	30 000
*includes 215 000 neonatal cases	

Fig. 34.25 Global deaths from eight vaccine-preventable diseases. Source: Global Alliance for Vaccines and Immunization, 2002.

KEY FACTS

- Vaccination aims to prime the adaptive immune system to the antigens of a particular microbe so that a first infection induces a secondary response.

- Vaccines are either live attenuated organisms, killed whole organisms, subcellular fractions or antigens produced artificially by gene cloning or chemical synthesis.

- In general, live vaccines are more effective than other types, but carry the risk of reverting to virulence or inducing disease in immunocompromised patients.

- The details of vaccine choice, route, dose and risks have to be considered for each disease individually, and there is room for considerable improvement in producing safe, effective and affordable vaccines.

- It is possible to calculate the percentage vaccine coverage necessary to eradicate infections in communities.

- Successful vaccination of the majority of a population may increase the age at which infection occurs in susceptibles, creating possible complications.

- Epidemiologic understanding can help resolve the conflicts between protecting individuals and protecting communities.

- Overall, vaccination is a very effective public health tool—but many challenges remain, including the effective implementation of existing vaccines worldwide and the design of new vaccines against those infections for which they are not yet available.

? QUESTIONS

1. Vaccines that consist of inactivated organisms are:*
   A. Good at inducing mucosal immunity
   B. Less stable than live vaccines
   C. Incapable of reverting to virulence
   D. Safer than live vaccines
   E. More immunogenic than live vaccines

2. Immunocompromised adult patients could safely be given:*
   A. Inactivated vaccines
   B. Live polio vaccine
   C. BCG vaccination
   D. Measles vaccine
   E. Tetanus vaccination
   F. DNA vaccines

3. p_c is a term used to define:*
   A. The percentage of a population that has been successfully vaccinated

   B. The vaccine coverage needed to eliminate infection
   C. The number of people subsequently infected by one infected individual
   D. A critical value at which there are too few susceptibles in a population to manintain transmission

4. The success of a vaccination campaign depends on:*
   A. Population density
   B. The ability of the vaccine to induce an appropriate immune response
   C. Whether 100% vaccination coverage is achieved
   D. The availability of a live attenuated vaccine

*Each question has more than one correct answer.

FURTHER READING

Epidemiology and prevention of vaccine-preventable diseases. The Pink Book, 7th edition, 2002. (also available on www.cdc.gov/nip/publications/pink)

Mims CA, White DO. *Viral Pathogenesis and Immunity*. Oxford: Blackwell Scientific, 1984

Vaccination: a series of expert reviews. *British Medical Bulletin* 2002; 62.

www.cdc.gov/nip/ Useful site with US vaccination schedules.

www.vaccinealliance.org/ Web site for GAVI, the Global Alliance for Vaccines and Immunization.

www.who.int/ith/ International Travel and Health 2002; good chapter on vaccine-preventable diseases, vaccines and vaccination.

Passive and non-specific immunotherapy

35

INTRODUCTION

An alternative to vaccination is needed for those who are already infected or are immunodeficient

The most dramatic and successful form of immunotherapy is vaccination, as described in the previous chapter. However, there are some situations where a different approach may be necessary. For instance:

- The patient may already be infected and so a more rapid build-up of immune effector mechanisms than occurs naturally may be needed.
- Alternatively, the patient's immune system may be inadequate and unable to respond either to the infection or to a vaccine, through immunodeficiency or some specially resistant property of the parasite.

This chapter deals with such situations.

PASSIVE IMMUNIZATION WITH ANTIBODY

Certain diseases are treated by a passive transfer of immunity, which can be life-saving

Before the introduction of antibiotics, acute infectious diseases were often treated by the injection of preformed antibody on the principle that the patient was already ill and it was too late for 'active' vaccination. Indeed, the demonstration that immunity to tetanus and diphtheria could be transferred to mice with serum from vaccinated rabbits was a key experiment in the discovery of antibody in the 1890s. Subsequently, the production of antiserum for the passive treatment of diphtheria, tetanus and pneumococcal pneumonia, and against the toxic effects of streptococci and staphylococci, became an important industry, and generations of horses that had retired from active duty were kept on as the source of 'immune serum'. The introduction of antitetanus serum in the early months of the First World War reduced the incidence of tetanus dramatically by up to 30-fold *(Fig. 35.1)*.

The advent of penicillin and other antibiotics has, of course, changed the picture considerably, and passive immunotherapy is now used for only a select group of diseases *(Fig. 35.2)*. The serum may be specific or non-specific and of human or animal origin.

The use of antiserum raised in animals can cause serum sickness

The use of antiserum raised in horses or rabbits has largely been abandoned because of the complications resulting from the immune response to the antibody, which is of course a foreign protein. These include progressively more rapid elimination (and therefore reduced clinical effectiveness) and, more seriously, serum sickness due to immune complex

deposition in for example the kidney and skin (see Chapter 17), and even anaphylaxis. These complications can be avoided by using human serum taken during convalescence or following vaccination—to prevent infection after exposure (e.g. rabies) or to minimize its severity (e.g. varicella in immunodeficient children).

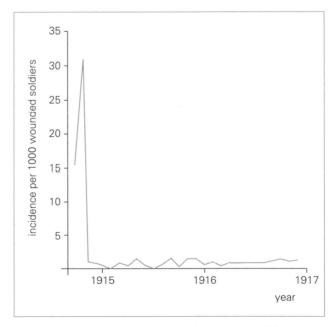

Fig. 35.1 Passive immunization significantly reduced the incidence of tetanus in the early months of the First World War. The figure shows the incidence of tetanus per 1000 wounded soldiers in British hospitals during 1914–1916. There was a dramatic fall after the introduction of antitetanus serum in October 1914.

SPECIFIC PASSIVE IMMUNOTHERAPY WITH ANTIBODY		
infection	source of antibody	indication
diphtheria	human, horse	prophylaxis, treatment
tetanus	human, horse	
varicella-zoster	human	prophylaxis in immunodeficiencies
gas gangrene	horse	
botulism		post exposure
snake bite		
scorpion bite		
rabies	human	post-exposure (plus vaccine)
hepatitis B	human	post-exposure
hepatitis A	pooled human immunoglobulin	prophylaxis (travel)
measles		post-exposure

Fig. 35.2 Specific passive immunotherapy with antibody. Although not so commonly used as 50 years ago, passive injections of specific antibody can still be a life-saving treatment.

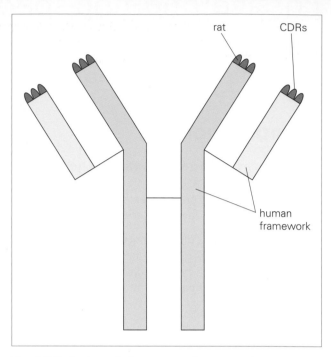

Fig. 35.3 Grafting of all six rat complementarity determining regions (CDRs) onto a human Ig framework to create a 'humanized' rat monoclonal antibody.

Theoretically the best form of specific antibody is a monoclonal antibody with a precisely known specificity

In practice, a mixture of several monoclonal antibodies might be required in situations where individual antigens are expressed in low quantities on the microbe or where binding to more than one epitope is required for full effectiveness. We have previously described the derivation of mouse mono-clonal antibodies, but a serious complication is that they are highly immunogenic in humans and give rise to human anti-mouse antibodies (HAMA) which accelerate clearance of the monoclonal from the blood and possibly cause hypersensitivity reactions; they also prevent the mouse antibody from reaching its target and, in some cases, block its binding to antigen. Logic points to removal of the xenogeneic (foreign) portions of the monoclonal antibody and their replacement by human Ig structures using recombinant DNA technology. One refined approach is to graft the six complementarity determining regions (CDR) of a high affinity rodent mono-clonal onto a completely human Ig framework without loss of specific reactivity (Fig. 35.3). This is not a trivial exercise, however, and the objective of fusing human B cells to make hybridomas is still appealing, taking into account not only the gross reduction in immunogenicity but also the fact that, within a species, antibodies can be made to subtle differences such as major histocompatibility complex (MHC) poly-morphic molecules and tumor-associated antigens on other individuals, whereas xenogeneic responses are more directed to immunodominant structures common to most subjects. Notwithstanding the difficulties in finding good fusion partners, large numbers of human monoclonals have been established.

A radically different approach involves the production of transgenic xenomouse strains in which megabase size unrearranged human Ig *H* and *k* light chain loci have been introduced into mice whose endogenous murine Ig genes have been inactivated. Immunization of these mice yields high affinity (10^{-10}–10^{-11}M) human antibodies which can then be isolated using hybridoma or recombinant approaches. Potent anti-inflammatory (anti-IL-8) and antitumor (anti-epidermal growth factor receptor) therapeutic agents have already been obtained using such mice. There is still a snag in that even human antibodies can provoke anti-idiotype responses; these may have to be circumvented by using engineered antibodies bearing different idiotypes for subsequent injections. Many human monoclonals are being evaluated for clinical use; one can cite IgG anti-RhD for the prevention of rhesus disease of the newborn, and highly potent monoclonals for protection against varicella-zoster, cytomegalovirus, group B streptococci and lipopolysaccharide endotoxins of Gram-negative bacteria.

Engineering antibodies

There are other ways around the problems associated with the production of human monoclonals which exploit the wiles of modern molecular biology. Reference has already been made to the 'humanizing' of rodent antibodies, but an important new strategy based upon bacteriophage expression and *selection* has achieved a prominent position. In essence, mRNA, preferably from primed human B cells, is converted to cDNA, and the antibody genes, or fragments therefrom, are expanded by the polymerase chain reaction (PCR). Single constructs are then made in which the light and heavy chain genes are allowed to combine randomly as Fab or single chain Fv (scFv) fragments in tandem with the bacteriophage coat protein gene (Fig. 35.4). This *combinatorial library* encodes a huge repertoire of antibody fragments expressed as fusion

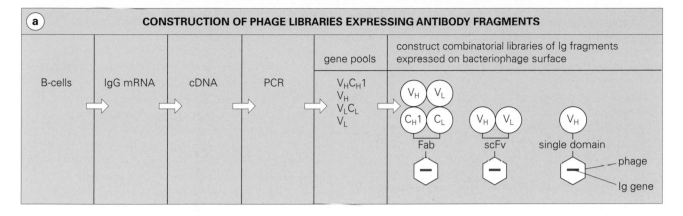

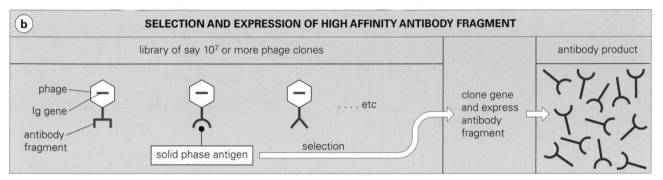

Fig. 35.4 Pools of genes encoding Ig domains derived from IgG mRNA are randomly combined and expressed either as Fab or single chain Fv (scFv) fragments on the surface of the bacteriophage. Libraries expressing single domains of the heavy chain variable region (V_H) (human or llama usually) can also be constructed. Phage clones containing genes encoding high affinity antibody fragments can be selected from these extremely large libraries using solid phage antigen. The appropriate Ig genes can then be cloned and expressed in suitable vectors to produce abundant antibody fragments.

proteins with a filamentous coat protein on the bacteriophage surface. The extremely high number of phages produced by *Escherichia coli* infection can now be panned on solid phase antigen to select those bearing the highest affinity antibodies attached to their surface *(Fig. 35.4)*. Because the genes which encode these highest affinity antibodies are already present within the selected phage, they can readily be cloned and the antibody fragment expressed in bulk.

It should be recognized that this selection procedure has an enormous advantage over techniques which employ *screening*, because the number of phages which can be examined is several logs higher. Although a 'test-tube' operation, this approach to the generation of specific antibodies does resemble the affinity maturation of the immune response in vivo in the sense that antigen is the determining factor in selecting out the highest affinity responders. In order to increase the affinities of antibodies produced by these techniques, antigen can be used to select higher affinity mutants produced by random mutagenesis (or even more effectively by site-directed replacements at mutational hot spots), again mimicking the natural immune response which involves random mutation and antigen selection. Phage libraries have been created which express just single heavy chain variable region domains whose affinity can be surprisingly high—sometimes in the low nanomolar range.

Not only can the genes for a monoclonal antibody be engineered for expression in bulk in the milk of lactating animals but plants can also be exploited for this purpose. So-called 'plantibodies' have been expressed in bananas, potatoes and tobacco plants. Just imagine a high-tech farmer with one field growing anti-tetanus toxoid, another anti-meningo-coccal polysaccharide, and so on—the very stuff of science fiction!

Antibody in pooled normal serum can provide protection against infection

With common infections, it can be assumed that most normal people have antibody to the pathogen in their serum. The clearest proof of this is that patients with hypogamma-globulinemia can be kept free of recurrent infection by regular injections of IgG from pooled normal serum, and that immunodeficient children can be protected against measles in the same way *(Fig. 35.5)*. Immunoglobulin is prepared from batches of plasma from 1000–6000 healthy donors after screening for hepatitis B and C and HIV. With improvements in methods of preparation, intravenous injection is now preferred to intramuscular injection in most cases. Dosages for this type of therapy range from 100–400 mg IgG/kg/month.

In healthy individuals the probability of contracting hepatitis A in an endemic area is enormously reduced by a single injection of as little as 5 ml of IgG. The immunity conferred by mothers on their newborn infants by placental transfer of IgG and subsequently by colostral IgA (though the latter is not absorbed, but remains in the intestine) is further evidence for the protective effect of relatively small amounts of antibody.

INDICATIONS FOR NORMAL IMMUNOGLOBULIN THERAPY
X-linked agammaglobulinemia/hypogammaglobulinemia
common variable deficiency
Wiskott–Aldrich syndrome
ataxia telangiectasia
IgG subclass deficiency with impaired antibody response
chronic lymphocytic leukemia
post-bone marrow transplantation (for CMV pneumonitis)
?AIDS

Fig. 35.5 Indications for normal immunoglobulin therapy. Sufficient antibody to protect immunocompromised patients against common infections can be obtained from pooled normal human plasma. (CMV, cytomegalovirus; HBsAg, hepatitis B surface antigen.)

NON-SPECIFIC CELLULAR IMMUNOSTIMULATION

Cytokines and other molecular mediators stimulate the immune system

The demonstration by William Coley almost one century ago that crude extracts of bacteria could induce remission and sometimes cure cancers indicated the extent to which the immune system can be non-specifically 'overstimulated', with potentially beneficial results. Until recently, many of the compounds used in this way have been of microbial origin, but current interest is directed mainly at cytokines and other molecular mediators, on the principle that their induction was probably the basis of action of the older crude materials *(Fig. 35.6)*.

Most of the applications of this type of immuno-stimulation have been in the tumor field, but some infectious diseases respond to treatment with cytokines *(Fig. 35.7)*. Foremost among these are the interferons (IFNs), notably IFNα, which is effective in a number of virus infections, though less than might have been predicted from the importance of its normal role in inhibiting viral replication. IFNγ has recently been found to benefit many cases of chronic granulomatous disease (CGD), though the mechanism is unclear. The unpleasant side effects of high dose therapy with interleukins, IFNs or tumor necrosis factor alpha (TNFα) restricts their casual use *(Fig. 35.8)*.

There is an interesting 'gray area' where immunostimulation and nutrition overlap

It has been claimed for many years that transfer factor (TF), a dialysed extract of peripheral leukocytes from normal patients,

NON-SPECIFIC IMMUNOSTIMULATORS	
microbial	Coley's toxin (filtered cultures of *Stretococci* and *Serratia marcescens* used against tumors) BCG (bacillus Calmette-Guérin) *Corynebacterium parvum* endotoxin (lipopolysaccharide) streptococcal-derived OK432
endogenous	thymus factors and hormones cytokines ?transfer factor

Fig. 35.6 A variety of foreign and endogenous materials have been used in an attempt to raise the general level of immunologic competence.

POTENTIALLY THERAPEUTIC CYTOKINES	
IFNα, IFNβ	hepatitis B (chronic) hepatitis C herpes zoster papillomavirus rhinovirus (prophylactic only) ?HIV warts
IFNγ	lepromatous leprosy leishmaniasis toxoplasmosis (brain) chronic granulomatous disease
IL-2	leprosy (local treatment) to skin lesions)
TNF	anti-TNF in septic shock
IL-1	receptor antagonist in septic shock
IL-10, TGFβ	septic shock
CSFs	bacterial infection due to neutropenia in irradiated patients

Fig. 35.7 Cytokines are increasingly used to improve immunity to infection as well as for some cancers and hematologic disorders. (CSF, colony stimulating factor; IFN, interferon; IL, interleukin; TGF, transforming growth factor; TNF, tumor necrosis factor.)

will restore T cell responses in unresponsive recipients, and some dramatic cures (e.g. of chronic mucocutaneous candidiasis) have been reported. Whether this restoration is antigen specific or non-specific has been the subject of great controversy, and in the absence of proper molecular characterization, TF is no longer regarded as an orthodox treatment.

SOME COMMON SIDE EFFECTS OF CYTOKINE THERAPY	
interferons	fever
	malaise
	fatigue
	muscle pains
	toxicity to: kidney
	liver
	bone marrow
	heart
IL-2	vascular leak syndrome
	hypotension
	edema
	ascites
	pulmonary edema
	renal failure
	hepatic failure
	mental changes; coma
TNFα	shock (as IL-2, with hypotension
	particularly marked)

Fig. 35.8 Treatment with cytokines, especially if prolonged, can lead to serious side effects. (IL, interleukin; TNFα, tumor necrosis factor alpha.)

Equally unorthodox, but attracting increasing attention, are a variety of plant products (e.g. saponins, ginseng, Chinese herbal remedies). These substances appear to improve resistance to infection and in some cases also act as adjuvants when combined with vaccines.

CORRECTION OF HOST IMMUNODEFICIENCY

Antibody defects are the easiest to treat

This subject is discussed in more detail in Chapter 30, and will only be briefly summarized here:

- Antibody defects are the easiest to treat, since immunoglobulin can be transferred and has a reasonably long half-life (about 3 weeks for IgG).
- Treatment of T cell defects is much less successful, though thymus or bone marrow grafting has been tried in certain cases (*Fig. 35.9*).
- Phagocytic defects are the most difficult to correct, and in practice antibiotics remain the mainstay of therapy, though the future may lie in gene replacement.

Gene defects have recently been identified in certain serious immunodeficiency diseases including hyper-IgM syndrome, CGD and Bruton's agammaglobulinemia.

TREATMENT OF IMMUNODEFICIENCY: AN OVERVIEW				
	B cell defects	**T cell defects**	**phagocyte defects**	**complement defects**
correction of defect	bone marrow graft (SCID)	thymus graft (DiGeorge) ?thymus hormones	?bone marrow graft (CGD)	—
replacement therapy	pooled normal IgG specific IgG	blood transfusion (ADA, PNP deficiency) ?cytokines ??transfer factor	?cytokines	not successful
symptomatic therapy	antibodies	antivirals	antibiotics	antibiotics steroids (for immune complex disease)

Fig. 35.9 The treatment of immunodeficiency depends upon a knowledge of the element at fault, some being more easily restored than others. (ADA, adenosine deaminase; CGD, chronic granulomatous disease; PNP, purine nucleoside phosphorylase; SCID, severe combined immunodeficiency.)

KEY FACTS

- Transfer of normal pooled IgG is the most widely practiced type of passive immunotherapy and is used to treat most forms of antibody deficiency.

- Specific antibodies can be used for certain defined conditions. Such antibodies can be produced as mouse or human monoclonals, as rodent complementarity determining regions (CDRs) grafted onto a human Ig framework, or selected as Fab, single chain Fv (scFv) or heavy chain variable region domain fragments from expression libraries of bacteriophages bearing the antibody fragments as a surface protein.

- Antibodies can be engineered for expression in bulk in conventional vectors in vitro, or in vivo in the milk of lactating animals or in plants.

- Non-specific stimulation of T-cell-mediated immunity is still experimental, but cytokines show some promise, particularly IFN for viral infections.

QUESTIONS

1. Which of the following could be described as 'passive' immunization?*
   A. Transplacental passage of maternal IgG
   B. Injection of an immunogen
   C. Injection of convalescent human Ig
   D. Injection of a human monoclonal antibody
   E. Injection of a bacterial lipopolysaccharide

2. Injection of horse anti-tetanus toxoid serum gives:*
   A. Protection against diphtheria toxin
   B. Active immunization against tetanus toxin
   C. Short term neutralization of tetanus toxin
   D. Serum sickness hypersensitivity reactions in some cases

3. Specific antibodies can be engineered for expression*
   A. As scFvs on the surface of bacteriophage
   B. As Fc fragments on the surface of bacteriophage
   C. As V_H domains on the surface of bacteriophage
   D. In *E. coli* of Ig heavy and light chain genes lacking the signal sequence
   E. In agammaglobulinemic mice lacking B and T cells

4. Interferon α is:
   A. Potentially therapeutic in streptococcal infections
   B. Lethal for *Candida albicans*
   C. Potentially of value for the treatment of hepatitis B infection
   D. An inhibitor of extracellular viral proliferation.

*Question has more than one correct answer

FURTHER READING

Allison AC. Immunopotentiation. In: Brostoff J, Scadding GK, Male D, Roitt IM, eds. *Clinical Immunology.* London: Gower Medical Publishing, 1991.

Coley WB. The therapeutic value of the mixed toxins of erysipelas and *Bacillus prodigiosus* in the treatment of inoperable malignant tumours. *Am J Med Sci* 1986; 112:251.

Parker MT, Collier LH, eds. *Topley and Wilson's Principles of Bacteriology, Virology and Immunity,* 9th edition, vol. 1. London: Edward Arnold, 1997.

INTRODUCTION

A nosocomial infection is any infection acquired while in hospital

Amassing a large number of sick people together under one roof has many advantages, but some disadvantages, notably the easier transmission of infection from one person to another. Hospital infection—also known as nosocomial infection—is defined as any infection acquired while in hospital (e.g. occurring 48 hours or more after admission and up to 48 hours after discharge). Most of these infections become obvious while the patient is in hospital, but some (as many as 50% of postoperative wound infections) are not recognized until after the patient has been discharged. Earlier discharges, encouraged to reduce costs, contribute to these unrecognized infections, although a shorter preoperative stay reduces the chance of acquiring hospital pathogens (see below).

Hospital infection may be acquired from:

- an exogenous source (e.g. from another patient—cross-infection—or from the environment);
- an endogenous source (i.e. another site within the patient—self- or auto-infection) *(Fig. 36.1)*.

An infection that is incubating in a patient when they are admitted into hospital is not a hospital infection. However, community-acquired infections brought into hospital by the patient may subsequently become hospital infections for other patients and hospital staff.

Many hospital infections are preventable

In 1850, Semmelweiss demonstrated that many hospital infections are preventable when he made the unpopular suggestion that puerperal fever (an infection in women who have just given birth, see Chapter 23) was carried on the hands of physicians who came directly from attending an autopsy to the delivery ward, without washing. A death rate of 8.3% was reduced to 2.3% by introducing the simple measure of handwashing before and after any clinical examination. Extensive studies in the USA in the 1970s showed that about

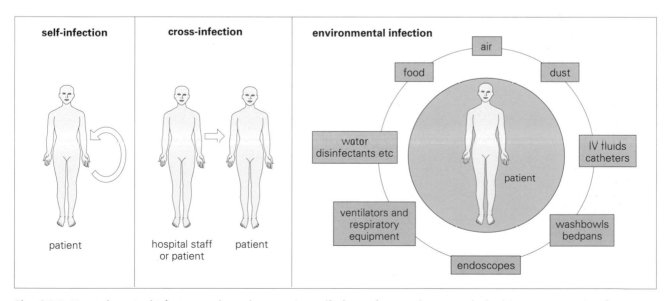

Fig. 36.1 Hospital-acquired infection can be endogenous (i.e. self-infection from another site in the body) or exogenous (i.e. from another person or from an environmental source). The sorts of organisms acquired from environmental sources depend upon the nature of the source, for example moist areas tend to be colonized with Gram-negative rods (e.g. *Escherichia coli, Klebsiella, Pseudomonas*) whereas air and dustborne organisms are those that can withstand drying (e.g. streptococci, staphylococci, mycobacteria and *Acinetobacter*). (IV, intravenous.)

35% of all infections acquired in hospital could be prevented. More recent US estimates place current costs arising from hospital infection at around 4.5 billion dollars/year, potentially contributing to 88 000 annual deaths.

COMMON HOSPITAL-ACQUIRED INFECTIONS

Urinary tract infections are the most common hospital-acquired infections

The infections most commonly acquired in hospitals are:

- surgical wound infection;
- respiratory tract infection;
- urinary tract infection (UTI);
- bacteremia.

The relative frequencies of these infections are illustrated in *Figure 36.2*. Each may be acquired from an exogenous or endogenous source, and even the 'self-source' may be derived from outside by the patient who becomes colonized with pathogens during his or her stay in hospital. Bacteremia may arise from a variety of sources and may be:

- primary—due to the direct introduction of organisms into the blood from, for example, contaminated intravenous fluids;
- secondary to a focus of infection already present in the body (e.g. UTI).

Other infections that may cause outbreaks in the hospital setting include gastroenteritis and hepatitis.

IMPORTANT CAUSES OF HOSPITAL INFECTION

Staphylococci and Escherichia coli *are the most common causes of hospital-acquired infection*

Almost any microbe can cause a hospital-acquired infection, though protozoal infections are rare. The pattern of hospital infection has changed over the years, reflecting advances in medicine and the development of antimicrobial agents. In the pre-antibiotic era the majority of infections were caused by Gram-positive organisms, particularly *Streptococcus pyogenes* and *Staphylococcus aureus*. With the advent of penicillin and other antibiotics active against staphylococci, Gram-negative organisms such as *Escherichia coli* and *Pseudomonas aeruginosa* emerged as important pathogens. More recently, the development of more potent and broad spectrum antimicrobials and the increase in invasive medical techniques has been accompanied by an increase in the incidence of:

- antibiotic-resistant Gram-positive organisms such as coagulase-negative staphylococci, enterococci and methicillin-resistant *Staph. aureus* (MRSA);
- multidrug-resistant Gram-negative organisms including those producing expanded spectrum beta-lactamases (ESBLs, see Chapter 33)
- *Candida*.

Many of these organisms are considered as 'opportunists'—microbes that are unable to cause disease in healthy people with intact defense mechanisms, but can cause infection in compromised patients or when introduced during the course of invasive procedures. Currently *E. coli* accounts overall for more hospital infections than any other single species, but staphylococci are a close second *(Fig. 36.3)*.

Viral infections probably account for more hospital-acquired infections than previously realized

These affect both patients and healthcare workers and include:

urinary tract infections
E. coli (other Gram-negatives to a lesser extent)
enterococci
staphylococci
Candida
surgical wound infections
staphylococci (*Staph. aureus* and coagulase-negative)
enterococci
E. coli, P. aeruginosa (other Gram-negatives to a lesser extent)
lower respiratory tract infections
P. aeruginosa (other Gram-negatives to a lesser extent)
Staph. aureus
bacteremia
staphylococci (*Staph. aureus* and coagulase-negative)
enterococci
Candida
E. coli (other Gram-negatives to a lesser extent)

Fig. 36.3 The general rank order of pathogen importance is listed for the different infection categories. Although a few species are the most important in all kinds of hospital infection, predominant pathogens vary in different infections. *Staphylococcus aureus* is very important in surgical wound infections and bacteremia, but much less important in urinary tract infections. The importance of Gram-negative rods has increased since the advent of broad spectrum antibiotics because these organisms often carry multiple antibiotic resistances.

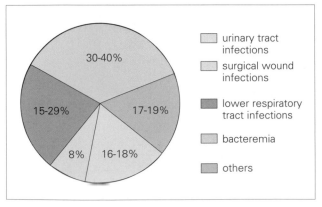

Fig. 36.2 The relative frequencies of different kinds of hospital infection vary in different patient groups, but urinary tract infections are the most common hospital-acquired infections.

- viruses acquired by the respiratory route, especially influenza, respiratory syncytial virus (RSV), parainfluenza, varicella-zoster virus (VZV); this may also include some of the viral causes of gastroenteritis;
- viruses acquired by contact with vesicular lesions such as VZV and herpes simplex virus (HSV);
- viruses acquired by contact with contaminated fomites such as noroviruses (previously referred to as Norwalk-like virus, NLV; small round structured virus, SRSV) and rotavirus;
- viruses acquired by contact with blood-contaminated fomites, needlestick injury or splash on mucous mem-

branes, such as hepatitis B virus (HBV), hepatitis C virus (HCV), HIV and human T cell lymphotropic virus (HTLV). These may also be acquired in countries where blood and blood products are not screened or in the rare instance where the blood donor was in the early incubation period of infection, thereby escaping detection by the screening assay. The latter is referred to as the window period and may be missed even if a viral genome detection method is used.

The risks of viral infections in hospital are summarized in *Figure 36.4*.

VIRUSES AS CAUSES OF HOSPITAL-ACQUIRED INFECTION			
virus	transmissibility	susceptibility of other patients and staff	resultant risk of hospital infection
influenza	++	+/−*	++
respiratory syncytial virus	++	++*	++
parainfluenza adenovirus rhinovirus	+	+*	+
varicella-zoster	++	−*	−
varicella-zoster (localized)	+	− −	− −
cytomegalovirus	−	+	− −†
rubella	++	+**	++
measles	++	− −	− −
exotic viruses (Lassa, Marburg, Ebola, rabies)	− −	++	− −
rotavirus	++	+	+
enteroviruses	+	+	+
hepatitis A	+	+	+
hepatitis B	++††	++	++
HIV (in countries where not screened)	++‡	++	++
hepatitis C	+††	++	++

*high in pediatric age group
**decreased since immunization program initiated
†except for blood transfusion and organ transplantation
††from needle-stick injuries and other exposure incidents
‡from blood or blood product

Fig. 36.4 Viruses are probably more important causes of hospital infection than generally recognized. The risk of hospital infection is a sum of the transmissibility of the virus and the susceptibility of the patient group. Some viruses, such as varicella-zoster, are of low risk in general, but very important in pediatric units and particularly in immunocompromised children.

SOURCES AND ROUTES OF SPREAD OF HOSPITAL INFECTION

Sources of hospital infection are people and contaminated objects

As stated above, the source of infection may be:

- human—from other patients or hospital staff, and occasionally visitors;
- environmental, from contaminated objects ('fomites'), food, water or air (see *Fig. 36.1*).

The source may become contaminated from an environmental reservoir of organisms, for example contaminated antiseptic solution distributed for use into sterile containers (*Fig. 36.5*). Eradication of the source will also require eradication of the reservoir.

Human sources may be:

- people who are themselves infected;
- people who are incubating an infection;
- healthy carriers.

The time period for which a human source is infectious varies with the disease (see Chapter 31). For example, some infections can be spread during their incubation period, others in the early stages of clinical disease, while others are characterized by a prolonged carrier state even after clinical cure (e.g. typhoid fever) (*Fig. 36.6*). Carriers of virulent strains of, for example, *Staph. aureus* or *Strep. pyogenes* may act as sources of hospital infection, although they themselves do not develop clinical disease. The carrier state may persist for a long time and go unnoticed unless there is an outbreak or, depending on the significance of the organism, a single case of infection that is traced to the carrier—e.g. a healthcare worker with chronic hepatitis B.

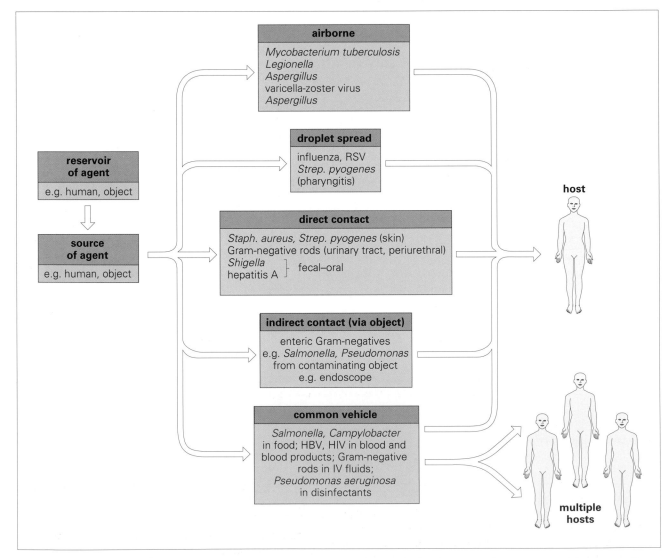

Fig. 36.5 Hospital infections are spread by the same routes as infections spread in the community. The reservoir and the source of infection may be human or inanimate and may be one and the same (e.g. a nurse with an infected skin lesion). If the reservoir and source are distinct (e.g. contaminated distilled water supply used to prepare a variety of pharmaceuticals), both must be eliminated if the spread of infection is to be halted, otherwise the reservoir may continue to contaminate new sources. (HBV, hepatitis B virus; IV, intravenous; RSV, respiratory syncytial virus.)

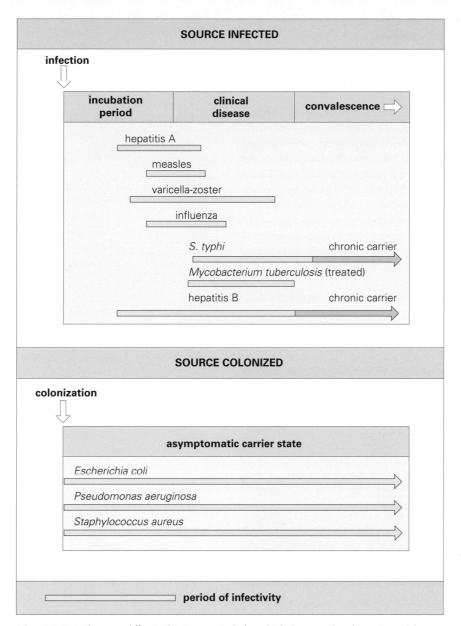

Fig. 36.6 Pathogens differ in the time periods for which they can be disseminated from an infected person. For some it is during the incubation period when infected people may not realize they are ill and infectious. Some people continue to carry organisms such as *Salmonella typhi* and hepatitis B virus long after they have recovered from the clinical disease. Opportunist pathogens are often members of the normal flora and may therefore be carried for long periods without the host experiencing any adverse effects.

Hospital infections are spread in the air and by contact and common vehicle

The important routes of spread of infection in hospitals are those common to all infections: airborne, contact and common vehicle. Examples of organisms spread by these routes in hospitals are illustrated in *Figure 36.5*. Although theoretically possible, vector-borne spread is very unusual in the hospital setting, as is sexually transmitted infection. It is important to remember that the same organism may be spread by more than one route. For example, *Strep. pyogenes* can be spread from patient to patient by the airborne route in droplets or dust, but is also transmitted by contact with infected lesions, for example on a nurse's hand. In addition, a

patient or healthcare worker with chickenpox can transmit VZV by the airborne route or by a susceptible person having direct contact with the vesicular lesions.

HOST FACTORS AND HOSPITAL INFECTION

Underlying disease, certain treatments and invasive procedures reduce host defenses

Host factors play a fundamental role in the infection equation, particularly in hospitals because of the high proportion of hospital patients with compromised natural defenses against infection. The spread of an infectious agent to a new host can result in a spectrum of responses: from colonization, through subclinical infection, to clinically apparent disease, which may be fatal. The degree of host response differs in different people depending upon their degree of compromise. The very young are particularly susceptible because of the immaturity of their immune system. Likewise, the elderly suffer a greater risk of infection because of predisposing underlying disease, impaired blood supply and immobility, which contribute to stasis and therefore to infection in, for example, the lungs. In all age groups, underlying disease and the treatment of that disease (e.g. cytotoxic drugs, steroids) may predispose to infection (*Fig. 36.7*), while invasive procedures allow organisms easier access to previously protected tissues (*Fig. 36.8*). The important host factors to be considered in hospital infection are summarized in *Figure 36.9*. Infections in the compromised host are discussed in more detail in Chapter 30.

A variety of factors predispose to wound infection

Wound infection or wound sepsis is characterized by the presence of inflammation, pus and discharge in addition to

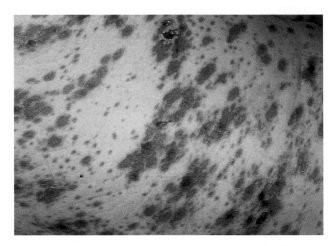

Fig. 36.7 Varicella in a patient with chronic myeloid leukemia resulting in purpuric confluent lesions on the trunk. (Courtesy of GDW McKendrick.)

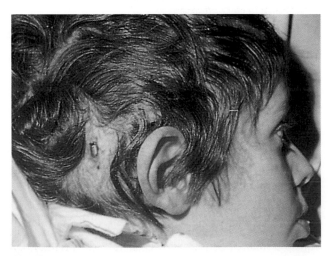

Fig. 36.8 Child with infected Spitz–Holter valve used to relieve hydrocephalus. (Courtesy of JA Innes.)

FACTORS WHICH PREDISPOSE PATIENTS TO HOSPITAL INFECTION		
age	patients at extremes of age are particularly susceptible	
specific immunity	patient may lack protective antibodies to e.g. measles, chickenpox, whooping cough	
underlying disease	other (non-infectious) diseases tend to lead to enhanced susceptibility to infection, e.g. hepatic disease, diabetes, cancer, skin disorders, renal failure, neutropenia (either as a result of disease or of treatment)	
other infections	HIV and other immunosuppressing virus infections; patients with influenza prone to secondary bacterial pneumonia; herpes virus lesions may become secondarily infected with staphylococci	
specific medicaments	cytotoxic drugs (including post-transplant immunosuppression) and steroids both lower host defenses; antibiotics disturb normal flora and predispose to invasion by resistant hospital pathogens	
trauma accidental	burns, stab or gunshot wounds, road traffic accidents	disturb natural host
intentional	surgery, intravenous and urinary catheters, peritoneal dialysis	defense mechanisms

Fig. 36.9 Hospital patients are not all at equal risk of infection. Some factors that predispose to infection can be influenced by, for example, treating underlying disease, improving specific immunity and avoiding inappropriate use of antibiotics. Other factors such as age are unalterable.

the isolation of organisms such as *Staph. aureus*. Extensive studies of postoperative wound infection have identified a number of predisposing factors:

- Prolonged preoperative stay increases the opportunity for the patient to become colonized with antibiotic-resistant hospital pathogens.
- The nature and length of the operation also have an effect (*Figs 36.10, 36.11*; see also Chapter 26).
- Wet or open wounds are more liable to secondary infection.

From these studies it has been possible to identify the patients and operations with greatest risk and apply preventive measures such as prophylactic antibiotic regimens and ultra-clean air in orthopedic operating theaters (see below).

RISK FACTORS FOR POSTOPERATIVE INFECTIONS	
length of preoperative stay	longer stay – more likely to become colonized with virulent and antibiotic-resistant hospital bacteria and fungi
presence of intercurrent infection	operating on an already infected site more likely to cause disseminated infection
length of operation	longer – greater risk of tissues becoming seeded with organisms from air, staff, other sites in patient
nature of operation	any operation which results in fecal soiling of tissues has higher risk of infection (e.g. postoperative gangrene), 'adventurous' surgery tends to carry greater risks
presence of foreign bodies	e.g. shunts, prostheses, impairs host defenses
state of tissues	poor blood supply encourages growth of anaerobes; inadequate drainage or presence of necrotic tissue predisposes to infection

Fig. 36.10 The risks of infection after surgery have been studied in considerable detail, and surgeons are consequently much more aware of the problems. However, 'high-tech' surgery is often long and difficult and predisposes the patient to postoperative infection.

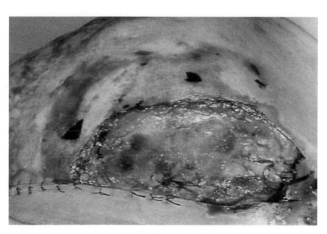

Fig. 36.11 Postoperative gangrenous cellulitis. There is a huge area of ulceration filled with gangrenous skin, with sloughing adjacent to the wound and surrounding cellulitis. (Courtesy of MJ Wood.)

CONSEQUENCES OF HOSPITAL INFECTION

Hospital infections affect both the patient and the community

Hospital infection may result in:

- serious illness or death;
- prolonged hospital stay, which costs money and results in a loss of earnings and hardship for the patient and their family;
- a need for additional antimicrobial therapy, which is costly, exposes the patient to additional risks of toxicity, and increases selective pressure for resistance to emerge among hospital pathogens;
- the infected patient becoming a source from which others may become infected, in hospital and in the community.

PREVENTION OF HOSPITAL INFECTION

There are three main strategies for preventing hospital infection

For the reasons outlined above, the prevention of hospital infection deserves a very high priority, and the three main strategies are:

- excluding sources of infection from the hospital environment;
- interrupting the transmission of infection from source to susceptible host (breaking the chain of infection);
- enhancing the host's ability to resist infection.

Exclusion of sources of infection

Exclusion of inanimate sources of infection is achievable, but it can be difficult to avoid contamination by humans

Exclusion of inanimate sources of infection is both desirable and to a large extent achievable. For example the provision of sterile instruments and dressings, sterile medicaments and intravenous fluids, clean linen and uncontaminated food, and the use of blood and blood products screened for infectious agents. However, many of the sources of infection are human or are objects that become contaminated by humans, in which case exclusion is more difficult. Hospitals must attempt to prevent patient contact with staff who are carriers of pathogens. The problem is the identification of staff who are carriers of pathogens and their relocation to less hazardous positions.

Staff must undergo health screening before employment and should have regular health checks (see *Fig. 36.12*). For example, students training to be healthcare workers in the UK are offered hepatitis B immunization and must know their post-immunization status before carrying out exposure prone

INFECTIOUS DISEASES WHERE STAFF CONTACT WITH PATIENTS SHOULD BE AVOIDED
diarrhea
hepatitis A
herpes simplex on hands (herpetic whitlow)
Streptococcus pyogenes infections
Staphylococcus aureus skin lesions
measles
mumps
whooping cough
rubella
varicella-zoster infections
upper respiratory tract infections (high-risk patients)

Fig. 36.12 Recommended work restrictions for staff with infectious diseases. In the event of a member of staff becoming infected either in the hospital or outside, he or she should be relieved from direct contact with patients. Kitchen staff should also be relieved from duty if they are suffering from diarrhea or hepatitis A, or have infected lesions on their hands.

procedures (EPPs). It is critical that those carrying out EPPs who either do not know their post-immunization status or have not responded to the hepatitis B vaccine are checked to ensure that they do not have a current HBV infection or have a protective level of hepatitis B surface antibody. This is because HBV could be transmitted to the patients if the healthcare worker carrying out EPPs is a hepatitis B carrier and also because the unprotected healthcare worker is at risk of infection from a hepatitis B carrier patient. Hospitals have bloodborne virus exposure policies for the management of healthcare workers and others exposed to viruses, including HBV, HCV, and HIV. Prophylaxis includes active and/or passive immunization against hepatitis B and a short course of antiretroviral therapy for HIV exposure.

In general, staff should be encouraged to report any incidences of infection (e.g. an infected cut or a bout of diarrhea). Appropriate immunizations should be offered and in some instances made mandatory. Work restrictions for personnel with selected infectious diseases are summarized in *Figure 36.12*. However, healthy carriers of, for example, virulent staphylococci are difficult to identify unless bacteriologic screening is undertaken, which is not feasible on a routine basis. In addition, staff are sources of opportunist organisms such as coagulase-negative staphylococci or enterobacteria, which are part of their normal flora and cannot be excluded.

Breaking the chain of infection

There are two elements to be considered in breaking the chain of infection: the structural and the human. The structure of the hospital and its equipment can play a role in preventing airborne spread of infection and in facilitating aseptic practices by the staff, but this is of no avail if staff do not use the facilities correctly and do not themselves act positively to prevent the spread of infection.

Control of airborne transmission of infection

Ventilation systems and air flow can play an important role in the dissemination of organisms by the airborne route

Wards comprising separate rooms have been shown to afford some protection against airborne spread, and rooms with controlled ventilation are even better. However, neither prevents the carriage of organisms into the room on staff and their clothing, and some studies suggest that this is a more important route of infection than airborne spread. There is no doubt, however, that *Legionella* infection is acquired by the airborne route, and air-conditioning systems throughout the hospital should be maintained so as to prevent the multiplication of these organisms (see Chapter 19). Hospital-acquired *Aspergillus* infection has been attributed to dissemination of the spores in hospital air, especially when building work is ongoing in the locality.

Ventilation systems in operating theaters must be properly installed and maintained to prevent the ingress of contaminated air and to minimize air currents carrying organisms from the staff in the operating room to the operation site. 'Ultra-clean' air is air passed through high efficiency filters to remove bacteria and other particles and has been shown to contribute positively to a reduction in the number of postoperative wound infections developing after long orthopedic operations.

Airborne transmission of infection can be reduced significantly by isolating patients

Patient isolation may be carried out:

- to protect a particularly susceptible patient from exposure to pathogens (i.e. protective isolation);
- to prevent the spread of pathogens from an infected patient to others on the ward (i.e. source isolation).

Isolation also helps to prevent the transmission of infection by other routes by limiting access to the patient and reminding staff of the importance of contact in the spread of infection.

Protective isolation can be provided by a single room on a ward or by enclosing the patient in a plastic isolator. With appropriate positive pressure ventilation, air should flow from the 'clean' patient area out of the room or isolator. Staff entering the room or in contact with the patient should wear sterile gowns, gloves and masks to prevent organisms they are carrying or have picked up from other patients from coming in contact with the patient.

Source isolation is ideally arranged by accommodation in an isolation unit in a separate building, hence the tuberculosis sanatoria of the past. In general, hospital isolation is more often arranged in a separate ward or in side rooms off the main ward. To prevent airborne transmission of organisms from the patient's room to the ward, air should flow from the ward to the isolation room. In practice it is difficult to maintain the correct air flows without sophisticated designs, including double doors and air locks.

Facilitation of aseptic behavior

A general state of cleanliness throughout the hospital is essential, and the design of hospital facilities affects the ease

CONTACT SPREAD OF OPPORTUNIST PATHOGENS		
patient	nursing activity	number of klebsiellae recovered per hand*
A	physiotherapy	10–100
	taking blood pressure and pulse	100–1000
	washing patient	10–100
	taking oral temperature	100–1000
B	taking radial pulse	100–1000
	touching shoulder	1000
	touching groin	100–1000
C	touching hand	10–100
D	extubation	100–1000
	touching tracheostomy	1000

*control handwashings taken prior to procedure yielded no klebsiellae

Fig. 36.13 Nursing procedures involving skin contact resulting in contamination of staff hands. These data are derived from experiments performed during an outbreak of *Klebsiella* infection among urology patients. (Data from Casewell MW, Phillips I, *Br Med J* 1977; 2:1315.)

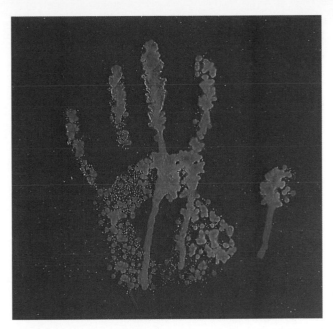

Fig. 36.14 Gram-negative rods are not usually part of the resident skin flora except in moist environments, but are readily carried on hands and can be transferred from a source to a susceptible patient. This picture shows an impression of a hand that was inoculated with approximately 1000 *Klebsiella aerogenes*.

with which the environment can be kept clean and the staff can practice good techniques.

Bacteriologically effective handwashing is one of the most important ways of controlling hospital infection

The hands of staff convey organisms to patients from septic lesions and healthy carrier sites of other patients, from equipment contaminated by these sources and from carrier sites of the staff themselves (*Figs 36.13, 36.14*).

Staff should therefore wash their hands:

- before any procedure for which gloves or forceps are necessary;
- after contact with an infected patient or one who is colonized with multiply-resistant bacteria;
- after touching infective material.

While soap and water are adequate in many circumstances, emphasis is shifting to the use of fast-drying alcohol-based gels and solutions which are easier to use and appear to have a more antibacterial result. A recent mandate from the United States Centers for Disease Control, for example, has put this approach into practice in US hospitals. Drying hands after any washing procedure is important. A more prolonged and thorough hand decontamination is required before commencing surgery.

The design of taps, soap dispensers and other washing facilities, including bedpan washers, has reached a high degree of sophistication. However, human behavior can be influenced by architectural design only to a limited degree, and there is often a disappointingly low compliance with the simple technique of handwashing. Therefore training and regular reinforcement in appropriate behavior is essential.

Enhancing the host's ability to resist infection

Host resistance can be enhanced by boosting immunity and reducing risk factors

Although attempts can and should be made to control and prevent hospital infection by removing sources of infection and preventing transmission from sources to susceptible hosts, neither of these strategies is failsafe. In addition, they do not protect the host from endogenous infection. A way of tipping the balance in favor of the host is to enhance his or her ability to resist infection, both by boosting specific immunity and by reducing personal risk factors. The following aspects should be considered:

- boosting specific immunity by active or passive immunization;
- the appropriate use of prophylactic antibiotics;
- care of invasive devices that breach the natural defenses (e.g. urinary catheters, intravenous lines);
- attention to the risks predisposing to postoperative infection.

Boosting specific immunity

Passive immunization provides short-term protection

Boosting specific immunity by immunization has been discussed in Chapters 34 and 35. The problem for the immunocompromised patient is that they may not be able to mount an antibody response. Passive immunization can afford short-term protection, for example with chickenpox

BOOSTING SPECIFIC IMMUNITY OF PATIENTS		
patient group	immunization	
	active	passive
elderly (especially those with multisystem disease)	influenza vaccine	–
pre-splenectomy pre-renal or bone marrow transplant	pneumococcal vaccine	–
hemodialysis patients	pneumococcal vaccine	–
infants born to HBsAg positive mothers	hepatitis B vaccine	hepatitis B immuno-globulin (especially if mother HBeAg positive)
immunocompromised: exposed to varicella-zoster virus (VZV)	live attenuated VZV vaccine in trials	zoster immune globulin as soon as possible after exposure (and within 7 days)
exposed to measles	–	normal human immune globulin within 5 days

Fig. 36.15 Many patients will have been protected against some infections by routine immunization during childhood, but sometimes it is helpful to boost specific immunity by immunization of patients at particular risk of infection.

exposure in susceptible patients who are neutropenic as a result of cytotoxic therapy and whose white cell count should recover after successful treatment. With the advent of efficacious hepatitis B vaccines, active immunization is recommended for all susceptible patients attending dialysis units. Other immunizations to protect hospital patients are summarized in *Figure 36.15*.

Appropriate use of prophylactic antibiotics

There are well-documented uses for prophylaxis, but antibiotics tend to be misused

This is discussed in Chapter 33. There are several well-documented uses for prophylactic antibiotics in 'dirty' surgery

and when the consequences of infection would be disastrous (e.g. in cardiac, neuro- and transplant surgery). However, there is a tendency to misuse antibiotics:

• first, by using them too often or for too long, thereby increasing the selection pressure for the emergence of resistant organisms;
• second, by choosing inappropriate agents.

Treatment (as opposed to prophylaxis) of patients and staff who are carriers of pathogens such as *Staph. aureus* or *Strep. pyogenes* has been used successfully to prevent endogenous infection and to control outbreaks of infection with these organisms. Topical preparations of antibiotics such as bacitracin, neomycin and fucidin have been used, but there is no doubt that the emergence of resistance is a problem. Pseudomonic acid (mupirocin), a fermentation product of *Pseudomonas fluorescens*, has been shown to be efficacious. It is unrelated to other classes of antibiotics in clinical use, diminishing concerns over the emergence of resistant strains with cross-resistance to other agents. Mupirocin is very active against Gram-positive cocci. In recent years it has played an important role in eradicating carriage of MRSA, but resistance (both low and high level) to the drug has occurred.

Gut decontamination regimens and selective bowel contamination aim to reduce the reservoir of potential pathogens in the gut

Gut decontamination regimens to reduce the aerobic Gram-negative flora of neutropenic patients has been practiced for some time. With some patients (e.g. liver transplant) in intensive care units (ICU) selective bowel decontamination (SBD) has been employed. The aim is to reduce the reservoir of potential pathogens in the gut by oral administration (or via a nasogastric tube) of a high concentration of a mixture of antibiotics. At the present time there is still controversy about the efficacy and safety of SBD.

Care of invasive devices

Care of invasive devices is essential to reduce the risk of endogenous infection

It is essential to take care of intravascular devices to reduce the risk of endogenous infection from skin organisms, and of catheters to reduce the risk that the periurethral flora will cause endogenous infection of the bladder in catheterized patients. Guidelines for the care of urinary catheters are discussed in Chapter 20.

The majority of hospital-acquired bacteremias and candidemias are infusion-related

These infusion-related bacteremias and candidemias derive mainly from vascular catheters. Most bacteremias associated with invasive devices are caused by the patient's own skin flora, although this may be a more resistant flora acquired during the patient's stay in hospital replacing the 'community-acquired' flora. Coagulase-negative staphylococci are the most common etiologic agents, but *Staph. aureus*, various Gram-negative rods, and *Candida* are also implicated. These infections are largely preventable if appropriate steps

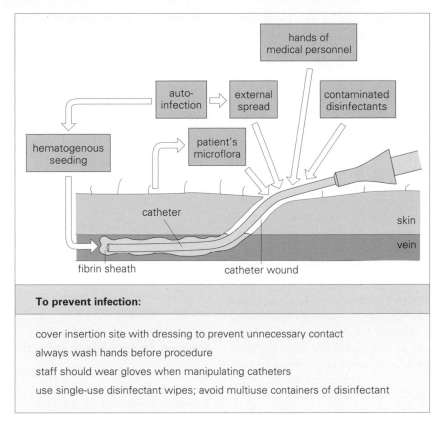

Fig. 36.16 Sources of intravascular device-related infection and opportunities for the prevention of infection.

are taken. The sources of infection and measures for prevention are shown in *Figure 36.16*.

Reducing the risks of postoperative infection

Prevention of postoperative infection involves minimizing the risks

Reducing the risks of postoperative infection involves an understanding of the risks and the ways in which they can be circumvented. For example:

- The preoperative length of stay in hospital should be kept to a minimum.
- Intercurrent infections should be treated appropriately before surgery whenever possible (e.g. treatment of UTI before resection of the prostate)
- Operations should be kept to the minimum duration consistent with good operating technique.
- Adequate debridement of dead and necrotic tissue is essential, together with adequate drainage and maintenance or re-establishment of a good blood supply to provide the body's natural defenses with optimum working conditions.
- Prevention of pressure sores and stasis by good nursing techniques and active physiotherapy minimizes the risks of developing respiratory tract infection or UTI.

INVESTIGATING HOSPITAL INFECTION

Many of the epidemiologic principles outlined in Chapter 31 apply to the investigation of hospital infection. Outbreaks within hospitals are *epidemics*—they are detected because the incidence of an infection is seen to be above normal levels for that institution. Investigation therefore must determine the extent of the problem, identify the source of infection and the way in which it is spread, identify those at risk, and propose effective methods for control. As with infectious diseases in general the application of statistical techniques (e.g. calculation of risk ratios) and mathematical modeling has helped to provide an analytical and predictive framework for such infections, but day-to-day investigations still require the application of proven microbiologic approaches.

Hospital-acquired infections, like community infections, can involve all the major groups of pathogens, from prions to arthropods. However, a particular problem with hospital infections, compared with those occurring in the community, is the transmission of antibiotic-resistant bacteria, the emergence of which, and their spread, is favored by the hospital environment. Epidemiologic investigations of these infections place great importance on typing to identify the causative organism. Such *molecular* epidemiology can make a very important contribution to tracking and controlling infection.

In many hospitals the responsibility for investigating hospital infection falls on the infection control committee, which includes an infection control officer (who may be a physician or microbiologist) and at least one nurse. The roles of the infection control committee include:

- the surveillance of hospital infection;
- the establishment and monitoring of policies and procedures designed to prevent infection (e.g. catheter care

policy, antibiotic policy, disinfectant policy, bloodborne virus exposure incidents, including needlesticks and blood splashes);
- the investigation of outbreaks—tracking the source and routes of transmission.

Surveillance

Surveillance allows early recognition of any change in the number or type of hospital infections

Although hospital infection has been recognized for many years, accurate records were not initiated until the late 1950s. Since then national and international surveys have highlighted the prevalence and importance of hospital infection. By maintaining local surveillance, the infection control team can establish the normal trends in their hospital and therefore recognize any change in the number or type of infections early. Sources of surveillance data are:

- Microbiology laboratory reports. These can be used for general surveillance, for example monitoring hemodialysis patients regularly for hepatitis B surface antigen and HCV antibody, as outbreaks of HBV and HCV infection have been reported in renal units around the world, or for monitoring 'sentinel' or 'alert' organisms such as *Staph. aureus*, *Strep. pyogenes*, *M. tuberculosis*, salmonellae and shigellae.
- Ward rounds. New cases of infection can be identified by direct inspection, and previously identified cases of infection can be followed up. Surveys can also be carried out on the wards (e.g. of wound infections after different practices or procedures).
- Other sources include autopsy reports, staff health records and surveys of patients after discharge from hospital.

Investigation of outbreaks

When an outbreak (or epidemic) occurs or when routine surveillance highlights an increase in the incidence of infection, the infection control team should initiate an investigation. There is no universally applicable routine for finding the cause of an outbreak, but in principle each investigation has an epidemiologic element and a microbiologic element.

There must be a description of an outbreak in epidemiologic terms

This involves obtaining information about a number of relevant factors:

- How many people are infected?
- When were they admitted?
- When did they develop their infection?
- Are they all on the same ward?
- Are they all treated by the same medical or surgical team?
- Have they all been exposed to the same treatments?

The causative organism needs to be isolated and/or detected in all patients in the outbreak

It is the role of the microbiology laboratory to attempt to isolate the causative organism and to show that it occurs in all patients in the outbreak (i.e. they are all infected with organisms that are indistinguishable—see below). The identity of the infecting organism can provide clues as to the possible source:

- Respiratory and intestinal viruses implicate the source of infection as a patient or attending medical staff.
- Hepatitis indicates spread via contaminated blood products or hypodermics.
- An outbreak of wound infection with *Staph. aureus* is likely to be associated with contact spread from staff in theater or on the ward.
- An outbreak of *Salmonella* gastroenteritis is more likely to originate in the kitchen.
- Infections with *Legionella* or *Pseudomonas* are likely to reflect environmental (especially water) contamination.

In addition, the location of the outbreak, whether in a general ward, a surgical ward, a pediatric unit or intensive care unit (once described as the epicenter of hospital infections) may also provide valuable clues.

Stages in tracking infection

Once the problem has been identified clinically, appropriate specimens should be collected from the patients and, if the indicators are that medical staff are involved, from hospital personnel (see Chapter 32). Likely sources of environmental contamination (surfaces, materials, equipment, water) should also be sampled. This is an important step, as data (using a non-infectious DNA marker as an experimental infectious organism) have shown that after release there is a rapid spread from hands of medical staff to almost all available surfaces (computers, charts, telephones, control knobs, door handles, heater controls, patient monitors). Once samples have been collected the microbiology laboratory then has the task of identifying and typing the organisms concerned.

While the investigation is proceeding, steps should be taken to contain the outbreak and prevent spread to other patients. Infected patients must be isolated and treated appropriately. Staff who show a similar infection, or who are subsequently found to be carriers, must be suspended from duty until they have been treated. At the end of the investigation the relevant procedures must be reviewed to try and prevent the reoccurrence of a similar outbreak.

Epidemiologic typing techniques

Bacteria are the commonest causes of nosocomial infections and of the greatest concern because of the prevalence of antibiotic resistance. For example, a 1999 survey of isolates from intensive care units in the USA showed 52% methicillin-resistant *Staph. aureus* and 25% vancomycin-resistant entero-cocci. Comparable UK data from 1998 were 34% and 24%, respectively, having risen from 3.8% for *Staph. aureus* and 6.3% for *E. faecium* in 1993. Coliform bacteria are the commonest hospital-acquired infection (about a third), *E. coli* being the most common of these. Tracking infection is therefore disproportionately concerned with this group of pathogens, although many of the molecular techniques used are also applied to the identification of virus infections.

A variety of phenotypic and genotypic characters are used to 'fingerprint' bacteria for epidemiologic purposes

In epidemiologic studies of the spread of hospital infections, as in the investigation of outbreaks in the community, it is necessary to identify isolates of the infectious organisms to determine whether or not they are distinct (it may not be possible to say that two organisms are the same, only that they are indistinguishable). In the case of bacteria, if the species is a regular member of the normal human flora or is found frequently in the environment, it is necessary to distinguish the 'outbreak' strain from other strains of the same species not involved in the outbreak, but that may also be isolated during the course of the investigation. Essentially, typing is used to look for evidence of a clonal spread of a particular pathogen.

To be valuable in this context, good typing techniques must:

- be discriminatory (i.e. able to show differences between strains of the same species);
- be reproducible (i.e. the same strain gives the same result when tested on different occasions and in different places);
- have a high degree of typability (i.e. capable of assigning a type to all strains).

Antibiotic susceptibility patterns and simple biotyping can be carried out in most routine diagnostic laboratories, whereas the specialized typing techniques are more commonly performed in reference laboratories. This has the advantage that quality assurance can be optimized, but also means that there is an inevitable delay in reporting the results and therefore in learning whether an outbreak of hospital infection is caused by a single strain.

Antibiotic susceptibility patterns and simple biotyping

These tests are performed readily in the diagnostic laboratory (see Chapter 32) and are useful as a preliminary clue as to whether two isolates are indistinguishable. However, discrimination is poor: many susceptibility patterns are common, and quite different strains may have the same pattern. Conversely, during an outbreak, strains may gain or lose plasmids carrying antibiotic resistance markers.

Biotyping involves typing organisms by their ability to grow on different substrates or produce different onzymoo

Ideally the biochemical test employed in a biotyping scheme should differ from those used to identify the organisms. Identification tests are chosen because they 'lump' similar organisms together; biotyping tests are chosen because they 'split' species into distinct strains. However, diagnostic laboratories often use the profiles from miniaturized multi-test identification systems as biotypes *(Fig. 36.17)*.

Specialized typing techniques

Serotyping distinguishes between strains, using specific antisera

This classical technique distinguishes between strains by a difference in their antigenic structure, which is recognized by

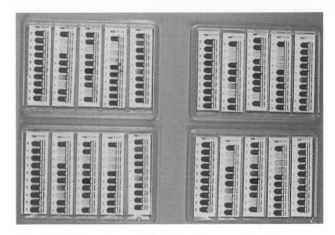

Fig. 36.17 Biotyping isolates of *Bacillus cereus* from an outbreak of infection in an intensive care unit. Biotyping schemes are based on the ability of different strains within a species to metabolize and grow on different substrates. Commercially available multi-test systems are designed primarily for identification purposes, but can also be used for biotyping. The strips contain a series of different biochemical tests. The isolate is inoculated into each well and, after incubation, a positive result is indicated by a color change. (Courtesy of S Dancer.)

reaction with specific antisera. The 'O' somatic antigens and 'H' flagellar antigens are therefore used to divide salmonellae into types (sometimes referred to as species; see Chapter 22). *Strep. pneumoniae, Neisseria meningitidis* and *Klebsiella aerogenes* can be typed on the basis of their capsular (K) antigens, and *Strep. pyogenes* on the basis of their M and T cell wall proteins. The established schemes use polyclonal antisera, but monoclonal reagents are now available. Serotyping requires the production and maintenance of appropriate banks of antisera, which is both time-consuming and costly. It is therefore usually restricted to reference laboratories.

Bacteriophage (phage) typing is used to type Staph. aureus, Staph. epidermidis *and* Salmonella typhi

This technique compares the pattern of lysis obtained when isolates (grown as lawns on agar plates) are exposed to a standard series of phage suspensions *(Fig. 36.18)*. In the past, this method has been important for typing *Staph. aureus, Staph. epidermidis* and *Salmonella typhi*, but has also been applied to other species such as *P. aeruginosa*. As with serotyping, phage typing requires the production, maintenance and testing of the standard phage suspensions and is usually carried out in reference laboratories rather than in the hospital diagnostic laboratory. In the United States, the Centers for Disease Control has forgone the use of bacteriophage typing in favor of molecular techniques such as pulsed field gel electrophoresis (PFGE) (see below).

Bacteriocin typing has been most successfully applied to P. aeruginosa *and* Shigella sonnei

Bacteriocins are small protein molecules produced by species of bacteria and lethal to other strains of the same or closely related species. The production of bacteriocins by the test strain produces a pattern of inhibition of growth of a standard

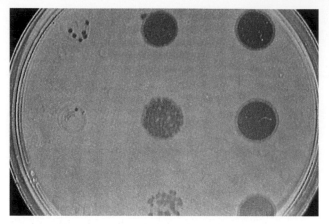

Fig. 36.18 Bacteriophage (phage) typing of staphylococci. After seeding the surface of an agar plate with the organism to be typed, suspensions of different phages are dropped onto the surface and the plate incubated. Phages that are able to lyse the strain will produce zones of clearing of the bacterial lawn. The patterns of lysis obtained with the same set of bacteriophages on different isolates of *Staph. aureus* collected, for example during an outbreak of wound infections, can be compared.

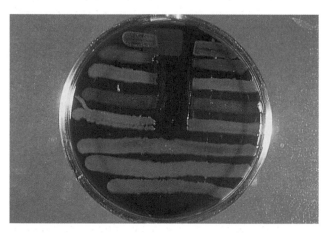

Fig. 36.19 Bacteriocin typing. The test isolate is grown in a band across the agar plate, and during this time bacteriocins produced by the isolate diffuse into the agar. After overnight incubation, the macroscopic growth is removed and the surface of the plate exposed to chloroform to kill remaining organisms (bacteriocins are resistant to the action of chloroform). Indicator strains are streaked across the plate at right angles to the original line and the plate incubated a second time. The pattern of inhibition of growth of the indicator is recorded and the strain assigned to a type.

set of indicator strains, which can be used to assign the test strain to a type *(Fig. 36.19)*. The method is potentially applicable to any species that produces bacteriocins (and most do). It has been most successfully applied to *P. aeruginosa* (pyocine typing, from the old name for the organism; *Pseudomonas pyocyaneus*) and *Shigella sonnei* (colicine typing, so-named because the species is genetically very similar to *E. coli* and sensitive to bacteriocins called colicines produced by that species).

Molecular typing

Molecular typing techniques involve characterizing an organism's DNA

The above methods have been of great use in the epidemiologic analysis of nosocomial pathogens but are all variations on the phenotypic characterization of isolates. Since the chromosome represents the most fundamental 'molecule of identity' in the cell, recent years have seen a trend toward more genotypic approaches to characterization, often referred to as 'molecular epidemiology'.

Plasmid profiles are an example of 'first generation' molecular epidemiology

Comparison of plasmid carriage in different isolates is only useful for species that carry a variety of plasmids and suffers from the drawback that what is actually being characterized is the plasmid and not the organism containing it. Different Gram-negative rods may acquire the same plasmids by conjugation between different species. However, this method has also been used to advantage to map the spread of antibiotic resistance plasmids among hospital pathogens *(Fig. 36.20)*.

Restriction enzymes and probes represent 'second generation' molecular epidemiology

Restriction-enzyme digestion of total cellular DNA from isolates results in a pattern of different-sized fragments which can be separated and compared by agarose gel electrophoresis—restriction-enzyme analysis (REA). All bacterial cells possess chromosomal DNA and can theoretically be analyzed by this process. However, the DNA sequences recognized by most restriction enzymes, such as *Eco*RI, *Hin*dIII, etc., are present in hundreds of copies throughout a typical bacterial chromosome. Thus, the challenge is to compare accurately electrophoretic patterns comprising hundreds of restriction fragments which often co-migrate in clusters of similar size, and may include resident plasmid DNA.

The principle of complementary DNA sequences hybridizing with each other (e.g. Southern hybridization; named after its inventor Ed Southern) has led to applications where specific DNA appropriately labeled 'probes', complementary to 'target' sequences found at various chromosomal locations, are hybridized against isolate REA patterns. Northern blotting is similar in principle but characterizes RNA sequences. Antibiotic resistance genes, and a variety of repeated sequences (e.g. transposons) have been especially useful targets in this context. The result is a pattern of hybridization with different restriction-fragments, commonly termed restriction-fragment length polymorphism (RFLP) analysis, corresponding to the chromosomal location of the probed sequences, which provides an indication of chromosomal relatedness between different isolates *(Fig. 36.21a)*. For example, copies of the genes for ribosomal RNA (5S, 16S and 23S rRNA) are found at different locations on the chromosome of many medically important bacteria. These highly conserved sequences (i.e. very similar sequences in different species) allow RFLP analysis using a common probe (i.e. ribotyping). However, discrimination between strains of the same species may be less because of the conserved nature of the target sequences.

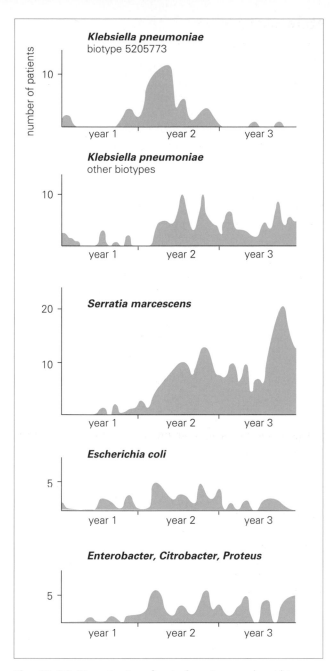

Fig. 36.20 Dissemination of a single resistance plasmid into several different strains and species of enterobacteria in one hospital. In year 1 in this hospital there were very few isolates of gentamicin-resistant enterobacteria. In the first 4 months of year 2, there was an outbreak of infection with a gentamicin-resistant *Klebsiella pneumoniae* belonging to a single biotype. Although this outbreak was contained, over subsequent months the same plasmid coding for the same aminoglycoside-modifying enzyme was found in other biotypes of the *Klebsiella* and in other Gram-negative species. (Adapted from O'Brien TE et al., *Antimicrob Agents Chemother* 1980; 17:537.)

The greatest success with RFLP analysis has primarily involved probes for insertion sequences that provide sufficient coverage (i.e. in number and diversity of chromosomal location) to reflect epidemiologically relevant interrelationships. The use of IS6110 probes in the RFLP analysis of *Mycobacterium tuberculosis* isolates is an example of a successful use of this approach. While superior to REA alone, RFLP analysis remains only moderately discriminatory for epidemiologic analysis.

PFGE and PCR are 'third generation' approaches to molecular epidemiology

Instead of using frequently-'cutting' restriction enzymes, chromosomal DNA may be digested using enzymes with rare recognition sites in bacterial chromosomes (e.g. *Not*I, *Sfi*I, *Spe*I and *Xba*I in most Gram-negatives; *Asc*I, *Rsr*II, *Sgr*AI and *Sma*I in most Gram-positives). The extremely large DNA fragments produced are too large to be separated by conventional agarose gel electrophoresis but may be resolved by electrophoretic current 'pulsed' in different directions for different lengths of time—pulsed field gel electrophoresis, (PFGE). PFGE has proved to be a powerful epidemiologic tool. The macro-restriction patterns produced by PFGE provide a sense of 'global' chromosomal monitoring—genetic events that affect distances between rare restriction-site sequences can be inferred from changes in restriction-fragment size *(Fig. 36.21b)*. To date, the major disadvantage to PFGE analysis has been extra time and effort involved in producing unbroken chromosomal molecules necessary for reproducible macro-restriction-fragment patterns. In general, the overall success with which PFGE analysis has been employed has made it the method of choice—the 'gold standard'—for the epidemiologic analysis of most pathogens of clinical concern.

Economy, speed and the relatively low level of technical expertise required by the polymerase chain reaction (PCR) (Chapter 32) have led to a wealth of amplification-based applications for epidemiologic analysis. One of the earliest and most common PCR-based approaches has been randomly amplified polymorphic DNA (RAPD), also called arbitrarily primed PCR (AP-PCR). The method is based on the use of relaxing conditions affecting the stringency (i.e. specificity) with which PCR primers bind to DNA templates. PCR primers are allowed to randomly bind to chromosomal sequences of varying homology, resulting in products which can be comparatively analyzed by agarose gel electrophoresis. A group of clinical isolates representing inter-patient transfer of a single strain would thus be expected to exhibit the same degree of 'randomness', resulting in identical PCR products *(Fig. 36.1c)*. However, several studies have shown that this method is especially prone to artifact and inter- and intra-laboratory variation. Nevertheless, the overall simplicity and utility of PCR continues to drive development and refinement of additional epidemiologic approaches which are beyond our ability to explore here.

'Fourth generation' molecular epidemiology is based on DNA sequence analysis

Since the chromosome is the most fundamental molecule of identity in the cell, a comparison of actual chromosomal sequences would seem the most fundamental means of assessing potential interrelationships in nosocomial isolates. Although still in its infancy as an epidemiologic approach, nucleotide sequence analysis is the basis for what one could consider fourth generation molecular epidemiology. How-

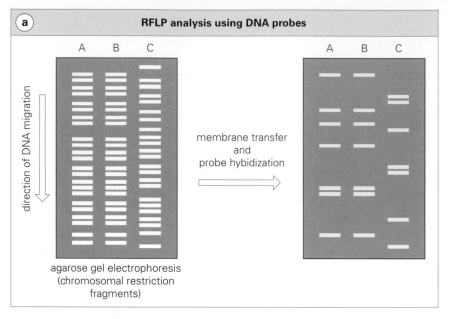

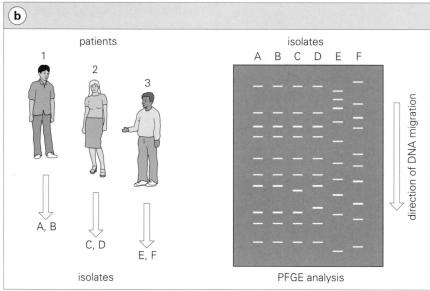

Fig. 36.21 (a) Restriction-fragment length polymorphism analysis using DNA probes. An illustration of three nosocomial isolates (A and B epidemiologically related; C unrelated) analyzed by restriction-enzyme analysis and subsequently by a specific DNA probe. (b) Pulsed field gel electrophoresis (PFGE) analysis of two bacterial isolates from each of three patients. Isolates in the first two patients are highly related (although slightly different in patient 2). Isolates from patient 3 are epidemiologically unrelated. (c) In the RAPD/AP-PCR approach to epidemiologic analysis, PCR products result from the random binding of PCR primers to chromosomal sequences, and the pattern is expected to be similar in epidemiologically related isolates. RAPD, randomly amplified polymorphic DNA; AP-PCR, arbitrarily primed polymerase chain reaction.

ever, issues related to the choice of epidemiologically relevant sequences, method of analysis, data output and interpretation remain to be resolved, a process being greatly facilitated by the current developments in bacterial genomics.

Molecular techniques for epidemiologic fingerprinting have many advantages

Although molecular techniques may require expertise and equipment that might not be routinely available, they have several advantages. They can be extremely precise, can be performed rapidly, do not involve handling infectious organisms and can be used to type all of the relevant isolates.

Investigation of viral infections

Nosocomial viral infections usually occur via the airborne route, contaminated fomites or blood-to-blood contact as outlined previously with, for example, RSV, noroviruses or hepatitis B, respectively. These are investigated mostly by

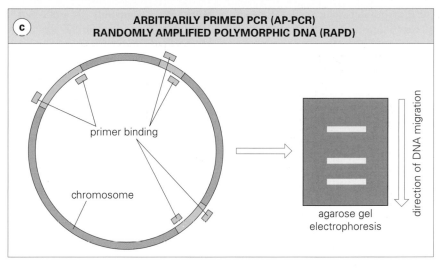

ARBITRARILY PRIMED PCR (AP-PCR)
RANDOMLY AMPLIFIED POLYMORPHIC DNA (RAPD)

primer binding

chromosome

agarose gel
electrophoresis

direction of DNA migration

Fig. 36.21, cont'd.

detecting virus in samples from symptomatic patients and then, depending on the clinical setting, collecting samples from asymptomatic patients when deciding whom to include in a cohort from whom isolates can be obtained. In general, only identification of the microbe as a virus is required in outbreaks of viral gastroenteritis, as the management is the same for all the viral causes of gastroenteritis. However, in an outbreak of respiratory infection, identification and typing of the virus is important. In influenza virus infections, considering both treatment and prophylaxis, only influenza A was susceptible to amantadine or rimantadine before the introduction of the neuraminidase inhibitor class of anti-influenza drugs. In addition, it is important to identify the circulating virus and match it with that season's vaccine components.

Molecular detection methods and typing methodologies such as sequencing may be required, usually for epidemiologic purposes rather than direct management of the patients. However, in a setting such as postoperative acute hepatitis B infection in a patient, an intensive investigation will be carried out covering the possible routes of transmission. This may include investigating blood products, healthcare workers who were involved in exposure-prone procedures, other patients on the operating list, sexual contacts, and other risk activities involving potentially blood-contaminated needles. Once the potential sources have been identified, serologic tests may be carried out to seek evidence of current, recent or past hepatitis B infection. Genome detection methods and sequencing of blood samples from the individual with acute hepatitis B as well as the potential source or sources will be carried out to confirm the transmission event or events.

Preventive measures

Once tracking is complete preventive measures can be introduced

Correct typing of the etiologic agent responsible for the outbreak, and knowledge of its characteristics and mode of transmission, allow preventive measures to be taken. What these include depends to a great extent on the pathogen involved, but all must aim to improve basic hygiene, from

more effective handwashing and improved general cleaning to more effectively regulated sterilization of equipment. Hygiene is a crucial factor—some 20–40% of nosocomial infections, particularly *Staph. aureus* and coliforms, are thought to be spread between patients by hospital staff. With some organisms that are widely distributed in the environment (e.g. *P. aeruginosa*) or occur in water supplies (e.g. *Legionella*), preventive measures may involve radical improvements to facilities.

STERILIZATION AND DISINFECTION

It is clear that the prevention of hospital infection depends in part upon the availability of clean, and where necessary, sterile equipment, instruments and dressings, isolation facilities and the safe disposal of infected material. Sterilization and disinfection are often talked about by microbiologists in relation to the production of sterile culture media and other laboratory activities, but it must be stressed that the concept of sterility is central to almost all areas of medical practice. An understanding of the rationale of sterilization and disinfection will aid intelligent use of the range of sterile equipment (from needles to protheses) and techniques (from surgery to handwashing) employed in medical practice.

Definitions

Sterilization is the process of killing or removing all viable organisms

An item that is sterile is free from all viable organisms—in this sense viable means capable of reproducing. Sterilization is achieved by physical or chemical means, either by the removal of organisms from an object or by killing the organisms in situ, sometimes leaving toxic breakdown products (pyrogens) in the object.

Disinfection is a process of removing or killing most, but not all, viable organisms

Disinfection employs either:

* a chemical 'disinfectant', which kills pathogens but may not kill viruses or spores;

- a physical process such as boiling water or low pressure steam, which reduces the bioburden (i.e. the load of viable organisms).

Antiseptics are used to reduce the number of viable organisms on the skin

Antiseptics are a particular group of disinfectants. Some act differentially, destroying the transient flora but leaving the normal skin flora deep in the skin pores and hair follicles untouched *(Fig. 36.22)*. It is impossible to sterilize the skin (except by burning!), but thorough washing with antiseptic soaps can reduce the numbers of organisms on the surface considerably and therefore reduce contact spread of infection (see above). However, the resident bacteria in the hair follicles and ducts of sweat glands can recolonize the skin surface within hours.

Pasteurization can be used to eliminate pathogens in heat-sensitive products

Pasteurization reduces the total numbers of viable microbes in bulk fluids such as milk and fruit juices without destroying

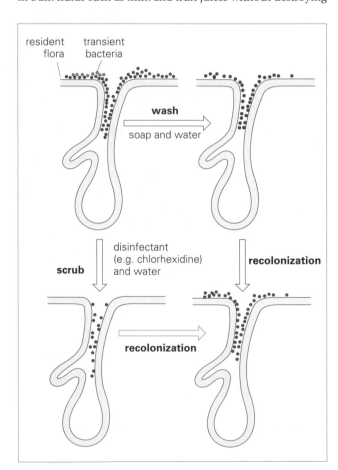

Fig. 36.22 Normal skin is colonized with bacteria both on the surface and deep in the pores and ducts of the sweat and sebaceous glands. In addition, bacteria may be carried transiently on the skin surface and may be transmitted from a contaminated source to a susceptible patient. Careful handwashing with soap and water removes the transient flora and some of the superficial resident flora. Scrubbing the hands with disinfectants removes more of the resident flora, but the skin surface is recolonized within hours from the normal flora deep in the skin pores.

flavor and palatability. It does not affect spores, but is effective against intracellular organisms such as *Brucella* and mycobacteria and many viruses.

Since the beginning of recorded history, various other techniques have been used to prevent the multiplication of microorganisms, such as drying and salting of food.

Deciding whether sterilization or disinfection should be used

Sterilization and disinfection processes are costly, and so it is important to choose the appropriate method and the one that causes the least damage to the material involved. A variety of considerations influence the choice of method. The detailed mechanisms of the death process of microorganisms may vary with the sterilizing technique used, but the net effect is similar in that essential cell constituents (nucleic acids or proteins) are inactivated.

It is easier to sterilize a clean object than a physically dirty one

This is because organic matter protects microbes and hinders penetration of heat or chemicals and may inactivate certain chemicals. In other words, a low bioburden is a prerequisite for cost-effective sterilization.

The rate of killing of microorganisms depends upon the concentration of the killing agent and time of exposure

The number of organisms surviving sterilization can be expressed by the equation: N is proportional to $1/CT$, where N is the number of survivors, C is the concentration of agent and T is time of exposure to the agent. If a population of microbes is exposed to a sterilizing technique, and the number of survivors expressed as a logarithm is plotted against time, the slope of the graph defines the death rate *(Fig. 36.23)*. These lines may be sigmoid or have shoulders, indicating that individual cells respond slightly differently, some being killed more easily than others. In the case of bacteria, the physiologic state of the organisms influences the shape of the killing curve; young, replicating cells are usually more vulnerable than stationary or decline-phase organisms or those that are sporing. Graphs like those shown in *Figure 36.23* can be used to predict the conditions necessary to achieve sterility. However, these experimental data are usually based on pure cultures in the laboratory (bacterial spores are often used as model systems) whereas in real life the bioburden is mixed. Therefore predictions from such data may be inappropriate for mixed populations.

Techniques for sterilization

Sterilization may be achieved by:

- heat;
- irradiation (gamma or ultraviolet);
- filtration;
- chemicals in liquid or gaseous phase.

Other techniques of doubtful efficiency include freezing and thawing, lysis, dessication, ultrasonication and the use of electrical discharges, but these are not applied in hospital practice.

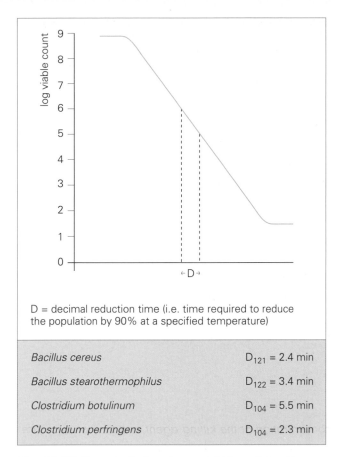

D = decimal reduction time (i.e. time required to reduce the population by 90% at a specified temperature)

Bacillus cereus	D_{121} = 2.4 min
Bacillus stearothermophilus	D_{122} = 3.4 min
Clostridium botulinum	D_{104} = 5.5 min
Clostridium perfringens	D_{104} = 2.3 min

Fig. 36.23 Theoretically there is a straight line relationship between the log viable count of a bacterial population and time when the population is exposed to a lethal temperature. In practice these lines are usually sigmoid. The D value is the time required to reduce the population by 90% at a specified temperature. *Bacillus stearothermophilus* spores are used as biologic indicators of effective heat sterilization by including filter paper strips carrying a standard number of spores into the autoclave cycle. The strips are then incubated to attempt to recover viable organisms. The usual autoclave cycle of 121°C for 15 minutes is adequate to kill *B. stearothermophilus* with a margin of safety.

Ultraviolet irradiation is inefficient as a sterilant, and its important uses in the hospital setting are in inhibiting growth of bacteria in water in complex apparatus such as auto-analyzers and in air in safety hoods in virology laboratories. The potential for damage to the cornea and skin precludes wider use of ultraviolet irradiation. It should be remembered that the agents of Creutzfeldt–Jakob disease (CJD), bovine spongiform encephalopathy (BSE) and scrapie are highly resistant and are not completely inactivated by formalin, ultraviolet irradiation, ionizing radiation or regular autoclaving. Sterilization can be achieved by boiling in 1N NaOH for 10 minutes at atmospheric pressure followed by autoclaving at a higher than normal temperature for a longer period than usual (134°C for 18 min), but obviously this technique cannot be applied to living tissues or materials that are damaged at high temperatures.

Heat

Heat, as a way of transferring energy, is the preferred choice for sterilization on the grounds of ease of use, controllability, cost and efficiency.

Dry heat sterilizes by oxidation of the cell components

Incineration and the use of the laboratory Bunsen burner are examples of sterilization by dry heat. Glassware can be sterilized in a hot air oven at 160–180°C for 1 hour.

The most effective agent for sterilization is saturated steam (moist heat) under pressure

This can be achieved using an autoclave. Steam under pressure aids penetration of heat into the material to be sterilized (such as dressings), and there is a direct relationship between temperature and steam pressure. Steam under pressure has a temperature in excess of 100°C, which results in increased killing of microbes.

Sterilizing efficiency is improved by evacuating all of the air from the autoclave chamber. The subsequent introduction of high pressure steam rapidly penetrates to all parts of the chamber and its load, and results in predictable rises in temperature in the center of articles to be sterilized. The length of an autoclave cycle is determined by the holding time plus a margin of safety, and is derived from the thermal death curves for heat-resistant pathogens such as clostridia. Therefore the usual cycle of 121°C for 15 minutes is sufficient to kill the spores of *Cl. botulinum* with an adequate margin of safety. However, the spores of some bacterial species, especially soil organisms, are able to withstand this temperature. The safety margin is reduced in the presence of large numbers of organisms because there is a greater probability of more heat-resistant individuals existing in a large population; hence the importance of cleaning instruments, whenever possible, before sterilization.

Moist heat in an autoclave is used to sterilize surgical instruments and dressings and heat-resistant pharmaceuticals. A method for the sterilization of heat-sensitive instruments such as endoscopes uses a combination of low temperature (subatmospheric) steam and formaldehyde.

All of these processes need to be carried out in a suitable pressure vessel and are therefore usually available in the hospital central sterile supply department.

Immersion in boiling water for a few minutes can be used as a rapid emergency measure to disinfect instruments

Immersion in boiling water for a few minutes will kill vegetative bacteria and many, but not all, spores. The addition of 2% sodium carbonate to the water potentiates the sporicidal effect.

Pasteurization uses heat at 62.8–65.6°C for 30 minutes

This technique was devised by Pasteur to prevent the spoilage of wine by heating it to 50–60°C. It is now used for fluids such as milk to reduce the number of bacteria. This helps to eliminate pathogens present in small numbers and to improve the shelf-life of milk. The fluid is held at a temperature of 62.8–65.6°C for 30 minutes or may be 'flash' pasteurized at 71.7°C for 15 seconds. After either process the fluid should be kept at a temperature below 10°C to minimize subsequent bacterial growth.

Irradiation

Gamma irradiation energy is used to sterilize large batches of small volume items

The use of gamma irradiation energy for sterilization is an industrial process that works well with products such as needles, syringes, intravenous lines, catheters and gloves. It can also be used for vaccines and to prevent food spoilage. Although the capital cost of the equipment is high, the process is continuous and 100% efficient. Articles are sterilized while sealed in their final packaging, without any heat gain. The process must be conducted in a suitably constructed building, usually at a location distinct from the hospital and usually outside the hospital administration. However, irradiation can cause materials to deteriorate and is thus not suitable for resterilization of equipment. The killing mechanism involves the production of free radicals, which break the bonds in DNA. Irradiation kills spores, but at a higher dose than vegetative cells because of the relative lack of water in spores.

Sterilization using ultraviolet irradiation is discussed above.

Filtration

Filters are used to produce particle- and pyrogen-free fluid

Solutions that are heat-sterilized will contain pyrogens. These heat-stable breakdown products of microbes are capable of inducing fever and are therefore undesirable in products such as intravenous fluids. Filtration or separation of the product from the contamination has a long history in the clarification of water and wine. Modern filters are composed of nitro-cellulose and work by electrostatic attraction and physical pore size to retain organisms or other particles. The resulting fluid should be particle-free. Filtration is used in some parts of the world to purify drinking water.

Filtration techniques are also used to recover very small numbers of organisms from very large volumes of fluid (e.g. *Legionella* from cooling tower water) and can be used as a method for quantifying bacteria in fluids.

Chemical agents

The gases ethylene oxide and formaldehyde kill by damaging proteins and nucleic acids

The need for sterilization by gaseous chemicals has been greatly reduced by the success of gamma irradiation (see above), but two alkylating gases, ethylene oxide and formaldehyde, are still used:

- Ethylene oxide is used in some centers to sterilize single use medical requisites such as heart valves. However, it is toxic and potentially explosive.
- Formaldehyde is not explosive, but has an extremely unpleasant odor and is an irritant to mucous membranes. It has been used as a disinfectant to decontaminate rooms (such as isolation rooms) and in the laboratory to disinfect exhaust-protective cabinets. A high relative humidity is essential for effective killing.

The liquid glutaraldehyde is used to disinfect heat-sensitive articles

Glutaraldehyde is less toxic than formaldehyde and can be stabilized in solution to remain active for up to several weeks at in-use concentration. It is used for the disinfection of, but does not sterilize, heat-sensitive articles such as endoscopes and for inanimate surfaces.

Many different antimicrobial chemicals are available, but few are sterilant

Some, like the derivatives of pine and turpentine, have been known since ancient times, and chloride of lime and coal tar fluids were in use before the germ theory of disease was established. Most fall into the category of disinfectant or antiseptic, but a few are capable of rendering articles sterile. Factors that affect their efficacy include:

- physical environment (e.g. porous or cracked surfaces);
- presence of moisture;
- temperature and pH;
- concentration of the agent;
- hardness of water;
- the bioburden on the object to be disinfected;
- the nature and state of the microbes in the bioburden;
- the ability of the microbes to inactivate the chemical agent.

It is obvious that the above factors are difficult to control in every circumstance. The main groups of chemical agents are shown in *Figure 36.24*. They act by causing chemical damage to proteins, nucleic acids or cell membrane lipids. The activity of a given disinfectant may result from more than one pathway of damage.

Controlling sterilization and disinfection

In general it is preferable to control the process rather than the product

This means that it is better to run checks on the technique while it is in operation rather than attempting to recognize process failure by isolating microorganisms from the product. Trying to discover whether one or a few viable organisms remain is analogous to trying to find a needle in a haystack. It is known that damaged bacteria can recover given time and special nutrient recovery media, but it may not be feasible to hold back a batch of product for such tests. In addition, how many samples of the product should be tested? If too few are examined, the likelihood of missing a failed sample is high; if too many are examined, too much of the batch is used up in quality control to be economically sensible.

The usual process controls are either physical or chemical checks on the technique, for example tests that show that the autoclave reached the desired temperature for the desired time. They do not show that there are no viable organisms remaining after the process, but this is assumed if the process satisfies the controls. However, the stringency of the controls can be altered intentionally or accidentally to give either an undersensitive or oversensitive test.

DISINFECTANTS FOR HOSPITAL USE		
group	**examples**	**advantages and disadvantages**
phenolics	clear-soluble phenolic compunds, white fluids	good general-purpose disinfectants, not readily inactivated by organic matter, active against wide range of organisms including mycobacteria, not sporicidal
	chloroxylenols	inactivated by hard water and organic matter, *Pseudomonas* grows readily in chloroxylenol solutions, limited activity against other Gram-negatives
halogens	hypochlorites (chloramine)	cheap, effective, act by release of free chlorine, active against viruses and therefore recommended for disinfection of equipment soiled with blood (because of hepatitis risk), inactivated by organic material, corrode metals
	iodine and iodophors	useful skin disinfectants, sporicidal
other heavy metals	mercuric chloride	used as topical skin preparation
quaternary ammonium compounds	benzalkonium chloride, cetavlon	have detergent properties, activity against Gram-negative << Gram-positive, improved by combination with diguanide, e.g. chlorhexidine, useful as skin disinfectants, inactivated by hard water and organic materials, contamination of stock solutions with Gram-negative rods can be a problem
diguanides	chlorhexidine	useful disinfectant for skin and mucous membranes, inactivated by many materials and too expensive for environmental use, alcoholic solutions are less easily contaminated, combinations of chlorhexidine and detergent highly effective for disinfection of hands
alcohols	ethyl alcohol, isopropyl alcohol	good choice for skin disinfection and for clean surfaces, sometimes used in combination with iodine or chlorhexidine (see above), water must be present for bacterial killing (i.e. 70% ethanol best), isopropyl preferred for skin and articles in contact with patient
aldehydes	formaldehyde/formalin glutaraldehyde	too irritant for use as general disinfectant kills vegetative organisms, including mycobacteria, slowly but effectively, more active, less toxic than formaldehyde, sporicidal (within 6 hours when fresh), slightly irritant, used in alkaline solution which is stable for 1–2 weeks, expensive, limited use, e.g. disinfection of endoscopes
hexachlorophene		activity against Gram-positive >> Gram-negative, used in soap or dusting powder as skin disinfectant (use restricted after potentially toxic blood levels found in infants who had hexachlorophene emulsion spread over whole body) introduced as substitute for hexachlorophene in soap, considerable antibacterial effect on repeated use

Fig. 36.24 Disinfectants for use in hospitals. Note that no one group of disinfectant has all the properties desirable for use both on skin and on inanimate surfaces.

Disinfectants can be monitored by microbiologic 'in-use' tests

These tests involve challenging the solution with a bacterial suspension and withdrawing samples, which are then treated to prevent carryover of the disinfectant and cultured. However, these tests are rarely performed in the hospital setting, where the use of disinfectants is guided largely by the manufacturer's recommendations.

KEY FACTS

- Any infection acquired in hospital is termed a hospital-acquired or nosocomial infection.

- Hospital infections often have serious consequences for the individual, for the hospital community and for the community at large. They may be caused by almost any organism, but a few species cause the vast majority of infections.

- The hospital environment favors the survival of resistant strains and therefore infections are often caused by organisms with limited antibiotic susceptibility.

- Most common hospital-acquired infections are UTIs, respiratory tract infections, surgical wound infections and bacteremia (septicemia).

- The most important bacterial causes are Gram-positive cocci (staphylococci and streptococci) and Gram-negative rods (e.g. *E. coli, Pseudomonas*). Multiply-antibiotic-resistant organisms are common. *Candida* is the significant fungal cause, and viruses probably cause more hospital-acquired infections than previously recognized.

- Infecting organisms originate from the patient's own flora (endogenous infection) or from other human or inanimate sources (exogenous or cross-infection). Airborne and contact spread are the most important routes of transmission.

- Host factors are of critical importance in determining susceptibility to infection.

- Surveillance should be an ongoing activity to facilitate early recognition of outbreaks of infection. Investigation of outbreaks involves both epidemiologic and microbiologic expertise. Molecular techniques to 'fingerprint' the causative organism are becoming increasingly sophisticated.

- Prevention of hospital-acquired infections by excluding sources, interrupting transmission and enhancing the patient's resistance is fundamental to improving patient care and reducing costs.

- Sterilization and disinfection are key processes in the control and prevention of hospital-acquired infections as well as being central to many areas of medical practice.

QUESTIONS

As a surgeon you are called by the nurses to see a patient who has developed a fever. Three days ago he underwent a colonic resection for carcinoma of the colon. The operation went smoothly, and he was progressing well on the ward. His past medical history before admission was unremarkable, although he is noted to be a smoker. On examination his temperature is 37.8°C, he is slightly dyspneic at rest and there are a few basal crackles in his chest at both bases. His abdominal wound is dressed and you are reluctant to disturb the dressings.

1. What are the common causes of postoperative infections in patients and what steps can be taken to reduce these problems?

2. What investigations would you order?

3. How would you treat him?

FURTHER READING

Bennett JV, Brachman PS, eds. *Hospital Infections,* 4th edition. Philadelphia: Lippincott-Raven, 1998.

Herwaldt LA, Decker MD, eds. *A Practical Handbook for Hospital Epidemiologists.* Thorofare, NJ: Slack, 1998.

Mayhall CG, ed. *Hospital Epidemiology and Infection Control.* Baltimore: Williams & Wilkins, 1999.

Wenzel RP, ed. *Prevention and Control of Nosocomial Infections,* 3rd edition. Baltimore: Williams & Wilkin, 1997.

Wenzel RP, Brewer TF, Butzler JP. *Guide to Infection Control in the Hospital.* Hamilton, Ontario: BC Decker, 2002.

Pathogen parade

See index for alphabetical listing of all organisms (includes Pathogen parade entries)

VIRUSES

ADENOVIRUSES

Characteristics	Virus family	Type	Envelope	Shape	Size (nm)	Nucleocapsid
	Adenoviridae	dsDNA	–	Icosahedral	70–90	Icosahedral

Fifty-one types, sharing a common group-specific antigen. Rod-like structures (fibers) topped with knobs project from the vertices of particles, and attach virus to the cell.

Replication
After attachment, endocytosis and uncoating, viral DNA is transcribed within the nucleus by cellular DNA-dependent RNA polymerase. RNA transcripts corresponding to several genes (less than the whole genome) undergo cleavage and splicing to form monocistronic mRNA. Early mRNA codes for enzymes needed for replication; late mRNA (after viral DNA synthesis) for structural proteins. Particles are assembled in the nucleus and released from the damaged cell.

Diseases
Cause pharyngoconjunctival fever; epidemics of acute respiratory disease, including pneumonia; intestinal illness (mesenteric adenitis, intussusceptions); keratoconjunctivitis; hepatitis and disseminated disease in immunosuppressed individuals. Can cause hemorrhagic cystitis or CNS disease.

Transmission
Via respiratory droplets, feces, and sometimes from eye to eye via contaminated hands, towels, or eye drops.

Pathogenesis
Adenoviruses infect epithelium of respiratory tract and eyes, and probably intestine. Spread to involve lymphoid tissues and can persist for long periods in tonsils and adenoids of children. Viral protein interferes with immune defences by blocking action of interferon and Tc cells.

Laboratory identification
Virus isolation in cell culture in samples including throat swabs, feces, and urine; detect antigen in nasopharyngeal aspirates by immunofluorescence; DNA detection in various samples by PCR; and virions in fecal samples by electron microscopy. Serology by detecting a rise in complement-fixing antibody titer.

Treatment and prevention
No specific antiviral treatment but some drugs such as ribavirin and cidofovir are under investigation. Live oral vaccine (types 3, 4, 7 in enteric-coated capsules) has been used in military recruits to prevent outbreaks of respiratory infection.

Organ systems and disease involvement
Gastrointestinal tract infections, 292; host-parasite relationship, 169, 175; immunocompromised host, 436; lower respiratory tract infection, 225-226; pathological consequences, 196

ARENAVIRUSES These include Lassa fever and lymphocytic choriomeningitis (LCM) viruses.

Characteristics	Virus family	Type	Envelope	Shape	Size (nm)	Nucleocapsid
	Arenaviridae	ssRNA –ve sense	+	Spherical	50–300	Helical

Virions are pleomorphic, containing two circular RNA segments, one negative and one ambisense, and in addition host ribosomes visible as granules inside the envelope (Latin *arena*, sand).

Replication
Viral RNA-dependent RNA polymerase produces positive strand RNA, which is translated to form a nucleoprotein and two glycoproteins. Maturation is by budding with no cytopathic effect on the cell.

Diseases	Febrile illness, sometimes complicated by aseptic meningitis (LCM), or by severe hemorrhagic disease (Lassa fever, Argentinian and Bolivian hemorrhagic fevers).
Transmission	Cause inapparent persistent infections in the natural rodent host and can result in zoonotic spread to humans via contact with rodent excreta. LCM virus occurs worldwide, comes from mice and hamsters; Lassa fever virus in West Africa from the bush rat *Mastomys natalensis*; Junin and Machupo viruses from bush mice (*Calomys* spp.) in South America causing Argentinian and Bolivian hemorrhagic fevers.
Pathogenesis	Natural rodent host is infected in utero or neonatally, and non-cytopathic virus remains in all tissues throughout life. In human host, virus spreads systemically causing meningitis or hemorrhagic disease by local or general replication plus immunopathology.
Laboratory identification	Specialist reference laboratory tests: detect specific antibody, viral RNA detection by PCR, and virus isolation.
Treatment and prevention	Ribavirin can be used as treatment and prophylaxis for Lassa fever. Vaccines for routine use are not available.
Organ systems and disease involvement	Immunocompromised host, 401-402

BUNYAVIRUSES

Characteristics	**Virus family**	**Type**	**Envelope**	**Shape**	**Size (nm)**	**Nucleocapsid**
	Bunyaviridae	ssRNA –ve sense	+	Spherical	80–120	Helical

Contains more than 100 different viruses. Bunyamwera is a locality in Africa where the prototype virus was isolated. Important human members are the hantaviruses (Southeast Asia, USA), Rift Valley Fever (RVF, Africa) virus, and La Crosse (Californian encephalitis) virus.

Replication	After attachment to cell receptors and endocytosis, nucleocapsid enters cytoplasm by fusion with endosomal membranes; the three segments of RNA are transcribed into mRNA and translated. Virus RNA is then transcribed and replicated. Glycoproteins are synthesized and glycosylated in endoplasmic reticulum, entering the Golgi complex, where budding takes place, with release by exocytosis or lysis of the cell.
Diseases	Cause febrile viremic illnesses; generally mild. RVF can cause hemorrhagic phenomena, sometimes with a lethal outcome; La Crosse virus can cause encephalitis; and hantaviruses can cause renal disease (Korean hemorrhagic fever) or a severe pulmonary syndrome.
Transmission	With the exception of the hantaviruses, which are acquired from urine of infected rodents, Bunyaviruses are transmitted by mosquitoes (or ticks or sandflies), and there is a bird or mammal reservoir.
Pathogenesis	After reaching the blood, virus disseminates to the CNS, liver, kidneys, and multiplies in vascular endothelium (hantaviruses).
Laboratory identification	Specialist reference laboratory tests: antibody detection, viral RNA detection and virus isolation.
Treatment and prevention	Ribavirin may be effective in hantavirus hemorrhagic fever with renal syndrome if given early. Prevention is by avoiding contact with arthropod vector (RVF virus, La Crosse virus) or with infected rodents (hantaviruses). Vaccines have been developed for RVF.

Organ systems and disease involvement	Lower respiratory tract infection, 220; multisystem zoonoses, 402

CORONAVIRUSES

Characteristics	**Virus family**	**Type**	**Envelope**	**Shape**	**Size (nm)**	**Nucleocapsid**
	Coronaviridae	ssRNA +ve sense	+	Spherical	120–160	Helical

Virions are pleomorphic but roughly symmetrical with a characteristic fringe of surface projections (Latin *corona*, crown).

Replication	Viral RNA-dependent RNA polymerase uses genomic positive strand to produce negative strand RNA, which acts as template for new positive strands. Nucleocapsids bud into endoplasmic reticulum from which they are released by exocytosis.
Diseases	Common cold-type illness (possibly gastroenteritis). Sudden acute respiratory syndrome (SARS)-associated coronavirus infection, severe lower respiratory tract infection.
Transmission	Respiratory droplets.
Pathogenesis	Replication in cells lining upper respiratory tract. Optimum growth temperature 33–35°C.
Laboratory identification	Not available routinely. Antibody tests, electron microscopic examination of various samples, and viral isolation. Became critical with the identification of SARS-associated coronavirus infection in China and Hong Kong.
Treatment and prevention	No antivirals or vaccines available.

Organ systems and disease involvement	Gastrointestinal tract infections, 292; lower respiratory tract infection, 230-231; upper respiratory tract infection, 201-202

FILOVIRUSES These include Ebola and Marburg viruses.

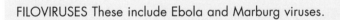

Characteristics	**Virus family**	**Type**	**Envelope**	**Shape**	**Size (nm)**	**Nucleocapsid**
	Filoviridae	ssRNA –ve sense	+	Tubular	80–14 000	Helical

Replication	Enters cell cytoplasm and is transcribed, resulting in subgenomic mRNAs.
Diseases	Hemorrhagic disease, conjunctivitis, neurological symptoms.
Transmission	Person-to person. Probable animal reservoir. Incubation period 3–9 days (Marburg) and 4–16 days (Ebola).
Pathogenesis	Virus spreads to multiple sites of the body. Generalized hemorrhage in most organs.
Laboratory identification	Specialist reference laboratory tests: antibody and antigen detection, viral RNA detection, virus isolation, electron microscopy.
Treatment and prevention	Supportive. Isolation of patients.

Organ systems and disease involvement	Multisystem zoonoses, 402-403

FLAVIVIRUSES These includes dengue, Japanese encephalitis, yellow fever, tick-borne encephalitis, West Nile, and hepatitis C viruses.

Characteristics	Virus family	Type	Envelope	Shape	Size (nm)	Nucleocapsid
	Flaviviridae	ssRNA +ve sense	+	Spherical	40–60	Icosahedral

The flaviviruses were assigned to their own family as sufficient differences were identified between this group of viruses and the alphaviruses, which together had come under the *Togaviridae*. The *Flavivirus*, *Pestivirus*, and *Hepacivirus* genera have been placed in the *Flaviviridae* family. Of these, it is only the members of the *Flavivirus* genus that are transmitted by arthropod vectors (**ar**thropod-**bo**rne **viruses** also called arboviruses). Hepatitis C virus has been placed in the *Hepacivirus* genus. Pestiviruses cause veterinary diseases around the world.

Replication

The positive strand RNA is translated into structural and non-structural proteins, the latter including the RNA-dependent RNA polymerase, which replicates the viral genome by directing the formation of a negative strand template and thus giving rise to positive strand progeny. Full length RNA is formed, with rapid cleavage of the resulting polyprotein. After assembly, the virus exits from the cell, budding from the endoplasmic reticulum.

Diseases

The arboviruses cause febrile illnesses, which may be severe when there is involvement of liver (yellow fever) or CNS (West Nile virus, Japanese and tick-borne encephalitides), or when there are immunopathologic complications (dengue hemorrhagic fever). Hepatitis C causes acute and chronic hepatitis (the former being mostly asymptomatic), cirrhosis, and hepatocellular carcinoma.

Transmission

Infected tick or mosquito bites for the arboviruses. Routes of transmission for hepatitis C include contaminated blood products, blood contaminated needles or equipment, i.e. injecting drug use, tattoos, body piercing. Vertical and sexual transmission infrequent.

Pathogenesis

Initial infection via skin (arboviruses) causes no detectable local lesion. Virus spreads to local lymph nodes and blood, liver (yellow fever), or CNS (mononuclear cells often infected in dengue). Immunopathology important in dengue hemorrhagic fever. Ingested virus infects gut epithelium of mosquitoes and ticks, and spreads to, and multiplies in, salivary glands. HCV-associated liver disease is probably due to direct cytopathic infection of hepatocytes in addition to the host immune/inflammatory responses.

Laboratory identification

Hepatitis C antibody and HCV RNA detection. HCV RNA load and genotype for monitoring disease progression and treatment response. Serological methods, viral RNA detection by PCR and, to a lesser extent, virus isolation are used to diagnose the arbovirus infections.

Treatment and prevention

There is no antiviral therapy for arbovirus infections. A live attenuated virus vaccine prevents yellow fever, tick-borne and Japanese encephalitis viruses. Vector control measures limit virus transmission. Hepatitis C can be treated with ribavirin and pegylated interferon.

Organ systems and disease involvement

General, 307-308; central nervous system (CNS), 336; diagnosis and control, 499-500, 504, 541; pathological consequences, 196; vaccination, 532; vector-borne, 383-386

HEPATITIS B

Characteristics	**Virus family**	**Type**	**Envelope**	**Shape**	**Size (nm)**	**Nucleocapsid**
	Hepadnaviridae	dsDNA	+	Spherical	42	Icosahedral (circular)

Infectious Dane particles consist of an envelope, the hepatitis B surface antigen (HBsAg), surrounding the core or nucleocapsid. There are a number of genotypes, A to G. The virus is unusual as it is the only human virus, other than the retroviruses, that encodes a reverse transcriptase.

Replication
After attachment to hepatocytes, particles are endocytosed and uncoated. In the nucleus, viral DNA polymerase converts viral DNA into a complete circular dsDNA. Negative strand DNA is transcribed by cellular RNA polymerase to form a single positive RNA strand, which moves to the cytoplasm, is translated into protein, and is then encapsulated into cores together with viral DNA polymerase. The positive RNA strand is then used to synthesize negative strand DNA (reverse transcriptase activity). A small fragment from the 5′ end of the positive RNA strand primes synthesis of all but about one-third of the positive DNA strand. Hence complete particles contain dsDNA with a ssDNA region. Release from cell is by budding. Viral DNA can be integrated into host DNA.

Diseases
Acute and chronic hepatitis including fulminant liver failure, cirrhosis, and hepatocellular carcinoma. Persistent infection known as the carrier state is common after infection in infancy or early childhood and non-icteric infection in adults. 350 million carriers worldwide.

Transmission
Spread via blood, for example by contaminated needles, by sexual routes and from mother to baby. Median incubation period 10–12 weeks, range 6 weeks to 6 months.

Pathogenesis
Virus spreads via blood to liver and replicates in hepatocytes. Immunopathological disease due to cytotoxic T cells lysing HBsAg-bearing hepatocytes. Immune complex formation can cause rash and arthritis.

Laboratory identification
Neutralizable HBsAg in blood indicates either acute or persistent infection. Detection of anti-HBc IgM assists diagnosis of recent infection. Presence of HBe antigen means blood is highly infectious. Detection of anti-HBc and anti-HBs in the absence of HBsAg indicates previous infection and immunity. Serum HBV DNA quantification assists monitoring of the carrier state and response to antiviral treatment. The virus cannot be grown in cell culture.

Treatment and prevention
Immunomodulators such as interferons, which were of moderate success, have been superseded by specific antiviral treatment with lamivudine and adefovir. The genetically engineered HBsAg-based vaccine is highly effective. Post-exposure prophylaxis also involves using hepatitis B immunoglobulin.

Organ systems and disease involvement
General 33, 34, 275; diagnosis and control, 499-500, 304, 541, 551-552; gastrointestinal tract infections, 304-307; host-parasite relationship, 132; immunocompromised host, 436; pathological consequences, 196; vaccination, 531-532

HEPATITIS D (DELTA)

Characteristics	**Virus family**	**Type**	**Envelope**	**Shape**	**Size (nm)**	**Nucleocapsid**
	Deltavirus	ssRNA	+ (HBsAg)	Spherical	38–43	Heterogeneous satellite

Classified as a satellite as it requires hepatitis B to provide the envelope proteins to assemble infectious virus.

Replication	RNA-directed RNA synthesis. Two forms of the delta antigen, small and large, required for genome replication and assembly of ribonucleoprotein particles into new virions.
Diseases	Acute and chronic hepatitis. Most HDV co-infections are cleared. Superinfections can result in chronic infection, cirrhosis, and liver failure.
Transmission	Spread via blood. Incubation period is 3–7 weeks.
Pathogenesis	Virus spreads via blood to liver and replicates in hepatocytes.
Laboratory identification	HDV specific IgM and IgG, detect delta antigen or viral RNA.
Treatment and prevention	Mostly indirect by treating hepatitis B. Prevented by hepatitis B immunization.
Organ systems and disease involvement	Gastrointestinal tract infections, 308

HEPATITIS E

Characteristics	Virus family	Type	Envelope	Shape	Size (nm)	Nucleocapsid
	Caliciviridae	ssRNA +ve sense	–	Icosahedral	32–34	Icosahedral

Replication	RNA-dependent RNA polymerase. Two subgenomic mRNAs are transcribed from the full length negative strand and the products undergo post-translational modifications.
Diseases	Sporadic acute and sometimes fulminant hepatitis. Epidemic enterically transmitted hepatitis.
Transmission	Spread via fecal–oral route. Mean incubation period is 6 weeks.
Pathogenesis	Virus spreads to liver and replicates in hepatocytes.
Laboratory identification	HEV-specific IgM and IgG.
Treatment and prevention	Supportive.
Organ systems and disease involvement	Gastrointestinal tract infections, 304

HERPESVIRUSES These include herpes simplex (HSV), varicella–zoster (VSV), cytomegalovirus (CMV), Epstein–Barr virus (EBV), human herpes virus (HHV) 6, 7 and 8.

Characteristics	Virus family	Type	Envelope	Shape	Size (nm)	Nucleocapsid
	Herpesviridae	dsDNA	+	Icosahedral	180–200	Icosahedral

Replication	Virus attaches to specific receptor on cell and enters by fusion of envelope with plasma membrane. Nucleocapsid moves to nucleus; viral DNA is uncoated at nuclear pores and then transcribed by cellular RNA polymerase so that the five sets of viral genes are sequentially activated. 'Immediate–early' gene products stimulate synthesis of second wave of 'early' gene products that are involved in genome replication and include the DNA polymerases. After DNA replication the remaining 'late' gene products are expressed and are involved in assembly. In the nucleus, viral DNA is inserted in capsids,

and resulting nucleocapsids attach to sites on inner nuclear membrane where envelope proteins are present and budding takes place between inner and outer nuclear membranes. Enveloped virus particles are transported through the cytoplasm and released by reverse phagocytosis. Replication cycle about 36 h. Generally persist for long periods in body, often in latent form (in neurones, monocytes, T cells, B cells), and can reactivate.

Diseases

Type	Clinical features include
HHV1 (HSV1)	Gingivostomatitis, cold sores, encephalitis
HHV2 (HSV2)	Genital herpes, cutaneous herpes, encephalitis, meningoencephalitis
HHV3 (VZV)	Varicella, zoster (shingles)
HHV4 (EBV)	Mononucleosis (glandular fever), hepatitis, encephalitis, Burkitt's lymphoma, nasopharyngeal carcinoma
HHV5 (CMV)	Mononucleosis, hepatitis, pneumonitis, congenital CMV
HHV6	Exanthem subitum, mild febrile illness
HHV7	Exanthem subitum, mild febrile illness
HHV8	Associated with Kaposi's sarcoma

Transmission

HSV: saliva, vesicle fluid, sexual contact, birth canal in neonate. VZV: respiratory droplets, vesicle fluid. EBV: saliva, organ transplants. CMV: saliva, urine, semen, cervical secretions, milk; also via organ transplants and across placenta. HHV6, 7: saliva. HHV8: semen.

Pathogenesis

HSV: vesicular lesions on mouth, skin, genitals; axonal travel to latency sites in sensory ganglia; reactivation (cold sores). VZV: respiratory infection, systemic spread to skin, axonal travel to latency sites in sensory ganglia; reactivation (zoster). EBV: pharyngeal infection, systemic spread, latency in B cells, epithelium; subclinical reactivation. CMV: pharyngeal infection, systemic spread, latency in mononuclear cells; reactivation. HHV6, 7: present in T cells. HHV8: infects endothelial cells in Kaposi's sarcoma.

Laboratory identification

Isolation of virus in cell culture for HSV, CMV and VZV. Detecting intranuclear inclusions in tissue biopsies, multinucleated cells. DNA detection by PCR methods using a range of samples. Lymphocytosis, atypical lymphocytes, heterophile antibody (Monospot) and VCA IgM for EBV, and CMV IgM.

Treatment and prevention

Aciclovir, valaciclovir, famciclovir (HSV, VZV); ganciclovir, valganciclovir, foscarnet (CMV). Varicella–zoster immune globulin (VZIG) is used to prevent or attenuate chickenpox when susceptible immunocompromised individuals are exposed to infection. Live attenuated varicella vaccine licensed for use.

Organ systems and disease involvement

General, 32-33, 317; central nervous system (CNS), 331-332; diagnosis and control, 499-500, 501-502; host-parasite relationship, 132, 148, 171, 175-176; immunocompromised host, 436; infection of skin, soft tissue, muscle and associated systems, 368-372; lower respiratory tract infection, 231; pathological consequences, 194-195; sexually transmitted disease, 263-264; upper respiratory tract infection, 202-208; vaccination, 533, 536

NOROVIRUSES

Characteristics

Virus family	Type	Envelope	Shape	Size (nm)	Nucleocapsid
Caliciviridae	ssRNA +ve sense	–	Spherical	27	Icosahedral

Norovirus is the genus name for the group of viruses previously called 'Norwalk-like viruses' (NLV) or Small Round Structured Viruses (SRSV).

Replication

RNA-dependent RNA polymerase. Subgenomic mRNAs are transcribed from the full length negative strand, and the products undergo post-translational modifications.

Diseases	Acute gastroenteritis, sporadic and outbreaks.
Transmission	Fecal–oral route. Incubation period is up to 48 h.
Pathogenesis	Replication in small intestine mucosal epithelium likely leading to flattened short villi. Mucosal cell damage, atrophic villi, loss of digestive enzymes, reduced absorption leads to diarrhea.
Laboratory identification	Fecal material: viral RNA detection; electron microscopy; antigen detection by ELISA.
Treatment and prevention	Supportive. Good hygiene and sanitary disposal of waste.
Organ systems and disease involvement	Gastrointestinal tract infections, 292

ORTHOMYXOVIRUSES Influenza viruses.

Characteristics	**Virus family**	**Type**	**Envelope**	**Shape**	**Size (nm)**	**Nucleocapsid**
	Orthomyxoviridae	ssRNA, linear, –ve sense, eight segments	+	Pleomorphic	80–120	Helical

Envelope glycoproteins: hemagglutinin (H) attaches virus to sialic-acid-containing receptor on cell and, after exposure to endosomal acid, acts as fusion protein; neuraminidase (N) cleaves sialic acid from glycoproteins and is involved in release of virus from cell surface.

Influenza A: widespread in birds, horses, pigs, humans. Genetic reassortments between animal and human strains produce subtypes with novel combinations of H and N genes referred to as antigenic shift; new strains can cause pandemics. Antigenic drift also occurs and is a gradual alteration by developing point mutations in H to generate new strains. Influenza B: occurs only in humans; undergoes antigenic drift and can cause epidemics. Influenza C: of doubtful pathogenicity in humans.

Replication	Virus binds to cell via its H, enters a vesicle, its envelope fusing with vesicle wall. After uncoating, viral polymerase transcribes genome into eight mRNAs, which are translated in the cytoplasm. Progeny RNA synthesized in nucleus and nucleocapsids assembled in cytoplasm. Viral matrix protein joins nucleocapsid to viral envelope components in the cell wall and maturation takes place by budding.
Diseases	Incubation period 1–2 days. Fever, myalgia, malaise, nasal discharge, sore throat, cough, pneumonia.
Transmission	Via respiratory droplets.
Pathogenesis	Mainly infection of respiratory tract but can cause neurological and other symptoms. Cytokines contribute to symptoms, and secondary bacterial infection is quite common.
Laboratory identification	Virus isolation in cell culture. Detection of viral antigen by immunofluorescence or viral RNA by PCR. Serology: acute and convalescent sera tested by complement fixation test.
Treatment and prevention	Amantadine can be used for treatment and prophylaxis for influenza A infection only. Neuraminidase inhibitors such as zanamivir and oseltamivir are effective against both influenza A and B viruses. A killed vaccine containing current circulating A and B strains prevents disease in susceptible at-risk individuals.

| **Organ systems and disease involvement** | Diagnosis and control, 504; general, 30-31, 32; host-parasite relationship, 172, 173; lower respiratory tract infection, 226-230; microbes as parasites, 10; vaccination, 533 |

PAPOVAVIRUSES These include papillomaviruses, JC and BK viruses.

Characteristics	**Virus family**	**Type**	**Envelope**	**Shape**	**Size (nm)**	**Nucleocapsid**
	Papovaviridae	dsDNA	–	Icosahedral	45–55	Icosahedral (circular)

Replication
Virus attaches via unknown receptor to epithelial cell; viral mRNA is transcribed in the nucleus by a cellular transcriptase; early gene products initiate viral DNA replication, transcription, transformation; late gene products are structural proteins. Of the early genes, T and t antigens are expressed in transformed cells. The Papovaviridae include papillomaviruses, polyomaviruses and simian vacuolating viruses (e.g. SV40), with at least 75 types of human papillomavirus genotypes and two polyomaviruses (BK and JC viruses). These viruses persist in latent form and can reactivate.

Diseases
Papillomaviruses cause warts on skin and genital regions. Sexually transmitted warts are strongly associated with carcinoma of cervix, HPV16 and HPV18, carcinoma of penis, vulva, rectum, and can cause laryngeal papilloma in children (infected via birth canal). Polyomaviruses on primary infection cause mild upper respiratory illness. In immunocompromised patients, JC virus causes progressive multifocal leukoencephalopathy (PML), and BK virus is excreted in urine and can cause nephropathy, in particular hematuria.

Transmission
Papillomaviruses: from skin to skin by direct or indirect contact, and between mucosae by sexual intercourse. Polyomaviruses: from the upper respiratory tract by droplets and perhaps by contact with infected urine.

Pathogenesis
Papillomavirus infection of epithelial cells and local multiplication results in a wart after an incubation period of up to 1–2 months. The wart regresses over the course of many months; there is no spread to deeper tissues, but viral DNA remains in basal epithelial cells and can reactivate. When genital warts undergo malignant change, viral genome remains in cell; cofactors are involved. Polyomaviruses spread from the upper respiratory tract and localize in tubular epithelium in the kidney (excretion in urine) or in oligodendrocytes to cause PML.

Laboratory identification
Serologic methods are unsatisfactory. Vacuolated or inclusion-bearing cells (koilocytosis) seen on Papanicolaou staining; virus particles visible (urine or tissues) by electron microscopy. Virus culture either difficult (polyomaviruses) or impossible (papillomaviruses). In specialist laboratories, tests for the viral antigens or viral DNA sequences, including in situ hybridization and PCR, can be carried out.

Treatment and prevention
No effective antivirals or vaccines available. Skin warts can be destroyed by freezing (liquid nitrogen) and areas of cervical dysplasia (genital warts) by laser treatment. Many slower methods are used (podophyllin, salicylic acid). Preventive measures include shoes for plantar warts and condoms for genital warts.

Organ systems and disease involvement
General, 34; immunocompromised host, 436; infection of skin, soft tissue, muscle and associated systems, 367-368; pathological consequences, 196; sexually transmitted disease, 264

PARAMYXOVIRUSES These include measles, mumps, respiratory syncytial virus (RSV), human metapneumovirus, Nipah virus and Hendra virus.

Characteristics	**Virus family**	**Type**	**Envelope**	**Shape**	**Size (nm)**	**Nucleocapsid**
	Paramyxoviridae	ssRNA, non-segmented, –ve sense	+	Pleomorphic	120–250	Helical

Envelope glycoproteins are H (hemagglutinin), N (neuraminidase), F (fusion), and G. H and N are combined (HN) in paramyxoviruses (mumps, parainfluenza 1–4), morbillivirus (measles) has H, and pneumovirus (RSV) has G (no H or N).

Replication Virus particle binds via its attachment protein (HN, H or G) to cell surface, penetrates and is uncoated. Viral polymerase transcribes genome into mRNAs, which are translated into viral proteins. Nucleocapsid is assembled and matrix protein joins it to the envelope proteins forming on the plasma membrane of the infected cell. Release then occurs by budding.

Diseases Measles: fever, nasal discharge, rash (very rarely encephalitis, subacute sclerosing panencephalitis); incubation period 10–14 days. Mumps: parotitis, aseptic meningitis (rarely orchitis, encephalitis); incubation period 18–24 days. Parainfluenza viruses: common cold; bronchiolitis, pneumonia; incubation period 3–6 days. RSV: common cold (adults), bronchiolitis, pneumonia (infants); incubation period 2–8 days. Metapneumovirus: mild upper respiratory tract disease, severe bronchiolitis and pneumonia in children. Nipah virus: encephalitis or pneumonia. Hendra virus: pneumonia and encephalitis.

Transmission Respiratory droplets. Contact with body fluids of infected animals, including urine and feces, for Nipah and Hendra viruses.

Pathogenesis Initial infection via respiratory tract. RSV and parainfluenza virus infections: local replication and disease. Measles and mumps: no lesions at site of initial infection, spread to local lymph nodes, blood and invasion of skin and mucosa (measles) or salivary glands, CNS (mumps). Zoonotic infection: contact with infected animals' body fluids (Hendra, Nipah).

Laboratory identification Virus isolation in cell culture. Demonstration of viral antigen by immunofluorescence in nasopharyngeal aspirates (RSV, parainfluenza) or viral RNA detection by PCR. Serology: measles and mumps IgM and IgG; complement-fixing tests for RSV.

Treatment and prevention Aerosolized ribavirin for infants and highly immunocompromised individuals with severe RSV infections, and symptomatic highly immunocompromised individuals with parainfluenza infection. Measles and mumps prevented by live attenuated virus vaccines. No vaccines in routine use for RSV and parainfluenza viruses.

 Organ systems and disease involvement General, 501; central nervous system (CNS), 333-335; infection of skin, soft tissue, muscle and associated systems, 374-375; lower respiratory tract infection, 219-220, 225, 226, 231; upper respiratory tract infection, 210-212, 214; vaccination, 525, 527, 528, 529-530

PARVOVIRUS

Characteristics	**Virus family**	**Type**	**Envelope**	**Shape**	**Size (nm)**	**Nucleocapsid**
	Parvoviridae	ssDNA	–	Icosahedral	18–26	Icosahedral

The family includes human parvovirus B19 (single serotype), and the adeno-associated viruses. The latter are defective, requiring concurrent infection of the cell with 'helper' adenovirus or herpes virus; positive DNA strands and negative DNA strands are carried in separate particles. The former are autonomous, but require mitotically active cells.

Replication	Occurs in the nucleus. Viral DNA replication takes place only when cell DNA replication is occurring (i.e. during the S phase of the cell cycle). Cellular transcriptase forms a cDNA strand to give dsDNA, and transcripts produce mRNAs.
Diseases	B19 parvovirus causes a mild disease, erythema infectiosum, in children, with a 'slapped cheek' rash. Aplastic crisis may occur in those with sickle cell anemia. Arthropathy is common in infected adults. Intrauterine infection may result in fetal death with hydrops fetalis. The adeno-associated viruses are not known to cause disease.
Transmission	Via respiratory droplets.
Pathogenesis	Virus spreads from respiratory tract and can infect hemopoietic cells in bone marrow.
Laboratory identification	Detection of parvovirus-specific IgM antibody or viral DNA.
Treatment and prevention	There is no specific antiviral treatment and no vaccine, although the parvovirus B19 host cell receptor has been identified. Supportive measures include fetal exchange transfusion in hydrops fetalis and using human intravenous immunoglobulin, which contains B19 IgG, to damp down viral replication in infected immunosuppressed patients with recurrent episodes of anemia.
Organ systems and disease involvement	General, 372

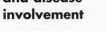

PICORNAVIRUSES These include enteroviruses, coxsackieviruses, echoviruses, polioviruses and hepatitis A virus.

Characteristics	**Virus family**	**Type**	**Envelope**	**Shape**	**Size (nm)**	**Nucleocapsid**
	Picornaviridae	ssRNA +ve sense	–	Icosahedral	25–30	Icosahedral

	Hepatitis A is the only member of the *Hepatovirus* genus of this family and is distinct from the other picornaviruses.
Replication	Virus binds to cell via receptor molecule intercellular adhesion molecule-1 (ICAM-1), resulting in endocytosis and uncoating. The positive sense viral ssRNA acts as mRNA, which is translated into a single polyprotein, cleaved by virus-coded protease into separate proteins. These include the RNA polymerase that makes negative-strand cRNA, which in turn acts as template for positive strands of viral RNA. RNA and capsid proteins assemble in the cytoplasm to form nucleocapsids, which are released on death of the cell. General features: four viral capsid proteins (VP1–VP4). There is no envelope.
Diseases	Rhinoviruses: more than 100 serotypes; common cold viruses.
	Enteroviruses:
	• Polioviruses, types 1–3: aseptic meningitis, paralytic poliomyelitis.
	• Echoviruses (enterocytopathic human orphan viruses): 32 types; aseptic meningitis, rashes.
	• Coxsackieviruses: 29 types; aseptic meningitis, herpangina, myopericarditis (coxsackievirus B).
	• Enteroviruses 68–71: conjunctivitis (enterovirus 70), polio-like illness (enterovirus 71)
	• Hepatitis A virus: hepatitis
Transmission	Respiratory droplet spread for rhinoviruses and certain group A coxsackieviruses. Other enteroviruses and hepatitis A spread by the fecal–oral route.
Pathogenesis	Rhinoviruses (acid-labile, optimal growth 33°C) replicate in upper respiratory tract. Enteroviruses (resist pH 3.0–9.0) replicate in pharynx and gastrointestinal tract, often with spread to lymph nodes and blood, and then to CNS (e.g. polio, echoviruses), heart and muscle (coxsackie B), or liver (hepatitis A).

Laboratory identification	Hepatitis A IgM detection. The rest of the picornavirus diagnoses involve virus isolation in cell culture from a range of samples and viral RNA detection by PCR. Serology of limited use because of multiple serotypes, mostly IgM tests.					

Treatment and prevention

No specific treatment. Poliomyelitis prevented by vaccination with live attenuated (Sabin) or killed (Salk) vaccine. Hepatitis A prevented by human normal immunoglobulin which contains hepatitis A IgG or inactivated virus vaccine. No vaccines for other picornaviruses.

Organ systems and disease involvement

Central nervous system (CNS), 332-333; diagnosis and control, 541; gastrointestinal tract infections, 303-304; host-parasite relationship, 172; infection of skin, soft tissue, muscle and associated systems, 372, 377; sexually transmitted disease, 273; upper respiratory tract infection, 201-202; vaccination, 516, 530-531, 532

POXVIRUSES

Characteristics	*Virus family*	*Type*	*Envelope*	*Shape*	*Size (nm)*	*Nucleocapsid*
	Poxviridae	dsDNA	+/–	Brick or ovoid	250 x 300	Complex structure

The largest viruses; dermatotrophic, causing 'pocks' on the skin.

Replication

Takes place in the cytoplasm (unlike other DNA viruses) and viral DNA-dependent RNA polymerase is used to synthesize mRNA. Transcripts are translated directly into proteins, some of which undergo post-translational cleavage to give functional molecules. After assembly, infectious virions are released as the cell disintegrates, some of them acquiring an envelope in the Golgi complex.

Diseases

Molluscum contagiosum causes a mild infection with nodular skin lesions. Cowpox or milkers' nodules virus lesions on cow udders can cause vesicular lesions on the skin of milkers. Orf virus is responsible for contagious pustular dermatitis in sheep, and those in contact with infected animals may develop vesicular skin lesions. After exposure to monkeys infected with monkeypox virus (monkeys are a favorite food in some parts of the Ivory Coast), humans develop a smallpox-like disease, which is distinguishable from smallpox by laboratory tests. Smallpox was eradicated in late 1979.

Transmission

By direct contact with virus from skin lesions. Molluscum contagiosum is transmitted between humans, but monkeypox, cowpox, orf, and milkers' nodules viruses are zoonoses, transmissible from the animal host to humans.

Pathogenesis

Infection generally initiated in skin with local replication to form virus-rich vesicles; limited spread to local lymph nodes. Smallpox infection was via the respiratory tract, and spread via blood to cause severe disease with disseminated skin and mucosal lesions.

Laboratory identification

Characteristic poxvirus particles are seen on electron microscopic examination of scrapings or biopsies of skin lesions. Cell culture methods for virus isolation, antibody tests, and DNA detection methods are not available routinely.

Treatment and prevention

In the past methisazone was used to treat the serious side effects very occasionally caused by vaccination against smallpox with live vaccinia virus. Vaccination was the principal method used to eradicate smallpox. Vaccinia was the first virus to be used as an expression vector for live recombinant vaccines.

Organ systems and disease involvement

Infection of skin, soft tissue, muscle and associated systems, 373; vaccination, 516

REOVIRUSES These include rotaviruses and Colorado tick fever virus.

Characteristics	Virus family	Type	Envelope	Shape	Size (nm)	Nucleocapsid
	Reoviridae	dsRNA, 10 (reo) or 11 (rota) segments	–	Icosahedral	75	Icosahedral (double layered)

Replication
Virion resists acid pH, drying, detergents. Host protease in intestinal phagolysosome cleaves outer capsid protein to produce a fully infectious particle, which binds to cell membrane via receptor. Core enters cytoplasm, viral RNA-dependent RNA polymerase (one molecule for each genome segment) synthesizes 10–11 mRNAs (not polyadenylated), which direct synthesis of proteins, one of which is an RNA polymerase. The latter produces negative strand viral RNA; positive strands are formed, and the assembled virus is released by cell lysis.

Diseases
Orthoreovirus (three types): few if any symptoms; the word reovirus derives from respiratory enteric orphan virus (orphan because initially not associated with any disease). Rotaviruses (types A–D): diarrheal illness, especially in infancy and childhood, and sometimes respiratory symptoms. Colorado tick fever virus endemic in the Rocky Mountains (orbivirus group): acute febrile illness, leukopenia, gastrointestinal and neurological symptoms, rash and, rarely, severe hemorrhagic disease.

Transmission
Orthoreoviruses: fecal–oral and possibly respiratory spread. Rotaviruses: fecal–oral spread (virus survives drying and stomach acid). Colorado tick fever virus: by bite of an infected tick, mostly rodent reservoir.

Pathogenesis
Orthoreoviruses: entry via respiratory or gastrointestinal tract (M cells) and spread to local lymphoid tissue. Rotaviruses: infection of enterocytes with no spread to deeper tissues; causes gastrointestinal illness with shortening and flattening of villi and interference with transport mechanisms. Colorado tick fever: virus enters skin via tick bite, spreads to local lymph nodes and blood, infects erythrocytes, and causes febrile illness.

Laboratory identification
Virus particles in feces by electron microscopy, viral antigen detection by ELISA or viral RNA. Detection of viral antigens on erythrocytes by immunofluorescence or specific IgM (Colorado tick fever). Virus isolation not generally used.

Treatment and prevention
No antiviral agents routinely available. Rotavirus diarrhea is treated supportively by replacing water and electrolytes. Cross infection prevented by improved hygiene. Live attenuated rotavirus vaccine. Anti-tick measures protect against Colorado tick fever.

Organ systems and disease involvement
Gastrointestinal tract infections, 290-292; vaccination, 534-535

RETROVIRUSES These include HIV-1, HIV-2, HTLV-1 and HTLV-2.

Characteristics	Virus family	Type	Envelope	Shape	Size (nm)	Nucleocapsid
	Retroviridae	ssRNA diploid +ve sense	+	Spherical	80–120	Icosahedral

Family includes HIV-1,HIV-2 (lentiviruses); HTLV-1, HTLV-2 (oncoviruses); human foamy virus (spumavirus), which causes foamy change in cells, but little else known; endogenous retroviruses, which exist as sequences in human genome.

Replication
HIV: binds to CD4 cell surface receptor and chemokine coreceptors, enters and is uncoated. Virion RNA-dependent DNA polymerase (reverse transcriptase) transcribes

viral genome into dsDNA (provirus), which is then integrated into host cell DNA by viral integrase. Transcription is by host RNA polymerase; genomic and viral mRNA are formed, and translated into structural and regulatory proteins. Viral genes *gag*, *pol*, *env* code for structural proteins, and other gene products have regulatory functions. Nucleocapsids assemble in cytoplasm and are released by budding.

Diseases

HIV: mild early illness with mononucleosis; sometimes aseptic meningitis; later (1) often after many years progressing to AIDS, with multiple opportunistic infections, Kaposi's sarcoma, (2) HIV-specific CNS disease (AIDS neuropathy, AIDS-related dementia), (3) intestinal syndrome, with diarrhea, weight loss ('slim' disease in Africa). HTLV-1: tropical spastic paraparesis, T cell leukemia. HTLV-2: neurological disease.

Transmission

HIV: via blood, semen, transplacental transfer. HIV-1 worldwide, HIV-2 mainly West Africa. HTLV-1: via milk and blood; occurs in certain islands in Caribbean and Japan, and in parts of South America, Africa. HTLV-2: via blood.

Pathogenesis

HIV: initial entry via mucosal route with infection of CD4-positive cells (helper T cells, dendritic cells, monocytes, macrophages). Spread through body including CNS, placenta. Action on immune cells results in severe immunosuppression leading to opportunist infections and reactivations (viral, bacterial, protozoal). Also Kaposi's sarcoma associated with presence of HHV8. HTLV-1: pathogenesis of CNS disease not clear. Leukemia (mean 30 years after infection) results from multistage process initiated by *tat* gene product in infected T cells stimulating transcription of host genes that control cell division.

Laboratory identification

HIV: combination assays detect antibodies and p24 antigen with type differentiation by immunoblot. HIV-1 RNA load assays to monitor disease progression and treatment responses. HIV-1 proviral DNA qualitative detection. Genotypic antiretroviral resistance tests. HTLV-1 and -2 antibody tests with type differentiation by immunoblot.

Treatment and prevention

HIV: various classes of drug inhibit virus replication and arrest disease progress without eliminating virus from body (viral DNA transcripts remain in infected cells). These are nucleoside, nucleotide, and non-nucleoside reverse transcriptase inhibitors (e.g. zidovudine, tenofovir and nevirapine, respectively), protease inhibitors (e.g. nelfinavir) and fusion inhibitors. Treatment of opportunist infections. Various vaccines are undergoing clinical trials. Prevention by avoiding bloodborne virus (e.g. needle exchange programs, treatment of blood and blood products) and practicing safe sex (e.g. education, condoms). HTLV-1 and -2: antiretroviral drug regimens under investigation.

Organ systems and disease involvement

Central nervous system (CNS), 336-337; congenital disease, 318; diagnosis and control, 450, 503; general, 32, 34-35; host-parasite relationship, 135, 137, 148, 154, 170, 173-174; immunocompromised host, 431; infection of skin, soft tissue, muscle and associated systems, 380; pathological consequences, 194; sexually transmitted disease, 264-273; vaccination, 522, 536

RHABDOVIRUS Rabies virus.

Characteristics

	Virus family	Type	Envelope	Shape	Size (nm)	Nucleocapsid
	Rhabdoviridae	ssRNA –ve sense	+	Bullet	180 x 75	Helical

Replication

Viral G protein attaches to acetylcholine receptor or other molecules on cell; virus is endocytosed and uncoated. Virion RNA polymerase synthesizes five mRNAs, and virus-coded RNA polymerase replicates viral RNA. After assembly of nucleocapsid the envelope is acquired by budding from the plasma membrane without detectable cell damage. Rabies virus can infect all mammals. Present in wild animals in all continents except Australia and Antarctica. Only one serotype.

Diseases	Incubation period 2–10 weeks. CNS symptoms and signs (excitement, confusion, lethargy, hydrophobia), progression to seizures, paralysis, coma and death.
Transmission	Via bite of infected dog, cat, skunk, raccoon, bat. Human-to-human transmission not a feature.
Pathogenesis	Virus replicates at site of bite, ascends axons to CNS where it spreads, and then descends down peripheral nerves to skin, salivary glands.
Laboratory identification	Brain tissue (at autopsy), corneal scrapings, biopsy of hair-bearing skin, examined for presence of inclusions (Negri bodies), rabies antigen by immunofluorescence, and viral RNA detection by PCR.
Treatment and prevention	No specific treatment. Post-exposure prophylaxis by washing wound, giving human rabies-specific immunoglobulin and vaccine. Disease prevented by inactivated vaccine produced in human diploid cells.
Organ systems and disease involvement	Central nervous system (CNS), 335-336; general, 32; host-parasite relationship, 161; vaccination, 532

TOGAVIRUSES These include rubella, Chikungunya, O'nyong-nyong, Ross River, Eastern and Western encephalitis viruses.

Characteristics	Virus family	Type	Envelope	Shape	Size (nm)	Nucleocapsid
	Togaviridae	ssRNA +ve sense	+	Spherical	60–70	Icosahedral

Human togaviruses include the non-arthropod-borne rubella virus (genus *Rubivirus*), and the arboviruses of the *Alphavirus* genus. The latter occur in all parts of the world, often have exotic names (Kyasanur Forest disease virus, India; Omsk hemorrhagic fever virus, Russia), and replicate in the arthropod vector as well as in the vertebrate host. Most have animal reservoirs. The alphaviruses include Western equine encephalomyelitis (WEE), Eastern equine encephalomyelitis (EEE), Ross River virus.

Replication	The positive strand RNA is translated into structural and non-structural proteins, the latter including the RNA-dependent RNA polymerase, which replicates the viral genome by directing the formation of a negative strand template and thus giving rise to positive strand progeny. Full length and subgenomic length RNA is formed. After assembly, the virus exits from the cell, budding from the plasma membrane.
Diseases	Rubella causes a mild rash. In adults it may be complicated by arthralgia, and a primary infection in pregnancy can result in fetal infection and congenital malformations. The remaining togaviruses cause febrile illnesses, which may be severe when there is involvement of the CNS (equine encephalitides).
Transmission	Rubella is transmitted between humans by respiratory droplets; the rest are transmitted by the bite of infected arthropods.
Pathogenesis	Initial infection via respiratory tract (rubella) or skin (arthropod-borne viruses) causes no detectable local lesion. Virus spreads to local lymph nodes and blood, multiplying in respiratory tract, placenta and fetus (rubella) or CNS (equine encephalitides). Mononuclear cells often infected (rubella). In mosquitoes, ingested virus infects gut epithelium, spreads to salivary glands, and multiplies there.
Laboratory identification	Rubella-specific IgM antibody indicates recent infection. Serological methods, viral RNA detection by PCR and to a lesser extent virus isolation are used to diagnose the arthropod-borne togavirus infections.

Treatment and prevention	There is no antiviral therapy. A live attenuated virus vaccine prevents rubella and, as a result, congenital rubella. Vaccines are not available for the other arthropod-transmitted togaviruses, but horses can be protected from WEE and EEE with veterinary vaccines.
Organteam systems and disease involvement	General, 315-316; central nervous system (CNS), 336; host-parasite relationship, 171; infection of skin, soft tissue, muscle and associated systems, 375-376; vaccination, 525, 526, 527, 529-530

HUMAN PRION DISEASES

Characteristics	Not viruses. Etiological agents of the four human prion diseases share the same general features. The diseases are Creutzfeldt–Jakob disease (CJD), kuru, Gerstmann–Straussler–Scheinker syndrome (GSS) and fatal familial insomnia (FFI). The prototype agent, scrapie, causes CNS disease in sheep. Structure and mode of replication unknown. Contain little or no nucleic acid. Host-coded prion (proteinaceous infectious particle) protein in slightly altered form (protease-resistant) is closely associated with infectivity. Highly resistant to heat (special autoclaving procedures required for destruction), chemical agents and irradiation. Very slow replication, very long incubation period (up to 20 years in humans). Infect a variety of mammals and can be transmitted to cows, mink, cats and mice for example when food contains infected material.
Diseases	'Spongiform encephalopathies', 'prion diseases'. Kuru: fatal neurologic diseases in Papua New Guinea, no longer seen. CJD: rare chronic encephalopathy, occurs worldwide; 10% cases familial with mutated prion protein gene. GSS and FFI.
Transmission	Kuru: from infected human brain by cannabalism. CJD: in most cases unknown; occasionally transmitted from infected human brain by medical and surgical procedures; familial cases genetically transmitted. Variant CJD (vCJD) from consumption of BSE (bovine spongiform encephalopathy) infected food.
Pathogenesis	Infectious agent replicates inexorably in lymphoid tissues, and then in brain cells, where it produces intracellular vacuoles and deposition of altered host prion protein. Uniformly fatal if host lives long enough.
Laboratory identification	Intracellular vacuoles (spongiform change) visible histologically in brain. Altered prion protein detectable in brain, but test not routinely available. Isolation of agent requires experimental animals and is lengthy, difficult and not undertaken. No specific immune responses.
Treatment and prevention	No treatment or vaccine. Kuru died out when cannibalism ceased. Iatrogenic transfer of CJD preventable (e.g. when genetically engineered growth hormone became available).
Organ systems and disease involvement	General, 53-55, 337-338; host-parasite relationship, 64

BACTERIA

GRAM-POSITIVE COCCI

GENUS STAPHYLOCOCCUS

Genus contains at least 16 different species, of which three are of greatest medical importance: *Staph. aureus, Staph. epidermidis, Staph. saprophyticus.*

MAJOR DISTINGUISHING FEATURES OF MEDICALLY IMPORTANT STAPHYLOCOCCI

Test	*Staph. aureus*	*Staph. epidermidis*	*Staph. saprophyticus*
Coagulase production*	+	–	–
Protein A on cell surface	+	–	–
Production of recognized exotoxins	+	–	–
Hemolysin production	+**	–**	+
Resistance to novobiocin (5 µg)	†	–	+

* Note that the coagulase-negative species *Staph. epidermidis* and *Staph. saprophyticus* and other less commonly isolated coagulase-negative species (e.g. *Staph. capitis* and *Staph. haemolyticus*) are often referred to simply as 'coagulase-negative staphylococci' without further identification.

** Usual result, but not for all strains.

† Useful for distinguishing between *Staph. epidermidis* and *Staph. saprophyticus.*

STAPHYLOCOCCUS AUREUS

Characteristics
Gram-positive coccus; cells in clusters (reflecting ability to divide in more than one plane); individual cells approximately 1 µm in diameter. Some strains produce capsules. Non-fastidious; capable of aerobic and anaerobic respiration.

Laboratory identification
White or golden colonies on blood agar. Catalase positive, coagulase positive; most strains ferment mannitol anaerobically. Kits available for biochemical characterization.

Diseases
Boils; skin sepsis; postoperative wound infection; scalded skin syndrome; catheter associated infection; foodborne infection; septicemia, endocarditis; toxic shock syndrome; osteomyelitis; pneumonia.

Transmission
Normal habitat: humans (and animals associated with them); skin, especially nose and perineum (carriage rates higher in hospital patients and staff). Spread is by contact and airborne routes. Organism survives drying; tolerant of salt and nitrites.

Epidemiologic analysis
Pulsed-field gel electrophoresis and other molecular techniques have largely replaced bacteriophage typing.

Pathogenesis
Virulence multifactorial, and most factors shown below are present in some strains.
Present in all strains:
- mucopeptide;
- coagulase.

Present in some strains:
- cell-associated—capsule, protein A, fibronectin-binding protein, collagen-binding proteins;
- extracellular products—enterotoxins, epidermolytic toxin, toxic shock syndrome toxin, membrane-damaging toxins (hemolysins), leukocidin, staphylokinase;
- Many strains have protein A bound to the mucopeptide of the cell wall. This protein interacts non-specifically with host IgG antibodies reducing opsonization and causing local activation of complement.

Treatment and prevention	Antibiotics of choice are beta-lactamase-stable penicillins; however, over 80% of hospital isolates are beta-lactamase producers. Multiple drug resistance (including methicillin and tolerance or resistance to vancomycin) is a worldwide problem. Mupirocin can be used for topical treatment of carriage. Prevention of spread by isolation and/or treatment of carriers in high-risk areas in hospital. No vaccine available.
Organ systems and disease involvement	Diagnosis and control, 475, 479, 484, 490, 546, 548, 550, 554; gastrointestinal tract infections, 292; immunocompromised host, 427-428; infection of skin, soft tissue, muscle and associated systems, 350-352; microbes as parasites, 17, 18

STAPHYLOCOCCUS EPIDERMIDIS

Characteristics	As for *Staph. aureus*.
Laboratory identification	White colonies on blood agar; catalase positive, coagulase negative, mannitol not fermented anaerobically. Kits available for biochemical characterization.
Diseases	Opportunist pathogen associated with device-related sepsis (e.g. catheter-related sepsis; prosthetic valve endocarditis; infection of artificial joints; shunt infections); urinary tract infection; sternal wound osteomyelitis.
Transmission	Normal habitat: skin (carriage rate approximately 100%). Spread by contact with self, other patients or hospital personnel. Almost all infections acquired in hospital, but may be endogenous. Survives drying; salt tolerant.
Epidemiologic analysis	Pulsed-field gel electrophoresis and other molecular techniques have largely replaced bacteriophage typing.
Pathogenesis	Extracellular slime production may be a marker of virulence and aid in the colonization of plastic implants (e.g. intravenous catheters and prostheses).
Treatment and prevention	Antibiotic resistance: often multiresistant (including penicillin and methicillin). Prevention of infection: catheter care; no vaccine available.
Organ systems and disease involvement	Diagnosis and control, 479, 484; immunocompromised host, 428

STAPHYLOCOCCUS SAPROPHYTICUS

Characteristics	As for *Staph. aureus*.
Laboratory identification	White colonies on blood agar; catalase negative, coagulase negative, mannitol not fermented anaerobically. Kits available for biochemical characterization.
Diseases	Urinary tract infection in previously healthy women (associated with intercourse).
Transmission	Normal habitat: skin and genitourinary mucosa. Endogenous spread to urinary tract in colonized women.
Epidemiologic analysis	Pulsed-field gel electrophoresis and other molecular techniques.
Pathogenesis	Virulence factors unknown, but organism has the ability to colonize periurethral skin and mucosa.
Treatment and prevention	Urination after intercourse helps to wash organisms out of the bladder and prevent infection.

| **Organ systems and disease involvement** | Urinary tract infection (UTI), 241 |

GENUS STREPTOCOCCUS

A large group of Gram-positive cocci distributed widely in man and animals, mostly forming part of the normal flora, but some species responsible for some major infections. Individual cells 0.5–1 µm diameter and, because they divide in one plane only, occur in pairs and chains. The medically significant streptococci may be conveniently divided on the basis of either hemolysis on blood agar (complete hemolysis, beta; partial hemolysis, alpha; no hemolysis, gamma) or by the presence or absence of a group-specific carbohydrate antigen (i.e. the Lancefield Group labeled alphabetically A to V).

BETA-HEMOLYTIC STREPTOCOCCI

STREPTOCOCCUS PYOGENES (GROUP A STREPTOCOCCUS)

Characteristics
Gram-positive cocci in chains, cells less than 1 µm diameter, non-motile, non-spore-forming.

Laboratory identification
Grown on blood agar. Pronounced hemolytic activity (enhanced anaerobically). Catalase negative. Bacitracin (0.04 units); all strains are susceptible; detection of group-specific carbohydrate; detection of L-pyrrolidonyl arylamidase (PYR)

Diseases
Infections of upper respiratory tract and of skin and soft tissue (e.g. pharyngitis, cellulitis, erysipelas, lymphadenitis). Toxic manifestations include scarlet fever. Non-suppurative sequelae (acute glomerulonephritis and rheumatic fever) are important complications of both skin and throat infections.

Transmission
Normal habitat is the human upper respiratory tract and skin. Spread by airborne droplets and by contact. Survival in dust may be important. Epidemiologic typing of strains (see below) useful in outbreaks.

Epidemiologic analysis
Acid extraction of antigen from cell wall reacting with specific antisera (rabbit) either in a grouping precipitin or latex agglutination reaction. In addition to this group-specific polysaccharide, type-specific M and T antigens can be detected and are used as a typing scheme for epidemiologic purposes. Pulsed-field gel electrophoresis and other molecular techniques are also helpful for epidemiologic analysis.

Pathogenesis
Strep. pyogenes elaborates many enzymes and exotoxins, which may play a role in infection: erythrogenic toxin (lysogenic phage mediated); streptolysins; streptokinase A and B (therapeutic applications); deoxyribonuclease; hyaluronidase ('spreading factor').

Treatment and prevention
Penicillin is drug of choice. Vaccines not available. Erythromycin is an alternative for penicillin-allergic patients, but resistance to erythromycin is increasing.

Organ systems and disease involvement
Diagnosis and control, 548, 554, 589; immunocompromised host, 427; infection of skin, soft tissue, muscle and associated systems, 352-354; upper respiratory tract infection, 209-210

STREPTOCOCCUS AGALACTIAE (GROUP B STREPTOCOCCI)

Characteristics	Gram-positive cocci in chains.
Laboratory identification	Beta-hemolytic on blood agar; colonies larger than *Strep. pyogenes* frequently pigmented after anaerobic incubation on Columbia agar (Islam's medium). Grow in the presence of bile on MacConkey agar. Biochemical tests include hippurate hydrolysis (positive), aesculin hydrolysis (negative). Possess Group B Lancefield capsular antigen. Group-specific carbohydrate and commercially available molecular probes for definitive identification. Positive CAMP (Christie, Atkins, Munch-Peterson) test.
Diseases	Neonatal meningitis and septicemia. Mastitis in bovines.
Transmission	Normal habitat; gut and vagina. Babies acquire organism from colonized mother at birth or by contact spread between babies in nursery after birth.
Pathogenesis	Virulence factors not clearly identified.
Treatment and prevention	Susceptible to penicillin, but less so than *Strep. pyogenes*; combination of penicillin and gentamicin for serious infections. Screening pregnant women recommended; prophylactic antibiotics may be given to babies (especially premature) of carriers.
Organ systems and disease involvement	Central nervous system (CNS), 241

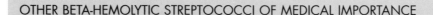

OTHER BETA-HEMOLYTIC STREPTOCOCCI OF MEDICAL IMPORTANCE

Streptococci of Lancefield Groups C and G may sometimes cause pharyngitis. Group D streptococci are now reclassified in the genus *Enterococcus* (see below).

STREPTOCOCCUS MILLERI GROUP

Microaerophilic streptococci that often form small colonies and carry Lancefield Group A, C, F or G antigens. Have a propensity for abscess formation (especially in liver and brain).

ALPHA-HEMOLYTIC STREPTOCOCCI

STREPTOCOCCUS PNEUMONIAE

Characteristics	Gram-positive coccus characteristically appearing in pairs (diplococci) in Gram films. Cells approximately 1 μm diameter, often capsulate. Requires blood or serum for growth. Capable of aerobic and anaerobic respiration; growth may be enhanced in CO_2.
Laboratory identification	On blood agar alpha-hemolytic 'draughtsman' colonies that may autolyse within 48 h at 35°C. Catalase negative. Susceptible to bile (bile solubility test) and optochin (ethyl hydrocuprein hydrochloride; available in paper disks). Polysaccharide capsules can be demonstrated by appropriate staining techniques. They are antigenic and in the presence of specific antiserum appear to swell (quellung reaction).
Diseases	Pneumonia, septicemia and meningitis. Otitis and related infections in children. Capsular type III frequently associated with pneumonia.
Transmission	Normal habitat is the human respiratory tract; ca. 5% of population may carry in small numbers. Transmission via droplet spread.

Pathogenesis	Capsule protects the organism from phagocytosis. Pneumolysin may have a role as a virulence factor, but to date no known exotoxins. Splenectomy may predispose to infection. Viral infection may be a precursor to pneumonia.
Treatment and prevention	Penicillin remains the antibiotic of choice, but resistance is increasing rapidly, and susceptibility test results should be used to guide therapy. Vaccine available.
Organ systems and disease involvement	Central nervous system (CNS), 328-329; host-parasite relationship, 151; lower respiratory tract infection, 220; microbes as parasites, 12; upper respiratory tract infection, 212-213; vaccination, 533-534

ORAL STREPTOCOCCI

There are several other species of alpha-hemolytic streptococci that in the past have been lumped together under the colloquial heading 'viridans streptococci'. These and some of the non-hemolytic streptococci have now been reclassified. Most species are commensals in the mouth. *Strep. mutans* is strongly associated with dental caries. Several species are capable of causing bacterial endocarditis. Most strains are susceptible to penicillin; however, moderate to high resistance has also been observed. Moderately resistant isolates may be treated with penicillin plus an aminoglycoside while highly resistant strains require a broad spectrum cephalosporin or vancomycin. It is important to distinguish these streptococci from *Strep. pneumoniae* in cultures from the respiratory tract.

GENUS ENTEROCOCCUS (FECAL STREPTOCOCCI)

	Formerly classified in the genus *Streptococcus*, with which they share many characteristics; there are currently 16 species of enterococci. *E. faecalis* and *E. faecium* are the most important clinically and are considered together.
Characteristics	Gram-positive cocci, cells often in pairs and chains; more ovate appearance than streptococci. Non-fastidious; capable of aerobic and anaerobic respiration.
Laboratory identification	On blood agar may produce alpha, beta or no hemolysis. Resistant to 40% bile salts and optochin; relatively heat tolerant (grow at 45°C), and salt tolerant (grow in 6.5% NaCl); hydrolyze esculin. Kits available for biochemical identification. Carry Lancefield's Group D antigen, but extraction of the antigen is more difficult than with streptococci (it is teichoic acid rather than polysaccharide).
Diseases	Urinary tract infection; endocarditis; infrequent, but severe septicemia after surgery and in the immunocompromised.
Transmission	Normal habitat is the gut of humans and animals. Most infections thought to be endogenously acquired, but cross-infection may occur in hospitalized patients.
Pathogenesis	No toxins or other virulence factors convincingly demonstrated. Plasmid-mediated hemolysin may play a role.
Treatment and prevention	Penicillins used in combination with aminoglycosides. Resistant to cephalosporins, and incidence of resistance to vancomycin is a problem. Some fluoroquinolones, linezolid and quinupristin/dalfopristin may be used in treatment. Patients with known heart defects should be given prophylactic antibiotics to prevent endocarditis before dentistry or surgery on gut or urinary tract.
Organ systems and disease involvement	Diagnosis and control, 481, 491

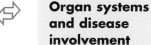

GRAM-POSITIVE RODS

GENUS CORYNEBACTERIUM

This genus contains many species, is widely distributed in nature, and is part of a spectrum, with *Mycobacterium* and *Nocardia*, having similar cell wall structure containing mycolic acids. The species of major importance is *C. diphtheriae*. This and other pathogens within the genus need to be distinguished from commensal corynebacteria.

CORYNEBACTERIUM DIPHTHERIAE

Characteristics
Gram-positive, non-capsulate, non-sporing, non-motile rods, 2–6 μm in length. In Gram-stained films, cells arranged as 'Chinese letters' or pallisades and showing irregular staining or granule formation are characterisitic. Non-fastidious, but growth enhanced by inspissated serum (Loeffler medium). Capable of aerobic and anaerobic respiration.

Laboratory identification
Grows on blood agar, but identification aided by a selective medium (e.g. blood tellurite) on which characteristic black colonies form within 48 h at 35°C (but many other organisms may produce black colonies). Three biotypes of *C. diphtheriae* are recognized: mitis, intermedius and gravis, and they have characteristic colony morphology. *C. diphtheriae* is catalase positive and reduces nitrate. Species identification on the basis of carbohydrate fermentation tests should be performed in serum base not peptone. Toxin production has been traditionally demonstrated by the Elek test. A polymerase chain reaction (PCR) assay for the toxin gene is now available. It is important to demonstrate toxigenicity to confirm diphtheria diagnosis, but non-toxigenic strains may also be associated with disease (e.g. septicemia, endocarditis).

Diseases
Diphtheria caused by toxigenic strains of *C. diphtheriae*. Focus of infection may be the throat or the skin.

Transmission
Normal habitat: usually nasopharynx, occasionally skin of humans. Infection is usually spread by aerosol. Patients may carry toxigenic organisms for up to 2–3 months after infection.

Pathogenesis
Disease is due to production of diphtheria toxin controlled by the *tox* gene, which is integrated into the bacterial chromosome on a lysogenic phage. When concentration of exogenous inorganic iron (Fe^{3+}) is very low, exotoxin production is maximal; the selective advantage to the organism is unknown. The mode of action of the toxin is to block protein synthesis of the host cells by inactivating an elongation factor.

Treatment and prevention
Urgent supportive therapy to maintain airway essential in throat diphtheria. Antitoxin neutralizes toxin, penicillin kills organisms; antibiotics have little effect since diffusion of toxin is not influenced by inhibition of organisms at local site. In outbreak, carriers treated with penicillin or erythromycin. Immunization effective in prevention of diphtheria; in areas where immunization rates reach 85%, herd immunity sufficient to protect whole population. Circulating antibody after immunization neutralizes test dose of standardized toxin (Schick test). Positive result (i.e. skin reaction) equates with insufficient antibody. Babies acquire immunity from immune mothers for a few months.

Organ systems and disease involvement
Microbes as parasites, 17; pathological consequences, 187; upper respiratory tract infection, 214-216; vaccination, 528

OTHER CORYNEBACTERIA

C. ulcerans has been found in diphtheria-like disease. It produces two toxins, one of which is neutralized by diphtheria antitoxin, the other is similar to that produced by *C. pseudotuberculosis*. *C. jeikeium* is being isolated increasingly from blood cultures and wounds in immunosuppressed patients. It is usually detected by its relative resistance to antibiotics other than glycopeptides such as vancomycin and teicoplanin. *C. pseudotuberculosis* is a significant pathogen of horses and sheep. *C. xerosis* and *C. pseudodiphtheriticum* are skin inhabitants, and many other coryneforms may also be found on skin. These, and other related genera such as *Brevibacterium* and *Rhodococcus*, are lipophilic and require lipids for optimal growth.

GENUS BACILLUS

This genus contains more than 50 species, most of which are soil organisms. There are two species of major medical importance: *B. anthracis* and *B. cereus*.

BACILLUS ANTHRACIS

Characteristics
Large (4–10 µm) Gram-positive spore-forming encapsulated rods. Spores are formed only after the organism is shed from the body. Respires aerobically.

Laboratory identification
In smears of body fluids the capsule can be stained with polychrome methylene blue (McFadyean reaction). This is diagnostic of *B. anthracis*. The species is non-fastidious; grows well on simple media. Characteristic colonies (Medusa head) are probably related to chaining of the long rods. Non-hemolytic on horse blood agar (many of the other species are hemolytic). Growth in CO_2 encourages the formation of the capsule and smooth colonies. Biochemical reactions are unhelpful except in expert hands.

Diseases
Anthrax is a significant disease in both domesticated and wild animals. It is a zoonosis and humans are usually infected by contact with infected hides or bones. Intestinal anthrax is rare in humans. Woolsorter's disease (i.e. respiratory or inhalation anthrax) is also rare. However, the potentially lethal effect of anthrax infections has especially attracted interest as an aspect of biological warfare.

Transmission
Soil organisms: *B. anthracis* can survive in competition with other organisms for many years depending on the temperature and humidity. The carcasses of animals dying with anthrax are buried 6 feet deep to prevent organisms being carried to the surface. Humans are accidental hosts, and infection is usually acquired when spores enter abrasions on the skin or are inhaled.

Pathogenesis
The polyglutamic acid capsule is antiphagocytic. In addition an exotoxin encoded on a temperature-sensitive plasmid is produced. Toxin has three components: edema factor, lethal factor and protective antigen. Individually the components have no biologic effect, but toxicity is produced by either of the first two factors together with the antigen. The toxin acts locally in the skin and lung. Pasteur used heat attenuation to produce a virulent strain that could be used as an attenuated vaccine.

Treatment and prevention
Ciprofloxacin is the drug of choice but (depending on susceptibility) penicillin, doxycycline, erythromycin, or chloramphenicol may also be used. Prevention includes control measures such as formalin disinfection of hides, strict control of infected domestic animals, and the immunization of veterinarians and laboratory workers at risk.

Organ systems and disease involvement
 Multisystem zoonoses, 404-405

BACILLUS CEREUS

Characteristics	Large Gram-positive spore-forming rod. This and many other *Bacillus* species are similar to *B. anthracis* in many respects except most are motile and non-capsulate. Respires aerobically.
Laboratory identification	Non-fastidious. Produces hemolysis on horse and sheep blood agar. Lecithinase production and inability to utilize mannitol are used as distinguishing features on a specially designed selective medium.
Diseases	*B. cereus* causes food poisoning, the commonest association being with reheated cooked rice and pulses. Two different syndromes are recognized, due to different toxins (see below). The organism is also a rare cause of bacteremia especially in immunocompromised hosts.
Transmission	*B. cereus* spores are found on many foods, especially rice, pulses and vegetables. Infection/symptoms occur following ingestion of organisms or toxin.
Pathogenesis	Some strains produce heat-stable toxin in food associated with spore germination; this gives rise to a syndrome of vomiting within 1–5 h of ingestion. Others produce a heat-labile enterotoxin after ingestion, which causes diarrhea within 10–15 h.
Treatment and prevention	The majority of illness is short-lived and self-limiting, and antibiotic treatment is not indicated. Bacteremia in immunocompromised patients and other *B. cereus* infections should be treated promptly with gentamicin, vancomycin, ciprofloxacin, or clindamycin. As with other foodborne infections, hygienic preparation of food is paramount. Cooked food should be stored in a refrigerator and reheated thoroughly before serving.
Organ systems and disease involvement	General, 288-289

GENUS LISTERIA

These organisms were included with the genus *Corynebacterium* in earlier classifications. They also share antigenic relationships with enterococci and lactobacilli. *L. monocytogenes* is the species of major medical importance.

LISTERIA MONOCYTOGENES

Characteristics	Short Gram-positive rods, often coccobacillary in clinical material (must avoid confusion with streptococci in chains); frequently Gram variable. Motile at 25°C with a characteristic 'tumbling' movement; non-motile at 37°C.
Laboratory identification	Hemolytic on sheep or horse blood agar. Selective medium aids recovery of these organisms, especially from food samples (fish, chicken and cheeses). Cold enrichment at +4°C for several weeks is also an effective selective technique. On translucent, non-blood-containing agar, colonies appear green-blue in oblique light. Catalase-positive, nitrate reduction negative; coupled with motility at room temperature these results are useful identifying features. Biochemical and serological tests provide definitive identification.
Diseases	Meningitis and sepsis in neonates. Infections in the immunocompromised (particularly meningitis) and in pregnant women.
Transmission	Widely distributed in nature, survives well in cold. Reaches food chain via silage as well as more directly via for example vegetables. Excreted in large numbers in cows' milk. Humans may carry *Listeria* in gut as normal flora. Infection may be acquired by

ingestion or transplacentally to the baby in utero. While 13 different serotypes exist, pulsed-field gel electrophoresis and other molecular techniques are routinely used to investigate outbreaks.

Pathogenesis

Virulent strains produce internalins (cell attachment factors), hemolysins, and a motility protein; organism can survive in phagocytes.

Treatment and prevention

Treatment with penicillin or ampicillin, often in combination with gentamicin. Widespread distribution of organism in nature makes prevention of acquisition difficult. Pregnant women have been advised against eating uncooked food thought to be of particular risk (e.g. coleslaw, paté, soft cheese, unpasteurized milk).

Organ systems and disease involvement

Central nervous system (CNS), 329; congenital disease, 318; gastrointestinal tract infections, 302-303; host-parasite relationship, 64

GENUS CLOSTRIDIUM

This genus contains many species of Gram-positive anaerobic spore-forming rods; a few are aerotolerant. Widely distributed in soil and in the gut of man and animals. The spores are resistant to environmental conditions. The major diseases associated with species of the genus are gangrene, tetanus, botulism, food poisoning and pseudomembranous colitis. In each of these the production of potent protein exotoxins is an important cause of pathology, and in several species the genes encoding toxins are carried by plasmids or bacteriophages.

CLOSTRIDIUM PERFRINGENS

Characteristics

Anaerobic Gram-positive rods; spore-forming, but spores rarely seen in infected material. More tolerant of oxygen than other clostridia.

Laboratory identification

Hemolytic colonies on blood agar incubated anaerobically. Identification confirmed by demonstration of alpha-toxin (lecithinase) production in the Nagler's test. Germination of heat-resistant spores (with subsequent toxin production) may be responsible for food poisoning. Five types of *C. perfringens* (A–E) identified on the basis of toxins produced; type A strains can be further divided into several serotypes.

Diseases

Gas gangrene resulting from infection of dirty ischemic wounds. Food poisoning following ingestion of food contaminated with enterotoxin-producing strains.

Transmission

Spores and vegetative organisms widespread in soil and normal flora of man and animals. Infection acquired by contact; may be endogenous (e.g. wound contaminated from patient's own fecal flora) or exogenous (e.g. contamination of a wound with soil, ingestion of contaminated food).

Pathogenesis

In ischemic wounds, production of various (at least 12) toxins and tissue-destroying enzymes allows organism to establish itself and multiply in wound. Local action of toxins produces necrosis thereby further impairing blood supply and keeping conditions anaerobic, and aiding spread of organism into adjacent tissues. Food poisoning results from the ingestion of large numbers of vegetative cells, which sporulate in the gut and release enterotoxin.

Treatment and prevention

Gangrene requires rapid intervention with extensive debridement of the wound. Penicillin is the antibiotic of choice (alternatively metronidazole, clindamycin or imipenem). Anti-alpha-toxin may be given. Hyperbaric oxygen may also be helpful. Food poisoning does not usually require specific treatment.

Organ systems and disease involvement	General, 288-289

CLOSTRIDIUM TETANI

Characteristics	Gram-positive spore-forming rod with terminal round spore (drumstick). Strict anaerobe.
Laboratory identification	Grows on blood agar in anaerobic conditions as a fine spreading colony; 'ground glass' appearance (hand lens inspection of cultures important). Has very little biochemical activity useful for identification purposes. Demonstration of toxin in a specimen is possible in a two-mouse model in which one animal is protected with antitoxin, the other unprotected (performed in Public Health reference laboratories).
Diseases	Tetanus (lockjaw). Severe disease characterized by tonic muscle spasms and hyperflexia, trismus, opisthotonos and convulsions.
Transmission	Organism widespread in soil. Acquired by man by implantation of contaminated soil into wound. Wound may be major (e.g. in war, in road traffic accident) or minor (e.g. a rose thorn puncture while gardening). No person-to-person spread.
Pathogenesis	Tetanus results from neurotoxin (tetanospasmin) produced by organisms in wound. Toxin genes are plasmid-encoded. The organism is non-invasive, but the toxin spreads from site of infection via bloodstream and acts by binding to ganglioside receptors and blocking release of inhibitory neurotransmitters. Causes convulsive contractions of voluntary muscles.
Treatment and prevention	Antitoxin is available (hyperimmune human gamma globulin; tetanus immune globulin). Penicillin (or metronidazole) and spasmolytic drugs indicated. Prevention readily available and effective in form of immunization with toxoid. Usually given in childhood, but if immunization status of injured patient is unknown, toxoid is given in addition to antitoxin.
Organ systems and disease involvement	Central nervous system (CNS), 339-340; infection of skin, soft tissue, muscle and associated systems, 355-356; pathological consequences, 187; vaccination, 529

CLOSTRIDIUM BOTULINUM

Characteristics	Anaerobic Gram-positive rods. Not easily cultivated in competition with other organisms. Produces most potent toxins known to man. Seven immunologically distinct toxins (A, B, Cα, Cβ, D, E and F) produced by different strains of *C. botulinum*. Types A, B and E (and in some cases F) are most commonly associated with human disease: serotypes A and B linked to a variety of foods (e.g. meat), serotype E especially associated with fish.
Laboratory identification	Requires strictly anaerobic conditions for isolation. Grows on blood agar, but very rarely isolated from human cases of disease. Detection of the toxin in the food or serum from the patient is the way of confirming the diagnosis.
Diseases	Major pathogen of birds and mammals, rare in humans. Botulism acquired by ingesting preformed toxin. Disease entirely due to effects of toxin. Infant botulism results from ingestion of organisms and production of toxin in infant's gut. Associated with feeding honey contaminated with spores of *C. botulinum*. Wound botulism: toxin produced by organisms infecting a wound. Extremely rare
Transmission	Soil is the normal habitat. Intoxication most often by ingestion of toxin in foods that have not been adequately sterilized (e.g. home-preserved foods) and improperly processed

cans of food. Toxin is associated with germination of spores. There is no person-to-person spread.

Pathogenesis	Toxin released from organism as inactive protein and cleaved by proteases to uncover active site. It is acid stable and survives passage through stomach. Taken up through stomach and intestinal mucosa into bloodstream. Acts at neuromuscular junctions inhibiting acetylcholine release. Results in muscle paralysis and death from respiratory failure.
Treatment and prevention	Supportive therapy is paramount. Trivalent antitoxin is available. In the rare cases of infant and wound botulism (i.e. when the organism is growing in vivo), penicillin is effective. Prevention relates to good manufacturing practice. The toxin is not heat stable, therefore adequate cooking of food before consumption will destroy it.
Organ systems and disease involvement	Central nervous system (CNS), 340; gastrointestinal tract infections, 292-293; pathological consequences, 187

CLOSTRIDIUM DIFFICILE

Characteristics	Slender Gram-positive anaerobic rod; spore-former; motile.
Laboratory identification	Difficult to isolate in ordinary culture because of overgrowth by other organisms; selective medium containing cefoxitin, cycloserine and fructose may be helpful; however, mere presence of the organism is not indicative of infection. Diagnosis by detection of toxin in feces (i.e. immunoassay or tissue culture cytotoxicity assay).
Diseases	Pseudomembranous colitis (antibiotic-associated diarrhea). Can be rapidly fatal especially in the compromised host.
Transmission	Component of normal gut flora; flourishes under selective pressure of antibiotics. May also be spread from person to person by the fecal–oral route.
Pathogenesis	Toxin-mediated damage to gut wall. Produces both an enterotoxin (toxin A) and cytotoxin (toxin B).
Treatment and prevention	Oral vancomycin or metronidazole. Other antibiotics should be withheld if possible. Prevention of cross-infection in hospitals depends upon scrupulous attention to hygiene.
Organ systems and disease involvement	Diagnosis and control, 481, 491; gastrointestinal tract infections, 289-290; host-parasite relationship, 59

GENUS MYCOBACTERIUM

	Mycobacteria are widespread both in the environment and in animals. The major human pathogens are M. tuberculosis and M. leprae, but awareness of the importance of other species (e.g. M. avium complex) is increasing with their recognition as pathogens in AIDS and other immunocompromised patients.
Characteristics	Aerobic rods with a Gram-positive cell wall structure, but stain with difficulty because of the long-chain fatty acids (mycolic acids) in the cell wall. Acid fastness can be demonstrated by resistance to decolorization by mineral acid and alcohol (Ziehl–Neelsen stain). Mycobacteria grow more slowly than many other bacteria of medical importance, but the genus can be divided into: rapid growers (form visible colonies within ca. 3–7 days); slow growers (form visible colonies only after ca. 2 weeks to 2 months' incubation).

Laboratory identification	Staining and microscopic examination of specimens for acid-fast rods is important because of the time required for culture results. All species except *M. leprae* can be grown in artificial culture, but they require complex media. Identification is based on rate of growth (rapid or slow), optimum temperature of growth and pigment production. Scotochromogenic species produce pigment in the absence of light whereas photochromogenic species require exposure to light before pigment becomes apparent. Further biochemical tests are required for full specification. Polymerase chain reaction methods, DNA probes and sequence-based approaches are available for identification purposes.
Diseases	*M. tuberculosis* causes tuberculosis in humans and animals. *M. leprae* is restricted to man and causes leprosy. Mycobacteria other than tuberculosis (MOTT) are associated with a range of conditions, usually in immunocompromised hosts. *M. avium-intracellulare* (*M. avium* complex) has important associations with AIDS patients in the US; in Africa *M. tuberculosis* is more common.
Transmission	Droplet spread aided by ability of organisms to survive in the environment (*M. tuberculosis, M. leprae*). Unpasteurized milk from cattle infected with *M. bovis* has been responsible for human infections in the past. Social and environmental factors and genetic predisposition all have a role. Leprosy requires close and prolonged contact for spread.
Pathogenesis	Both *M. tuberculosis* and *M. leprae* are intracellular parasites surviving within macrophages. They give rise to slowly developing, chronic conditions in which much of the pathology is attributable to host immune responsiveness rather than to direct bacterial toxicity.
Treatment and prevention	Prolonged treatment with combinations of antimycobacterial drugs is required. Bacille Calmette–Guérin (BCG) vaccination is valuable for prevention in endemic areas. Isoniazid (or rifampin and pyrazinamide) prophylaxis used for contacts of cases of tuberculosis. Pasteurization of milk and improvement of living conditions have played a major role in prevention.
Organ systems and disease involvement	Central nervous system (CNS), 329; diagnosis and control, 450, 496-497; host-parasite relationship, 152, 153, 157, 171, 175; immunocompromised host, 434-435; infection of skin, soft tissue, muscle and associated systems, 357-359; lower respiratory tract infection, 232-235; microbes as parasites, 11, 13; pathologic consequences, 184; urinary tract infection (UTI), 246; vaccination, 517, 524, 531

GENUS ACTINOMYCES

The actinomycetes are true bacteria, although they have in the past been considered to resemble fungi because they form branching filaments. They are related to the corynebacteria and mycobacteria in the chemical structure of their cell walls. It is important to differentiate them from fungi because infections with actinomycetes should respond to antibacterial agents whereas similar clinical presentations caused by fungi are resistant to antibacterials (and extremely refractory to treatment by antifungal agents). This genus contains many species, some of which are important to man as producers of antimicrobial agents. A few are pathogenic to man and animals; *A. israelii* causes actinomycosis.

ACTINOMYCES ISRAELII

Characteristics	Gram-positive anaerobic filamentous branching rods. Non-sporing, non-acid fast.
Laboratory identification	Forms 'sulfur granules' composed of a mass of bacterial filaments in pus. These can be identified by washing pus, squashing granules and observing in stained microscopic preparations. Gram-positive branching rods also visible in stained pus. Forms characteristic breadcrumb or 'molar tooth' colonies on blood agar after 3–7 days anaerobic incubation at 35°C
Diseases	Actinomycosis follows local trauma and invasion from normal flora. Hard non-tender swellings develop which drain pus through sinus tracts. Cervicofacial lesions are most common, but abdominal lesions after surgery and infection related to intrauterine contraceptive devices also occur.
Transmission	A. israelii is part of normal flora in mouth, gut and vagina. Infection is endogenous. There is no person-to-person spread.
Pathogenesis	Virulence factors not described.
Treatment and prevention	Penicillin is the drug of choice. Prolonged treatment is required, accompanied by surgical drainage.
Organ systems and disease involvement	Gastrointestinal tract infections, 310; immunocompromised host, 434

GENUS NOCARDIA

Characteristics	Aerobic Gram-positive rods that form thin branching filaments. Widespread in the environment. N. asteroides complex represents the important human pathogens.
Laboratory identification	Gram stains of pus may reveal Gram-positive filaments or rods. Sulfur granules not seen. Grow as 'breadcrumb' colonies on blood agar within 2–10 days' incubation. Often acid fast.
Diseases	N. asterioides complex are opportunistic pathogens especially infecting immunocompromised patients; primarily a pulmonary infection, but secondary spread to form abscesses in brain or kidney is common. N. brasiliensis is the cause of actinomycetoma in Central and South America.
Transmission	Infection is acquired from the soil by the airborne route. Outbreaks of infection in renal transplant units have been associated with local building work. Actinomycetoma is acquired by implantation of organisms into wounds and progressive destruction of skin, fascia, bone and muscle.
Pathogenesis	Appears to be related to organism's ability to survive the host's inflammatory responses. Infection is controlled by cell-mediated immunity, but this may be defective in immunocompromised patients.
Treatment and prevention	Nocardiosis is often difficult to treat, but most regimens include sulfonamides as the drug of choice.
Organ systems and disease involvement	Immunocompromised host, 434

GRAM-NEGATIVE RODS

ENTEROBACTERIACEAE

Most numerous facultative anaerobes in the human gut, comprising approximately 10^9/g of feces. Outnumbered only by Gram-negative anaerobes (e.g. *Bacteroides*), which are present in numbers approximately ten times those of the enterobacteria. Genera of the family Enterobacteriaceae share features that distinguish them from other families; can be distinguished from each other by biochemical tests.

GENUS ESCHERICHIA

Genus contains only one species of medical importance: *E. coli*.

ESCHERICHIA COLI

Characteristics	Gram-negative rod; motile; with or without capsule; non-fastidious, facultative anaerobe; bile tolerant; capable of growth at 44°C.
Laboratory identification	Grows readily on routine laboratory media and on bile-containing selective media. Lactose fermenter. Kits available for full identification.
Diseases	Urinary tract infection; diarrheal diseases; neonatal meningitis; septicemia.
Transmission	Normal habitat is gut of man and animals; may colonize lower end of urethra and vagina. Spread is by contact and ingestion (fecal–oral route); may be food-associated; may be endogenous. Possesses O (somatic), H (flagellar), K (capsular) and F (fimbrial) antigens, which can be used to characterize strains by serotyping (e.g. O157:H7 EHEC strains, see below). Colicin (bacteriocin) typing also possible but pulsed-field gel electrophoresis most often used for epidemiologic analysis.
Pathogenesis	A variety of virulence factors have been identified, particularly in strains associated with diarrheal disease:

- endotoxin: present in all strains;
- adhesins—P fimbriae (pili) associated with urinary tract infection; colonization factors (e.g. CFA I, II and III, K88, K99) associated with gastrointestinal tract infection in humans and animals;
- capsule present in some strains; may be associated with adhesion. K1 capsular type associated with neonatal meningitis;
- enterotoxins associated with diarrheal disease: ETEC (enterotoxigenic *E. coli*) produce heat-stable (ST) and cholera-like heat-labile (LT) toxins; EIEC (enteroinvasive *E. coli*) produce shiga-like cytotoxin; EHEC (enterohemorrhagic *E. coli*) produce verotoxin—associated with hemolytic uremic syndrome.

Treatment and prevention	Wide range of antibacterial agents potentially available, but incidence of resistance variable and often plasmid-mediated; must be determined by susceptibility testing. Specific treatment of diarrheal disease usually not required. No currently available vaccine.

Organ systems and disease involvement	Diagnosis and control, 546; gastrointestinal tract infections, 280-282; microbes as parasites, 12-13, 18, 23; urinary tract infection (UTI), 241; vaccination, 535

GENUS *PROTEUS*

Genus contains several species, of which two are of medical importance: *P. mirabilis* and *P. vulgaris*.

Characteristics
Gram-negative rod; non-fastidious; facultative anaerobe; bile tolerant; likes alkaline pH; characteristic unpleasant odor; highly motile and swarms on some media.

Laboratory identification
Lactose non-fermenter; produces urease; kits available for full identification. Species can be distinguished by indole test: *P. mirabilis*, indole-negative; *P. vulgaris*, indole-positive. O (somatic) and H (flagellar) antigens characterize. *P. vulgaris* strains OX-19, OX-2 and OX-K share antigens with rickettsiae in the typhus and spotted fever groups and are agglutinated by antibodies produced by patients with these rickettsial infections (Weil–Felix test). Serologic response to *Proteus* infection not useful diagnostically.

Diseases
Urinary tract infection; hospital-acquired wound infection, septicemia, pneumonia in the compromised host.

Transmission
Normal habitat is human gut, soil and water. Contact spread; infection often endogenous.

Pathogenesis
Characterized virulence factors include endotoxin, urease; possible role for bacteriocins.

Treatment and prevention
Range of agents available, but *P. vulgaris* commonly more resistant to antibacterials than *P. mirabilis*. Prevention is by good aseptic technique in hospitals. No vaccine available.

Organ systems and disease involvement
Antimicrobial agents, 496; obstetric and perinatal infections, 318; upper respiratory tract infection, 241, 244, 247; urinary tract infection (UTI), 241, 244, 247

GENUS *KLEBSIELLA* AND RELATED ENTEROBACTERIA *SERRATIA* AND *ENTEROBACTER*

Unlike *E. coli*, species of the genera *Klebsiella*, *Serratia* and *Enterobacter* are rarely associated with infection except as opportunists in compromised patients.

Characteristics
Gram-negative rods, sometimes capsulate (usual for *Klebsiella*), non-fastidious growth requirements. Capable of aerobic and anaerobic respiration.

Laboratory identification
Lactose-fermenting, bile-tolerant organisms. Grow readily on routine laboratory media. Oxidase negative. Full identification based on biochemical reactions (commercial kits available).

Diseases
Opportunist infections in the compromised (usually hospitalized) host. Urinary and respiratory tracts most common sites of infection. Distinction between colonization and infection can sometimes be difficult.

Transmission
Normal habitat is gut of man and animals and moist inanimate environments, especially soil and water. Infection may be endogenous or acquired by contact spread. *Klebsiella* have remarkable capacity for survival on hands. Pulsed-field gel electrophoresis most commonly used for epidemiologic investigation of hospital-acquired infection.

Pathogenesis
All possess endotoxin and fimbriae or other adhesins. Capsules, where present, are important in inhibiting phagocytosis.

Treatment and prevention
Multiple antibiotic resistance, usually plasmid-mediated, is common, and susceptibility must be determined by laboratory tests if treatment is indicated. Prevention depends upon scrupulous attention to aseptic techniques and to hand washing in hospitals.

Organ systems and disease involvement
Klebsiella: sexually transmitted disease, 262; *Serratia:* urinary tract infections (UTI), 318; *Enterobacter:* antimicrobial agents, 476, 492-493; gastrointestinal tract infections, 283, 288, 302, 310; hospital infection 552, 559, 241; urinary tract infection (UTI), 241

GENUS *SALMONELLA*

Unlike other members of the Enterobacteriaceae, *Salmonella* and *Shigella* are not normal inhabitants of the human gut (except in post-infection carriers). Both genera are responsible for diarrheal disease, which may be severe; *Salmonella* may also cause bacteremia (most commonly associated with *S. typhi*, *S. paratyphi* and *S. choleraesuis*).

Regarding taxonomy, the Kauffmann–White classification recognizes each serologically distinct salmonella (of which there are over 2000) as a species (a convention also retained here). These designations are arranged in groups based on the serologic identification of O (somatic) and H (flagellar) antigens. DNA hybridization studies now indicate only two *Salmonella* species. Within *S. enterica* (the most important for human infection) six subgroups (A, B, C1, C2, D and E) can be distinguished. Distinction on basis of infection is between *S. typhi*, *S. paratyphyi*, *S. schottmuelleri* (formerly *S. paratyphi* B) and *S. hirshfeldii* (formerly *S. paratyphi* C), which cause enteric fevers, and other serotypes (e.g. *S. enteritidis*) which cause diarrheal disease.

KAUFFMANN–WHITE CLASSIFICATION				
Group	Name*	Somatic (O) antigen	Flagella (H) antigen Phase I	Flagella (H) antigen Phase II
A	*S. paratyphi* A	1,2,12	a	–
B	*S. schottmuelleri*	1,3,5,12	b	1,2
	S. typhimurium	1,4,5,12	i	1,2
C1	*S. hirshfeldii*	6,7, Vi	c	1,5
	S. choleraesuis	6,7	c	1,5
	S. virchow	6,7	r	1,2
D	*S. typhi*	9, 12, Vi	d	–
	S. enteritidis	1,9,12	g,m	–

* Examples of a few important species only

Characteristics
Gram-negative, motile non-sporing rods. All except *S. typhi* are non-capsulate. Capable of aerobic and anaerobic respiration.

Laboratory identification
Bile tolerant. Non-fastidious. Oxidase negative. Lactose non-fermenters. Produce acid and gas from glucose (except *S. typhi*, which is anaerogenic). Combination of biochemistry (commercial kits available) and serotyping required for full identification; important to distinguish enteric fever salmonellae from others. Detection of circulating antibody (Widal test) may aid diagnosis of enteric fevers. While serotyping (and phage typing of most important serotypes) is useful for investigation of outbreaks, molecular approaches such as pulsed field gel electrophoresis are more definitive.

Diseases
Vast majority cause diarrheal disease; very occasionally invasive (particularly *S. choleraesuis*). Sickle cell disease predisposes to osteomyelitis. *S. typhi*, *S. paratyphi*, *S. schottmuelleri* (formerly *S. paratyphi* B), and *S. hirshfeldii* (formerly *S. paratyphi* C) cause systemic disease, typhoid and paratyphoid (enteric fevers).

Transmission
Widespread in animals; encountered in food chain (especially in poultry, eggs, meat, milk and cream). Acquired by ingestion of contaminated food or person to person via fecal–oral route. *S. typhi* and *S. paratyphi* are human pathogens only. Spread via fecal–oral route, usually via contaminated water or food. Carriers are important source of organisms.

Treatment and prevention	*S. typhi* and *S. paratyphi* infections should be treated with systemic antibiotics based on susceptibility tests. Antibiotic resistance is an increasing problem in many countries (important implications for travelers). Salmonella diarrhea should not be treated with antibiotics unless there is evidence of invasive disease. Prevention depends upon interrupting fecal–oral transmission and on eliminating opportunities for transmission via the food chain. Vaccines are available to protect against *S. typhi* and *S. paratyphi*.
Organ systems and disease involvement	Gastrointestinal tract infections, 282-283, 301-302; host-parasite relationship, 129, 132; sexually transmitted disease, 273; vaccination, 519, 534

GENUS *SHIGELLA*

	Contains four species of importance to man as causes of bacillary dysentery: *S. dysenteriae*, *S. boydii*, *S. flexneri* and *S. sonnei* (in descending order of severity of symptoms).
Characteristics	Gram-negative rods. Non-motile (in contrast to salmonellae). Non-capsulate. Capable of aerobic and anaerobic respiration.
Laboratory identification	Non-fastidious, bile-tolerant. Lactose non-fermenters. Full identification requires use of biochemistry (commercial kits available) and serologic tests for O antigens. Serodiagnosis of disease not applicable.
Diseases	Bacillary dysentery.
Transmission	Human pathogens spread by fecal–oral route, especially in crowded conditions. Small infective dose.
Pathogenesis	Invasion of ileum and colon causes damage, which results in diarrhea. Intense inflammatory response involving neutrophils and macrophages characteristic. *S. dysenteriae* produces an exotoxin (Shiga toxin) causing damage to intestinal epithelial cells. In fewer instances, the toxin results in damage to glomerular endothelial cells, leading to hemolytic uremic syndrome (HUS).
Treatment and prevention	Antibiotic therapy (e.g. fluoroquinolones, trimethoprim–sulfamethoxazole) should only be given for severe diarrhea; usually not required. Many strains carry multiple antibiotic resistances, usually on plasmids; thus susceptibility testing is important. Prevention depends upon interrupting fecal–oral spread; hand hygiene important. No vaccine available.
Organ systems and disease involvement	Diagnosis and control, 495; gastrointestinal tract infections, 287-288; host-parasite relationship, 126, 132; sexually transmitted disease, 273; vaccination, 535

GENUS *PSEUDOMONAS* AND RELATED ORGANISMS *BURKHOLDERIA, STENOTROPHOMONAS* AND *ACINETOBACTER*

This group contains a large number of species, a few of which are human pathogens, some are animal pathogens and others are important pathogens of plants. Species also widely distributed and may contaminate the hospital environment and cause opportunist infections. Most important in humans are:

P. aeruginosa, important opportunist in compromised patients;

Burkholderia pseudomallei, cause of melioidosis, a disease of restricted geographic distribution;

Burkholderia cepacia, commonly associated with nosocomial infection and respiratory tract infections in cystic fibrosis patients;

Stenotrophomonas maltophili, an opportunistic pathogen also commonly associated with nosocomial infection;

Acinetobacter baumannii (and other species), opportunistic pathogens causing a variety of infections (e.g. wound, respiratory tract, urinary tract); frequently antibiotic resistant.

PSEUDOMONAS AERUGINOSA

Characteristics
Aerobic Gram-negative rod, motile by means of polar flagella. Able to utilize a very wide range of carbon and energy sources and to grow over a wide temperature range. Does not ferment carbohydrates. Does not grow anaerobically (except when nitrate is provided as a terminal electron acceptor).

Laboratory identification
Grows readily on routine media including bile-containing selective media. Produces irregular iridescent colonies and a characteristic smell. Most strains produce a blue-green pigment (pyocyanin; unique to *P. aeruginosa*) and a yellow-green pigment (pyoverdin). Pigment production is enhanced on special media (King's A and B); oxidase positive.

Diseases
P. aeruginosa is an opportunist pathogen that can infect almost any body site given the right predisposing conditions. It causes infections of skin and burns, it is a major lung pathogen in cystic fibrosis and can cause pneumonia in intubated patients. It can also cause urinary tract infections, septicemia, osteomyelitis and endocarditis.

Transmission
Carriage as part of the normal gut flora occurs in a small percentage of normal healthy people and in a higher proportion of hospital inpatients. Thus endogenous infection may occur in compromised patients. *P. aeruginosa* is widespread in moist areas in the environment; patients usually become infected by contact spread, directly or indirectly, from these environmental sites.

Pathogenesis
A number of virulence factors have been identified, including endotoxin and exotoxin A, which acts as an inhibitor of elongation factor in eukaryotic protein synthesis. Extracellular polysaccharide capsule helps to prevent phagocytosis (e.g. massive amounts of alginate produced by strains specifically in cystic fibrosis patients). Pigments may have a role in pathogenicity, and pyoverdin acts as a siderophore.

Treatment and prevention
Resistant to many antibacterial agents; propensity to develop resistance during therapy. Combination antimicrobial chemotherapy based on susceptibility testing is required (e.g. aminoglycoside and beta-lactam antibiotic). Prevention depends upon good aseptic practice in hospitals, avoidance of unnecessary or prolonged broad spectrum antibiotic treatment and prophylaxis.

Organ systems and disease involvement
Diagnosis and control, 485, 493, 495, 546; immunocompromised host, 426-427

CURVED GRAM-NEGATIVE RODS

There are several genera of curved Gram-negative rods that contain species that occur in humans as pathogens. Three of the most important are *Vibrio*, *Campylobacter* and *Helicobacter*.

GENUS VIBRIO

Most important species is *V. cholerae.*

Characteristics

Curved Gram-negative rods, highly motile by means of single polar flagellum. Capable of aerobic and anaerobic respiration (facultatively anaerobic). Many species are salt (NaCl) tolerant; some salt-requiring.

Laboratory identification

Grow in alkaline conditions (can be selected from other gut flora in alkaline peptone water). Oxidase positive. Grow on thiosulfate citrate bile salts sucrose (TCBS) medium to form yellow colonies (*V. cholerae*) or green colonies (other species). Biochemical tests and use of specific antisera required for complete identification.

Diseases

Cholera caused by *V. cholerae*. *V. parahaemolyticus* causes diarrheal disease. *V. vulnificus* causes wound infections and bacteremia.

Transmission

V. cholerae is a human pathogen; no animal reservoir, but El Tor biotype survives better in the inanimate environment than classicial *V. cholerae*. Infection is acquired from contaminated water (usually) or food (sometimes). *V. parahaemolyticus* and *V. vulnificus* acquired from consumption of contaminated fish and seafood.

Pathogenesis

V. cholerae possesses several virulence factors (e.g. mucinase, adhesins and, most importantly, enterotoxin). Chromosomally encoded subunit toxin produced after cells bind to intestinal epithelium, enters cells and binds to ganglioside receptors activating adenyl cyclase and causing fluid loss, resulting in massive watery diarrhea. *V. parahaemolyticus* produces a cytotoxin (which also hemolyzes human red blood cells—the Kanagawa test). *V. vulnificus* produces cytolytic compounds and antiphagocytic polysaccharides.

Treatment and prevention

For cholera, fluid replacement (oral rehydration therapy: ORT) is of prime importance. Tetracycline shortens symptoms and duration of carriage. Some protection with oral vaccine. Prevention of cholera depends upon provision of a clean (chlorinated) water supply and adequate sewage disposal. Specific treatment not indicated for *V. parahaemolyticus* diarrhea. Tetracycline or aminoglycosides used in treatment of *V. vulnificus*. *V. parahaemolyticus* and *V. vulnificus* infections can be prevented by adequate cooking of seafood.

Organ systems and disease involvement

Gastrointestinal tract infections, 285-287, 288; host-parasite relationship, 126, 127, 129; microbes as parasites, 8, 17; pathological consequences, 187; vaccination, 518, 534

GENUS CAMPYLOBACTER

Curved Gram-negative rods, once classified as vibrios, campylobacters are primarily pathogens of animals, but several species also cause infections in man. *C. jejuni* is a major cause of bacterial gastroenteritis in developed countries. At a much lower frequency, *C. coli* also causes gastroenteritis. The infections caused by these organisms have an essentially identical clinical presentation, and laboratories generally do not distinguish between them.

CAMPYLOBACTER JEJUNI

Characteristics

Slender, curved (seagull-shaped) Gram-negative rods. Motile by means of a polar flagellum at one or both ends. Microaerophiles. Do not utilize carbohydrate.

Laboratory identification

Require enriched media and moist microaerophilic environment (10% O_2) for growth. Incubation at 42°C for 24–72 h. Colonies resemble water drops. Full identification by biochemical tests and characteristic antibiotic susceptibility pattern.

Diseases	Diarrhea. Can invade to give septicemia.
Transmission	Animal reservoir. Organisms acquired from contaminated food and milk (but do not multiply in these vehicles). Person-to-person spread rare.
Pathogenesis	Little known, but cytotoxin implicated. Also invasion and local destruction of gut mucosa.
Treatment and prevention	No specific treatment necessary for diarrhea. Erythromycin for invasive disease. Prevention depends upon good food hygiene. No vaccine.
Organ systems and disease involvement	Antimicrobial agents, 489; gastrointestinal tract infections, 283, 284, 285

HELICOBACTER PYLORI

Characteristics	Associated with gastritis and duodenal ulcers; originally named *C. pylori* but now moved into the genus *Helicobacter*. Overall cellular morphology similar to *Campylobacter*.
Laboratory identification	Require enriched media and moist microaerophilic environment (10% O_2) for growth. Incubation at 37°C for 24–72 h produces translucent colonies. Differentiated from *Campylobacter* by tests such as nitrate reduction (*C. jejuni*, positive; *H. pylori*, negative) and urease (*C. jejuni*, negative; *H. pylori*, positive). Full identification by biochemical tests and characteristic antibiotic susceptibility pattern. Organism in endoscopic biopsy specimens; positive urease test from endoscopic biopsy specimens or labeled urea breath test also very useful.
Diseases	Gastritis and duodenal ulcers, associated with gastric carcinoma.
Transmission	Person-to-person transmission (fecal–oral) likely. Infections observed in multiple family members.
Pathogenesis	Little known, but both bacterial and host factors involved. Protease affects gastric mucosa; urease produces ammonia and buffers stomach acid. Some invasion of intestinal epithelium.
Treatment and prevention	Proton pump inhibitor plus antibiotics (e.g. clarithromycin, metronidazole, tetracycline).
Organ systems and disease involvement	Host-parasite relationship, 128, 129

GRAM-NEGATIVE NON-SPORE-FORMING ANAEROBES

Historically, all short Gram-negative anaerobic rods or coccobacilli have been classified in the genus *Bacteroides* and longer rods with tapering ends in the genus *Fusobacterium*. Recent applications of new techniques to the *Bacteroides* have resulted in the definition of two additional genera: *Porphyromonas* and *Prevotella*. The genus *Bacteroides* is now restricted to species found among the normal gut flora. *Prevotella* contains saccharolytic oral and genitourinary species, including *P. melaninogenica* (formerly *B. melaninogenicus*), which produces a characteristic black-brown pigment. The genus *Porphyromonas* contains asaccharolytic pigmented species, which form part of the normal mouth flora (*P. gingivalis*) and may be involved in endogenous infection within the oral cavity. The most important non-sporing anaerobe causing infection is *B. fragilis* although others are much more common (e.g. in gingivitis and other endogenous oral infections).

BACTEROIDES FRAGILIS

Characteristics	Small pleomorphic Gram-negative rods or coccobacilli. Capable only of anaerobic respiration. Non-spore forming, non-motile.
Laboratory identification	Grows on blood agar incubated anaerobically and in other media designed for isolation of anaerobes. Plates may require up to 48 h incubation at 35°C for colonies to become visible. Cultures have a foul odor due to the fatty acid endproducts of metabolism. These can be used as identifying characteristics by analysis of culture supernates by gas–liquid chromatography (GLC). The major products of *Bacteroides* are acetate and succinate. Full identification in the diagnostic laboratory is based on biochemical tests and antibiogram. Commercial kits are available.
Diseases	Intra-abdominal sepsis; liver abscesses; aspiration pneumonia; brain abscesses; wound infections. Infections often mixed with aerobic and microaerophilic bacteria.
Transmission	Endogenous infection arising from contamination by gut contents or feces is most common route of acquisition.
Pathogenesis	Little is known about the virulence factors of *B. fragilis*. A polysaccharide capsule and production of extracellular enzymes are probably important features. An anaerobic environment is essential and in mixed infections growth of aerobic organisms probably helps the growth of *Bacteroides* by using up available oxygen.
Treatment and prevention	Metronidazole well-established as the drug of choice for *Bacteroides* infections. Many strains produce beta-lactamases and thus susceptibility to penicillin and ampicillin is unreliable. Prevention of endogenous infection difficult; good surgical technique and appropriate use of prophylactic antibiotics important in abdominal surgery.
Organ systems and disease involvement	Gastrointestinal tract infections, 310

GRAM-NEGATIVE COCCI

GENUS NEISSERIA

	This genus contains several more or less fastidious species of which two, *N. gonorrhoeae* and *N. meningitidis*, are important human pathogens.
Characteristics	Non-motile Gram-negative diplococci with fastidious growth requirements: capnophilic; *N. meningitidis* is capsulate, *N. gonorrhoeae* is not.
Laboratory identification	Gram stains of pus or cerebrospinal fluid may reveal Gram-negative kidney-shaped diplococci, often intracellular (in polymorphs). Require supplemented media for growth (chocolate agar). *N. gonorrhoeae* easier to isolate on enriched media containing antibiotics to inhibit other organisms of normal flora from sample sites. The two species are differentiated by sugar utilization pattern. Kits available to detect *N. gonorrhoeae* nucleic acid in specimens. Latex agglutination test for *N. meningitidis* types A and C.
Diseases	*N. gonorrhoeae*: gonorrhea, and pelvic inflammatory disease and salpingitis in females; ophthalmia neonatorum in infants born to infected mothers. *N. meningitidis*: meningitis; occasionally septicemia in absence of meningitis.
Transmission	Human pathogens; no animal reservoir. *N. gonorrhoeae* may be carried in genital tract, nasopharynx and anus. Spread by sexual or intimate contact. *N. meningitidis* carried in pharynx. Carriage rate in population increases during epidemics. Droplet spread. *N. meningitidis* has several immunologically distinct capsular types (e.g. A, B, C, Y, W135).

Pathogenesis	Several virulence factors have been identified. *N. gonorrhoeae*: pili or fimbriae act as adhesins; endotoxin; outer membrane proteins; protease production; resistance to lytic activity of serum; IgA proteases. *N. meningitidis*: the polysaccharide capsule is antiphagocytic; endotoxin and IgA protease also implicated.
Treatment and prevention	*N. gonorrhoeae*: resistance to first line drugs now widespread; usual choice is beta-lactamase-stable cephalosporin (e.g. ceftriaxone). *N. meningitidis*: penicillin or ceftriaxone (or equivalent cephalosporin); can be combined with chloramphenicol. Prevention of gonorrhea requires education, contact tracing. No vaccine available. Rifampicin is used for prophylaxis of close contacts of *N. meningitidis* meningitis. Tetravalent vaccine available (types A, C, Y, W135).
Organ systems and disease involvement	Central nervous system (CNS), 325-327; host-parasite relationship, 173; sexually transmitted disease, 256-258; vaccination, 534

GENUS MORAXELLA

Moraxella catarrhalis, previously classified as *Branhamella catarrhalis*, is a Gram-negative coccus morphologically similar to *Neisseria*, but with less fastidious growth requirements. Formerly regarded as a commensal in the respiratory tract, it has been associated with a variety of infections, including bronchitis, bronchopneumonia, sinusitis and otitis media. The majority of strains produce beta-lactamase and may be involved in the 'protection' of more obvious pathogens, especially in the respiratory tract, by destroying penicillin or ampicillin administered as treatment.

GENUS HAEMOPHILUS

The genus contains many species; *H. influenzae* and *H. ducreyi* are of medical importance.

HAEMOPHILUS INFLUENZAE

Characteristics	Small Gram-negative rods, frequently coccobacillary. Non-motile. Fastidious, capnophilic, facultative anaerobe. May be capsulate when isolated from site of infection.
Laboratory identification	Requires both hematin (X factor) and NADP (V factor) for growth (other species require one factor only). Grows on blood containing enriched media. Larger colonies around colonies of other organisms that secrete V factor (e.g. *Staph. aureus*) (satellitism). Dependence on X and V used as indicator of identity. *H. influenzae* can also be distinguished from other species by its inability to produce porphyrin. Six antigenically distinct capsular types recognized (a–f). Type b has been most frequently found in disease although this is changing with the introduction of vaccines against the type b strains. Capsulate organisms can be agglutinated by specific antisera and detected directly (e.g. by latex agglutination) in specimens.
Diseases	Capsular type b *H. influenzae* causes meningitis, osteomyelitis, epiglottitis, otitis. All are more common in children than older age groups. Non-capsulate strains associated with acute exacerbations of chronic bronchitis. Invasive disease due to type c and f isolates increasing.
Transmission	Normal habitat is upper respiratory tract in humans and associated animals. Transmitted from person to person by airborne route. Osteomyelitis probably follows septicemia from respiratory focus.

Pathogenesis Polysaccharide capsule is important virulence factor. Outer membrane proteins and endotoxin may play a part, but no known exotoxin.

Treatment and prevention Beta-lactamase-producing strains increasing. Ampicillin (or amoxicillin) may be used if isolates are susceptible. Third generation cephalosporin (e.g. cefotaxime or ceftriaxone) are usual alternatives. All children should be immunized with Hib vaccine. Rifampicin prophylaxis recommended for close contacts of *Haemophilus* meningitis.

Organ systems and disease involvement Central nervous system (CNS), 327-328; upper respiratory tract infection, 212-213; vaccination, 518, 534

HAEMOPHILUS DUCREYI

Cause of the genital tract infection 'soft chancre'. Slender Gram-negative rods appearing in pairs or chains. Direct microscopic examination of smear from chancre can be diagnostic. Organism very susceptible to dehydration; inoculate plates in clinic. Requires enriched medium (as for *H. influenzae,* but with addition of antibiotics to inhibit growth of other genital tract organisms).

GENUS BORDETELLA

There are three species, of which one, *B. pertussis*, is of medical importance.

Characteristics Small Gram-negative coccobacilli. Slow growing and fastidious in its growth requirements.

Laboratory identification Requires enriched medium (e.g. Bordet–Gengou or blood charcoal agar). Intolerant of fatty acids in medium. Fails to grow on routine blood agar (i.e. 5–7% blood). Requires 3–7 days incubation in moist atmosphere. Irridescent bisected pearl colony type characteristic on Bordet–Gengou. Further identification by reaction with specific antisera.

Diseases Whooping cough (pertussis).

Transmission Human pathogen spread by airborne route from cases of disease (healthy carriage not documented).

Pathogenesis Several virulence factors, including tracheal cytotoxin, fimbrial antigen and endotoxin. Stimulates a lymphocytic response.

Treatment and prevention Erythromycin is the drug of choice for cases and close contacts of whooping cough. Antibacterial therapy has little effect on clinical course, but may reduce infectivity and incidence of superinfection. Whole cell inactivated vaccine administered to young children in three doses together with diphtheria and tetanus toxoids. Newer subunit vaccines also effective.

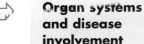

Organ systems and disease involvement Host-parasite relationship, 125, 152, 172; lower respiratory tract infection, 217; microbes as parasites, 17; vaccination, 518, 529

GENUS BRUCELLA

There are several species of the genus *Brucella*, each characteristically associated with an animal species. Four species—*B. abortus* from cattle, *B. suis* from pigs, *B. canis* from dogs, and *B. melitensis* from goats—are most often found causing human zoonotic infections.

Characteristics	Small Gram-negative coccobacilli. Intracellular pathogens. Growth enhanced by erythritol in placenta of animals (not in man).
Laboratory identification	Some strains slow-growing and fastidious, requiring complex growth media. Isolation from blood cultures improved by use of biphasic systems (e.g. Castenada bottles containing both broth and agar). Usually require 3–5 days' incubation in CO_2-enriched environment, but some strains of *B. abortus* may take up to 4 weeks—important in investigation of fever of unknown origin (FUO). Identification is by biochemical reactions, patterns of resistance to certain dyes, and serologic tests. The disease may be diagnosed by examination of patient's serum for antibodies.
Diseases	Undulant fever (brucellosis). Patients frequently present with FUO. Infection may become chronic if not adequately treated.
Transmission	Zoonotic infections transmitted to man through consumption of contaminated milk or other unpasteurized dairy products (increasingly seen in individuals who prefer untreated products) and by direct contact (occupational hazard for veterinarians, abbatoir workers and farmers).
Pathogenesis	Virulence associated with ability to survive intracellularly, especially in bone marrow, liver and spleen, and thus 'hide' from host defenses. Erythritol is a growth stimulant for the organism in animals and accounts for the tropism of the organisms to the placenta and fetus. This is not true in humans.
Treatment and prevention	Doxycycline alone or in combination (e.g. with streptomycin or rifampin). Tetracyclines may not be tolerated during long treatment courses required (combinations with fluoroquinolone or trimethoprim–sulfamethoxazole also effective). Recrudescence of infection is common. Prevention depends upon eliminating the disease from domestic animals by vaccination and pasteurization of milk. Vaccination is available for persons at risk in some countries, but is not used in USA or UK.
Organ systems and disease involvement	Multisystem zoonoses, 407-408

FRANCISELLA TULARENSIS

Characteristics	Small Gram-negative coccobacilli. Strict aerobe. Intracellular pathogen. The organism is found worldwide and occurs in a variety of wild and domestic animals.
Laboratory identification	Requires specialized medium (e.g. chocolate agar plates supplemented with cysteine) and lengthy incubation. Identification is by reaction with specific (i.e. anti-Francisella) antiserum. The diagnosis of disease may be aided by examination of patient's serum for antibodies. However, the long-term persistence of antibody may cloud discrimination of current from past disease. Antibody against Brucella may cross react with Francisella.
Diseases	*Francisella tularensis* causes tularemia (also known as glandular fever, deerfly fever or tick fever). Human disease is most commonly acquired from bite of an infected tick or contact with an infected animal (e.g. infected squirrels and rabbits). Tularemia quickly develops after a short period of incubation (e.g. 3–4 days), potentially leading to high fever, chills, myalgia, malaise depending on the specific form of the disease (i.e. ulceroglandular, glandular, oculoglandular, oropharyngeal, pneumonic, gastrointestinal, and typhoidal).
Transmission	Zoonotic infections transmitted to humans through contact with infected animals, the bite of infected fleas or ticks, or ingestion of contaminated meat.

Pathogenesis	Virulence associated with an antiphagocytic capsule and the ability to survive intracellularly in macrophages. *Francisella tularensis* is highly infectious with as few as 10 organisms causing disease. For this reason the public health agencies such as the World Health Organization and the US Centers for Disease Control have expressed concern about its potential use as an agent of bioterrorism.
Treatment and prevention	Streptomycin or gentamicin. Prevention depends upon avoiding the vectors and reservoirs of infection and use of protective clothing and gloves. In the United States, a live attenuated vaccine is available for at-risk individuals (e.g. laboratory workers, hunters, trappers, etc.).
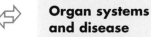 **Organ systems and disease involvement**	Multisystem zoonoses, 407

PASTEURELLA MULTOCIDA

Characteristics	Facultatively anaerobic, small Gram-negative coccobacilli. Occurs as a commensal in the upper respiratory tract of many animals including livestock, poultry, and domestic pets.
Laboratory identification	Gram stain of pus or other fluid specimen. Organisms grow well on ordinary bacteriologic media at 37°C. Oxidase-positive and catalase-positive. Bipolar staining enhanced by Wright, Giemsa, or Wayson stains.
Diseases	Infected animal (e.g. cat or dog) bite. Acute onset of redness, pain, and swelling.
Transmission	Zoonotic (animal bite) infection.
Pathogenesis	Capsule.
Treatment and prevention	Treat animal bite as polymicrobial infection (e.g. a beta-lactam antibiotic such as amoxicillin combined with a beta-lactam inhibitor).
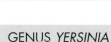 **Organ systems and disease involvement**	Multisystem zoonoses, 407

GENUS YERSINIA

A member of the family Enterobacteriaceae. This genus contains a variety of species, only a few of which are considered important human pathogens.

YERSINIA PESTIS

Characteristics	Gram-negative rods, facultatively anaerobic, zoonotic.
Laboratory identification	Exhibits bipolar staining with special (e.g. Wright-Giemsa, Wayson's) stains. Grows best on media containing blood or tissue fluids. Tentative identification by biochemical reactions. Definitive identification by immunofluorescence.
Diseases	Bubonic plague results from multiplication within monocytes with production of antiphagocytic proteins. Reaching the lymph nodes an intense hemorrhagic inflammation develops. Dissemination via the bloodstream leads to hemorrhagic and necrotic lesions in multiple organs. Pneumonic plague results from inhalation leading to hemorrhagic consolidation and sepsis.

Transmission	Zoonotic infection transmitted to humans through the bite of fleas carried by rodents.
Pathogenesis	Multiple virulence factors including lipopolysaccharides with endotoxic activity, antiphagocytic envelope protein, and plasmid-encoded virulence factors. Concern has been expressed regarding the possible use of this organism as an agent of bioterrorism.
Treatment and prevention	Streptomycin is the drug of choice with tetracycline as an alternative. Vaccine available for those at risk. Control and eradication of infected animals is important.
Organ systems and disease involvement	Multisystem zoonoses, 405-407

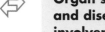

YERSINIA ENTEROCOLITICA

Characteristics	Gram-negative rods, zoonotic. A multitude of serotypes exist however, depending on geographic origin, most causing human disease are serotype 03, 08, or 09.
Laboratory identification	Non-lactose-fermenting Gram-negative rods; urease-positive and oxidase-negative. Bipolar staining. Facultative anaerobe that grows best and is motile at 25°C but non-motile at 37°C. Diagnosis involves isolation of the organism from the patient's feces or other body fluid (blood, vomit, etc.). Confirmation by biochemical and serological tests.
Diseases	*Y. enterocolitica* most commonly causes enterocolitis although extraintestinal infections may also (rarely) occur.
Transmission	Infection results from ingestion of contaminated food and drink (e.g. unpasteurized milk, raw pork, etc.). The organism adheres to and penetrates the terminal ileum leading to non-specific ileocolitis with potential lymph node infection and bacteremia. Symptoms include fever, abdominal pain and diarrhea which may be watery or bloody. *Y. enterocolitica* can grow at refrigeration temperatures and transmission by blood transfusion has been observed.
Pathogenesis	Multiple virulence factors including plasmid-encoded proteins related to adherence and invasion.
Treatment and prevention	Most enteric infections are self-limited. When necessary, treatment is usually with aminoglycosides, trimethoprim–sulfamethoxazole, or third-generation cephalosporins. Prevention includes avoiding contaminated food and drink.
Organ systems and disease involvement	Gastrointestinal tract infections, 283, 284, 288

GENUS LEGIONELLA

This is one of the newer discoveries in microbiology history, originally demonstrated by techniques used for virus isolation (e.g. growth in embryonated hens' eggs). In free-living state, can grow in water, but difficult to cultivate on routine laboratory media. *L. pneumophila* is the pathogen of greatest medical importance.

LEGIONELLA PNEUMOPHILA

Characteristics	In tissue appear as Gram-negative coccobacilli; pleomorphic on laboratory media; stain poorly with Gram's stain (and therefore easily missed). Fastidious growth requirements in laboratory.

Laboratory identification	Direct fluorescent antibody tests performed on sputum samples have the advantage of specificity, distinguishing *L. pneumophila* from environmental contaminants. However, relatively few organisms may be present in expectorated sputum. Silver staining techniques are better than standard Gram staining method. Require enriched media containing iron and cysteine and absorbents to remove fatty acids. Most require incubation for 3–5 days for growth. Produces small tenacious colonies. Further identification based on requirement for cysteine and serologic characteristics. Diagnosis is often based on antibody detection rather than culture.
Diseases	Legionnaires' disease; one of the causes of atypical pneumonia. Pontiac fever which may be caused by other species is a less severe flu-like illness.
Transmission	Environmental saprophyte acquired by inhalation of contaminated water from showers, air conditioning systems, cooling towers.
Pathogenesis	Virulence factors unclear, but intracellular survival in alveolar macrophages important. Host prediposition (e.g. immunocompromise, chronic lung disease) important.
Treatment and prevention	Erythromycin (may be combined with rifampicin or ciprofloxacin); levofloxacin or azithromycin in more serious (e.g. immunocompromised) cases. No vaccine available; prevention depends upon maintenance of hot water and air-conditioning systems, particularly in large buildings such as offices, hospitals and hotels.
Organ systems and disease involvement	Antimicrobial agents, 489; lower respiratory tract infection, 223, 224

GARDNERELLA VAGINALIS

Characteristics	Formerly known as *Haemophilus vaginalis* and *Corynebacterium vaginalis*. Gram-variable facultatively anaerobic rods.
Laboratory identification	Special culture requirements (e.g. increased levels of carbon dioxide). Vaginal epithelial cells covered with 'clue cells' (Gram-variable coccobacilli) and the amine or 'whiff' test (i.e. presence of fishy odor after addition of potassium hydroxide to a sample of vaginal discharge) helpful in diagnosis.
Diseases	Cause a variety of genitourinary infections but one of a number of organisms commonly associated with bacterial vaginosis. To a lesser extent may also be associated with genitourinary infections (i.e. lower urinary tract) in men.
Transmission	Transmitted by sexual contact.
Pathogenesis	Poorly understood.
Treatment and prevention	Metronidazole, clindamycin. Condom use may aid in prevention.
Organ systems and disease involvement	Sexually transmitted disease, 263

SPIRAL BACTERIA

There are three genera of medical importance: *Treponema*, *Leptospira* and *Borrelia*.

GENUS TREPONEMA

Regularly coiled spirochetes with a longer wavelength than *Leptospira*. Several species and subspecies are important human pathogens; others are members of the normal flora, especially in the mouth. *T. pallidum* and its subspecies *pertenue,* and *T. carateum* are the most important species.

Characteristics	Individual cells too small to visualize by direct light microscopy; can be seen with dark ground (darkfield) illumination or after silver impregnation or immunofluorescent staining. Cells are actively motile by means of flagella contained within the periplasmic sheath.
Laboratory identification	*T. pallidum* and closely related species cannot be grown in artificial media; diagnosis of infection depends upon microscopic examination of fluid from primary lesions and on serology.
Diseases	*T. pallidum*: syphilis. *T. pallidum–pertenue* and *T. carateum*: the non-sexually transmitted treponematoses, yaws and pinta.
Transmission	Very susceptible to heat and drying, so successful transmission depends upon very close contact. *T. pallidum* is spread by close sexual contact and may also be vertically transmitted in utero. Yaws and pinta spread by direct contact from infected skin lesions. No animal reservoir.
Pathogenesis	Study of virulence factors hampered by the inability to grow *T. pallidum* in artificial culture media. Disease presents characteristically in three phases: after local primary infection, organisms widely disseminated in the body and may become quiescent for months or years. Immunopathology plays a major role in causing damage to the host, particularly in the tertiary stage of disease.
Treatment and prevention	Penicillin is the treatment of choice for syphilis. Tetracycline may be given to penicillin-allergic patients. Prevention depends upon detection and treatment of cases, contact tracing and serologic testing of pregnant women. Possible cross-reactions between *T. pallidum* and the species causing yaws and pinta must be noted.
Organ systems and disease involvement	Congenital infections, 317-318; sexually transmitted disease, 251-256

GENUS LEPTOSPIRA

Two species: *L. interrogans* and *L. biflexa*; the former is parasitic, the latter contains free-living species. Within the species *interrogans* there are several different serogroups and serovars responsible for disease in humans and animals.

LEPTOSPIRA INTERROGANS

Characteristics	Finely coiled spirochetes with hooked ends. Cells 0.1–0.2 μm in diameter, up to 20 μm in length. Not visible by direct light microscopy unless stained by silver impregnation or immunofluorescent methods. Dark ground (darkfield) microscopy reveals rotational and directional motility by means of periplasmic flagella.
Laboratory identification	Direct microscopy of blood and urine possible, but difficult to interpret. Leptospira can be grown, with difficulty, in special serum-containing media. Serologic diagnosis is usual.
Diseases	Leptospirosis or Weil's disease in humans and animals.
Transmission	Leptospirosis in humans is a zoonosis, usual hosts being rodents, bats, cattle, sheep, goats and other domestic animals. Leptospires excreted in urine contaminate food and water. Infection occurs by contact either through occupation (e.g. sewer workers,

farmers, abbatoir workers) or recreation (e.g. canoeing, windsurfing on inland waters). Organisms may penetrate unabraded skin and conjunctiva.

Pathogenesis	After initial invasion there is hematogenous spread before the organisms localize in various organs including the liver and kidney. Subclinical infection is common in endemic areas.
Treatment and prevention	Penicillin; doxycycline in penicillin-allergic patients. Disease may be prevented after exposure by doxycycline.
Organ systems and disease involvement	Multisystem zoonoses, 407-408

GENUS BORRELIA

Two species of Borrelia are of importance in humans: *B. burgdorferi* causes Lyme disease; *B. recurrentis* causes relapsing fever.

Characteristics	Less finely coiled than the leptospires. Cells 0.2–0.5 μm in diameter; stain readily, so are visible by light microscopy.
Laboratory identification	Microaerophilic, complex nutritional requirements, long growth time (weeks) thus culture is not routinely used for identification. *B. recurrentis* demonstrated in blood smears by staining with Giemsa or acridine orange. *B. burgdorferi* much more difficult to visualize. Culture from biopsy material possible, but difficult; diagnosis usually by serology.
Diseases	In relapsing fever the relapsing element may be due to antigen switching. Lyme disease slowly progressive rather than relapsing. Characteristic 'bull's eye' skin lesion (erythema chronicum migrans) commonly occurs. Joint pains and fatigue common and later, in untreated cases, neurologic and cardiac manifestations.
Transmission	*B. recurrentis* spread from person to person by lice. Lyme disease is a zoonosis transmitted to humans by hard ticks (*Ixodes* spp.) associated with deer. Ticks are found on bracken and undergrowth and attach to exposed skin. Tick bite is often unnoticed, but less than a minute is required for the organisms to enter the host.
Pathogenesis	Little known about pathogenesis of either disease. Antigen switching in *B. recurrentis* presumably allows evasion of host's antibody response.
Treatment and prevention	Doxycycline; but erythromycin and penicillin have both been used successfully. Prevention depends upon avoiding contact with vectors (e.g. protective clothing for walkers and forestry workers).
Organ systems and disease involvement	Host-parasite relationship, 173; vector-borne, 389-391

OTHER BACTERIA

MYCOPLASMAS

Characteristics	Distinguished from other prokaryotes and placed in the class Mollicutes because they lack a true cell wall and consequent rigidity. This is a stable characteristic exhibited by genera such as *Mycoplasma* and *Ureaplasma* and is distinct from cell wall-deficient and L-forms of other species. The outer membrane, the outermost layer, functions as the major antigenic interface. It is a flexible triple-layered structure of proteins and lipids. Many

species also contain cholesterol in the membrane, which is absent from other bacterial cells. The important species is *M. pneumoniae*, but *M. hominis* and *U. urealyticum* may cause genital tract infections.

Laboratory identification
Many species are fastidious, and complex media and soft agar may be required for satisfactory culture. Cultures incubated for at least 7 days, although some species (e.g. *M. hominis*) grow readily on moist blood agar plates within 48 h. Cells variable in size (up to 100 μm but many smaller than 0.5 μm) and morphology; cannot be stained by Gram's stain (no cell wall), but impressions of colonies can be stained with Dienes' or Romanowsky's stains. Diagnosis of infection based on serology because of difficulties of culture.

Diseases
M. pneumoniae is an important cause of 'atypical pneumonia'. Mycoplasmas are also associated with genital infections (e.g. non-gonococcal urethritis) and with joint and other inflammatory infections. Other mycoplasmas are important pathogens of animals and birds.

Transmission
Transmission of *M. pneumoniae* is from person to person by airborne route. Other mycoplasmas and ureaplasmas can be transmitted by sexual contact.

Pathogenesis
Surface protein adhesin binds *M. pneumoniae* to sialogycolipids on respiratory epithelium of host. Other virulence factors are not yet clearly understood.

Treatment and prevention
Tetracycline or erythromycin (note that the lack of cell wall target means lack of susceptibility to beta-lactams). No vaccine currently available. Prevention by interruption of spread is difficult.

 Organ systems and disease involvement
Sexually transmitted disease, 262

RICKETTSIAE

Characteristics
These organisms have requirement for coenzyme A, NAD and ATP, which they cannot supply themselves, and are therefore obligate intracellullar parasites; with rare exceptions they need to be grown in cell cultures or experimental animals.

Laboratory identification
Small (0.7–2 μm diameter), Gram-negative bacteria. Isolation in laboratory is difficult for the reasons outlined above (and may carry a high risk of laboratory-acquired infection); therefore rarely attempted outside specialized facilities. Diagnosis of infection based on serology.

Diseases
Typhus; Rocky Mountain, Mediterranean and other spotted fevers; Q fever.

Transmission
Maintained in animal reservoirs and transmitted by bites of ticks, fleas, mites and lice. In contrast, *Coxiella burnetii* (a related organism now moved to a separate genus) survives drying and is transmitted in aerosols from animals or materials contaminated by infected animals and inhaled.

Pathogenesis
Mechanisms unclear, but organisms have a predilection for endothelial cells, giving rise to characteristic primary skin lesion (in spotted fevers) and vasculitis. The intracellular habitat is important to the organism's survival in the face of host defenses.

Treatment and prevention
Tetracycline, fluoroquinolones, or chloramphenicol. Beta-lactams ineffective. Infection prevented by avoiding contact with vectors. Vaccines available for at-risk groups (e.g. veterinarians, farm workers).

 Organ systems and disease involvement
Diagnosis and control, 463-464; gastrointestinal tract infections, 300-302; multisystem zoonoses, 403-404; vector-borne, 386-389

CHLAMYDIAE

Characteristics	Obligate intracellular parasites (unable to synthesize ATP) with distinct lifecycle involving elementary bodies and reticulate bodies. Small cells with genome approximately 25% of that of *E. coli*. Important species are *Chlaymdia trachomatis*, *Chlamydophila psittaci* and *Chlamydophila pneumoniae*.
Laboratory identification	Must be grown in cell culture, so cultural techniques are limited to specialized laboratories. In cell cultures, *C. trachomatis* forms characteristic, glycogen-containing inclusion bodies, which can be stained with iodine. Both *C. psittaci* and *C. trachomatis* contain specific surface antigens that allow detection by immunofluorescent antibody techniques. *C. pneumoniae* currently detectable only by serology.
Diseases	*C. trachomatis* causes trachoma (eye infection), urethritis and other infections of the genital tract, and pneumonitis in newborns, acquired during birth from infected mothers. *C. pneumoniae*, described more recently, now recognized as important cause of atypical pneumonia. *C. psittaci* causes the atypical pneumonia, psittacosis.
Transmission	*C. pneumoniae* and *C. psittaci* are acquired by inhalation, the latter from infected birds or contaminated bird litter. *C. trachomatis* is spread by direct contact and is sexually transmitted.
Pathogenesis	Virulence factors remain unclear, but the intracellular habitat and different lifecycle forms help organisms to evade host defenses. Uptake into cells may be by parasite-encoded mechanisms.
Treatment and prevention	Tetracyclines, erythromycin (tetracyline should not be used in children) or fluoroquinolones are effective. Vaccines not available and may not be useful because of the immunopathologic element of the infections.
Organ systems and disease involvement	Diagnosis and control, 460, 463-464; eye infections, 343-345; host-parasite relationship, 129; sexually transmitted disease, 258-261

FUNGI

SUPERFICIAL MYCOSES

DERMATOPHYTES

	General term for species invading superficial layers of skin. Of the many species involved, those belonging to *Epidermophyton*, *Microsporum* and *Trichophyton* are of greatest importance.
Characteristics	Filamentous fungi invading surface keratinized structures—skin, hair, nails. Hyphae penetrate between cells.
Laboratory identification	Examination of KOH-treated skin scrapings for hyphae; fluorescence under Wood's lamp. Culture on media useful in identifying species. Both Sabouraud dextrose agar (SDA) and dermatophyte test medium (DTM) can be used.
Diseases	Tinea, ringworm, athlete's foot.
Transmission	By fungal material on skin scales.
Pathogenesis	Skin inflammation, pruritus—sometimes localized hypersensitivity reactions.
Treatment and prevention	Topical antifungal agents (griseofulvin). Improved skin care and hygiene.
Organ systems and disease involvement	Host-parasite relationship, 135-136; infection of skin, soft tissue, muscle and associated systems, 360-363

SPOROTHRIX SCHENCKII

Characteristics	Dimorphic fungus (capable of growing as both single-celled yeast and multicelled hyphae). Occurs in external environment. Invades subcutaneous tissues.
Laboratory identification	Budding cells in inflammatory exudate from lesions. Culture on SDA.
Diseases	Sporotrichosis.
Transmission	Direct fungal contamination of wounds in skin (e.g. those made by thorns).
Pathogenesis	Ulceration or abcess formation in draining lymphatics.
Treatment and prevention	Potassium iodide, ketoconazole. Protection of skin.
Organ systems and disease involvement	Infection of skin, soft tissue, muscle and associated systems, 363

DEEP MYCOSES

ASPERGILLUS

	A. fumigatus is the most important of three common species, the others being *A. flavus* and *A. niger*.
Characteristics	Filamentous fungi causing opportunistic infections in immunocompromised patients. Occur widely in external environment. Invade lungs and blood vessels.
Laboratory identification	Presence of hyphae in tissues. Culture on SDA. Serology.
Diseases	Aspergillosis.
Transmission	Inhalation of airborne stages (conidia).
Pathogenesis	Causes thrombosis and infarction when blood vessels invaded. Partial blockage of airways from fungal mass. Allergic bronchopulmonary reactions.
Treatment and prevention	Amphotericin B.
Organ systems and disease involvement	Diagnosis and control, 552; general, 39-40; immunocompromised host, 433; lower respiratory tract infection, 235

BLASTOMYCES DERMATITIDIS

Characteristics	Dimorphic fungus. Invades through lungs, can become widely disseminated in body.
Laboratory identification	Yeast cells in sputum or skin lesions. Culture on SDA.
Diseases	Blastomycosis.
Transmission	Inhalation of airborne spores.
Pathogenesis	Fungal infection in lungs. Presentation may be confused with tuberculosis. Can produce abscesses.

Treatment and prevention	Ketoconazole.
Organ systems and disease involvement	Infection of skin, soft tissue, muscle and associated systems, 364

CANDIDA ALBICANS

Characteristics	Dimorphic fungus, occurring as yeast on mucosal surfaces as component of normal flora, but forms hyphae when invasive. Produces opportunistic infections in stressed, suppressed and antibiotic-treated individuals. *Paracoccidioides brasiliensis* in central and South America has many similarities.
Laboratory identification	Fungal stages in tissues. Culture on SDA.
Diseases	Candidiasis, thrush.
Transmission	Part of normal flora of skin, mouth and intestine.
Pathogenesis	Localized mucocutaneous lesions; invasion of all major organs in the disseminated condition.
Treatment and prevention	Oral and topical antifungals (e.g. nystatin, miconazole). Ketoconazole, amphotericin B, fluconazole, and flucytosine for disseminated disease.
Organ systems and disease involvement	General, 40; host-parasite relationship, 57, 58-59; immunocompromised host, 431-432; infection of skin, soft tissue, muscle and associated systems, 363; sexually transmitted disease, 262-263; upper respiratory tract infection, 213

COCCIDIOIDES IMMITIS

Characteristics	Dimorphic fungus, growing as hyphae in soils, but as yeast-like endospores within capsules (spherules) in tissues. Invasion through lungs; can become widely disseminated in body.
Laboratory identification	In sputum or tissues. Culture on SDA. Serology.
Diseases	Coccidioidomycosis. Indigenous to the Americas.
Transmission	Inhalation of airborne stages (arthroconidia).
Pathogenesis	Lung infections give mild, influenza-like condition, but serious illness may follow dissemination.
Treatment and prevention	Amphotericin B, ketoconazole.
Organ systems and disease involvement	Central nervous system (CNS), 329; infection of skin, soft tissue, muscle and associated systems, 364

CRYPTOCOCCUS NEOFORMANS

Characteristics	Encapsulated yeast-like fungus common in soils where there are bird droppings. Invades through lungs; can spread to CNS.

Laboratory identification	Encapsulated yeast cells in sputum or cerebrospinal fluid. Culture on SDA. Serology.
Diseases	Cryptococcosis.
Transmission	Inhalation of airborne cells.
Pathogenesis	Lung infection may result in influenza-like condition or pneumonia. In immunocompromised patients, CNS involvement leads to meningitis.
Treatment and prevention	Amphotericin B and flucytosine.
Organ systems and disease involvement	Central nervous system (CNS), 329; general, 39, 40; immunocompromised host, 432-433, 435; infection of skin, soft tissue, muscle and associated systems, 364

HISTOPLASMA CAPSULATUM

Characteristics	Dimorphic fungus, growing as hyphae in soil where there are bird droppings. Invades through lungs and grows as yeast cells, which can survive intracellularly after phagocytosis. Can become widely disseminated in body.
Laboratory identification	Yeast cells in sputum or tissues. Culture on SDA. Serology.
Diseases	Histoplasmosis.
Transmission	Inhalation of airborne spores.
Pathogenesis	Can produce acute and chronic pulmonary disease. Serious illness results from dissemination into other organs.
Treatment and prevention	Amphotericin B, ketoconazole.
Organ systems and disease involvement	General, 39; immunocompromised host, 433

PNEUMOCYSTIS (JIROVECI) CARINII

Characteristics	Respiratory organism previously classed as a sporozoan protozoan, now classified as a fungus. Lives extracellularly within alveoli.
Laboratory identification	Histologic identification of organism in tissues.
Diseases	Pneumonia-like condition, severe in immunocompromised patients. Worldwide distribution.
Transmission	Assumed to be by droplets.
Pathogenesis	Inflammation in lung.
Treatment and prevention	Trimethoprim–sulfamethoxazole or pentamidine.
Organ systems and disease involvement	General, 495-496; immunocompromised host, 433-434; lower respiratory tract infection, 235

PROTOZOA

CRYPTOSPORIDIUM PARVUM

Characteristics	Intestinal sporozoan, invades and reproduces in epithelial cells of small intestine. Forms oocysts, which are passed in feces.
Laboratory identification	Small (5 μm) oocysts in feces, detected by flotation and acid-fast staining.
Diseases	Cryptosporidiosis. Worldwide distribution.
Transmission	Fecal–oral. Swallowing infective oocysts, usually in contaminated water. Animal reservoirs of infection.
Pathogenesis	Invasion of epithelial cells causes diarrhea; can be profuse in immunocompromised patients.
Treatment and prevention	No routine treatment available; spiramycin can be used in immunocompromised patients. Improved sanitation.
Organ systems and disease involvement	Gastrointestinal tract infections, 297; general, 43

CYCLOSPORA CAYETANENSIS

Characteristics	Intestinal sporozoan. Forms oocysts, which are passed in feces.
Laboratory identification	8–10 mm oocysts with two sporocysts found in feces, detected by flotation and acid-fast staining.
Diseases	Cyclosporosis
Transmission	Fecal–oral. Swallowing infective oocysts in contaminated food. Birds may act as reservoir hosts.
Pathogenesis	Diarrhea. Infection can be serious in immunocompromised patients.
Treatment and prevention	Trimethoprim–sulfamethoxazole. Washing of fruit and vegetables.
Organ systems and disease involvement	Gastrointestinal tract infections, 297

ENTAMOEBA HISTOLYTICA

Characteristics	Intestinal ameba, lives in intestine as trophozoite; produces resistant cysts, which are passed in feces.
Laboratory identification	Motile trophozoites or four-nucleate cysts in feces, detected in fresh or fixed stained smears.
Diseases	Amebic dysentery, liver abscess. Worldwide distribution, commonest in tropical and subtropical countries.
Transmission	Fecal–oral. Swallowing cysts in contaminated water or food.
Pathogenesis	Invasion of large bowel mucosa causes ulceration and diarrhea, often bloody. Spread to liver causes formation of sterile abscess.

Treatment and prevention	Metronidazole, tinidazole. Hygiene and sanitation.
Organ systems and disease involvement	Gastrointestinal tract infections, 294-296

NAEGLERIA FOWLERI

Characteristics	An ameba commonly found in the soil and in warm bodies of fresh water (e.g. lakes, rivers, and unchlorinated swimming pools). *N. fowleri* is the cause of primary amebic meningoencephalitis (PAM).
Laboratory identification	Motile trophozoites present in CSF which must not be confused with white blood cells.
Diseases	PAM is characterized by meningoencephalitic symptoms (e.g. headache, fever, nausea, etc.).
Transmission	Infection is rare but occurs (e.g. during swimming) when the ameba enters the nose and subsequently moves to the brain and spinal cord. Infection is most common during summer months when water is warm.
Pathogenesis	*N. fowleri* trophozoites invade the olfactory mucosa, ultimately moving to the subarachnoid space. Protein and glucose in CSF support growth and invasion of brain parenchyma. Medical care complicated by the rarity of the disease and difficult early diagnosis. Without treatment death results within 7–10 days.
Treatment and prevention	Amphotericin B. Only swimming in uncontaminated bodies of water (e.g. chlorinated swimming pools, etc.).
Organ systems and disease involvement	Host-parasite relationship, 64

GIARDIA LAMBLIA

Characteristics	Intestinal flagellate; lives on mucosa of small bowel. Produces cysts, which are passed in feces.
Laboratory identification	Four-nucleate cysts in feces, detected in fixed stained smears. Direct recovery of binucleate trophozoites from bowel.
Diseases	Giardiasis. Wordwide distribution.
Transmission	Fecal–oral. Swallowing cysts, usually in contaminated water. Animal reservoirs of infection.
Pathogenesis	Large numbers of trophozoites can cause severe diarrhea and impaired absorption. Most severe in immunocompromised patients.
Treatment and prevention	Metronidazole, tinidazole. Improved sanitation, water treatment.
Organ systems and disease Involvement	General, 273; gastrointestinal tract infections, 296-297; host-parasite relationship, 126

GENUS LEISHMANIA

Genus contains several species, of which *L. brasiliensis*, *L. donovani* and *L. tropica* cause major disease.

Characteristics	Sporozoa living intracellularly in macrophages as amastigote stage. Transmitted by phlebotomine sandflies.
Laboratory identification	Clinical signs, presence of amastigotes in stained biopsy material, in-vitro culture of tissue specimens to obtain promastigotes.
Diseases	Visceral (donovani), cutaneous (tropica) and mucocutaneous (brasiliensis) leishmaniasis. Disease also known by many local names (e.g. kala-azar, Oriental sore, espundia). Commonest in tropical and subtropical countries.
Transmission	By bite of infected sandfly.
Pathogenesis	Visceral: hepatosplenomegaly from invasion of macrophages in liver and spleen; allergic reactions after treatment causing dermal nodules. Cutaneous: localized ulcers, which resolve. Mucocutaneous: progressive invasion of mucocutaneous tissues in nose and mouth.
Treatment and prevention	Antimonials, pentamidine. Avoidance of vectors.
Organ systems and disease involvement	Diagnosis and control, 463; host-parasite relationship, 152; infection of skin, soft tissue, muscle and associated systems, 364-365; vaccination, 536; vector-borne, 396-397

GENUS PLASMODIUM

Genus contains four species causing disease: *P. falciparum*, *P. malariae*, *P. ovale* and *P. vivax*. *P. falciparum* and *P. vivax* are commonest.

Characteristics	Sporozoa living intracellularly in liver and primarily in red blood cells.
Laboratory identification	Parasites in red blood cells in stained blood smear.
Diseases	Malaria. Commonest in tropical and subtropical countries.
Transmission	By bite of infected anopheline mosquito.
Pathogenesis	Bursting of infected red cells causes periodic fevers. In falciparum malaria, sequestration of infected cells in brain capillaries can cause fatal cerebral malaria; this infection is sometimes associated with intravascular hemolysis. Infection with *P. malariae* can lead to nephritis due to immune complex deposition.
Treatment and prevention	Many antimalarial drugs, but parasites show considerable drug resistance. Avoidance of vectors. Mosquito control.
Organ systems and disease involvement	Central nervous system (CNS), 338; diagnosis and control, 507; host-parasite relationship, 162; pathological consequences, 189, 190; vector-borne (malaria), 391-394

TOXOPLASMA GONDII

Characteristics	Sporozoan living intracellularly, forming large tissue cysts. Natural host is cat, where parasite has enteric cycle, producing oocysts in feces. In humans organisms can invade many tissues.

Laboratory identification	Serology; need repeated tests to establish current infection.
Diseases	Toxoplasmosis. Worldwide distribution.
Transmission	Swallowing oocysts passed by cats; ingestion of tissue cysts in raw or undercooked meat; transplacental.
Pathogenesis	In adults causes mild influenza-like disease; lymph nodes may be enlarged. Symptoms more severe in immunocompromised patients. Congenital infections can damage eye or brain and prove fatal.
Treatment and prevention	Pyrimethamine, sulfadiazine. Hygiene, cooking of meat.
Organ systems and disease involvement	General, 318; central nervous system (CNS), 338; eye infections, 345-346

TRICHOMONAS VAGINALIS

Characteristics	Flagellate living in urogenital system of females and, occasionally, males. Trophozoite form only, no cyst.
Laboratory identification	Identification of trophozoites in stained material from vaginal smears.
Diseases	Trichomoniasis. Worldwide distribution.
Transmission	Venereal.
Pathogenesis	Mild in males; causes vaginitis with discharge in females.
Treatment and prevention	Metronidazole, tinidazole. Use of condoms.
Organ systems and disease involvement	Diagnosis and control, 463, 496; sexually transmitted disease, 263

GENUS TRYPANOSOMA

	Genus contains three species that cause disease: *T. gambiense*, *T. rhodesiense* (African trypanosomiasis) and *T. cruzi* (American trypanosomiasis).
Characteristics	Flagellates living in blood and tissues. *T. cruzi* has intracellular stages.
Laboratory identification	Organisms in blood or cerebrospinal fluid (African) or blood, biopsy or culture (American). Serology.
Diseases	African trypanosomiasis (sleeping sickness): sub-Saharan Africa. American trypanosomiais (Chagas' disease): South America.
Transmission	By bite of infected insect vector: tsetse fly (African) or reduviid bug (American).
Pathogenesis	African: infection of CNS causing meningoencephalitis. American: destruction of infected cells, especially neurones, megacolon, megaesophagus, cardiac failure.
Treatment and prevention	Arsenicals. Avoidance of vectors. Vector control.

Organ systems and disease involvement	Diagnosis and control, 463; infection of skin, soft tissue, muscle and associated systems, 377-378; vector-borne, 394-396

MICROSPORIDIA (CONTAINS A NUMBER OF SPECIES)

Characteristics	Intracellular pathogens, in intestine and other organs, characteristic spores.
Laboratory identification	Detection of organisms in biopsies, CSF and urine. Gram, acid-fast and other stains can be used.
Diseases	Microsporidiosis.
Pathogenesis	Diarrhea, other symptoms dependent on organ infected. Infection can be serious in immunocompromised patients.
Treatment and prevention	Metronidazole. Hygiene and sanitation.
Organ systems and disease involvement	Gastrointestinal tract infections, 294, 297

ISOSPORA BELLI

Characteristics	A protozoal coccidian parasite infecting epithelial cells of the small intestine.
Laboratory identification	Diagnosis of infection based on observation of oocysts in feces. Internal morphology of the oocyst helpful in identification. Final identification generally possible only after oocyst sporulation.
Diseases	Chronic intestinal disease especially in immunocompromised patients. Symptoms of infection include diarrhea, headache, fever, malaise, and abdominal pain.
Transmission	Infection occurs by ingestion of oocysts from the feces of another host.
Pathogenesis	Invasion of epithelial cells in the small intestine. Cycles of reproduction (asexual to sexual reproduction) with additional epithelial cell invasion and further production of oocysts which are excreted in the stool.
Treatment and prevention	Trimethoprim–sulfamethoxazole.
Organ systems and disease involvement	Gastrointestinal tract infections, 297; immunocompromised host, 435

HELMINTHS

TAPEWORMS

DIPHYLLOBOTHRIUM LATUM

Characteristics	Large adult tapeworm in intestine. Scolex with sucking grooves not suckers. Eggs released and passed in feces.
Laboratory identification	Fecal smears, fresh or stained. Eggs in feces have characteristic operculum (lid).

Diseases	Diphyllobothriasis (fish tapeworm). Worldwide distribution. Commonest where fish eaten raw.
Transmission	Larval stages in fish. Adult worm acquired when infected fish eaten raw or undercooked.
Pathogenesis	Usually harmless; may be associated with vitamin B_{12} deficiency.
Treatment and prevention	Niclosamide, praziquantel. Cooking of fish. Sanitation.
Organ systems and disease involvement	Gastrointestinal tract infections, 300

ECHINOCOCCUS GRANULOSUS

Characteristics	Large fluid-filled (hydatid) cysts, in abdomen, liver, lungs, CNS.
Laboratory identification	Scans, serology.
Diseases	Hydatidosis, hydatid disease. Worldwide distribution, commonest in sheep-rearing countries.
Transmission	Swallowing eggs released from adult tapeworms in dogs. Natural cycle is adult (dog), larval cysts (sheep).
Pathogenesis	Cysts exert pressure on internal organs. Release of cyst fluid can cause anaphylaxis.
Treatment and prevention	Mebendazole, albendazole. Surgical removal of cysts. Prevention of dogs eating infected viscera from sheep. Hygiene after handling dogs.
Organ systems and disease involvement	Central nervous system (CNS), 338-339; host-parasite relationship, 170; multisystem zoonoses, 410-411

HYMENOLEPIS NANA

Characteristics	Small (2–4 cm) adult tapeworms in intestine. Scolex with suckers and hooks. Eggs passed in feces. Lifecycle can be direct or via insect intermediate host.
Laboratory identification	Fecal smears, fresh or stained. Thin-shelled eggs in feces.
Diseases	Hymenolepiasis (dwarf tapeworm). Worldwide distribution.
Transmission	Swallowing eggs. Accidental ingestion of larvae in insects.
Pathogenesis	Usually harmless. Numbers of worms can build up by autoinfection (direct hatching of eggs from adult worms in intestine) and enteritis may result.
Treatment and prevention	Niclosamide, praziquantel. Hygiene and sanitation.
Organ systems and disease involvement	Gastrointestinal tract infections, 300

GENUS TAENIA

	Two species of this genus infect humans: *T. saginata* and *T. solium*.
Characteristics	Large (meters) adult tapeworms in intestine. Scolices with suckers (*saginata*) or suckers and hooks (*saginata* and *solium*). Proglottids (segments) passed in feces. Small cysts (larval stages of *solium*) in muscles, CNS and eyes.
Laboratory identification	Proglottids in feces. Species identifiable on basis of number of branches to uterus (*T. saginata* 15–20; *T. solium* 5–10).
Diseases	Taeniasis (beef and pork tapeworms). Cysticercosis (*T. solium* only). Worldwide distribution.
Transmission	Adult worms acquired by eating raw or undercooked meat (beef, saginata; pork, solium) from animals infected with larval stages. *T. solium* eggs can hatch in humans, allowing cysts to develop.
Pathogenesis	Adult worms essentially harmless. In cysticercosis, cysts in brain can result in neurologic symptoms.
Treatment and prevention	Niclosamide, praziquantel. Adequate cooking of meat. Prevention of human feces contaminating grazing and feeding areas of cattle and pigs.
Organ systems and disease involvement	Central nervous system (CNS), 339; gastrointestinal tract infections, 300; infection of skin, soft tissue, muscle and associated systems, 378; zoonoses, 410

FLUKES

CLONORCHIS SINENSIS

Characteristics	Liver fluke. Narrow elongated worms in bile ducts.
Laboratory identification	Fecal smears, fresh or stained. Eggs in feces.
Diseases	Clonorchiasis (Asia).
Transmission	Larval stages in fish; adult flukes acquired when infected fish eaten raw or undercooked.
Pathogenesis	Damage to liver, inflammation of bile ducts.
Treatment and prevention	Praziquantel. Cooking of fish. Sanitation.
Organ systems and disease involvement	Gastrointestinal tract infections, 309

PARAGONIMUS WESTERMANII

Characteristics	Lung fluke. Thick fleshy worms living as pairs in cysts.
Laboratory identification	Eggs in sputum or feces.
Diseases	Paragonimiasis (Asia).
Transmission	Larval stages in crabs; adult flukes acquired when infected crab meat eaten raw or undercooked.

Pathogenesis	Inflammation of lungs, secondary bacterial infections.
Treatment and prevention	Praziquantel. Cooking of crab meat. Sanitation.
Organ systems and disease involvement	Lower respiratory tract infection, 237

GENUS SCHISTOSOMA

	Genus contains several species able to infect humans. Three are of major importance: *S. haematobium*, *S. japonicum* and *S. mansoni*.
Characteristics	Blood flukes; adult worms in blood vessels around intestine (*S. japonicum*, *S. mansoni*) or bladder (*S. haematobium*). Eggs in tissues.
Laboratory identification	Fecal smears, fresh or stained. Spined eggs in feces (*S. japonicum*, small lateral spine; *S. mansoni*, large lateral spine). Eggs in urine (*S. haematobium*, terminal spine).
Diseases	Schistosomiasis. Widely distributed in tropical/subtropical countries (*S. mansoni*, Africa, S. America; *S. haematobium*, Africa, Middle East; *S. japonicum*, Asia).
Transmission	Larvae released from eggs infect aquatic snails. These release infective cercariae larvae, which actively penetrate human skin.
Pathogenesis	Hypersensitivity responses to eggs cause inflammation, granuloma formation, fibrosis and obstructive disease in intestine, bladder and liver.
Treatment and prevention	Praziquantel. Avoidance of infected waters. Removal of snails. Sanitation.
Organ systems and disease involvement	General, 49; host-parasite relationship, 170; infection of skin, soft tissue, muscle and associated systems, 365; pathological consequences, 193; urinary tract infections (UTI), 246; vector-borne, 397-398

NEMATODES

ASCARIS LUMBRICOIDES

Characteristics	Large (up to 30 cm) intestinal roundworm; migratory stages pass through liver and lungs.
Laboratory identification	Fecal smears, fresh or stained. Thick-shelled eggs in feces; worms also passed occasionally.
Diseases	Ascariasis. Worldwide distribution. Commonest in tropical and subtropical countries.
Transmission	Swallowing infective eggs in contaminated soil, food or water.
Pathogenesis	Migrating larvae cause pneumonia-like symptoms. Adults can obstruct intestine, interfere with digestion and absorption of food, migrate in bile duct. Allergic symptoms common.
Treatment and prevention	Mebendazole, pyrantel, piperazine. Hygiene and sanitation.
Organ systems and disease involvement	Gastrointestinal tract infections, 298-300; host-parasite relationship, 126; pathological consequences, 190

ENTEROBIUS VERMICULARIS

Characteristics	Small (1 cm) roundworm in large bowel. Worms emerge from anus at night to lay eggs.
Laboratory identification	Eggs recovered from perianal skin; adult worms in feces.
Diseases	Enterobiasis, pinworm. Worldwide distribution. Commonest in children.
Transmission	Swallowing eggs, which can be carried on fingers and in dust. Eggs infective when laid, so direct reinfection is common.
Pathogenesis	Perianal pruritus.
Treatment and prevention	Mebendazole, pyrantel, piperazine. Hygiene.
Organ systems and disease involvement	Gastrointestinal tract infections, 297-298

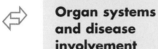

FILARIAL NEMATODES

	Large group. Most important species living in lymphatic tissues (*Wuchereria bancrofti*, *Brugia malayi*) or in skin (*Onchocerca volvulus*).
Characteristics	Adults very long, thin worms, living in lymphatics with microfilariae larvae in blood (*Wuchereria, Brugia*) or in subcutaneous nodules with microfilariae in skin (*Onchocerca*).
Laboratory identification	Detection of microfilariae in stained blood smear or fresh skin snip.
Diseases	Lymphatic filariasis (*Wuchereria, Brugia*). Onchocerciasis or river blindness (*Onchocerca*).
Transmission	Microfilariae taken up by blood-feeding insects (mosquitoes, *Wuchereria, Brugia*; Simulium blackflies, *Onchocerca*), develop to infective stage and reintroduced into humans at the next blood meal. Widely distributed in tropical and subtropical countries.
Pathogenesis	In lymphatic filariasis, adult worms cause inflammation of lymph nodes and blockage of lymphatics, sometimes causing elephantiasis (big leg). In onchocerciasis, hypersensitivity to microfilariae larvae leads to skin and eye lesions.
Treatment and prevention	Diethyl carbamazine (lymphatic) and ivermectin (onchocerciasis). Avoidance of vectors. Vector control.
Organ systems and disease involvement	Eye infections, 346; infection of skin, soft tissue, muscle and associated systems, 365; vector-borne, 398

HOOKWORMS

	General term for intestinal bloodsucking worms. Two major species: *Ancylostoma duodenale* and *Necator americanus*.
Characteristics	Small (1 cm) intestinal roundworms; migratory stages pass through skin and lungs. Adult worms have expanded mouths for attachment to intestinal mucosa.
Laboratory identification	Fecal smears, fresh or stained. Thin-shelled eggs in feces. Culture of feces, eggs hatching after 24 h to release larvae.

Diseases	Hookworm disease (ancylostomiasis, necatoriasis). Widespread in tropical and subtropical countries.
Transmission	Infective larvae penetrate skin (both species) or mucous membranes after ingestion (*Ancylostoma*).
Pathogenesis	Bloodsucking of worms can lead to anemia and protein loss. Larval penetration associated with dermatitis.
Treatment and prevention	Mebendazole, pyrantel. Hygiene and sanitation.
Organ systems and disease involvement	Gastrointestinal tract infections, 299; infection of skin, soft tissue, muscle and associated systems, 365

STRONGYLOIDES STERCORALIS

Characteristics	Minute (2 mm) intestinal roundworm, living in humans only as larvae and parthenogenetic females. Migratory stages pass through skin and (possibly) lungs. Eggs hatch in intestine; larvae in feces may become infective directly or initiate a free-living generation in soil, from which infective larvae develop.
Laboratory identification	Larvae in fresh fecal specimens.
Diseases	Strongyloidiasis. Widespread in tropical and subtropical countries.
Transmission	Infective larvae penetrate skin.
Pathogenesis	In immunocompromised patients, repeated autoinfection (development of larvae released from females in the intestine) can lead to hyperinfection (disseminated strongyloidiasis), with larvae invading all body tissues. Hyperinfection can be fatal. Diarrhea and malabsorption accompany heavy intestinal infections.
Treatment and prevention	Tiabendazole (thiabendazole). Hygiene and sanitation.
Organ systems and disease involvement	Gastrointestinal tract infections, 298-300; general, 47; host-parasite relationship, 64; multisystem zoonoses, 411-412

TOXOCARA CANIS

Characteristics	Invasion of larvae of roundworm species normally maturing in intestine of dogs.
Laboratory identification	Serology.
Diseases	Toxocariasis, visceral larva migrans. Worldwide distribution.
Transmission	Swallowing infective eggs passed by dogs in contaminated soil, food or water.
Pathogenesis	Invasion of body tissues causing granulomatous inflammatory responses. Larvae in CNS may cause epilepsy-like condition; in the eye granulomas may cause blindness.
Treatment and prevention	Tiabendazole (thiabendazole). Hygiene. Routine deworming of puppies and pregnant bitches.

| **Organ systems and disease involvement** | Central nervous system (CNS), 338; eye infections, 346; pathological consequences, 193 |

TRICHINELLA SPIRALIS

Characteristics	Minute (2–3 mm) roundworms, living as adults in the intestine. Coiled larvae in muscles. Low host specificity; infects and matures in wide variety of mammals.
Laboratory identification	Clinical signs, serology, muscle biopsy.
Diseases	Trichinellosis (trichinosis). Worldwide distribution.
Transmission	Acquired by eating raw or undercooked meat (usually pork) containing infective larvae.
Pathogenesis	Diarrhea during intestinal phase. Allergic symptoms, muscle pain, cardiac effects during muscle invasion; last phase can be fatal.
Treatment and prevention	Mebendazole. Cooking of meat.
Organ systems and disease involvement	Diagnosis and control, 1; host-parasite relationship, 126; infection of skin, soft tissue, muscle and associated systems, 378; multisystem zoonoses, 411

 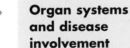

TRICHURIS TRICHIURA

Characteristics	Medium size (0.75 cm) roundworms in large bowel. Body of characteristic 'whipworm' form, with long thin anterior and short, thicker posterior.
Laboratory identification	Fecal smears, fresh or stained. Eggs in feces have characteristic shape, oval with plug at each pole. Endoscopy.
Diseases	Trichuriasis. Worldwide distribution. Commonest in tropical and subtropical countries.
Transmission	Swallowing infective eggs in contaminated soil, food or water.
Pathogenesis	Diarrhea, intestinal inflammation, occasionally rectal prolapse.
Treatment and prevention	Mebendazole. Hygiene and sanitation.
Organ systems and disease involvement	Gastrointestinal tract infections, 298-300; host-parasite relationship, 126

Answers

A contemporary approach to microbiology

1. Viruses, bacteria, fungi, protozoa, worms, arthropods (prions are not organisms in a conventional sense)
2. Acute respiratory infections, AIDS, diarrheal diseases, TB, malaria
3. Hanta virus, human herpes virus 8, hepatits E–G, *Escherichia coli* O157, *Borrelia burgdorferi*, *Helicobacter*, toxin-producing *Staphylocccus aureus*
4. Increased travel, new patterns of food production, distribution and use, new agricultural practices, changes in sexual behaviour, medical interventions, antibiotic overuse, social, economic, political and possibly climatic change.

CHAPTER 1

Microbes as Parasites

1. In prokaryotes there is no distinct nucleus, DNA occurs in a single circular chromosome and is also present in plasmids, transcription and translation are simultaneous. In eukaryotes there is a distinct, membrane-bound nucleus, DNA is present in several chromosomes, translation requires mRNA and occurs on ribosomes in the cytoplasm, the cytoplasm is rich in organelles.
2. Microparasites are generally microscopic in size, can live within cells, can replicate in the host and can increase in number rapidly after a single infection event. Macroparasites are generally larger (>1 mm), live outside cells, most cannot replicate within the host, so increases in number require repeated infection events.
3. Use of the host's genetic machinery, use of intercellular nutrient pools, protection from some of the host's defensive mechanisms.
4. Observational (shape, size, staining), biochemical (respiratory patterns, production of enzymes, toxins), immunologic (responses to antibodies), molecular (analysis of DNA, response to probes).

CHAPTER 2

The Bacteria

1. B – Lipopolysaccharide
2. C – Staphylococcus
3. E – Every 30 minutes
4. E – All of these
5. D – Mutation
6. B – Transposons

CHAPTER 3

The Viruses

1. B – Influenza virus
2. C – Vaccinia virus
3. A – Sialic acid
4. D – Human T cell lymphotropic virus

CHAPTER 4

The Fungi

1. C – *Candida*
2. D – Dead skin

CHAPTER 5

The Protozoa

1. B – Malaria
2. D – *Toxoplasma*
3. D – *Giardia*

CHAPTER 6

The Helminths and Arthropods

1. D – *Taenia solium*
2. C – *Wuchereria bancrofti*
3. B – Transmission involves an aquatic snail
4. E – All of these

CHAPTER 7

Prions

1. D – Bite of a contaminated insect vector
2. E – None of these
3. B – Treatment with sodium hydroxide and sodium hypochlorite

CHAPTER 8

The Host–Parasite Relationship

1. E – All of these
2. C – In the large intestine
3. D – They always cause disease
4. E – All of these

CHAPTER 9

The Innate Defenses of the Body

1. D – Salivary amylase
2. A – Monocytes; B – Kupffer cells; D – Lymph node medullary macrophages
3. A – Generates reactive oxygen intermediates; C – Contains microbicidal cytoplasmic granules; D – Is a professional phagocytic cell
4. C – Opsonizes bacteria
5. A – Respond to interferon; B – Contain perforin; C – Contain granzymes
6. A – C-reactive protein; B – Mannose binding protein; C – Lysozyme; E – Complement

CHAPTER 10

Adaptive Responses Provide a 'Quantum Leap' in Effective Defense

1. B – C3bBb; E – C42
2. E – C3
3. A – synthesize and secrete antibody; C – Are derived from B cells; E – Have a high RNA content
4. A – Antibody of similar specificity to that on the surface of the parent B cell
5. B – MHC; E – Peptides derived from intracellular processing of proteins
6. B – Antigen
7. A – T cells
8. B – Cytotoxic T cells

CHAPTER 11

The Cellular Basis of Adaptive Immune Responses

1. A – Tolerance
2. A – By binding to specific receptors
3. D – IL-4
4. B – Antigen-specific IgM; C – Antigen neutralization

CHAPTER 12

Background to the Infectious Diseases

1. (a) Show that diabetes occured only in people infected with the virus, either by antibody tests or by prospective studies of populations.
   (b) Isolate the virus or detect virus 'footprints' (nucleic acid sequences, antigens) from the pancreas of diabetics but not from non-diabetics.
   Note: It might be difficult to prove if:
   1. the virus turned out to be *a* cause rather than *the* cause of diabetes
   2. the virus infected nearly everyone but only caused diabetes in an occasional individual
   3. the disease did not appear until 10–20 years after the infection.
2. Rabies spreads directly from animal to animal via saliva, and infection of humans is not necessary for its maintenance in nature.
3. The steps are listed in Figure 12.1. Attachment/entry, multiplication, and shedding are the most important.
4. (a) Delete the gene from the virus by molecular engineering and see if it is then less virulent.
   (b) Produce antibody to the gene product(s) and see if passive administration of the antibody reduces virulence.
   (c) Attempt to replace the interfered-with cytokine or other components of the immune system. This is less likely to be successful.
5. Microbes that have to spread through the body step by step (Fig. 12.3) take a least a week to do so.
6. Because microbes have developed strategies to interfere with phagocytic function, for instance by inhibiting phagocytosis or by inhibiting phagolysosomal fusion.

CHAPTER 13

Entry, Exit and Transmission

1. Respiratory, fecal–oral, sexual, zoonoses.
2. Because the infection is not shed from body surfaces (see Fig. 13.1) or not in sufficient amounts to infect other people. In many cases human infection is not needed for the maintenance and spread of the microbe.
3. No. Certain infections are spread via urine (leptospirosis or Lassa fever, from animals to humans) but for efficient person-to-person spread the microbe would need to be very infectious and resistant to drying.
4. Yes. Common colds can be spread by hands and handkerchiefs.
5. The routes are:
   • *prenatal* (placenta): blood cells and vascular endothelium of mother and fetus, plus trophoblast cells in placenta
   • *perinatal*: blood cells and mucosal cells of cervix and vagina of mother, plus conjunctival and respiratory epithelial cells of infant
   • *postnatal*: maternal blood cells and cells lining mammary gland and ducts
   • *germline*: ova and sperm.
6. If there are receptors on respiratory epithelial cells to which microbes can attach, it could infect these cells. Gonococci, for example, can infect conjunctival cells.

CHAPTER 14

Immune Defenses in Action

1. A – Reactive oxygen intermediates; C – Cytotoxic lipid peroxides; E – Nitric oxide
2. B – Inhibiting virus assembly; C – Inhibiting viral RNA translation
3. A – Opsonizing the parasite for subsequent phagocytosis; D – Blocking microbial entry into the host cell; E – Inducing antibody-dependent cellular cytotoxicity
4. A – Antigen-specific T cells; B – Production of cytokines such as IFN

CHAPTER 15

Spread and Replication

1. (a) Salivary glands are reached from the blood after passage across vascular endothelium (mumps) or via peripheral nerves (rabies virus).
   (b) The liver is reached from the blood after transit through Kupffer cells or vascular endothelium, in sinusoids.
2. Yes. In the case of:
   (a) herpes simplex and varicella-zoster viruses (the basis for reactivation and renewed shedding)
   (b) rabies virus (spread via nerves to salivary gland and transmission in saliva of animals).
3. (a) Polioviruses. This means exposure to circulating antibody.

(b) Herpesviruses. This mean protection from circulating antibody and possible carriage of infection into organs by migrating leukocytes.

4. Because they replicate very slowly (doubling time measured in days).

5. Sickle cell gene and susceptibility to malaria.

CHAPTER 16

Parasite Survival Strategies and Persistent Infections

1. No. Commoner with short amino acid sequences.

2. Because the outer surface is the main target for host defense and therefore more likely to undergo variation as an avoidance strategy.

3. (a) – No; (b) – No

4. If antiviral lymphocytes and antibodies had increased access to epidermal cells, i.e. during local inflammation.

CHAPTER 18

Upper Respiratory Tract Infections

1. **Diagnosis**

Acute otitis media.

2. **Most likely pathogens**

Haemophilus influenzae and *Streptococcus pneumoniae* are the most common pathogens. Less commonly *Moraxella catarrhalis*, Group A β-hemolytic streptococci, and *Staphylococcus aureus* are implicated. Acute otitis media often follows a viral upper respiratory tract infection. Congestion of the eustachian tubes results in fluid stasis within the middle ear and secondary bacterial infection. The pressure building up within the anatomic constraints of the middle ear causes pain, and may lead to perforation of the tympanic membrane, with a discharge of pus.

3. **Treatment**

Treatment should involve antibiotics, usually oral unless the child is vomiting. Options include amoxicillin either alone or in combination with a beta-lactamase inhibitor such as clavulanic acid to cover the increasing proportion of *H. influenzae* that are beta-lactamase positive. Alternatives include orally active second and third generation cephalosporins. Penicillin-allergic patients should be given co-trimoxazole or a new macrolide with increased activity against *H. influenzae*.

4. **Possible complications**

Complications include acute mastoiditis, which is rare since the advent of antibiotic therapy, and recurrent infections leading to chronic exudative otitis media (glue ear), which is a much more common problem.

CHAPTER 19

Lower Respiratory Tract Infections

1. **Differential diagnosis**

This case is suggestive of an atypical pneumonia. Causes are:

- Chlamydial infections such as *Chlamydophila pneumoniae* (also referred to as TWAR) and *Chlamydophila psittaci*.

- *Mycoplasma pneumoniae*.
- *Legionella pneumophila*.
- *Coxiella burnetii* (Q fever).

2. **Other questions particularly relevant to the differential diagnosis to ask**

- What is your occupation?
- Have you traveled recently?
- Do you have any pets at home or any hobbies?

These questions are always an important part of the history, but may be especially relevant with regard to *C. psittaci* (contact with infected birds), *L. pneumophila* (air conditioning systems) and *C. burnetii* (Q fever, contact with infected sheep/cattle).

3. **Further investigations**

Serology

- To detect *Mycoplasma pneumoniae* – particle agglutination test (IgM and IgG) and complement fixation test (CFT) on paired acute and convalescent sera collected 10–14 days apart, or test the acute serum specimen taken at least 10 days after the illness. The hematology laboratory should also test for the presence of cold agglutinins.

- To detect chlamydiae – microimmunofluorescence for type-specific IgM/IgG or enzyme-linked immunosorbent assay (ELISA), and CFT on paired acute and convalescent sera collected 10–14 days apart, or test the acute serum taken at least 10 days after the illness. The CFT uses the chlamydial group-specific antigen.

- To detect *L. pneumophila* – urine sample for legionella antigen serum sample to detect the presence of antibody is less sensitive.

- To detect *C. burnetii* – CFT of paired acute and convalescent sera collected 10–14 days apart, or test the acute serum specimen taken at least 10 days after the illness. Phase 1 antibody is detected in chronic Q fever infection. Phase 2 antibody is detected in acute and chronic Q fever infection.

Culture for chlamydiae, mycoplasma, and *Legionella* may be attempted, depending upon available laboratory facilities.

4. **Diagnosis**

Mycoplasma pneumoniae infection on the basis of a fourfold rise in CFT, a positive agglutination test titer having diluted the serum 1 in 1024, and positive cold agglutinins.

5. **Treatment**

The antibiotic of choice is erythromycin or tetracycline.

CHAPTER 20

Urinary Tract Infections

1. **Significance of bacterial count**

This patient's urine specimen shows a bacterial count $>10^5$ per ml of urine.

2. **Why urine is screened for infection in pregnancy**

Pregnant women have an increased risk of developing a urinary tract infection because the ureters dilate under the action of progesterone. This allows the urine to remain static and infection to ascend from the bladder. In the early stages of infection the patient may be asymptomatic, hence the need to screen the urine for the presence of infection. The risk of pyelonephritis is greater in the pregnant woman with a positive urine culture. Both urinary tract infection and pyelonephritis may cause septicemia, which may result in premature labor. It is therefore necessary to identify and treat urinary tract infections in pregnancy promptly.

3. The three most likely causes of this patient's infection
In the light of the culture result showing 'coliforms' the most likely causes are *Escherichia coli* followed by *Proteus mirabilis*. Other Gram-negative rods such as *Klebsiella* or *Pseudomonas* would be very unlikely unless the patient had a history of recurrent infection or previous instrumentation of the urinary tract.

4. Antimicrobials suitable for treating this infection in pregnancy
It may be possible to treat a simple urinary tract infection with a urinary sterilizing agent such as nitrofurantoin. Ampicillin is a suitable first-line antibiotic in areas where there is a low prevalence of resistant *Escherichia coli*. Where the prevalence of resistance is high, it may be necessary to use an oral cephalosporin. If the patient is unwell and requires parenteral antibiotics, an injectable cephalosporin can be given.

CHAPTER 21

Sexually Transmitted Diseases

1. Most likely diagnosis
Pneumocystis carinii pneumonia (PCP) in a person with HIV1 infection.

2. Further investigations
- Arterial blood gas analysis.
- Induced sputum or bronchoscopy and bronchoalveolar lavage for PCP examination.
- HIV1 and HIV2 antibody screening assay: this is positive and therefore a further confirmatory test is performed and demonstrates the presence of antibody to HIV1. In addition, *Pneumocystis* cysts are seen on cytology.

3. Management
The diagnosis should be discussed sensitively with the patient and a further serum specimen collected to confirm the diagnosis. A second specimen should always be retested to ensure that no errors in the collection, labeling of the specimen, dispatch, or handling of the specimen in the laboratory have occurred. The laboratory should have tested both the serum from the original specimen and repeated the test on any remaining serum in the original tube containing the blood clot.

First line treatment for PCP, which would have already been started on clinical suspicion, generally comprises oxygen and co-trimoxazole, and in severe cases methylprednisolone. If the patient develops an allergy to the sulfa-containing drugs such as co-trimoxazole, intravenous pentamidine treatment should be instituted. Clinicians will be guided by the clinical signs and symptoms as well as the results of the blood gas analysis.

4. Prognosis and follow-up
This patient has an AIDS-defining diagnosis (i.e. PCP) and her prognosis in terms of survival duration is variable. Baseline CD4 counts and a p24 antigen test would be performed as would a syphilis and viral hepatitis screen.

Regular PCP prophylaxis with co-trimoxazole should be instituted and she should be followed up regularly. She should be monitored clinically, and CD4 counts should be repeated at regular intervals. A decision about whether to start antiretroviral treatment should be discussed.

Other issues include a discussion regarding her partner and HIV testing, safe sex, and whether she has or is planning to have children. Counseling about the wider aspects and implications of her diagnosis with a health advisor should be arranged.

CHAPTER 22

Gastrointestinal Tract Infections (a)

1. Most likely diagnosis and differential diagnosis
The most likely diagnosis is acute hepatitis B infection (HBV). The differential diagnosis includes hepatitis A, hepatitis C, delta hepatitis (as a hepatitis B coinfection/superinfection), cytomegalovirus (CMV) infection, and Epstein–Barr virus (EBV) infection.

2. Investigations
- Collect a clotted blood specimen for hepatitis B surface antigen (HBsAg) testing and markers of HBV infection (see below).
- HBsAg testing: using enzyme-linked immunosorbent assay (ELISA) or similar tests:
  - Anti-HB core IgM
  - Anti-HB core (total IgM and IgG)
  - HBeAg.

The results of these investigations are as follows: HBsAg enzyme immunoassay (EIA) positive (confirmed by specific neutralization with immune serum containing antibody to the HBsAg); anti-HB core IgM positive; anti-HB core (total IgM and IgG) positive; HBeAg positive.

These results are consistent with an acute HBV infection.

If the sample is HBsAg negative, test for HAV IgM and HCV antibody. HCV antibody would not be detected at this early stage by EIA because anti-HCV seroconversion may be delayed for several months after an acute HCV infection. The test is usually repeated 2 months later if clinically indicated.

3. Management
- Repeat the HBV serology in 1, 3 and 6 months to see whether the infection resolves. If HBsAg is still present after 6 months this man is a hepatitis B carrier and should be followed up regularly because he may develop complications of chronic HBV infection (i.e. chronic active hepatitis, chronic persistent hepatitis, hepatocellular carcinoma). In addition, some individuals switch from being HBeAg positive to anti-HBe positive and some lose their HBsAg and become anti-HBs positive.
- Advise the patient to avoid alcohol and strenuous exercise.
- This man is also at risk of other infectious diseases because of his intravenous drug abuse and this should be discussed with him in the general context of health counseling.

4. Control of infection
HBV infection is a notifiable disease in the UK. Sexual partners or individuals with whom this man has shared needles should be followed up, counseled and tested to see whether they have serologic evidence of a past hepatitis B infection as a matter of urgency. If there is no evidence of past HBV infection these individuals should be offered a course of

hepatitis B immunization together with an injection of hepatitis B hyperimmune globulin (HBIG) to attenuate, modify or prevent HBV infection.

Gastrointestinal Tract Infections (b)

1. Immediate management.
- Admit to a source isolation room in the ward.
- Collect blood for urea and electrolyte determination.
- Rehydrate orally unless she is vomiting, in which case intravenous fluids are needed.
- Send a stool sample to bacteriology and virology for analysis.

2. Most likely viral causes of the diarrhea
Viral gastroenteritis can be divided into sporadic infantile gastroenteritis and epidemic viral gastroenteritis. The most common cause of sporadic infantile gastroenteritis is a rotavirus infection. Adenovirus infections are the second most common cause.

3. Diagnosis of a viral infection
- Electron microscopy (using phosphotungstic acid as a negative stain) is the method of choice because in this setting it is a 'catch-all' method that allows detection of a variety of viruses for which there are no generally available specific tests for detecting viral antigen or antibody to that antigen.
- There is a particle agglutination test that is specific for rotavirus infection. This is widely used, but may miss some rotavirus infections.
- In specialized laboratories enzyme-linked immunosorbent assays (ELISAs), radioimmunoassays (RIAs), or nucleic acid detection methods are available for some of the viruses associated with gastroenteritis.

Wheel-like particles which are 65 nm diameter, are demonstrated by electron microscopy and rotaviral infection is diagnosed.

4. Natural course of the infection
If the child is dehydrated, fluid replacement therapy is needed. There is no specific treatment for any of the viral causes of diarrhea, and rotaviral excretion should decrease within a week. Avoid lactose-based fluids as the loss of the distal parts of the intestinal villi due to viral infection results in a disaccharidase deficiency and therefore lactose intolerance/malabsorption.

The most important measures to prevent nosocomial infection are to place the child in source isolation and maintain high standards of hygiene, in particular thorough handwashing after contact with the child by any member of staff.

CHAPTER 23

Obstetric and Perinatal Infections

1a. Likely diagnosis and likely pathogens
The baby is septicemic. The most likely pathogens responsible for septicemia in the newborn are organisms acquired from the mother's genital tract. Group B streptococci are the most common, but *Escherichia coli* and *Listeria monocytogenes* are also important pathogens in this age group.

1b. Investigation

The baby should have a septic screen. In particular, this involves a blood culture and cerebrospinal fluid (CSF) sample. Deep ear swabs and a gastric aspirate may help to identify the pathogen responsible. A maternal vaginal swab should also be taken. Antimicrobial therapy should be started before the results of cultures are known and there are many different regimens which may be used. Common combinations are cefotaxime and benzylpenicillin, or ampicillin and gentamicin. The use of aminoglycosides requires careful monitoring of pre- and post-dose serum levels to minimize toxicity. Once the pathogen has been identified, the antibiotic regimen can be tailored accordingly.

Group B streptococci were isolated from this baby's blood culture and he was treated with intravenous benzylpenicillin and gentamicin.

1c. Risk factors in the mother's history
- Early rupture of membranes – Yes.
- Maternal pyrexia – No.
- A long and difficult labor – Yes.

CHAPTER 24

Central Nervous System Infections

1. Urgent investigations
A computerized tomographic (CT) scan of the patient's head followed by a lumbar puncture if the CT scan does not demonstrate raised intracranial pressure.

2. Diagnoses
It is important to rule out a subarachnoid hemorrhage, a subdural hemorrhage (both are unlikely in the absence of red blood cells and xanthochromic appearance in the CSF), a cranial space-occupying lesion including a cerebral abscess, metabolic causes of seizures, and meningitis.

The presentation and findings are more consistent with an encephalitic process and the most common causes of a viral encephalitis include herpes simplex virus (HSV), mumps, and enteroviruses. More detailed clinical examination revealed the presence of genital ulcers.

3. Management and treatment
There is enough evidence to implicate HSV infection as the cause of the encephalitis and so intravenous aciclovir should be started immediately together with other general supportive measures. It is important that this patient is treated with aciclovir for at least 2 weeks to prevent a relapse. Finding diffuse slow wave activity on an electroencephalogram (EEG) would further assist in making a diagnosis. A genital swab should be collected for viral isolation and cerebrospinal fluid (CSF) should be cultured, although it is extremely unusual to isolate HSV from CSF. Finally, it is possible to detect HSV DNA in CSF specimens using the polymerase chain reaction (PCR) technology and this service may be available in some laboratories.

CHAPTER 25

Infections of the Eye

1. Infections associated with a choroidoretinitis
Cytomegalovirus (CMV), *Toxoplasma gondii*, *Toxocara* (*canis* or *catis*), *Mycobacterium tuberculosis*, or acute retinal necrosis,

which is thought to be associated with varicella–zoster virus.

2. How would you make the diagnosis?

The diagnosis is almost invariably clinical and is made with the assistance of an ophthalmologist. In such a patient it can sometimes be difficult to differentiate between *Toxoplasma* and CMV. CMV retinitis sometimes has a classical appearance referred to as tomato ketchup and cottage cheese! Serology may be helpful in the diagnosis of *Toxoplasma* infection. In addition, in certain centers vitreous fluid from the affected eye can be collected. Detection of CMV DNA in this sample can be performed using a nested polymerase chain reaction approach involving two sets of primers, one set internal to the other, which increases the sensitivity of the test.

3. Treatment for CMV retinitis

Commence with a treatment course of intravenous ganciclovir while monitoring the hemoglobin, white cell count, and platelet count because this antiviral drug is myelosuppressive. If bone marrow suppression occurs, an alternative drug is foscarnet (which is nephrotoxic). It is best to site permanent intravenous access as this patient will need maintenance therapy with either of these drugs together with regular ophthalmologic follow-up to detect and prevent reactivation.

CHAPTER 26

Infections of the Skin, Muscle, Joints, Bone and Hemopoietic System (a)

Infections of the Skin, Muscle, Joints, Bone and Hemopoietic System (b)

1. Likely diagnosis

The most likely diagnosis is an acute osteomyelitis. In children of this age, it may be accompanied with a history of minor trauma. It can be difficult to diagnose, particularly if vomiting is a major part of the illness.

2. Investigations

Investigations that should be performed are:
- full blood count
- blood cultures
- radiographs of the affected area.

In acute osteomyelitis, radiographic changes usually lag behind the clinical picture. The most common pathogen in such cases is *Staphylococcus aureus*.

3. Treatment

Treatment should be commenced using intravenous flucloxacillin and oral fusidic acid (or other equivalent anti-staphylococcal treatment) while the results of cultures are awaited. Intravenous fluids and nasogastric aspiration should also be started. The limb should be immobilized by splinting, and traction will reduce the pain. Pain relief and antipyretics should also be given as appropriate. If the patient's temperature does not settle, it may be necessary to drain any collection of pus operatively. Any pus should be sent to microbiology for culture.

Infections of the Skin, Muscle, Joints, Bone and Hemopoietic System (c)

1. Differential diagnosis

- Roseola infantum (also called exanthema subitum) due to human herpes virus 6 (HHV 6).

- Enteroviral infections (i.e. due to echoviruses, coxsackieviruses).
- Fifth disease due to erythrovirus B19, which is unlikely because the classical presentation is red, slapped cheeks together with a fine rash.
- Measles and rubella, which are unlikely because of the clinical findings and she is up to date with her immunization schedule.

2. Investigations

- Collect a throat swab and stool specimen for viral isolation, in particular for the enteroviruses.
- Collect a serum specimen for the following tests: HHV 6 IgM (reference laboratory test), erythrovirus B19 IgM, measles-specific IgM, rubella-specific IgM, and enterovirus-specific IgM.

Her fever subsided over 3 days and HHV 6 specific IgM was detected in the serum specimen.

CHAPTER 27

Vector-borne Infections

1A. Differential diagnosis

Malaria, viral hemorrhagic fever and typhoid fever.

If someone has a history of travel to an area such as Sierra Leone (West Africa) and develops this clinical picture within 3 weeks of their return, then the risk of having a viral hemorrhagic fever must be considered. This is important as these patients are placed in a category of suspicion of illness risk, which is graded as minimal, moderate or strong. The type of hospital isolation unit to which the patient is admitted depends upon this risk assessment. This patient was graded as a medium risk and was admitted to a high security unit in which he could be investigated and treated. In addition, any individuals in close contact with him should be contacted as they may be at risk.

1B. Immediate investigations

After the patient is transferred to the high security isolation unit, which contains its own laboratory, a full blood count including a differential cell count and thick and thin films, blood urea, electrolytes and glucose, an electrocardiogram, a midstream urine (MSU) specimen and stool and blood cultures should be collected.

A picture of a hemolytic anemia, leukopenia and a slightly lowered platelet count was seen in this case. The thin film revealed normal size, multiple infected red blood cells and approximately 10% of the red blood cells contained flimsy ring forms (malarial trophozoites). A diagnosis of falciparum malaria was made.

A serum sample should be sent for arboviral serology as individuals from endemic areas can present with dual infections.

1C. Management

Management comprises full supportive care and treatment with intravenous quinine. Hematologic and biochemical parameters should be monitored, and in particular the level of parasitemia in response to treatment, blood glucose and renal function.

This patient made an uneventful recovery and was found to have had chloroquine-resistant falciparum malaria.

2. D – Lyme disease
3. A – Lymphatic filariasis
4. E – The parasites develop first in the liver

CHAPTER 28

Multisystem Zoonoses

1. D – Brucellosis

CHAPTER 29

Fever of Unknown Origin

1. Probable diagnosis and critical further investigations

It is probable that this patient has infectious endocarditis. She has an artificial aortic valve, which makes this diagnosis highly likely given the presence of a fever and a murmur. In these circumstances it is important to take blood cultures to identify the pathogen responsible. At least three sets of cultures should be taken on three separate occasions to ensure the highest chances of isolating the organism. An echocardiogram, which is most sensitive if performed by a transesophageal approach should be performed. The presence of vegetations on echocardiography are diagnostic, although their absence does not exclude the diagnosis.

2. Most common pathogen

Streptococci, usually of the viridans type and found as part of the normal flora of the mouth, are the most common organisms responsible for endocarditis. However, with the increasing use of cardiac surgery to replace damaged valves, staphylococci, both *Staphylococcus aureus* and coagulase-negative staphylococci (CNS), are important. CNS are especially implicated in prosthetic valvular endocarditis. Many other organisms have been implicated as the cause of endocarditis, including some fastidious Gram-negative rods, and more unusually, fungi.

The majority of cases of endocarditis used to be due to rheumatic valve disease as a consequence of rheumatic fever. An increasing number of cases are associated with prosthetic valves, and staphylococci are the most prominent organisms found in this group of patients. Infection can be acquired at the time of surgery, when it will present within the first few months postoperatively and usually manifests within a few weeks. Alternatively it may present later, as in this case, when it is the result of organisms settling on the valve during a bacteremia. The classic signs of endocarditis may not be present in this group of patients and the presentation may be more acute.

This patient's blood cultures revealed *Staphylococcus aureus* in all three sets.

3. Crucial components of management

It is essential that a physician, a surgeon, and a microbiologist are involved at an early stage. It may be necessary to remove an infected valve surgically if there is no response to antimicrobial therapy. A multidisciplinary team is best placed to make such a decision for each individual case.

4. Possible complications

The most serious complications include abscess formation within the valve and endocardium. Infected tissue embolizing from an infected valve on the left side of the heart may result in cerebral, renal, or more unusually, bone abscesses.

5. Guidelines to reduce the risk of this disease occurring

In the UK, guidelines are available from the British Heart Foundation in conjunction with the British Society for Antimicrobial Agents and Chemotherapy on the use of antimicrobial prophylaxis before dentistry. Prophylactic and therapeutic guidelines are available in most countries.

Although there is little evidence that the majority of cases of endocarditis are due to dental manipulation, litigation has ensued where a dentist has failed to give prophylaxis to patients known to be at risk of endocarditis.

CHAPTER 30

Infections in the Compromised Host

1. Most likely diagnosis and diagnostic tests

The most likely diagnosis is *Cryptococcus neoformans* (fungal) infection. The serum can be immediately tested for cryptococcal antigen and an Indian ink or nigrosin stain performed on the cerebrospinal fluid (CSF) deposit. Rapid detection of cryptococcal antigen in CSF and serum may be performed using a latex particle agglutination test.

2. Other confirmatory investigations

Culture of *C. neoformans* together with antifungal sensitivity tests, which are usually performed in reference laboratories. Cryptococcal antigen was detected in both the serum and the CSF and capsulated yeasts were seen in the CSF.

3. Management

- Treat with antiemetics, analgesics, and intravenous amphotericin B (with or without 5 flucytosine) or fluconazole depending upon the clinical picture.
- Continue fluconazole maintenance therapy to prevent recurrences after recovery.
- Consider that this patient now has two AIDS-defining diagnoses and this has prognostic implications.
- Repeat the cryptococcal antigen tests monthly for 6 months or if the patient is symptomatic. Lumbar punctures may be repeated at 1 and 6 months to monitor recovery.

CHAPTER 31

Strategies for Control: An Introduction

2. D – Pandemic
3. A – The maximum reproductive rate of an infectious organism
4. C – Measles is transmitted by respired droplets
5. B – Measles
6. E – All of these

CHAPTER 33

Attacking the Enemy: Antimicrobial Agents and Chemotherapy

1. Main classes of antibacterial agents

The major classes fo antibacterial agents (with examples) are: inhibitors of cell wall synthesis (penicillins, cephalosporins, glycopeptides); inhibitors of protein synthesis (aminoglycosides, tetracyclines, chloramphenicol, macrolides, lincosamides, streptogramins, oxazolidinones, fusidic acid); inhibitors of nucleic acid synthesis (quinolones, rifampicin, sulfonamides, trimethoprim, co-trimoxazole); inhibitors of cytoplasmic membrane function (polymyxins).

2. Mechanisms of resistance to antibacterials

The target site may be altered (altered cell wall, methicillin resistance); access to the target site may be altered due to altered uptake or increased exit (tetracycline efflux); enzymes may be produced that modify or destroy the antibacterial agent (beta-lactamases, aminoglycoside-modifying enzymes).

3. Selective toxicity

Fungi and parasites are eukaryotic, as is their human host, thus making selective targets (which do not adversely affect the host) more difficult to locate and interfere with. Viruses pose a similar problem since they have no cellular structure of their own but instead use host-cell resources (enzymes, etc.) to infect and reproduce.

CHAPTER 34

Vaccination

1. C – Incapable of reverting to virulence; D – Safer than live vaccines
2. A – Inactivated vaccines; E – Tetanus vaccination; F – DNA vaccines
3. B – The vaccine coverage needed to eliminate infection; D – A critical value at which there are too few susceptibles in a population to maintain transmission
4. A – Population density; B – The ability of the vaccine to induce an appropriate immune response

CHAPTER 35

Passive and Non-specific Immunotherapy

1. A – Transplacental passage of maternal IgG; C – Injection of convalescent human Ig; D – Injection of a human monoclonal antibody
2. C – Short term neutralization of tetanus toxin; D – Serum sickness hypersensitivity reactions in some cases
3. A – As scFvs on the surface of bacteriophage; C – As V_H domains on the surface of bacteriophage
4. C – Potentially of value for the treatment of hepatitis B infection

CHAPTER 36

Hospital Infection: Sterilization and Disinfection

1. Common causes of postoperative infections in patients and steps to reduce these problems

The most common cause of a postoperative pyrexia is a wound infection. Other causes of pyrexia include chest and urinary infections. Chest infections are particularly common after abdominal surgery because the patient is in pain and finds coughing difficult. Urinary infections are often a result of catheterization. Non-infectious causes of postoperative pyrexia include deep venous thrombosis.

Surgical wound infections are substantially reduced by giving prophylactic antibiotics, which should be effective against the most common pathogens responsible for infection in the type of surgery being used.

2. Investigations

It is important that the wound dressing is removed so that the wound can be examined and a swab is taken. Sputum culture and urine culture should also be sent. A chest radiograph is needed if there is clinical evidence of a chest infection.

This man's wound is red and discharging small amounts of pus at the lower end and a wound swab grows *Staphylococcus aureus*.

3. Treatment

Initially this patient would be treated with flucloxacillin. The laboratory will have the results of antibiotic sensitivity testing the following day. Methicillin is used in the laboratory to detect flucloxacillin resistance. The organism is resistant to flucloxacillin and is referred to as a 'methicillin-resistant *Staphylococcus aureus*' or MRSA strain.

The patient should be source isolated in a side room and staff should be made aware of the risks of carrying the organism on their hands. *Staph. aureus* is carried on a variety of sites on the body, including the nose, hair, axillae, wrists and hands, and the perineum. Swabs should be collected from these sites in this patient to check for carriage.

The carriage rate is higher in hospitals than in the community. MRSA ward outbreaks may occur, especially as the organism survives in dry environments. In this case, the most likely source of the MRSA is the patient's skin or nose.

The following measures should be taken to reduce the chance of the MRSA spreading: these include isolating the patient and careful wound dressing technique and good handwashing technique by any member of staff attending him. In addition, he should be treated with a glycopeptide antibiotic, either vancomycin or teicoplanin. If vancomycin is used, the serum concentration must be monitored.

Index

This index is in letter-by-letter order, whereby hyphens and spaces within index headings are ignored in the alphabetization. Characters in brackets are excluded from initial alphabetisation.
(PP) following the page number refer to entries from the Pathogen Parade.

Abbreviations, used in subentries:
CMV - Cytomegalovirus
EBV - Epstein-Barr virus
FUO - Fever of unknown origin
HBV - Hepatitis B virus
HIV - Human immunodeficiency virus
HSV - Herpes simplex virus
MHC - Major histocompatibility complex
RSV - Respiratory syncytial virus
SARS - Severe acute respiratory syndrome
STD - Sexually transmitted diseases
UTIs - Urinary tract infections
VZV - Varicella-zoster virus

A

abacavir 503
abdominal pain, in bacterial diarrheal disease 284
'abdominal policeman' (omentum) 162
abortion, spontaneous, in animals 409
abscess 350
  amebic liver 310
  brain 212, 339, 340
  breast 319
  computerized tomography 417
  epidural 329
  formation 350
  intra-abdominal 277, 417
  liver 310
  lung 220–225, 236–237
  in lymphogranuloma venereum 261
  peritonsillar (quinsy) 209
  renal 244
  skin, due to *Staphylococcus aureus* 350–351, 424
Acanthamoeba 345
acetylcholine, release inhibition by botulinum toxin 340
aciclovir (acycloguanosine) 501–502
  action 502
  genital herpes 264
  HSV infection 264, 369
  mode of action 501–502
  structure 501
  topical/systemic use 502
acid-fast bacteria 11, 358, 359, 456–457
acne 356–357, 357
  treatment 357
acquired immune deficiency syndrome *see* AIDS
actin-myosin contractile system 75
Actinobacillus, periodontal disease 214
Actinomyces 434, 596(PP)
  peritonitis 310
Actinomyces israelii 597(PP)
Actinomyces viscosus, periodontal disease 214

actinomycosis 310, 434
acute phase proteins 80, 82, 144
  see also C-reactive protein
acyclovir (acycloguanosine) *see* aciclovir
Addisonian crisis 327
adeno-associated viruses 372
adenosine diphosphate (ADP) ribosylation 187
adenoviruses 569(PP)
  antigen concealment 169
  attachment 205
  interference with MHC class I expression 175
  transformation of cells in culture 196
  types/clinical effects 225
  vaccine 226
adenovirus infections 225–226
  diarrhea 292
  hemorrhagic cystitis 242
  in immunodeficiency 436
  pneumonia 225–226, 227
  upper respiratory tract 205
adenylate cyclase toxin 217
adhesins 12–13, 220
  microbial attachment in respiratory tract 125
adjuvants 522–523
  Freund's 523
adult respiratory distress syndrome (ARDS) 189
adult T cell leukemia 194, 380
Aedes aegypti 384
aerobic respiration 13
aflatoxins 39
African trypanosomiasis *see* trypanosomiasis, African
agammaglobulinemia
  Bruton-type 424
  measles in 375
agarose gel electrophoresis–restriction-enzyme analysis 558
age 3
  incidence of childhood viral infections 525
  pneumonia etiology 221
  susceptibility to infections 165
  hospital-acquired 550
  vaccination programs 524
  zoster predisposition 371
  see also elderly
age at infection 443, 444
  age at vaccination relationship 447
age at vaccination relationship 447
agglutination 150
  bacterial agglutination tests 150, 151
  latex particles 150, 151, 458, 459, 467
  red blood cells (hemagglutination) 467, 468
AIDS 252
  case number/infection route in UK 274
  cryptosporidiosis 297
  definition 272, 431
  diarrhea/diarrheal disease 435
  discovery 447
  factors causing progression to 270
  historical aspects 447
  Kaposi's sarcoma 436
  mycobacterial infections 434–435
  opportunistic fungi 40
  opportunistic infections 272, 429, 431
    prophylaxis 272
  opportunistic tumors 272

prophylaxis 272
  pathogenesis 268, 270
  toxoplasmosis 338
  treatment 272
  tuberculosis 234–235
  see also HIV infection
AIDS-related complex (ARC) 265
air, microorganism numbers in 125, 201
airborne spread of infection 132, 133, 134, 201, 220, 552
air conditioning, transmission of infections 134, 552
air travel, SARS infection 231
alcohol-fast bacteria 456
alcohols, disinfectants 565
allergic bronchopulmonary aspergillosis 234, 235
allergic reactions
  beta-lactams 480
  to helminths 190
  in schistosomiasis 397–398
  type I hypersensitivity 190
  see also hypersensitivity
alpha toxin 356
alphaviruses 385, 386
aluminum salts 522–523
alum-precipitated antigens 522–523
alveolar macrophage 72, 74
  microbial avoidance 125–126
alveolitis, extrinsic allergic 191
amantadine 501, 504, 561
  influenza management 2 230
amebae 294
  free-living, meningitis due to 300
  immune evasion 43
  spread via olfactory nerves 161
  see also Entamoeba histolytica
amebiasis *see Entamoeba histolytica* infection
amebic liver abscess 310
American trypanosomiasis (Chagas' disease) 377–378, 395–396
amikacin 485
aminoglycoside(s) 485
  adverse effects 485
  endocarditis treatment 419–420
  indications 487
  resistance 485
  routes of administration 485
  structure 487, 488
  see also individual drugs
amoxicillin 247
  sinusitis 213
amphotericin B 433, 505
ampicillin 247
  Haemophilus influenzae meningitis 326
  Pasteurella multocida infection 407
  peritonitis 310
  sinusitis 213
  typhoid 301
amprenavir 503
amputations 356
amyloid plaques, prions/prion infections 53, 54
anaerobic bacteria
  metronidazole 496
  normal flora 57, 58
anaerobic infections
  burn wounds 426
  cellulitis 354–355, 355
  lung abscess 234
  necrotizing fasciitis 355–356
  periodontal disease 214
  peritonitis 310
  traumatic/surgical wounds 355

anaerobic respiration 13
anal intercourse 273
anal pruritus 299
anaphylactoid reaction 189
anaphylaxis 190
anaphylotoxins (C3a and C5a) 77–78, 88, 189
Ancylostoma duodenale 48
  clinical features of infection 299
  cutaneous larval migrans 365
  eggs 299
  gastrointestinal tract infections 297
  infection via skin 124, 298
  transmission/life cycle 298
anemia
  hemolytic 190
  iron-deficiency 299
  in malaria 190, 394
  microorganisms causing 381
  parvovirus infections 372
anergy 106, 152, 171
anesthesia, local, in leprosy 358
animals, transmission of infections from 137–141
ankylosing spondylitis 379
Anopheles mosquitoes 391–392
anthelmintic drugs 411
anthrax 404–405
antibacterial agents
  aminoglycosides 485
  antibiotic assays 499, 500
  appropriate use 507
  bactericidal/bacteriostatic 474
  bacteriophage therapy 19
  beta-lactams 478–480
  cell wall synthesis inhibitors 14, 478–485
    see also individual agents
  chloramphenicol 487–489
  classification 474–475, 477, 479
  combinations 498–499, 500
  co-trimoxazole 495–496
  cytoplasmic membrane function inhibitors 496
  diarrhea associated 59, 289–290
  ethambutol 497
  fusidic acid 491–492
  glycopeptides 480–481, 484–485
  isoniazid 497
  killing rate (killing curves) 562, 563
  lincosamides 489, 490–491
  long-term, acne treatment 357
  macrolides 489–490
  microorganism/host interactions 473, 510
  minimum bactericidal concentration (MBC) 419, 498, 499
  minimum inhibitory concentration (MIC) 419, 498, 499
  nitroimidazoles 496
  nucleic acid synthesis inhibitors 14, 15, 492–496
  oxazolidinones 491
  polymyxins 496
  prophylactic 420
    nosocomial infections 554
  protein synthesis inhibitors 485–492
  pyrazinamide 497
  quinolones 492–493
  resistance *see* antibacterial agents, resistance
  rifamycins 493–494
  streptogramins 489, 491
  sulfonamides 494–495

antibacterial agents (cont'd)
 susceptibility testing 464, 466, 497–499
  patterns in hospitals 557
 targets/sites of action 474–475
  cell wall synthesis inhibitors 14, 478–485
  cytoplasmic membrane function inhibitors 496
  nucleic acid synthesis inhibitors 14, 15, 492–496
  protein synthesis inhibitors 485–492
 tetracyclines 485, 487
 therapeutic index 499
 trimethoprim 495–496
 use/misuse 507
 see also antimicrobial agents; specific infections
antibacterial agents, resistance 25, 450, 475–477, 478, 489
 aminoglycosides 485
 appropriate use 507
 bacteriophage therapy 19
 beta-lactams 479
 catheter-associated infections 428
 chloramphenicol 488–489
 development/acquisition 65, 66, 475–476, 477
 erythromycin 489
 evolutionary aspects 113, 476
 genetics 475–477
 glycopeptides 481, 484
 integrons 476–477
 macrolides 489
 mechanisms/targets 478
 methicillin-resistant staphylococci 479, 546, 556
 metronidazole 496
 mutation(s) 475
 plasmid-mediated 18, 475–476
 quinolones 492
 resistance cassettes 476–477
 rifamycins 494
 tetracyclines 485, 487
 vancomycin 484
 see also specific bacterial species
antibiotic resistance see antibacterial agents, resistance
antibiotics see antibacterial agents; antimicrobial agents
antibodies
 affinity 150
 antibody-mediated immunity 148–151
 anti-idiotype, as vaccines 520
 autoantibodies see autoantibodies
 classes/subclasses (isotypes) 150
  see also immunoglobulin(s)
 deficiency/defects 424, 426
  see also immunodeficiency
 detection, diagnosis of infections 453, 454, 466–468
 enhancing 385
 maternal, optimum age to vaccinate 225
 monoclonal see monoclonal antibodies
 neutralizing 150, 220
 opsonization 151
 in type II hypersensitivity 190
 see also immunoglobulin(s)
antibody–antigen complexes see immune complex(es)
antibody-dependent cell-mediated cytotoxicity (ADCC) 93, 94, 96
antibody-mediated immunity 148–152
 see also humoral immune response
antifungal agents 504–505, 506
 adverse effects 505, 506
 classification by structure/target 504–505
 resistance 505

therapeutic applications 506
antigen(s)
 alum-precipitated 522–523
 bacterial cell walls 7
 challenge 468–469
 concealment 169–170
 concentration, control of immune response 106
 detection 458–460
 'H' (flagellar) 12, 557
 'K' (capsular) 557
 mimicking host antigens see molecular mimicry
 'O' (somatic) 11, 557
 pathogen-associated molecular patterns (PAMPs) 75, 82
 polyclonal activators 104, 105
 polysaccharide, in vaccination 521
 presented on spherical structures, vaccines 523
 receptors 102
 recognition 87, 104
 serotyping 557
 superantigens 174–175
 'surrogate' 520
 T-independent 104
antigen–antibody complexes see immune complex(es)
antigen-antibody reaction, serologic tests 466–468
antigenic drift 172–173
 influenza viruses 227
antigenic shift 227, 533
antigenic variation 172–173
 bacteria 13
 spirochetes causing relapsing fever 389
 trypanosomes 43
antigen-presenting cells (APC) 104, 105
antigen-specific immunosuppression 173
anti-idiotype vaccines 520
antimicrobial agents 2, 473–511
 administration 449
 appropriate use 507
 discovery 473, 475
 ideal properties 473, 475
 rational design 473, 475
 resistance see antibacterial agents, resistance; resistance
 selective toxicity 473
 specificity 447–449
 targets/sites of action 448, 450
 toxicity 450
 use/misuse 507
 see also antibacterial agents; antifungal agents; antiparasitic agents; antiviral agents
antimicrobial chemicals 564, 565
antimicrobial peptides, skin 143
antimonial compounds 397
antimyocardial antibody 190
antiparasitic agents 508–509
 drug targets 505–506
 metronidazole 496, 508
 resistance 506–507
antisense oligonucleotides, antiviral therapy 504
antiseptics 562
 urinary tract 496
antiserum see immunization, passive
anti-streptolysin O 468
anti-streptolysin O antibody 210
anti-streptolysin O test 469
antituberculous drugs 234, 496–497
antiviral agents 270–272, 450, 499–504, 501
 CMV infection 204
 drug development 504
 influenza virus inhibitors 504
 interferon therapy 504
 protease inhibitors 503–504

resistance 271, 499, 503
 reverse transcriptase inhibitors 503
 sites of action 502
apoptosis 83, 153
 virus induced 175–176
appendicitis 299
arbitrarily primed polymerase chain reaction (AP-PCR) 559
arboviruses 383
 infection cycle/route 383
 vertical transmission 383
arbovirus infections 383–386
 encephalitic 385–386
 hemorrhagic fevers 386
 multisystem 383–384
 vaccines 532–533
arenaviruses 401–402, 569–570(PP)
 infections 401–402, 504
 serologic diagnosis 401
arsenical drugs 395, 396
artemisin 394, 507
arthralgia 378–379
arthritis
 Lyme disease 390–391
 post-infectious 378–379
 reactive 378–379
 septic 257, 378–379
 viral 378–379
arthropod(s) 49–51, 383
 biting, infection via skin 124, 138
 control 383, 384
 genital infestations 275
 skin infestations 365–366
 viruses transmitted by see arboviruses
arthropod-borne infections 383–399
 bloodsucking vectors 138–140
 diseases/organisms transmitted 49, 51, 139
 transmission routes/methods 133, 138–140, 383
arthropod-borne viruses see arboviruses
arthrospores 360–361, 362, 363
Arthus reaction 192
Ascaris, identification 466
Ascaris lumbricoides 626(PP)
 eggs 297, 298, 299
 transmission/life cycle 298
Ascaris lumbricoides infection
 clinical features 298–299
 gastrointestinal tract 297
 hypersensitivity 298
 pneumonitis/respiratory distress 298
 pulmonary eosinophilia 237
Aschoff's nodules 210
aseptic behavior 552–553
aspergilloma 235
aspergillosis 235
 allergic bronchopulmonary 234, 235
 antifungal agents for 433, 506
 cerebral 433
 invasive 433
 transmission 433, 552
Aspergillus 616(PP)
Aspergillus flavus 39–40
Aspergillus fumigatus 234, 238, 433
 bronchopulmonary aspergillosis 234, 235
 exotoxin 185
astroviruses 292
attenuation, vaccines 516–517
auramine stain 358, 456, 457
autoantibodies
 antimyocardial 190
 EBV infection 206
 in type II hypersensitivity 190
autoclaving 563
 see also sterilization

autoimmunity, vaccines inducing 521
 DNA vaccines 520
autoinfection 411–412
 strongyloidiasis 298, 299
azidothymidine (AZT; zidovudine) 501, 503
azole antifungals 505
AZT (azidothymidine) 501, 503

B

Babesia, effect on hemopoietic system 381
bacille Calmette–Guérin see BCG (bacille Calmette–Guérin) vaccine
Bacillus 404, 591–592(PP)
Bacillus anthracis 404–405, 591(PP)
 anthrax toxin 185, 404
 infection via skin 124
 spores 404
Bacillus cereus 592(PP)
 diarrhea due to 284, 288–289
 lipid storage granules 457
bacteremia 159, 160
 hospital-acquired 546, 554
 infective endocarditis 417–418, 419
bacteria 11–28
 adaptation to environment 15
 aerobic/anaerobic metabolism 13
 antibiotic resistance see antibacterial agents, resistance
 antibiotic susceptibility testing 464, 466, 497–499
 antigenic variation 13
 attachment 12–13, 125, 126, 127
 capsules 12, 167
 cell division 14
 cell wall see cell walls
 chromosome 11
 classification 9–10, 11–13
 colonial characteristics 464
 conjugation 22–23
 culture 462–463
 DNA replication 13–14
 endospores 24
 enzymes produced 185–186, 464
 evasion of host defenses see host defense evasion
 exotoxins see exotoxins
 extrachromosomal elements 17–19
 fermentative/non-fermentative 464
 flagella 12, 90
 gene expression 14–17
  see also gene expression
 generation times 113
 gene transfer 19, 21–24
 genome replication 13–14
 genome sequences 24–27
 Gram-negative see Gram-negative bacteria
 Gram-positive see Gram-positive bacteria
 growth curves 13
 growth/division 13–14
 growth requirements 462–463, 464
 'H' (flagellar) antigens 12
 identification schemes 464–466, 465
 iron-binding proteins 167
 killing rate (killing curves) 562, 563
 mutation 19–24
 normal flora see flora, normal
 nutrient uptake/transport 13
 'O' (somatic) antigens 11
 pili (fimbriae) 12–13
 plasmids 17–19
  see also plasmids

as prokaryotes 7
randomly-induced attenuation 517
recombination 21, 22
replication rate 158
  and host immune response 150
septation (cell division) 14
size comparisons 1
structure 11–13
survival under adverse conditions 24
toxins *see* toxins
transcription 14–15
transduction 21–22
transformation 21, 22
translation 15
transposition 23–24
as vectors for genes, vaccine development 519
virulence *see* virulence
zoonoses 140
bacterial infections
  FUO 416
  incubation, latency/infectious periods 443
  muscle 350–357
  opportunistic 429, 434–435
  oropharyngeal invasion 130
  perinatal 318
  persistent 177
  pharyngitis 207
  via skin 124
  skin rashes due to 194
  systemic, skin manifestations 352
  in transplant recipients 429, 430
  urinary tract invasion 130
  see also specific infections
bacterial overgrowth 60
bacterial vaginosis 263
bactericidal agents 474
  see also antibacterial agents
bactericidins 72
bacteriocins, typing 557–558
bacteriophage 19
  combinatorial libraries 540–541
  lytic cycle 19
  temperate/lysogenic 19, 22
  as therapeutics 19
  transduction by 21–22
  typing 557, 558
bacteriostatic agents 474
bacteriuria 130, 244
  asymptomatic 244, 246
  laboratory diagnosis 246
  significant 245
Bacteroides
  commensalism/mutualism 61
  normal flora of intestine 58
  periodontal disease 214
  in vagina 263
Bacteroides fragilis 605(PP)
  otitis/sinusitis 212
  peritonitis 310
Baghdad boil (Oriental sores) 396, 536
balanitis, *Candida albicans* 252, 263
Bartonella brucelliformis 381
basic (case) reproductive rate (R₀) 441–444
  estimation 443
basophil 79
  morphology 80
B cell(s) (B lymphocytes) 87, 99
  antibody synthesis 102
  antigen receptors 102
  clonal expansion 102, 104, 106
  defects 424
  differentiation 102–103
  EBV infection 206
  epitopes 519–520
  helper T cells role 104, 106
  in malnutrition 427
  memory cells 102–104
  polyclonal activators 176
  self-tolerance induced by vaccines 449

surface markers 100, 102
T-independent antigen recognition 104, 105
  see also lymphocytes
B cell lymphomas, EBV association 208
BCG (bacille Calmette–Guérin) vaccine 235, 531
  controlled trials 531
  current schedules/practices 531
  development 517
  genetic deletions 517
  leprosy prevention 359, 531, 535
  problems 152, 531
  as vector for vaccines 519
beef tapeworm (*Taenia saginata*) 300
behavior
  host-parasite relationship changes 66
  sexual *see* sexual behavior
  spread of infections influenced 444
benzylpenicillin, neurotoxicity 480
beta-lactamases 479, 482
  inhibitors 479, 484
beta-lactams 478–480, 481
  adverse effects 479–480
  allergy 480
  characteristics 483–484
  mode of action 478–480
  resistance 479
  route of administration 478–479
  structures 481
  see also individual antibiotics
bile, microbial evasion mechanism 128, 129
bilharzia 49
  see also schistosomiasis
biliary tract infections 310
biopsy, lung 204, 231
bioterrorism 3
  smallpox 373
  vaccination 536–537
biotyping 557
birds, transmission of infections 141
bites
  human, anaerobic cellulitis from 355
  insect *see* arthropod-borne infections
  Pasteurella multocida transmission 407, 609(PP)
  rats 408–409
BK virus 242, 436
Black Death 406
black eschar 404
blackheads 357
blackwater fever 190, 394
bladder
  cancer 242, 397
  catheterization 243, 248
  defense mechanisms 129
  incomplete emptying 242
  obstruction 243
  see also urinary tract infections (UTIs)
Blastomyces dermatitidis 364, 616–617(PP)
blastomycosis
  antifungal agents for 506
  skin infections 364
blindness
  Chlamydia trachomatis causing 343–344, 345
  Onchocerca volvulus causing 345, 346
  Toxoplasma gondii causing 345–346
blood
  donors, screening 273, 307, 547
  films, malaria diagnosis 394
  spread of infection from 137, 160
  spread of infection to 159–160

transfusions, hepatitis C associated 307
blood-brain barrier 323
blood-cerebrospinal fluid barrier 162, 323
blood culture, infective endocarditis 418
blue tongue 135
B lymphocytes *see* B cell(s) (B lymphocytes)
body lice 365–366, 386
  epidemic typhus transmission 388
  relapsing fever transmission 387, 389
body temperature *see* temperature
boils 350–351
Bolivian hemorrhagic fever 401, 403
  ecology 403
bone infection 378–380
bone marrow
  stem cells 99
  transplant recipients, infections 429
Bordetella 607(PP)
Bordetella pertussis 238
  BvgS/BvgA proteins 17
  interference with host ciliary activity 125, 126
  lymphocytosis 380
  toxins 185, 217
  see also pertussis (whooping cough)
Bornholm disease (pleurodynia; epidemic myalgia) 377
Borrelia 613(PP)
  infections 389
  variable major protein (VMP) 389
Borrelia burgdorferi 253, 331, 390
  septic arthritis 379
  see also Lyme disease
Borrelia recurrentis 253, 389, 390
  gene switching 173
  morphology 389
Borrelia vincenti, pharyngitis 208
botulinum toxin 185, 292
  antitoxin 293
  mechanism of action 186, 187, 340
  types 292–293
botulism 292–293, 340
  antitoxin 293
  clinical features 340
  foodborne 293, 340
  infants 293, 340
  laboratory diagnosis 293
  prevention 293, 340
  treatment 340
bovine spongiform encephalopathy (BSE) 7, 53, 54, 338, 563
  transmission 54
  see also prions/prion infections
brain
  abscess 212, 339
    infections causing 340
  cysticercosis 339
  damage, pertussis vaccine causing 529
  granulomas 338
  hydatid cysts 338
  influence on immune response 163–164
  tuberculoma 417
Branhamella catarrhalis (*Moraxella catarrhalis*) 223, 606(PP)
Branhamella catarrhalis (*Moraxella catarrhalis*) 223
Brazilian purpuric fever (BPF) 344
breast abscess 319
breast feeding, HIV vertical transmission 314
breast milk
  acquisition of normal flora 57
  HTLV1 transmission 380

transmission of infections 136–137, 319
Brill–Zinsser disease 389
broadfish tapeworm (*Diphyllobothrium latum*) 300
bronchiolitis 219, 238
bronchitis 238
  acute 218
  chronic 218–219
    acute exacerbation 218–219
bronchopneumonia 220, 221
Brucella 607–608(PP)
Brucella abortus 409
Brucella melitensis 409
Brucella suis 409
brucellosis (Malta fever; undulant fever) 409–410
  clinical features 409–410
  prevention 410
  relapsing persistent course 173
  serologic diagnosis/treatment 410
Brugia 398
  microfilariae in lung 237
Brugia malayi 50, 398
Bruton-type agammaglobulinemia 424
buboes 261, 406
bubonic plague 405
'bull neck' appearance 215
bunyaviruses 385, 386, 570(PP)
Burkitt's lymphoma 148
  EBV 195, 208
  malaria as cofactor 148, 195, 208, 394
burns 423
  wound infections 124, 426–427
Buruli ulcers 359
B virus, encephalitis associated 332

C

C3 convertase 77, 88, 90
C3d receptor (CR₂) 123
caliciviruses
  diarrhea 292
  hepatitis E 303, 304
California encephalitis virus 385
Calymmatobacterium granulomatis 252, 262
Campylobacter 283–285, 603(PP)
  animal reservoir/transmission 284–285
  culture from feces 285
  diarrhea 283–285
Campylobacter jejuni 284–285, 603–604(PP)
  inflammatory enteritis 285
Campylobacter pylori see Helicobacter pylori (*Campylobacter pylori*)
cancer
  bladder 242, 397
  cervical *see* cervical cancer
  gastric 197, 293
  liver 195, 196, 307
  nasopharyngeal 194–195
  skin 195, 196
  virus inducing 34, 35, 120, 194–197, 208
Candida 39, 130
  infections *see* candidiasis/*Candida* infections
  moisture requirement 363
Candida albicans 252, 262–263, 617(PP)
candidemia, hospital-acquired 554
candidiasis/*Candida* infections
  antifungal agents for 506
  balanitis 252, 263
  chronic mucocutaneous 363, 431
  cutaneous 363, 364
  disseminated 431–342
  eye infections 432
  gastrointestinal 431
  hospital-acquired 554
  infective endocarditis 431

candidiasis/*Candida* infections (*cont'd*)
  nails 77
  opportunistic infections 431–432
  oral 213
  oropharyngeal/esophageal 130, 431
  otitis externa 213
  vaginitis/vaginal thrush 58–59, 252, 262–263
candidin 152
capsomeres 32
capsule
  bacteria 12, 167
  'K' antigens 557
carbapenems 481, 484
carbenicillin, adverse effects 480
carbuncles 350
cardiolipin 254
caries, dental 57–58, 214
carriers 445
  cholera 285, 286–287
  enteric fevers 301, 302
  HBV 305–307, 548–549
  healthcare workers 285
  Salmonella typhi 301, 302, 548–549
  Staphylococcus aureus 350, 351, 548–549
  Staphylococcus pyogenes 548–549
case control studies 445
case definition 447
caspases 83, 84
catabolite activation protein (CAP) 17
cataract, congenital rubella 316, 317
cathelicidins 143
cathepsin G 76, 77
catheterization, bladder 243, 248
catheters
  dialysis, infections 428
  urinary *see* urinary catheters
cats
  Pasteurella multocida transmission 407, 609(PP)
  zoonoses transmitted from 140, 338
CD molecules 100, 102
CD4 cells
  HIV infection 270
    decrease in 267–268
    treatment 271
  see also helper-T cells
CD4 molecule 123, 267
CD8 cells 267
  see also cytotoxic T cells (CTL)
cefaclor 247
cefalexin 247
cefotaxime 478
ceftriaxone
  chancroid 262
  gonorrhea 258
cefuroxime 247
cell culture techniques 463–464
cell lines 463
cell lysis
  by complement 79–80, 81, 151, 154
  direct effects of microorganisms 184
  by natural killer (NK) cells 83, 84, 154
cell-mediated immune response 99–110, 151–154
  DNA vaccines 520
  fetus 313
  in HIV infection 267–268
  impaired
    CMV infection 202–203
    Cryptococcus neoformans infection 432
    fungal meningitis 329
    Pneumocystis carinii infection 433–434
    reactivation of CMV 203
  leprosy 358

measles 374
  protective/pathologic effects 193
  tuberculosis 232–233
  type IV hypersensitivity 190, 193
  see also T cell(s)
cell membranes (plasma membrane) 7
cellulitis 350, 354–355
  anaerobic 355
  Pasteurella multocida 407
  postoperative gangrenous 551
cell walls, bacterial 7, 11–12
  synthesis 478, 480
    antibacterial agents inhibiting 478–485
  see also lipopolysaccharide (LPS); peptidoglycan
central nervous system
  host defenses 131, 323
  infection/invasion routes 160–162, 323–324
  microbial evasion of defenses 131
  spread of infection via 160–162, 325
  tumors, zoster predisposition 371
central nervous system infections 323–341
  African trypanosomiasis 395
  helminthic 338–339
  host response 324–325
  parasitic 338–339
  pathologic consequences 324–325
  see also encephalitis; meningitis
cephalexin 247
cephalosporins 478, 483
  structure 481
cephamycins 481, 484
cerebellar hypoplasia
cerebral aspergillosis 433
cerebral malaria 331, 338, 394
cerebrospinal fluid (CSF)
  cell count increase in infections 324, 325
  culture 327
  normal composition 325
  spread of infection via 162
cervical cancer 367
  HSV2 cocarcinogenic role 195, 196
  human papillomaviruses 196, 367
cervical dysplasia 265
cervical secretions, CMV transmission 202
cervicitis, chlamydial 260
cesarean section, HIV vertical transmission 314
cestodes *see* tapeworms
Chagas' disease (American trypanosomiasis) 377–378, 395–396
  antiprotozoal drugs 508
chagoma 395
chancre
  African trypanosomiasis 395
  primary syphilis 254
  soft (chancroid) 252, 261–262
chancroid (soft chancre) 252, 261–262
chemical agents, sterilization 504
chemiluminescence 458
chemokines 106
chemotactic factors (C3a and C5a) 77–78, 189
chemotaxis
  bacterial flagella 12
  phagocytes 77, 89, 90
chemotherapy 473–511
  disadvantages 449–450
  vaccination comparison 447–450
  see also antimicrobial agents
chest radiographs
  pneumonia 221, 223, 224
  tuberculosis 233
  whooping cough 218

chickenpox *see* varicella (chickenpox)
chiclero ulcer 396
chiggers 49, 389
childbed fever (puerperal sepsis) 319
children
  bronchiolitis 219
  diarrheal disease mortality 277, 279
  HBV 306
  HIV infection 269
  measles 374, 375
  meningitis 325, 326, 327–328
  mixing patterns/infection transmission 446
  pneumonia 221
  shigellosis (bacillary dysentery) 287
  urine samples 245
  see also infants
Chlamydia 8, 258–261, 615(PP)
  cell/tissue culture 260, 463–464
  characteristics/life cycle 258–259, 259
  diseases associated 259
  elementary body (EB)/reticulate body (RB) 259, 260
  inclusion bodies 260
  infection route/receptors 260
  persistent infections 177
  prevention/treatment of infections 260–261, 344
Chlamydia pneumoniae 259
  pneumonia 223
Chlamydia psittaci 259
Chlamydia trachomatis
  attachment 343
  microscopy 260
  serotypes A, B and C 259
  serotypes D-K 252, 259
  serotypes L1, L2 and L3 252, 259, 261
Chlamydia trachomatis infection
  asymptomatic 259–260, 260
  cervicitis 260
  clinical syndromes/complications 259
  diagnosis 260, 460, 462
  genital 252
  inclusion conjunctivitis 343
  inflammatory response/damage 260
  laboratory diagnosis/tests 260
  lymphogranuloma venereum 252, 259
  neonatal 344
  trachoma 343–344, 345
  transmission 259–260
  treatment/prevention 260–261, 344
  urethritis 252, 260
chloramphenicol 487–489
  adverse effects 489
  mode of action 487
  resistance 488–489
  rickettsial infections 387
  routes of administration 487
  structure 487
  typhoid 302
chloroquine 394, 508
  resistance 450, 507
chlortetracycline 485
cholera 285–287
  diagnosis/carrier detection 285, 286–287
  management/prevention 287
  symptoms/pathogenesis 286
  transmission/factors associated 285–287
  vaccine 287
  see also Vibrio cholerae
cholera toxin
  B subunit in vaccine 518
  mechanism of action 186
  subunits 187

chorea 210
chorioretinitis 345–346
  Toxoplasma gondii 345–346
chronic fatigue syndrome 377
chronic granulomatous disease (CGD) 145–146, 423
  IFNα therapy 542
ciclopirox 505
cilia, activity and microbial inhibition 125, 126
ciprofloxacin
  gonorrhea 258
  typhoid 302
  UTIs 247
cirrhosis
  HBV complication 307
  hepatitis 303
  pipe-stem 309
  portal in schistosomiasis 309
classification systems 9–10
clavulanic acid 479, 484
climate change 3
clindamycin 490–491
  diarrhea associated 59, 289–290
  see also lincosamides
clofazimine 359
clonal selection and expansion 102–103
cloning vectors, plasmids 18–19
Clonorchis sinensis 49, 625(PP)
  infections 309
Clostridium 593–595(PP)
  traumatic/surgical wound infections 355–356
Clostridium botulinum 594–595(PP)
  exotoxin *see* botulinum toxin
  spores 340
  see also botulism
Clostridium difficile 59, 289–290, 595(PP)
Clostridium perfringens 593–594(PP)
  acute necrotizing disease (pig-bel) 289
  diarrhea due to 284, 288–289
  enterotoxins and β toxin 288
  exotoxin 185, 186
  gas gangrene 350, 355–356
  lecithinase (α-toxin) 185, 356
  Nagler reaction 356
  puerpural sepsis due to 319
Clostridium tetani 594(PP)
  endospores 24
  exotoxin 185, 186, 339–340
  traumatic/surgical wounds 355–356
  see also tetanus
cloxacillin
  burns infections 427
  endocarditis 420
  Staphylococcus aureus infections 427
clue cells 263
c-*myc* 34, 195, 208
coagulase 185–186
coagulation
  defects, yellow fever 384
  disseminated intravascular (DIC) 189
co-amoxiclav, UTIs 247
Coccidioides immitis 617(PP)
  meningitis 329
Cockayne syndrome 21
codons
  START 15
  STOP 15
cohort studies 445
cold chain, for vaccines 515
colds *see* common cold
cold sores 177, 368, 369
  genital 264
  pathogenesis 368
Coley's toxin 542
colicins 72, 558
colitis
  amebic 294, 295
  antibiotic-associated 289–290

hemorrhagic 281
pseudomembranous 289
collectins 144
Colorado tick fever virus 381, 386
Combivir 503
comedones 357
commensalism 61
commensal organisms see flora, normal
common cold 201–202
  clinical features/treatment 202
  pathogenesis 201–202, 206
  transmission 134, 201
  viruses causing 201, 205
complement
  activation
    by antigen–antibody complexes 87, 88, 89, 90
    by lipopolysaccharide 189
    by microorganisms 77–80
  acute inflammatory response 77–79
  alternative pathway 77, 78, 88, 90, 143–144
  assays 468, 470
  C1 component 88
  C3a and C5a components 77–78, 88, 189
  C3 component and cleavage 77, 79
  C9 component 79–80
  cell lysis mechanism 79–80
  classical pathway 77, 88
  deficiency 424
    disseminated gonorrhea in 258
    Neisseria meningitidis bacteremia 326
  fixation tests 387, 467, 469
  lytic mechanism compared with cytotoxic cells 154
  membrane attack complex (MAC) 79–80, 81, 82, 88
  microbial escape strategies 114, 167, 169
  tissue-damaging reactions 189
complete Freund's adjuvant (CFA) 523
compromised hosts see immunocompromised hosts
computerized tomography (CT)
  abscess 417
  brucellosis 409
  FUO 417
concanavalin A 469
Concorde study 270–271
condoms 251, 273
condylomata acuminata (genital warts) 252, 264, 265, 367
congenital infections 171, 313–318
  CMV 317
  HIV 318
  infection route 319
  listeriosis 302–303, 318
  rubella 315–316, 317, 526, 527
  syphilis see syphilis
  toxoplasmosis 318, 345, 346
congenital malformations 313–318
Congo-Crimean hemorrhagic fever virus 386
conjugation, bacterial 22–23
conjunctiva, infection route 124–125, 343
conjunctival hemorrhage 408
conjunctival infections 343–345
  causative organisms 343
  transmission 343, 345
conjunctivitis 343–345
  chlamydial 343–344
  HSV 368
  inclusion 343
  in measles 374
  staphylococcal, in neonates 319–320
contact lenses, infections associated 345
contact tracing 256, 258, 307

contagious pustular dermatitis (orf) 368
control of infections
  community-based by vaccination 524–526
  eradication vs. 450–451
  population mixing patterns 446
  public health 528
  strategies 447–450
  see also antimicrobial agents; epidemiology; vaccination
convulsions
  pertussis vaccine side effect 218
  rabies 335
cornea, dendritic ulcer 345, 368
coronary artery aneurysms 377
coronaviruses 230–231, 571(PP)
  attachment 205
  common colds due to 201, 205
  diarrhea 292
corticosteroids 424–425
Corynebacterium 590–591(PP)
  staining 457
Corynebacterium diphtheriae 590(PP)
  adhesion mechanisms 214–215
  diphtheria due to 214–216
  exotoxin 185, 186
  pharyngitis due to 208
  regulation of toxin production 17
  repressor protein (DtxR) action 17
co-trimoxazole 494, 495–496, 498
  brucellosis 410
  chancroid 262
  Pneumocystis carinii pneumonia 434
  typhoid 302
  UTIs 247
cough
  acute bronchitis 218
  transmission of infections 132, 134
  'whoop' see pertussis (whooping cough)
'cough plates' 217
Coxiella burnetii 387, 403
  pneumonia 223
  Q fever 387, 403–404
  transmission 404
coxsackie A virus
  attachment 125, 205
  common cold due to 205
  pharyngitis 202
  rashes due to 372
  ulcers 207
coxsackie B virus
  myocarditis and pericarditis 377
  postviral fatigue syndrome 377
coxsackieviruses
  isolation/detection 377
  transmission/infection route 377
crab louse (Phthirus pubis) 252, 275
C-reactive protein (CRP) 80, 82, 88, 144
  actions/role 144
'creeping eruption' 365
Creutzfeldt–Jakob disease (CJD) 53, 54, 337–338, 563
  hereditary aspects 338
  sporadic (sCJD) 54
  transmission 337–338
  variant (vCJD) 53, 338
  see also prions/prion infections
croup 214, 225
'crowing' 214
Cryptococcus neoformans 40, 432–433, 617–618(PP)
  cell-mediated immune response impaired 432
  encephalitis 331
  meningitis 326, 329
  opportunistic infection 432–433
  skin infections 364
  treatment of infections 432
cryptosporidiosis
  AIDS in 297

diagnosis 297
diarrhea 297
Cryptosporidium
  identification 466
  opportunistic infection 435
  reproduction 43
Cryptosporidium parvum 297, 619(PP)
  distribution/life cycle 297
cultivation of organisms see culture of organisms
culture media
  bacteria 462–463
  fungi 462–463
  selective 463
culture of organisms 453, 462–464
  Campylobacter 285
  chlamydia and rickettsia 463–464
  pure cultures 462
  Salmonella 283, 302
  specimens for 454
  time required 454
  urine 246
  viruses 463–464
cutaneous larva migrans 365
cyclic AMP (cAMP) 187, 217
cyclooxygenase pathway 78, 79
cyclospora 297
Cyclospora cayetanensis 619(PP)
cyst(s)
  calcified, Taenia solium 378
  Entamoeba histolytica 294
  Giardia lamblia 256, 295, 296
  hydatid see hydatid cyst(s)
  lung 237
  Pneumocystis carinii 434
cysticercosis 339, 410
cystic fibrosis 235–236, 238
  lung infections 235–236, 428
  Pseudomonas aeruginosa colonization of lung 236
cystitis
  acute 244
  hemorrhagic, adenoviruses causing 242
  treatment 247
cytokines 104–106, 147–148
  actions/sources 104–106, 107, 108
  as adjuvants for vaccines 523
  assessment 470–471
  control of infection 147
  definition 104
  fever due to 144
  induced by endotoxins 188, 189
  interferons (IFNs) see interferons (IFNs)
  in malaria 393
  microbial strategies against 114–115
  pathogenesis of shock 189
  side-effects of therapy 543
  therapeutic immunostimulation 153, 542–543
  in type IV hypersensitivity 193
  virus-encoded and evasion 175
  see also tumor necrosis factor (TNF); individual interleukins
cytomegalovirus (CMV) 208
  attachment/reactivation 177
  reactivation 203
  shedding in urine 242
  transmission 202
cytomegalovirus (CMV) infection
  antiviral treatment 204
  bone marrow transplant recipients 429
  cell-mediated immunity impairment 202–203
  clinical diagnosis 204
  clinical effects 208
  congenital 317
  effect on hemopoietic system 381
  encephalitis 333
  eye infections 345

fetal infection 204
  in immunodeficiency 204, 435
  immunosuppression due to 174
  interstitial pneumonia 231
  intrauterine 171
  pregnancy 202
  reactivation
    in immunodeficiency 435
    in pregnancy 317
  retinitis 345
  transmission in saliva 202
  treatment 502
  urinary tract 242
cytopathic effect (CPE) 464, 466
cytoplasmic membrane, antimicrobials inhibiting functions 496, 504–505
cytotoxic agents 424
cytotoxicity
  by activated macrophage 80
  antibody-dependent cell-mediated (ADCC) 93, 94, 96
  antibody-mediated in type II hypersensitivity 190
  by NK cells 83, 145
  T cell and NK cell comparison with complement 154
  by tumor necrosis factor (TNF) 80
  virus-infected cells 83
cytotoxic molecules 156
cytotoxic T cells (CTL) 91, 94, 107
  activity measurement 470
  killing mechanism 152–154
  live attenuated vaccines 520–521
  recognition 175

D

dalfopristin 491
Dane particle 305, 307
dapsone, leprosy 359, 494
deafness, congenital rubella 315
defensins 77
β-defensins 143
delayed-type hypersensitivity (cell-mediated) 152, 154, 190, 193, 469, 470
  absence in HIV infection 267–268
Delhi boil (Oriental sores) 396, 536
delta antigen 308
Delta study 271
delta virus (hepatitis D virus) 303, 308
dementia, in HIV infection 336–337
dendritic cells 104, 105
  as adjuvants for vaccines 523
dendritic ulcers 345, 368
dengue 386
  myalgia 377
dengue fever 150, 189, 384–385
dengue hemorrhagic fever shock syndrome 384–385
dengue virus 384–385
dental caries (decay) 57–58, 214
dental plaque 57–58, 214
deoxycytidine (ddC; zalcitabine) 503
deoxyinosine (ddI; didanosine) 503
dermatitis
  contagious pustular (orf) 368
  schistosomes causing 365, 397
dermatophyte infections 360–362
  clinical features 360–362
  diagnosis/identification 362, 364
  skin/hair/nails 360–362
  transmission 135–136, 360–361
  treatment 363
dermatophytes 360, 615(PP)
  arthrospores 360–361, 363
  colonial characteristics and structures 362–363, 364

dermatophytes (*cont'd*)
distribution/hosts 360, 361
fluorescence under ultraviolet light 362
dermatophytid reactions 361–362
dermicidins 143
developing countries 2
bowel flora 57
diarrheal diseases 277, 279, 281–282, 290
Escherichia coli infections 281–282
HIV infection 266–267
measles complications 375
diabetes mellitus
anaerobic cellulitis of feet 355
insulin-dependent, rubella causing 315
pyelonephritis and UTIs 243
diagnosis of infections 453–472
antibody detection 453, 454, 466–468
cultural techniques *see* culture of organisms
diagnostic routes (flow-chart) 455
FUO 417
gene probes 460–462
genomic methods 25
non-cultural techniques 455–462
toxin detection 458, 459
see also microscopy; serologic diagnosis/tests
dialysis catheters, infections 428
diarrhea/diarrheal disease 277–292
in AIDS 435
antibiotic-associated 59, 289–290
bacterial causes 280–289
Bacillus cereus 284
Campylobacter 283–285
Clostridium perfringens 284, 288–289
enterotoxigenic *E. coli* in children 281–282
Escherichia coli 280–282
features and comparisons 284
other causes 284–285, 288–289
Salmonella 282–283
Shigella 287–288
Vibrio cholerae 285–287
bloody/mucus 287, 295
children 277, 279, 281–282
definition/terminology 278
helminths (worms) causing 297–300
strongyloidiasis 299
Trichuris trichiura 298
illness/mortality in children 277, 279, 290
infectious causes 187
mechanism 187
protein absorption 129
protozoa causing 293–300
Cryptosporidium parvum 297, 435
Entamoeba histolytica 295
Giardia lamblia 296
Isospora belli 435
role in infection transmission 132, 134, 187
viral causes 290–292
rotaviruses 290–292
watery, in cholera 286, 287
see also food-associated infections; food poisoning
didanosine (deoxyinosine; ddi) 503
didehydrodideoxyuridine (d4T, stavudine) 503
diethylcarbamazine 398
diffusion tests, antibiotic susceptibility 497–498
Digenea *see* flukes
DiGeorge syndrome 424, 522
diguanides, disinfectants 565

dihydroxypropoxy-methylguanine (DHPG) *see* ganciclovir
dilution test, antibiotic susceptibility 498
diphtheria 214–216
anterior nasal 215
antitoxin 215
nasopharyngeal 215
respiratory obstruction 213, 215
time course/incubation period 443
treatment 215
vaccine 216, 518
diphtheria toxin 17, 214, 215
detection 467
fragments A and B 215
mode of action 187, 215
diphtheria toxoid 214, 518
vaccination practice 528
diphtheria, pertussis and tetanus (DPT) vaccine 218, 518
current practice/schedule 528–529
see also pertussis (whooping cough), vaccination/vaccines
Diphyllobothrium latum (fish tapeworm) 300, 623–624(PP)
disease
definition 445
detection/diagnosis 447
new outbreaks 447
disinfectants 565
monitoring effectiveness 565
disinfection 561–565
choice of method 562–565
control 564–565
definition 561–562
disseminated intravascular coagulation (DIC) 189
DNA
amplification 462
see also polymerase chain reaction (PCR)
repair 20–21
replication *see* DNA replication
sequence analysis 559–560
synthesis
antibacterial agents inhibiting 492–496
antifungal agents inhibiting 504, 505
antiviral agents inhibiting 503–504
typing techniques 558–560
see also gene expression
DNA chips 26–27
DNA microarrays 26–27
DNA polymerase 13–14
viral, inhibition 501, 502
DNA probes 25, 455, 460–462, 558
DNA replication
bacteria 13–14
frequency/accuracy 13–14
origin of replication (OriC) 13
plasmids 17–18
replication forks 13
rolling circle model 17
DNA vaccines 520
DNA viruses 36
cancers associated 194–197
classification/groups 9
disruption of antimicrobial response 175
genome integration into host 196
mRNA synthesis 31
transformation of cells 196–197
dogs
Pasteurella multocida transmission 407, 609(PP)
rabies transmission 335
Strongyloides infections 411
toxocara infection from 338
zoonoses transmitted from 140–141
dog tapeworm *see* *Echinococcus*

granulosus (dog tapeworm)
dog ticks, rickettsial infections transmitted 387
Donovan bodies 262
donovanosis 262
dorsal root ganglion 325, 368
double diffusion test 467
doxycycline 485
chlamydial infection 260–261
lymphogranuloma venereum 261
syphilis 256
see also tetracyclines
droplet transmission 132, 133, 134, 229–230
drug misusers
HBV transmission 305
infective endocarditis 417
drug resistance *see* resistance
drying, microbial resistance 132
Duffy antigen 393
duodenal ulcers 293
dust, transmission of infections 136
dwarf tapeworm (*Hymenolepis nana*) 300
dysentery 278
amebic 295
bacillary comparison 295
bacillary *see* shigellosis
dysuria 244

E

Eastern equine encephalitis virus 332, 333, 385
Ebola hemorrhagic fever 402–403
Ebola virus 402–403
echinocandins 505
echinococcosis *see* hydatid disease
Echinococcus, life cycle 410
Echinococcus granulosus (dog tapeworm) 309, 378, 624(PP)
hydatid cysts *see* hydatid cyst(s)
ocular infection 345, 346
see also hydatid disease
Echinococcus multilocularis 410
echoviruses
attachment 205
common colds due to 205
rashes due to 372
ecthyma gangrenosum 426, 427
ectothrix infection 362, 363
eczema herpeticum 368, 370
edema 79
efavirenz 503
effective reproductive rate (R) 441–444
egg antigens, in vaccines, hypersensitivity 521
Ehrlich, Paul 473, 474
Ehrlichia, effect on hemopoietic system 381
ehrlichiosis 381, 387
elastase, *Pseudomonas* 176
elderly
hospital-acquired infection risk 550
meningitis 328
zoster 371
electrolytes, replacement 283, 287, 292
electron microscopy 457–458
electroporation 21
Elek test 467
elephantiasis 398
ELISA *see* enzyme-linked immunosorbent assay (ELISA)
emerging diseases 2–3
empyema 237
enanthem 372
encephalitis, viral 331–337
arbovirus 336, 385–386
B virus 332
causes 333

herpes simplex virus (HSV) *see* herpes simplex virus (HSV)
measles 337, 527
mumps 333, 375
Murray valley 385
Nipah virus 333–335
pathogenesis 334
poliovirus 332
postinfectious 337
postvaccinial 337
retroviruses 336–337
St Louis 337, 385
subacute, in HIV infection 336
togaviruses 336
VZV 333
encephalitis (non-viral), toxoplasmosis 333
Encephalitozoon intestinalis 297
encephalomyelitis
influenza complication 230
myalgic (postviral fatigue syndrome) 377
pathogenesis 334
viral 324
encephalopathy
pertussis vaccine side effect 218
scrapie-type agents causing 337–338
spongiform 337–338
endemic infections 445
endocarditis
infective *see* infective endocarditis
treatment 419–420
endocytosis, parasite-directed/induced 129
endophthalmitis, *Candida* 431
endospores 24
endothelial cell leukocyte adhesion molecule-1 (ELAM-1) 79
endothrix infection 362, 363
endotoxins 11, 129, 188–189
actions 188
Bordetella pertussis 217
detection 459
host responses 144, 188–189
organisms producing and cytokines induced 189
see also lipopolysaccharide (LPS)
endotoxin shock (septic shock) 188–189, 540, 542
Entamoeba histolytica 8, 295, 619–620(PP)
cysts 294
exotoxin 185
life cycle 294
Entamoeba histolytica infection 294–296
amebic liver abscess 310
dysentery 295
laboratory diagnosis 295
lung 237
opportunistic STD 273
enteric fevers 301–302
carriers 301, 302
clinical features 301
diagnosis 302
treatment/prevention 302
see also typhoid fever
Enterobacter 599(PP)
UTIs 241
Enterobacteriaceae 598(PP)
Enterobius vermicularis (pinworm; threadworm) 297, 627(PP)
clinical features of infection 300
eggs 300
identification 466
Enterococcus 589(PP)
vancomycin resistance 484, 556
enterocolitis, definition/terminology 278
enterotoxins
Clostridium perfringens 288
Escherichia coli 281
Staphylococcus aureus 292
Vibrio cholerae 286

enteroviruses
  myocarditis and pericarditis 377
  pharyngitis 202
  see also hepatitis A virus (HAV)
Enterozoon bieneusi 297
environmental infections, hospital-acquired 545, 548–549
enzyme-linked immunosorbent assay (ELISA) 458, 460, 468
  Chlamydia 260
eosinophil(s)
  extracellular killing of parasites 83–84
  granules/contents 84, 146, 147
eosinophilia, tropical pulmonary (Weingarten's syndrome) 237
epidemic myalgia (Bornholm disease) 377
epidemics 445
  surveillance systems 447
epidemiological typing, hospital-acquired infections 556–557
epidemiology 445
  analytical 445
  concepts/principles 441–447
  descriptive 445
  detection/diagnosis 447
  experimental 445
  genomic methods 25
  hospital-acquired infections 555–556
  host populations 442
  ribosomal RNA sequencing 25
  surveillance systems 447
  terminology 445
  tuberculosis 559
  vaccination program design 528
epidermodysplasia verruciformis 196, 368
Epidermophyton 360
epidural abscess 329
epiglottitis, acute 213
  emergency treatment 213
episomes 23
epitopes 519–520
Epstein–Barr virus (EBV)
  antigens 204–205
  cancers associated 208
  DNA 195
  immune cells signaling interference 175
  latency 206
  receptor 123
  replication in B cells 206
  transmission 204–205
Epstein–Barr virus (EBV) infection 204–208
  autoantibodies 206
  B cell lymphomas 208
  B cell proliferation inhibited by TNF 148
  Burkitt's lymphoma 148, 195, 208
  clinical features 205–206
  effect on hemopoietic system 381
  HIV-associated lymphomas 195
  immunologic events 205–206
  immunosuppression due to 174
  infectious mononucleosis 205
    see also infectious mononucleosis
  laboratory diagnosis 206–207
  latent 206
  myalgic encephalomyelitis 377
  nasopharyngeal carcinoma 194–195, 208
  post-transplant lymphoproliferative disorder 436
  reactivation 177, 206
  sore throats due to 202, 204–208
  transmission 135, 204–205
  treatment 208
  tumor development 436
eradication of infections 513

control *vs.* 450–451
  factors favoring 451
  measles 525, 529–530
  smallpox 2, 373, 450, 451
  two-stage vaccination program 525
  vaccination coverage 525, 526
  vaccination strategies 525
erysipelas 350, 352, 354
Erysipelothrix rhusiopathiae, cellulitis 355
erythema 79
erythema chronicum migrans 390, 391
erythema infectiosum 372, 381
erythrocytes *see* red blood cells
erythromycin 489, 490
  acne 357
  adverse effects 489
  burns 427
  Campylobacter diarrhea 285
  chancroid 262
  resistance 489
  syphilis 256
  whooping cough 218
  see also macrolides
escape mutants 173
eschar 404, 426
Escherichia coli 598(PP)
  adhesion mechanisms 281
  capsular acid polysaccharide (K) antigens 243
  characteristics of strains/groups 280, 281
  colonization of urinary tract 243
  diffuse-aggregative (DAEC) 281
  enteroaggregative (EAEC) 281
  enterohemorrhagic (EHEC) 281
  enteroinvasive (EIEC) 280, 281
  enteropathogenic (EPEC) 280, 281
  enterotoxins 281
  exotoxins 185, 186
  fimbriae (pili) 12–13, 243, 281
  growth/division 13–14
  hemolysin production 244
  lac operon and gene regulation 16, 17
  vaccine development 535
  verotoxin 281
  verotoxin-producing (EHEC) 280, 281
Escherichia coli infections
  diarrheal disease 280–282
    incidence in developing countries 281–282
    laboratory diagnosis 280, 281, 282
    treatment 282
  hospital-acquired infection 546, 556
  meningitis 326, 327, 329
  puerpural sepsis due to 319
  UTIs 241, 243–244
esophageal cancer, *Helicobacter pylori* protection 293
esophageal varices 398
esophagitis, *Candida* 431
espundia 398
ethambutol 497
ethionamide, leprosy 359
ethylene oxide 564
eukaryotes 7
  evolution 63–64
  mitochondrion evolution 64
evasion of host defenses *see* host defense evasion
evolution
  bacteria 113
  evasion of host defenses 64–65, 113–116
  mitochondria 64
  parasitism 63–67
  pressure of infection as influence 65
exanthems *see* rashes

exanthem subitum (roseola infantum) 372
exotoxins 17, 129, 184
  detection 459
  of importance in disease 185
  modes of action/consequences 184, 185
  subunit structure 185, 186–187
  see also specific bacterial genera
extracellular pathogens, host defenses against 8–9, 93–94
  antibody-dependent cell-mediated cytotoxicity 93, 94, 96
  eosinophil action against 83–84
  humoral immunity 97
  innate immune response 83–84
  opsonization/phagocytosis 97
  see also antibodies; complement; natural killer (NK) cells; phagocytosis
extrinsic allergic alveolitis 191
eye
  congenital rubella 315
  defense mechanisms 345
eye infections 343–347
  Candida 432
  of deep layers 345–346
  HSV 368
  ophthalmia neonatorum 256, 257, 320, 344
  ophthalmic zoster 371
  Pseudomonas aeruginosa 345
  see also blindness; conjunctivitis
eyelid infections 343

F

Factor VIII 273
fasciitis 350
  necrotizing 355–356
Fasciola hepatica 309
fatal familial insomnia 54, 338
fatigue, chronic fatigue syndrome 377
Fc receptors, production by microbes 172, 176
fecal contamination, urine samples 245
fecal-oral spread of infection 132, 133, 134, 303–304
  helminths 47
feces
  Giardia lamblia detection 296
  parasite transmission 293–294
  protozoan cysts 296, 297
  rice water stool 286, 287
feet
  anaerobic cellulitis in diabetics 355
  dermatophyte infections 361
fermentation 13
Fernandez reaction 470
fetus
  cell-mediated immune response 313
  congenital infections *see* congenital infections
  failure of mother to reject 313
  immune defenses 297, 313
  malformations 313–315
    CMV infection 204
  routes of infection 319
  VZV infection 371
fever 188
  continuous/intermittent types 413
  definition 413
  enteric *see* enteric fevers
  factitious 413
  hemorrhagic *see* hemorrhagic fevers
  malaria 393
  mechanisms and cytokines involved 144, 188, 413
  puerperal 319

relapsing *see* relapsing fever
  swinging 413
  tumor necrosis factor (TNF) 188
  undulant, in brucellosis 409
fever of unknown origin (FUO) 413–421
  bacterial infections 416
  classical 415, 416
  definition 413
  early enteric fever 301
  endocarditis *see* infective endocarditis
  HIV-associated 415, 416, 418
  infective causes 413–414, 416
  investigations (by stage) 414–415
  neutropenic 415, 416, 418
  non-infectious causes 413
  nosocomial 415, 416, 418
  parasitic 416
  specific patient groups 415–416, 418
  treatment 415
fifth disease 372
filarial nematodes 48, 398, 627(PP)
  infection via skin 124
filariasis 398
  lymphatic 398
  treatment/prevention 398
filoviruses 402–403, 571(PP)
filtration, sterilization 564
fimbriae (pili) 12–13, 22–23
fingerprinting, epidemiological 557, 560
fish-tank granuloma 359, 360
fish tapeworm (*Diphyllobothrium latum*) 300
flagella
  bacterial 12, 90
  'H' antigens 12, 557
flagellins 12
flatworms *see* flukes; tapeworms
flaviviruses 384–385, 385, 572(PP)
fleas
  plague transmission 405
  see also arthropod-borne infections
flora, normal 57–60, 123
  absence 60
  advantages/disadvantages 59–61
  anaerobic bacteria 57, 58
  bacterial distribution/frequency 57–58
  bacterial number 57
  gastrointestinal tract 58, 59, 290
  genitourinary tract 58–59
  germ-free animals 60
  neonates, acquisition 57
  oral cavity 57, 213
  organisms by site 58, 454
  postnatal acquisition and changes 57
  prevention of colonization by pathogens 59–60, 72
  respiratory tract 57–58, 202
  skin 57, 123, 349, 554
  specimen handling/interpretation
flow cytofluorimetry 468, 470
fluconazole 505
flucytosine (5-fluorocytosine) 504
fluid
  loss in cholera 286
  replacement 283, 292
flukes (trematodes)
  blood *see Schistosoma*
  infections 48
    anthelminthic drugs 506, 509
    gastrointestinal tract 300
  liver 309
  see also Schistosoma; schistosomiasis
fluorescence microscopy 457
fluorescent antibody test, *Chlamydia* 260
fluorescent treponemal antibody absorption (FTA-ABS) test 255, 256

5-fluorocytosine 504
fluoroquinolones 492, 493
folliculitis 350, 353
fomites 548
food, spore-contaminated 288, 289
food-associated infections
  definition/terminology 277
  hepatitis A 303–304
  listeriosis 302
  pathogens 278
  tapeworms 378
  see also diarrhea/diarrheal disease
food poisoning 292–293
  Bacillus cereus 288–289, 292
  botulism 293, 340
  causes and diarrhea in 187
  definition/terminology 187, 277
  Staphylococcus aureus 292
foot-and-mouth disease 135
foreign bodies 416, 424
  susceptibility to infections 165
foreskin, increased infection risk
  129, 130
formaldehyde 518, 564
foscarnet (phosphonoformate) 502
  CMV 204
F plasmid (F factor) 23
fractures, zoster predisposition 371
Francisella tularensis 407, 608(PP)
Frei skin test 261
Freund's adjuvants 523
fungal infections 39–40
  antifungal agents 505–506
    mechanism of action 504–505
  burns 426, 427
  cutaneous 39, 40
  cutaneous/subcutaneous 39, 40
  deep/systemic 39, 40
  FUO 416
  in hematological malignancies
    429
  infective endocarditis 419
  meningitis 326, 329, 340
  occupational hazards 191, 360
  opportunistic 39, 40, 429,
    431–434
  skin 353, 359–364
  subcutaneous 39, 40, 363–364
  superficial 39, 40, 360–363, 505,
    506
  systemic 364, 505, 506
    skin manifestations 352, 364
  in transplant recipients 429, 430
fungi 39–41
  cell morphology 466
  classification 39–40
  colonial characteristics 466
  culture 462–463
  dimorphic 39
  exotoxins produced 185
  filamentous 39, 40
  groups 39–40
  growth forms 39, 40
  growth requirements 462–463,
    466
  identification 466
  inhalation, occupational diseases
    191
  reproduction/budding 39
  shedding from skin 135–136
  skin infection 124
  skin rashes due to 194
  structure/characteristics 39
  toxins 39
  yeast-like forms 39
  zoonoses 140
fusidic acid 491–492
  adverse effects 492
  mode of action 491

G

gallbladder, *Salmonella* infection
  301
gallium scan 417

gamma irradiation, sterilization by
  564
ganciclovir 501, 502
  CMV 204
  structure 501
gangrene 350, 354–355
  gas 350, 355–356
  synergistic bacterial 355
Gardnerella vaginalis 263, 611(PP)
  bacterial vaginosis/vaginitis 252,
    263
gas gangrene 350, 355–356
gas liquid chromatography,
    microbial product detection
    459
gastric acid, microbial evasion
    mechanism 127, 129
gastric cancer, *Helicobacter pylori*
    protection 197, 293
gastric ulcers 293
gastritis, *Helicobacter pylori* 293
gastroenteritis
  definition/terminology 278
  neonatal 320
  viral 290–292, 561
  see also diarrhea/diarrheal disease
gastrointestinal enzymes 129
gastrointestinal hemorrhage
  schistosomiasis 398
  yellow fever 384
gastrointestinal tract
  attachment of microorganisms
    126
  defense mechanisms 126–129,
    127, 131, 278
  microbial success strategies 128,
    131, 277
  normal flora 58, 59
    antibiotic-associated changes
      59, 60, 290
  obstruction, *Ascaris lumbricoides*
    causing 298
gastrointestinal tract infections 187,
    277–312, 279
  Ancylostoma duodenale 297
  bacterial 280–289, 300–303
  candidiasis 431
  damage caused by 279
  diarrhea due to 187, 277
    see also diarrhea/diarrheal
      disease
  flukes 300
  Helicobacter pylori 293, 604(PP)
  helminths 293–294
  localized or invasive 277, 279
  pathogens 277, 278
  protozoan 44, 293–300
  systemic/disseminated 279,
    300–310
  tapeworms 300
  viral 290–292, 303–308
  worms (nematodes) 297–300
'gay bowel syndrome' 273
gene cloning
  vaccine development 518–519,
    519–520
  HBV 532
  viruses as vectors 518–519, 519
gene expression
  activation (positive regulation)
    16, 17
  bacterial 14, 17
  DNA microarrays 26–27
  lac operon in *E. coli* 16, 17
  mRNA transcriptional regulation
    15–17
  operators and operator sites 16
  operons 14–15
  regulation in bacteria 15–17
  repression (negative regulation)
    16, 17
gene probes 25, 460–462, 558
gene switching 173
'generation time' of infections 441,
    442
genetic determinants

host susceptibility to disease
  162–163
  microbial, virulence/pathogenicity
    162–163
genetic recombination 173
genetic shift 173
genital cold sores 264
genital herpes 252, 263–264, 368
genital tract
  host defenses 131
  infection route 129
  microbial evasion of defenses
    129–130, 131
genital tract infections
  Candida albicans 252, 262–263
  chlamydial 252, 258–261
  HSV 252, 263–264, 368
  inguinal lymphadenopathy 261
  transmission 134
  see also sexually transmitted
    diseases (STDs); specific
    infections
genital ulcers
  chancroid 261–262
  donovanosis 262
  HIV increased transmission risk
    269
  HSV 263–264
genital warts 252, 264, 265, 368
genome sequences, bacterial 25
genomics, bacterial 24–27
  applications 25
  DNA microarrays 26–27
gentamicin 485, 487, 498
  burns 427
  peritonitis 310
  see also aminoglycoside(s)
germ-free animals 60
germ theory of disease 119
Gerstmann–Sträussler–Scheinker
    syndrome 54, 338
Ghon complex/focus 233
giant cell pneumonia 231, 375
Giardia lamblia 296, 620(PP)
  attachment in intestinal tract
    126, 127
  cysts 256, 295, 296
  infection see giardiasis
  life cycle 296
  opportunistic STD 273
  transmission 296
  trophozoites 295, 296
giardiasis
  diagnosis 296
  diarrhea 296
  treatment 296–297, 496, 509
gingival crevice 214
gingivitis 214
Global Polio Eradication Initiative
    531
glomerulonephritis
  acute
    immune complex(es) 210
    streptococcal infection
      complications 190
    Streptococcus pyogenes causing
      210, 354
  chronic 190
  in malaria 394
  type III hypersensitivity 190, 192
glucocorticoids 163
glue ear 212
glutaraldehyde 564
glycopeptides 480–481, 484–485
  adverse effects 484–485
  mode of action 481
  resistance 481, 484
  route of administration 481
  see also individual drugs
goblet cells 95, 96
gonococcus see *Neisseria gonorrhoeae*
gonorrhea 252, 256–258
  asymptomatic 256, 257
  damage due to inflammatory
    response 256
  disseminated infection 258

laboratory diagnosis 258
  symptoms/complications
    256–257
  treatment/follow-up 258
  see also Neisseria gonorrhoeae
Gram-negative bacteria 7, 456
  burns infections 426–427
  cell wall structure 11, 12
  diarrhea due to 280–288
  endotoxins 188
  infections in neutropenia 429
  opportunistic, otitis externa 213
  outer membrane 11
  periplasmic space 13
  UTIs 241
Gram-positive bacteria 7, 456
  cell wall structure 11–12
  classification 9
  cocci 355, 585(PP)
  diarrhea due to 288–289
  infections in neutropenia 429
  pus in impetigo 354, 355
  UTIs 241
Gram stain 11, 456
granuloma
  brain 338
  fish-tank 359, 360
  formation 193
  leprosy 359
  non-infective causes 417
  retina 338
  rheumatic fever 210
  schistosomiasis 398
  swimming pool 359
  Toxocara infections 338
  tuberculosis 232, 233
  see also chronic granulomatous
    disease (CGD)
granuloma inguinale (donovanosis)
    262
granulomatous reactions, chronic
    261–262
granuloma venereum (donovanosis)
    262
granzymes 83, 153, 154
'gray baby syndrome' 489
griseofulvin 504, 505
Guillain–Barré syndrome 230, 337
gut decontamination 554

H

Haemophilus 606(PP)
Haemophilus ducreyi 252, 607(PP)
  chancroid (soft chancre) 252,
    261–262
  characteristics/culture 261–262
Haemophilus influenzae
    606–607(PP)
  antibodies to 328
  attachment 125
  capsulated/unencapsulated strains
    328
  infections
    bronchitis 218
    influenza 230
    lung infections in cystic fibrosis
      235
    meningitis 326, 327–328
    otitis and sinusitis 212–213
    pneumonia 223
    septic arthritis 379
  virulence factors 326, 327
Haemophilus influenzae biotype
    aegyptius 344
Haemophilus influenzae type b 328
  acute epiglottitis 213
  Hib vaccine 328, 518, 534
  pharyngitis 187, 208
hair
  dermatophyte infections
    360–362
  loss 361, 362
hairy T cell leukemia 194
hairy tongue 206

halogens, disinfectants 565
haloprogin 505
hand, foot and mouth disease 372
　ulcers 207
handwashing 545, 553, 561
Hansen's disease see leprosy
Hantaan virus 402
hantavirus
　pulmonary disease 220
　renal disease 242
'H' (flagellar) antigens 12, 557
head lice 365–366
heart
　congenital rubella 315
　defects, prophylactic antibiotics
　　420
　granulomas in rheumatic fever
　　210
heart disease, rheumatic 210
heart failure
　Chagas' disease 378, 395
　diphtheria toxin causing 215
heart murmurs 418
heart valves
　prosthetic 419, 428
　streptococcal infections 417–418
heat-shock proteins 95, 144
heat sterilization 563
helicase 13
Helicobacter pylori (Campylobacter
　pylori) 283, 293, 603(PP)
　cancer association 197, 293
helminths 47–49
　allergic reactions 190
　anthelminthic drugs 506, 509
　CNS infection 338–339
　eosinophil action against 83–84
　host antibody responses 150
　identification 466
　infections 47–48
　　gastrointestinal tract 293–294
　　multisystem 410–412
　　opportunistic 299, 411, 435
　　vector-borne 397–398
　reproduction 48
　soil-transmitted 298
　surfaces as host-parasite interface
　　47–48
　transmission 47–48
　zoonoses 140
　see also flukes; nematodes;
　　parasites; tapeworms
helper T-cells (TH cells) 93,
　104–106, 108
　antibody production 104
　HIV infection 267–268
　TH1 and TH2 91, 93
　　imbalance 171–172
　see also CD4 cells
helper viruses 35
hemagglutination tests 467, 468
hemagglutinin, influenza virus 30,
　227
hematological malignancy,
　infections in 429
　Candida 431
　see also leukemia; lymphoma
hematuria 244, 246
hemoglobinopathies 66
hemolysins 186, 244
hemolytic anemia, in malaria 190
hemolytic streptococci
　α-hemolytic 58
　β-hemolytic see streptococci
hemolytic-uremic syndrome (HUS)
　281
hemophiliacs, HIV and AIDS 270
hemopoietic system, infections 380
hemorrhagic cystitis 436
hemorrhagic fevers 386
　arboviruses causing 386
　zoonotic 402–403
hemorrhagic shock syndrome
　532–533
hepadnaviruses 304
　see also hepatitis B virus (HBV)

hepatitis 303–308
　chronic active 308
　directly targeting the liver 303
　EBV infection 205
　nonA-nonB
　　enteric(hepatitis E) 304
　　transfusion-associated
　　　(hepatitis C) 307
　　viruses causing 303
　see also specific types of viral hepatitis
hepatitis A 303–304, 305
　clinical/virological course 304
　immunoglobulin therapy 541
　opportunistic STD 273
　vaccine 303, 532
hepatitis A virus (HAV) 303–304
　laboratory diagnosis 304
　transmission 303–304
hepatitis B 252, 303, 304–307
　arthritis 379
　clinical/virologic course 306
　complications 307
　detection/diagnosis 307
　in immunodeficiency 436
　incubation periods 442
　neonatal infection 319
　pathology/immune response 306
　persistent infection 33, 307
　therapy (antiviral) 307
　vaccines 303, 307, 531–532
　　indications/for high-risk groups
　　　532, 551–552
　　recombinant DNA 532
hepatitis B immunoglobulin (HBIg)
　307
hepatitis B virus (HBV) 252,
　304–307, 573(PP)
　antigens/antibodies 304–305,
　　306, 307
　as candidate for eradication 532
　carriers 305–307, 548–549
　children 306
　HBeAg 304, 306, 307
　HBsAg 304–305, 306, 307, 531
　　vaccine development 518,
　　　531–532
　hepatocellular carcinoma and
　　196
　in semen 135
　transmission 275, 305–306
　yellow fever vaccine
　　contamination 163
hepatitis C 303, 307–308
　bone marrow transplant
　　recipients 436
hepatitis C virus (HCV) 307–308
　hepatocellular carcinoma and
　　196
　transmission 307–308
hepatitis D 303, 308
hepatitis D virus (HDV) 308,
　573–574(PP)
hepatitis E 303, 304
hepatitis E virus (HEV) 304,
　574(PP)
hepatitis viruses 303
hepatocellular carcinoma 196, 307
hepatosplenomegaly
　brucellosis 409
　in schistosomiasis 309, 398
herbivores, anthrax 404
herd immunity 513, 525
herpes gladiatorum 368
herpes simplex virus (HSV)
　gC (glycoprotein C) formation
　　175
　isolation for vesicle fluid 369
　type 1 (HSV1) 263–264, 368
　　pathogenicity 164
　　transmission 263, 368
　type 2 (HSV2) 263–264, 368
　　cocarcinogenic role in cervical
　　　cancer 195, 196
　　transmission 263, 368
herpes simplex virus (HSV)
　infection

acyclovir (acycloguanosine) 264
　CNS 368
　conjunctival 345
　diagnosis 202
　　PCR 463
　encephalitis 264, 331–332, 334,
　　368
　genital herpes 252, 263–264, 368
　latent 176, 368
　meningitis 332
　mucocutaneous 368–369
　neonatal 319, 368
　oral 368
　pharyngitis 202
　reactivation 176–177, 368
　　factors provoking 368
　　in immunodeficiency 435–436
　transmission 368, 547
　treatment 369, 501
herpesviruses 574–575(PP)
　interference with MHC class I
　　expression 175
　vaccines 536
herpes zoster see zoster (shingles)
herpetic whitlow 368
hexachlorophene 565
Hib vaccine 328, 518, 534
highly active antiretroviral therapy
　(HAART) 271
　Pneumocystis (carinii) jiroveci 235
　side effects 271
histiocytes 159
Histoplasma capsulatum 433,
　618(PP)
histoplasmosis
　antifungal agents for 433, 506
　disseminated infection 433
history, infectious diseases 1, 2
history-taking, FUO 414, 416
HIV 264–273
　antibodies and detection of 272
　antibody responses 270
　antigenic drift 173
　apoptosis inhibition 176
　drug resistance 271
　gp41 (fusion protein) 174, 267,
　　503
　gp120 267
　HIV1 266
　HIV2 266, 269
　infection process 267–268
　isolation/discovery 265
　origin/development 266
　receptor 123, 267
　replication 266, 267, 272
　in semen 135
　structure and genetic map 266
　tat and rev genes 265, 266
　transmission, vertical 314
　viral load, decrease 271
HIV infection 264–273
　associated encephalopathy 270
　cell-mediated immune response
　　267–268
　children 269
　clinical features/progression 270
　congenital 318
　dementia 336–337
　developing countries 266–267
　drug-resistant 271
　FUO associated 415, 416, 418
　global impact/incidence 2, 251
　immune system/response
　　267–268
　immunosuppression in 173–174,
　　174, 268–269
　incidence 268, 269
　incubation period 267–268
　laboratory tests 272–273
　lymphoma associated 195
　meningitis 332
　monitoring 273
　mononucleosis-type illness 270
　opportunist infections and
　　tumors associated 271
　origin/global spread 266–267

partner mixing matrix 444
　prevalence 269
　reactivation of persistent
　　infections 180
　subacute encephalitis and
　　dementia in 336–337
　TNF increase 148
　transmission 269–270
　　genital ulcers 269
　　heterosexual 269–270
　　homosexual 269
　　injecting drug users 270
　　measures to control 273
　　monitoring 273
　　needle stick injury 270
　　vertical 269
　treatment 270–272
　　antiretroviral therapy 270–271
　　compliance 271
　　drug resistance 271
　vaccine prospects 273, 536
　see also AIDS
HLA, disease susceptibility 66, 162
homosexual behavior 251, 273
hookworms 627–628(PP)
　attachment in intestinal tract
　　126, 127
　cutaneous larval migrans 365
　eggs 298, 299
　in gastrointestinal tract 297
　iron-deficiency anemia 299
　transmission/life cycle 298
　see also Ancylostoma duodenale;
　　Necator americanus
hordeolum 343
horizontal transmission 35
hormones, susceptibility to
　infections and 165
hospital-acquired infections
　545–561
　age/risk 550
　candidiasis/Candida infections
　　554
　causes 546–547
　common infections 546
　consequences 551
　epidemiological typing 556–557
　frequencies by patient group 546
　FUO 415, 416, 418
　host factors influencing 549–551
　human sources 548–549
　　hospital staff 551–552, 556
　　normal flora 60
　　time period of infectivity 549
　hygiene measures 561
　identification 556–557
　infection control committees
　　555–556
　invasive devices associated 550,
　　554
　investigations 555–561
　outbreak investigation 556, 561
　pneumonia 221, 222, 223
　postoperative infections 555
　predisposing factors 549–550
　prevention 551–555, 561
　sources/route of spread 548–549
　staff as sources 551–552, 556
　surveillance 556
　viral 546–547
hospital staff
　as carriers of pathogens 551–552,
　　556
　handwashing 553
　infected, restrictions 552
host
　adaptation, for parasite changes
　　66
　classes of populations 442
　compromised see
　　immunocompromised hosts
　direct damage by organisms
　　184–187
　pathogen relationships 8–9
　responses
　　to endotoxins 188–189

host (cont'd)
  evolution of parasite
    adaptations 64–65, 66, 155
  as series of body
    surfaces/infection sites 123
  susceptibility 162
host defense(s) 423
  after microbial penetration
    72–85, 143–156
  apoptotic responses 175–176
  assessment 468–471
  biochemical/physical barriers
    71–72, 123, 131, 159, 201
    antimicrobial peptides 143
  disruption 423–424
  evasion see host defense evasion
  extracellular pathogens see
    extracellular pathogens, host
    defenses against
  failure in persistent infections
    176
  gastrointestinal tract 126–129,
    127, 131, 278
  innate see immune system/
    response, innate (natural)
  intestinal parasites 8–9
  intracellular pathogens 8
    see also intracellular pathogens
  microbial spread to lymph/blood
    159, 160, 160
  mucosal surfaces 72, 94–95
  oropharyngeal 130
  reduced, hospital-acquired
    infections 549–551
  respiratory tract 125–126, 143,
    201
  speed of response against microbe
    113, 117, 150
  types and microbial answers to
    114–116
  urinogenital tract 129–130
  vaginal 129
  see also complement; cytotoxicity;
    immune system/response;
    phagocytes; specific
    anatomical regions
host defense evasion 114–116, 131,
    167–181
  of adaptive immune defenses
    167
    see also immune evasion
    mechanisms/strategies
  of antiphagocytic devices 114
  bile 128, 129
  evolution 64–65, 113–116
  gastrointestinal tract 127, 129,
    131
  of immediate natural defenses
    114–115
  infection route/mechanisms 131
  of innate immune defenses
    114–115
  by intracellular pathogens 169
  of mechanical barriers 114, 125
  respiratory tract 125–126, 131
  STDs 253
  strategies 66, 167
host-microbe associations 60–62
  symbiotic associations 60–62
host-parasite interactions 1–2,
    57–68, 117–118
  adaptation for balanced
    relationships 117–118
  changing nature 64–66
  helminths 47–48
  social/behavioral changes
    affecting 66, 67
  see also parasitism
human anti-mouse antibodies
    (HAMA) 540
human foamy virus 265
human genome viruses 265
human herpesvirus 1 (HHV1) see
    herpes simplex virus (HSV),
    type 1 (HSV1)
human herpesvirus 2 (HHV2) see

herpes simplex virus (HSV),
    type 2 (HSV2)
human herpesvirus 3 (HHV3) see
    varicella-zoster virus (VZV)
human herpesvirus 4 (HHV4) see
    Epstein–Barr virus (EBV)
human herpesvirus 5 (HHV5) see
    cytomegalovirus (CMV)
human herpesvirus 6 (HHV6)
  encephalitis associated 332
  infection 372
  re-infection/reactivation in
    transplant recipients 436
human herpesvirus 7 (HHV7)
  infection 372
  re-infection/reactivation in
    transplant recipients 436
human herpesvirus 8 (HHV8) 197,
    373
  infection 373
human immunodeficiency virus see
    HIV
human papillomaviruses
  E6 and E7 genes 196
  electron micrograph 458
  transmission 135, 264, 367
  types/characteristics 367–368
  see also individual viruses
human papillomavirus infection
  basal layers of skin 351, 367
  cervical cancer 195, 264, 367
  diagnosis/treatment 367
  genital warts 252, 264, 265
  immune responses 367
  mucocutaneous lesions 367–368
  route 124
  skin cancer 195, 196
  as STD 252
  vulva/penis/rectum 367
human parvoviruses see parvoviruses
human placental viruses 265
human T cell lymphotropic virus 1
    (HTLV1) 34, 265
  infections 380
  lymphomas and leukemias 194,
    195, 380
  tax protein 380
  transmission 380
  tropical spastic paraparesis 337
human T cell lymphotropic virus 2
    (HTLV2) 34, 265
  infections 380
  leukemia associated 194
humoral immune response
    148–152
  microbial strategies against 115
  primary/secondary 103–104, 150
  urinary tract defenses 244
  see also antibodies; B cell(s)
    (B lymphocytes)
hydatid cyst(s) 170, 338, 410
  brain 338
  lung 170, 237
  rupture and type I hypersensitivity
    190
hydatid disease 310, 338–339, 378,
    410–411
  liver lesions 310
  transmission 141, 410
  see also Echinococcus granulosus
hydrocele 398
hydrogen peroxide 76
hydrophobia 335
hydroxyl radicals 76
hygiene 561
  chlamydial infections prevention
    344
  handwashing 545, 553, 561
Hymenolepis nana (dwarf tapeworm)
    300, 624(PP)
  life cycle 48
hypersensitivity 189–193
  type I (allergic/anaphylactic/
    immediate) 190, 191
  type II (cytotoxic) 190, 191
  type III (immune complex)

190–191, 191, 193
  type IV (cell-mediated) 191, 193,
    469, 470
  to vaccines 521–522
hypogammaglobulinemia 541
  transient 424, 426
hypoglycemia, in malaria 394

I

identification of organisms 453
  bacteria 464–466
  fungi 466
  genomic methods 25
  hospital-acquired infections
    556–557
  protozoa/helminths 466
  specialized typing methods
    556–557
  viruses 466
idiotype 106
idiotype network 520
idoxuridine (IDU) 501
immune complex(es)
  acute glomerulonephritis 190
  complement activation 87, 88,
    89, 90
  deposition 190, 191
    hepatitis B 307
    malaria 394
  immune tolerance due t 171
  phagocytic cell activation 89, 91
  type III hypersensitivity 190–191,
    193
immune complex disease 190, 191
immune evasion mechanisms/
    strategies 115–116, 167–181
  antigenic variation 172–173
  concealment of antigens 169–170
  immunosuppression 174–176
  local interference with immune
    response 176
  persistence advantage 177, 179
  signaling interference between
    immune cells 175–176
  see also host defense evasion
immune system/response
  abnormalities after burns 426
  adaptive (acquired) 71, 87–98,
    143, 151–154
    compromised 423
    deficiency see
      immunodeficiency
    overactivity 189–193
    vaccination principle 513
    see also antibodies; humoral
      immune response
  boosting, hospital-acquired
    infection prevention
    553–554
  cell-mediated see cell-mediated
    immune response
  cellular basis 99–110
  CNS infections 324–325
  cytokine actions 104–106, 107,
    108
  depression in infections 173–174
  developing, effect of vaccination
    524
  dual role in tuberculosis 233
  evasion see immune evasion
    mechanisms/strategies
  evolution of parasites to
    overcome 64–67
  fetus 297, 313
  'gaps' and microbial exploitation
    171
  influence of brain on 163–164
  innate (natural) 71–86, 87,
    143–151
    compromised 423
    overactivity 187–188
    primary defects 423
    secondary defects 423–424,
    426–428

see also complement;
    eosinophil(s); interferons
    (IFNs); phagocytes
  innate/adaptive systems
    integration 97
  innate vs. adaptive 71, 87
  pathological effects of organisms
    187–193
  race between host and
    microorganism 113
  regulatory mechanisms 106, 109
  surface vs. systemic infections 157
  susceptibility to infections and
    162
  see also host defense(s)
immune tolerance 105, 106–107,
    108
  induced by microbes 171–172
immunization
  active see vaccination; vaccines
  passive 539–541, 553–554
immunoassay 458–460
  antibiotics 499, 500
  ELISA see enzyme-linked
    immunosorbent assay
    (ELISA)
immunocompromised hosts
    423–437
  bacterial meningitis 329
  causes 423
  contraindication to live vaccine
    522
  cryptosporidiosis 297
  innate immunity defective 423
  interstitial pneumonia 231
  microorganisms infecting 425
  papillomaviruses infection of skin
    367
  pneumonia 220
  reactivation of infections 176
  treatment of infections 432
  zoster 371
  see also immunodeficiency;
    immunosuppression
immunodeficiency
  acquired, syndrome see AIDS
  CMV infection 204
  common variable 424
  leishmaniasis 396–397
  primary 423, 424, 425
  secondary/acquired 423,
    424–425
    infections associated 429–431
  severe combined (SCID) 424
  treatment 543
  vaccination contraindications
    522
  see also immunocompromised
    hosts
immunofluorescence 457, 458, 470
  RSV infection diagnosis 220
immunoglobulin(s)
  class switching 103, 150
  structure/properties 87, 88, 89
  therapy 541–542
  uptake by microbes for immune
    evasion 170
  see also antibodies
immunoglobulin A (IgA) 89
  in colostrum 541
  secretory piece 88, 94
  structure 88
  synthesis/structure 94
immunoglobulin D (IgD) 89
immunoglobulin E (IgE) 88–89
  binding to mast cells 94
  in worm infections 190
immunoglobulin G (IgG) 89
  immune response regulation 106
  structure 88
  in type II hypersensitivity 190,
    191
immunoglobulin M (IgM) 89, 150
  detection in diagnosis of infection
    467
  immune response regulation 106

monomeric 103
rubella, in cord blood 315–316
structure 88, 151
immunoglobulin (normal) therapy
541
indications 542
immunological memory 71, 150,
154
induction by vaccines 514
role/nature of response 102–104
immunopathology 183, 189
immunoprecipitation 467
immunostimulation, non-specific
cellular 542–543
immunosuppression
drugs/chemotherapy causing
424–425, 429
in HIV infection 268–269
infections/microbes causing
174–176, 424
in malaria 394
opportunistic infections in 2,
429, 430
reactivation of infections 180
skin cancer linked to
papillomaviruses in 195,
196
strongyloidiasis in 299
virus infections causing 174
immunotherapy
non-specific cellular 542–543
passive 539–541, 553–554
impetigo 350, 354, 355, 370
streptococcal 352
incidence of infections 445
peaks and seasonal 447
incomplete Freund's adjuvant (IFA)
523
incubation period 168, 441, 442,
443, 445
indinavir 503
infants
botulism 293, 340
mortality due to gastroenteritis
290
RSV infections 219–220
see also neonatal infections
infection
acute 178
agents that are major killers 513
biological response gradient
120–121
causes/discovery 118–120
conflicts between host/microbes
113
see also host defense(s); host
defense evasion
control see control of infections
definition 445
global eradication see eradication
of infections
'hit-and-run' 157, 158, 168
'iceberg' concept 120, 121
incidence 445
latent see latent infections
multisystem 401–412
obligatory steps 113
persistent see persistent infections
problems in assigning etiology
119–120
receptors/attachment process 123
recovery from 154–155
routes/sites of entry 123–130
severity/variations 120–121
spread see spread of infections
surface, rapid replication in 158
surface vs. systemic 157–158
systemic, stepwise spread 158
transmission see transmission of
infections
types 118, 119
infection control, hospitals
555–556
see also hospital-acquired
infections
infectious mononucleosis 205, 381

laboratory diagnosis 206–207
see also Epstein–Barr virus (EBV)
infection
infective doses 132
infective endocarditis 416–420
antibiotic prophylaxis 420
blood culture 418
Candida 431
mortality 418–419
pathogenesis 418
rat bite fever 408
signs/symptoms 418
staphylococcal 417–418, 419–420
streptococcal 417–418, 419
treatment 419–420
infertility, women 256–257
inflammation, bacteria causing
159–160
inflammatory response, acute 85,
183
acute phase proteins 80, 82, 144
antibody-mediated 87–89
complement/phagocyte synergism
77–79
initiation by antibody bound to
mast cells 88–89, 94–95
macrophage role in initiation 79,
81, 144
pathology 79
influenza
acute bronchitis 218
CNS complications 230
diagnosis/serology 230
epidemics/pandemics 227–228,
229
influenza virus inhibitors 504,
561
management/prevention 230
myalgia 377
myocarditis and pericarditis 377
neuraminidase inhibitors 504,
561
pneumonia 227
secondary bacterial infections
230
symptoms/pathogenesis 230
time course 443
transmission 229–230
upper respiratory tract infection
205
vaccines 230, 533
development 518, 533
DNA vaccines 520
killed/inactivated 533
live cold-adapted strains 533
recombinant RNA 533
influenza A virus 226–227, 228,
561
amantadine action 504
genetic recombination 173
influenza viruses 226–230, 228,
238
antigenic drift/antigenic shift
227, 533
attachment process 30, 125, 205
genome 227
inhibitors 504
mutations 172–173
nomenclature 227
structure/budding 227
types 226–227, 229
see also individual viruses
infusion-related bacteremia 554
innate immunity see immune
system/response, innate
insect vectors 383
transmission of infections 47,
138–140
insertion sequences (ISs) 23–24
integrons 476–477
inter-epidemic period 446–447
interferons (IFNs) 82–83, 148
adverse effects 504, 543
IFNα 82, 148
chronic granulomatous disease
therapy 542

hepatitis C treatment 308
therapeutic immunostimulation
542
IFNβ 82, 148
IFNγ 144, 148
as adjuvant for vaccines 523
microbial strategies against 115,
148, 167
molecular basis of action 82–83,
149
release by T cells 91, 92, 94, 105
synthesis in viral infections
82–83
therapeutic applications 504
viral hepatitis treatment 504
viral infections 149
interleukin-1 (IL-1)
as adjuvant for vaccines 523
fever mechanism 188
interleukin-2 (IL-2) 105
as adjuvant for vaccines 523
receptor 105
therapy 542, 543
interleukin-4 (IL-4), release by T
cells 105
intestinal epithelial cells, cholera
toxin action 186
intestinal tract see gastrointestinal
tract
intra-abdominal abscess 277, 417
intra-abdominal sepsis 310
intracellular pathogens 8
antigen concealment/immune
evasion 169
host defense(s) 8
immune defense mechanisms
89–93
inhibition of viral replication by T
cells 91–93
killing by phagocytes 75–77
obligate, Chlamydia 258–259,
260
spread from blood 160
T cell-induced killing by
macrophage 91
intradermal challenge 468
intrauterine infections see congenital
infections
invasive devices, care 554–555
invertebrate vectors 138–140
bloodsucking arthropods
138–140
molluscs/crustacea 139–140
iodine, disinfectants 565
iron-deficiency anemia 299
irradiation, sterilization by 564
irradiation therapy 425
ISCOMs (immune-stimulating
complexes) 523, 533
isolation of patients 552
isoniazid (isonicotinic acid
hydrazide) 235, 497
isospora 297
Isospora belli 297, 623(PP)
Isospora belli infection 435
ivermectin 398

J

Japanese encephalitis virus 332,
333, 336, 385
vaccine 532
jaundice 303
hepatitis 303
JC virus 324
infection 336, 436
infection route/reactivation 242
shedding in urine 242
Jenner, Edward 515
'jock itch' 362
joint
infections 378–380
prostheses, infections 428
'jumping genes' see transposons
Junin virus 402

K

kala-azar 396
Kaletra 503
Kaposi's sarcoma 197, 373
in AIDS 436
HHV8 association 197, 373
Kawasaki syndrome 377
keratin 123
keratitis 345
ketoconazole 505
kidney
abscess 244
disease 242
failure
acute, in hemolytic-uremic
syndrome 281
leptospirosis 408
histological appearance 245
infections see pyelonephritis
stones 243
strictures 243
transplantation
infections 430
post-transplant
lymphoproliferative disorder
(PTLD) 436
tumors 243
see also entries beginning renal
killing curves 498, 500, 562, 563
'kissing' bug (reduviid) 395
Klebsiella 599(PP)
ankylosing spondylitis association
379
UTIs 241
Klebsiella aerogenes, serotyping 557
Klebsiella pneumoniae, attachment
125
Koch, Robert 119
Koch's postulates 119
Koplik's spots 374, 375
Korean hemorrhagic fever 242, 402
Kupffer cells 72, 74
Kuru 7, 53, 54, 338
see also prions/prion infections
kwashiorkor 287, 424
Kyasanur forest virus 386

L

labor, neonatal infections during
319, 320
laboratory diagnosis see diagnosis of
infections; serologic
diagnosis/tests
lac operon 14
gene regulation 16, 17
La Crosse virus 386
β-lactams see beta-lactams
lactic acid 129
lactic acidosis, in malaria 394
Lactobacillus aerophilus 58
lactoferrin 77, 80
Lamivudine (3TC; thiacytidine) 503
Langerhans' cells, HIV infection
267
large granular lymphocyte (LGL) 83
see also natural killer (NK) cells
larva migrans, cutaneous 365
laryngitis 214
laryngotracheobronchitis, acute 225
Lassa fever 155, 401, 402, 504
Lassa fever virus 401
latency-associated transcripts 176
latent infections 33–34, 168, 176,
178
HSV 176, 368
varicella-zoster virus (VZV) 176,
370
latent period 441, 442, 443
latex particle agglutination 458,
459, 467
LD50 162
lecithinase 186, 356

Legionella 610–611(PP)
  transmission 552
Legionella pneumophila 224, 225, 610–611(PP)
  exotoxin 185
  pneumonia 223
Legionnaires' disease 223, 224, 225, 331
Leishmania 621(PP)
  evasion of host defenses 43, 396
  intracellular parasite 396
  pathogenicity 164
  promastigotes 536
  species/distribution/diseases 396
Leishmania braziliensis 397
Leishmania donovani 164, 466
leishmaniasis 396–397
  cutaneous 364–365, 396
    vaccine approaches 536
  cytokines 152, 153
  diagnosis/treatment 397
  drug targets 505, 508
  mucocutaneous 365
  New World 364–365, 396
  Old World 365, 396
  vaccine prospects 397, 536
  visceral 396
'leishmanization' 536
leonine facial appearance 358, 359
leprosy 357–359
  BCG (bacille Calmette-Guérin) vaccine 359, 531, 535
  cell-mediated immune response 358
  clinical features 358
  granulomas/histology 359
  immune response 358
  lepromatous (LL) 152, 358, 359
  prophylaxis 359
  T-cell immunity 152
  treatment 359, 494, 497
  tuberculoid (TT) 358, 359
  vaccine development 359
  see also Mycobacterium leprae
Leptospira 407–408, 612(PP)
Leptospira icterohaemorrhagiae 253
Leptospira interrogans 407–408, 612–613(PP)
  serogroups 408
  transmission 407–408
leptospirosis 407–408
leukemia
  adult T cell 194, 380
  aspergillosis in 433
  chronic myeloid, varicella in 550
  hairy T cell 194
  HTLV1 causing 194, 380
  infections associated 429
  reactivation of persistent infections 180
  varicella (chickenpox) in 371
leukoencephalopathy, progressive multifocal 436
levofloxacin 247
lice
  head 365–366
  Phthirus pubis (crab louse) 252
  see also body lice
ligand-binding assays 460
light microscopy 456–457
lincosamides 489, 490–491
linezolid 491
lipid A 11, 188
lipid peroxidation 146
lipodystrophy 271
lipopolysaccharide (LPS) 7, 11, 144, 188
  complement activation 189
  composition 188
  mast cell degranulation 189
  pathogen-associated molecular patterns (PAMPs) 75
  see also endotoxins
lipopolysaccharide binding protein 144
liposomes 523

lipoxygenase pathway 78, 79
Listeria 592–593(PP)
Listeria monocytogenes 302–303, 318, 592–593(PP)
  exotoxin 185
  isolation 318
  meningitis 302, 326, 329
  transmission 302, 318
listeriosis 302–303
  congenital/neonatal 302–303, 318
  prevalence 318
liver
  abscesses 310
  cancer 195, 196, 307
  damage
    hepatitis 303
    yellow fever 384
  failure, leptospirosis 407–408
  host defense/microbial evasion 131
  parasitic infections 308–310
  viral infections *see* hepatitis
liver flukes 49
  infections 309
  see also flukes (trematodes); helminths
lockjaw *see* tetanus
louping ill virus 332, 333
lower respiratory tract infections 217–232
  acute 217–232
  chronic 232–237
  hospital-acquired 546
  parasitic 237
Lubeck disaster 163, 515
lumbar puncture, brain abscess 339
lung
  abscess 220, 236–237, 237
  biopsy 231
    CMV 204
  caseous necrosis 232, 233
  consolidation in pneumonia 220, 224
  hydatid cysts 237
  infection route 220
  microorganism number in 125
  see also under pulmonary; respiratory tract
lung fluke 49, 237
  see also flukes (trematodes); helminths
lupus vulgaris 359
Lyell's disease (staphylococcal scalded skin syndrome) 320, 351, 353
Lyme disease 331, 390–391
  arthritis in 390–391
  clinical features 391
  diagnosis/treatment 391
  transmission 389–391, 390
  see also Borrelia burgdorferi
lymph, spread of microorganisms 159–160
lymphadenitis, inguinal 406
lymphadenopathy
  cervical, in African trypanosomiasis 395
  inguinal 261
  retroperitoneal 417
  in tularemia 407
lymphangitis 398
lymphatic filariasis 399
lymphatic system 159–160
lymph nodes 101, 159–160
  anatomy 100
  filarial nematodes in 398, 627(PP)
lymphocytes
  in CNS infections 324–325
  counting 468, 470
  surface markers, detection 468, 470
  see also B cell(s) (B lymphocytes); T cell(s) (T lymphocytes)
lymphocytic choriomeningitis (LCM) 332, 401, 402

lymphocytic choriomeningitis (LCM) virus 401
lymphocytosis 380
lymphogranuloma venereum 259, 261
lymphoid tissue 99, 101
lymphokines
lymphoma
  Burkitt's *see* Burkitt's lymphoma
  in HIV infection 195
  HTLV1 and HTLV2 viruses 194
lysozyme 11, 77, 80, 143
lytic infections 33

M

Machupo virus 402, 403
macrolide-lincosamide-streptogramin resistance 489
macrolides 489–490
  resistance 489
  structure 489, 490
  see also erythromycin
macroparasites 7–8, 441
  basic reproductive rate (R_0) 443
  see also arthropod(s); helminths
macrophage 72–73
  activation 91, 154
  acute inflammation initiation 79, 81
  alveolar *see* alveolar macrophage
  cytotoxicity of virus-infected cells 80
  granules/contents 146, 147
  inflammatory response initiation 144
  intracellular organisms 160
    Leishmania 396
    salmonellae 301
    T cell-induced killing of 91, 154
  origin/distribution 72–73, 72–74
  phagocytosis *see* phagocytosis
  polymorphonuclear leukocyte (PMN) *vs.* 147
  spleen and lymph node sinuses 72, 74
  Toll-like receptors 144
  types 72, 74
macules 351
maculopapular rashes
  measles 374, 375
  viral 366–367
maggots 365
major basic protein (MBP) 83–84
major histocompatibility complex (MHC) 91
  class I molecules 92
  class II molecules 92, 104
  disease susceptibility and 162
  T cell restriction 91, 104, 521
    vaccine non-responders 520, 521
malaria 2, 43, 66, 391–394
  anemia 190
  cerebral 331, 394
  clinical features 393
  cofactor in Burkitt's lymphoma 195, 208, 394
  complications 393–394
  diagnosis 394
  effect on pneumococcal/meningococcal vaccines 534
  immune complex deposition 190
  immunity 394
  immunosuppressive effects 394
  malignant tertian (*P. falciparum*) 190, 394
  prevention/treatment 394
    antiprotozoal drugs 505, 508
    DNA vaccines 520
    drug resistance 507
    vaccine development and trials 535–536
  quartan, nephropathy 190

resistance in sickle cell disease 393
sickle cell anemia 162, 393
TNF role and pathology due to 393, 394
transmission 138, 391–392
tumor necrosis factor (TNF) 148, 393, 394
UK case number 416
see also Plasmodium
Malassezia furfur 360
malignant pustule 404
malignant transfromation *see* transformation, malignant
malnutrition
  reduced immunopathology in 194
  shigellosis (bacillary dysentery) 287
  Strongyloides infections in 411–412
  susceptibility to infections 165
  T and B cell levels 424, 427
Malta fever *see* brucellosis
mannose binding protein 80, 82, 88
Mantoux reaction 152, 154, 234, 531
marasmus 424
Marburg hemorrhagic fever 402–403
Marburg virus 402
margination 79
mast cell 80
  degranulation 77–79, 80, 90, 189
  mediators released 79, 89, 90
  at submucosal surfaces 94, 95
mathematical modeling 445
Mazzotti reaction 398
M cells 127, 129, 282–283
measles 374–375
  agammaglobulinemia 375
  age at infection 444, 527
  annual notification 443
  cell-mediated immune response 374
  children 374, 375
  clinical features 231, 374
  clinical impact 374
  complications 375
    age-dependent risks 527
    encephalitis after 337, 527
    immunosuppression due to 174
    secondary bacterial pneumonia 231
  diagnosis/treatment/prevention 375
  etiology/transmission 374–375
  global eradication 525, 529–530
  inter-epidemic period 447
  lung biopsy 231
  pathogenesis/time course 158, 159, 443
  persistence as survival strategy 174, 176, 194
  resistance to reinfection 374
  vaccination/vaccines 231
    effect on incidence 374, 514
    killed hypersensitivity 321
    practice/schedule 529–530
measles, mumps and rubella (MMR) vaccine 211, 231, 316
  current practice/schedule 529–530
  effect on measles incidence 374
  in immunocompromised patients 521
  mass vaccination, serious disease risk 526
  optimum age to vaccinate 521
measles virus
  attachment 125
  F (fusion) protein 521
  transmission 374
Mediterranean spotted fever 387

membrane attack complex (MAC) 79–80, 81, 82, 88
meningitis 323
  aseptic, leptospirosis causing 408
  bacterial 325–329
    chronic 340
    diagnosis/identification 327
    emergency treatment 325, 326, 327
    Escherichia coli 326, 327, 329
    Haemophilus influenzae 326, 327–328
    histology 325
    Listeria monocytogenes 302, 326, 329
    meningococcal 325–327
    Mycobacterium tuberculosis 329, 331
    neonatal 329
    prevention 326
    sequelae 327, 328, 329
    Streptococcus pneumoniae 326, 327, 328–329
    transmission 326
  children 325, 326, 327–328
  chronic 340
    infections causing 340
  CSF changes 324, 325
  detection of causative agents 458
  elderly 328
  fungal 326, 329, 340
  lymphocytic 401
  mumps associated 333
  neonatal 319
  parasitic 338–339
  protozoal 330
  rashes 326, 327
  treatment 326
  vaccine 327
  viral 330–331, 332, 336–337
meningitis C conjugate vaccine 327
meningococcal infections, transmission 134
meningococcal meningitis 325–327
meningococcal septicemia 327
mercuric chloride, disinfectants 565
messenger RNA (mRNA)
  antisense oligonucleotides 504
    bacteria 14–17
    monocistronic 14, 32
    synthesis, inhibition, rifamycins 493
    viral 31–32
      translation 32
  synthesis
    DNA viruses 31
    retroviruses 31–32
    RNA viruses 31–32
Metchnikoff, Elie 72, 73
methenamine 496
methicillin-resistant staphylococci 479, 546, 556
methicillin-resistant *Staphylococcus aureus* (MRSA) 479, 556
methicillin-resistant *Staphylococcus epidermidis* 479
metronidazole 296, 496
  adverse effects 496
  Entamoeba histolytica infection 296
  giardiasis 296
  lung abscess 237
  mode of action 496
  peritonitis 310
  resistance 496
  Trichomonas vaginalis infections 263
microbes
  cell structure 7
  classification systems 9–10
  direct damage to host tissues 184
  entry sites/routes 123–130
  exit from host and transmission 123, 130–132
  receptors for 123
  size comparisons 1

stability in environment 131–132
  terminology 1
microbial evasion of host defense *see* host defense evasion
microbiology 3
  approaches 1–4
  see also specific methods/techniques
microcephaly 317
microfilarial infections 346, 398
  respiratory tract 237
microglia 73
microimmunofluorescence tests 387
microorganisms *see* microbes
microparasites 7–8, 441
  basic reproductive rate (R₀) 441–443
  host populations 441
  incubation/latency/infectious periods 442
  see also bacteria; fungi; protozoa; viruses
microphage *see* neutrophils
microphthalmia 345
microscopy 456–458
  applications in microbiology 456
  bright field 456
  dark field (dark ground) 457
  electron 457–458
  fluorescence 457
  light 456–457
  phase contrast 457
  staining methods 456–457
  syphilis diagnosis 254
  urine specimens 246
  wet preparations 456
Microsporidia 623(PP)
microsporidians 297
Microsporum 360, 362
Microsporum canis 360, 466
Microsporum gypseum 360
midges 49
miliary tuberculosis 232
milk
  pasteurization 409, 410, 562, 563
  transmission of infections 136–137
  see also breast milk
minimum bactericidal concentration (MBC) 419, 498, 499
minimum inhibitory concentration (MIC) 419, 498, 499
minocycline 485
  see also tetracyclines
mites
  scabies 366
  scrub typhus transmission 389
  transmission of infections 49, 51, 138–140
  see also arthropod-borne infections
mitochondria, evolution of 64
molecular epidemiology 558–560
molecular mimicry 170, 190, 521
  examples 171
molecular typing methods 558–560
molluscs, transmission of infection 139–140
molluscum contagiosum 367–368
monkeypox 373
monobactams, structure 481
monoclonal antibodies
  anti-idiotype responses 540
  anti-idiotype vaccines 520
  'humanized' 501, 540
  passive immunotherapy 540
    serum sickness 193, 539–540
  production 461
  species/strain detection using 458, 460
  transgenic xenomouse strains 540
monocytes 72, 74
  dengue virus infection 384–385
  HIV infection 267, 270

morphology/granules 146, 147
mononuclear phagocyte system 72, 73, 74
mononucleosis, infectious 205, 206–207, 381
Montenegro test 397
Moraxella catarrhalis (Branhamella catarrhalis) 223, 606(PP)
mortality, infectious disease 2, 3
mosquitoes 49, 51
  control and drug resistance problems 391–392
  infection transmission 124
  lymphatic filariasis transmission 398
  malaria transmission 391–392
  yellow fever transmission 384
mouth *see* oral cavity
mRNA *see* messenger RNA (mRNA)
mucinase 127, 128
mucocutaneous infections, pathogenesis 349, 351
mucocutaneous lesions, virus-induced 366–373
mucosal-associated lymphoid tissue (MALT) 94, 101
mucosal surfaces, host defense mechanism 72, 94–95
mucus
  barrier against infections 72
  microbial evasion mechanism 127
mumps 210–211
  age at infection 210–211, 444
    complication risk 527
  arthritis associated 379
  clinical consequences 211
  diagnosis 211
  encephalitis associated 333, 375
  inter-epidemic period 447
  meningitis associated 333
  myocarditis and pericarditis 377
  pathogenesis 211
  time course/incubation period 443
  treatment/prevention 211
  vaccines/vaccination 211
    current practice/schedule 530
    effect on incidence 514
    Jeryl Lynn 528
    risk of serious disease 528
    Urabe Am 9 528
mumps virus 210–211
  replication 211
  transmission 210
mupirocin 351, 554
muramyl dipeptide (MDP) 523
Murray valley encephalitis 385
muscle
  bacterial infections 350–357
  parasitic infections 377–378
  spasms 335, 340
  viral infections 377
mutation(s) 163
  antibiotic resistance due to 475
  antigenic variation by 172
  DNA microarrays 26
  DNA repair 20–21
  point 21, 26
  single nucleotide polymorphisms (SNPs) 26–27
  site-directed 517
mutualism 61
myalgia 377
  epidemic (Bornholm disease) 377
myalgic encephalomyelitis 377
Mycobacterium 595–596(PP)
  adjuvanticity 523
  atypical 232, 359
  cell wall structure 11–12
  cross-reacting antigens 152
  other than tuberculosis (MOTT) 232, 435
  species 232
  Ziehl-Neelsen staining 234, 358, 359, 456

Mycobacterium avium complex (MAC) 435
Mycobacterium avium-intracellulare 434–435
Mycobacterium bovis, attenuation 163
Mycobacterium infections 232
  in AIDS 434–435
  skin 357–359
  treatment 234, 496–497
Mycobacterium leprae 357–359
  acid-fast rod identification 358
  animal models 358
  immunosuppression due to 174
  replication rate 159, 497
  transmission 357
  see also leprosy
Mycobacterium marinum infection 359
Mycobacterium tuberculosis 232
  brain abscess 339
  cross-reacting antigens 152
  drug-resistance 497
  evasion of host defenses 125, 128
  immune cells signaling interference 175
  kidney infection 244
  meningitis due to 326, 329, 331
  peritonitis due to 310
  replication rate 159, 497
  septic arthritis due to 379
  skin infection 359
  treatment 496–497
  urine samples for detecting 246
  see also tuberculosis
Mycobacterium ulcerans infection 359
Mycoplasma 485, 613–614(PP)
  T strains 252, 262
  urethritis due to 252, 262
Mycoplasma hominis
  non-gonococcal urethritis 262
  septic arthritis 379
Mycoplasma pneumoniae
  acute bronchitis 218
  attachment 125
  pneumonia 223
mycoses *see* fungal infections
myiasis 365
myocardial antibodies, streptococcal infections 190
myocarditis
  Chagas' disease 378, 395
  diphtheria 215
  Trichinella spiralis infection 378
  viral etiology 377
myonecrosis 350, 355–356
  clostridial (gas gangrene) 350, 355–356
myositis, viral 377
myxomatosis 66, 118
myxomavirus 66, 118

N

Naegleria 64, 330, 620(PP)
nafcillin 351
naftifine 505
Nagler reaction 356
nails, dermatophyte infections 360–362
nalidixic acid 492
  UTIs 247
nasal mucosa and septum, in leprosy 358, 359
nasopharyngeal carcinoma 194–195
  EBV infection associated 208
natural killer (NK) cells 83–84, 92, 94, 144–145
  cytotoxicity 144–145
  cytotoxic T cell and complement comparison 154
  killing mechanism 83–84

natural killer (cont'd)
  reduced activity in HIV infection 267
  target recognition 144–145
Necator americanus
  cutaneous larva migrans 365
  eggs 299
  gastrointestinal tract infection 297, 299
  infection via skin 124, 297
  transmission/life cycle 298
necrotizing fasciitis 355–356
necrotizing infections of skin 350
Negri bodies 336
Neisseria 605–606(PP)
  complement action against 143–144
Neisseria gonorrhoeae
  antibiotic resistance 258
  attachment mechanisms 129, 173, 256
  gene switching 173
  ophthalmia neonatorum due to 256, 257, 320, 344
  pathogenicity, molecular basis 164
  pharyngitis due to 208
  sensitivity to drying 258
  septic arthritis due to 379
  spread/features associated 256, 257
  transmission/reservoirs 256
  virulence factors 256
  see also gonorrhea
Neisseria meningitidis 57, 325–326
  meningitis 325–327
  serotypes 534
  transmission 134
  vaccines 534
  virulence factors 326, 327
nelfinavir 503
nematodes
  classification 48
  evolution of parasitism 64
  expulsion from gut 95, 96
  filarial 398, 627(PP)
  infections 49
    anthelminthic drugs 505–506, 507, 509
    gastrointestinal tract 297–300
    lower respiratory tract 237
    ocular 346
    infection via skin 124
    structure/life cycle 48
    zoonoses 50
neomycin 487
neonatal infections
  acquired from birth canal 319, 320
  bacterial meningitis 329, 330
  Chlamydia trachomatis 344
  conjunctival 344
  gastroenteritis 320
  HIV infection diagnosis 273
  HSV infection 319, 368
  meningitis 329
  pneumonia 221
  routes of infection 319
  septicemia/meningitis 319
  tetanus 320, 339
neonatal vaccination, effect on immune system 524
neonates
  acquisition of normal flora 57
  conferred immunity 541
neoplasia, secondary immunodeficiency in 424
nerves
  botulinum toxin action 187
  peripheral, CNS infections from 324
  spread of infection via 160–161
netilmicin 485
neuralgia, postherpetic 371
neuraminidase, influenza virus 227
neuraminidase inhibitors 504, 561

neurologic disease, viral etiology 337
neutropenia 429
  FUO 415, 416, 418
  infections, treatment 432
  opportunistic pathogens 429
neutrophils 72, 73, 75
  activation 75
  in Arthus reaction 192
  chemotaxis 77
  dysfunction after burns 426
  in fungal infections 40
  granules 73, 75, 146
  killing process 75–77, 145–147
  lack/reduced numbers 429
    adult respiratory distress syndrome 189
  macrophage comparison 147
  nitroblue tetrazolium (NBT) test 468, 470
nevirapine 503
new variant CJD see Creutzfeldt–Jakob disease (CJD)
nifurtimox 378
Nipah virus encephalitis 333–335
nitric oxide 77, 147
nitroblue tetrazolium (NBT) test 468, 470
nitrofurantoin 496
  UTIs 247
nitroimidazoles 496
'nits' 275
Nocardia 597(PP)
Nocardia asteroides 434
nocardiosis, pulmonary 434
non-nucleoside reverse transcriptase inhibitors (NNRTIs) 270–271
noroviruses 292, 547, 575–576(PP)
northern blotting 558
Norwalk-like virus 292, 547, 575–576(PP)
Norwalk virus 292
Norwegian scabies 366
nose, normal flora 57
nosocomial infections see hospital-acquired infections
nucleic acid(s)
  hybridization 462
  see also DNA; RNA
nucleic acid probes 25, 460–462, 558
nucleocapsids 29
nucleoid 11
nucleoside analogues 503–504
nucleoside reverse transcriptase inhibitors (NRTIs) 270–271
nucleotide sequence analysis 559–560
nurse cells 378
nutrition
  bacteria 13
  immunostimulation overlap 542–543
nystatin 505

O

'O' (somatic) antigens 11, 557
obstetric infections see pregnancy
'obstruction leads to infection' 424, 428
occupational diseases
  fungal infections 191, 360
  Q fever 387, 403–404
  skin infections 360
  sporotrichosis 364, 365
  see also individual diseases/infections
ocular infections see eye infections
'ocular promiscuity' 344
olfactory nerves, spread of infection via 161
omentum 162
Onchocerca volvulus 365, 398
onchocerciasis (river blindness) 345, 346, 365

hypersensitivity to larval antigens 365
  ocular damage 346
  treatment 346
oncogenes 34–35, 194, 195
operator (in operons) 16
operons 14–15, 477
ophthalmia neonatorum 256, 257, 320, 344
Opisthorchis 309
opportunistic infections 2
  in AIDS see AIDS; HIV infection
  bone marrow transplant recipients 429
  hospital-acquired 546
  HTLV1 infection 380
  in neutropenia 429
  respiratory tract 201, 205
opportunistic pathogens 425
  bacteria 429, 434–435
  fungal 39, 40, 429, 431–434
  protozoa/helminths 299, 411, 429, 435
  viruses 429, 435–436
opsonic activity, assays 468, 470
opsonins 77, 82
opsonization 89, 97, 151
oral cavity
  candidiasis 213
  HSV infection 368
  infections 213–214
  normal flora 57, 213
oral rehydration 283, 287, 292
orf (contagious pustular dermatitis) 368
organs, blockage due to microorganism effects 184
Oriental sores (Baghdad boil) 396, 536
Orientia tsutsugamushi 388, 389
oropharynx
  infection route/defense evasion 130
  infections 202
    transmission 135
oroya fever 381
orthomyxoviruses 576–577(PP)
oseltamivir 504
Osler's nodes 418, 419
osteomyelitis 160, 379–380
  treatment 379–380
otitis 211–213
  causative organisms 211–213
otitis externa 213
otitis media 212–213
owl's eye inclusion body 231
oxygen, singlet 76
oxytetracycline 485

P

pacemakers, infections 428
palate, ulcers 207
palivizumab 501
pandemics 445
papilloma 351
  skin see warts
papillomaviruses see human papillomaviruses
papovaviruses 577(PP)
papules 351
Paragonimus westermani 49, 625–626(PP)
  lung infections 237
parainfluenza virus
  attachment 125, 205
  types/clinical effects 225
parainfluenza virus infections
  laryngitis 214
  pneumonia 225, 227
  upper respiratory tract 205
paralysis
  botulism 187, 340
  rabies 335–336
paramyxoviruses 578(PP)

see also individual viruses
parasites 1, 383
  adaptation to host 64–66, 117–118
  cultivation 463
  host response see host-parasite interactions
  survival strategies 167–172
  see also immune evasion mechanisms/strategies
parasitic infections
  CNS 338–339
  CNS disease 338–339
  FUO 416
  gastrointestinal tract 293–300
  host relations see host-parasite interactions
  immune evasion strategies 65
  intestinal
    host defense(s) 8–9
    transmission 294
  liver 308–310
  lower respiratory tract 237
  muscle 377–378
  skin 364–366, 396
  in transplant recipients 429, 430
  UTIs 242
  see also individual diseases/infections
parasitism 60, 61–62
  advantages 62
  disadvantages 63
  evolution 63–67, 64–67
  host control 63
  origin of mitochondria 64
  parasitic dependency spectrum 62–63
  see also host-parasite interactions
paratyphoid 300–302
parotid gland, in mumps 212
parotitis 210–211
parvovirus B19, rashes due to 372
parvoviruses 120, 372, 578–579(PP)
  anemia 372
  arthritis due to 379
  defective 372
  diarrhea due to 292
  effect on hemopoietic system 381
Pasteur, Louis 449
Pasteurella multocida 407, 609(PP)
pasteurization 410, 562, 563
pathogen-associated molecular patterns (PAMPs) 75, 82
pathogenicity
  genetic determinants 162–163
  molecular basis 164
  role of correct classification 9, 10
pathogenicity islands 24
pathologic consequences of infections 183–197
  activation of natural immune system 187–189
  direct effects of microbes 183–187
  malignant transformation 34, 35, 194–197
  overactivity of adaptive immune system 187–188, 189–193
  rashes 193–194
  see also individual diseases/infections
patients, isolation 552
Paul–Bunnell test 210
pediculosis 365–366
Pediculus spp 275, 365–366
pelvic inflammatory disease 257, 258
penicillin 483
  allergy 480
    alternatives to 481, 489
  anthrax 405
  gonorrhea 258
  hypersensitivity 450
  infective endocarditis 419
  leptospirosis 408
  Lyme disease 391
  meningitis 326

Pasteurella multocida infection 407
pneumonia 225, 226
rat bite fever 409
resistance 450
Streptococcus pyogenes skin
infections 354
structure 478, 481
syphilis 256
penicillin-binding proteins (PBPs)
475, 478, 482
methicillin-resistant staphylococci
479
Penicillium, microscopy 466
penis
chancre 254
genital herpes 264
human papillomavirus infection
367
pentamidine
leishmaniasis 397
Pneumocystis carinii pneumonia
434
trypanosomiasis 395
peptides, cloned, as vaccines
519–520
peptidoglycan 7, 11
synthesis 478, 480
penicillin-binding proteins
(PBPs) 482
perforin 83, 84, 153, 154
pericarditis, viral etiology 377
perinatal infections 318–321
transmission 135
periodontal disease 214
periosteal reactions 379
peripheral nerves, CNS infections
from 324
peritoneal cavity, spread of infection
via 162
peritonitis 277, 310
peritonsillar abscess (quinsy) 209
perivascular cuffing 395
permethrin 275
persistent infections 33–34, 167,
176–180
hepatitis B 33
survival advantage for microbe
176, 179
pertussis (whooping cough)
217–218
age at infection 444
chest radiographs 218
clinical features/complications
217
inter-epidemic period 447
management 217–218
time course/incubation period
443
toxin 217, 529
transmission 217
vaccination/vaccines 218
complications 218, 522, 529
development 218
effect on case number 529
two-component and new 529
see also Bordetella pertussis
pets
diseases from 66, 67, 140–141
see also cats; dogs
Peyer's patches 101, 129, 301
phage *see* bacteriophage
phagocytes
acute inflammatory response 77,
79
antimicrobial factors in 75–77
chemotaxis 89, 90
congenital defects 423
defects, treatment 543
discovery 72, 73
immune complexes activating 89,
91
intracellular killing of organisms
75–77
'professional' 72
recruitment/chemotaxis 77
see also macrophage; neutrophils

phagocytosis 89, 91
activity, nitroblue tetrazolium
(NBT) test 468, 470
discovery 73
killing process/mechanisms
75–77, 145–147
non-oxidative 76, 146–147
oxidative 76, 145–146
microbial strategies against 13,
114, 167
opsonization 89, 97, 151
rate after 97, 151
phagolysosome 75
phagosome 75
pharyngitis 202–210
causative organisms 207
laboratory diagnosis 210
pharynx, normal flora 58
phase contrast microscopy 457
phenolic disinfectants 565
phosphonoformate (foscarnet) *see*
foscarnet
(phosphonoformate)
Phthirus pubis (crab louse) 252, 275
phytohemagglutinin 469
picornaviruses 579–580(PP)
see also individual viruses
pig-bel (acute necrotizing disease)
289
pili (fimbriae) 12–13, 22–23
pinworm *see Enterobius vermicularis*
(pinworm: threadworm)
piperazine 299
pityriasis versicolor 360
Pityrosporum (*Malassezia*) *furfur* 360
plague 405–407
Black Death 406
bubonic 405, 406
pneumonic 405, 406
plantar warts 367
plant products, immunostimulation
by 543
plants, edible, vaccination delivery
537
plasma cells 99
plasmids 11, 17–19, 163
antibiotic resistance 18, 475–476
dissemination 558, 559
as cloning vectors 18–19
conjugative/non-conjugative
22–23
copy number 17–18
exotoxins encoded 18, 184
replication 17–18
R plasmids 18
virulence genes 18
Plasmodium 391–392, 621(PP)
effect on hemopoietic system
381, 393
immune evasion 43
invasion of red blood cells 381,
393
life cycle 392, 393, 394, 535
see also malaria
Plasmodium falciparum 66, 391–392
cerebral malaria 338
drug resistance 507, 508
life cycle 392, 393
malaria *see* malaria
replication rate 159
Plasmodium malariae 391, 393, 394
malarial nephropathy due to 190
Plasmodium ovale 391, 393, 394
Plasmodium vivax 391, 393, 394
plastic prostheses/devices, infections
428
platyhelminths *see* flukes
pleural cavity, spread of infection via
162
pleural effusion 237
pleurodynia (Bornholm disease;
epidemic myalgia) 377
pneumococcal vaccine 225,
533–534, 534
pneumococcus *see Streptococcus
pneumoniae*

Pneumocystis carinii 40, 58, 231,
235, 433–434, 495, 618(PP)
cysts 434
pneumonia 434
transmission 235
pneumonia 220–225, 238
in adults 221, 222, 223, 224, 225
causative organisms 221–222,
222, 223, 225
bacterial 223–225
CMV 204
measles 231
plague 405, 406
Pneumocystis carinii 434
rat bite fever 408
RSV 219–220
cause of death 220, 224
in children 221
complications 224
diagnosis 224
chest radiograph 221, 223, 224
lung biopsy 231
serologic 225
sputum samples 224
infection route 220, 225
interstitial 220, 221, 226
varicella complication 370
signs/symptoms 223
treatment/prevention 225, 226
types 220, 221
community-acquired 222
'giant cell' 231
hospital-acquired 221, 222,
223
lobar 150, 151, 220, 221
necrotizing (lung abscess) 220,
221, 236, 237
primary atypical 223, 225
secondary bacterial 230, 231
viral 225–231, 227
bacterial *vs.* 221
pneumonic plague 405, 406
pneumonitis, *Ascaris* causing 298
poliomyelitis 332
age at infection 444
global eradication program 531
inter-epidemic period 447
pathogenesis/pathology 324–325
time course/incubation period
443
vaccination/vaccines 2, 521
advantages of types 530–531
current schedules/practices
530–531
effect on incidence 514
killed/inactivated (IPV; Salk)
530–531
live attenuated oral (OPV;
Sabin) 516–517, 530–531
poliovirus
capsid protein 334
CNS infection route 323, 324
encephalitis associated 332, 333
meningitis associated 332
structure 334
pollution, susceptibility to
infections 165
polyclonal activators 104, 105
polyene antifungals 505
polymerase chain reaction (PCR)
463
applications 25, 27, 455, 462
disease etiology 120
epidemiology 559
nested PCR 463
primers 462, 463
single nucleotide polymorphisms
27
polymorphonuclear granulocytes
(polymorphs) *see* neutrophils
polymorphs *see* neutrophils
polymyxins 496
mode of action 496
route of administration 496
polyneuritis 215, 230
polyomaviruses 196

infection in
immunocompromised hosts
436
UTIs 242
see also individual viruses
polysaccharide capsules 167
population density, vaccination
success 527
population mixing patterns 446
porins 11, 479
pork tapeworm *see Taenia solium*
portal fibrosis 398
portal hypertension 398
postabortal fever 262
postherpetic neuralgia 371
postinfectious encephalitis 337
post-kala-azar dermal leishmaniasis
(PKDL) 396
postnatal infections *see* neonatal
infections
postpartum fever 262
post-transplant lymphoproliferative
disorder (PTLD),
EBV-associated 436
postvaccinial encephalitis 337
postviral fatigue syndrome 377
Powassan virus 385
poxviruses 580(PP)
molluscum contagiosum
367–368
orf (contagious pustular
dermatitis) 368
smallpox 373
see also individual viruses
praziquantel
hydatid disease 410
schistosomiasis 398
precipitation tests 467
pregnancy 313
bacteriuria/UTI 243, 247
bladder outflow obstruction 243
failure to reject fetus 313
infections 314
bacterial 317–318, 318
CMV 202, 317
congenital *see* congenital
infections
listeriosis 302, 318
peripartum 318–321
reactivation 180, 314, 317
susceptibility 165, 313
varicella-zoster virus 318, 371
rubella risk 526
rubella vaccination 526
prevalence 445
prions/prion infections 7, 53–55,
337–338, 584(PP)
amyloid plaques 53, 54
cell damage 54
characteristics 53
crossing species barriers 54
development 54
diagnosis 54
genetic influences 53
inactivation 563
medical problems 54–55
molecular strain types 53
pathogenesis 53
PrP^C and PrP^{Sc} proteins 53, 54,
55
interactions 53
'rogue protein' pathogenesis 53
structure 53
susceptibility determinants 53
transmission 54
treatment 54
see also individual diseases
pristinamycin 489
privileged sites 169–170
proctitis, chlamydia causing 261
prokaryotes 7
prophages 19, 22
Propionibacterium acnes 57, 356–357
prostatic hypertrophy 243
prostatitis, acute/chronic 244
prostheses, infections 428, 494

protease, IgA cleavage 176
protease inhibitors 270–271,
    503–504
protein(s)
    absorption 129
    prion 'rogue proteins' 53
    synthesis *see* protein synthesis
    viral 32
    see also individual proteins
protein A 176
protein-energy malnutrition (PEM)
    424, 426
    measles 375
protein synthesis
    antibacterial agents inhibiting
        485–492
    bacterial toxins inhibiting 187
    viruses 32
Proteus 599(PP)
    urease production 244
Proteus mirabilis, UTIs 241
Proteus vulgaris 387
proto-oncogenes 34
protozoa 43–45
    attachment in intestinal tract
        126, 127
    exotoxins produced 185
    identification 466
    immune evasion 43
    intracellular/extracellular species
        43
    location/diseases due to 43–44
    reproduction 43
    size comparisons 1
    transmission 43–44, 391–392
    see also individual species
protozoal infections
    arthropod-borne 391–397
    drug treatment 505–507
    gastrointestinal tract 44, 293–300
    meningitis 330
    opportunistic 429, 435
    persistent 177
    skin rashes due to 194
    zoonoses 140
    see also individual diseases/infections
pseudomembranous colitis 59, 485,
    491
Pseudomonas, elastase 176
Pseudomonas aeruginosa 235,
    426–427, 602(PP)
    antibiotic resistance 427
    bacteriocin typing 557–558
    exotoxin 185
    virulence factors 427
Pseudomonas aeruginosa infections
    236
    burn wounds 426–427
    in cystic fibrosis 235, 236
    eye 345
    host defenses, lysozyme 143
    liver abscesses 310
    prevention 427
    septic arthritis 379
    urinary tract 241
Pseudomonas cepacia 236
pseudomonic acid (mupirocin)
    554
public education, food-associated
    diarrhea prevention 284
public health, infection control 528
puerperal fever/sepsis 319, 545
pulmonary aspiration 237
pulmonary tuberculosis 234
pulsed field gel electrophoresis
    (PFGE) 559, 560
purified protein derivative (PPD)
    232
pyelonephritis 243, 244–245
    acute 245
    treatment 247–248
pyocines 558
pyocines 558
pyrazinamide 497
pyrexia *see* fever
pyrogens 413, 564
pyuria 244, 246

Q

Q fever 387, 403–404
quarantine 406
quaternary ammonium compounds,
    disinfectants 565
QUIL A 523
quinghaosu 394
quinine 394, 507
quinolones 492–493
    contraindications 493
    mode of action 492
    resistance 492
    structure 492, 493
    see also individual drugs
quinsy 209
quinupristin 491

R

rabies 335–336
    antigen detection/diagnosis 336
    clinical features 335–336
    immunoglobulin 336, 539
    incubation period/pathogenesis
        335
    raccoon 335
    vaccination/vaccines 336, 532
rabies virus 334
    CNS infection 324, 325
    infection route 124
'rales' 223
randomly amplified polymorphic
    DNA (RAPD) 559, 561
rapid plasma reagin (RPR) test 254
rashes
    bacterial infections 194
    'butterfly-wing' 354
    causes/types/character 194
    chickenpox (varicella) 370, 371
    coxsackieviruses 372
    distribution 366–367
    echoviruses 372
    immunologic basis 193–194,
        194
    maculopapular 351, 372
        rickettsial infection 387, 388
    measles 374–375, 375
    meningococcal meningitis 326,
        327
    parvovirus B19 causing 372
    protozoal infections 194
    rickettsial infections 387, 388
    rubella 376
    scarlet fever 210
    smallpox 373
    zoster 371
    see also skin infections
rat bite fever 408–409
rats, plague transmission 405
reactivation of infections 176–177
    circumstances/organisms/sites
        180
    pregnancy 180, 314, 317
    stages 180
reactive arthritis 378–379
reactive nitrogen intermediates
    (RNIs) 147
reactive oxygen metabolites 76, 77,
    83, 84
    oxidative killing mechanism 77,
        83, 145–146
receptors, on host cells 31, 123
recombination 21, 22
rectum, human papillomavirus
    infection 367
red blood cells
    organisms replicating in 381
    Plasmodium in 160, 381, 393
'red-man' syndrome 484
reduviid ('kissing') bug 395
regulons 16
relapsing fever 389–390
    clinical course 390

    diagnosis/treatment 390
    endemic form 389
    transmission 387, 389
renal calculi 243
reoviruses 581(PP)
replication of organisms 157–166
    bacteria 13–14
    fungi 39
    genetic determinants 162–163
    rates 150, 159
    viruses 170
repressors 16, 17
resistance
    antibacterial agents *see*
        antibacterial agents,
        resistance
    antifungal agents 505
    antiparasitic agents 506–507
    antiviral agents 499, 503
respiratory burst 75–77, 145, 146
respiratory obstruction, diphtheria
    213, 215
respiratory syncytial virus (RSV)
    attachment 125, 205, 219
    infection route 219
    vaccine, hypersensitivity 522
respiratory syncytial virus (RSV)
    infection 201, 219–220, 501
    bronchiolitis 219
    common colds 205
    diagnosis/treatment 220
    immunopathologic basis 220
    infants 219–220, 504
    pneumonia 219–220
respiratory tract
    as continuum 201, 203
    infection via 125
    microbial attachment/infection
        125
    microbial evasion of defenses
        126, 131
    normal flora 57–58, 201
respiratory tract infections 201–216,
    217–232
    defense/cleaning mechanisms
        125, 131, 143, 201
    compromised 428
    hospital-acquired 547, 561
    lower tract *see* lower respiratory
        tract infections
    microorganisms 125–126, 201,
        203, 205
    'professional' *vs.* 'secondary'
        organisms 201, 204
    Pseudomonas aeruginosa in cystic
        fibrosis 235–236, 236
    responses 220, 223
    surface epithelium-restricted 201,
        203
    transmission 132, 134
    upper tract infections 201–216
restriction enzymes, molecular
    typing 558
restriction-fragment length
    polymorphism (RFLP)
    analysis 558–559, 560
retina
    detachment 346
    granulomas 338
retinitis, CMV 204
Retrovir 503
retroviruses 581–582(PP)
    endogenous 170
    genome integration 170
    meningitis and encephalitis
        336–337
    mRNA synthesis 31–32
    oncogenes 34–35
    transmission 137
    types/diseases associated 265
    see also individual viruses
reverse transcriptase 170, 266
    inhibitors 503
rhabdoviruses 582–583(PP)
    see also individual viruses
rheumatic fever 210, 354

rheumatic heart disease 210
rhinoviruses
    attachment 125, 205
    common cold due to 201
    infective doses 132
rhodamine stain 457
ribavirin (tribavirin) 401, 503–504
    hepatitis C 308
    RSV infection 220
    structure 501
ribosomes 11
    aminoglycoside resistance and
        485
    RNA sequencing 25
ribotyping 558
rice water stools 286, 287
ricin 185
Rickettsia 8, 386, 485, 614(PP)
    cell/tissue culture 463–464
    infection via skin 124, 386
    transmission/reservoirs 386
Rickettsia, infections 386–389
    characteristics/features 387
    clinical features 387
    infection route/process 124, 386,
        387
    persistent 177
    rashes/skin lesions 376
    serologic tests 387
    treatment 387
Rickettsia akari 388
Rickettsia conorii 388
rickettsialpox 387
Rickettsia prowazekii 386, 388
Rickettsia rickettsii 124, 388
Rickettsia typhi 388, 389
rifabutin 493
rifampin
    bacterial meningitis prophylaxis
        326
    leprosy 359
rifamycins 493–494
rifapentine 493
Rift Valley fever virus 386
    vaccine 532
rimantadine 504, 561
    influenza management 230
ringworm (tinea) 360–362
    antifungal agents for 506
risus sardonicus 321, 340
ritonavir 503
Ritter's disease (staphylococcal
    scalded skin syndrome) 320,
    351, 353
Ritter's disease (staphylococcal
    scalded skin syndrome: toxic
    epidermal necrolysis) 320,
    351, 353
river blindness *see* onchocerciasis
RNA, messenger *see* messenger RNA
    (mRNA)
RNA polymerase 15
RNA viruses 36, 37
    dsRNA 32
    mRNA synthesis 31–32
    negative single-stranded 31, 32,
        33
    positive single-stranded 31, 32,
        33
Rocky Mountain spotted fever 376,
    387, 388
rodents, plague transmission 405
'rogue protein' prions 53
roseola infantum (exanthem
    subitum) 372
rose spots 301
Ross river virus 379, 386
rotaviruses 290–292
    attachment in intestinal tract
        126, 127
    diarrhea due to 290–292
        mechanism 290–291
    electron microscopy 291–292
    vaccine development 534–535
    see also individual viruses
roundworms *see* nematodes

Rous sarcoma virus 34–35
rubella 372, 375–376
  age at infection 444
  age-dependent risks 527
  arthritis 379
  CNS infection 337
  congenital 315–316, 317, 526, 527
  fetal impact 375–376
  intrauterine infection 171
  myocarditis 376
  ocular infections 345
  pathogenesis 376
  serologic diagnosis 376
  time course/incubation period 376, 443
  vaccination/vaccines 316
    current practice/schedule 530
    effect on incidence 514
    optimum age to vaccinate 526
    risk of serious disease 526
    virus attenuation 163
    see also measles, mumps and rubella (MMR) vaccine

S

Sabouraud agar 362
saliva
  CMV transmission 202
  defense/cleansing mechanism 130, 213
  EBV transmission 204–205
  reduced and infections 130, 213
  transmission of infections 136
Salmonella 600–601(PP)
  culture of organisms 283, 302
  infection route 282–283, 301
  opportunistic STD 273
  passage through body 283
  recycling 282
  septic arthritis due to 379
  species/serotypes/antigens 282, 557
  transmission/reservoirs 282–283
  transport in macrophage 301
Salmonella diarrhea 282–283
  clinical features 284–285
  excretion, infection prevention 283
  infection route/spread 282–283
  laboratory diagnosis/culture 283
  treatment 283
Salmonella enteritidis 283
Salmonella paratyphi 282, 283, 300
  vaccine 302, 534
Salmonella typhi 282, 283, 300, 301
  carriers 301, 302, 548–549
  enzyme-deficient strains 534
  infection route/transport 301
  infective dose 129
  vaccine 302, 534
    polysaccharide (Vi antigen) 534
    Ty21a (live attenuated) 517, 534
  as vector for vaccines 519
  see also enteric fevers; typhoid fever
Salmonella typhimurium 159
sandfly, leishmaniasis transmission 396
sandfly fever 386
saquinavir 503
sarcoidosis 417
Sarcoptes scabiei 252, 275
SARS (severe acute respiratory syndrome) 230–231
SARS-associated coronavirus infection (SARS CoV) 230–231
scabies 365–366
  genital 275
scalded skin syndrome (Ritter's

disease) 320, 351, 353
scalp infections 360–362, 363
scarlet fever 210, 353
Schistosoma 626(PP)
  host antigen uptake 170
  immune evasion 170
  larvae, respiratory symptoms 237
  life cycle 48, 397, 398
  species 49
  transmission 124, 140
Schistosoma haematobium 49, 309, 397
  bladder cancer association 242, 397
  urine samples for detecting 246
Schistosoma japonicum 49, 397
  intestinal infections 300
Schistosoma mansoni 49, 193, 397
  intestinal infections 300
  life cycle 309
  liver damage 309
schistosomiasis 309, 397–398
  allergic reactions 397–398
  cell-mediated immunity 193
  clinical features 193, 397–398
  dermatitis 365, 397
  granulomas 398
  treatment 398
  urinary 397
school, mixing patterns and infection transmission 446
'Scotch tape' test 299
scrapie 7, 53, 54, 337
  spread between species 54
scrapie-type agents 337–338, 563
scrofuloderma 359
scrub typhus 388, 389
scrum pox 368
seasonal incidence of infections 134, 447
  bronchiolitis due to RSV 219
sebum, increased production 356–357
selective bowel decontamination 554
selenium sulphide 363
semen
  CMV transmission 202
  transmission of infections 135
sensory nerves
  HSV infections 368, 369
  VZV reactivation and zoster 368, 369, 371
sepsis
  intra-abdominal 310
  puerperal 319, 545
septic arthritis 257, 378–379
septicemia 188, 189
  burns patients 426
  neonatal 319
septic shock (endotoxin shock) 188–189, 540, 542
seroconversion 445, 467
serologic diagnosis/tests 466–468
  arenavirus infections 401
  brucellosis 410
  Chagas' disease 396
  EBV infection 206–207
  FUO 414–415
  gonorrhea 258
  HIV infection 272–273
  Lyme disease 391
  pneumonia 225
  rickettsial infections 387
  syphilis 254–255
  virus identification 458, 466–468
serologic surveys 443, 444
seroprevalence 445
serotyping 557
Serratia 599(PP)
  UTIs 241
serum sickness 191, 193, 539–540
severe combined immunodeficiency (SCID) 145, 424
sewage disposal 134, 285
sexual behavior 135, 251, 444

control of HIV infection 273
partner number, frequency distribution of numbers 446
transmission of infections 251, 444
transmission of STDs 444
urinary tract infection risk factor 242
sexually transmitted diseases (STDs) 129, 133, 134–135, 251–276
  basic (case) reproductive rate (R₀) 444
  behavioral/spatial factors 444
  common diseases, etiology/treatment 252
  control 444
  genital herpes 252, 263–264, 368
  HIV infection increased transmission risk 269
  host factors influencing 251, 253
  incidence/reasons for increase 135, 251
  inguinal lymphadenopathy 261
  less common diseases 252
  microbial evasion of host defenses 254
  opportunistic 273, 275
  sexual behavior and 135, 251, 444
  transmission 134–135, 251, 253
    possible mechanisms/types 135
  see also individual diseases/infections
shedding, of microorganisms 131, 159
  urine 242
  viruses 136, 169, 177
shellfish, transmission of infection 139, 285, 304
  hepatitis A 304
Shigella 601(PP)
  antibiotic resistance 287–288
  molecular basis of pathogenicity 164
  opportunistic STD 273
  vaccine development 535
Shigella boydii 287
Shigella dysenteriae 287
  exotoxin 185
  infections see shigellosis (bacillary dysentery)
  infective doses 132
Shigella flexneri 287
Shigella sonnei 287
  bacteriocin typing 557–558
shigellosis (bacillary dysentery) 287–288
  amebic dysentery comparison 295
  children 287
  diarrhea and features 284–285, 287
  management 287–288
Shine–Dalgarno sequence 15
shingles see zoster (shingles)
shock
  cytokine role in pathogenesis 189
  endotoxin (septic) 188–189, 540, 542
sickle cell anemia
  malaria resistance and 162, 393
  parvovirus infections 372
  pneumococcal immunization 225
sickle cell gene 162
sigma factor 14
'silent grief,' in African trypanosomiasis 395
simian vacuolating virus 40 (SV40) 197
Simulium 346
sinusitis 211–213
skin
  anatomy 350
  antimicrobial peptides 143
  barrier against infections 72, 131, 349

antimicrobial peptides 143
  microbial evasion 131, 349
cancer, papillomaviruses associated 195, 196
colonization and antiseptics action 562
grafts, infections 428
lesions, gonorrhea 257
microorganisms infecting via 124
normal flora 57, 123, 349, 554, 562
rashes see rashes
toxin-mediated damage 349
transmission of infections 135–136
skin infections 349
  in anthrax 404
  arthropod 365–366
  bacterial 194, 349, 350–357, 353
  fungal 353, 359–364
  grafts 428
  manifestation of systemic infections 350
  mycobacterial 357–359
  occupational hazards 360
  parasitic 364–366
  pathogenesis 349, 350, 351
  viral 366–373
  yeasts 360
  see also rashes
skin patches, vaccination delivery 537
slapped cheek syndrome 372
sleeping sickness see trypanosomiasis, African
'slim' disease 270
slow virus infections 333, 337
smallpox 373
  bioterrorism threat 373
  global eradication campaign 2, 373, 450, 451
small round-structured viruses 292, 547, 575–576(PP)
snails, schistosomiasis transmission 397
sneezing, transmission of infections 132, 133, 201
social changes, host-parasite relationship changes 66, 67
soft tissue infections, bacterial 350–357
Southern hybridization 558
species 9
specificity, concept 447–449
specimens
  for antibody detection 453, 467
  for antigen detection 458, 459
  collecting/processing 245, 453–455
  culture of organisms from 453, 462–463
  electron microscopy 457
  for microscopy 456–458
  processing 453–455
    protocols 455, 471
  transport 245
  urine 245–246
spectinomycin, gonorrhea 258
spiramycin 297
  congenital toxoplasmosis 318
  cryptosporidiosis 297
spirillar fever 409
Spirillum minor 408–409
spirochetes 251, 253
  antigenic variation 389
  dark field microscopy 457
  see also individual organisms
spleen 101
  anatomy 100
splenectomy, pneumococcal immunization after 225
splenomegaly
  brucellosis 409
  kala-azar 396
splinter hemorrhages 418, 419
spondylitis, ankylosing 379

spongiform encephalopathies 53, 337–338
sporadic Creutzfeldt–Jakob disease (sCJD) 54
spores, heat sterilization 563
Sporothrix schenckii 364, 616(PP)
  septic arthritis 379
sporotrichosis 364, 365
spotted fevers 388
spread of infections 157–166
  from blood 160
  via cerebrospinal fluid 162
  genetic determinants 162–163
  hospital-acquired infections 549
  mechanisms 160
  via nerves 160–161
  other routes/factors 162, 163–164
  systemic 157, 158
sputum
  pneumonia 224
  Ziehl-Neelsen staining 234
squamous cell carcinoma of skin 196
src oncogene 34–35
staining methods
  for electron microscopy 457
  Gram stain 11, 456
staphylococcal scalded skin
    syndrome (toxic epidermal
    necrolysis: Ritter's disease)
    320, 351, 353
staphylococci
  coagulase-negative 417, 428, 484
  glycopeptide resistance 484
  infections
    dialysis catheters 428
    infective endocarditis 417–418, 419–420
    neonatal 320
    via skin 124
  methicillin-resistant 479, 546, 556
  toxins, as superantigens 174–175
Staphylococcus aureus 585–586(PP)
  antibiotic resistance/sensitivity
    351, 475, 476, 479
  carriers 350, 351, 548–549
  colony appearance 464
  enterotoxins and food poisoning 292
  exotoxins 17, 185, 186
  methicillin-resistant 479, 556
  normal flora of skin
Staphylococcus aureus infections
  abscesses 320, 350–351, 424
  breast abscess 320
  burn wounds 427
  cellulitis 355
  conjunctival 344
  eyelid 343
  hospital-acquired 546
  infective endocarditis 419
  lung, in cystic fibrosis 235
  osteomyelitis 160, 379
  otitis externa 213
  scalded skin syndrome 351, 353
  septic arthritis 379
  skin 350–351, 427
    treatment 351
  surgical wound infections 427–428
  toxic shock syndrome 352, 353
Staphylococcus epidermidis 586(PP)
  antibiotic resistance 428
  infections 428
    septicemia 429
    urinary tract 241
  methicillin-resistant 479
  normal flora of skin 57
Staphylococcus pyogenes, carriers 548–549
Staphylococcus saprophyticus 586–587(PP)
  UTIs 241
stavudine (d4T, didehydrodideoxy-uridine) 503

stem cells 99, 105
sterilization 561–565
  chemical agents 564
  choice of method 562–565
  control 564–565
  definition 561
  filtration 564
  heat 563
  irradiation 564
  prion protein resistance 563
  techniques 562–565
Stevens–Johnson syndrome 495
'sticky eye' 319–320
St Louis encephalitis (SLE) virus 336, 385
stools *see* feces
streptobacillary fever 409
Streptobacillus moniliformis 408–409
streptococci
  α-hemolytic 58
  β-hemolytic 58, 427, 464, 587(PP)
    antimyocardial antibody 190
    neonatal infection 319
    puerpural sepsis 319
  group A 190, 319
    skin infections 352–354
  group B 319
    neonatal meningitis 329, 330
  infections
    burn wounds 427
    infective endocarditis 417–418, 419
    via skin 124
  oral 58, 417, 589(PP)
Streptococcus agalactiae 588(PP)
Streptococcus mitis 417
Streptococcus mutans 57, 214
Streptococcus oralis 417
Streptococcus pneumoniae 57, 328–329, 588–589(PP)
  attachment 125
  infection
    bronchitis 218, 219
    meningitis 326, 327, 328–329
    otitis and sinusitis 212–213
    pneumonia 223, 224, 225
  serotypes/antigenic diversity 533, 557
  sputum smears in pneumonia 224
  vaccine 225, 533–534
  virulence factors 326, 327, 328
Streptococcus pyogenes 57, 464, 587(PP)
  antibiotic resistance 210
  colony appearance 464
  erythrogenic toxin 185, 353
  exotoxins 185
  M and T proteins 164, 352, 557
  M types 210
Streptococcus pyogenes infections
  burn wounds 427
  cellulitis 355
  complications 209–210
  diagnosis 210, 354
  erysipelas 352, 354
  glomerulonephritis 354
  impetigo 352, 354, 355
  pathogenicity mechanism 164
  pharyngitis 208
  rheumatic fever/heart disease 210
  scarlet fever 210
  skin 354, 427
  tonsillitis 208, 210
  transmissibility 427
Streptococcus sanguis 417
streptogramins 489, 491
streptomycin 487
  brucellosis 410
  plague 406
  rat bite fever 409
  tularemia 407
stress, influence on susceptibility 163, 165
stress proteins 144

Strongyloides stercoralis 64, 411–412, 628(PP)
  eggs 411
  life cycle/transmission 298, 411
strongyloidiasis 411–412
  autoinfection and reactivation 47, 298, 299, 435
  clinical features 299, 411–412
  disseminated/hyperinfection 298, 411–412, 435
  gastrointestinal tract 298
  immunocompromised hosts 299, 435
  pulmonary eosinophilia 237
stye 343
subacute sclerosing panencephalitis (SSPE) 325, 337, 375
'suicide inhibitors' 479
sulfonamides 494–495
  mode of action 494, 495
  nocardiosis 434
  structure 494
  see also individual drugs
superantigens 174–175
superoxide anion 76, 145
superoxide dismutase 76
suramin 398
surgical wound infections 427–428
  Clostridium 355–356
  hospital-acquired 546, 550–551
  predisposing factors 550
  surveillance 445
survival strategies of microbes *see*
    immune evasion
    mechanisms/strategies;
    persistent infections
susceptible people, density 444
SV40 197
sweating, in malaria 393
swimmer's itch 190, 365
swimming pool granuloma 359
symbiotic associations 60–62
Symmer's pipestem fibrosis 398
symptoms of infections, cause 183
syphilis 251–256
  chancre 254
  congenital 254, 314, 317–318, 345
  prevention 256
  'fever therapy' 144
  incidence 253
  laboratory diagnosis/tests 254–255
    serological tests 256
  pathogenesis 254, 255
  stages 254
  transmission 253
  treatment 256
  see also Treponema pallidum

T

Taenia 625(PP)
Taenia saginata (beef tapeworm) 300
Taenia solium (pork tapeworm) 410
  calcified cysts 378
  cysticercosis 339, 378, 410
  larval stages 378
  muscle infection 378
  transmission and eggs 378
tapeworms 48, 378
  anthelminthic drugs 506, 509
  attachment in intestinal tract 126, 127
  beef (*Taenia saginata*) 300
  fish (*Diphyllobothrium latum*) 300
  infections 300
    sites/hosts 378
  larvae 378
  ocular damage 346
  lifecycle 48
  transmission 48, 49, 378
  see also individual species
T cell(s) (T lymphocytes) 89–95, 99

activation 91, 155
anergy 106, 152
antigen recognition 91, 102, 104
autoreactive 106–107
CD8-positive 153, 267–268
clonal expansion 102–103
cross-priming 154
cytokines released 91, 104–106, 107, 108
cytotoxic (CTL) *see* cytotoxic T cells (CTL)
defects/deficiency 424
  contraindication to live vaccine 522
  Strongyloides infections 411
  treatment 543
deletion 106, 152
EBV infection 205
epitopes, peptide vaccines 519
helper *see* helper T-cells (TH cells)
HIV infection 173–174
HTLV1 infection 379
interferon release 91, 92, 94, 105, 152
killing of intracellular parasites 91, 154
in malnutrition 424, 427
memory cells 102–104
MHC restriction 91
polyclonal activators 175, 469–470
  superantigens 174–175
proliferation assays 468–471
receptor (TCR) 91, 93, 102, 104, 152
  genetic rearrangements 102
recognition of intracellular organisms 91, 93
responsiveness, assays 468–471
self-tolerance induced by vaccines 449
skin lesions mediated by 194
suppressor (Ts) cells 109
surface markers 100, 102
virus replication inhibition 91–93
see also lymphocytes
teeth, decay 214
teicoplanin 480
  see also glycopeptides
temperature
  increased *see* fever
  regulation 413
  sensitivity of organisms 157
temperature-sensitive mutants, vaccine development 517, 533
tenofovir 503
teratogenic viruses 314, 316
tetanospasmin 185
tetanus 339–340
  antitetanus immunoglobulin 340
  neonatal 320, 339
  toxoid 104, 150, 340, 518
    current practice/schedule 529
  vaccine 518
  see also Clostridium tetani
tetracyclines 487
  acne 357
  chlamydial infection 260–261
  cholera 287
  contraindications 487
  donovanosis 262
  leptospirosis 408
  Lyme disease 391
  lymphogranuloma venereum 261
  mode of action 485, 486
  plague prophylaxis 407
  Q fever 404
  relapsing fever 390
  resistance 485, 487
  rickettsial infections 387
  structure 488
therapeutic index 450
thermoregulation 413
thiabendazole 412

thiacytidine (3TC; lamivudine) 503
thorns, fungal infections after
    363–364
threadworm see Enterobius
    vermicularis (pinworm:
    threadworm)
throat
    gonococcal infection 257
    sore 202–210
thrombocytopenia
    microorganisms causing 381
    varicella complication 371
thrush 58–59
    oral 214
    vaginal 252, 262–263
    see also candidiasis/Candida
        infections
tick-borne encephalitis virus 385
ticks 138–140
    Lyme disease transmission 390
    relapsing fever transmission 389
    rickettsial infections transmission
        387
    skin lesions caused by 365–366
tinea capitis 360–361, 362
tinea corporis 360–361, 362
tinea cruris 362
tinea imbricata 362
tinea manuum 362
tinea pedis 361, 362
tinidazole 296
tissue culture 463–464
tissue damage 155, 184, 189
T lymphocytes see T cell(s) (T
    lymphocytes)
tobramycin 426, 485, 487
togaviruses 379, 583–584(PP)
    meningitis and encephalitis 336
    see also individual viruses
tolerance see immune tolerance
Toll-like receptors 144
tolnaftate 505
tongue, in scarlet fever 210
tonsillitis 202–210
topoisomerase 13
toxic epidermal necrolysis
    (staphylococcal scalded skin
    syndrome: Ritter's disease)
    320, 351, 352
toxic shock syndrome 188
    Staphylococcus aureus 352, 353
toxic shock syndrome toxin (TSST1)
    188
toxins
    antibody blocking 89, 91
    detection 458, 459
    food poisoning 277, 292–293
    as immunosuppressants 174
    pathologic consequences
        184–186
    see also endotoxins; enterotoxins;
        exotoxins
Toxocara canis 48, 338, 410,
    628–629(PP)
    larval infection of eye 345, 346
Toxocara cati 338
toxocariasis 140, 410
    ocular 345, 346
toxoids 104, 184–185, 518
    see also diphtheria toxoid; tetanus
Toxoplasma gondii 318, 338,
    621–622(PP)
    blindness 345–346
    evasion of host defenses 43
toxoplasmosis 66, 140, 345–346
    AIDS 338
    antiprotozoal drugs 505, 508
    central nervous system (CNS)
        infection 338
    chorioretinitis 345–346
    congenital 318, 345, 346
    encephalitis 333
trachea, normal flora 58
tracheal cytotoxin 217
tracheitis 214
trachoma 343–344, 345

transcription
    activators 16
    bacteria 14–15
    initiation/termination 14
    repressors 16, 17
    as target for antimicrobial agents
        15
    see also messenger RNA (mRNA)
transfer factor (TF) 543
transformation, bacteria 21, 22
transformation, malignant 195,
    196–197
    changes induced 195
    by viruses 34, 35, 120, 194–197
translation 15
    viral proteins 32
transmission of infections 123,
    130–132, 383, 445
    airborne 132, 133, 134, 201, 220,
        552
    animals 137–141
    arthropods see arthropod-borne
        infections
    behavioral/spatial factors 444
    blood 137, 225, 241
    control vs. eradication 450–451
    droplet 132, 133, 134, 229–230
    dynamics and serologic surveys
        443–444
    factors influencing 130–132
    fecal-oral 132, 133, 134,
        303–304
    gastrointestinal tract 134
    between groups 444, 446
    hematogenous 137, 225, 241
    horizontal 137, 138
    hospitals see hospital-acquired
        infections
    milk 136–137
    oro-anal 263, 273
    oropharynx 135
    prevention by vector control 383,
        384
    respiratory tract 132, 134, 201,
        220, 225
    skin 135–136
    success
        age at infection 447
        reduced by mass vaccination
            447, 526
    transplacental 137
    two-stage vaccination program
        525
    types 132–137
    urinogenital 135, 241
    vector importance 383
    vertical 137, 138, 383
    zoonoses 133, 140–141
    see also individual diseases/infections
transmission potential (R₀)
    441–444
transplant
    donors
        pre-transplantation serology
            435
        screening 435
            CMV IgG 435
    recipients, infections 429–431,
        435–436
        CMV infection 435
        HSV infection 435–436
        screening 435
        serology baseline 435
        time-course 430
transposition 23–24
transposons 24, 476
traumatic injuries 423, 427–428
    Clostridium infections 355–356
    subcutaneous fungal infections
        363–364
travelers 2
    malaria 392, 394
    Salmonella typhi vaccination 302
traveler's diarrhea 297
trematodes see flukes
trench fever 388

Treponema 612(PP)
    species/diseases associated 253
Treponema pallidum 252
    characteristics 254
    infection route 124
    replication rate 150, 159
    transmission 253
    see also syphilis
Treponema pallidum
    hemagglutination assay
        (TPHA) 255
Treponema pallidum inhibition (TPI)
    test 468
Treponema pertenue 124
tribavirin see ribavirin (tribavirin)
Trichinella spiralis 1, 8, 378, 410,
    629(PP)
    transmission/life cycle 378, 411
trichinosis (trichinellosis) 1, 299,
    411
    muscle infections 378, 411
Trichomonas vaginalis 59, 622(PP)
    transmission 263
trichomoniasis
    treatment 496
    urethritis 242, 252
    vaginitis 252, 263
Trichophyton 360, 361–362
    infection via skin 124
Trichophyton rubrum 361
Trichophyton tonsurans 361
Trichophyton verrucosum 360
trichothiodystrophy 21
trichuriasis 298–299
Trichuris trichiura (whipworm)
    629(PP)
    eggs 298, 299
    transmission/life cycle 298
trigeminal ganglion 368
trigeminal nerve, ophthalmic zoster
    371
trimethoprim 494, 495–496
    mode of action 495
    resistance 496
    route of administration 495
    structure 495
    UTIs 247
triple vaccine see diphtheria,
    pertussis and tetanus (DPT)
    vaccine
trismus see tetanus
Trizivir 503
Tropheryma whippelii 120
tropical infections 2
tropical pulmonary eosinophilia
    (TPE; Weingarten's
    syndrome) 237
tropical spastic paraparesis 337,
    380
Trypanosoma 622(PP)
Trypanosoma brucei gambiense 173,
    395
Trypanosoma brucei rhodesiense 173,
    395
Trypanosoma cruzi 377–378, 395
trypanosomes, African
    antigenic variation 43, 172, 395
    evolution of parasitism 64
    gene switching 173
trypanosomiasis, African 395
    antiprotozoal drugs 505, 508
trypanosomiasis, American see
    Chagas' disease
tsetse fly, trypanosomiasis
    transmission 395
tubercles 233
tuberculin reaction/test 234, 470,
    531
tuberculoma 417
tuberculosis 2, 232–235, 238, 331
    AIDS in 234–235
    cell-mediated immune response
        232–233
    chest radiographs 233
    complications/spread 233–234
    diagnosis 152, 234

drug resistance 497
    epidemiology 559
    joints/bones 380
    meningitis 326, 329, 331, 497
    miliary 232, 233, 329, 331, 497
    pathogenesis 232
    pathology 232, 233
    primary 234
    pulmonary 234
    secondary 234
    spinal 329, 380
    susceptibility
        genetic determinants 162
        racial 171
    transmission 232
    treatment/prevention 234
    in twins 163
    vaccine see BCG (bacille
        Calmette–Guérin) vaccine
    see also Mycobacterium tuberculosis
tuberculous meningitis 326, 329,
    331
tularemia 407
tumor see cancer
tumor necrosis factor (TNF) 80
    action in septicemia/meningitis
        188
    fever mechanism 188
    increase in HIV infection 148
    in malaria 148, 393, 394
    therapy and side-effects 542, 543
tumor viruses 120, 194–197
twins, tuberculosis 163
typhoid fever 300–302
    pathogenesis 159
    transmission 134
    vaccination see Salmonella typhi
    see also enteric fevers; Salmonella
        typhi
Typhoid Mary 301
typhus
    endemic 388, 389
    epidemic 388–389
    rash 376
    scrub 388, 389

U

ulcers 351
    Buruli 359
    chiclero 396
    cutaneous leishmaniasis 396
    dendritic 345, 368
    duodenal/gastric 293
    genital see genital ulcers
    hand, foot and mouth disease
        207
ultraviolet light/radiation 518, 563
umbilicus, Clostridium tetani
    contamination 320
undulant fever see brucellosis
upper respiratory tract infections
    201–216
    see also specific infections/anatomical
        regions
urea breath test 293
Ureaplasma urealyticum 262
urethra
    defense mechanisms 129–130
    female, UTIs 130, 242
    gonococcal infection 258
    gonorrheal discharge 256
    normal flora 58
urethritis, causative agents 242,
    252, 262
    Chlamydia trachomatis 252, 260
    gonococcal 257
    non-gonococcal 260, 262
    trichomoniasis 242, 252
urinary catheters
    guidelines for care 248
    infective organisms 428
    urine samples from 246
urinary tract
    antiseptics 496

urinary tract (*cont'd*)
host defense mechanism 131, 244
microbial evasion 129–130, 131
resistance to bacterial colonization 244
urinary tract infections (UTIs) 241–249
acquisition/etiology 241–242
infection route 129–130
acute lower tract 244
bacteria causing 241, 242
catheters causing 428
clinical features/complications 244–245
CMV infection 242
complicated 247–248
hospital-acquired 247, 546
laboratory diagnosis 245–246
males/females 130, 241, 242
obstruction 428
parasites causing 242
pathogenesis 242–244
predisposing factors 242, 243, 428
prevention 248, 496
recurrent 244, 247–248, 248
schistosomiasis 397
specimens (diagnostic) 245–246, 246
transmission 134–135
treatment 247–248, 496
quinolones 492–493
sulfonamides and trimethoprim 495–496
uncomplicated 247
upper tract 244–245
viral etiology 241–242
virulence of pathogens 243–244
urinary urgency and frequency 244
urine
'bag' 245
CMV transmission 202
culture media/methods 246
infection *vs.* contamination 245
inhibition of bacterial growth 244
microscopy 246
midstream (MSU) 245
residual, infections due to 243
specimens/collection 245–246, 246
suprapubic aspiration 245, 246
urinogenital tract *see* genital tract; urinary tract
uroepithelial cells, bacteria adhesion 243

V

vaccination 513–538
age
age at infection relationship 525
current vaccine practices 524, 528–537
optimum age to vaccinate 525
aims 513
bacterial meningitis 327
bioterrorism 536–537
chemotherapy comparison 447–450
community-based control 524–526
coverage 525, 526
epidemiological analysis 528
epidemiological effects 524–526
transmission reduction 526
viral disease incidence 514
factors influencing success 527–528
global deaths from preventable disease 537
historical aspects 515

mass 447, 525, 526
coverage for infection eradication 525, 526
impact 526
increased risk of serious disease 526
indirect effects 526
methods of delivery 537
newborns, effect on immune system 524
post-exposure, in rabies 532
principle 514
risk, relationship to infection risks 527–528
schedules 524
smallpox eradication 373
two-stage program 525
see also immunization, passive; *individual diseases/infections*
vaccines 2
adjuvants 522–523
awaited 536–537
complications 218, 337, 449–450, 514–515, 515, 521–522, 529
autoimmunity 521
contamination 163
encephalitis after 337
genetic susceptibility to disease 163
hypersensitivity 450, 521
non-responders 521
resistance to 450
toxicity 450
costs 515–516
duration of response 514
experimental 534–536
in general use 528–534
heterologous 516, 534–535
immunogenic 528
inactivated toxins (toxoids) 518
killed ('inactivated') 517–518, 518
advantages/disadvantages 520–521
immunocompromised patients 522
live attenuated 375, 515, 516–517
advantages/disadvantages 520–521
contamination 521
contraindications 522
measles, mumps and rubella (MMR) 211
'octopus' molecule 520
pathological consequences 521–522
primary/secondary immune responses 103–104
requirements 514–516
smallpox 373
specificity 449
stability 515
target 449
types 516–520
antigens presented on spherical structures 523
attenuated strains 163
cloned/synthetic peptides 519–520
DNA vaccines 518–519, 520, 532
inactivated toxins (toxoids) 184–185, 518
killed ('inactivated') *see above*
live attenuated *see above*
site-directed/deletion mutants 517
subcellular fractions 518
vectors for cloned genes 518–519
see also individual diseases/infections
vaccinia virus 516, 518
vagina
Bacteroides 263
Candida infection 252, 262–263

defense mechanisms 129
discharges 256, 258, 262
normal flora 58–59
pH 129
secretions 129
vaginitis 263
Gardnerella vaginalis 252, 263
Trichomonas vaginalis 252, 263
vaginosis, bacterial 263
vancomycin 480
infective endocarditis 419–420
resistance 481, 484, 556
variant Creutzfeldt–Jakob disease (vCJD) 53, 338
varicella (chickenpox) 369–372
age at infection 444
clinical features 370
complications 370–371, 550
diagnosis/treatment 371–372
in leukemia 371, 550
time course/incubation period 370, 443
varicella-zoster virus (VZV) 369–372
isolation difficulty 371
persistence as survival strategy 179
spread via nerves 160–161, 370
varicella-zoster virus (VZV) infection 369–372
CNS infection 324
encephalitis 332, 333
immunosuppression due to 174
latent 176, 370
pregnancy 318, 371
primary infection 370
reactivation 368, 369, 370, 371
treatment 372
vaccines 533
see also varicella (chickenpox); zoster (shingles)
variola *see* smallpox
vascular permeability 77–79
vasculitis, Kawasaki syndrome 377
vector-borne infections 3, 383–399
helminth 397–398
protozoal 391–397
viruses *see* arboviruses
see also arthropod-borne infections; *Borrelia*; *Rickettsia*, infections
vectors
for cloned genes 518–519
control 384
importance in infection transmission 383
lifespan, effect on disease transmission 383
see also arthropod(s)
Venereal Disease Research Lab (VDRL) test 254
venereal spread of infections *see* sexually transmitted diseases (STDs)
Venezuelan equine encephalitis (VEE) virus 385
ventilation systems, hospitals 552
verotoxins, *Escherichia coli* 281
vertebrates, transmission of infections 133, 140–141
multisystem infections 401–412
vertical transmission 35, 137, 138, 383
vesicles 351, 366
HSV infections 368
zoster 370
vesicoureteral reflux 243
Vibrio 603(PP)
Vibrio alginolyticus 355
Vibrio cholerae 285
attachment in intestinal tract 126, 127
enterotoxin 286
exotoxin 185, 186
infective dose 129
mucinase 127

serotypes and O antigens 285–286
non-O1 285–286
O1, El Tor and classical 285, 286
O139 285–286
vaccines 534
virulence gene expression 17
see also cholera
Vibrio parahaemolyticus 286
diarrhea due to 284, 288
Vibrio vulnificus, cellulitis 355
vidarabine 501
virion 29
virulence 162
detection 460
virulence, bacterial
genes 162–163
in bacteriophage 19
expression 15, 17
pathogenicity islands 24
on plasmids 18
prophage conversion 19
regulation 17
transposons 24
prophage conversion 19
urinary tract pathogens 243–244
viruses 1, 29–38
attachment process 30, 125, 126, 127
as drug target 504
host cell membrane receptors 30, 31
host immune defenses 150
cancer-inducing 34, 35, 120, 194–197, 208, 314, 316
cell/tissue culture 463–464
classification 9–10, 35–37
enveloped 29, 32–33
cytopathic effect (CPE) 464, 466
evolution/origin 64, 83
extracellular killing by NK cells 83–84
helper 35
host specificity 30
identification by serologic tests 458, 466, 467
immune evasion 168, 176
infection process 29–31
via skin 124
latency 168, 176
major groups 35–37
monotypic 228–229
mRNA *see* messenger RNA (mRNA)
nucleic acid 29
replication 32
organization/structure 29
oncogenes 34–35
pharyngitis 207
replication 31–33, 170
assembly 32–33
budding/release 32–33, 157, 158
genome integration into host 120, 170
inhibition 91–93
protein synthesis 32
rate 150, 159
shedding 136, 169, 177
size comparisons 1
spread to lymph/blood 159–160
transmission routes 29, 30, 319
tropism 123
as vectors for genes, vaccine development 518–519
zoonoses 140
see also DNA viruses; RNA viruses; *individual viruses*
virus infections
cytotoxic T cell action 91–93, 154
detection using serologic tests 466–468
FUO 416
hospital-acquired 546–547, 560–561
immunosuppression due to 174

incubation/latency/infectious periods 443
interferon synthesis/action 82–83, 148, 149
latent *see* latent infections
lytic 33–34
mucocutaneous lesions due to 366–373
muscle 377
natural killer (NK) cell action 83
opportunistic 429, 435–436
outcome 33–35
perinatal 318
persistent 33–34, 169, 177
reactivation 176–177
silent infections 168
skin rashes due to 194
in transplant recipients 429, 430
vaccination, effect on incidence 514
see also antiviral agents; *specific infections*
visceral larva migrans *see* toxocariasis
vitamin B, production by gut flora 60
vitamin C deficiency, gum infections 213
vitamin K, production by gut flora 60
v-*myc* 34
volutin (polyphosphate) storage granules 457
vomiting 284, 289
vulva, human papillomavirus infection 367

W

warts 351, 367
genital 252, 264, 265, 367
plantar 367
types 367
virus replication 170
see also human papillomaviruses
waterborne infection 134
cryptosporidiosis 297
Giardia lamblia 296
leptospirosis 407–408
pathogens 278
Salmonella 282
typhoid 300–301, 302
water contamination
cholera 285
hepatitis A 303
Waterhouse–Friedrichsen syndrome 327
Weil–Felix test 387
Weil's disease 408
Weingarten's syndrome (tropical pulmonary eosinophilia) 237
Western equine encephalitis (WEE) virus 332, 333, 336, 385
Whipple's disease 120
whipworm *see* Trichuris trichiura (whipworm)
white blood cells, in urine 246
Whitfield's ointment 363, 505
whitlow, herpetic 368
whooping cough *see* pertussis (whooping cough)

Widal test 302
Winterbottom's sign 395
winter vomiting disease 292
woodchuck hepatitis virus 196, 305–306
woolsorter's disease 404
World Health Organization (WHO)
disease detection/diagnosis 447
SARS 230
worm infections *see* helminths, infections
wound infections
burns 426–427
Clostridium 355–356
infection site 124
predisposing factors 550–551
surgical *see* surgical wound infections
see also traumatic injuries
Wuchereria bancroftii 398
microfilariae in lung 237

X

xeroderma pigmentosum 21

Y

yeasts 39
skin infections 360
yellow fever 303, 384, 386
hemorrhagic phenomena 189
urban and jungle 384

vaccine 384, 532
HBV contamination 163
yellow fever virus 383, 384
Yersinia enterocolitica 284, 288, 610(PP)
diarrhea 288, 407
pathogenicity mechanism 164
Yersinia pestis 405, 609–610(PP)
infection via skin 124
virulence factors 405

Z

zalcitabine (deoxycytidine; ddC) 503
zanamivir 504
zidovudine (azidothymidine; AZT) 503
Ziehl–Neelsen stain 234, 358, 359, 456
zoonoses 49, 50, 155, 401
definition 140
hemorrhagic fevers 402–403
multisystem 401–412
pathogens/vectors/diseases 140–141
transmission 133
zoster (shingles) 370–371
ophthalmic 371
pathogenesis 369, 371
reactivation in immunodeficiency 436
zygomycosis, antifungal agents for 506